D1759106

Oxford Textbook of

Public Mental Health

Oxford Textbook of
Public Mental Health

Edited by

Dinesh Bhugra
Centre for Affective Disorders
Institute of Psychiatry, Psychology and Neuroscience
King's College London
London, UK

Kamaldeep Bhui
Centre for Psychiatry
Wolfson Institute of Preventive Medicine
Barts and The London, Queen Mary University of London
London, UK

Samuel Y. S. Wong
Jockey Club School of Public Health and Primary Care
Chinese University of Hong Kong
Hong Kong, China

Stephen E. Gilman
Department of Social and Behavioral Sciences
Department of Epidemiology
Harvard TH Chan School of Public Health
Boston, MA, USA

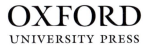

OXFORD
UNIVERSITY PRESS

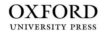

OXFORD
UNIVERSITY PRESS

Great Clarendon Street, Oxford, OX2 6DP,
United Kingdom

Oxford University Press is a department of the University of Oxford.
It furthers the University's objective of excellence in research, scholarship,
and education by publishing worldwide. Oxford is a registered trade mark of
Oxford University Press in the UK and in certain other countries

Published in the United States of America by Oxford University Press
198 Madison Avenue, New York, NY 10016, United States of America

British Library Cataloguing in Publication Data
Data available

Library of Congress Control Number: 2018947924

ISBN 978–0–19–879299–4

Printed and bound by
Bell & Bain Ltd, Glasgow

Oxford University Press makes no representation, express or implied, that the
drug dosages in this book are correct. Readers must therefore always check
the product information and clinical procedures with the most up-to-date
published product information and data sheets provided by the manufacturers
and the most recent codes of conduct and safety regulations. The authors and
the publishers do not accept responsibility or legal liability for any errors in the
text or for the misuse or misapplication of material in this work. Except where
otherwise stated, drug dosages and recommendations are for the non-pregnant
adult who is not breast-feeding

Links to third party websites are provided by Oxford in good faith and
for information only. Oxford disclaims any responsibility for the materials
contained in any third party website referenced in this work.

Preface

Whereas public health in its own right as a medical speciality has a long history, in many parts of the world public mental health has come into its own as a speciality of psychiatry and thus of medicine only in the last two decades or so. There is no doubt that evidence for the prevention of mental illness and promotion of mental health is getting stronger by the day and yet there appears to be a reluctance among clinicians, in general, and mental health care professionals, in particular, to take on the role of educators and advocates for public mental health. One reason often given by clinicians for this lapse is that there is a lack of training at both undergraduate and postgraduate levels, which focuses on diagnosis and management of illness. However, even in countries where preventive and social medicine has a major presence in the curriculum, the focus is often on infection control and immunization rather than on mental health, especially on mental health promotion and prevention of mental illness. Furthermore, resources in healthcare services around the globe are on management and treatment and cure rather than on prevention. Health budgets on public health, if indeed they exist, are only a fraction of the whole health budget, and very little consideration is given to mental health. Mental health promotion and prevention of mental illness are not only linked, but also provide a very different focus.

There is little doubt that the global burden of disease due to mental illness is increasing rapidly. However, it is well recognized that three-quarters of psychiatric disorders in adulthood start before the age of 24 years and nearly half below the age of 15 years. Conduct disorder in childhood is related to later personality disorder and subsequent criminal activity. Emotional disorders in childhood are linked with self-harm, sexual dysfunction, and eating disorders, as well as depression in later life. Hence it is imperative that every effort is made to improve school mental health. Parenting skills take on a major role in the prevention of many disorders. Experiences in the past are represented in the patient's memory and operate in the present to trigger psychiatric illnesses and sometimes precipitate these and in others produce relapse. Working with children at preschool level and school-based health promotion focusing on a number of initiatives can lead to reduced rates of conduct disorder. Educating individuals, families, and societies is at the core of public health. An understanding of the role that social factors play in the precipitation and perpetuation of psychiatric illnesses is critical in developing any educational activities.

There is little doubt that positive mental health can lead to social and economic benefits, including better educational attainment, better productivity, better physical health and lower mortality and improved resilience to adversity. Mental health promotion and prevention of mental illness are effective means and strategies to improve functioning of individuals and also reduce the burden of disease. It is possible to prevent between a quarter and a half of adult lifetime prevalence of mental illness. This includes addictions and common mental disorders.

In addition to looking at vulnerability, we also need to study resilience and protective factors. Apart from genetic vulnerabilities, social inequalities as evidenced by unemployment, poor housing, overcrowding, and poverty contribute to the genesis of mental illness. Social determinants of mental health are significant and many of these factors can be avoided by governments taking appropriate actions. Clinicians have a major role to play by advocating for change both as members of the profession and as members of society. Gender, interpersonal violence, and abuse and age are important factors in the causation of mental ill health. Social capital and networks, emotional and social literacy, and good physical health can enable individuals to develop resilience. Child abuse—physical, emotional, or sexual—can contribute to deteriorating mental health in childhood, as well as in adulthood. One-parent families, overuse of alcohol, violence, parental unemployment, and other developmental factors have been identified as vulnerabilities that can lead to mental illness. The role of the family and of upbringing cannot be underestimated. In this day and age social media plays a significant role in the genesis of mental ill health. High-risk-taking behaviours such as smoking, drug use, lack of physical exercise, and unhealthy eating and obesity can further contribute to the genesis of mental illness. Various vulnerable groups have been identified, and include minority ethnic groups, children in care, those with intellectual disability, elderly, LGBTQI individuals, and prisoners. Thus, special attention is needed to develop public mental health models for these groups.

Taking into account cultural factors and cultural patterns of child rearing and child development, it becomes obvious that psychiatry has to be at the heart of public mental health and any educational strategies. Encouraging social and community cohesion and green spaces can add to self worth and self-esteem, and a sense of belonging. This is particularly relevant for individuals who are socio-centric in their outlooks.

Another reason why public mental health is needed is to link physical illness and mental health care aspects of the care in a closer context in order to teach holistic coping strategies. Effective strategies must use social paradigms at individual, familial, cultural, and social levels. This volume is divided into four broad sections: general principles of public mental health; evidence; needs of special vulnerable groups; and interventions. We have been blessed with a group of experienced authors who, in spite of their busy schedules, provided their expert contributions for this volume. Our grateful thanks to them all. In particular, we would like to thank Sarah Stewart-Brown for her advice and steer.

We are grateful to staff at Oxford University Press, especially Peter Stevenson, Lauren Tiley, and Rachel Goldsworthy, for their support.

Finally, no amount of thanks can convey our gratitude to Andrea Livingstone, who worked hard on the volume, coordinating and chasing authors in a wonderfully understated manner. This project would not have come to fruition without her strength, her commitment, and help.

Dinesh Bhugra
Kamaldeep Bhui
Samuel Y. S. Wong
Stephen E. Gilman

Contents

Abbreviations

ACE	Adverse childhood experiences
ACT	Assertive Community Treatment
ACTH	Adrenocorticotropic hormone
AD	Alzheimer's disease
ADAS-Cog	Alzheimer's Disease Cognitive Assessment Scale Cognitive Subscale
ADHD	Attention deficit hyperactivity disorder
AESOP	Aetiology and Ethnicity in Schizophrenia and Other Psychoses
APMS	Adult Psychiatric Morbidity Survey
AOR	Adjusted odds ratio
ART	Antiretroviral treatment
ASD	Autism spectrum disorder
AUDIT	Alcohol Use Disorders Identification Test
BA	Behavioural activation
BC-IYSI	British Columbia Integrated Youth Services Initiative
BD	Bipolar disorder
BDNF	Brain-derived neurotrophic factor
BFT	Behavioural family therapy
BHPS	British Household Panel Survey
CAFES	Coffee and Family Education and Support
CAH	Congenital adrenal hyperplasia
CAIS	Complete androgene insensitivity syndrome
CES-D	Centre for Epidemiological Scale for Depression
CBT	Cognitive–behavioural therapy
CHeW	Charity Evaluation Working Group
CI	Confidence interval
CIPOLD	Confidential Inquiry into Premature Deaths of People with Learning Disabilities
CMD	Common mental disorders
CNS	Central nervous system
COA	Clinical outcome assessment
CRH	Corticotropin-releasing hormone
CSDH	Commission on Social Determinants of Health
CTT	Classical test theory
CYP	Cytochrome P450
DALY	Disability-adjusted life year
DCS	Demand–control–support
DFID	Department for International Development
DHSS	Department of Health and Social Security
DSD	Disorders of sex development
D-SIB	Direct self-injurious behaviour
DSM	*Diagnostic and Statistical Manual of Mental Disorders*
DUP	Duration of untreated psychosis
DV	Domestic violence
DVO	Domestic violence officers
EAP	Employee-assistance programme
ECA	Epidemiologic Catchment Area
ED	Emergency Department
EFT	Emotionally focused therapy
EMDR	Eye movement desensitization and reprocessing
EMI	Extramarital involvement
EPA	Eicosapentaenoic acid
EPDS	Edinburgh Postnatal Depression Scale
EPPIC	Early Psychosis Prevention and Intervention Centre
ERI	Effort–reward imbalance
ESPAD	European School Survey Project on Alcohol and Other Drugs
EU	European Union
FASD	Fetal alcohol spectrum disorder
FEP	First-episode psychosis
FGA	First-generation antipsychotic
fMRI	Functional magnetic resonance imaging
FSW	Female sex workers
GAF	Global Assessment of Functioning
GBD	Global Burden of Disease study
GBG	Good Behavior Game
GDP	Gross domestic product
GHQ	General Health Questionnaire
GLADS	Glasgow Level of Ability and Development
GSA	Gay–straight alliances
GWAS	Genome-wide association studies
HHSRS	Housing Health and Safety Rating System
HPA	Hypothalamic–pituitary–adrenal
HR	Hazard ratio
HSE	Health and Safety Executive
IAPT	Improving Access to Psychological Therapies
IBA	Identification and brief advice
ICD	*International Classification of Diseases*
ICM	Intensive Case Management
ID	Intellectual disability
IHME	Institute for Health Metrics and Evaluation
IPS	Individual Placement and Support
IPT	Interpersonal psychotherapy
IPV	Intimate partner violence
IRF	Item response function
IRT	Item response theory
LAI	long-lasting (injectable) antipsychotics

LAMIC	Low- and middle-income country	QPR	Question Persuade and Refer
LEDS	Life Events and Difficulties Schedule	RCT	Randomized controlled trial
LGB	Lesbian, gay, and bisexual	RDoC	Research Domain Criteria
LGBTI	Lesbian, gay, bisexual, transgender, and intersex	RE-AIM	Reach, Effectiveness, Adoption, Implementation and Maintenance
LGBTQI	Lesbian, gay, bisexual, transgender, queer, and intersex	RMT	Rasch measurement theory
LTC	Long-term condition	RR	Relative risk
MDD	Major depressive disorder	SAMe	S-adenosyl methionine
MDG	Millennium Development Goal	SAMHSA	Substance Abuse and Mental Health Services Administration
MeSH	Medical subject heading	SD	Standard deviation
MET-h	Metabolic equivalent of task-hours	SDG	Sustainable Development Goal
mhGAP	Mental Health Gap Action Programme	SEAL	Social and emotional aspects of learning
MHS	Military Health System	SEL	Social and emotional learning
MFT	Marriage and family therapy	SEWA	Self-Employed Women's Association
MGMH	Movement for Global Mental Health	SES	Socio-economic status
MHIN	Mental Health Innovation Network	SEP	Socio-economic position
MHPPS	Mental Health and Psychosocial Support Network	SEYLE	Saving and Empowering Young Lives in Europe
MI	Motivational interviewing	SF	Short form
MMHA	Maternal Mental Health Alliance	SGA	Second-generation antipsychotic
MMT	Methadone maintenance treatment	SMR	Standard mortality ratio
MSM	Men who have sex with men	SNS	Social networking site
MUP	Minimum price per unit of alcohol	SOS	Signs of Suicide
MYM	Master Your Mood	S/R	Spirituality and religion
NAIRU	Non-Accelerating Inflation Rate of Unemployment	SSD	Schizophrenia spectrum disorders
NCS	National Comorbidity Surveys	SUDEP	Sudden unexpected death in epilepsy
NCS-R	NCS-replication	SWB	Subjective well-being
NDD	Neurodevelopmental disabilities	TaMHS	Targeted Mental Health in Schools
NET	Narrative exposure therapy	TasP	Treatment as prevention
NGO	Non-governmental organization	TAU	Treatment as usual
NHS	National Health Service	TM	Transtheoretical Model of Behavior Change
NIMH	National Institute of Mental Health	TrkB	Tyrosine kinase B
NSSI	Non-suicidal self-injury	25(OH)D	25-Hydroxyvitamin D
OCD	Obsessive–compulsive disorder	UAI	Unprotected anal intercourse
OECD	Organisation for Economic Co-operation and Development	UHC	Urban health centre
OH	Occupational health	UN	United Nations
OJ	Organizational justice	UNCRPD	United Nations Convention on the Rights of Persons with Disability
ONS	Office for National Statistics	UNODC	Unit Nations Office on Drugs and Crime
OR	Odds ratio	UV	Ultraviolet
PAH	Polycyclic aromatic hydrocarbons	VHA	Veterans Health Administration
PANSS	Positive and Negative Syndrome Scale	WEMWBS	Warwick-Edinburgh Mental Well-being Scale
PAR	Population attributable risk	WFC	Work–family conflicts
PCB	Polychlorinated biphenyls	WHA	World Health Assembly
PFLAG	Parents and Friends of Lesbians and Gays	WHO	World Health Organization
PLWH	People living with HIV	WHO-5	Five-item WHO Well-Being Index
PHC	Primary health centre	WMA	World Medical Association
PPI	Positive psychology interventions	YAM	Youth Aware of Mental Health
PrEP	Pre-exposure prophylaxis	YLD	Years lived with disability
PROM	Patient-reported outcome measures	YLL	Years of life lost
PST	Problem-solving therapy	YRBS	Youth Risk Behavior Surveillance
PTSD	Post-traumatic Stress Disorder		

Contributors

Syed Masud Ahmed, Centre of Excellence for Health System and Universal Health Coverage, BRAC James P. Grant School of Public Health, BRAC University, Dhaka, Bangladesh

Paulo Amarante, Laboratory of Studies and Research in Mental Health and Psychosocial Care, Oswaldo Cruz Foundation, Rio de Janeiro, Brazil

Kenneth L. Appelbaum, Department of Psychiatry, University of Massachusetts Medical School, Worcester, MA, USA

Skye P. Barbic, Department of Occupational Science and Occupational Therapy, University of British Columbia, Vancouver, BC, Canada

Katie Blissard Barnes, Harrogate and District NHS Foundation Trust, Harrogate, UK

Mel Bartley, Institute of Epidemiology and Health, University College London, London, UK

Ruth Bell, Department of Epidemiology and Public Health, Institute of Health Equity, University College London, London, UK

Ingvar A. Bergdahl, Occupational and Environmental Medicine, Department of Public Health and Clinical Medicine, Umeå University, Umeå, Sweden

Sabyasachi Bhaumik, Leicestershire Partnership NHS Trust and University of Leicester, Leicester, UK

Vishal Bhavsar, Department of Psychosis Studies, Institute of Psychiatry, Psychology and Neuroscience, King's College London, London, UK

Dinesh Bhugra, Centre for Affective Disorders, Institute of Psychiatry, Psychology and Neuroscience, King's College, London, UK

Kamaldeep Bhui, Centre for Psychiatry, Wolfson Institute of Preventive Medicine, Barts and The London, Queen Mary University of London, London, UK

Jed Boardman, Institute of Psychiatry, Psychology and Neuroscience, King's College London and Centre for Mental Health, London, UK

Philip Boyce, Westmead Clinical School, Sydney Medical School, University of Sydney and Department of Psychiatry, Westmead Hospital, Sydney, Australia

M. Harvey Brenner, Department of Health Behavior and Health Systems, University of North Texas Health Science Center, School of Public Health, Fort Worth, TX, USA; Department of Health Policy and Management, Johns Hopkins University, Bloomberg School of Public Health, Baltimore, MD, USA

Katherine Brown, Institute of Alcohol Studies, London, UK

Stefan J. Cano, Modus Outcomes, Letchworth Garden City, UK

Vladimir Carli, National Centre for Suicide Research and Prevention of Mental Ill-Health, Karolinska Institute, Stockholm, Sweden

Mauro Giovanni Carta, Department of Public Health, Clinical and Molecular Medicine, University of Cagliari, Italy; Center for Consultation-Liaison Psychiatry and Psychosomatics, Department of Public Health, St. John's Hospital, Sardinia, Italy

David J. Castle, St. Vincent's Hospital Melbourne and Department of Psychiatry, University of Melbourne, Melbourne, Australia

Wai Chi Chan, Department of Psychiatry, University of Hong Kong, Hong Kong, China

Prabha S. Chandra, Department of Psychiatry, National Institute of Mental Health and Neurosciences (NIMHANS), Bangalore, India

Fiona J. Charlson, University of Queensland School of Public Health, Herston, QLD, Australia; Queensland Centre for Mental Health Research, Wacol, QLD, Australia; Institute for Health Metrics and Evaluation, University of Washington, Seattle, WA, USA

Mirai Chatterjee, SEWA –Self Employed Women's Association, Ahmedabad, India

Prabha S. Chandra, Department of Psychiatry, University of Montreal and Research Center, CHU Sainte-Justine, FRSQ and Fondation Julien/Marcelle and Social and Community Paediatrics, Montreal, QC, Canada

Christopher C. H. Cook, Department of Theology and Religion, Durham University and Tees, Esk and Wear Valleys NHS Foundation Trust, Durham, UK

Patricia Conrod, Department of Psychiatry, University of Montreal Senior Research Fellow, CHU Ste-Justine, FRSQ; Fondation Julien/Marcelle and Jean Coutu Chair in Social and Community Pediatrics Research Center, Montreal, QC, Canada

Giulia Cossu, Department of Public Health, Clinical and Molecular Medicine, University of Cagliari, Italy; Center for Consultation-Liaison Psychiatry and Psychosomatics, Department of Public Health, St. John's Hospital, Sardinia, Italy

Giuseppe Costa, Department of Clinical and Biological Sciences, University of Turin, Turin, Italy

Tom K. J. Craig, Health Service and Population Research Department, Institute of Psychiatry, Psychology and Neuroscience, King's College London, London, UK

Sandra K. Davidson, Department of General Practice, University of Melbourne, Melbourne, Australia

Tanya Deb, Health Service and Population Research Department, Institute of Psychiatry, Psychology and Neuroscience, King's College London, London, UK

Angelo d'Errico, Department of Epidemiology, Local Health Company of Collegno and Pinerolo, Piedmont Region, Grugliasco, Italy

Geetha Desai, Department of Psychiatry, National Institute of Mental Health and Neuro Sciences (NIMHANS), Bangalore, India

Keshav Desiraju, Formerly Ministry of Health and Family Welfare, Government of India, New Delhi, India

Jennifer Dykxhoorn, PsyLife Group, University College London, Division of Psychiatry, London, UK

Jenny Edwards, Mental Health Foundation, London, UK

Iris Elliott, Mental Health Foundation, London, UK

Holly E. Erskine, University of Queensland School of Public Health, Herston, QLD, Australia; University of Queensland Centre for Clinical Research, Herston, QLD, Australia; Queensland Centre for Mental Health Research, Wacol, QLD, Australia; Institute for Health Metrics and Evaluation, University of Washington, Seattle, WA, USA

Alize J. Ferrari, University of Queensland School of Public Health, Herston, QLD, Australia; Queensland Centre for Mental Health Research, Wacol, QLD, Australia; Institute for Health Metrics and Evaluation, University of Washington, Seattle, WA, USA

Susan L. Fletcher, Department of General Practice, University of Melbourne, Melbourne, Australia

Megan Galbally, School of Medicine, University of Notre Dame, Perth, Australia

Shweta Gangavati, Leicestershire Partnership NHS Trust, Leicester, UK

Stephen E. Gilman, Department of Social and Behavioral Sciences and Department of Epidemiology, Harvard TH Chan School of Public Health, Boston, MA, USA

Ian Gilmore, School of Medicine, University of Liverpool, Liverpool, UK; National Drug Research Institute, Faculty of Health Sciences, Curtin University, Perth, Australia

William Gilmore, National Drug Research Institute, Faculty of Health Sciences, Curtin University, Perth, Australia

Alain Gregoire, Maternal Mental Health Alliance UK, Global Alliance for Maternal Mental Health, University of Southampton, Southampton, UK

Petra C. Gronholm, Health Service and Population Research Department, Institute of Psychiatry, Psychology and Neuroscience, King's College London, London, UK

Jane M. Gunn, Department of General Practice, University of Melbourne, Melbourne, Australia

Hideki Hashimoto, Department of Health and Social Behaviour, University of Tokyo School of Public Health, Tokyo, Japan

Claire Henderson, Health Service and Population Research Department, Institute of Psychiatry, Psychology and Neuroscience, King's College London, London, UK

Max Henderson, Leeds and York Partnership NHS Foundation Trust, Leeds, UK

Avinash Hiremath, Leicestershire Partnership NHS Trust, Leicester, UK

Mohammad Didar Hossain, BRAC James P. Grant School of Public Health, BRAC University, Dhaka, Bangladesh

Felicia A. Huppert, The Well-being Institute, University of Cambridge, Cambridge, UK; Institute for Positive Psychology and Education, Australian Catholic University, Sydney, Australia

Miriam Iosue, Department of Medicine and Health Sciences, University of Molise, Campobasso, Italy

Amala Jesu, South Staffordshire and Shropshire Healthcare NHS Foundation Trust, Stafford, UK

Pallavi Karnatak, Trimbos International Department, Trimbos Institute, Utrecht, The Netherlands

Norito Kawakami, Department of Mental Health, University of Tokyo School of Public Health, Tokyo, Japan

Reza Kiani, Leicestershire Partnership NHS Trust and University of Leicester, Leicester, UK

Yoo Na Kim, Jockey Club School of Public Health and Primary Care, Chinese University of Hong Kong, Hong Kong, China

James B. Kirkbride, PsyLife Group, University College London Division of Psychiatry, London, UK

Christina Blanner Kristiansen, Psychiatric Department and Psychiatric Research Academy Odense, Odense University Hospital, Denmark

Linda Chiu Wa Lam, Department of Psychiatry, Chinese University of Hong Kong, Hong Kong, China

Joseph T. F. LAU, The Jockey Club School of Public Health and Primary Care, Faculty of Medicine, The Chinese University of Hong Kong, Shatin, Hong Kong, China; School of Public Health, Zhejiang University School of Medicine, Hangzhou, Zhejiang, China

Annisa Lee, School of Journalism and Communication, Chinese University of Hong Kong, Hong Kong, China

Che Kin Lee, Department of Psychiatry, Kowloon Hospital, Hong Kong, China

Janni Leung, University of Queensland School of Public Health, Herston, QLD, Australia; Queensland Centre for Mental Health Research, Wacol, QLD, Australia; Institute for Health Metrics and Evaluation, University of Washington, Seattle, WA, USA

Bennett L. Leventhal, Department of Psychiatry, Langley Porter Psychiatric Institute, Weill Institute for Neuroscience, University of California San Francisco, San Francisco, CA, USA

Jinghua Li, 1. School of Public Health, Sun Yat-sen University, Guangzhou, China; Sun Yat-sen Global Health Institute, Sun Yat-sen University, Guangzhou, China

2. Sun Yat-sen Global Health Institute, Sun Yat-sen University, Guangzhou, China

Ana Lusicic, Orygen Youth Health, NorthWestern Mental Health, Melbourne, Australia

Lieselotte Mahler, Charité University Clinic for Psychiatry and Psychotherapy, Berlin, Germany

Michael Marmot, Department of Epidemiology and Public Health, Institute of Health Equity, University College London, London, UK

Lydia Matoke, Herbalists Society of Kenya, Nakuru, Kenya

Mike McHugh, Consultant in Public Health, Leicestershire County Council, Leicester, UK

Kwame McKenzie, Wellesley Institute, Centre for Addiction and Mental Health, Department of Psychiatry, University of Toronto, Toronto, ON, Canada

Dasari Mohan Michael, Humber NHS Foundation Trust, Willerby, UK

Daniel Miranda, Oswaldo Cruz Foundation: Politics, Science and Culture in Health, Petrópolis, Brazil

Matthew Mishkind, University of Colorado Anchutz Medical Campus, Helen and Arthur E. Johnson Depression Center, Denver, CO, USA

Richard Montoro, Department of Psychiatry and Sexual Identity Centre, McGill University, Montreal, QC, Canada

Joshua Moses, Department of Anthropology and Department of Environmental Studies, Haverford College, Haverford, PA, USA

Olive Mukamana, Research Center, CHU Sainte-Justine, Montreal, QC, Canada

Götz Mundle, Center for Mental Health, Oberberg City, Berlin, Germany

Povl Munk-Jørgensen, Psychiatric Department, Odense University Hospital, Denmark

Christine W. Musyimi, Africa Mental Health Foundation, Nairobi, Kenya; Free University Amsterdam, Amsterdam, The Netherlands

Victoria N. Mutiso, Africa Mental Health Foundation, Nairobi, Kenya

Erick S. Nandoya, Africa Mental Health Foundation, Nairobi, Kenya

David M. Ndetei, Africa Mental Health Foundation and Department of Psychiatry, University of Nairobi, Nairobi, Kenya

Roger M. K. Ng, Department of Psychiatry, Kowloon Hospital, Hong Kong, China

Wai Ching Ng, Association for Concern for Legal Rights of Victims of Domestic Violence, Department of Social Work, Chinese University of Hong Kong, Hong Kong, China

Timo O. Nieder, Department for Sex Research and Forensic Psychiatry, Interdisciplinary Transgender Health Care Center Hamburg, University Medical Center Hamburg-Eppendorf, Hamburg, Germany

Niels Okkels, Department of Affective Disorders and Psychiatric Research Academy Aarhus, Aarhus University Hospital Risskov, Denmark

D. Padmavathy, Department of Nursing, National Institute of Mental Health and Neurosciences (NIMHANS), Bangalore, India

Anita Patel, Anita Patel Health Economics Consulting Ltd, London, UK

Soumitra Pathare, Centre for Mental Health Law and Policy, Indian Law Society, Pune, India

Melissa Petrakis, St. Vincent's Hospital Melbourne, Mental Health Service and Department of Social Work, Medicine, Nursing and Health Sciences, Monash University, Caulfield East, Australia

Jessica L. Plauché, Department of Psychiatry, Zuckerberg San Francisco General Hospital and Trauma Center, University of California at San Francisco, San Francisco, CA, USA

Martin Plöderl, Department of Crisis Intervention and Suicide Prevention and Department of Clinical Psychology, Christian Doppler Clinic, Paracelsus Medical University, Salzburg, Austria

Antonio Preti, Department of Public Health, Clinical and Molecular Medicine, University of Cagliari, Center for Consultation-Liaison Psychiatry and Psychosomatics, Department of Public Health, St. John's Hospital, Sardinia, Italy

Marguerite Regan, Mental Health Foundation, London, UK; Public Health England, London, UK

Felix J. Rosenberg, Oswaldo Cruz Foundation: Itaborai Forum: Politics, Science and Culture in Health, Petrópolis, Brazil

Kai Ruggeri, Policy Research Group, Department of Psychology, University of Cambridge, Cambridge, UK, and Department of Health Policy & Management, Mailman School of Public Health, Columbia University, New York, USA

Damian F. Santomauro, University of Queensland School of Public Health, Herston, QLD, Australia; Queensland Centre for Mental Health Research, Wacol, QLD, Australia; Institute for Health Metrics and Evaluation, University of Washington, Seattle, WA, USA

Veena A. Satyanarayana, Department of Clinical Psychology, National Institute of Mental Health and Neuro Sciences (NIMHANS), Bangalore, India

Stephen Scott, Department of Child and Adolescent Psychiatry, Institute of Psychiatry, Psychology and Neuroscience, King's College London, London, UK

Anne Scully-Hill, Faculty of Law, Chinese University of Hong Kong, Hong Kong, China

Edward Shaw, Institute of Health and Wellbeing, University of Glasgow, Glasgow, UK

Rui She, Jockey Club School of Public Health and Primary Care, Chinese University of Hong Kong, Hong Kong, China

Laura Shields, Trimbos International Department, Trimbos Institute, Utrecht, The Netherlands

Jay H. Shore, University of Colorado Anschutz Medical Campus, Helen and Arthur E. Johnson Depression Center, Denver, CO, USA

Fasli Sidheek, Department of Clinical Psychology, National Institute of Mental Health and Neuro Sciences (NIMHANS), Bangalore, India

Morton Silverman, University of Colorado Denver School of Medicine, Aurora, CO, USA

Daniel J. Smith, Institute of Health and Wellbeing, University of Glasgow, Glasgow, UK

Sarah Stewart-Brown, Warwick Medical School-Statistics and Epidemiology, University of Warwick, Coventry, UK

Stephan Stiller, School of Journalism and Communication, Chinese University of Hong Kong, Hong Kong, China

Supraja T. A, Department of Psychiatric Social Work, National Institute of Mental Health and Neurosciences (NIMHANS), Bangalore, India

Graham Thornicroft, Health Service and Population Research Department , Institute of Psychiatry, Psychology and Neuroscience, King's College London, London, UK

Eduardo Torre, Laboratory of Studies and Research in Mental Health and Psychosocial Care, Oswaldo Cruz Foundation, Rio de Janeiro, Brazil

Lakshmi Vijayakumar, SNEHA – Suicide Prevention Centre and HOD – Voluntary Health Services, Chennai, India; University of Griffith, Brisbane, Australia; University of Melbourne, Melbourne, Australia

Danuta Wasserman, National Centre for Suicide Research and Prevention of Mental Ill-Health, Karolinska Institute, Stockholm, Sweden

Maryann Waugh, University of Colorado Anschutz Medical Campus, School of Medicine, Helen and Arthur E. Johnson Depression Center, Colorado Access, Denver, CO, USA

Katherine Weare, Southampton Education School, University of Southampton, Southampton, UK

Ursula Werneke, Department of Clinical Sciences, Psychiatry, Sunderby Research Unit, Umeå University, Umeå, Sweden

Nathan H. White, Institute for Faith and Resilience, Lafayette, LA, USA

Harvey A. Whiteford, School of Public Health, University of Queensland, Australia; Queensland Centre for Mental Health Research, Wacol, QLD, Australia; Institute for Health Metrics and Evaluation, University of Washington, Seattle, WA, USA

Rob Whitley, Department of Psychiatry, McGill University, Montreal, QC, Canada

Carmen Wong, Centre for Research and Promotion of Women's Health, Jockey Club School of Public Health and Primary Care, Chinese University of Hong Kong, Hong Kong, China

Samuel Y. S. Wong, Jockey Club School of Public Health and Primary Care, Chinese University of Hong Kong, Hong Kong, China

Dexing Zhang, School of Public Health and Primary Care, Chinese University of Hong Kong, Hong Kong, China

Shuo Zhang, Health Service and Population Research Department, Institute of Psychiatry, Psychology and Neuroscience, King's College London, London, UK

Hua Zhong, Pearl River Delta Social Research Centre, Department of Sociology, Chinese University of Hong Kong, Hong Kong, China

Introduction

Dinesh Bhugra

Public health has contributed in a major and successful way in controlling infectious diseases and educating people to look after their health and well-being in a more pragmatic manner. There is no doubt that public health contributions to physical health have been more prominent thus far. Public health established itself as a medical speciality centuries ago. The elimination of smallpox from the world and a reduction in cases of poliomyelitis reflect this shift and eradication. However, public mental health has become a more robust sub-speciality in the past few decades only. This volume reflects its coming of age.

The principles of public health are well recognised and well known. Some of these principles are equally and easily applicable in mental health. One of major challenges in many parts of the world has been the mind–body dualism that has often excluded mental health from any dialogue about health. Even when infectious diseases strike, such as the Ebola epidemic, the mental health of survivors and those who recover and grief over losses has to be taken into account. There is considerable evidence to suggest that social determinants affect the mental, as well as the physical, health of populations. Poverty, unemployment, and overcrowding are some of the key factors that affect mental health. Challenges to mental health are both integrated with physical ill health, as well as separately and occasionally in isolation. This means in practicality that some fresh principles may be needed and some older ones may need to be modified. A major challenge is to identify what is meant by mental health and whether it is an absence of diseases, as the World Health Organization defines it. This means that many chronic or co-morbid conditions can produce permanent states of ill health, which cannot be the case.

In this volume, Patel reminds us that the economic costs of mental illness are substantial and extend far beyond those related simply to mental health care. Of course, studies looking at economic costs may not always take into account social costs. She provides a cautionary note in that simple knowledge of costs is not always very helpful for a number of reasons. As epidemiologists move towards a web of causation of disorders, it is inevitable that costs will have to be looked at in a similar way. In times of economic difficulties and the always-rising costs of health care and competing demands, difficult decisions about resource allocation have to take into account alternative care options. Efficacy and efficiency need to be understood together.

It is unimaginable to conceive of a good and just society that would not put health and equal access to health as central concerns. Equally, in the field of mental health and mental illness, social justice and human rights cannot but be central concerns but are often ignored [1]. Health, including mental health, is a fundamental human right, but, regrettably, in many societies it is not seen as such. This is despite the fact that health is important to individuals and the society on a daily basis and healthy individuals are a major asset to any society. A tragedy of policy is that society often focuses on illness and ill individuals, rather than on health itself. The challenge for any society is to deliver health—which is a personal good—to the society as a whole thereby benefiting the society as a whole. Promoting individual health requires societal-level transformations, whereas treating illness in individuals very often requires individual-level actions and the focus on public mental health is often on the whole population level, ignoring vulnerable and individual levels.

Venkatapuram [2] argues that every human being has a moral entitlement to a capability to be healthy, especially to a level that is commensurate with equal human dignity in the contemporary world. The capability to be healthy carries with it both a moral and social basis. To this end, it is crucial that clinicians, researchers, and policymakers understand what this capability means and its relationship with key social and cultural factors.

The capabilities approach to health is an evaluative analytic framework that makes interpersonal comparisons possible, especially for making public policy and can be used to create and share the concepts of social justice [3–8]. Such a way of looking at health places the emphasis on individual responsibility to maintain health, and society or the culture have a responsibility to provide the right levels of information.

Prevention of mental illness

There is considerable evidence that mental illness in adulthood, in a majority of cases, starts below the age of 24 years [9], and in nearly half starts below the age of 15 years. Thereby, it is a moral imperative that mental health promotion and education about prevention should start at an early age. Complicating the development of such an approach are the distinctions between disease and illness and the underlying explanatory models that patients and their carers have about their symptoms and experiences. Disease refers to underlying pathology and illness is the social consequence of disease as experienced by the 'patient' for which they seek treatment [10], whereas clinicians are trained in diagnosing and dealing with disease, thereby creating a conflict within the therapeutic encounter. Nordenfelt and colleagues argue that health should be seen as an ability to achieve certain goals and ambitions and should not be seen as simple absence of disease as more and more people are living with complex co-morbidities [11, 12]. Therefore, it would appear that we need to redefine health [13]. Huber et al. [13] suggest that physical, social, and mental health need to be understood in their proper context.

Venkatapuram argues that the health of the individual should be understood as the ability to achieve a basic cluster of beings and doings [2]. This is the ability to achieve a set of interrelated 'capabilities and functionings'. In this context, capabilities refer to real practical possibilities of being or doing something that will have a functional outcome contributing to a recovery approach. The paradox is that measurement of health and health outcomes is about resulting achievements or the inability to have these. This raises important questions for broader society, as well as for (mental) health professionals. Linking multiple capabilities to achieve certain beings and doings gives a way forward, especially looking at outcomes. In psychiatry such an approach rises above the traditional biomedical model by linking it with socio-cultural and spiritual approaches, thus confirming an interlinking strategy of understanding health capabilities and creating potential for interventions. In psychiatry, the notions of illness create a tension between what is understood as disease and whether there is an underlying basis for a physical template causing mental illness. Statistical variations, behavioural variations, or good subjective well-being are strongly defined by cultures and societies within which we live, work, and age. Venkatapuram challenges Boorse's assumption that mental illness can be defined through the tabulation of normal distribution of mental functioning [2, 14–17]. It is also refutable that biomedical systems are not affected by social determinants. Nordenfelt argues that health is about positive ability (and absence of disability) [11, 12], which means that the concept of disability may take precedence over health. His conclusion is that a person's health reflects the person's second-order abilities to achieve various vital goals, which include living a normal life span, (with) good health, bodily integrity, use of the senses, imagination and thought, emotions and emotional attachments, conception of good, meaningful, and respectful social affiliations, concerns for other species, ability to play, and control over one's material and political environment. Above all, the capabilities approach is a set of ideas that question and provide an alternative view on well-being of individuals and society. The focus on capabilities and equity is at the heart of capabilities approach [2]. This approach focuses on nurturing, protecting, providing, and expanding the capabilities of individuals to enable them to conceive, pursue, and revise their life plans [4, 8]. Capability to achieve something is a real opportunity and health is critical to achieving economic and material well-being. Thus, the capabilities approach to mental health is an individual's ability to achieve a group of capabilities and functionings, allowing an individual in the modern world to lead a life full of equal human dignity. Adopting this approach changes the strategies for public health and especially public mental health.

If this capabilities approach to mental health were to be applied to public mental health agenda, it is quite likely that stigma, which has dogged mentally ill individuals, may be reduced if the focus appears to be on health and not illness. If the integrated approach, as developed and advocated by Venkatapuram [2], is to be applied, then the message on intervention will have to focus on what human beings are capable of. This would have a tremendous impact on the lives of those who may have intellectual disability [18]. Capability to be mentally healthy will be seen in the context of social justice and equity in terms of resources for service development, as well as research. Thus, there is a framework for reaching social justice that will ensure that individuals have equitable capabilities building on basic capabilities. The focus on basic human dignity and helping

develop a capabilities framework cannot be seen in isolation with economic systems, which will also affect resources and funding. It is also likely to vary between socio-centric and ego-centric societies.

Taking into account what individuals are capable of achieving offers a real opportunity to deliver possibilities of better prevention strategies, as well as ensuring that those who develop illness will have the maximum number of opportunities to achieve their full potential with full human dignity. A capabilities approach to health will also enable us to manage recovery and create an environment in which individuals can reach their maximum abilities and lead a fulfilled life. The possibilities of using such an approach are endless.

Social inequalities, across social, economic, environmental dimensions, and inequalities in mental health, are at the heart of mental health services. Stewart-Brown, in Chapter 1, provides a helpful overview of public health principles in the context of public health. Social determinants of health, including mental health, are critical in our understanding of providing public mental health interventions. In Chapter 2, Bell and Marmot present a framework for thinking about the lifetime causes of inequalities in mental health and how such a framework can be used to explore how experiences and conditions affect mental health across the life course. They focus on factors that affect child development because of the importance of child developmental outcomes for future mental and physical health, and on life chances. As advocates, psychiatrists and public health professionals alike need to heed Bell and Marmot's clarion call to address the causes of social inequalities in mental health through multiple types of policies and interventions. Ferrari and colleagues (Chapter 4) look at global burden of disease and provide an overview of the findings from the Global Burden of Disease Study, once again confirming that mental illness carries with it a huge burden.

In Chapter 9, Dykxhoorn and Kirkbride highlight the epidemiological tools needed in order to quantify the burden of psychiatric disorders Epidemiological data help us understand the aetiology and health needs of the population and also the burden of disease. They point out that the incidence and prevalence of these disorders varies by person and place, with a particular focus on the patterns of psychiatric disorders by ethnicity. However, in Chapter 10, Rosenberg and Miranda draw our attention to critical epidemiology as the science of understanding and describing the distribution of health as socially determined and of contributing to the achievement of the universal right to it. They argue that as formal epidemiology segregates quantitative phenomena from concrete reality, it cannot reach the essence of the social determination of health and disease as a process. They suggest that as direct and indirect causation, distant, intermediate, or proximate levels of organization of the epidemiological interrelations are all part of an integrated totality that is constructed from the historically changing dialectic relationship between particular social classes and their lived spaces. It is important to understand 'spaces of exclusion', which, indeed, may contribute to mental ill health. They see critical epidemiology as the means to understand this relationship and to select the 'spaces of social exclusion' as the prioritized targets for a participative construction of new health models leading to the effective reduction of health inequities. They believe that such an approach will universalize the right to health in all its objective and subjective meanings.

Plauché and Leventhal (see Chapter 28) remind us that child and adolescent mental health has become a pressing, international public health crisis. The rates of various psychiatric disorders are high and nearly half of psychiatric disorders in adulthood start before the age of 15 years, resulting in a tremendous adverse impact on children and the young people, families, and communities. They highlight five principal features: developmental epidemiology, healthy development and well-being, access to care, the effects of adverse childhood experiences, and paediatric psychopharmacology. Their concluding remarks include strategies to promote healthy child and adolescent development, as well as for the prevention, early identification, and early intervention for child and adolescent mental disorders. At the other end of the age spectrum, argue Lam and Chan in Chapter 29, that with increasing longevity around the globe, multiple complex co-morbidities start to appear, adding to the burden of disease and reminding clinicians that dementia is now a public mental health priority. Clinicians and researchers need to collect data from large-scale studies and policymakers need to take these findings into account when planning services.

There is no doubt that genetic vulnerabilities and their interactions with environmental and social factors influence development of various psychiatric disorders. In Chapter 6, Shaw and Smith highlight that public mental health is influenced by a wide range of social, political, and economic factors, and most forms of psychiatric disorder have an important underlying genetic component. Any advance in public mental health needs to be cognisant of the important role of genetics in determining mental health and well-being. Shaw and Smith propose that there are key ethical challenges in discovering genetic risk factors for psychiatric disorders across the lifespan with consideration of the role of epigenetic processes during development. They remind us that the public health significance of psychiatric genetics within the context of ongoing global efforts to understand more fully the causes of mental illness and how this work might lead to new approaches to diagnosis, classification, and treatment across the world.

In Chapter 5, McKenzie describes models of causation of mental illness, which are, indeed, complex. He highlights that we need to understand how diagnoses are made and what a mental illness actually is. Research into causation and the interaction between biological and social theories of mental illness provide a way forward. Using schizophrenia and other psychoses as a lens to see through aetiology, McKenzie explores what is known about the different mechanisms through which mental illness may be caused. The four dimensions of causation, individual, ecological, and interactions and time are offered as a simple framework for organizing complex aetiological theories.

Moses and Whitley, in Chapter 7, chart the contributions of anthropology to public mental health. They reinforce the message that there are three main traditions in anthropological practice: (i) individual-level approaches, investigating mental health beliefs, behaviours, and illness narratives; (ii) meso-level approaches, assessing the provision, nature, and practice of mental health care systems; and (iii) macro-level approaches, examining the mental health impact of societal structures, including political and economic structures. They emphasize that public mental health needs to look at the three level approaches. Other factors such as climate change need to be considered and public mental health challenges using these traditions need a multi-scale, interdisciplinary ecological approach.

The impact of economic downturn on the mental health of populations has been significant. The Great Depression, nearly a

century ago, evidenced increasingly higher rates of mental disorder at successively lower social class levels. These findings have been replicated several times. Dynamic interpretations of these relations have concentrated on vulnerability to economic crises, especially recessions, resulting in major increases in mental hospitalization and suicide. Brenner argues in Chapter 18 that psychiatric morbidity and suicide are very strongly influenced by unemployment and income loss, creating a paradigm of relating economic crises to social class and the interrelationship between physical and mental health. New multivariate analyses, using gross domestic product declines and unemployment increases as the main recessional indicators, find that world suicide and industrialized country overall mortality rates increased as a result of the Great Recession and government austerity. There may be a circular relation linking economic crises, social class, and the interactive relations of mental and physical health. In Chapter 38, Vijayakumar and Silverman describe that although methods and rates of suicide differ across cultures, some common threads can emerge. Risk factors also include economic difficulties. They identify ease of access to certain means, which can be managed by political or legal action such as reducing the number of over-the-counter painkillers, such as aspirin or paracetamol, and reduced access to pesticides.

Fletcher and colleagues remind us in Chapter 45 of the role that stress can play in biological triggering of symptoms, even if some stress is needed to function effectively in some settings; however, inevitably, sustained stress is not good for one's health. They describe models of stress and the role of stressful events in developing psychiatric disorders and prevalence of stress in the community. They argue persuasively that our reactions can be moulded by a number of factors and there needs to be effective strategies for managing and preventing stress.

The social environment plays a significant role in the onset, course, and outcome of mental disorders. The impact has been conceptualized in two broad ways. The first is in terms of unspecified aspects of the physical and emotional structure of the society, such as higher rates of psychiatric disorders in many urban populations and among minority communities. The second task is to drill down to the essence of what aspects of these environments are toxic—typically exploring associations between illness and stressful experiences, especially those involving abusive and bullying interactions. Both models also suggest preventive and restorative social interventions that could modify how mental health care is delivered. Poverty, low education, unemployment, and overcrowding do play a role in the genesis of poor mental health. For people of low-income countries, poverty is all pervasive and affects physical, as well as mental, health in various ways.

Whereas Craig and Boardman point out in Chapter 17 that the quality of housing and mental illness is well established, in Chapter 47 Werneke and Bergdahl focus on environmental and dietary toxins. Once again it may not be a uni-directional link, and complex factors may play a role. However, people who already have serious mental illness and are living in poor circumstances may experience stress, which contributes to their poor recovery. Craig and Boardman recommend an early step-wise approach through progressively more independent settings, from hospital to group home. They illustrate this with the example of 'housing first' approaches that bypass the traditional rehabilitation model placing people directly into permanent housing with the flexible support they need to maintain it.

Werneke and Bergdahl remind us that dietary and environmental factors are also likely to affect mental health. It is becoming increasingly clear that many nutritional constituents, such as omega-3 fatty acids, vitamins, and minerals, have a major impact on mental health. Dietary and environmental factors are more likely to influence neurodevelopmental disorders, depression, and psychosis. Potential interactions between foodstuffs and psychotropic medicines are worth bearing in mind. Toxic substances such as lead, methylmercury, and various organic compounds can affect populations. In Chapter 23, Amarante and Tore discuss the effects of environmental contaminants and agrochemicals on mental health, relating this discussion to the issue of the right to health and the critique of the paradigm of chemicalization of life. Food insecurity, rights, and institutional neglect all affect the chemicalization of life, including intoxication of the population, environmental injustice, and human rights violations, and strengthen the renewal of interests of the 'disease industry' and the medicalization processes.

Various groups who are vulnerable to mental illness include women, LGBTQI (lesbian, gay, bisexual, transgender, queer, and intersex), those with intellectual disability, prisoners, and others. Health equity means that everyone who needs mental health care has easy access and the services are funded properly and that there are no unnecessary and unavoidable disparities in health consequences and/or access to resources and opportunities in order to achieve health in the context of individual's needs so that the society could realize justice as a whole. What exactly should be achieved for equity depends on referred ethical basis. Mental ill health can be a consequence and a cause of health inequity. It reviews how inequity in socio-economic conditions and capabilities, including—but not limited to—access to healthcare services, affect people's risk of mental ill health from the life course perspective. It also reviews that social stigma and subsequent social exclusion of those with mental ill health further precludes health equity. Finally, it reviews the concept of 'social determinants of health' as a policy agenda to realize health equity in public mental health provision.

In Chapter 15, Huppert and Ruggeri note that until recently the biomedical model dominated thinking about both physical health and mental health. It is now more useful to frame health as an integrated totality, one that includes our physiological functioning, our behaviour, and all of the influences on the two. Evidence now tells us that by strengthening mental health and well-being we not only reduce the risk of mental illness, but in doing so we enhance population health in its widest sense. Equally, improving physical health and well-being have a significantly positive influence on population mental health. It is now vitally important that we exploit our understanding of this positive feedback loop and it's potential to tackle some of the pressing health and well-being challenges we face. In Chapter 34, Zhang and Wong draw our attention to the benefits of healthy lifestyles on physical health and disease prevention but point out that similar findings are relatively lacking for mental health. They provide an overview on the impact of lifestyles on mental health. At last, we now have a clear opportunity to meaningfully draw physical and mental health together as a mutually dependent, integrated whole. In many respects this journey is just beginning.

In Chapter 37, Lau et al. cover the patterns of HIV spread and its prevention and care. HIV is called a social disease as the transmission is related to risky behaviours and its co-occurrence with other conditions of mental illness and substance use. This obviously brings with it a moral dimension. Mental health problems are prevalent both among key populations for HIV prevention and people living with HIV, and can influence HIV-related risk behaviors, interact synergistically, and compromise the effectiveness of HIV prevention, treatment, and care. Lau et al. explore and describe some new promising approaches, such as positive psychology interventions.

Mukamana and Conrod provide, in Chapter 36, an overview of substance use disorders and review various risk factors for drug addiction, both at the individual and environmental level, in the context of prevalence of these conditions and resulting burden. Of course, prevention strategies include universal interventions in which drug supply control policies, and psychosocial and educational interventions are directed at the general population—interventions targeting high-risk populations and brief interventions for those already experiencing problematic drug use. They illustrate these with examples of effective interventions in each category and make recommendations for research and practice based on the available evidence. They go on to provide a comprehensive and developmentally appropriate approach to prevention as a promising strategy to integrate effective interventions that target the multiple factors implicated in the development of drug addiction.

Violence against women, including intimate partner violence, unemployment, unhygienic living and work environment, and social capital play a significant role in precipitating common mental disorders throughout the lifespan. Wong et al. (Chapter 49) and Supraja et al. (Chapter 50) review the key aspects of interpersonal violence against women. Women generally show higher rates of many psychiatric disorders. In addition, they also look after ill members of the family, thereby adding to their distress, as well as stress. They are also more likely to face poor social conditions, such as overcrowding, poverty, insecure employment, and so on. Social determinants of mental health are an important aspect in identifying mental ill health and illness. An integration between public health and primary care is a possible option and step forward. Policymakers and legislators need to work with civil society and local people in order to develop and deliver, will have to develop ways in which the social determinants of mental health can be addressed, and work with people, especially women, at the centre of all our efforts. In Chapter 24, Sidheek and colleagues highlight that family is a unit tied together with a system of unique heritage, shared history, a set of values, and shared internalized perceptions and assumptions about the world. Families also provide a sense of togetherness and we-ness, along with a sense of shared purpose. By and large a family provides psychological and social milieu for character formation of its individual members and within which children are born and brought up, thereby making the unit a prime example of helping develop the world view. This set of relationships becomes immensely important in the developmental course of an individual, especially for their sense of well-being, which also goes on throughout one's lifespan. Of course, life-cycle stages are not linear, where a family moves from one stage to the next after having cleared the previous stage. There is also an overlap, which means that at any given time, members of the families can be going through different life stages based on a number of factors.

Other vulnerable groups have their own needs and require different strategies in public mental health.

In Chapter 25, Appelbaum illustrates how incarceration can affect public mental health and safety and describes the benefits of mental health treatment during and after incarceration for individual patients and for society. In his review he points out that the conditions of confinement can make inmates either better or worse, including the detrimental effects that harsh prison environments can have on future criminal behaviours. His evidence emphasizes how mass incarceration has, in many countries, had great fiscal and social costs but has had very limited beneficial effects on crime rates. There are often opportunities and alternatives to incarceration that may be better for individual offenders, family members, and the broader community.

Montoro, in Chapter 27, focuses on the sexual minority youths, whereas Plöderl and colleagues highlight, in Chapter 26, the overall picture of mental health needs of LGBTQI individuals. There is no doubt that in many cultures LGBTI individuals face specific mental health challenges. Rates of psychiatric disorders are much greater in these groups when compared with their heterosexual counterparts. Fewer studies are available for trans(-gender) and inter(-sex) individuals, but the available data illustrate that a majority reported increased levels of mental health problems compared with their cisgendered or non-inter counterparts. Current explanatory models center on the pathogenic effect of homonegativity, transnegativity, and internegativity. These are further complicated by rigid gender roles and gender-role expectations, resulting in minority stressors that LGBTI individuals and those who are perceived as LGBTI are faced with. These authors describe that such experienced or internalized minority stress can explain mental health disparities well. This contrasts with the medical view still held in many countries that LGBTI conditions are inherently pathological. Evidence-based LGBTI-specific prevention and intervention programmes are beginning to emerge. Montoro points out that the term used to describe sexual minority youth is broad and includes adolescents from both sexual orientation and gender minorities. As a major task of adolescence is identity formation, sexual minority youth are particularly vulnerable during this period of self-definition ('coming out') both because of societal stigma and traditionally poor parental support. He defines these terms used and, indeed, preferred by the diverse identities in this population and outlines basic concepts in sexual orientation and gender identity. The stigma experienced by LGBTQI individuals in their day-to-day lives further contributes not only to an increased risk of mental ill health, but also to delays in help-seeking. This is further complicated by the further creation of mental health disparities of sexual minority youth. Stigma is present at individual, interpersonal, and structural levels, the chapter will conclude with a discussion of the multiple multi-level interventions necessary to have an impact on these disparities. Policymakers and clinicians are uniquely positioned to have a powerful impact on the mental health disparities of sexual minority youth. Human rights-based equity is critical and, as Shields and colleagues remind us in Chapter 57, these rights have to be protected in these uncertain times.

Those individuals who have intellectual disability are also likely to experience high rates of psychiatric disorders and, in addition, also face further health inequalities. In Chapter 30, Bhaumik and colleagues describe the global prevalence of intellectual disability with special emphasis on the prevalence of mental health problems. There is no doubt that this population also experiences a lack of resources and barriers to accessibility. Those with intellectual disability are also likely to face premature mortality. Preventive

strategies and health promotional aspects are necessary with better training in order to improve quality of health care.

The health, social, and economic effects of alcohol use are not only experienced directly by those who drink, but also indirectly by their families, communities, and society at large. Alcohol use is associated with many health conditions, including liver disease, cardiovascular disease, cancers, and a range of mental health problems, and is strongly linked to violence, accidents, self-harm, suicide, and fetal alcohol spectrum disorder. Gilmore et al., in Chapter 35, outline both primary and secondary prevention approaches to reduce alcohol-related harm that are evidence-based. Primary prevention approaches include regulating alcohol affordability, availability, and promotion, and providing information and education. Secondary prevention relies on early intervention.

Schools are often an underutilized source for improving public mental health. In many countries students attempt or commit suicide after examination results come out. In Chapter 42, Weare suggests that schools are increasingly concerned with the well-being and mental health of their students. However, we now know a great deal about 'what works' from a growing evidence base of evaluations of specific programmes and of broader strategies and approaches. She recommends that schools that are successful in engaging their students use a 'whole-school approach' right across the organization, with a base of universal work to promote the well-being of all staff and students from which targeted approaches gain coherence and support. She points out that the school and classroom climate/ethos is supportive, warm, connected, and safe, and there are active steps to tackle stigma and prejudice around mental health. 'Difficult' student behaviour is seen as meaningful, having deeper roots, and as an opportunity for learning and growth, as well as needing proportionate and helpful consequences. The students are encouraged and facilitated to develop the resilience to resist adverse circumstances. Of course, students have to work across families, parents, and others rather than in isolation by getting them involved and 'heard', and through engaging positively in school life. Specific programmes and interventions, for example to address social and emotional skills, underpin this ethos. It is important that programmes have clear aims and programme fidelity, and have to have a long-term perspective along with having robust and clear processes to identify early, refer, and treat those with greater levels of mental health difficulty. These approaches must be integrated into the whole-school approach, involving the young person and their family, liaising closely with specialist services, and with easy and transparent pathways to timely and effective interventions.

There is increasing understanding about the interplay and impact of poor mental health on society and the opportunities both to prevent mental health problems from developing and escalating, and to recover from mental health problems. Despite this, mental health is still, for the most part, a neglected issue in countries' public health services and non-governmental organization (NGO)-related work. NGOs are well placed to play a transformative role in improving the lives of people living with mental health problems. They can be central to improving the mental health of communities, particularly those with higher exposure to risk and fewer opportunities to protect and promote their mental health. This is strongly evident in low- and middle-income countries where poverty compounds the issue, and there is a lack of mental health clinicians, limited services, and high levels of mental health stigma and discrimination. In Chapter 51, Regan and colleagues remind us that in recent times biomedical models of mental illness have given way to more environmental and social factors. These determinants of health play a major role in sustainability of mental health and their impact on society needs further detailed scrutiny. It is agreed fairly commonly that mental health remains neglected in many countries. They rightly point out that under these circumstances public health services and NGOs can play a transformative role in improving the lives of people living with mental health problems but, equally importantly, in prevention of mental illness through education and mental health promotion. They can thus be the key to improving the mental health of communities, particularly those with higher exposure to risk and fewer opportunities to protect and promote their mental health, especially in low- and middle-income countries where poverty compounds the issue, and there is a lack of mental health clinicians and resources. In Chapter 48, Chatterjee illustrates this with the example of a well-functioning NGO, the Self Employed Women's Association, which was established nearly 50 years ago. The organization supports and empowers women, and, using case examples, Chatterjee makes some observations that may help others in low- and middle-income countries.

In Chapter 53, Stewart-Brown emphasizes that resilience and well-being are closely related. However, she reminds us that these two concepts are relatively new in the field of public health and psychiatry and the research. She argues, using research evidence, that resilience is both a product and a marker of mental well-being. As a consequence approaches to enhancing resilience and well-being are the same. Of course, ideally these should start with relational support in infancy and childhood and carry on throughout the life course with programmes to support personal development.

Building on the theme, Cook and White, in Chapter 54, using ideas about both concepts resilience and the role of spirituality, address the importance of spirituality in positive adaptation to adversity, often called resilience. Recognition of the significance of spirituality for clinical and public mental health applications is growing, yet has often been under-recognized. Cook and White suggest that spirituality is well placed to provide both valuable perspective on resilient adaption and resources for supporting that adaptation. As an environmental influence, spirituality exerts itself at personal and communal levels through a number of associated constructs, such as self-efficacy, meaning, and transcendence. On the whole, research indicates that spirituality is positively correlated with health and inversely correlated with psychopathology, although negative associations with spirituality may also occur. Owing to the significance of spirituality in resilient adaptation, Cook and White recommend that clinicians and public mental health policymakers alike are to be encouraged in supporting existing personal and communal spiritual strengths in the promotion of well-being.

In Chapter 14, McKenzie describes the models and importance of social capital. Social capital is a theory that focuses on and describes features of the fabric of society. These factors include levels of civic participation, social networks, and levels of trust because such forces enable shaping of the quality and quantity of social interactions and the institutions that underpin society. The role of social capital in the genesis of mental ill health and its importance in helping the resilience need further study. McKenzie suggests that there appears to be an association between higher levels of some types of social capital and a lower risk of mental health problems.

Stewart-Brown points out in Chapter 53 that research is the key to our understanding of the causation of psychiatric disorders and subsequent application not only in clinical settings, but also in public mental health. There are several methods and modes of research applicable to different disciplines and settings. Of course, once these methods have been developed and performed their use can spread across other disciplines. It is inevitable that in many cases these research methods can be extremely complex and will therefore require careful evaluation and interpretation. She reminds us that more complex research methods have evolved. And also that research is heavily influenced by the questions asked, the method and the interpretation in tune with the mindsets of the researchers and what they regard as good evidence. She goes on to emphasize that public mental health as a new area of practice and many of its attributes—the need for a focus on the positive, complexity, and holism—demand a new level of consciousness in research.

Ndetei and colleagues illustrate in Chapter 59 the use of faith healers and traditional healers as co-players in delivery of services that patients may find useful and acceptable. They remind us that traditional healers have a unique role and by training them professional health sector can improve engagement and get the targets right.

In Chapter 15, Huppert and Ruggeri also challenge the reluctance of some members of the psychiatry and public health communities to take well-being seriously They examine unresolved issues such as how precisely to define and measure well-being in its true sense, and how to address doubts and barriers to accepting the value and public health benefits of improving well-being in the population. They outline the health economic case for the financial benefits of promoting well-being in the population.

Occupational health plays a wide-ranging role in optimizing the health of the workforce and the workplace. In Chapter 12, Barnes and Henderson highlight the importance and the role the workplace can play for improving public mental health. Of course, not all work is good and not stressful and can thereby further contribute to further health inequalities. Poor mental health can have deleterious effect on the workplace at a number of levels, such as on an individual, organizational, and wider economic levels.

Healthy lifestyles can also influence mental health. McHugh's chapter (Chapter 21) explains the interaction between physical and mental health and it is evident that healthy lifestyles are essential for improving both physical and mental health and prevention of ill health.

Social media and telemental health are incredible advances of the twenty-first century, but their role in healthcare has so far been rather limited. Telemental health is a term for health care that includes audio and video telecommunications technologies such as video-teleconferencing, computers, mobile devices, the Internet, telephones, and broadband connectivity to provide mental health services across time and physical distance. Telemental health can, indeed, make a significant and positive impact on public mental health by its ability to not only increase access to care, but also more effectively tailor mental health services to individual or community-wide health care needs, as described by Waugh and colleagues in Chapter 56. However, ethical aspects of such approaches need to be remembered. Waugh and colleagues illustrate ways in which telemental health is currently being used to influence and deliver mental health promotion, prevention, and treatment.

Where next?

There is no doubt that mental health is an integral part of an individual's well-being and health, although sometimes there have been difficulties in defining it. Mental health and mental illness should not be seen as two ends of a spectrum and we need a clearer definition and identified links between the two. Sartorius defined mental health as a state of the organism that allows the full performance of all its functions [19]. He also sees mental health as a state of balance within oneself and between an individual and their physical and social (and cultural) environment. Maslow defines it as an ability to function well and in so doing meet the needs of food, shelter, survival, and so forth [20]. However, his hierarchy describes basic human needs at a more primitive level. Mental health is related to feelings of self-worth and contributes to the self-esteem of the individual. Therefore, a mixture of physical, social, and psychological well-being defines mental health and well-being. An individual has links with external wider culture and society, which helps them perform certain functions as a member of the group and other functions as an individual. Interactions between the individual and that person's immediate family and peers and society at large will allow them to function effectively and successfully. Bhugra et al. see mental health as a state of equipoise [21], where the individual is at peace with their self and functions effectively socially. The individuals are able to look after their needs.

Psychiatry by definition and history has often focused too much on mental illness and not enough on mental health. Training and the curricula both at undergraduate and postgraduate levels may cover some aspects of preventive and social medicine but often do not deal with mental health and well-being. In addition, in order to obtain the best health both physical and mental health aspects must be integrated.

Public mental health has to focus not only on primary prevention, but also on mental health promotion. Hopefully, this volume will start the process of discussion and draw attention to the core principles of public mental health. It is important that clinicians and policymakers start to take a long-term intergenerational view thereby ensuring that general population and vulnerable individuals get the right evidence-based prevention strategies.

References

1. Bhugra D. Social justice for people with mental illness. *Int Rev Psychiatry* 2016; 28: 335–419.
2. Venkatapuram S. *Health Justice*. Cambridge: Polity Press, 2011.
3. Sen A. *Choice, Welfare and Measurement*. Cambridge, MA: MIT Press, 1982.
4. Sen A. *Development as Freedom*. New York: Knopf, 1999.
5. Sen A. *The Idea of Justice*. London: Allen Lane, 2009.
6. Nussbaum M, Sen A. *The Quality of Life*. New York: Clarendon Press, 1993.
7. Nussbaum M. *Women and Human Development: The Capabilities Approach*. New York: Cambridge University Press, 2000.
8. Nussbaum M. *Frontiers of Justice: Disability, Nationality, Species Membership*. Cambridge, MA: Bellknap Press, 2006.
9. Campion J, Bhui K, Bhugra D. EPA guidance on prevention of mental illness. *Eur Psychiatry* 2012; 27: 68–80.
10. Eisenberg L. Disease and illness. *Culture Med Psychiatry* 1977; 1: 9–23.
11. Nordenfelt L. *On the Nature of Health: An Action-Theoretic Approach*. Dordrecht: D Reidel, 1987.
12. Nordenfelt L, Khushf G, Fulford KWM. *Health, Science and Ordinary Language*. Amsterdam: Rodopi, 2001.
13. Huber M, Knottnerus JA, Green L, et al. How should we define health? *BMJ* 2011; 343: d4163.
14. Boorse C. On the distinction between disease and illness. *Philos Public Aff* 1975; 5: 49–68.
15. Boorse C. What a theory of mental health should be. *J Theory Soc Behav* 1976; 6: 61–84.
16. Boorse C. Wright on Functions. *Philos Rev* 1976; 85: 70–86.
17. Boorse C. A rebuttal on health. In: Hunter JM, Almeder RF (eds). *Biomedical Ethics Reviews: What is Disease*. Clifton, NJ: Humana Press, 1977, pp. 1–134.
18. Venkatapuram S, Ventriglio A, Bhugra D. Capability to be healthy—implications for prevention. *Int J Soc Psychiatry* 2015; 61: 518–520.
19. Sartorius N. *Fighting for Mental Health*. Cambridge: Cambridge University Press, 2002.
20. Maslow A. *Towards a Psychology of Being*. New York: Van Nostrand, 1968.
21. Bhugra D, Till A, Sartorius N. What is mental health. *Int J Soc Psychiatry*. 2013; 59: 3–4.

SECTION I

Background and general principles

CHAPTER 1

Principles of public health
Application to public mental health

Sarah Stewart-Brown

Context of public health practice

Public health principles have a long history, being evident in the archaeological finds and surviving texts of ancient Greece and Rome [1], as well as in the Middle and Far East. In the modern Western world over the last two centuries, public health has come to be recognized as a specific discipline with profoundly beneficial effects. But public health initiatives have rarely been enacted without debate, and often years of controversy. This is because these initiatives, while improving health, saving lives, and reducing costly health care in the longer term, usually incur a cost to the public purse or to private corporations, and often demand a change in beliefs, attitudes, and behaviour from citizens and policymakers. It took 40 years from the first scientific reports of the health effects of tobacco to begin the serious implementation of tobacco-control policies [2], and new policies covering a wide range of environments and sectors continue to be put in place to the present day. Once in place, policies tend to become rapidly accepted by the public and in the great majority of cases have the expected positive effect on health and health behaviours. Occasionally, they have unexpected and negative effects.

Seat belt-wearing laws are another good example of the introduction of public health policy. Intense public debate for over ten years preceded legislation. This debate made a valuable contribution in its own right because media coverage had an educating effect. By the time legislation was introduced in 1983, 40% of the public had already decided to do the safe thing and buckle up. After legislation was enacted the rates of use shot up to 95% and have remained there ever since [3]. Rear seat belt legislation was introduced without public debate. Wearing rates of rear seat belts increased much more slowly and still lag behind front seat belt rates. Both seat belt wearing and tobacco control illustrate the fact that successful public health initiatives work best when a high proportion of the public supports them. They are usually multifaceted, often need to be enacted in more than one sector over a long period of time, and may need legislative backing.

The practice of public health, as defined in 1988 by the then-President of the UK Faculty of Public Health Medicine, Donald Acheson, is thus the 'the art and science of preventing disease, prolonging life and promoting health through the organised efforts of society'. Previously, in 1920, in the USA, C.E.A. Winslow had offered a fuller definition in which he added 'the informed choices of society, organisations, public and private, communities and individuals' to 'the organised efforts of society' [4]. Like any artistic endeavour, no two public health initiatives are the same and in planning and developing an approach to tackling public health issues, well-established public health principles are valuable.

Public mental health

Until very recently public health focused on physical illnesses, initially communicable diseases and, more recently, the 'lifestyle' diseases of coronary heart disease and cancer. There have been occasional initiatives aiming to reduce suicide, like changes in domestic gas supplies and appliances, and changes in the prescribing and packaging of medicines, but the practice of public mental health is very new. One reason for this stems from the routine statistics in which public health practice is grounded (see the next section). Until recently those that have been readily available were mortality statistics, which systematically under-represent the importance of illnesses that disable but rarely kill. Several things have conspired to bring public mental health to the fore in the twenty-first century; these include:

♦ from a scientific perspective, the estimation of quality-adjusted life years has enabled the relative importance of mental illness to be highlighted;

♦ from a societal perspective, the taboo associated with mental illness is beginning to be challenged—now that well-respected public figures are speaking out about their illnesses and the effect they have on their lives, it is less easy to turn a blind eye to mental illness;

♦ finally, recognition is dawning in public health that many of the determinants of physical illness have their origins in mental or psychological drivers of health-risk behaviours, therefore further progress in eliminating, for example heart disease or cancer, is going to depend on addressing mental health.

Public health principles

Most of the principles of public health are directly applicable to public mental health and pertain to both the art and the science. The former have evolved from experience of practice, of trying to get change implemented in the face of opposition from those with a vested interest in the status quo, and the research on these principles is primarily observational and qualitative. The latter derive almost entirely from quantitative investigation. To enable improvements in public health it is essential to grasp both the art and the science. In the UK, public health has been recognized as having four components: health promotion, disease prevention, health protection, and healthcare quality. This chapter will focus primarily on the first two.

Epidemiology

Public health practice is grounded in the quantitative science of epidemiology—the study of disease in populations. Its starting point is an agreed definition of the disease and clarity about the population under study.

Populations

The two most basic epidemiological statistics are prevalence and incidence, and both depend on accurate population statistic. *Prevalence* is the number of people with a disease in a defined population at one point in time and the prevalence of illness varies according to the population being studied. It is usually important to base prevalence statistics on the general population and calculating these rates involves population surveys like the British Psychiatric Morbidity Surveys [5]. But general population surveys have to consider places where adults with mental illness are likely to be over-represented, for example institutions caring for people with mental illness, homeless people, and prisoners, as well as adults in private households. Children and adolescents need to be surveyed as well as adults and this requires a different sampling frame, depending on the age group. The ideal in all surveys is to include a randomly selected sample, one that is most likely to accurately represent the whole population. Non-response bias, owing to the fact that people who do not want to take part in studies are usually different in both subtle and not-so-subtle ways from people who do take part, is ubiquitous in surveys. The effect of random sampling biases can be estimated with statistical methods, but other types of bias cannot. Understanding the population under study and the biases inherent in the sampling methods is fundamental to the interpretation of epidemiological statistics.

Incidence is the number of new cases of a disease in a defined population over a defined period of time. *Event rate statistics*, like mortality rates, are similar—the number of deaths in a defined population over a defined period of time. Like prevalence rates, these statistics depend for interpretation on accurate knowledge of the population and are effected by biases in data collection. Unlike prevalence statistics they demand a monitoring system like notification of communicable disease or registration of deaths. The first attempts to count deaths in the UK started in 1665 when the Bills of Mortality were introduced in London to monitor the progress of the plague. The systematic UK-wide registration of births and deaths began only in 1836 and William Farr, the father of epidemiology, developed a basic classification system to aid reporting of these deaths. For the next century epidemiology was based on these statistics relating to cause of death and initiatives to prevent disease would be prioritized on the basis of the number of deaths due to that disease. Until the beginning of the twentieth century they focused on communicable disease. With advances in sanitation and medicine, communicable disease incidence and mortality declined and public health attention turned to cardiovascular disease and then to cancer. Although it is now well known that mental illness is a powerful risk factor for premature death [6], it is only counted as the primary cause of death when that death was unequivocally

a suicide. As a result, it has taken until the twenty-first century for the public health community to wake up to the importance of mental health

Definition of disease

Both prevalence and incidence statistics are also dependent on a clear definition of disease. Communicable disease is perhaps the easiest to define because the bacterium or virus is either present or not. Cancer is, in theory, easy to define, but as methods of detection become more sophisticated cancerous cells can be detected at a point where they may not go on to develop into disease and the recorded incidence of cancer has increased since cancer screening programmes were introduced simply because abnormalities that would have resolved spontaneously are now labelled as cancer [7, 8].

The diagnosis of mental illness depends on the observations of clinicians and the identification of patterns of behaviour and affect. Observations about what is and is not important change over time and new classifications of patterns of behaviour and affect appear in response to new interventions and structures. What constitutes normal and abnormal behaviour and affect varies over time and from one culture to another [9]. The stigma of mental illness and the relative ignorance of the general population about its nature mean that a more than half of those with mental illness are not in contact with mental health services [10]. Psychiatric epidemiology is therefore challenging and estimates of the proportion of the population with mental illness vary widely from 38% in a recent study in the European Union [11] to 18% in the most recent Adult Psychiatric Morbidity survey in the UK [10]. The variation in prevalence statistics for mental illness makes comparison with other diseases difficult, but the development of the common metric *the disability-adjusted life year* (DALY) has been helpful in this respect. Based on clinicians' knowledge of the impact of different diseases on quality of life, the DALY has enabled statistics on premature mortality to be combined with statistics on estimates of disability to show that mental illness is responsible for more DALYs lost (23%) than cardiovascular disease (16%) or cancer (16%) [12]. Asking the general public, in anonymous surveys, about health problems and how they impact on daily life provides another basis for estimating the impact of mental health problems. These take into account non-diagnosed mental illness and the impact of mental health problems that fall short of a diagnosis. Studies like this suggest that mental health problems are a more important cause of disability than all physical health problems put together [13].

Cross-sectional studies providing estimates of prevalence ignore the dynamic nature of mental health. Surveys pick up people who currently meet the criteria for mental illness, but cohort and panel studies, which follow people over time, are needed to make calculations of lifetime risk. These studies suggest that more than twice as many people experience depression over the course of their lifetime as are identified as having depression at any one point in time [14]. The nature of these diseases is essentially one of remission and relapse. Cohort studies have also been important in demonstrating that the great majority of mental illness first makes itself known in childhood [15].

Health and well-being

Medicine is based on dichotomy, dividing the population into those with disease and those without; and the focus of interest is disease. Epidemiology is grounded in this medical model. Many authorities, from the World Health Organization (WHO) onwards [16], have pointed out that health is more than the absence of disease. The WHO first introduced the concept of health as well-being [16], and continues to define mental health as a positive concept [17]. Because of the ubiquitous use of the description 'health services' to describe services to treat illness, the WHO approach to labelling creates problems. It is preferable to allow the term mental health to cover the spectrum from illness to wellness and to look for another term to define the positive. In the UK the term 'mental well-being' is used. The nature of mental well-being has been debated and described by philosophers and spiritual traditions over the course of several millennia [18]; more recently, other disciplines like psychologists and social scientists have contributed [19, 20], and there is now a broad measure of agreement that mental well-being covers positive feelings (affect) and positive functioning (behaviour) [21] (see Chapters 15 and 53), in much the same way that the diagnosis of mental illness is based on negative affect and behaviours. Description and classification of the various dimensions of mental well-being is in its infancy compared with mental illness, and understanding will become more sophisticated as more interest is paid and research done. But as health promotion (see 'Health promotion' section later) focuses on health, wellness, or well-being, it requires measures of the positive end of the mental health spectrum. In the absence of clear agreement about the level of mental health constituting well-being, researchers use a variety of measures and cut-off points, for example the point separating the top 15% or 20% of the population from the rest. This relatively arbitrary approach works well enough to begin studying the epidemiology of mental well-being, in the same way as studies of the importance of cholesterol in heart disease aetiology were valuable before the optimum level of cholesterol was defined.

Causality and risk

Because measurement of prevalence or incidence often reveals systematic differences over time, place, and demographic sectors of the population, epidemiology opens the door to studying the causes of disease. The communicable disease model, which had dominated thinking in medicine for most of the last century, is based on finding an organism that is always present when the disease occurs. Epidemiology is very good at identifying factors or agents associated with a specific disease to a certain degree. The classic research establishing the risk model as fundamental to public health was that describing the association between lung cancer and smoking [22]. This association is strong: smoking increases risk by a factor of 40. However, cases occur in non-smokers and heavy smokers do not always get the disease. Unlike bacterial causes of disease, tobacco smoking was neither sufficient nor necessary, but it clearly played a key role in disease causation and public health measures to curtail tobacco have reduced the prevalence of this disease, and many others that turned out to be associated with smoking. The concept of risk based on probability of association was born and with it the need to develop criteria to decide if an association between a factor and a disease was incidental to the causal pathway or part of it. Bradford Hill proposed a set of criteria that, with only small adjustments, have stood the test of time (Table 1.1)

Table 1.1 Criteria for causation

Criteria	Comments
There is a strong relationship between the factor and the disease	The strength of the relationship is measured as relative risk (cohort studies) or odds ratio (case–control studies) and the statistical probability of observing this
There is a consistent relationship between the factor and the disease	Different studies in different populations using different methodologies all demonstrate the association
The relationship is specific, i.e. the factor causes only one disease and the only one factor is associated with the disease, e.g. exposure to asbestos and mesothelioma	Specificity is a valuable criterion when present, but its absence is no longer regarded as necessary to establish a causal role
The putative cause precedes the putative effect or disease	This criterion is fundamental to establishing causality and requires evidence from cohort studies where the putative cause has been measured at one point in time and the effect at a later time. Cohort studies are expensive and take a very long time. Because their size has to be limited by cost, they are not good at establishing the causes of rare diseases. Case–control studies work better for rare diseases but provide less precise estimates of risk
Demonstrating a biological gradient (dose–response relationship) is a strong indicator of causality; the more of the factor present the greater the risk of disease	Not essential to establishing causality: some factors only cause disease above a certain level and are safe below that level. Some non-causal associations can show this pattern, e.g. birth order and Down syndrome. The causal factor is maternal age, which is strongly correlated with birth order
The association is coherent with what is already known of the natural history and biology of disease; a similar causal relationship is already established; and/or a biological explanation exists for the association	All these factors provide support for causality but none is essential. The biological mechanisms for smoking causing cancer came a long time after the epidemiological evidence was secure. We still do not know the biological mechanisms behind prone sleeping and cot death
Experiential evidence; demonstrating that it is possible to change the incidence or prevalence of disease by changing the level of exposure to the factor or agent	This is the most powerful evidence in support of causality. It can be regarded as a test of causality rather than a criterion and in many instances evidence of this kind is unavailable.

Source: Data from Detels, R, McEwen J, Beaglehole R, Tanaka H, Oxford Textbook of Public Health, Third Edition, Copyright (1997), Oxford University Press.

[23]. A factor that is associated with an outcome but does not fulfil the criteria for causality is called a confounding factor.

The role of social inequality as a cause of mental illness represents a good exemplar for examining causality in mental health. Numerous cross-sectional studies produced over a long period of time have shown a consistent gradient in mental health according to indicators of social position: income, education, and social class [24, 25]. Cohort studies show that social position in childhood predicts mental health in later life, including depression and substance use, as well as cognitive development [26]. So from many points of view social inequality fulfils the criteria for causality. Yet there is also a strong effect of mental illness on social position as mental illness leads to unemployment, lower income [27], and lower educational attainment [28]. Therefore, the relationship is bidirectional, making it difficult to untangle the extent of causality and impossible to do so in cross-sectional studies. Evidence is also emerging that mental well-being is less strongly associated with social position than mental illness [29], suggesting that the relationship is complex. The regression analyses (see Chapter 58) that are used to estimate risk start from the assumption of a linear relationship and work best when estimating the risk of a single causative factor on a single illness. In mental health research such analyses are used to compare the strength of association of a number of possible causal factors; the factors that are independently predictive are believed to be the causal ones. But in mental health research risk factors are often related to each other in a causal chain, or one factor may potentiate another or protect against problems and some factors may be easier to measure accurately than others.

The criterion that it is necessary to establish that the putative cause existed before the putative effect is a very important one in establishing causality. This research demands longitudinal or cohort studies, which are both expensive and time consuming. While essential for epidemiology, cohort studies do not get round the issues present in mental health research that risk factors interact with protective and potentiating factors throughout the life course in complex causal pathways, which are beyond the scope of regression analyses commonly used to estimate risk. It is not uncommon to find studies that adjust for risk factors that are part of the causal chain, potentiate other factors, or protect against disease. These can distort the results. Potent causal factors for mental illness, like attachment security in infancy, abusive and neglectful parenting, and parental mental illness are themselves associated with social inequality. They are also hard to measure accurately so their effects in regression models are almost always underestimated and may appear less strong than the social inequality measures, which are usually easy to measure. Psychologists have recognized complex causal pathways and use path analyses or structural equation modelling in an attempt to untangle cause and effect. A further complication that besets epidemiological studies of specific mental illnesses is that discrete illnesses rarely occur in isolation; comorbidity—the presence of more than one psychiatric diagnosis—is the norm [30]. And risk factors for one discrete mental illness usually increase the risk of others.

Epidemiology is valuable as a method of researching mental illness, but many of the criteria and principles of epidemiology are challenged by mental health research and the approaches commonly used may offer less precise estimates than we are led to believe. Epidemiological approaches need to be used with care and insight in this field and new approaches and methods developed to allow for the complexity encountered in this field.

Health needs assessment

One of the practical uses of epidemiology is in estimating health need [31]. But health needs are not always conceptually simple. Needs can be felt—that is, the individual perceives poor health and a need for services, which may or not be articulated. This is particularly pertinent in mental health services, where under-diagnosis is common and a high proportion of the population might benefit from services if they expressed their needs. Expressed needs are felt needs that have been articulated and for which services are demanded, but not necessarily available; carers of patients with mental illness may express the need for respite care, which is not available. Normative needs are those defined in relation to an objective norm of health care usually by a professional; all those with clinical depression should receive cognitive behaviour therapy, for example. Comparative needs attempt to assess whether one set of needs is more or less important than another, based on the severity and extent of the problem and range of services available. Suicide prevention would rank highly in a comparative needs assessment on the grounds of severity but not so high on the grounds of frequency.

Ideally, need for services would be balanced by demand and supply, but this is not usually the case (Fig. 1.1). There are unmet needs for which services are available; there are services for which there is little demand and demand for services which are both available and unavailable. Healthcare needs also need to be distinguished from health needs in that the first need to be met with health services and the second might be met with wider social and environmental services or action.

Health needs assessment not only takes into account the different types of need described, but also uses information gathered using different methods (Fig. 1.2).

Epidemiological needs assessment provides estimates of the numbers of people in the population with the health problem or disease and thus the need for services. This information may depend on accurate survey data. Through randomized controlled trials and systematic reviews, evidence is provided of the effectiveness of services to meet the need, and an estimate of currently available services is provided through health services statistics. This type of needs assessment starts from the assumption that if there is no effective intervention there is no legitimate health need.

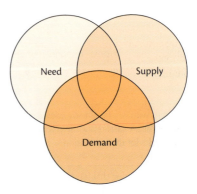

Fig. 1.1 The interrelationship of need, supply, and demand.

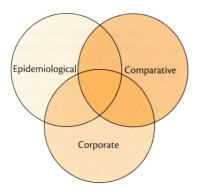

Fig. 1.2 Approaches to health needs assessment.

Comparative needs assessment is based on statistics related to up-take of health services: number of outpatient visits, home visits, in-patient stays, or drugs prescribed. Actual need for health services is assumed to be the same in different places. The value of services to patients is not considered. The latter is perhaps the crudest way of estimating need for services, but in practice is the most common approach considered by managers because the data are readily available.

Corporate needs assessment gathers the views, desires, and knowledge of a range of stakeholders, including patients, carers, and providers. It can provide a radically different perspective from the other approaches and may identify services that do not seem to be meeting any need and also needs that were previously unrecognized and where research to identify effective intervention is needed. Users and carers of mental health services may identify the need for services that focus on their well-being rather than just their illness. Such needs would not be picked up in any of the other approaches.

Rapid appraisal is an approach to establishing health needs in places where information is scarce and action is felt to be needed in the near future [32]. It has its origins in the developing world but has been applied effectively in the UK and involves:

◆ interviews with a wide range of local informants;

◆ examining existing data and records for the area;

◆ observations made in the neighbourhood or in the homes of interviewees;

◆ triangulation of one set of data against another.

Participatory needs assessment puts the emphasis on action *by* rather than *for* or *to* communities [32]. It has its basis in community development and aims to address issues known to the community by encouraging communities to tackle problems by harnessing community resources. It is ideally suited to community-based action to promote mental health and prevent mental illness.

Health impact assessment

Health impact assessment emerged from environmental impact assessment and is used to assess the likely impact of all proposals for development on the health of the community [32]. Mental Health Impact Assessment (MHIA) is now a well-established tool [33]. It is being used as a training resource to introduce the concept of public mental health and to begin consideration

of its determinants. Although the WHO Europe, in conjunction with the Mental Health Foundation, has recommended that every policy should be scrutinized for its impact on mental health and well-being, this has yet to happen in any significant way. In the meantime, MHIA remains valuable as a way of starting the process of mental health improvement, both nationally and locally.

Disease prevention

As the name implies disease prevention aims to reduce the prevalence and incidence of specific diseases. The starting point is therefore always epidemiological information about a specific disease and its causes.

Approaches to disease prevention are categorized as primary, secondary, or tertiary.

Primary prevention aims to prevent a disease appearing in the first place. Immunization to prevent communicable disease, fluoridation of the water supplies to prevent dental caries, and stop-smoking clinics to prevent cancer and heart disease are classic examples.

Secondary prevention aims to identify disease at an early stage when the disease process can be reversed by intervention. Screening programmes are secondary prevention; safeguarding legislation and services that aim to remove children from abusive or neglectful homes before they damage their mental or physical health are another. Identification and intervention in postnatal depression is secondary prevention for the mother but primary prevention for the infant

Tertiary prevention aims to slow the progress or mitigate the consequences of established disease. Programmes to increase the chances of employment in populations with mental illness would fall into this category. Programmes that remove children from homes where abuse and neglect have already caused damage would be tertiary prevention.

Many initiatives in public mental health have components of all three approaches. For example, school and workplace mental health programmes are often multicomponent. They aim to put in place policies that could prevent mental illness in those who are currently well, for example establishing policies to prevent bullying; or to educate and sensitize staff to the early signs of mental health problems in colleagues so that support can be provided early to those who need it; and to offer facilities, such as workplace counselling services, for people with established mental health problems.

Screening programmes offer a seemingly attractive approach to finding people with mental health problems and offering them services. But screening programmes can do harm through over-diagnosis and treatment and need to be thoroughly evaluated before being put into place [34]. There are good reasons why screening programmes tend to be ineffective in mental health.

Screening in mental health

The most successful screening programmes—for example those offered in the neonatal period, screening for hypothyroidism—are ones where there is a clear biological basis for the problem, a clear demarcation between the biological markers of the diseased and well population, and a clear intervention that can change the course of the disease.

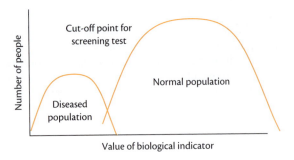

Fig. 1.3 Diagram to illustrate optimal indicators for screening programmes.

In a situation like that shown in Fig. 1.3, the optimum cut-off point falls where the distribution of the factor in the well population intersects with the distribution in the diseased population. It is a clear point where the number of individuals whose values fall below the cut-off point but do not have the problems (false positives) and the number whose values fall above but do have the problem (false negatives) are minimized.

Unfortunately, no measure of mental health has ever shown a bipolar distribution like this. Every measure that has been validated in general populations is continuous and unipolar, as Fig. 1.4 illustrates for one common measure of mental health, the 12-item General Health Questionnaire (GHQ-12).

The GHQ-12 is regarded as a good indicator of mental illness for use in in surveys of the adult population, but has not been found to be helpful in clinical screening because its sensitivity and specificity are not adequate.

The criteria for effective screening programmes, first described by Wilson and Junger in 1968 [35], and with minor modifications still in use today [8], are shown in Box 1.1. Those related to the condition, the test, and the treatment derive from Wilson and Junger. Those related to the screening programme have been developed in the UK by the National Screening Committee from experience of managing large-scale screening programmes and the things that can go wrong with them

With regard to the conditions, mental illnesses fulfil most of the criteria in that many are common and disabling and there are long-term studies to understand the natural history of the conditions. Some might argue that many potential preventive measures have not been put in place, but the number of these for which there are reliable studies showing cost-effectiveness is quite small. The problems for mental illness screening programmes derive in large part from the test criteria. Screening instruments are based on proxy or self-report, and while these are safe they are subject to social desirability bias in reporting and depend on self-awareness. They are therefore imprecise. And cut-off points in a continuous distribution are somewhat arbitrary (see Fig. 1.4). These factors mean that the test sensitivity

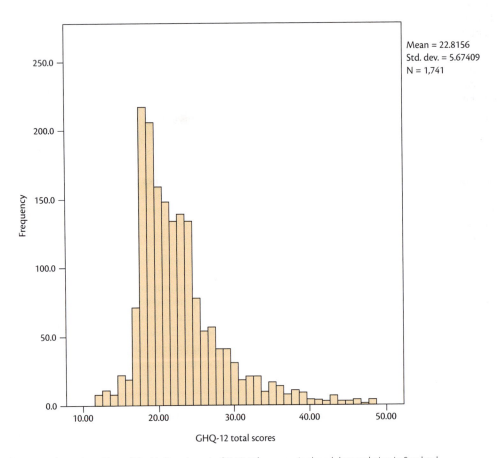

Fig. 1.4 Distribution of scores on the 12-item General Health Questionnaire (GHQ-12) measure in the adult population in Scotland.
Source: data from Tennant R, Fishwick R, Platt S, Joseph S, Stewart-Brown S, Monitoring positive mental health in Scotland: validating the Affectometer 2 scale and developing the Warwick-Edinburgh Mental Well-being Scale for the UK, Copyright (2006), NHS Health Scotland, University of Warwick, and University of Edinburgh

---

Box 1.1 Criteria for effective screening programmes

The condition

- Should be an important public health problem—common and disabling

- The epidemiology and natural history of the condition should be well understood and there should be detectable risk factor disease marker latent period or early symptomatic stage

- All cost-effective primary prevention should have been implemented as far as possible

The test

- There should be a simple, safe, precise, and validated tool

- The distribution of the test values in the target population should be known and a suitable cut-off level defined

- The test should be acceptable to the general population

- There should be an agreed policy on further diagnostic investigation of individuals with a positive test result and the choices available to these individuals

The treatment

- There should be an effective treatment of intervention for patients identified through early detection with evidence of early treatment leading to better outcome than later treatment

- There should be agreed evidence-based policies covering which individuals should be offered treatment and the appropriate treatment to be offered

- Clinical management of the condition and patient outcomes should be optimized by all healthcare providers prior to participation in a screening programme

The screening programme

- There should be evidence from high-quality randomized controlled trials that the screening programme is effective in reducing mortality or morbidity

- There should be evidence that the complete screening programme (test, diagnostic procedures, treatment/intervention) is clinically socially and ethically acceptable to health professionals and the public

- The benefits of the screening programme should outweigh the physical and psychological harm (caused by the test, diagnostic procedures and treatment)

- The opportunity costs of the screening programme (including testing diagnosis and treatment) should be economically balanced in relation to expenditure on medical care as a whole

- There should be a plan for managing and monitoring the screening programme and an agreed set of quality-assurance standards

- Adequate staffing and facilities for testing diagnosis and treat and programme management should be available prior to the commencement of the screening programme

- All other options for managing the condition should have been considered (e.g. improving treatment, providing other services)

Source: Data from UK National Screening Committee, Guidance Criteria for appraising the viability, effectiveness and appropriateness of a screening programme, Copyright (2010), Public Health England.

---

and specificity of instruments that could be used to screen for mental illness is very likely to be poor.

Tables 1.2 and 1.3 define the four key parameters for judging the quality of a screening test. Special studies need to be undertaken to estimate their values. Simple programme evaluations do not identify false negatives and so can only be used calculate positive predictive value. Sensitivity in the region of 80% is regarded as acceptable, although many cases will be missed. Specificity needs to be in the region of 90% to prevent the harms and costs that accrue from false-positive cases.

Issues to do with provision of treatment only need to be considered if the test passes these criteria, but in this section, too, there are problems. Mental health services in the UK are currently insufficient to cope with appropriate demand for services and could not cope with the doubling in the number of patients who would need treatment if effective screening programmes could be put in place. Clear cut-off points defining who should and should not be treated would remain difficult to define.

Ultimately, screening programmes should be tested in very expensive, large randomized controlled trials in which the overall health of the screened population is shown to be better than that of an unscreened population, but even such robust studies fail to take all the possible issues into account. Screening programmes speak to a medical model of illness, one in which people with illness simply need to be found and referred to doctors for all to be well. One subtle cost of screening that is very rarely evaluated, is the implicit message these programmes give to the public—that health is determined by a biological test and treatment from a health service if there is a problem. This contrasts with the key public health message that health is most often determined by self-awareness and self-care. A second subtle cost is that they apparently absolve other people from responsibility. Mental illness may be caused by toxic systems or by other people—bullying in schools and workplaces being prime examples—and system-wide change involving everyone may be needed to change this.

Table 1.2 Parameters of screening programmes

Screening test	Disease	
	Present	Absent
Positive	a	b
Negative	c	d

a = true positive; b = false positive; c = false negative; d = true negative

Table 1.3 Definition of sensitivity and specificity positive predictive and negative predictive value

Term	Definition	Formula
Sensitivity	The % of people with the disease who test positive	a/a = c
Specificity	The % of those without the disease who test negative	d/d + b
Positive predictive value	The % of those who test positive who have the disease	a/a + b
Negative predictive value	The % of those who test negative who do not have the disease	d/d = c

Putting in place a screening programme that refers people with problems elsewhere can prevent this and thus act counter to primary prevention.

Case finding

Screening needs to be distinguished from case finding. The latter aims to increase knowledge and skills in the general population, managers, teachers, and healthcare professionals so that they are able to recognize the signs and symptoms of mental illness and to act appropriately. Several well-established programmes, like Mental Health Literacy [36] and Mental Health First Aid [37], aim to do this. Acting appropriately may be having a conversation with the person identified and putting in place some simple measures to change the stressors that can be changed. It could also mean encouraging the person to seek help from their doctor. In the latter situation the 'case' retains control, whereas in screening programmes control rests with the programme

Targeting and the population paradox

Demonstration of systematic variation in disease prevalence by demographic group or by place mean that it is, in theory, possible to target preventive initiatives to particular population groups in which a high prevalence has been demonstrated. Targeting on the basis of social indicators is common in public health and attractive because it concentrates resources where they are most needed. The Increasing Access to Psychological Therapies (IAPT) initiative was targeted at people living in less affluent areas. Sure Start Children's Centres were initially provided only to deprived communities.

While this may be a valuable approach, there are also pitfalls, as Fig. 1.5(a, b) shows. The former shows the social class distribution of childhood behaviour problems. The prevalence is 5–6 times greater in social class V and the non-working population than it is in social classes I and II. Fig. 1.5(b) illustrates the same data in a different way. It shows the number of children with behaviour problems in each group. This depends on both the prevalence and the size of the population. The two figures together demonstrate that targeting services at the population with the highest prevalence may only reach a small percentage of those with problems because the larger social groups have more children with problems, even though the prevalence is lower. This phenomenon, known as the population paradox, always needs to be thought through in proposals to target services

The Rose hypothesis and the prevention paradox

Professor Geoffrey Rose proposed in the 1980s that the prevention of diseases or health problems that were continuously distributed in the population was most efficiently addressed with whole-population approaches [38]. He showed how a very small change in blood pressure across an entire population would have a greater effect on the prevalence and incidence of diseases for which hypertension was a determinant than a big change in those at risk. Such small changes can sometimes be achieved in public health by introducing low-cost initiatives like reducing salt levels in processed foods. Rose called this the 'prevention paradox' and showed that it applied to mental health, as well as physical health [39]. The issues he raised are illustrated in Fig. 1.6.

If a population strategy could shift the distribution of mental health from the first curve to the second one—the proportion of the population falling in the tail of the distribution—the illness side of psychiatric diagnosis—would fall. Studies in both child and adult populations have shown that the mean level of mental health is correlated with the proportion of that population with diagnosed illness [40–43], and it follows that if the mean can be shifted towards health and well-being the number with illness will fall. So the hypothesis holds true for the common mental illnesses studied—namely depression and childhood behaviour problems. Whether it holds true for severe and enduring mental illness has yet to be demonstrated, partly because it is difficult to show a change in prevalence of relatively rare illness in population studies without very large numbers.

For common mental health problems, it remains only to be shown that it is possible to shift the mean levels of mental health in a positive direction in studies carried out in general populations. General population studies of mindfulness [44], singing [45], and approaches to reducing loneliness in the elderly [46] have proved positive and it can be safely assumed that if these were offered to the general population prevalence levels of common mental disorders would fall. Interestingly Geoffrey Rose's conclusions mirror those researching school-based [47] and parenting support programmes [48, 49], where multiple systematic reviews have concluded that the combination of universal and targeted approaches work best. Rose's words derived from research on a variety of conditions: 'the population carries a collective responsibility for its own health and wellbeing, including that of its deviants' speak to another public health principle that as members of the general population 'those practicing public health are part of the problem as well as part of the solution'. In this way, public health is very different from clinical practice in that practitioners recognize themselves to be part of the public and expect to be changed themselves by public health initiatives.

Behaviour change

In the current era where 'lifestyle' diseases dominate public health, disease prevention often depends on enabling people to change their health-related behaviour. Early thinking—that it was simply a matter of telling people that a certain lifestyle was bad for their health (health education)—was rapidly superseded by more sophisticated thinking, which recognized the extent of addiction

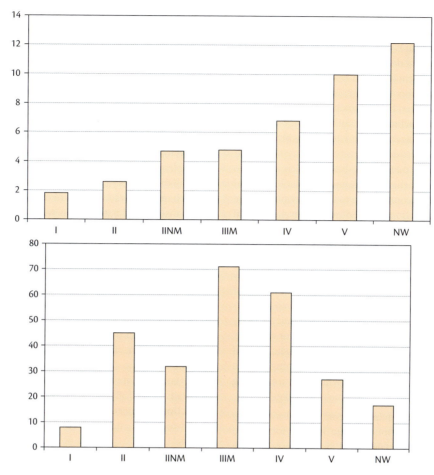

Fig. 1.5 (a) Distribution (%) of antisocial behaviour across social class: children aged 5–10 years. (b) Distribution (*n*) of antisocial behaviour across social class: children aged 5–10 years.

Source: Data from Meltzer H, Gatward R, Mental health of children and adolescents in Great Britain, Copyright (1999), Office for National Statistics.

and personal gain afforded by unhealthy lifestyles. Various models have been described.

The health belief model is the earliest model, developed in the 1950s [50]. It attempts to predict health-related behaviour in terms of patterns of belief. Motivation to change behaviour covers three things: individual perceptions, modifying factors, and likelihood

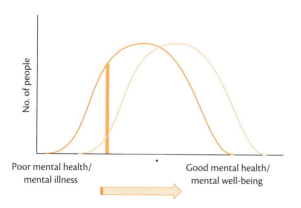

Fig. 1.6 The Rose hypothesis.

Source: Adapted from Slade M, Oades L, Jarden A, Wellbeing, Recovery and Mental Health, Copyright (2017), with permission from Cambridge University Press.

of action. Individual perceptions are factors that affect the perception of illness or disease; they deal with the importance of health to the individual, perceived susceptibility to illness, and perceived severity. Modifying factors include demographic variables, perceived threat, and cues to action. Likelihood of action is influenced by the above and by barriers to action, which may include structural and psychosocial factors

The ***transtheorectical model*** dates from 1984 [51], and covers three organizing constructs: the stages of change, the processes of change, and the levels of change. Stages of change include pre-contemplation, contemplation, preparation, action, maintenance, and relapse. Wider understanding of the stages of change enabled by this model has had a profound effect on disease prevention. It suggests that the helper's role is first to identify and enable movement from pre-contemplation into contemplation, then to help in planning and supporting the change with an expectation that relapse is common and not a reason to give up.

The ***theory of planned behaviour*** was also introduced in the 1980s [52], building on the Theory of Reasoned Action by adding a new component: perceived behavioural control. The latter is the degree to which a person believes that they control their own behaviour. People are much more likely to intend to change when they feel that they could do so successfully. Perceived behavioural control requires both self-efficacy (belief in one's own ability to succeed in the task) and controllability (the extent of belief that outside factors have control over the behaviour).

The more sophisticated models recognize that behaviour is influenced by more than information and reason. It starts to take account of psychological barriers to change, including recognizing that most negative health-related behaviours have short-term positive effects on mental states, which is in part why they are addictive. It also links to personal agency—the extent to which people believe they can influence outside factors. In this way behaviour change starts to be related to mental well-being, which is held to include both agency and self-beliefs. Improving population mental well-being can thus be seen as contributing to the behaviour change agenda and makes the connection between behaviour change and health promotion (see the next section).

Nudge is not only a popular idea at present in government circles, but also a principle that has been recognized in health promotion practice for many years [53]. It is a way of supporting health by 'making healthy choices the easy choices'. A nudge is any aspect of the 'choice architecture' that alters people's behaviour in a predictable way. A nudge is not a mandate; it is simple, cheap, and also easy to avoid: displaying healthy food like fruit at eye level, for example, or sweets somewhere less visible. It requires an understanding of the influences on personal choice, making the 'do nothing' option the healthiest, giving feedback to tell people when they are making unhealthy choices, and expecting people to make mistakes.

Social marketing applies the principles of commercial marketing tools to health and social behaviour change [54]. It focuses on high-risk groups and tailors campaigns and awareness raising on consumer research and health insights. Social marketing can help move people from pre-contemplation to contemplation in the transtheoretical model described earlier.

Health promotion

Health promotion evolved from health education—a discipline that was connected to, but distinct from, public health. While in the UK the disciplines are now closely aligned, there have often been tensions between them because of the different starting points and theoretical perspectives. Public health has often adopted the medical, negatively focused model and enjoyed greater power and influence because of its medical roots. Health promotion is based on a salutogenic model of health [55], one that aims to examine and provide that which supports health and well-being. It has grown from the practice of health education, which has different roots from public health and is based as much on art as science. While much quantitative and experimental research has been carried out, health promotion is often supported by qualitative research and by learning from experience of practice. It is interesting and reassuring that this discipline has come to the same conclusions as Geoffrey Rose, who started from disease prevention and worked from an essentially quantitative, theoretical base.

Like public health, in the past the principle focus of health promotion has been tackling issues and factors that were known to be important to physical health. There may have been more concentration on the positive (physical activity and healthy eating)—than the negative (enabling people to give up smoking and drink sensibly), but the orientation was risk factors for disease. Both disciplines have worked with awareness of the extent to which the physical and social environment influence the lives of individuals but there was more awareness in health promotion of the holistic nature of health and more sympathy for psychological influences.

Mental health promotion emerged within health promotion like public mental health emerged within public health [56]. And both disciplines are now meeting up with positive psychology, which has turned the traditional negative approach of psychology around and discovered that starting from a positive perspective, focusing individuals on what is going right in their lives, on solutions, and the development of strengths, can be more effective than focusing on problems [57].

For all disciplines in making this transition to the positive, one of the tensions relates to the nature of health and well-being. The nature of disease and pathology is well studied and for the most part well understood. The nature of health and well-being has received much less attention and much of what is known in some disciplines is not common knowledge in medicine or among the general public. Embarking on a programme when the direction of travel is known but before the end point is crystal clear is something that sits comfortably within the principles of public health. It is clear, for example, that a more active population would be healthier, but exactly what level of what type of exercise is healthiest for whom is not yet known. It is accepted that this will emerge as the programme evolves.

The components of health promotion were described in the Ottowa Charter [58]. These recognize, as an underlying principle, that action that needs to be taken in many different ways in many sectors to enable change to come about. These were categoriszd as follows.

Developing healthy policy. Supportive policies are an important part of health promotion; policymakers need to be on board, but as many health ministers have discovered, policy does not effect change on its own.

Create supportive environments. In unhealthy environments with no green spaces, traffic pollution, damp housing, limited access to employment, healthy foods, and opportunities for physical activity it is difficult to implement positive behavioural change. Changing the environment makes health possible

Community action. Engaging communities in promoting their own health has been recognized as more effective than making changes on the community's behalf. It brings people together and gives them ownership of endeavours and destinies. This type of community development means addressing the community's priorities, which may not necessarily align with those of the health authorities. Asset-based approaches that start from building a picture of the community's strengths work better than those based on deficits [59]. Enabling community development is definitely an art. A set of principles and approaches has been described, but as every community is different there is no set of rules to follow, and working with and responding to what emerges on the ground is necessary. If successful, community development empowers communities to take charge of their own destiny through collective political endeavour and the development of social capital. It thus promotes the mental health and well-being of individuals who become involved.

Develop personal skills. Provision of information and education for health and life is the health education component of health promotion and is an essential starting point. But personal development involves something beyond this. It enables individuals to develop more control over their own lives and their environment. The ways to support behaviour change have been described earlier and have traditionally been focused on health-related lifestyles. Public mental health would add a new range of skills, including the development of emotional literacy and social skills; self-regulation, conflict resolution, and anger management; and self-esteem and self-awareness building. Well-respected, evidence-based mental health approaches like cognitive behaviour therapy and mindfulness-based stress reduction can support many of these endeavours. Ultimately, individuals can move from being passive recipients of health care to being actively engaged in developing their own well-being. Diseases can be prevented and treated by doing things to people. Well-being development depends on the individual taking control of their own lives. Helping people make this transition is another art, one that is well respected in some psychotherapeutic services, but is not, to date, an art that is well developed in medical or social services.

Reorient services. The final plank of health promotion described in the Ottowa Charter calls for a reorientation of health services towards a more salutogenic approach, one that focuses on the positive, and encourages and supports personal development and engagement in health. Patient groups are calling for such a reorientation of mental health services. They would like to see a greater focus on well-being, and personal strengths and a greater focus on recovery [60]. Getting the balance right between caring for and, if necessary, controlling those who are seriously mentally ill and supporting the development of personal control and engagement is not simple. This service development aspect of public mental health will require skill development on the part of mental health professionals.

Settings. Health promotion is carried out in different settings: schools, workplaces, communities, and families, as well as health services, and requires a knowledge of practice in those settings. It is impossible to enable the implementation of a programme in a school unless the way that school works is well understood. If the head teacher and staff are not on board with the changes they will not be sustained. Each setting has its own set of principles and approaches to practice based on experience in those settings.

Complexity. Ultimately, health promotion is about dealing with complexity. Trying to achieve change in a complex system requires a dynamic interplay and balancing of the need for support and challenge, between changing the environment and enabling individuals to change, doing things for or to others, and enabling others to learn that they can do things themselves. Some skills, like understanding human beings and their needs, and understanding organizations and how they work are transferable from one setting to another, but some skills are setting specific

Management and leadership for public health

The principles of management and leadership are, like health promotion, part of the art of public health practice [61]. They are both disciplines in their own right with a large supporting literature and it is not possible to do more than touch on them here. Both are

mentioned here because they are very important for public mental health. Making the case with clarity and persuasion for a change in mindset amongst diverse groups and disciplines is fundamental to progress. So, too, is the courage to tackle outdated views and practices and absorb negative reactions without giving up. Long time frames and patience are also a given.

Leadership

The literature on leadership started from the tenet that leaders were born, not made. But leadership skills can be developed and honed during training to practice public health. Someone needs to have a grasp of what needs to change and how, based on the research literature, experience, and insight, and to convey that vision to many others. Leaders are not necessarily senior managers or policymakers, and the skills for these roles are rather different.

The qualities of leaders have been described as:

- initiative and perception;
- self-assurance, courage, and integrity;
- being able to see the bigger picture and longer time frame;
- goal orientation;
- good communication skills and the ability to work with a wide range of individuals;
- high energy levels;
- above-average intelligence.

To the above list may be added emotional intelligence and the capacity to read other people, resilience, and the capacity not to be daunted by failure. Few people have all of these and, ultimately, to be successful individuals need the self-awareness to play to their own strengths and to build and support teams that are skilled in different ways.

Leaders have been classified as transformational—those who enable change—and transactional—leaders who preserve the status quo. Both are important in public health. Transformational leaders need to understand change and the different theories of change. They need to understand advocacy and to be comfortable working with the media, using both positive and negative press coverage to enable change. In public health they need to work with a wide range of other stakeholders.

Both types need to understand teams and the different types of organization, but for transactional leaders this is fundamental. In public health, transactional managers need to be good at building and sustaining partnerships and in encouraging and developing individuals

Leaders are not necessarily managers and vice versa. There is an important management role in 'keeping the show on the road', which involves many skills. With change being inevitable in organizations and societies managers also need to be able to manage change and may end up managing the changes brought about by transformational leaders.

Sustainability

Changing the public's health depends on initiatives and programmes that can be sustained, and public health is littered with programmes that have come and gone. Achieving sustainable change is another important art.

It is possible for charismatic leaders to achieve change through force of personality. Unless the organization wants the change or is persuaded that it is valuable, when the leader moves on the changes will be lost. It is easier for those with power over resources or staff to bring in changes. Two remarkable initiatives in public mental health have recently been introduced in the UK by politicians or civil servants working with or in the Treasury. The first, Sure Start, was a visionary initiative to transform the lives of families and children in deprived areas. It was widely valued by the third sector, which was given power in the development and management of Sure Start Children's Centres. The potential for these centres to impact on health, educational achievement, crime, and many other outcomes of great importance for government and societies was great. Sadly, the civil servant who lead this vision died suddenly and prematurely, and in the face of an evaluation that showed only that unrealistic expectations had not been achieved, there was no one to champion these centres. The third sector was not powerful enough to prevent widespread closure of these centres in the face of austerity measures.

The introduction of the new service to provide more primary mental healthcare in deprived areas, known as Increasing Access to Psychological Therapies (IAPT), was another example of a charismatic leader, a peer of the realm, and an academic economist, persuading the then Chancellor to fund a specific initiative. So far, IAPT has survived and may end up being incorporated into primary care or mental health services, but initiatives like this are on fragile territory

Gradual change, building on years of work changing the mindsets of relevant stakeholders, introduced at a steady, manageable pace is more likely to be sustainable. Achieving this requires public health leaders to have very long time frames and much patience and resilience. The latter requires an organizational stability that has not been a feature of public health practice in the UK over the last 50 years.

Bringing to bear all the potential benefits of public mental health will require very high levels of leadership sustained over long periods of time. Understanding the principles of public health and how these can be applied to public mental health is an important starting point for the development of such leaders.

References

1. Hippocrates (400BC) The Book of Prognostics. Available at: http://pinkmonkey.com/dl/library1/hipp10.pdf (accessed 5 March 2018).
2. Cancer Research UK. 50 years of life-saving tobacco control. Available at: http://scienceblog.cancerresearchuk.org/2014/01/11/50-years-of-life-saving-tobacco-control/ (accessed 20 March 2017).
3. Road Safety Observatory. Seat Belts: Key Facts. Available at: http://www.roadsafetyobservatory.com/KeyFacts/vehicles/seat-belts (accessed 20 March 2017).
4. Winslow, Charles-Edward Amory. Available at: https://www.encyclopedia.com/education/encyclopedias-almanacs-transcripts-and-maps/winslow-charles-edward-amory (accessed 5 March 2018).
5. NHS Digital. Adult Psychiatric Morbidity Survey: Survey of Mental Health and Wellbeing, England, 2014. Available at: http://content.digital.nhs.uk/catalogue/PUB21748
6. Wahlbeck K, Westman J, Nordentoft M, Gissler M, Munk Laursen T. Outcomes of Nordic mental health systems: life expectancy of patients with mental disorders. Br J Psychiatry 2011; 199: 453–8.
7. Raffle AE, Alden B, Quinn M, Babb PJ, Brett MT. Outcomes of screening to prevent cancer: analysis of cumulative incidence of cervical abnormality and modelling of cases and deaths prevented. BMJ 2003; 326: 901.
8. Raffle AE, Muir Gray JA. Screening: Evidence and Practice. Oxford: Oxford University Press, 2007.
9. Elder-Vass D. The Reality of Social Construction. Cambridge: Cambridge University Press, 2013.
10. Adult Psychiatric Morbidity Survey. Survey of Mental Health and Wellbeing, England, 2014. Available at: http://content.digital.nhs.uk/catalogue/PUB21748/apms-2014-full-rpt.pdf
11. Wittchen HU, Jacobi F, Rehm J, Gustavarsson A, Svensson M, Jonsson B, et al. The size and burden of mental disorder and other disorders of the brain in Europe. Eur Neuropsych Pharmacol 2011; 21: 655–78.
12. Murray CJL, Lopez Ad (eds). The Global Burden of Disease and Injury Series, Volume 1: A Comprehensive Assessment of Mortality and Disability from Diseases, Injuries, and Risk Factors in 1990 and Project to 2020. Cambridge, MA: Harvard University Press, 1996.
13. Stewart-Brown L, Layte R. Emotional health problems are the most important cause of disability in adults of working age. J Epidemiol Commun Health 1997; 51: 672–5.
14. Andrews G, Poulton R, Skoog I. Lifetime risk of depression: restricted to a minority or waiting for most? Br J Psychiatry 2005; 187: 495–6.
15. Department of Health. No health without mental health: supporting document- The economic case for improving efficiency and quality in mental health. Available at: https://www.gov.uk/government/uploads/system/uploads/attachment_data/file/215808/dh_123993.pdf (accessed 16 September 2013).
16. World Health Organization (WHO). Preamble to the Constitution of the World Health Organization. Geneva: WHO, 1948.
17. World Health Organization (WHO). The World Health Report—Mental Health: New Understanding New Hope. Geneva: WHO, 2001.
18. Schoch R. The Secrets of Happiness: Three Thousand Years of Searching for the Good Life. New York: Simon and Schuster, 2008.
19. Jahoda M. Current Concepts of Positive Mental Health. New York: Basic Books, 1958.
20. Kahneman D, Diener E, Schwarz N (eds). Well-Being: Foundations of Hedonic Psychology. New York: Russell Sage Foundation, 1999.
21. Huppert FA, Ruggieri K. Controversies in wellbeing: confronting and resolving the challenges. In: Bhugra D, Bhui K, Wong SYS, Gilman SE. (eds). Oxford Textbook of Public Mental Health. Oxford: Oxford University Press, 2018, pp. 130–40.
22. Doll R, Hill AB. The mortality of doctors in relation to their smoking habits. BMJ 1954; 1: 1451–5
23. Bradford Hill A. The environment and disease: association or causation? Proc R Soc Med 1965; 58: 295–300
24. World Health Organization (WHO). Review of Social Determinants and the Health Divide in the European Union. Geneva: WHO, 2013.
25. World Health Organization. Social determinants of mental health. Available at: http://apps.who.int/iris/bitstream/10665/112828/1/9789241506809_eng.pdf (accessed 5 March 2018).
26. Luo Y, Waite LJ. The impact of childhood and adult SES on physical, mental, and cognitive well-being in later life. J Gerontol B Psychol Sci Soc Sci 2005; 60: S93–S101.
27. Kessler RC, Heeringa S, Lakoma MD, et al. Individual and societal effects of mental disorders on earnings in the United States: results from the National Comorbidity Survey Replication. Am J Psychiatry 2008; 165: 703–11.
28. Broidy LM, Tremblay RE, Brame B, et al. Developmental trajectories of childhood disruptive behaviors and adolescent delinquency: a six-site, cross-national study. Dev Psychol 2003; 39: 222–66.
29. Stewart-Brown S, Chandimali Samaraweera P, Taggart F, Stranges S. Socio-economic gradients and mental health: implications for public health. Br J Psychiatry 2015; 206: 461–5.
30. Substance Abuse and Mental Health Services Administration (SAMHSA). 2014 National Survey on Drug Use and Health (NSDUH). Rockville, MD: SAMHSA, 2014.
31. Gillam S, Yates J, Badrinath P. Health needs assesment. In: Gillam S, Yates J, Badrinath P (eds) Essential Public Health Theory and Practice. Cambridge: Cambridge University Press, 2012, pp. 111–123.

32. Blair M, Stewart-Brown S, Waterston T, Crowther R. *Child Public Health*. Oxford: Oxford University Press, 2010.

33. Adler University. Mental Health Impact Assessement. Available at: https://www.adler.edu/resources/content/4/5/documents/Adler_ISE_MHIA_130328.pdf (accessed 5 March 2018).

34. Stewart-Brown S, Farmer A. Screening could seriously damage your health. *BMJ* 1997; 314: 533.

35. Wilson JMG, Junger G. *Principles and Practice of Screening for Disease*. Geneva: World Health Organization, 1968.

36. Kutcher S, Wei Y, Coniglio C, Mental health literacy: past, present, and future. *Can J Psychiatry* 2016; 61: 154–8.

37. Mental Health First Aid USA. Available at: https://www.mentalhealthfirstaid.org/

38. Rose G. *The Strategy of Preventive Medicine*. Oxford: Oxford University Press, 1992.

39. Rose G. The mental health of populations. In: Williams P, Wilkinson G, Rawnsley K (eds) *The Scope of Epidemiological Psychiatry: Essays in Honour of Michael Shepherd*. Florence, KY: Taylor & Frances/Routledge,1989, pp. 77–85.

40. Veerman JL, Dowrick C, Ayuso-Mateos JL, Dunn G, Barendregt JJ. Population prevalence of depression and mean Beck Depression Inventory score. *Br J Psychiatry* 2009; 195: 516–19.

41. Goodman A, Goodman R. Population mean scores predict child mental disorder rates: validation SDQ prevalence estimators in Britain. *J Child Psychol Psychiatry* 2011; 52: 100–8.

42. Rose G, Day S. The population mean predicts the number of deviant individuals. *BMJ* 1990, 301, 1031–4.

43. Whittington JE, Huppert FA. Changes in the prevalence of psychiatric disorder in a community are related to changes in the mean level of psychiatric symptoms. *Psychol Med* 1996; 26: 1253–60.

44. de Vibe M, Bjørndal A, Tipton E, Hammerstrøm K, Kowalski K. Mindfulness Based Stress Reduction (MBSR) for improving health, quality of life, and social functioning in adults. *Campbell Syst Rev* 2012: 3: 1–127.

45. What Works Wellbeing Centre. Policy Briefing 2016 Music Singing and Wellbeing in Healthy Adults. Available at: https://whatworkswellbeing.files.wordpress.com/2016/11/wellbeing-singing-music-diagnosed-conditions-dec2016.pdf (accessed 5 March 2018).

46. Cattan M, White M, Bond J, Learmouth A. Preventing social isolation and loneliness among older people: a systematic review of health promotion interventions. *Ageing Soc* 2005; 25: 41–67.

47. Weare K, Nind M. Mental health promotion and problem prevention in schools: what does the evidence say? *Health Promot Int* 2011; 26(Suppl. 1): i29–69.

48. Stewart-Brown S, Scharder-McMillan A. Parenting for mental health: what does the evidence say we need to do? Report of Workpackage 2 of the DataPrev project. *Health Promot Int* 2011; 26: i10–28.

49. Prinz RJ1, Sanders MR, Shapiro CJ, Whitaker DJ, Lutzker JR. Population-based prevention of child maltreatment: the U.S. Triple p system population trial. *Prev Sci* 2009; 10: 1–12.

50. Rosenstock I. Historical origins of the health belief model. *Health Educ Behav* 1974; 2: 328–35.

51. DiClemente CC, Prochaska JO. Toward a comprehensive, transtheoretical model of change: stages of change and addictive behaviors. In: Miller WR, Heather N (eds) *Treating Addictive Behaviors*, 2nd ed. New York: Plenum Press, 1998, pp. 3–24.

52. Ajzen I. The theory of planned behavior. *Organ Behav Hum Decis Process* 1991; 50: 179–211.

53. Thaler R, Sunstein C. *Nudge*. New York: Penguin Books, 2008.

54. French J, Blair-Stevens C, McVey D, Merritt R. *Social Marketing and Public Health: Theory and Practice*. Oxford: Oxford University Press, 2009.

55. Antonovsky A. *Unravelling The Mystery of Health—How People Manage Stress and Stay Well*. San Francisco, CA: Jossey-Bass Publishers, 1987.

56. Tudor K. *Mental Health Promotion: Paradigms and Practice*. London: Routledge, 1996.

57. Sin NL, Lyubomirsky S. Enhancing wellbeing and alleviating depressive symptoms with positive psychology interventions. *J Clin Psychol* 2008; 65: 467–87.

58. World Health Organization (WHO). The Ottawa Charter for Health Promotion. Available at: http://www.who.int/healthpromotion/conferences/previous/ottawa/en/ (accessed 2 February 2018).

59. Kretzmann J, McKnight J. *Building Communities From the Inside Out: A Path Toward Finding and Mobilizing a Community's Assets*, 3rd ed. Chicago, IL: ACTA Publications. 1993.

60. Crepaz-Keay D (ed.) *Mental Health Today ... And Tomorrow: Exploring Current and Future Trends in Mental Health*. Hove: Mental Health Foundation; Pavilion Publishing and Media Limited, 2015.

61. Gillam S, Yates J. Management, leadership and change. In: Gillam S, Yates J, Badrinath P (eds) *Essential Public Health Theory and Practice*. Cambridge: Cambridge University of Press, 2012, pp. 13–28.

CHAPTER 2

Social inequalities and mental health

Ruth Bell and Michael Marmot

Social inequalities and mental health deserve to be at the top of the public health agenda in countries around the world. There are at least four reasons. Firstly, mental disorders, including depression, anxiety, and drug use, among others, are some of the leading causes of poor health and disability around the world [1–3]. Secondly, social inequalities in the distribution of mental health exist [4]. Thirdly, mental disorders contribute to further inequalities that can deepen and entrench existing socio-economic inequalities[5]. Fourthly, these issues have major consequences for population health.

In this chapter we discuss evidence linking social inequalities, across social, economic, and environmental dimensions to inequalities in mental health. We present a framework for thinking about the lifetime causes of inequalities in mental health and we use this framework to discuss how experiences and conditions affect mental health across the life course. We focus particularly on factors that affect child development because of the importance of child developmental outcomes for future mental and physical health, and on life chances. There is widespread agreement among experts that 'giving every child the best possible start will generate the greatest societal and mental health benefits' [6]. Finally, we discuss the need for more attention to be focused on addressing the causes of social inequalities in mental health through multiple types of policies and interventions.

Social inequalities in the distribution of mental health

Evidence is consistent across countries that socio-economic disadvantage is associated with increased risk of mental disorders. Fryers et al. definitively demonstrated the ubiquity of the association in research that brought together 25 years of European population surveys and relevant population studies [7]. They found that in Europe and other developed areas relatively high levels of common mental disorders (CMDs) are associated with poor education, material disadvantage, and unemployment [7].

Studies in low- and middle-income countries also provide convincing evidence for the association of social disadvantage with CMDs. A systematic review of evidence about the association of poverty and CMDs in low- and middle-income countries found that poverty, measured in various ways, was associated with CMDs [8].

Inequalities in mental health are well documented in England by the Adult Psychiatric Morbidity Survey—a general population survey that has been carried out four times, starting in 1983. While the survey is cross-sectional, it gives periodic insights into the mental health of the population. Fig. 2.1 shows data from the 2007 survey: there is evidence of a social gradient in CMDs by household income, with lower income associated with higher prevalence of CMDs, and with women more likely than men to have CMDs at all levels of household income [9]. A population study in the UK found that the association between low income and mental disorders may largely be accounted for by debt [10].

The 2014 Adult Psychiatric Morbidity Survey found that one in six people have a CMD. Gender differences are evident: among women, one in five have a CMD; among men the estimated prevalence is one in eight. The 2014 survey also corroborates the finding that social disadvantage is associated with poor mental health, and additionally finds evidence that the prevalence of CMD among women has grown in England since 2000, whereas among men there has been little change [11]. In particular, women aged 16–24 years are at highest risk of mental disorders, including CMDs, self-harm, and positive screenings for post-traumatic stress disorder and bipolar disorder [11]. Explanations for the gender differences in mental health are not well understood. There are two research questions here: why is there more mental illness in women than men; and why is it getting worse in women? The influence of societal and cultural factors on women and men is one area of research. Another strand of research focuses on how psychological distress manifests in men and women. According to this, women are more likely to internalize responses to psychological distress and to develop anxiety and depressive symptoms, and men are more likely to externalize responses and to develop substance abuse and social behaviour problems [12].

Turning from the UK to the USA: mortality in middle-aged, white, non-Hispanic Americans has shown an alarming increase between 1999 and 2013, after years of decline. By contrast, mortality among US Hispanics and six comparison countries has been steadily declining since the 1990s (Fig. 2.2) [13]. Case and Deaton find that this increase in mortality is largely accounted for by increasing death rates from drug and alcohol poisonings, suicide, and alcohol-related diseases (chronic liver diseases and cirrhosis)—all of which are related to poor mental health

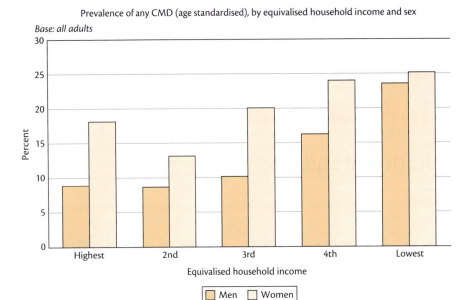

Fig. 2.1 Prevalence of any common mental disorder (age standardized) by household income and sex; England.

Source: Reproduced from The NHS Information Centre for health and social care, McManus, S, Meltzer,H, Brugha,T, et al. [eds], Adult psychiatric morbidity in England, 2007: Results of a household survey, Copyright (2009), Crown Copyright.

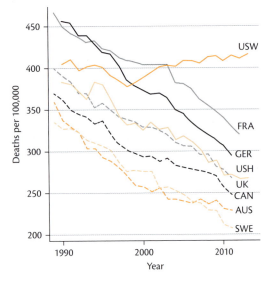

Fig. 2.2 All-cause mortality, ages 45–54 years, for US white non-Hispanics, US Hispanics, and six comparison countries.

Note: USW: US White non-Hispanics; USH: US Hispanics; FRA: France; GER: Germany; UK: United Kingdom; CAN: Canada; AUS: Australia; SWE: Sweden.

Source: Reproduced from Proc Natl Acad Sci U S A, 112(49), Case, A, Deaton A, Rising morbidity and mortality in midlife among white non-Hispanic Americans in the 21st century, pp. 15078-83, Copyright (2015), with permission from National Academy of Sciences.

[13]. While the study does not separate out the data for men and women, the study found that the increase in mortality among non-Hispanic whites in midlife was mostly driven by higher mortality rates among the least educated—the lower the education the steeper the rise; thus, the gradient became steeper. This is compelling evidence of the importance of social inequalities in mental health to population health. Increasing midlife mortality in midlife, white, non-Hispanic Americans

represents what Case and Deaton describe as an 'epidemic of pain, suicide, and drug overdoses' that reflect growing levels of psychological distress [13]. The authors point to economic insecurity as a possible driver of this 'epidemic'. Looking also at the major causes of morbidity in the USA, Case and Deaton find 'declines in self-reported health, mental health, and ability to work, increased reports of pain, and deteriorating measures of liver function' [13].

Understanding the causes of population-level misery on this scale requires a different approach from that required for understanding the causes of psychological distress at the individual level. Our perspective on social inequalities and mental health[1] is not only rooted in evidence from social epidemiology and public health, but it also applies research from other disciplines [16].

Other lines of evidence identify the differential vulnerabilities of subgroups of the population to macro-level influences. The break-up of the Soviet Union in 1991 precipitated deep social and economic changes in the countries affected. In the following years (1992–2001) there were an estimated 2.5–3 million more deaths in the Russian Federation than expected, based on the 1991 mortality level [17]. Study evidence points to the influence of the effects of hazardous alcohol consumption on Russian mortality in the 1990s [18], and to psychological distress in former Soviet Union countries [19]. A study by Murphy et al. found that the mortality increase in Russia in 1990s was mainly accounted for by mortality increases among men and women with low educational attainment, whereas mortality among university-educated people

---

[1] In this context, mental health is broadly understood as more than the absence of mental illness; good mental health enables people to function effectively in all areas of their lives [14, 15]. Within this broad understanding, there are several validated instruments to assess mental health that are designed for use in different contexts.

improved, resulting in an increase in educational inequalities in mortality [20].

The causes of socio-economic inequalities in mental health

Given the major contribution that social inequalities and mental health make to population health globally and within countries there is an urgent need for further research and policy attention on these areas [4]. The World Health Organization (WHO) Commission on Social Determinants of Health (CSDH) laid out a conceptual framework for thinking about the causes of health inequalities [21]. The CSDH presented evidence and arguments about the need to take a life course approach, by improving the conditions in which people are born, grow, live, work, and age. It demonstrated that health inequalities flow from differential experiences and exposures arising from level of education, income, wealth, occupation, ethnicity, and gender. The CSDH argued that differential conditions of daily life are shaped by the distribution on power, money, and resources. Further work examining the social determinants of mental health emphasizes that mental health and many CMDs are shaped to a great extent by the social, economic, and physical environments in which people live [6].

Theories about how levels of social disadvantage influence mental health focus on material and psychosocial pathways. Those lower in the social hierarchy are more likely to experience adverse social, economic, and environmental conditions that not only have direct effects on health, but also create psychological stress. Stressors may include relationship problems, ill health, working and employment conditions, debt, poor neighbourhood environment, and housing conditions, among other factors. The effects of psychological stressors can be buffered by individual-level characteristics, including self-efficacy, control, and resilience, as well as by social support, in the form of emotional support, material support, and information. These protective factors are themselves socially graded according to level of socio-economic disadvantage [6]. However, individual-level characteristics, including control and resilience, and social support are protective at all levels of society. Evidence shows that social disadvantage starts before birth and accumulates throughout life [22].

Early life and adolescence

The mental health of men and women and the social distribution of mental health are important issues not only for public health in their own right, but also because of the effect of adult mental health on children in the household, and consequently on the children's life chances and mental health. In the family context, child mental health may also influence parental mental health [23]. This section looks at three things: (i) mental illness among parents and carers as a risk to good child development; (ii) social influences on early child development, which influence inequalities in mental and physical health in adulthood; and (iii) adverse childhood experiences and their influence on adult mental health

Maternal depression has been identified as a global threat to children's health and development [24]. Poor maternal mental health affects children even before birth. A meta-analysis of prospective studies of depression during pregnancy and preterm birth and low birthweight found that women with depression during pregnancy are at increased risk of giving birth preterm

and having low birthweight babies. There was heterogeneity in the methods of measurement of depression and in the findings of the studies analysed. Overall, the meta-analysis found that risk of preterm and low birthweight was higher for depressed mothers in developing countries than in the USA and other developed countries, and it was higher among socio-economically disadvantaged women in developing countries, and among low-income mothers in the USA versus middle- or high-income mothers in the USA [25]. Socially disadvantaged women are also more likely to have antenatal depression than more advantaged women [25], which reflects the social distribution of prevalence of CMD across society.

The impact of poor maternal mental health on children after birth creates risks for child development. These may include delayed language development and higher levels of behaviour difficulties, which reflect socio-emotional problems. Marryat and Martin undertook a major longitudinal study in Scotland of maternal mental health and child development with annual visits and assessments over 4 years [26]. The first visits were in 1995–96 when babies were 10 months old. The researchers found that four times as many women in the lowest income group had repeated mental health problems than those in the highest income group (24% vs 6%). Where no-one in the household had paid employment women's mental health was worse than when someone in household was in employment. The study also found that children's developmental outcomes across socio-emotional and cognitive domains were worse when mothers had repeated episodes of poor mental health than when mothers had a brief episode of poor mental health. Even when mothers had a brief episode of poor mental health child development outcomes were worse than when women had no episodes of poor mental health. Separating out the effects of poor maternal mental health and other factors that affect child development, the study found that poor maternal mental health is significantly independently associated with the following outcomes for children: worse peer relations, emotional well-being, and behaviour [26].

The association between social disadvantage and early child development outcomes follows a social gradient. Maternal low educational attainment was associated with poorer cognitive outcomes among children, living in a deprived area was associated with worse behavioural and cognitive outcomes, low household income was associated with worse emotional well-being and peer relations, persistent poverty was associated with worse behavioural and cognitive outcomes, living in a household with poor relationships between the parenting couple was associated with worse emotional well-being and peer relationships, and where mothers had low social support there was an association with worse behavioural outcomes [26].

Poor child development outcomes have lifelong effects on mental and physical health, on educational attainment and subsequent employment opportunities, and on social outcomes. Clearly, the factors affecting maternal mental health and child development are complex and interrelated. Efforts to address maternal mental health and efforts to improve children's outcomes need to address these social, economic, and environmental determinants in a holistic way.

There is study evidence that the social patterning of socio-emotional difficulties and behavioural problems is apparent among children as young as 3 years of age. Kelly et al. used data from the Millennium Birth Cohort Study, a longitudinal study of around 19,000 children born in the UK in 2000–01 [27]. They assessed

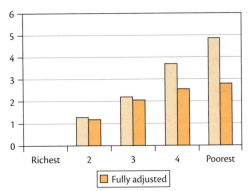

Fig. 2.3 Socio-emotional difficulties at 3 years of age: Millennium Cohort Study.
Source: Reproduced from Arch Dis Child, 96(9), Kelly, Y, et al, What role for the home learning environment and parenting in reducing the socioeconomic gradient in child development? Findings from the Millennium Cohort Study, pp. 832-837, Copyright (2011), with permission from BMJ Publishing Group Ltd.

socio-emotional difficulties, which manifest as behavioural problems, and verbal ability in children at the age of 3 and 5 years. The results for socio-emotional ability are shown in Fig. 2.3.

In Fig. 2.3, the paler bars show the social gradient pattern: those from poorer families are more likely to have behavioural difficulties than those from higher-income households, and the effect is incremental by increasing level of household poverty. However, the darker bars show the pattern when the data are adjusted for parenting activities and psychosocial markers. When someone reads stories to the child, and teaches the child songs, the alphabet, and counting; the child does painting activities at home; the child is taken to the library; the child has regular meal and bed times—basically a variety of supportive parenting activities—there is still a gradient, but the outcomes for all children are better at all household incomes, but especially for children from the poorest households. Kelly et al. found similar patterns when they focused on language skills, assessed by verbal ability as an indicator of cognitive development. By the age of 3 years, children living in poverty are, on average, 8 months behind their peers in language and 9 months behind in school readiness [27].

Behavioural problems in childhood predict a range of poor social, economic, and health outcomes in adulthood. Fergusson et al. analysed data from a 25-year longitudinal study of a birth cohort of young people in New Zealand [28]. Information was collected on child conduct problems at the age of 7–9 years and subsequently on a wide range of outcomes in early adulthood, including crime, substance use, mental health, suicide, sexual/partner relationships, and education/employment. The study found that the 5% of children with the most disturbed behavior at the age of 7–9 years were four times as likely as those in the top 50% to have committed a violent offence by the age of 25 years, three times as likely to have attempted suicide, and nearly three times as likely to have become a teenage parent, after controlling for other potential influences, including intelligence and socio-economic disadvantage at the age of 7–9 years, and nearly 1.5 times more likely to have no qualifications [28].

Turning to adverse experiences in early life, these have lifelong effects on health-damaging behaviours, namely binge drinking, poor diet, smoking, violence perpetration, heroin/crack cocaine use, and unintended teenage pregnancy, some of which are associated with poor mental health. Bellis et al. set out to find the levels of childhood adverse experiences in England and the proportion of health-damaging behaviours that are potentially avoidable if adversity in childhood were addressed [29]. To do this the researchers carried out a nationally representative survey of nearly 4000 adults aged 18–69 years that asked questions about adverse experiences while growing up before the age of 18 years, and about current health behaviours. Childhood adverse experiences included verbal, physical, and sexual abuse, and parental separation, domestic violence, mental illness, alcohol abuse, drug use, and parental incarceration. Nearly half of all respondents had experienced at least one of these adverse experiences and 9% had experienced four or more. Reporting of four or more adverse childhood experiences was higher among those from deprived areas than those from more affluent areas. Based on the findings of the survey, the researchers modelled the proportion of health-damaging behaviours that could be attributable to adverse childhood experiences: 12% of binge drinking, 14% of poor diet, 23% of smoking, 52% of violence perpetration, 59% of heroin/crack cocaine use, and 38% of unintended teenage pregnancy [29]. Support for families and children has the potential to improve parental mental health and to reduce adverse experiences for children, with potentially enormous benefits to mental and physical health.

While poor mental health can affect any young person, those who are poorer are disproportionally affected. Evidence from a systematic review of the literature of depressed mood and anxiety by socio-economic position among young people aged 10–15 years found that prevalence of depressed mood or anxiety was 2.5 times higher in those of low socio-economic status than those of high socio-economic status [30]. Evidence from the Millennium Birth Cohort shows that the length of time lived in poverty affects children's mental health. Children aged 11 years who were in poverty at four or five waves of the survey were more likely to have socio-emotional problems than who had experienced fewer episodes of poverty [31].

While socio-economic disadvantage during early life and adolescence can have lasting effects on mental health, social deprivation at any stage of life, early life, adolescence, and adult life is associated with depressive symptoms. Nicholson et al. examined which was more important for depressive symptoms in adult life in Eastern Europe: social deprivation experienced in early life, in adolescence, or in adult life [32]. They analysed data from a cross-sectional study including 12,053 men and 13,582 women from Russia, Poland, and the Czech Republic. The study assessed depressive symptoms in relation to socio-economic circumstances during childhood (assessed by recall of household amenities and father's education); participants' own level of education; and current circumstances (assessed by financial difficulties and possession of household items). The findings were different in the three countries. They found that depression was largely influenced by adult socio-economic adversity rather than by conditions in early life or education. However, the effects of current conditions on depressive symptoms were stronger for men than among women, and they were stronger among men from Poland and Russia, countries that had recently experienced social changes, than from the Czech Republic [32]. As previously discussed, macro-level socio-economic changes can have powerful effects on mental health, especially of disadvantaged groups.

Employment, lack of employment, and mental health

Employment is generally good for mental health, provided employment and working conditions are good [33].

Financial security is one element of good employment that exerts influence on mental health. Good employment also provides opportunities to use and develop skills, to increase self-esteem, to develop and widen social networks, to exercise control, and to develop social standing, all of which potentially support mental well-being. These beneficial effects are dependent on the quality of working and employment conditions. Being in work does not necessarily create financial security; evidence from the Joseph Rowntree Foundation shows that in the UK there were 3.8 million workers living in poverty, which is 12% of all workers (2014–15 data) [34].

Stress at work poses significant risk for mental and physical health. The Labour Force Survey in Great Britain is a quarterly household survey of around 38,000 households. Respondents are asked to report on various factors, including their experience of work-related stress, anxiety, and depression. In 2015–16, 488,000 people reported work-related stress at a level they believed was making them ill (1510 per 100,000 workers), which is 37% of all work-related ill health. Workload was most commonly reported as the cause, followed by lack of support, harassment or bullying, and changes at work [35].

Two main models of stress at work have been examined in epidemiological studies: the control–demand model, where work stress is characterized by high demands and low control [36], and the effort–reward model, which is characterized by an imbalance between effort and reward at work [37]. These models of work stress are associated with higher risk of mental illness. Both types of stress at work follow a social gradient with those in lower occupational classes at higher risk than those in higher occupational classes [38]. Additional factors influencing stress at work may be

protective, such as supportive managers and co-workers, or adverse, such as organizational injustice, and harassment or bullying. Preventive measures to reduce stress at work are feasible, and workplace interventions can help [39].

Insecure employment, an increasingly prevalent feature of the labour market in many countries, also creates risks for mental health. Researchers from Hamburg carried out a systematic review of studies to find out if having an insecure job is better for health than having no job at all. The researchers found that having an insecure job was as bad for mental health as being unemployed [40].

Turning to unemployment, there is consistent evidence that unemployment is bad for mental health [41]. Analysis of data from countries in Europe between 1970 and 2007, a period when there was a series of economic ups and downs, shows that every 1% increase in unemployment was associated with a 0.79% rise in suicides among those under 65 years of age [42].

Studies are still examining the health effects of the global financial crisis of 2008. A study on rates of suicide after the 2008 financial crisis in countries in Europe and the Americas found that suicide rates increased, especially among men and in countries with higher levels of job loss [43]. A systematic review of research on health outcomes and the 2008 financial crisis in Europe found consistent evidence of an association between the financial crisis and an increase in suicides, especially among men, and with worsening mental health [44].

The consequences of economic crises on employment and consequently on financial security and other benefits of employment have been investigated as possible contributory factors to worsening mental health. A longitudinal study using health data from the Health and Retirement Survey in the USA and the Survey of Health, Ageing and Retirement in Europe, covering the years 2004–2010 on people aged 50–64 years who were in employment when they were recruited to the survey cohorts, found that depressive scores increased after job loss (Fig. 2.4) [45].

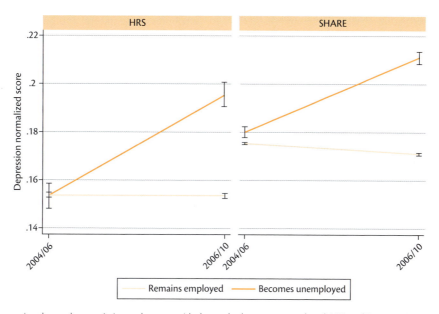

Fig. 2.4 Depression scores comparing those who remain in employment with those who become unemployed, USA and European Union, 2004–10.

Note: Displaced workers (top line) and continually employed workers (bottom line) over the period 2004–10; ages 50–64 years, HRS and SHARE. HRS is a study in the USA; SHARE is a study in Europe.

Source: Reproduced from Int J Epidemiol, 43(5), Riumallo-Herl, C, et al, Job loss, wealth and depression during the Great Recession in the USA and Europe, pp. 1508-17, Copyright (2014), with permission from Oxford University Press

Do the more generous social welfare systems in European countries help protect mental health? The study found that among US workers in the study, but not among workers from the 13 European countries, the effect of job loss on depressive symptoms was weaker among workers who had greater wealth before becoming unemployed than among those who had less wealth before becoming unemployed [45]. Therefore, individual wealth mattered less for mental health among people who became unemployed in the European Union countries than in the USA.

A study in Europe that examined the association of welfare generosity with self-reported health and the distribution of self-reported health found that educational inequalities in self-rated health are lower in countries with more generous welfare systems [46]. The evidence suggests that more generous welfare spending is associated with better health for the least educated, which contributes to lower health inequalities. A possible mechanism is that more generous welfare spending provides financial security, especially for those with the least education, which helps protect against risks to mental health associated with social disadvantage.

Unemployment is associated with poor mental health, especially in times of economic recession or labour market transitions, and when prospects of finding another job are not good [47]. The socio-economically disadvantaged and those with low educational attainment are disproportionately affected. The evidence supports calls for the effects on mental health to be considered in all labour policies [48].

Older ages

Early life, life history, and present living conditions all affect the mental health of older people. Cumulative experience of adverse and protective factors across the life course contribute to social inequalities in the risk of poor mental health at older ages. Additionally, older people are more at risk of social isolation and loneliness, and evidence shows that social isolation, lack of mental stimulation, and low levels of physical activity increase risks of poor mental health among older people [49].

The built and natural environment

Aspects of the built and natural environment can affect mental health. Poor-quality housing contributes to social inequalities in mental health. There is a social gradient in fuel poverty and cold homes in the UK, with lower-income households more likely to be at risk of fuel poverty and living in cold homes than high-income households. An evidence review by the University College London Institute of Health Equity found that living in cold homes has a significant effect on the mental health of adults and young people [50].

Living in overcrowded homes is also associated with poor mental health. Overcrowding affects the quality of relationships between those living together as families, creates stress, and is a risk for mental health. Among children, overcrowded living conditions are a risk for poorer socio-emotional development and educational outcomes [51, 52].

There has been growing interest and research in the benefits of the natural environment and 'green and blue' spaces for mental health. Spending more time in green spaces is positively associated with better self-reported mental health [53]. In England there are inequalities in access to green space as more deprived areas have fewer green spaces than less deprived areas [54]. Intrinsic benefits to mental health may accrue through spending time in natural environments, and benefits may be associated with engagement in social activities and with physical activities in natural environments [55].

Taking a social determinants approach to address social inequalities in mental health

Given the size of the problem of poor mental health, the extent of social inequalities in mental health, and the consequences of poor mental health for individuals, families, and societies, it is clear that more attention needs to be focused on addressing the causes of social inequalities in mental health.

As part of the WHO Gulbenkian initiative on mental health, we reported on the social determinants of mental health and how they could be addressed. We applied learning from previous work on social determinants of health [21, 56], and described the following multi-level framework for strategies and interventions to reduce mental disorders and promote mental well-being [6].

Life-course: interventions to address risk factors during prenatal, pregnancy, and perinatal periods; early childhood; adolescence; working and family-building years; older ages; and also address gender-related issues at all life course stages.

Parents, families, and households: interventions to improve parenting behaviours; material conditions (income, access to resources, food/nutrition, water, sanitation, housing, employment); employment conditions and unemployment; parental physical and mental health; pregnancy and maternal care; social support.

Community: interventions to address neighbourhood trust and safety; community-based participation; violence/crime; attributes of the natural and built environment; neighbourhood deprivation.

Local services: early years' care and education provision; schools; youth/adolescent services; health care; social services; clean water and sanitation.

Country-level factors: interventions to address poverty; inequality; discrimination; governance; human rights; armed conflict; national policies to promote access to education; employment; health care; housing and services proportionate to need; social protection policies that are universal and proportionate to need.

There are no simple causal pathways to mental health. Rather, there are a multiplicity of inter-related risks and protective factors. Addressing social inequalities requires a systems-wide approach that addresses the social determinants of mental health at multiple levels.

References

1. Whiteford HA, Degenhardt L, Rehm J, et al. Global Burden of disease attributable to mental and substance use disorders: findings from the Global Burden of Disease Study 2010. *Lancet* 2013; 382: 1575–86.
2. Vigo D, Thornicroft G, Atun R. Estimating the true global burden of mental illness. *Lancet Psychiatry* 2016; 3: 171–8.

3. Global Burden of Disease Study 2013 Collaborators. Global, regional, and national incidence, prevalence, and years lived with disability for 301 acute and chronic diseases and injuries in 188 countries, 1990–2013: a systematic analysis for the Global Burden of Disease Study 2013. *Lancet* 2015; 386: 743–800.

4. Allen J, Balfour R, Bell R. Social determinants of mental health. *Int Rev Psychiatry* 2014; 26: 392–407.

5. Campion J, Bhugra D, Bailey S, Marmot M. Inequality and mental disorders: opportunities for action. *Lancet* 2013; 382: 183–184.

6. World Health Organization (WHO) and Calouste Gulbenkian Foundation. *Social Determinants of Mental Health.* Geneva: WHO, 2014.

7. Fryers T, Melzer D, Jenkins R, Brugha T. The distribution of the common mental disorders: social inequalities in Europe. *Clin Pract Epidemiol Ment Health* 2005; 1: 14.

8. Lund C, Breen A, Flisher AJ, et al. Poverty and common mental disorders in low and middle income countries: a systematic review. *Soc Sci Med* 2010; 71: 517–28.

9. McManus S, Meltzer H, Brugha T, Bebbington P, Jenkins R (eds). *Adult Psychiatric Morbidity in England, 2007: Results of a Household Survey.* London: The Health & Social Care Information Centre, 2009.

10. Jenkins R, Bhugra D, Bebbington P, et al. Debt, income and mental disorder in the general population. *Psychol Med* 2008; 38: 1485–93.

11. McManus S, Bebbington P, Jenkins R, Brugha T (eds). *Mental Health and Wellbeing in England: Adult Psychiatric Morbidity Survey 2014.* Leeds: NHS Digital, 2016.

12. Eaton NR, Keyes KM, Krueger RF, et al. An invariant dimensional liability model of gender differences in mental disorder prevalence: evidence from a national sample. *J Abnorm Psychol* 2012; 121: 282–8.

13. Case A, Deaton A. Rising morbidity and mortality in midlife among white non-Hispanic Americans in the 21st century. *Proc Natl Acad Sci U S A* 2015; 112: 15078–83.

14. Department of Health. *No Health Without Mental Health: A Cross-government Mental Health Outcomes Strategy for People of All Ages.* London: HMG, 2011.

15. World Health Organization (WHO). *Promoting Mental Health: Concepts, Emerging Evidence, Practice: Summary Report.* Geneva: WHO, 2004.

16. Marmot M, Bell R. Social inequalities in health: a proper concern of epidemiology. *Ann Epidemiol* 2016; 26: 238–40.

17. Men T, Brennan P, Boffetta P, Zaridze D. Russian mortality trends for 1991–2001: analysis by cause and region. *BMJ* 2003; 327: 964.

18. Leon DA, Saburova L, Tomkins S, et al. Hazardous alcohol drinking and premature mortality in Russia: a population based case-control study. *Lancet* 2007; 369: 2001–9.

19. Roberts B, Abbott P, McKee M. Levels and determinants of psychological distress in eight countries of the former Soviet Union. *J Public Ment Health* 2010; 9: 17–26.

20. Murphy M, Bobak M, Nicholson A, Rose R, Marmot M. The widening gap in mortality by educational level in the Russian Federation, 1980–2001. *Am J Public Health* 2006; 96: 1293–9.

21. Commission on Social Determinants of Health. *Closing the Gap in a Generation—Health Equity Through Action on the Social Determinants of Health.* Geneva: World Health Organization, 2008.

22. Marmot Review Team. *Fair society, healthy lives: strategic review of health inequalities in England post-2010.* Available at: www.instituteofhealthequity.org (2012, accessed 3 August 2012).

23. Webb E, Panico L, Bécares L, McMunn A, Kelly Y, Sacker A. The inter-relationship of adolescent unhappiness and parental mental distress. *J Adolesc Health* 2017; 60: 196–203.

24. Wachs TD, Black MM, Engle PL. Maternal depression: a global threat to children's health, development, and behavior and to human rights. *Child Dev Perspect* 2009; 3: 51–9.

25. Grote NK, Bridge JA, Gavin AR, Melville JL, Iyengar S, Katon WJ. A meta-analysis of depression during pregnancy and the risk of preterm birth, low birth weight, and intrauterine growth restriction. *Arch Gen Psychiatry* 2010; 67: 1012–24.

26. Marryat L, Martin C. *Growing Up in Scotland: Maternal Mental Health and its Impact on Child Behaviour and Development.* Edinburgh: Scottish Government, 2010.

27. Kelly Y, Sacker A, Del Bono E, Francesconi M, Marmot M. What role for the home learning environment and parenting in reducing the socioeconomic gradient in child development? Findings from the Millennium Cohort Study. *Arch Dis Child* 2011; 96: 832–837.

28. Fergusson DM, Horwood LJ, Ridder EM. Show me the child at seven: the consequences of conduct problems in childhood for psychosocial functioning in adulthood. *J Child Psychol Psychiatry* 2005; 46: 837–49.

29. Bellis MA, Hughes K, Leckenby N, Parkins C, Lowey H. National household survey of adverse childhood experiences and their relationship with resilience to health-harming behaviors in England. *BMC Med* 2014; 12: 72.

30. Lemstra M, Neudorf C, D'Arcy C, Kunst A, Warren LM, Bennett NR. A systematic review of depressed mood and anxiety by SES in youth aged 10–15 years. *Can J Public Health* 2008; 99: 125–9.

31. Taylor-Robinson D, Wickham S, Barr B, et al. *Consultation Response: Child Poverty and Health—the Impact of the Welfare Reform and Work Bill 2015–2016.* Liverpool: University of Liverpool, Institute of Psychology, Health and Society, 2016.

32. Nicholson A, Pikhart H, Pajak A, et al. Socio-economic status over the life-course and depressive symptoms in men and women in Eastern Europe. *J Affect Disord* 2008; 105: 125–36.

33. van der Noordt M, IJzelenberg H, Droomers M, Proper KI. Health effects of employment: a systematic review of prospective studies. *Occup Environ Med* 2014; 71: 730–736.

34. Tinson A, Ayrton C, Barker K, Born TB, Aldridge H, Kenway P. *Monitoring Poverty and Social Exclusion 2016.* York: Joseph Rowntree Foundation, 2016.

35. Health and Safety Executive. Work related Stress, Anxiety and Depression Statistics in Great Britain 2016. Available at: http://www.hse.gov.uk/statistics/causdis/stress/stress.pdf?pdf=stress (last accessed 6 February 2018).

36. Karasek RA, Theorell T. *Healthy Work: Productivity and the Reconstruction of Working Life.* New York: Basic Books, 1992.

37. Siegrist J. Adverse health effects of high-effort/low-reward conditions. *J Occup Health Psychol* 1996; 1: 27–41.

38. Wahrendorf M, Dragano N, Siegrist J. Social position, workstress, and retirement intentions: a study with older employees from 11 European countries. *Eur Sociol Rev* 2013; 29: 792–802.

39. Tan L, Wang MJ, Modini M, et al. Preventing the development of depression at work: a systematic review and meta-analysis of universal interventions in the workplace. *BMC Med* 2014; 12: 74.

40. Kim TJ, von dem Knesebeck O. Is an insecure job better for health than having no job at all? A systematic review of studies investigating the health-related risks of both job insecurity and unemployment. *BMC Public Health* 2015; 15: 985.

41. Paul KI, Moser K. Unemployment impairs mental health: meta-analyses. *J Vocat Behav* 2009; 74: 264–82.

42. World Health Organization (WHO) Regional Office for Europe. *Impact of Economic Crises on Mental Health.* Copenhagen: WHO, 2011.

43. Chang SS, Stuckler D, Yip P, Gunnell D. Impact of 2008 global economic crisis on suicide: time trend study in 54 countries. *BMJ* 2013; 347: f5239.

44. Parmar D, Stavropoulou C, Ioannidis JP. Health outcomes during the 2008 financial crisis in Europe: systematic literature review. *BMJ* 2016; 354: i4588.

45. Riumallo-Herl C, Basu S, Stuckler D, Courtin E, Avendano M. Job loss, wealth and depression during the Great Recession in the USA and Europe. *Int J Epidemiol* 2014; 43: 1508–17.

46. Dahl E, van der Wel KA. Educational inequalities in health in European welfare states: a social expenditure approach. *Soc Sci Med* 2013; 81: 60–9.

47. Frasquilho D, Matos MG, Salonna F, et al. Mental health outcomes in times of economic recession: a systematic literature review. *BMC Public Health* 2015; 16: 115.

48. Joint Action for Mental health and Wellbeing. Mental Health in all Policies. Available at: http://www.mentalhealthandwellbeing.eu/mental-health-in-all-policies (last accessed 6 February 2018).

49. UCL Institute of Health Equity. *Inequalities in Mental Health, Cognitive Impairment and Dementia Among Older People*. London: UCL Insitute of Health Equity, 2016.

50. UCL Institute of Health Equity. *Fuel Poverty and Cold Home-related Health Problems*. Available at: https://www.gov.uk/government/uploads/system/uploads/attachment_data/file/355790/Briefing7_Fuel_poverty_health_inequalities.pdf (last accessed 6 February 2018).

51. Solari CD, Mare RD. Housing crowding effects on children's wellbeing. *Soc Sci Res* 2012; 41: 464–76.

52. Chartered Institute of Envionmental Health. Mental health and housing—key issues. Available at: http://www.cieh-housing-and-health-resource.co.uk/mental-health-and-housing/key-issues/ (last accessed 6 February 2018).

53. van den Berg M, van Poppel M, van Kamp I, et al. Visiting green space is associated with mental health and vitality: a cross-sectional study in four european cities. *Health Place* 2016; 38: 8–15.

54. UCL Institute of Health Equity. Improving access to green spaces. Available at: https://www.gov.uk/government/uploads/system/uploads/attachment_data/file/357411/Review8_Green_spaces_health_inequalities.pdf (last accessed 6 February 2018).

55. Bowler DE, Buyung-Ali LM, Knight TM, Pullin AS. A systematic review of evidence for the added benefits to health of exposure to natural environments. *BMC Public Health* 2010; 10: 456.

56. World Health Organization (WHO). *Review of Social Determinants and the Health Divide in the WHO European Region: Final Report*. Copenhagen: WHO.

CHAPTER 3

Economic costs of mental illness

Anita Patel

Introduction: the place of economics in public mental health

The breadth of coverage in this book highlights both the substantial and multidimensional burdens of mental health problems worldwide: epidemiological, clinical, quality of life, personal, family, social, political, and so on. Each of these are connected to another important dimension, the economic burden. The importance of the economic burden is underlined by the simple fact that all healthcare systems need to tackle a gap between the resources that are available (which are always finite) and healthcare needs and wants (which continue to grow). Such gaps are of concern as they represent some level of unmet need, which, in turn, can be associated with a variety of further negative consequences. This supply–demand gap is naturally more obvious in contexts where resources are particularly low and/or demands particularly high, for example in low- and middle-income countries, where both human and financial resources available for health care are low (in both absolute and relative terms) and the treatment gap is a global concern [1].

A range of evolving factors over time (e.g. demographic changes, epidemiological trends, increased availability of expensive treatments, and general financial pressures on national and global economies) have led to acute challenges in doing ever more with less. Such challenges essentially necessitate difficult decisions about how to best use our limited physical and financial resources. A range of information is required to inform such decisions.

A common starting point is to understand the full impact of a condition, whether it is physical or mental ill health or both together, by identifying and quantifying the range of its multiple impacts. Each impact will have an economic dimension or consequence, so cost can be a convenient common metric or weight to represent a range of different impacts. Such monetary weighting can then enable comparisons (across various populations, sub-group, or areas otherwise defined) to identify and prioritize areas for further investment or intervention. For example, calls for greater emphasis on early intervention and preventative approaches to mental health care are often underpinned, among other arguments, by demonstrations of the substantial and potentially avoidable economic burdens associated with mental illness. A mental health strategy published by the UK government in 2011 is a clear illustration of this [2].

This chapter describes the nature of economic burdens, the potential uses and limitations of cost-of-illness information for resource allocation decisions, and the importance of giving consideration to the value associated with alternative resource allocation options.

Economic dimensions of mental illness

An example

In thinking about the economic dimensions and costs of mental illness, it is helpful to do so in relation to a typical scenario of mental illness experience:

> Maya had previously thrown away a packet of prescribed antidepressants. During the few weeks she had taken them, she had felt worse rather than better and could not imagine how she would ever return to her normal self. Now, after taking a different type of antidepressant for over 2 months, she felt more hopeful. She had been feeling increasingly low for many months and, although she visited her doctor once to ask for something to help her sleep, it wasn't until a long time later that she had felt able to also mention how difficult things felt during the daytime, especially at work. There had been some mornings when, after being awake half of the night, she couldn't bring herself to get up and dressed. She had, at first, tried some herbal remedies for insomnia but she still lacked sleep, resulting in several days off work and many more when she struggled to engage with her work or colleagues. She had confided in no one about her difficulties until 2 weeks into taking the antidepressants first prescribed to her. She had been due to attend her sister's birthday party but felt nauseous and simply couldn't face the effort needed. Although she had worried about disappointing her sister, calling her to tell her why she couldn't come ended up being a key turning point. Appalled to learn how Maya had been feeling, her sister had insisted Maya return to her doctor, and accompanied her for support. Since then, she has also been trying to drop off some cooked meals for Maya a couple of times a week, knowing that Maya often can't face going to the shops.

Now, let's look at this same scenario again, with a focus on its economic dimensions (highlighted in bold text):

> Maya had previously **thrown away** a packet of **prescribed antidepressants**. During the few weeks she had taken them, she had **felt worse** rather than better and could not imagine how she would ever **return to her normal** self. Now, after taking a **different type of antidepressant** for **over 2 months**, she felt more hopeful. She had been feeling increasingly low for **many months** and, although she **visited her doctor once** to ask for **something to help her sleep**, it wasn't until **a long time later** that she had felt able to **also mention how difficult things felt** during the daytime, especially at **work**. There had been some mornings when, after being awake half of the night, she couldn't bring herself to get up and dressed. She had, at first, tried some **herbal remedies** for insomnia but she still lacked sleep, resulting in **several days off work** and many more when she **struggled to engage with her**

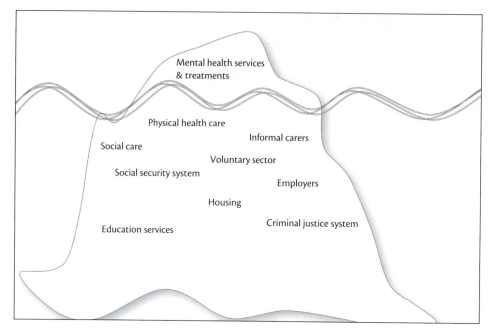

Fig. 3.1 Contributions to mental health care.

work or colleagues. She had **confided in no one** about her difficulties until 2 weeks into taking the antidepressants first prescribed to her. She had been due to attend her sister's birthday party but felt nauseous and simply couldn't face the effort needed. Although she had worried about disappointing her sister, calling her to tell her why she couldn't come ended up being a key turning point. Appalled to learn how Maya had been feeling, her sister had insisted Maya **return to her doctor**, and **accompanied her** for support. Since then, she has also been trying to **drop off some cooked meals** for Maya a couple of times a week, knowing that Maya often **can't face going to the shops**.

Those elements highlighted above represent a very diverse set of economic impacts that are not confined to those related to formal care inputs, and care is certainly not confined to the healthcare sector. Instead, health care is just the tip of the iceberg when it comes to economic impacts. The multiple dimensions of mental illness necessitate a complex set of involvements from multiple agents and agencies—for example, families, the criminal justice system, the housing sector, schools, and employers—as illustrated in Fig. 3.1. This was referred to as the 'mixed economy of care' by Knapp [3], who highlighted the crossover of care and budgets across public, voluntary, private, and informal care sectors. This complexity can present access issues for those suffering mental illnesses and challenges in identifying where both burdens and responsibilities fall. Evans-Lacko et al. outline the influence of the context surrounding formal care by illustrating international examples of programmes and actions outside of health services that have positively influenced mental health outcomes [4].

Costs of mental illness: examples and uses of estimates

Such multiple economic dimensions of illnesses are often summarized in the form of 'cost-of-illness' or 'burden-of-illness' estimates. These are generated by identifying the various consequences of an illness and attaching monetary valuations to

each. Knowing the size of the economic burden associated with an illness, especially relative to other illnesses, serves various uses. For example:

♦ identifying potential areas in which to achieve savings through some intervention, e.g. early intervention to change the course of an illness;

♦ highlighting inappropriate treatment levels as an indicator of unmet needs or avoidable clinical/economic burdens;

♦ more generally drawing greater attention to the illness, to increase public awareness of the illness, argue for greater investment or reprioritization of resources, and so on.

It is thus common to see public health campaigns or major cases for service change underpinned with estimates of economic burden [2, 5, 6]. Table 3.1 illustrates cost-of-illness estimates that were gathered from a range of sources and summarized in a Department of Health document [6]. Unsurprisingly, the significant impacts of mental illness beyond the individual and the healthcare system, in combination with high prevalence, generate some startling estimates of total economic burden.

Estimates of total burden associated with all mental illness are, expectedly, yet more staggering. For example, McCrone et al. [7] estimated total costs of services and lost earnings alone at £48 billion for the year 2007 (a contrast to the estimate of £32 billion generated 10 years earlier by Patel and Knapp for a broader set of impacts [8]) with an anticipated rise to £88 billion after accounting for population, pay, and price effects over time. A subsequent estimate of total costs of mental illness for England estimated annual costs at £105 billion (€122 billion), including costs of services, lost productivity at work, and reduced quality of life [9].

On a larger scale, the economic cost of mental health problems has been estimated to represent between 3% and 4% of gross national product in Member States of the European Union [10]. Cost estimates from Gustavsson et al. [11] highlight that mental

Table 3.1 Summary of cost statements reported by the Department of Health*

Author (year)	Stated condition	Stated inclusions/perspectives	Estimates of costs (£)					Cost year	Country	Time horizon	Unit (population vs average per person)
			Total	Services	Productivity loss	Families	Other				
Suhrcke et al. (2008) [58]	Mental illness	–	11,030–59,130	–	–	–	–	–	UK	1 year	Per child
Friedli and Parsonage (2007) [59]	Conduct disorder	–	5.2 billion	–	–	–	–	–	–	Lifetime	1-year cohort of children with conduct disorder
Sainsbury Centre for Mental Health (2005) [60]	Conduct disorder	–	–	–	–	–	60 million for crime	–	England and Wales	1 year	Adults who had conduct problems in childhood
McCrone et al. (2008) [7]	Depression	Total excluding informal care and other public service costs	7.5 billion	1.7 billion	Further 1.7–2.8 billion	–	5.8 billion for lost earnings; further human costs of 9.9–12.4 billion	2007	England	1 year	Population
McCrone et al. (2008) [7]	Anxiety	Health service and lost employment	8.9 billion	1.2 billion	7.7 billion (deduced from statement)	–	–	2007	–	–	Population
Bermingham et a. (2010) [61]	Medically unexplained symptoms	NHS, lost productivity and reduced quality of life	17.6 billion (deduced from statement)	3.1 billion	5.2 billion	–	Reduced QoL cost of 9.3 billion	2008–09	England	Annual	Population
Mangalore and Knapp (2007) [62]	Schizophrenia	Treatment and care, welfare benefits, families, lost productivity	6.7 billion	2 billion	3.4 billion including unemployment, work absence, and premature mortality	615 million for informal care and private expenditure	570 million for welfare	2004–05	England	Annual	Population
Knapp et al. (2007) [63]	Dementia	Accommodation, health services, social care services, informal care, lost employment	17 billion	8% for health services, 15% for social services	36% for lost employment and informal care combined	–	41% for accommodation	2007 (deduced)	UK	Annual	Population
Krapp et al. (2011) [5]; Platt et al. (2006) [64]; Kennelly et al. (2005) [65]	Suicide	–	1.7 million in England, 1.3 million in Scotland, 1.5 million in Ireland	–	–	–	–	–	England, Scotland, and Ireland	–	Average per suicide
Department of Health (2008) [66]	Alcohol misuse	Health service, lost productivity, crime, and antisocial behaviour, social support for people misusing alcohol and their families	17.7–25.1 billion	2.7 billion	6.0–7.3 billion due to work absence, reduced employment, and premature death	–	9–15 billion for crime	–	–	Annual	Population

*See 'Annex, page 19: Costs of different mental disorders across the life course.' Note that Table 3.1 summarizes only the information contained in the Annex statements, without reference to further details provided elsewhere; reasons for this will be discussed in the section 'Costs versus value: the need to consider outcomes'.

Note: NHS: National Health Service; QoL: quality of life.

health (and other) problems create a huge economic impact in very many countries and that immediate actions (more research, more treatment, and prevention) are needed to alleviate this burden.

Interpreting cost-of-illness estimates

On seeing these various estimates of the costs of mental illness, it may have become apparent that these headline figures might raise more questions than answers. For example:

◆ Exactly what population do they refer to?

◆ Do costs represent per-person costs or population-level costs?

◆ What type of cost impacts do they include/exclude?

◆ Whose views did they consider?

◆ Whose budgets do these costs fall upon?

◆ What were the data sources and their quality?

◆ Can they be compared against each other?

So, in looking back at Table 3.1, without further details it is unclear who is bearing the accommodation-related costs attributed to dementia and whether the health service costs estimated for alcohol misuse and anxiety considered the same range of services.

The significance of underlying details is often brought to light when there is a need to draw comparisons. This is illustrated by Jin and Mosweu [12], who recently reviewed the societal costs of schizophrenia. They examined 19 studies from around the world and found annual costs per patient ranged between around $US6000 in Thailand to $US95,000 in Norway (2015 values). Expectedly, they found that estimates of costs were influenced by patient-level factors, such as demographics and severity of illness, and that the main cost drivers for total costs were direct healthcare costs (which are necessarily influenced by differing healthcare systems and surrounding contextual factors) and lost productivity. However, they also found that cost variations were related to methodological differences between studies, such as how costs of productivity losses and co-morbidities were calculated.

Therefore, the questions noted above are among many recognized as valid ones to ask of cost-of-illness estimates. In the following, the main nuances to bear in mind when interpreting estimates for any health condition are highlighted.

In examining details underlying cost-of-illness estimates, it is interesting to note *when estimates were produced*. Estimates are influenced by both care availability and data availability, so can become less relevant over time. An early example comes from a governmental discussion document from England, entitled *Burdens of Disease* [13], published with the purpose of 'helping to inform debate and decision-making about priorities and resources within the NHS [National Health Service]'. Their general approach to estimation was to look at total national expenditure on health and social services and then to allocate this to the immediate cause. This 'top-down' approach means that the expenditure burden described was often lower than estimated in other burden of disease studies, which tended to also include costs of associated secondary diseases. However, use of such a method in *Burdens of Disease* [13] would have had the danger of double-counting. In more recent times, the availability and accessibility of information and data has vastly expanded. This helps produce estimates that are not only broad in their coverage, but also potentially more accurate. For example,

increased access to individual-level data for populations enables potentially more accurate 'bottom-up' approaches to identify costs associated with specifically defined sub-populations. Wittchen et al. [14] and Gustavsson et al. [11] demonstrated the drawing together of a vast range of epidemiological, economic, and other data to determine the cost of brain disorders (very broadly defined) for the whole of Europe. This was an update of previous estimates to take advantage of increased data availability [15]. However, as their remit was so ambitious—European-wide estimates for a range of brain disorders—they still faced data gaps that necessitated some assumptions and data imputations.

Whether an *incidence or prevalence* approach is taken for cost estimation is a fundamental factor to ascertain. Naturally, the two approaches can lead to very different cost-of-illness estimates as they essentially define two different types of populations. Further, given the large prevalence of mental illnesses, the need for robust estimates is vital as these form the basis of extrapolations or data cuts that are likely to be made. However, in the context of mental illness, population definition may be problematic owing to illness heterogeneity and the well-established stigma surrounding presentation, diagnosis, and treatment [16].

Co-morbidity, of both a mental and a physical nature, requires attention more generally given its high prevalence among those with mental illness. Rates of psychiatric co-morbidity alone can range from 21% to 81% in people with different mental illnesses [17], and the coexistence of more than one mental health problem has been demonstrated to increase the probability of service use [18]. This can lead to complex patterns of resource use and difficulties in attribution of resource use/costs to particular conditions. Recording practices or analytical approaches can either prevent identification of all relevant cases with the health condition of interest (thus underestimating costs) or double-count costs across conditions (and thus overestimate). For example, some datasets/estimates may utilize hierarchies of illness—as illustrated in the aforementioned NHS Executive estimate [13], which assigned costs only to immediate cause.

The long and undulating *course* of so many mental health conditions is of particular interest from an economic perspective given that this generates multiple and broad ranging disruptions in sufferers' lives. This is evident in the area of employment. Mental illnesses are prevalent in those of working age and cause difficulties in both securing and maintaining employment [19]. This, in turn, generates substantial cumulative income losses for the individuals concerned, plus a production loss for society more generally, which carries a high economic value [20]. Two further contributors to lost productivity are worth highlighting. Firstly, the premature mortality associated with high rates of suicide among those with mental illness [21]. Secondly, the premature mortality associated with mental ill health itself or the risk it presents for co-morbid conditions [22, 23].

Productivity losses as described earlier are not confined to those with mental illness. Such conditions also place significant *burdens on families and friends*, which impact on their quality of life and normal activities, including employment opportunities. While lost productivity receives much attention owing to its size and its importance to agendas related to national/global economic performance, other important impacts include a *disproportionate representation of mental illness among homeless and prison populations* [24, 25].

The range of costs that may or may not be considered in cost-of-illness studies is related to the *perspective* that is adopted. This is essentially a matter of whose point of view is being considered. Inclusion/exclusion of particular cost perspectives or items may sometimes be contentious. For example, welfare payments can have a substantial influence on cost-of-illness estimates given the size of welfare support in many countries. Also, level of welfare provision across different contexts will likely influence other aspects of the economy of care. Some argue that welfare payments should be excluded from cost estimates because they are a redistribution of purchasing power from one part of the economy to another, with no goods or services exchanged in return. However, others argue that this public expenditure could be used in other ways and thus should be included when considering a public sector perspective to the burden of an illness [26]. The potentially differential impacts on costs by stakeholders are illustrated by Andrews et al. [27], who examine costs of schizophrenia, and potential savings through effective interventions, from societal and public sector perspectives. Social welfare burden is, of course, an economic concern in itself for many governments. An example of attempts to reduce such burden specifically in relation to mental illness is provided by the implementation of the 'Improving Access to Psychological Therapies' programme in England. This aimed to widen access to effective psychological therapies, with the expectation that there would be a subsequent increase in employment rates and an associated reduction in welfare payments [28]. However, there have been various critiques of the approach and questions concerning whether the anticipated outcomes actually transpired [29, 30].

Level of analysis is also another aspect of perspective that can convey very different messages related to the costs of illness. Some conditions cost more per person than others—for example, at an individual level, costs associated with schizophrenia can be greater than for depression—but aggregate pictures differ as a result of differences in incidence/prevalence. The two types of estimates can thus serve very different purposes.

Time horizon is a major influence on the size of estimates. Many cost-of-illness studies aim to estimate 1-year, or annual, costs. As well as being straightforward to understand, this also brings advantages in data access and handling as many of the cross-sectional data required for cost-of-illness estimates tend to relate to financial reporting periods or short-term studies. However, examining longer periods of time is, perhaps, more relevant when it comes to long-term conditions. It is particularly important in the context of making a case for prevention/early intervention and in life-course approaches to illness management. Such estimates require a broader set of data, which brings its own challenges, and may rely on a greater number of assumptions. This may especially be the case where future trajectories of (as yet unknown) costs are attempted [7].

In highlighting just these few considerations, three things are clear. Firstly, as with any health-related data, any comparisons of cost-of-illness estimates should be undertaken with extreme care, particularly across different healthcare systems. Smith and Wright reviewed costs of mental illness studies in just one national context and found notable variations in prevalence/incidence rates, service coverage, unit costs applied to resource use, and inclusion/exclusion criteria [31]. Secondly, again as with any study, the reliability of the estimates depends on the appropriateness of the design for the question in hand and on data quality. Methodological variation does not in itself suggest weakness but can potentially suggest divergence between the original purpose of generating the estimate and the uses to which it is subsequently put. Finally, given the variations in design and underlying data, cost-of-illness estimates (particularly those with broader perspectives and relating to complex sets of burdens such as for mental illness) should generally be viewed as indicative, rather than definitive.

Costs versus value: the need to consider outcomes

While cost-of-illness estimates can highlight the size of problems, and, in turn, serve political and planning purposes [32], some (see, e.g., [31]) question their usefulness. Balancing limited healthcare resources against the demands placed on them requires recognition that resources are not an end in themselves but routes through which the health and welfare of populations can be improved. Optimality of resource allocation can be considered using a multitude of criteria related to the overall goals of healthcare systems—which can be multidimensional and variable, depending on funding systems—and other broader (and possibly conflicting) societal goals, such as equity or moral responsibility. One such criterion for such assessments is that of *value*. This concerns the relationship between what resources are expended and what outcomes result from the expenditure. Smith and Wright thus argued that rather than assessing just the costs of illness, it is more valuable to examine both costs *and effectiveness* of alternative methods of preventing or treating diseases to inform decisions about how best to use limited resources [31]. Such *value* or *efficiency* considerations are usually formulated in the form of *economic evaluations*, which identify, measure, value, and compare all relevant inputs (costs) and outputs (outcomes) for relevant alternative approaches. Fig. 3.2 illustrates this standard conceptual framework. A similar approach can also be used to determine which resources can be freed up from their existing use (i.e. disinvested), although such considerations have had relatively little attention overall in high-income settings, where the focus has instead been whether or not to adopt new treatments [33].

Types of economic evaluation

Several different types of economic evaluation follow this framework [34]; these are summarized in Table 3.2. All approaches have two keys features: they include a consideration of *outcomes*, as well as costs; and they are *comparative* in their nature, i.e. examine a treatment against at least one other. This enables a consideration of relative value and some sense of the *opportunity cost* of choosing one treatment rather than another. The examination of inputs/costs is standard across all approaches and they differ only in the nature and handling of outcomes information.

Cost-effectiveness analysis and cost-utility analysis, which each focus on one specific predefined outcome of interest, have long been widely used and adopted within various national-level decision-making processes about what interventions provide best value. However, the focus on one outcome does not lend itself well to assessments of complex conditions or public health interventions, which are likely to have multiple stakeholders involved, and a consequently broader set of costs and outcomes to consider. The cost–benefit analysis approach fits such situations better because it aims to place monetary values on the

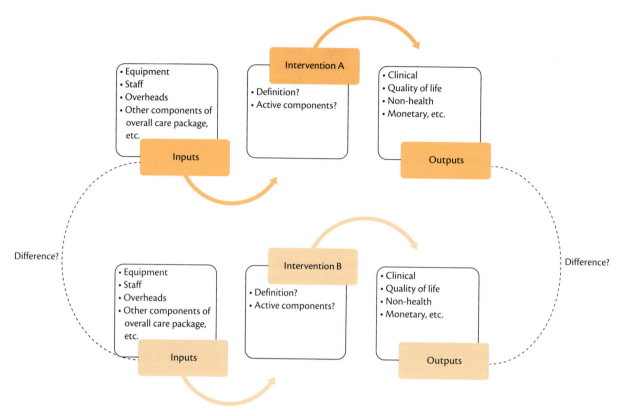

Fig. 3.2 Standard conceptual framework for economic evaluation.

outcomes of interest; as discussed earlier, using money as a common unit conveniently enables the summation of multiple dimensions into one summary figure. However, appropriately and reliably estimating monetary values for non-monetary outcomes is a challenge. Methods currently available to do this for public health economic evaluations are described by McIntosh et al. [35].

Table 3.2 Types of economic evaluation

Type of economic evaluation	Type of cost–outcome consideration
Cost-minimization analysis	For treatments providing the *same outcomes*, which approach costs less?
Cost-effectiveness analysis	Which treatment has the best combination of cost and *primary outcome*?
Cost-utility analysis	Which treatment has the best combination of cost and *quality-weighted length of life*?
Cost-benefit analysis	Which treatment maximizes the net *monetary benefit*?
Cost-consequences analysis	Which treatment has the best combination of cost and *all outcomes*?

In addition, there are some 'hybrid' or partial approaches to economic evaluation that adopt elements from the classic approaches, for example estimates and comparisons of future *monetary returns, pay-offs*, or *cost offsets* from current investments. These are often used when assessing longer-term impacts and, where the impacts are likely to be too far in the future to formally measure, assumptions can be made drawing on external information, such as relevant literature or expert opinion. Examples of such evaluations are provided by Knapp et al. [5], who used available evidence for 15 mental health promotion, prevention, or early interventions to estimate (using economic modelling techniques) their current costs and future economic pay-offs. Using this approach, they demonstrated that a number of effective and low-cost interventions addressing childhood mental health problems would be self-financing over time with pay-offs to the public sector and elsewhere (e.g. better educational performance, improved employment/earnings, reduced crime). Similarly, it has been estimated that each euro spent on mental health *research* could deliver a €0.37 return each year [36].

While there are sometimes conflicting views on the evidence base for preventative approaches (see, e.g. [37]), it is evident that the long-term nature of many mental health conditions necessitate interventions that aim to improve symptoms, long-term health, and quality of life, rather than cure. For particularly complex conditions such as schizophrenia, an appropriate treatment may be defined by broad packages of care to meet potentially diverse and long-term needs. Thus, low treatment costs might indicate the presence of unmet need, rather than efficiency, as low costs may be associated with inferior outcomes over time. This highlights the necessity for assessments of efficiency to cover all relevant costs and outcomes.

Economic evaluations of mental health care

There is now a substantial literature on the cost-effectiveness of a range of mental health care. For some conditions, the body of evidence is large enough to warrant systematic reviews or overviews (see [38] and [39] for some examples). While the quantity of economic evaluations may be too numerous to cover in any detail, it is worth noting here the type of interventions and treatment approaches that have been the focus of such evaluations—these largely represent the key developments in mental health care over the past few decades.

Medications have become the first-line treatment for many mental health problems owing to the development of numerous new medications and their relatively wider and easier reach than other types of interventions. Unsurprisingly, the ongoing costs associated with long-term medication use generated close interest in the cost-effectiveness of such medications, especially when priced highly while under patent protection. During that time, it was common to see economic arguments based on the increased acquisition costs of newer and more expensive drugs being offset by savings in hospitalization costs owing to better outcomes, relapse reduction, and so on. However, this argument is more nuanced [40, 41], given the interplay between medication, side effects, patient characteristics, surrounding packages of care, and so on (and, of course, commercial interests).

Another major care development that sparked a rise in economic evaluation is the growth and development of *psychological treatments*. These generate a range of economic considerations owing to their potential application across a range of conditions, labour intensity related to not only delivery, but also training and supervision (although online versions and delivery by less-qualified staff are now more commonly available), and variations in approach, content, setting, and format (e.g. brief vs long, individual vs group).

As discussed earlier, mental health care can comprise a wide range of treatments and support spread across numerous sectors (Fig. 3.1). Thus, besides economic evaluations of specific treatments, a number of economic evaluations have centred on assessing the cost-effectiveness of *alternative care configuration or settings*. Notably, the last half century or so has seen substantial shifts in many countries, away from long-term/hospital/residential care towards home/community-based care. As with the mixed evidence on new medications, this changing care pattern carries similar nuances in cost-effectiveness owing, for example, to the potentially more intensive care inputs that might be required to deliver effective care in the community and complexities in funding arrangements [42].

Finally, despite early debates on the cost-effectiveness of community-based care versus institutional care, the ongoing shift towards community-based care resulted in many innovations in *community care arrangements* (e.g. 'assertive community treatment', 'case management', 'care programmes', and 'home treatment'), which became the subject of economic evaluations.

Complexities and challenges for economic evaluation of mental health care interventions

While there is a relatively large and growing body of economic evidence concerning mental health care, and the rise of 'big data' represents a huge leap in what's possible for cost estimation and evaluation, mental health conditions and care carry some specific features that will continually necessitate some particular care and attention.

Firstly, given the array of effects that people with mental illness can experience (e.g. psychiatric, psychological, physical, employment, social, and quality of life), it is often inadequate or misleading for an economic evaluation to focus on a single *outcome measure*. Therefore, while many evaluations in this area may have a primary outcome measure, it is common for there to be a range of other relevant outcome measures that may be equally important. There are some combined measures of outcome, such as disability- or quality-adjusted life years, which bring together length and quality-of-life outcomes. Their general nature has led to their increased use in policy-making as they allow cost-effectiveness comparisons between different health areas. However, such approaches require credible data for individuals and multiple measures over time. While this may be feasible in some groups (see [43]), it may not be for others, for example those with cognitive impairment and communication difficulties [44, 45], or those difficult to follow-up. Further, the measures themselves may be problematic in particular patient groups [46, 47]. The cost-consequences approach mentioned in Table 3.2 allows the examination of multiple outcomes alongside costs and, rather than providing a definitive 'answer' regarding cost-effectiveness, it is a more disaggregated presentation approach that might better suit evaluations of mental health care.

Secondly, non-pharmacological treatments for mental illness are recognized as *complex interventions*, not just in terms of their nature, but also their implementation and evaluation. Given that mental health care is delivered by a range of agencies and services, parallels can be drawn with the delivery and evaluation of public health care. For example, Rychetnik et al. discuss that public health interventions require multiple, flexible, and community-driven strategies, and that where intervention evaluations show lack of effect, then an important question is whether the intervention itself did not work (i.e. the concept or theory of the intervention) or whether it was just poorly implemented [48]. For example, psychological therapies may not be delivered as planned and/or implementation may vary across therapists, patients, or other contexts, even when manualized.

Thirdly, the broad-ranging inputs to mental health 'care' can cause difficulties in defining the nature of the *comparator*, as the diversity of care is more likely to lead to variations in 'usual care' from setting to setting. Patel provides a visual representation of such variations in an international context [49], but such variations can exist even in narrowly defined service or geographical locations. Heterogeneity of service delivery interventions, and the difficulties this causes for their evaluation, is well documented [50].

Finally, economic studies of mental illness are likely to be of greater use to policymakers if they obtain the broadest possible perspective on costs [51]. However, the complex, interconnected and long-running nature of the bundle of inputs that make up mental health care naturally present a set of challenges for *data collection* to estimate total care costs. It is near impossible to collect either prospective or retrospective data from all relevant care providers or funders. Thus, data are commonly collected directly from study participants, rather than service-provider records. Some may question the reliability of self-reported data owing to the aforementioned cognitive problems, and so on. However, there is evidence of the (admittedly nuanced) reliability of such approaches [52–54], and self-report remains a crucial route through which to capture the richness and fullness of economic impacts that would otherwise be difficult to assess by other means, for example lost productivity and out-of-pocket expenses. There is nevertheless a need to remain focused on what's important to assess. This is illustrated by an analysis of data from five mental health service evaluations, which found that the costs of the five most expensive measured services within each study contributed to between 90% and 98% of total care costs [55].

These are just some of the issues that might warrant more attention in mental health care evaluations. There are, of course, many *general issues* relevant to any evaluation. Altogether, these generate many methodological variations between studies. So, just as discussed in relation to cost-of-illness studies, estimates from economic evaluations can similarly be challenging to bring together for the purposes of comparison or overview. Inconsistent findings may thus simply be due to differences in study populations, treatments, health systems, and other contextual factors, and so on. For example, when the National Institute for Health and Care Excellence in England produced clinical guidelines for antipsychotic medication for the treatment of schizophrenia [56], they reviewed 31 published economic evaluations from a number of different countries and found they included different categories of costs and assumptions about treatment outcomes, creating challenges in drawing comparisons and preventing examination of cost-effectiveness between new treatments.

Conclusion

The economic burden of mental illness falls upon a range of individuals, organizations, and sectors of society. While many physical health conditions similarly carry economic dimensions, mental illnesses have some notable features that have a particular bearing on the diversity and size of costs. Consequently, mental illness represents a substantial societal and monetary burden. Regardless of the many issues related to generating and interpreting information on the costs of illnesses, it is clear that treatment costs form only a small proportion of the total economic burden of mental illness. Taking broad perspectives in estimating such figures helps highlight mental health as a concern extending beyond the healthcare sector.

Of concern to many, such costs could double in just a couple of decades [7]. The scarcity of resources for health care requires difficult decisions concerning their distribution across different illnesses, populations, care approaches, and numerous other dividing lines. Various criteria—clinical, social, ethical, and moral, and so on—can be deployed for such decisions; value for money is an important one, especially in times such as now with enormous economic pressures on all sectors of society [57].

Assessments of value can take several forms, but all necessitate examining the relationship between inputs to, and outcome of, care. For evaluations of mental health care, such inputs and outcomes need to be considered in their widest sense to embody the breadth of care and impacts associated with mental health problems. There are related measurement problems, but none insurmountable; consequently, there is a substantial and growing body of high-quality evidence to better inform decisions about delivering cost-effective mental health care.

Importantly, there is opportunity and evidence for preventative approaches, in both mental and physical health care arenas and beyond the healthcare system. This could divert current trajectories of future care costs and bring economic advantages to many stakeholders.

References

1. Lancet Global Mental Health Group. Scale up services for mental disorders: a call for action. *Lancet* 2007; 370: 1241–52.
2. Department of Health. No health without mental health: a cross-government mental health outcomes strategy for people of all ages. Available at: https://www.gov.uk/government/uploads/system/uploads/attachment_data/file/213761/dh_124058.pdf (2011, accessed 22 December 2016).
3. Knapp M. *The Economic Evaluation of Mental Health Care.* Aldershot: Arena, 1995.
4. Evans-Lacko S, Ribeiro W, Brietzke E, et al. Lean economies and innovation in mental health systems. *Lancet* 2016; 387: 1356–8.
5. Knapp MRJ, McDaid D, Parsonage M (eds). *Mental Health Promotion and Mental Illness Prevention: The Economic Case.* London: Department of Health, 2011.
6. Department of Health. No health without mental health: a cross-government mental health outcomes strategy for people of all ages. Supporting document—the economic case for improving efficiency and quality in mental health. Available at: https://www.gov.uk/government/uploads/system/uploads/attachment_data/file/215808/dh_123993.pdf (2011, accessed 25 January 2017).
7. McCrone P, Dhanasiri S, Patel A, Knapp M, Lawton-Smith S. *Paying the Price: The Cost of Mental Health Care in England to 2026.* London: King's Fund, 2008.
8. Patel A, Knapp M. Costs of mental illness in England. *Mental Health Res Rev* 1998; 5: 4–10.
9. Centre for Mental Health. The economic and social costs of mental health problems in 2009/10. Available at: https://www.centreformentalhealth.org.uk/economic-and-social-costs-2009 (2010, accessed 22 December 2016).
10. European Commission. The State of Mental Health in the European Union. Available at: http://www.msssi.gob.es/organizacion/sns/planCalidadSNS/pdf/excelencia/salud_mental/opsc_est18.pdf.pdf (2004, accessed 22 December 2016).
11. Gustavsson A, Svensson M, Jacobi F, et al., on behalf of on behalf of the CDBE2010 Study Group. Cost of disorders of the brain in Europe 2010. *Eur Neuropsychopharmacol* 2011; 21: 718–79.
12. Jin H, Mosweu I. The societal cost of schizophrenia: a systematic review. *Pharmacoeconomics* 2017; 35: 25–42.
13. NHS Executive (NHSE). *Burdens of Disease.* Leeds: NHSE, 1996.
14. Wittchen HU, Jacobi F, Rehm J, et al. The size and burden of mental disorders and other disorders of the brain in Europe 2010. *Eur Neuropsychopharmacol* 2011; 21: 655–79.
15. Andlin-Sobocki P, Jonsson B, Wittchen HU, Olesen J. Cost of disorders of the brain in Europe. *Eur J Neurol* 2005; 12(Suppl. 1): 1–27.
16. Veen ND, Selten J-P, Schols DLW, Hoek HW, van der Tweel I, Kahn RS. Diagnostic stability in a Dutch psychosis incidence cohort. *Br J Psychiatry* 2004; 185: 460–4.

17. The ESEMeD/MHEDEA 2000 Investigators. 12-month comorbidity patterns and associated factors in Europe: results from the European Study of the Epidemiology of Mental Disorders (ESEMeD) project. *Acta Psychiatr Scand* 2004; 109: 28–37.

18. The ESEMeD/MHEDEA 2000 Investigators. Use of mental health services in Europe: results from the European Study of the Epidemiology of Mental Disorders (ESEMeD) project. *Acta Psychiatr Scand* 2004; 109: 47–54.

19. Jarvisalo J, Andersson B, Boedeker W, Houtman I. Mental disorders as a major challenge in prevention of work disability. European Commission Social Security and Health Reports, No 66. Available at: http://www.kela.fi/in/internet/liite.nsf/NET/150305153403SV/$File/Katsaus66_netti.pdf (2005, accessed 12 December 2016).

20. Thomas CM, Morris S. Costs of depression among adults in England in 2000. *Br J Psychiatry* 2003; 183: 514–19.

21. Centre for Suicide Prevention. The cost of suicide. SEIC Alert #74. Available at: http://csp.cloud8.ionlinehosting.net/LinkClick.aspx?fileticket=Jz_OfDJ9HUc%3D&tabid=538 (2010, accessed 12 December 2016).

22. Osborn DJ, Levy G, Nazareth I, Petersen I, Islam A, King MB. Relative risk of cardiovascular and cancer mortality in people with severe mental illness from the United Kingdom's general practice research database. *Arch Gen Psychiatry* 2007; 64: 242–9.

23. Saha S, Chant D, McGrath J. A systematic review of mortality in schizophrenia: is the differential mortality gap worsening over time? *Arch Gen Psychiatry* 2007; 64: 1123–31.

24. Fazel S, Khosla V, Doll H, Geddes J. The prevalence of mental disorders among the homeless in western countries: systematic review and meta-regression analysis. *PLOS Med* 2008; 5: e225.

25. Bebbington P, Jakobowitz S, McKenzie N, et al. Assessing needs for psychiatric treatment in prisoners: 1. Prevalence of disorder. *Soc Psychiatry Psychiatr Epidemiol* 2017; 52: 221–9.

26. Raftery J. Have the 'lunatics taken over the asylums'? The rising cost of psychiatric services in England and Wales, 1860–1886. In: Knapp M (ed.). *The economic Evaluation of Mental Health Care*. Aldershot: Arena, 1995, pp. 215–228.

27. Andrews A, Knapp M, McCrone P, Parsonage M, Trachtenberg M. Effective interventions in schizophrenia: the economic case. A report prepared for the Schizophrenia Commission. Available at: https://www.rethink.org/media/514083/LSE_economic_report_16nov.pdf (2012, accessed 22 December 2016).

28. Layard R, Clark D, Knapp M, Mayraz G. Cost-benefit analysis of psychological therapy. *Natl Inst Econ Rev* 2007; 202: 90–8.

29. Fitzpatrick M. A miscalculation of sublime dimensions. *Br J Gen Pract* 2006; 1; 56: 729.

30. Hawkes N. Talking therapies: can the centre hold? *BMJ* 2011; 342; 578.

31. Smith K, Wright K. Costs of mental illness in Britain. *Health Policy* 1996; 35: 61–73.

32. Tarricone R. Cost-of-illness analysis. What room in health economics? *Health Policy* 2006; 77: 51–63.

33. Hughes DA, Wood EM, Tuersley L. NICE recommendations: why no disinvestment recommendations to offset investment decisions? *BMJ* 2015; 350: 2656.

34. Drummond MF, Sculpher MJ, Stoddart GL, Torrance GW. *Methods for the Economic Evaluation of Health Care Programmes*. 4th ed. Oxford: Oxford University Press, 2015.

35. McIntosh E, Clarke P, Frew E, Louviere J (eds). *Applied Methods of Cost-Benefit Analysis in Health Care*. Oxford: Oxford University Press, 2010.

36. Haro JM, Wykes T. A road map for mental health research in Europe: developing mental health and well-being research priorities for Europe. Available at: http://www.gamian.eu/wp-content/uploads/2015/01/IG-20150120-Roamer.pdf (2015, accessed 22 December 2016).

37. Pelosi A. Is early intervention in the major psychiatric disorders justified? No. *BMJ* 2008; 337: a710.

38. Bereza BG, Machado M, Einarson TR. Systematic review and quality assessment of economic evaluations and quality-of-life studies related to generalized anxiety disorder. *Clin Ther* 2009; 31: 1279–308.

39. Knapp M, Barrett B, Romeo R, et al. An international review of cost-effectiveness studies for mental disorders. Working Paper No. 36, November 2004, Disease Control Priorities Project (a joint effort of the World Bank, The Fogarty International Center of the National Institutes of Health, the Bill & Melinda Gates Foundation, and the World Health Organization).

40. Cohen LJ. Looking beyond the formulary budget in cost-benefit analysis. *Am J Manag Care* 1997; 3: S11–17.

41. King D, Knapp M, Patel A, et al. The impact of non-adherence to medication in patients with schizophrenia on health, social care and societal costs—analysis of the QUATRO study. *Epidemiol Psychiatr Sci* 2014; 23: 61–70.

42. Walsh KK, Kastner TA, Gentlesk Green R. Cost comparisons of community and institutional residential settings: historical review of selected research. *Ment Retard* 2003; 41: 103–22.

43. Voruganti L, Heslegrave R, Awad AG, Seeman MV. Quality of life measurement in schizophrenia: reconciling the quest for subjectivity with the question of reliability. *Psychol Med* 1998; 28: 165–72.

44. Neumann PJ. Methods of cost-effectiveness analysis in the evaluation of new antipsychotics: implications for schizophrenia treatment. *J Clin Psychiatry* 1999; 60: 9–14.

45. Awad AG, Voruganti LN, Heslegrave RJ. Measuring quality of life in patients with schizophrenia. *Pharmacoeconomics* 1997; 11: 32–47.

46. McCrone P, Patel A, Knapp M, et al. A comparison of SF-6D and EQ-5D utility scores in a study of patients with schizophrenia. *J Ment Health Policy Econ* 2009; 12: 27–31.

47. Brazier J, Connell J, Papaioannou D, et al. A systematic review, psychometric analysis and qualitative assessment of generic preference-based measures of health in mental health populations and the estimation of mapping functions from widely used specific measures. *Health Technol Assess* 2014; 18: vii–viii, xiii–xxv, 1–188.

48. Rychetnik L, Frommer M, Hawe P, Shiell A. Criteria for evaluating evidence on public health interventions. *J Epidmiol Commun Health* 2002; 56: 119–27.

49. Patel A. Guest editorial: conducting and interpreting multi-national economic evaluations: the measurement of costs. In: Curtis L, Netten A (eds). *Unit Costs of Health and Social Care*. Kent: University of Kent, 2006, pp. 9–15.

50. Catty J, Burns T, Knapp M, et al. Home treatment for mental health problems: a systematic review. *Psychol Med* 2002; 32: 383–401.

51. Patel A. The promises and pitfalls of pharmacoeconomics in schizophrenia. *Eur Psychiatry* 2003; 18: S62–7.

52. Cheung AH, Dewa CS, Wasylenki D. Impact on cost estimates of differences in reports of service use among clients, caseworkers, and hospital records. *Psychiatr Serv* 2003; 54: 1328–30.

53. Goldberg RW, Seybolt DC, Lehman A. Reliable self-report of health service use by individuals with serious mental illness. *Psychiatr Serv* 2002; 53: 879–81.

54. Mirandola M, Bisoffi G, Bonizzato P, Amaddeo F. Collecting psychiatric resources utilisation data to calculate costs of care: a comparison between a service receipt interview and a case register. *Soc Psychiatry Psychiatr Epidemiol* 1999; 34: 541–7.

55. Knapp M, Beecham J. Reduced-list costings: examination of an informed short-cut in mental health research. *Health Econ* 1993; 2: 313–22.

56. National Institute for Clinical Excellence. *Guidance on the Use of Newer (Atypical) Antipsychotic Drugs for the Treatment of Schizophrenia. Technology Assessment Guidance—No. 43*. London: National Institute for Clinical Excellence, 2002.

57. Patel A. The inevitable pursuit of efficiency. *J Ment Health* 2013; 22: 89–92.

58. Suhrcke M, Pillas D, Selai C. *Economic Aspects of Mental Health in Children and Adolescents*. Copenhagen: WHO Regional Office for Europe, 2008.

59. Friedli L, Parsonage M. Mental Health Promotion: Building an Economic Case. Belfast: Northern Ireland Association for Mental Health, 2007.

60. Sainsbury Centre for Mental Health (SCMH) The chance of a Lifetime. Preventing Early Conduct Problems and Reducing Crime. Available at: http://www.scmh.org.uk/pdfs/chance_of_a_lifetime.pdf (2009, accessed 6 March 2018).

61. Bermingham S, Cohen A, Hague J, Parsonage M. The cost of somatisation among the working-age population in England for the year 2008/09. *Ment Health Fam Med* 2010; 7: 71–84.

62. Mangalore R, Knapp M. Cost of schizophrenia in England. *J Ment Health Policy Econ* 2007; 10: 23–41.

63. Knapp M, Prince M, Albanese E, et al. *Dementia UK: A Report into the Prevalence and Cost of Dementia*. London: Alzheimer's Society, 2007.

64. Platt S, McLean J, McCollam A, et al. *Evaluation of the First Phase of Choose Life: The National Strategy and Action Plan to Prevent Suicide in Scotland*. Edinburgh: Scottish Executive Social Research, 2006.

65. Kennelly B, Ennis J, O'Shea E. *Economic Cost of Suicide and Deliberate Self-harm. Reach Out: National Strategy for Action on Suicide Prevention 2005–2014*. Dublin: Department of Health and Children, 2005.

66. Department of Health. *Safe, Sensible, Social – Consultation on Further Action: Impact Assessments*. London: Department of Health, 2008.

CHAPTER 4

The global burden of mental and substance use disorders

A review of methods, findings, and applications of data from the Global Burden of Disease Study

Alize J. Ferrari, Holly E. Erskine, Fiona J. Charlson, Damian F. Santomauro, Janni Leung, and Harvey A. Whiteford

The history of burden of disease estimation

The term 'disease burden' refers to the impact diseases and injuries have on population health [1]. Estimates of disease burden can be used in a number of way but, ultimately, their purpose is to provide information that can inform the design of health systems and public health policies. If a health system is to be sufficiently aligned with the health needs of the population then policymakers need access to information that allows them to compare the relative health impact of different diseases and injuries. Estimates of disease burden and, in turn policy-making and service provision, were originally based on mortality statistics [1]. Consequently, communicable diseases, such as cholera, tuberculosis, and smallpox, were prioritized in health agendas owing to their high rates of mortality. In the twentieth century, a transition in global demographics and population health began to emerge. There was a significant global decline in deaths (particularly infant and child mortality) occurring as a result of declines in infectious diseases, improved nutrition, and better maternal health. Furthermore, a larger proportion of the population began to live longer and reach ages where chronic, non-communicable diseases were prevalent. This epidemiological transition meant that the relative importance of conditions resulting in loss of health (i.e. disability) rather than just loss of life (i.e. mortality) increased and needed to be considered in global health agendas.

The introduction of the disability-adjusted life year (DALY) as a metric for measuring disease burden became central to this effort. In 1993, the largest lender for health in the developing world, the World Bank, dedicated its 1993 World Development Report to health [1] and used the DALY as a new measure of disease burden. The DALY was novel in its approach as it quantified the burden imposed by both mortality and disability for a given condition. DALYs represent a 'health gap', with each DALY equating to the loss of one healthy year of life to a disease or injury. They indicate the state of a population's health relative to a gold standard of all individuals in that population living in perfect health for the entire duration of the standard life expectancy [2–4]. As shown in Fig. 4.1, DALYs are estimated by summing years lived with disability (YLDs) and years of life lost due to premature mortality (YLLs), the non-fatal and fatal burden associated with a health condition, respectively.

To estimate YLDs, the prevalence of a health condition in a population is multiplied by the average amount of disability associated with that condition. Disability is quantified using a 'disability weight', ranging from 0 (perfect health) to 1 (death), and represents 'within-the-skin' losses of health-related functioning (e.g. bodily functions, senses, cognition, and ambulation) [2]. To estimate YLLs, the total number of deaths attributable to the health condition is multiplied by the standard life expectancy at the age of death [4].

After the publication of the 1993 World Development Report, the World Bank commissioned the Global Burden of Disease Study 1990 (GBD 1990), which was led by the World Health Organization (WHO) and Harvard University. GBD 1990 estimated DALYs for 107 diseases and injuries across eight world regions [5]. One of the most influential findings from GBD 1990 was the large proportion of global disease burden due to certain non-communicable diseases (e.g. mental and substance use disorders), which did not feature in league mortality tables previously used to identify the most significant diseases. GBD 1990 reported that neuropsychiatric disorders accounted for a quarter of the world's YLDs and 9% of total DALYs. Five mental disorders featured in the top-ten leading causes of YLDs worldwide: major depression, alcohol use disorders, bipolar disorder, schizophrenia, and obsessive-compulsive disorder [5]. This finding had a significant impact on the public health community and global health agenda, bringing attention to what was previously a hidden or neglected health challenge [6]. While addressing the burden imposed by conditions responsible for large amounts of premature mortality remained important from

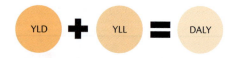

Fig. 4.1 The disability-adjusted life year (DALY).
Note: YLD: years lived with disability; YLL: years of life lost.

both ethical and economic standpoints, policymakers now needed to account for the disability imposed by non-communicable conditions, such as mental and substance use disorders.

GBD 1990 findings have been cited over 4000 times since they were published. However, the findings were not without controversy. Disease-specific advocates argued that the study had underestimated burden for their relevant health conditions. There was also debate around the use of age weighting and discounting. Age weighting placed greater weighting on burden estimates derived for those aged between 9 and 55 years in order to represent the greater social responsibility of youth and middle adulthood. Age discounting reflected the societal preference for a year of life saved now versus a year of life saved at some point in the future [5]. Additionally, some questioned the use of expert judgement to estimate disability weights. GBD 1990 disability weights were based on the views of an international group of health professionals. It was argued that health professionals made judgements based on the clinical presentation of diseases, which is typically more severe than the presentation of these diseases in the general population, thereby overestimating disability and burden [5, 7]. For mental and substance use disorders specifically, the aggregated cause group used for some disorders such as 'drug use' and 'unipolar depression' was deemed to be too heterogeneous. The failure to capture childhood mental disorders was also criticized, particularly for low-income regions such as Sub-Saharan Africa, where children constitute up to 40% of the total population [8].

After the release of GBD 1990, the burden estimation process continued to evolve as DALYs were updated to reflect new epidemiological data and methods. The WHO released updated DALYs for 2000 and 2005 [9], and again for 2011 [10] over 30 countries led their own national burden of disease studies from which subnational estimates of burden were generated. However, the most comprehensive effort to update the GBD framework since GBD 1990 was led by the Institute for Health Metrics and Evaluation (IHME) at the University of Washington. IHME is the coordinating centre for GBD, involving an international network of GBD contributors, and has continued to lead regular updates of GBD estimates. IHME led the Global Burden of Disease Study 2010 (GBD 2010), published in 2012, which estimated DALYs for 291 diseases and injuries (including 20 mental and substance use disorders) across 21 regions and 187 countries [11]. This was then updated in the 2013 iteration, the Global Burden of Disease Study 2013 (GBD 2013), published in 2015 [12–14]. This update of the study was expanded to incorporate a total of 306 diseases and injuries and re-estimated all burden estimates, including those for previous years. This meant that the findings of GBD 2013 superseded the findings of GBD 2010. This occurred again in the Global Burden of Disease Study 2015 (GBD 2015), which is discussed in greater detail in the next section [2–4, 15].

Global Burden of Disease Study 2015 burden estimation methodology for mental and substance use disorders

GBD 2015 maintained many of the founding principles that guided GBD 1990. For instance, it made use of comparable metrics (YLDs, YLLs, and DALYs) to estimate the fatal, non-fatal, and overall burden of diseases and injuries on the population [2–4, 15]. It was also designed to ensure that the science behind burden estimates was not prejudiced by advocacy. In response to the criticisms of GBD 1990 methodology, burden estimation underwent a number of changes in consultation with international groups of health professionals, philosophers, ethicists, and economists. These changes included the removal of age weighting and discounting, estimation of new disability weights from population-representative surveys, and propagation of 95% uncertainty intervals around all burden estimates to improve transparency of the limitations and interpretation of the findings. Narrow bounds of uncertainty indicated that the evidence surrounding that estimate was strong, and wider bounds of uncertainty indicated that the evidence was weaker and estimates needed to be interpreted with caution. Finally, the study was much broader in scope, estimating burden for a significantly expanded list of causes, which featured 20 mental and substance use disorders [7]. These changes were first made in GBD 2010 and maintained throughout GBD 2013 and GBD 2015.

The mental and substance use disorders included in GBD 2015 are listed below. To allow for comparability in measurement, case definitions adhered to diagnostic criteria presented in the Diagnostic and Statistical Manual of Mental Disorders (DSM) and the International Classification of Diseases (ICD) [16, 17]:

- depressive disorders: major depressive disorder and dysthymia;
- anxiety disorders;
- bipolar disorder;
- schizophrenia;
- attention-deficit/hyperactivity disorder;
- conduct disorder;
- autism spectrum disorders: autism, and Asperger's syndrome and other autism spectrum disorders;
- eating disorders: anorexia nervosa and bulimia nervosa;
- alcohol use disorders: alcohol dependence and fetal alcohol syndrome;
- cannabis use disorders;
- amphetamine use disorders;
- cocaine use disorders;
- opioid use disorders;
- idiopathic developmental intellectual disability;
- residual groups of 'other mental disorders' and 'other drug use disorders'.

GBD 2015 included a complete epidemiological reassessment of each disorder. YLDs were derived from systematic reviews of the epidemiological literature designed to capture population-representative data on the prevalence, incidence, remission, and excess mortality associated with each disorder [18–31]. A Bayesian meta-regression modelling strategy [32], DisMod-MR 2.1, was used to pool all the available data into a consistent epidemiological disease model, and estimate prevalence by disorder, age, sex, year, and location [2]. This allowed the estimation of prevalence and corresponding uncertainty for all geographies, regardless of data availability. Population surveys in Bangladesh, Indonesia, Peru, Tanzania, the USA, Hungary, Italy, Sweden, and the Netherlands, and an open-access Internet survey available in English, Spanish, and Mandarin, were used to derive disability weights for a range of health states, which together reflected all contributors to non-fatal burden in GBD 2015. In each survey, participants were presented with multiple pairings of health state descriptions and asked which of the two they considered the healthiest. Responses were anchored on a scale of 0 (perfect health) to 1 (death) using some supplementary questions which compared the benefit of lifesaving and disease prevention programmes for a subgroup of health states [33, 34]. Given that individuals may experience multiple health conditions at the same time, burden estimates were corrected for comorbidity. Micro-simulation techniques were used whereby hypothetical populations were exposed to the independent probability of experiencing any disease sequelae featured in GBD 2015. A multiplicative function was used to estimate a combined disability weight for individuals experiencing two or more sequelae. The difference between the average disability weight in those experiencing one sequela and the multiplicatively combined disability weight in those experiencing more than one sequelae became the 'comorbidity correction' [2].

YLLs were estimated by multiplying cause-specific death estimates by the reference standard life expectancy at the age the death occurred. Life expectancy data were obtained from standard model life tables generated for GBD 2015. Cause-specific death estimates were obtained from a comprehensive search of verbal autopsies, vital registries, and other mortally surveillance systems in all countries. Within each of these databases, cause-of-death codes from the ICD cause of death directory were matched to a cause within the GBD 2015 cause list. Deaths assigned to unclear or inaccurate diagnoses were reassigned using standard algorithms. A selection of modelling strategies was used to estimate cause-specific deaths by country, age, sex, and year, the most common of which was cause of death ensemble modelling (CODEm) [4]. Deaths and YLLs were estimated for schizophrenia, alcohol use disorders, drug use disorders, and eating disorders [4]. Although there is strong evidence to suggest that many of the remaining mental disorders are associated with an increased risk of mortality, there were insufficient data to allocate of deaths to these causes and estimate YLLs [35]. This issue is discussed further in upcoming sections.

More comprehensive explanation of the method used to estimate burden for mental and substance use disorders has been presented in greater detail elsewhere [2–4, 15, 36, 37].

A summary of Global Burden of Disease Study 2015 findings for mental and substance use disorders

GBD 2015 estimated that mental and substance use disorders accounted for 162.4 million (95% uncertainty interval: 121.0–205.6 million) DALYs across the globe. As a group, they were the leading cause of YLDs worldwide and the sixth leading cause of DALYs in 2015 (see Table 4.1).

Fig. 4.2 shows proportion of DALYs, YLDs, and YLLs explained by each disorder within the mental and substance use disorder group, globally in 2015. Depressive disorders accounted for the largest proportion of burden and contributed 33.6% of the mental and substance use disorder DALYs (see Fig. 4.2a). Anxiety disorders accounted for the second largest proportion of mental and substance use disorder DALYs (15.2%), followed by drug use disorders (10.2%) and schizophrenia (9.5%).

Mental and substance use disorders were the leading disorder category for non-fatal disease burden in 2015, accounting for 150.0 million (108.7–193.1 million) YLDs globally. YLDs accounted for the majority of mental and substance use disorder DALYs

Table 4.1 Proportion of years lived with disability (YLDs), years of life lost (YLLs), and disability-adjusted life years (DALYs) explained by the ten leading causes of global burden in 2015

GBD cause group	% DALYs (95% UI)		% YLDs (95% UI)		% YLLs (95% UI)	
Cardiovascular diseases	14.1	(13.1–15.1)	3.2	(2.9–3.6)	19.2	(18.9–19.7)
Diarrhea, lower respiratory, and other common infectious diseases	9.9	(9.1–10.7)	1.9	(1.7–2.1)	13.6	(12.9–14.3)
Neoplasms	8.5	(7.8–9.2)	1.1	(1.0–1.2)	12.0	(11.8–12.2)
Neonatal disorders	8.0	(7.3–8.8)	1.4	(1.0–1.8)	11.2	(10.8–11.6)
Other non-communicable diseases	7.8	(6.5–9.5)	17.5	(14.6–21.3)	3.2	(2.9–3.5)
Mental and substance use disorders	6.6	(5.2–7.8)	19.0	(16.0–23.3)	0.7	(0.7–0.8)
Musculoskeletal disorders	6.0	(4.7–7.4)	18.5	(16.4–21.0)	0.1	(0.1–0.1)
Diabetes, urogenital, blood, and endocrine diseases	5.9	(5.5–6.4)	8.3	(7.5–9.0)	4.8	(4.6–5.1)
Unintentional injuries	4.4	(4.0–4.6)	3.9	(3.5–4.2)	4.6	(4.1–4.9)
HIV/AIDS and tuberculosis	4.3	(3.9–4.8)	0.8	(0.7–1.0)	6.0	(5.6–6.6)

Note: Each proportion presented as a percentage of total global DALYs, YLDs, and YLLs. GBD: Global Burden of Disease Study; UI: 95% uncertainty interval.
Source: Data from Global Burden of Disease Study 2015.

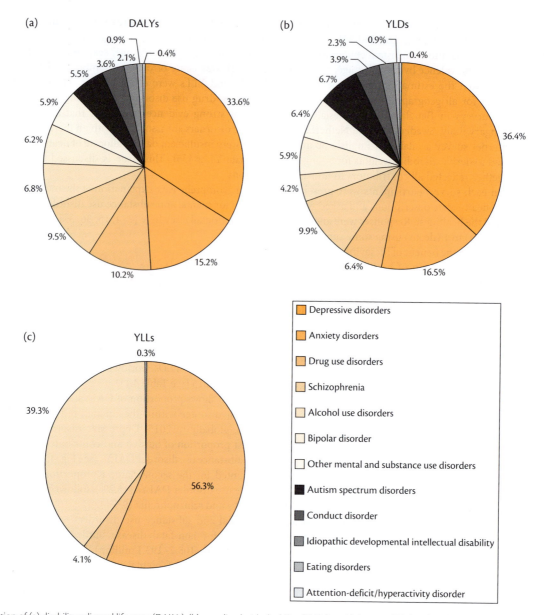

Fig. 4.2 Proportion of (a) disability-adjusted life years (DALYs), (b) years lived with disability (YLDs), and (c) years of life lost (YLLs) explained by each mental and substance use disorder, globally in 2015.

Source: Reproduced from Institute for Health Metrics and Evaluation (IHME), GBD Compare, Copyright (2015), with permission from University of Washington. Available from http://vizhub. healthdata.org/gbd-compare

(92.3%), and so the distribution of mental and substance use disorder YLDs largely mirrored that of DALYs (Fig. 4.2b). Depressive disorders accounted for the largest proportion of mental and substance use disorder YLDs (36.4%) followed by anxiety disorders (16.5%), schizophrenia (9.9%), and drug use disorders (6.4%). Mental and substance use disorders accounted for comparatively fewer global YLLs (12.5 million and 11.8–13.1 million, respectively). The vast majority of this fatal burden was attributed to drug use disorders (56.3%) and alcohol use disorders (39.3%) (Fig. 4.2c).

Overall, 85.1 million (64.4–106.1 million; 52.4%) DALYs globally were attributed to mental and substance use disorder in males and 77.3 million (57.1–99.1 million; 47.6%) in females. Males accounted for slightly more YLDs than females, with 75.4 million YLDs (54.9–96.2 million; 50.2%) attributed to mental and substance use

disorders in males versus 74.6 million YLDs (54.6–96.4 million; 49.8%) in females. Fatal burden differed to a greater extent between the sexes. Males accounted for 9.8 million (9.2–10.3 million; 78.5%) YLLs, whereas females accounted for 2.7 million (2.5–2.8 million; 21.5%) YLLs attributable to mental and substance use disorders.

Fig. 4.3 illustrates the pattern of absolute DALYs attributed to mental and substance use disorders across sex and age. Under the age of 15 years, males accounted for a greater proportion of DALYs than females. This is due to the greater amount of burden attributable to conduct disorder and autism spectrum disorders in this age group, which were more prevalent in males. This difference between males and females decreased from 15 years onwards, and the burden of mental and substance use disorders was higher for females than for males from 50 years of age onwards. This is due to

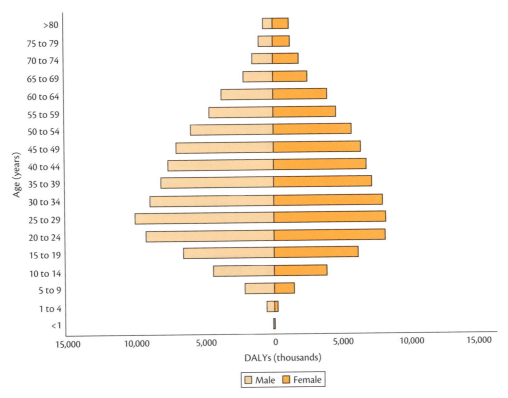

Fig. 4.3 Absolute disability-adjusted life years (DALYs) for all mental and substance use disorders in 2015 by age and sex.
Source: Reproduced from Institute for Health Metrics and Evaluation (IHME), GBD Compare, Copyright (2015), with permission from University of Washington. Available from http://vizhub. healthdata.org/gbd-compare

the increased burden of depressive disorders and anxiety disorders in adulthood, which were more prevalent in females.

Fig. 4.4 illustrates the global variation in age-standardized DALY rates per 100,000 in 2015, grouped by tenth percentiles. The global age-standardized DALY rate was 2183.3 per 100,000 (1627.1– 2766.3 per 100,000). No countries varied significantly from the global mean, with the exception of Russia, which had the highest rate of mental and substance use disorder DALYs (3437.4 DALYs per 100,000 and 2772.3–4134.9 per 100,000, respectively). This was largely due to the high burden attributable to alcohol use disorders and opioid use disorders.

Limitations in the burden estimation process for mental and substance use disorders

The interpretation and application of GBD findings require an understanding of the strengths and limitations of the burden estimation methodology. GBD methodology requires epidemiological data in order to estimate YLDs and, subsequently, DALYs. However, the available data for mental and substance use disorders are limited with some geographies and age groups having no data for any mental or substance use disorder whatsoever [38, 39]. Compared with prevalence, data for incidence, remission, and excess mortality are even more limited with only a handful of studies available for the majority of mental and substance use disorders. This lack of data means that a greater onus is placed on the statistical modelling techniques used to impute missing data [32]. Given that

the aim of GBD is to compare disease burden between countries, the imputation of missing data is considered preferable to the alternative, which is to completely exclude countries or age groups with no available raw data, thus assuming zero prevalence of mental and substance use disorders in these groups or locations. The lack of data is reflected in the large bounds of 95% uncertainty intervals accompanying the majority of mental and substance use disorder burden estimates. Large uncertainty intervals make it difficult to interpret differences in burden between countries and, importantly, track trends in burden over time which would be expected from changes in mental health treatment coverage or intervention effectiveness.

Within the available data, the definition of mental and substance use disorders themselves can prove problematic. To be included in GBD, studies reporting mental and substance use disorder epidemiology must define disorders according to DSM or ICD diagnostic criteria. This restriction ensures that disorders are consistently defined between studies and that burden reflects clinically significant presentations of disorders rather than psychological distress. Nonetheless, it can lead to fewer data being included in GBD analyses given that many epidemiological studies make use of instruments which measure symptoms of mental disorders (i.e. symptom scales) rather than diagnoses. Symptom scales typically overestimate the prevalence of disorders and can only be included in GBD analyses when there is sufficient data to generate a cross-walk from the symptom scale data to the level required to meet a diagnostic threshold. There is also debate as to whether the diagnostic criteria specified by DSM and ICD adequately reflect

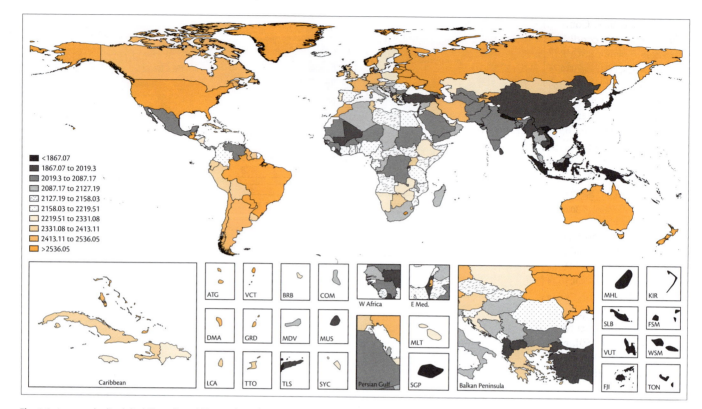

Fig. 4.4 Age-standardized disability-adjusted life year (DALY) rates per 100,000 individuals for mental and substance use disorders, 2015.
Note: DALY rates per 100,000 grouped by tenth percentiles.
Source: Reproduced from Institute for Health Metrics and Evaluation (IHME), GBD Compare, Copyright (2015), with permission from University of Washington. Available from http://vizhub.healthdata.org/gbd-compare

differences in disorder presentations across cultures. For example, certain cultures are more likely to describe the somatic symptoms of anxiety and depressive disorders, which may not be as easily detected by survey instruments using DSM and ICD criteria [40]. This could lead to an underestimate of mental and substance use disorders in certain cultures. While the inclusion criteria applied to all studies used in burden estimation helps ensure mental and substance use disorders are consistently defined in GBD, issues with definition and presentation across cultures must be considered when interpreting results.

As well as issues relating to data availability and case definition, a significant limitation of GBD 2015 was the lack of representation of the increased risk of mortality due to mental and substance use disorders in the YLL estimation process. As per GBD methodology, the cause of death data used for calculating YLLs followed ICD coding guidelines and only accounted for the direct cause of death as recorded in the various data sources [4]. This meant that most deaths in individuals with mental disorders were attributed to the direct physical cause of death, rather than the underlying mental disorder that may have led to the physical cause [37]. For instance, the GBD classification system places suicide in the injuries cause group. Supplementary analyses of GBD 2010 results demonstrated that the inclusion of attributable suicide DALYs would have increased the overall burden of mental and substance use disorders from 7.4% to 8.3% of global DALYs and increased their ranking from the fifth to the third leading cause of DALYs in 2010 [41]. Given the recognized link between mental and substance use

disorders and decreased life expectancy [42, 43], YLL estimates cannot be used as the only source of information for mortality in mental and substance use disorders.

More general limitations in GBD methodology must also be considered when interpreting the burden of mental and substance use disorders. GBD defines disability as 'within-the-skin' health loss encountered by the individual. Any non-health loss, future health or non-health loss, or impact on caregivers is not represented in the burden estimations. This is problematic for mental and substance use disorders, which tend to have their onset during the first quarter of life [44]. For example, a child with attention-deficit/hyperactivity disorder experiences not only the current 'within-the-skin' health loss measured by GBD, but is also likely to experience lower levels of academic achievement and economic success than their peers both during childhood and into adulthood [45]. Furthermore, their disorder inevitably impacts their parents and caregivers. As such, the burden measured by GBD only represents one component of the true impact of a disorder.

Related to the issue of the definition of disability is the methodology for estimating disability weights. In GBD 1990, disability weights were based on the judgement of health professionals with the assumption that their clinical knowledge would allow them to make accurate comparative judgements. From GBD 2010 onwards, disability weights were derived from surveys administered to the general population [34, 46]. Short, non-clinical descriptions were used to describe the health states and the name of the disorder in question was not included for the majority of mental disorders in order to avoid bias. Concerns were raised over the low disability weights for certain conditions considered very severe by clinicians, for example profound intellectual disability, and the wording of particular descriptions, for example the term 'violent' in the description for conduct disorder may have led participants to rate the disorder as more severe [18]. The extent to which the health loss and severity of different disorders was accurately communicated and the comprehension of the lay participants is unclear and disability weights remain an area for further exploration and improvement in the future.

Accessing GBD data for mental and substance use disorders

IHME, the institution that leads GBD, has created a suite of interactive visualization to allow researchers, policymakers, the public, and other interested parties to freely access GBD estimates [47]. All epidemiological data sources and outputs used in the estimation of YLDs and YLLs for GBD 2015 can be accessed via the Global Health Data Exchange, IHME's database of health and demographic data [48]. Other tools, such as 'GBD Compare' [49] and the 'GBD Results Tool' [50], enable users to view estimates of deaths, YLDs, YLLs, and DALYs and make comparisons by cause, location, age, sex, and year. The data can also be exported for further use.

Applications of burden estimates for mental and substance use disorders

A key challenge for researchers is to bridge the gap between psychiatric epidemiology and services by using epidemiological research to inform mental health planning and policy. As discussed earlier in this chapter, core burden of disease metrics facilitate the direct comparison of health loss across disease categories, geographies, sex, and age. However, GBD also produces modelled estimates of prevalence, incidence, remission, and excess mortality, which have a greater potential for practical application beyond being inputs for burden of disease estimation.

Modelled epidemiological estimates have been applied (generally as data inputs) in work conducted by the WHO and others. Examples include assessments of mental health workforce gaps [51] and development of models for scaling-up recommended packages of care for priority mental and substance use disorders [52], as well as cost-effectiveness analyses of mental health intervention packages [53–55]. Here, we provide examples of ways in which epidemiological estimates of mental and substance use disorders can inform the targeted scale-up and optimization of mental health services.

Projections

Each iteration of GBD (GBD 2010, GBD 2013, GBD 2015, and further iterations) provides us with revised epidemiological and burden estimates for earlier years, from 1990 onwards. Arguably though, it is the ability to use the data to estimate future burden of disease that is most useful in guiding mental health service planning, particularly in regions of the world where rapid epidemiological transitions are taking place (e.g. Sub-Saharan Africa) [56]. Creating projections of burden estimates is a complex task and involves many assumptions including projected trends in disease epidemiology (e.g. prevalence and mortality), as well as

demographic shifts in the population. For many of the mental disorders however, the assumptions underlying burden of disease estimate projection are simplified by the epidemiology of these disorders. Firstly, outputs from GBD have demonstrated that the prevalence rates of most mental disorders are relatively stable over time. Secondly, only three mental disorders included in GBD currently have a fatal burden component (YLLs). This simplifies being able to make projections for prevalence and mortality and, consequently, burden of disease estimates. Those mental disorders without a fatal component in GBD can be projected by combining existing prevalence rates and disability weights with projected population data. This method has been demonstrated in published work pertaining to the Pacific Islands and Sub-Saharan Africa [56, 57].

Service requirements

The incorporation of age- and sex-specific epidemiological estimates into health economic models, such as the WHO's mhGAP tool [55], demonstrates how epidemiological estimates can be used to estimate and plan for the development of mental health services, such as inpatient beds and workforce, in low- and middle-income countries. By drawing upon disorder-specific packages of care, target treatment coverage rates, and other context-specific parameters, mental health service requirements can be estimated to reflect a scaled-up delivery of services over time. An application of this approach detailing the implications for a scale-up of mental health services has been undertaken for post-conflict Syria [58], presenting estimated service contacts and workforce requirements (full-time equivalent) for selected disorders.

Cost-effectiveness models

Of particular interest from a policy perspective is the economic modelling of the potential health benefits of implementing and scaling-up cost-effective interventions [59, 60]. Health benefit analysis incorporates epidemiological estimates of prevalence, incidence, remission, and excess mortality (which reflect transitions between health states [healthy, diseased, and dead]) to estimate the disease burden avertable by selected intervention packages with known efficacy applied at nominated target coverage rate scenarios (e.g. no treatment and 50% treatment coverage). An example of the methodology employing a multiple cohort Markov model to model the disease dynamics of several multi-age cohorts in a given population has been published [58, 61].

Treatment gaps

In recent years, there have been signs of renewed global commitment to reduce the ubiquitous burden caused by mental and substance disorders. However, health information systems in many countries are not equipped to regularly collect information pertaining to key mental health indicators (e.g. treatment coverage) from which progress can be measured. Population-representative treatment rates for mental and substance use disorders captured in epidemiological surveys can be combined with GBD estimates of prevalence to calculate treated prevalence and treatment gaps, i.e. the difference between the total number of prevalent cases and the number in contact with services. Importantly, treatment gaps are affected not only by the unavailability of services, but also by other factors such as stigma faced by those with mental and substance use disorders. Treatment coverage has been identified as a key indicator for progress in mental health and towards universal health coverage in the 2030 Agenda for Sustainable Development [62, 63].

Burden of disease re-estimation

An important caveat when working with epidemiological estimates, such as those derived from GBD, is to acknowledge that these estimates reflect health loss at the country or regional level (unless otherwise specified). As such, subpopulations within a country that may experience rates different from the overall population (e.g. refugees) are not well represented by national GBD estimates. Subsequently, applying GBD data using methods outlined above is unlikely to represent the reality or needs of subpopulations. GBD methodology can be used with subpopulation prevalence estimates to re-estimate burden of disease to more accurately reflect health loss attributable to mental and substance use disorders in specific populations. For example, the epidemiology of mental disorders in populations exposed to armed conflict is known to differ from that of non-exposed populations and a re-estimation of burden estimates has been previously conducted [58].

Conclusion

GBD has made a valuable contribution to the global health field, given its ability to capture both fatal and non-fatal burden and compare this burden across location, age, sex, and time. The findings from GBD have aided in our understanding of the relative contribution of mental and substance use disorders to loss of health across the globe. A concerted effort is needed to scale-up health systems, especially in low- and middle-income countries, to address this burden by implementing evidence-based, cost-effective interventions [64]. The wealth of data generated by GBD can assist in this effort while also providing the foundation for the development of better prevention and treatment strategies.

References

1. World Bank. *World Development Report 1993: Investing in Health.* Washington, DC: Oxford University Press, 1993.
2. Vos T, Allen C, Arora M, et al. Global, regional, and national incidence, prevalence, and years lived with disability for 310 diseases and injuries, 1990–2015: a systematic analysis for the Global Burden of Disease Study 2015. *Lancet* 2016; 388: 1545–602.
3. Kassebaum NJ, Arora M, Barber RM, et al. Global, regional, and national disability-adjusted life-years (DALYs) for 315 diseases and injuries and healthy life expectancy (HALE), 1990–2015: a systematic analysis for the Global Burden of Disease Study 2015. *Lancet* 2016; 388: 1603–58.
4. Wang H, Naghavi M, Allen C, et al. Global, regional, and national life expectancy, all-cause mortality, and cause-specific mortality for 249 causes of death, 1980–2015: a systematic analysis for the Global Burden of Disease Study 2015. *Lancet* 2016; 388: 1459–544.
5. Murray CJL, Lopez AD (eds). *The Global Burden of Disease: A Comprehensive Assessment of Mortality and Disability From Diseases, Injuries, and Risk Factors in 1990 and Projected to 2020.* Cambridge, MA: Harvard University Press, 1996.
6. Prince M, Patel V, Saxena S, et al. No health without mental health. *Lancet* 2007; 370: 859–77.
7. Baxter AJ, Ferrari AJ, Erskine HE, Charlson FJ, Degenhardt L, Whiteford HA. The global burden of mental and substance use disorders: changes in estimating burden between GBD1990 and GBD2010. *Epidemiol Psychiatr Sci* 2014; 23: 239–49.
8. United Nations (UN). *World Population Prospects—The 2010 Revision.* New York: UN, 2011.
9. World Health Organization (WHO). *The Global Burden of Disease: 2004 Update.* Geneva: WHO, 2008.
10. World Health Organization (WHO). *WHO Methods and Data Sources for Global Burden of Disease Estimates 2000–2011. Global Health Estimates Technical Paper WHO/HIS/HSI/GHE/2013.4.* Geneva: Department of Health Statistics and Information Systems, WHO, 2013.
11. Murray CJL, Vos T, Lozano R, et al. Disability-adjusted life years (DALYs) for 291 diseases and injuries in 21 regions, 1990–2010: a systematic analysis for the Global Burden of Disease Study 2010. *Lancet* 2012; 380: 2197–223.
12. GBD 2013 DALYs and HALE Collaborators. Global, regional, and national disability-adjusted life years (DALYs) for 306 diseases and injuries and healthy life expectancy (HALE) for 188 countries, 1990–2013: quantifying the epidemiological transition. *Lancet* 2015; 386: 2145–91.
13. GBD 2013 Mortality and Causes of Death Collaborators. Global, regional, and national age–sex specific all-cause and cause-specific mortality for 240 causes of death, 1990–2013: a systematic analysis for the Global Burden of Disease Study 2013. *Lancet* 2015; 385: 117–71.
14. GBD 2013 Risk Factors Collaborators. Global, regional, and national comparative risk assessment of 79 behavioural, environmental and occupational, and metabolic risks or clusters of risks in 188 countries, 1990–2013: a systematic analysis for the Global Burden of Disease Study 2013. *Lancet* 2015; 386: 2287–323.
15. Forouzanfar MH, Afshin A, Alexander LT, et al. Global, regional, and national comparative risk assessment of 79 behavioural, environmental and occupational, and metabolic risks or clusters of risks, 1990–2015: a systematic analysis for the Global Burden of Disease Study 2015. *Lancet* 2016; 388: 1659–724.
16. American Psychiatric Association (APA). *Diagnostic and Statistical Manual of Mental Disorders (DSM-IV-TR).* 4th ed., text revision ed. Washington, DC: APA, 2000.
17. World Health Organization (WHO). *The ICD-10 Classification of Mental and Behavioural Disorders. Clinical Descriptions and Diagnostic Guidelines.* Geneva: WHO, 1992.
18. Erskine HE, Ferrari AJ, Polanczyk GV, et al. The global burden of conduct disorder and attention-deficit/hyperactivity disorder in 2010. *J Child Psychol Psychiatry* 2014; 55: 328–36.
19. Ferrari AJ, Baxter AJ, Whiteford HA. A systematic review of the global distribution and availability of prevalence data for bipolar disorder. *J Affect Disord* 2011; 134: 1–13.
20. Baxter AJ, Scott KM, Vos T, Whiteford HA. Global prevalence of anxiety disorders: a systematic review and meta-regression. *Psychol Med* 2013; 43: 897–910.
21. Charlson FJ, Ferrari AJ, Flaxman AD, Whiteford HA. The epidemiological modelling of dysthymia: application for the Global Burden of Disease Study 2010. *J Affect Disord* 2013; 151: 111–20.
22. Degenhardt L, Ferrari AJ, Calabria B, et al. The global epidemiology and contribution of cannabis use and dependence to the global burden of disease: results from the GBD 2010 study. *PLOS ONE* 2013; 8: e76635.
23. Erskine HE, Ferrari AJ, Nelson P, et al. Epidemiological modelling of attention-deficit/hyperactivity disorder and conduct disorder for the Global Burden of Disease Study 2010. *J Child Psychol Psychiatry* 2013; 54: 1263–74.
24. Ferrari AJ, Charlson FJ, Norman RE, et al. Burden of depressive disorders by country, sex, age, and year: findings from the Global Burden of Disease Study 2010. *PLOS Med* 2013; 10: e1001547.
25. Ferrari AJ, Somerville AJ, Baxter AJ, et al. Global variation in the prevalence and incidence of major depressive disorder: a systematic review of the epidemiological literature. *Psychol Med* 2013; 43: 471–81.
26. Baxter AJ, Vos T, Scott KM, Ferrari AJ, Whiteford HA. The global burden of anxiety disorders in 2010. *Psychol Med* 2014; 44: 2363–74.

27. Degenhardt L, Baxter AJ, Lee YY, et al. The global epidemiology and burden of psychostimulant dependence: findings from the Global Burden of Disease Study 2010. *Drug Alcohol Depend* 2014; 137: 36–47.

28. Degenhardt L, Charlson F, Mathers B, et al. The global epidemiology and burden of opioid dependence: results from the global burden of disease 2010 study. *Addiction* 2014; 109: 1320–33.

29. Baxter AJ, Brugha TS, Erskine HE, Scheurer RW, Vos T, Scott JG. The epidemiology and global burden of autism spectrum disorders. *Psychol Med* 2015; 45: 601–13.

30. Charlson FJ, Baxter AJ, Dua T, Degenhardt L, Whiteford HA, Vos T. Excess mortality from mental, neurological and substance use disorders in the Global Burden of Disease Study 2010. *Epidemiol Psychiatr Sci* 2015; 24: 121–40.

31. Degenhardt L, Bucello C, Calabria B, et al. What data are available on the extent of illicit drug use and dependence globally? Results of four systematic reviews. *Drug Alcohol Depend* 2011; 117: 85–101.

32. Flaxman AD, Vos T, Murray CJL (eds). *An Integrative Metaregression Framework For Descriptive Epidemiology*. Washington, DC: University of Washington Press, 2015.

33. Haagsma JA, Noordhout C, Polinder S, et al. Assessing disability weights based on the responses of 30,660 people from four European countries. *Popul Health Metr* 2015; 13: 10.

34. Salomon JA, Haagsma JA, Davis A, et al. Disability weights for the Global Burden of Disease 2013 study. *Lancet Glob Health* 2015; 3: e712–23.

35. Charlson FJ, Baxter AJ, Dua T, Degenhardt L, Whiteford HA, Vos T. Excess mortality from mental, neurological and substance use disorders in the Global Burden of Disease Study 2010. *Epidemiol Psychiatr Sci* 2015; 24: 121–40.

36. Degenhardt L, Whiteford HA, Ferrari AJ, et al. Global burden of disease attributable to illicit drug use and dependence: findings from the Global Burden of Disease Study 2010. *Lancet* 2013; 382: 1564–74.

37. Whiteford HA, Degenhardt L, Rehm J, et al. Global burden of disease attributable to mental and substance use disorders: findings from the Global Burden of Disease Study 2010. *Lancet* 2013; 382: 1575–86.

38. Baxter AJ, Patton G, Scott KM, Degenhardt L, Whiteford HA. Global epidemiology of mental disorders: what are we missing? *PLOS ONE* 2013; 8: e65514.

39. Erskine HE, Baxter AJ, Patton G, et al. The global coverage of prevalence data for mental disorders in children and adolescents. *Epidemiol Psychiatr Sci* 2017; 26: 395–402.

40. Kirmayer LJ. Cultural variations in the clinical presentation of depression and anxiety: implications for diagnosis and treatment. *J Clin Psychiatry* 2001; 62(Suppl. 13): 22–8.

41. Ferrari AJ, Norman RE, Freedman G, et al. The burden attributable to mental and substance use disorders as risk factors for suicide: findings from the Global Burden of Disease Study 2010. *PLOS ONE* 2014; 9: e91936.

42. Chang C-K, Hayes RD, Perera G, et al. Life expectancy at birth for people with serious mental illness and other major disorders from a secondary mental health care case register in London. *PLOS ONE* 2011; 6: e19590.

43. Wahlbeck K, Westman J, Nordentoft M, Gissler M, Laursen TM. Outcomes of Nordic mental health systems: life expectancy of patients with mental disorders. *Br J Psychiatry* 2011; 199: 453–8.

44. Erskine HE, Moffitt TE, Copeland WE, et al. A heavy burden on young minds: the global burden of mental and substance use disorders in children and youth. *Psychol Medicine* 2015; 45: 1551–63.

45. Erskine HE, Norman RE, Ferrari AJ, et al. Long-term outcomes of attention-deficit/hyperactivity disorder and conduct disorder: a systematic review and meta-analysis. *J Am Acad Child Adolesc Psychiatry* 2016; 55: 841–50.

46. Salomon JA, Vos T, Hogan DR, et al. Common values in assessing health outcomes from disease and injury: disability weights measurement study for the Global Burden of Disease Study 2010. *Lancet* 2012; 380: 2129–43.

47. Institute for Health Metrics and Evaluation. GBD Data Visualizations. Available at: http://www.healthdata.org/gbd/data-visualizations (2016, accessed 8 February 2018).

48. Institute for Health Metrics and Evaluation (IHME). *Global Health Data Exchange.* Seattle, WA: IHME, 2016.

49. Institute for Health Metrics and Evaluation. GBD Compare. Available at: http://www.healthdata.org/data-visualization/gbd-compare (2016, accessed 8 February 2018).

50. Institute for Health Metrics and Evaluation. GBD Results Tool. Available at: http://ghdx.healthdata.org/gbd-results-tool (2016, accessed 8 February 2018).

51. Bruckner TA, Scheffler RM, Shen G, et al. The mental health workforce gap in low-and middle-income countries: a needs-based approach. *Bull World Health Organ* 2011; 89: 184–94.

52. Patel V, Thornicroft G. Packages of care for mental, neurological, and substance use disorders in low-and middle-income countries: *PLOS Med* 2009; 6: e1000160.

53. Chisholm D, Lund C, Saxena S. Cost of scaling up mental healthcare in low- and middle-income countries. *Br J Psychiatry* 2007; 191: 528–35.

54. Chisholm D, Saxena S. Cost effectiveness of strategies to combat neuropsychiatric conditions in sub-Saharan Africa and South East Asia: mathematical modelling study. *BMJ* 2012; 344: e609.

55. Chisholm D, Burman-Roy S, Fekadu A, et al. Estimating the cost of implementing district mental healthcare plans in five low- and middle-income countries: the PRIME study. *Br J Psychiatry* 2016; 208(Suppl. 56): s71–8.

56. Charlson FJ, Diminic S, Lund C, Degenhardt L, Whiteford HA. Mental and substance use disorders in Sub-Saharan Africa: predictions of epidemiological changes and mental health workforce requirements for the next 40 years. *PLOS ONE* 2014; 9: e110208.

57. Charlson FJ, Diminic S, Whiteford HA. The rising tide of mental disorders in the Pacific region: forecasts of disease burden and service requirements from 2010 to 2050. *Asia Pacific Policy Stud* 2015; 2: 280–92.

58. Charlson FJ, Lee YY, Diminic S, Whiteford H. Applications of the epidemiological modelling outputs for targeted mental health planning in conflict-affected populations: the Syria case-study. *Glob Ment Health (Camb)* 2016; 3: e8.

59. Chisholm D, Lund C, Saxena S. Cost of scaling up mental healthcare in low- and middle-income countries. *Br J Psychiatry* 2007; 191: 528–35.

60. Chisholm D, Burman-Roy S, Fekadu A, et al. Estimating the cost of implementing district mental healthcare plans in five low-and middle-income countries: the PRIME study. *Br J Psychiatry* 2016; 208(s56): s71–8.

61. Habbema JDF, Boer R, Barendregt JJ. Chronic disease modelling. In: Killewo J, Heggenhougen HK, Quah SR (eds). *Epidemiology and Demography in Public Health.* San Diego, CA: Academic Press, 2010, pp. 173–8.

62. World Health Organization (WHO). *Mental Health and Substance Use. Health in 2015: From MDGs, Millennium Development Goals to SDGs, Sustainable Development Goals.* Geneva: WHO, 2015.

63. United Nations. Sustainable Development Goals. Available at: http://www.un.org/sustainabledevelopment/sustainable-development-goals/ (2016, accessed 8 February 2018).

64. Patel V, Chisholm D, Parikh R, et al. Addressing the burden of mental, neurological, and substance use disorders: key messages from Disease Control Priorities, 3rd edition. *Lancet* 2016; 387: 1672–85.

CHAPTER 5

Models of causation of mental illness

Kwame McKenzie

Introduction

Psychiatry has found it more difficult than other areas of medicine to identify the causes of illnesses. This may reflect the way that mental illnesses are diagnosed, our ability to understand the human brain and the mind, as well as turf battles between researchers arguing about whether biological or social factors are more important.

Psychiatry is making significant progress on all of these fronts. We are in an exciting time. From an aetiological perspective, many of the elements are in place that could revolutionize the way we think about mental illness and our ability to treat and prevent it.

The research is being undertaken by different groups around the world. It has rarely been collated. Pulling these disparate strands together in one place could help us to see new possibilities.

Our understanding of the causation of the most severe mental illnesses—schizophrenia and the other psychoses—has increased. Our understanding of the biological mechanisms that link individual and societal risk to actual psychosis are clearer than ever. Despite this, we have not had as much traction as we could in public health. It may be that the development of a more focused way to present complex theory could help to improve our ability to move from theory to change.

Diagnosing mental illness

Understanding how mental illnesses are diagnosed is important if we are to understand their aetiology. A useful starting point for investigating the cause of an illness is being clear how we know who has the illness. Diagnosis of mental health problems is strategic and political. In physical health all countries use the same World Health Organization (WHO) diagnoses, but in mental health the USA and China continue to use and refine their own systems.

There are three dominant systems of diagnosis used worldwide:

◆ the International Classification of Diseases (ICD), published by the WHO [1];

◆ the Diagnostic and Statistical Manual of Mental Disorders (DSM), published by the American Psychiatric Association [2];

◆ since the late 1970s China has developed its own diagnostic system [3].

There are many critiques of psychiatric diagnoses, but the central difficulty is that diagnoses are based on a system of description of symptoms, chronology, and epidemiology. There are no physical tests to support them. Psychiatric diagnoses are groups of symptoms that are linked together by statistical associations clinical experience and theory.

Unlike physical illnesses, where there is often general agreement, the three mental illness manuals have significant differences and they change over time.

A further issue is that because diagnoses are based on symptoms rather than clear physical pathology, each symptom cluster could contain a number of different illnesses with different causes. Using an example from physical medicine to illustrate the problem this causes; a common symptom like a headache may be caused by many different illnesses from muscle tension through vascular issues and even intracranial hemorrhage and tumors. Each of these problems has a different cause. Of course, there are clinical histories and particular symptoms that we know are characteristic of specific illnesses. But we tend to have confirmed this through laboratory tests and autopsies. The problem for psychiatry is that in the absence of clear biological substrates it is difficult to know which symptoms signify a group of problems and which are pathognomic.

The fact that diagnoses are linked to context and social norms could also offer challenges to the identification of causation [4]. The same set of symptoms in one jurisdiction may be considered an illness and in another jurisdiction it may not. However, as science has started to demonstrate the important of the environment in both the development of the brain and the way that problems are expressed, it increasingly seems that it is impossible to ignore context and social norms and these are likely to continue to be of relevance to making a diagnosis.

It would seem vital to keep in mind that mental illnesses tend to be syndromes (collections of symptoms) rather than illnesses. Because of this they may have multiple causes.

Theories of aetiology

The history of theories of aetiology of mental illness are reflected in the way we make diagnoses. We have moved from psychodynamic theories, through theories based on place and more recently to more biological theories. When I started in psychiatry 25 years ago there was a clear schism between those who consider mental health problems to be neurological diseases and those who think of them as sociological. These lines of demarcation remain for many. I will outline how we got to this dichotomy and how new ways of thinking will lead us out of it. To understand the problem, one has to understand theories of causation, in general, and then causation in mental illness, specifically.

A brief history of causation

Theories of causation have changed over time. Prior to the current theories of modern medicine the cause of disease was attributed to spiritual or environmental causes. Illnesses were thought to be due to the elements, humours, or miasma (bad air arising out of dirt and decaying organic matter) [5].

The theories that evolved into early public health medicine in high-income countries were built on these theories. Initial theories of causation were place-based. Poor areas, rather than people being poor, were considered to be the cause of many illnesses. Increased rates of illness were because of where you lived rather than who you were. In this way, early public health was environmental and ecological. It focused on urban areas and aimed to improve and sanitize the slums.

The ideas led to an improvement in living standards and life expectancy, which is unparalleled. The theories were not based on a sound understanding of what exactly was causing illness, but, nevertheless, they had a profound impact on our lives. They helped to ensure that there was clean water, sewage systems, safe food, and improved living conditions. The sanitary movement had a more profound impact on life expectancy than many subsequent health interventions [5].

Early public health theories were changed by the discovery of viruses and bacteria but this was linked to efforts to refine place based solutions to health. Based on current theories of the importance of place. John Snow, considered the father of modern epidemiology, was trying to map the cholera outbreak in Soho, London, England [6]. He found a small group of people who were outliers—they lived in Hampstead, North London, six miles from where most other cases of cholera were. He discovered that these North Londoners liked the taste of the water from Soho and so got it brought to them. He was then able to identify a specific water pump in Soho that they sent their staff to—it was at the epicentre of the outbreak. Removal of the handle of the Broad Street pump not only stopped the outbreak and saved lives, it also led to increased momentum for scientists trying to identify what was in substances such as water that made people sick.

The discovery of infectious agents has been one of the triumphs of medical science. However, germ theory, based on the discovery of viruses and bacteria, in some ways initially led to a simplification of theories of causation.

The intense study of germs moved the focus of the investigation of causation out of the field and the environment and into the laboratory. In some ways, initially more disconnected theories of causation based on laboratory findings were developed.

Over time it became clear that mono-causal germ theory had its problems. Some of the most profound were the fact that exposure did not always lead to illness. Exposure to a particular germ was necessary for a particular illness, but it was not always sufficient. Because of this, other factors needed to be taken into consideration. In addition, exposure depended on how you lived and where you lived.

The epidemiological triangle approach built on germ theory [7]. It asserted that disease was a product of an interaction between the agent (the germ), the host (the person), and the environment. The host and the environment determined both the levels of

exposure and or susceptibility to the actions of the particular germ. If you wanted to understand the aetiology of a specific illness, you needed to understand the germ, the environment, and the person. Laboratory-based investigation was important but so was the study of the environment.

With the introduction of penicillin and immunization, the importance of infections in high-income countries started to diminish. In their place, chronic diseases started to be seen as more significant public health issues. The epidemiological triangle is useful for infections, but its utility diminishes when trying to produce aetiological theories for chronic diseases, such as diabetes or schizophrenia, or degenerative disease. This is, in part, because these illnesses are characterized by the lack of a single specific agent.

A different approach is often used. The web-of-causation theory argues that for many chronic illnesses there is no specific agent. There are many different exposures, over time, which produce complex interactions of many factors. These different risks and exposures form interlocking events. Essentially, a person has a number of exposures (or agents) and each has a context (environment). Each person, exposure, and context triad forms an epidemiological triangle. For chronic diseases there are multiple exposures that are part of the creation of a disease process. Each of these exposures forms an epidemiological triangle. Each of these triangles link to another to form the web of causation for a particular disease [5].

It is rare, in chronic diseases, that any particular exposure by itself leads directly to an illness. Generally, exposures change the risk of developing an illness and change the risk of exposure to other risk factors. Increased risk can not only be directly linked to a particular exposure, but can also be indirect through the impact that one epidemiological triangle has on others in the web of causation. Just like a spider's web, if you move one corner you have an impact on the integrity of the whole.

Germ theory, the epidemiological triangle, and the web of causation have changed the focus from the solely ecological (area) towards the individual (whether it is their vulnerability, or their exposure to a germ or a risk factor) and the environment (what in a particular area makes people sick).

An important development on the journey towards the understanding of causations has been an appreciation that the agent in chronic disease can be a behaviour or a lifestyle choice rather than an external agent such as a bacteria. Because of this, the risk of an illness is linked very closely to how a person lives and who they are. The environment is included, but the environment is often linked to the individual.

This has led to theories of causation based mainly at the individual level and subsequently there has been a reaction to this because individual approaches by themselves may not do justice to the importance of context in the development of illness. A number of alternate approaches to considering causation have emerged. One group contains the general theories of susceptibility. These do not identify single or multiple risk factors associated with specific disorders but seek to understand why some social groups are more at risk than others. The assertion is that because some groups are at generally greater risk to multiple disorders there needs to be a theory to explain this at a group level rather than at an individual level. The question that these theories try to answer is: is there something about what is happening to the group or at the group level that could be causing differences in rates of illness and therefore differences in risk of illness for an individual?

The theory of fundamental social causes is a good example of a general theory of susceptibility. It neatly links the various theories of disease aetiology together and comes full circle to re-invigorate ecological perspectives [8].

The example of health disparities is an accessible way of introducing and considering the fundamental social causes theory.

In high-income countries, 100 years ago, disparities in life expectancy between rich and poor were mainly because of infectious diseases. Put simply, the poor lived in situations such as the rat-infested, overcrowded slums of cities where they were more likely to be exposed to and to contract infectious diseases. In addition, they were less likely to get effective treatment.

The impact of infectious diseases, and the disparities in life expectancy because of them, have been decreased with the advent of modern sewage systems, clean water, vaccination, and the development of antibiotics. However, disparities such as the difference in morbidity and mortality between rich and poor with in high-income countries have remained.

Instead of differences in lifespan and rates of illness being due to infectious diseases, they are now linked to chronic diseases such as diabetes, high blood pressure, cardiac problems, and cancer.

The fundamental social causes theory of aetiology states that disparities between the rich and poor are due to social factors such as power, money, and access to information. Increased rates of specific diseases may be considered to be linked to the action of specific agents, behaviours, lifestyles, or exposures, but the underlying factors leading to disparities are the fundamental social causes. Germs, behaviours, or choices of individuals are important mechanisms leading to illness, but the differential action of these mechanisms are linked to the fundamental social causes.

One of the utilities of the concept of fundamental social causes as a driver of disparities is that it allows a focus on what needs to be done at a group level to decrease the rates of illness. The risk of an individual can be modelled as being because of who they are and what they do, but who they are and what they do is determined, in part, by the structure of society.

A further, and important issue that flows from this theory is that ignoring the fundamental social causes leads to ineffective intervention. It is possible to produce successful interventions against the diseases currently linked to disparities, but over time there may be little impact on disparities between groups. There are many reasons for this; one is that many public health interventions (e.g. screening tests and preventive medicine) are more likely to be taken up by those with power money and access to information. Another issue is that the fundamental social causes will find another avenue through which to express themselves. Treating current problems may decrease the impact of that particular illness, but new problems may ensure that disparities continue—as happened when chronic diseases took over from infections as the main cause of differences in life expectancy in high-income countries.

General theories of susceptibility are useful but challenging. This may be, in part because the most successful aetiological theories seem to have been to build on previous theories. Rather than producing theories that are in opposition to each other, producing a new theory that encompasses previous theories has proved more profitable. For instance, early public health theories of causation were built on prior place-based theories and it could be argued that the web of causation was built on the epidemiological triangle.

Given this, linking theories that focus on the individual and theories that focus on the group or ecological level could be a useful way of better understanding causation in a complex world.

An elegant theory that pulls these different strands together is the Chinese Box or Russian Doll model of causation [9].

This theory posits that rather than being a group of epidemiological triangles or risks at the same level, a disease is caused by interconnected but separate levels of causation. Each of these levels of causation can be considered a Russian Doll.

The theory in its essence is that, rather than being a single web of causation, there are a number of webs working at different levels. Each of these levels can be thought of as a Russian Doll. Each fits inside the other. Levels move from lower, more internal levels such as our molecular biology, through numerous different levels, for instance genes, organs, organ systems, individuals, and interpersonal space, and higher levels such as societal factors. These levels have different sciences and are investigated in different ways: using methods in molecular genetics to investigate urban policy decisions may not prove that fruitful. In general, the amount of variance at a lower level is constrained by the level of variance the level above it. So, although there are some diseases in which the individual genetic risk outweighs most other factors, for chronic diseases with complex aetiologies, the impact of the environment and context on the rates of illness are often greater than biological processes.

Because of the way scientists tend to work, our understanding of how the different levels interact is underdeveloped. This is partly because there are difficulties in getting different sciences to speak to each other, but also because understanding how different types of science interact is challenging.

A further nuance to the Russian Doll theory comes from the four-dimensions model [10]. This model understands that, for practical purposes, it may be worth dividing the different levels of the Russian Doll model into two: individual and ecological. It then specifically acknowledges and includes the possibility that ecological influences, such as fundamental social causes, can have an impact on individual causes. And then includes the concept of time.

The four dimensions are: individual, ecological, interactions, and time.

The simplification aims to focus discussion on the different elements of an aetiological process and to produce an architecture for investigation, as well as a simplified model, which may help intervention. It aims to be practical.

Different levels of causation have been discussed earlier in the chapter when outlining the Russian Doll theory. The fact that levels may interact may be obvious, but specifically allowing for it aims to ensure that it is not forgotten. Time is considered important because different processes may have different chronologies: for instance, there may be periods or ages in which people or groups of people are particularly sensitive to certain environmental exposures (e.g. when you are young or when you are old), there may be different lengths of exposure needed to cause a problem, there may be a lag time between exposure and the development of an illness, and, of course, different process at different levels may have different 'time spans'. The understanding of causation may, in part, be helped by understanding how these different chronologies overlap. Moreover, there may be times when the environment is particularly sensitive to the actions of people and that may change the risk of illness. The current impacts of humans on global warming are more acute now than they previously were. Similarly, the impact of the actions of humans on the social environment changes at different times in the history of a country.

In summary, the history has been that public health was 'ecological' in its origins; the advent of germ theory led to a unicausal theory of disease. Initially, the environment as a whole was considered, then specific factors within the environment that promoted illness. There had been a progressive individualization of risk a perpetuation of the idea that risk is individually determined and a dissociation of risk from social contexts. Modern theories have tried to balance individual risk-factor analysis with ecological analyses of causation. Including time allows for a deeper understanding of the multi-level causation of illness in an environmental and historical context.

Mental illness, biology, and environment

The history of causation offers a useful backdrop for considering the aetiology of mental illnesses. It offers a multi-level platform on which to consider cause. For many mental illnesses the idea that there are biological, social and psychological factors that contribute is not considered contentious.

Most people are happy to accept that more common mental illnesses such as depression and anxiety may run in a family. This would imply a genetic contribution. Most people would also likely agree that certain drugs might cause depression and that hormonal changes, for instance at puberty or at menopause, can also spark a depression. Few would have a problem with the idea that you can become depressed because of a physical illness. The list of agreed biological causes is long and not contentious.

Similarly, the list of social factors that are considered possible causes of depression is extensive. They are essentially 'loss' events and include being fired from work, being evicted, being imprisoned, breaking up with your partner, and loss of other family members.

Other theories suggest that there can be a mindset that promotes depression. The idea of negative thinking is one populous iteration of a number of possible psychological processes that may increase vulnerability to depression.

If asked to reflect I would imagine that many would have little problem with the assertion that depression and anxiety can be caused by a complex array of biological, social, and psychological factors. This is well reflected in the Wikepedia page on the causes of mental illness [11].

There is less agreement on the contribution of biological, psychological, and social factors to mental illnesses that are often more persistent and severe, such as schizophrenia and other psychoses. Again, this disagreement is well reflected in the Wikepedia page [12].

However, surprisingly, understanding the current scientific directions and findings of the causation of schizophrenia and other psychoses gives an exciting lens to the way that social factors get under the skin, and allows exploration of how the newer models of causation work in the real world.

Schizophrenia

Schizophrenia and other psychoses are substantial public health problems that impose a profound impact on national economies, health and social systems, affected individuals, and their families and carers.

Schizophrenia is a chronic illness with a 0.5–1% risk in lifetime. Its huge costs to society are often linked to healthcare and welfare costs, but the major impact is on individuals and families.

Schizophrenia is as much a concept or syndrome as an illness. There are no physical tests to diagnose schizophrenia or other psychoses. The diagnosis is based on the symptoms that are presented and the lack of a physical cause for the problems. The symptoms found in schizophrenia can be caused by many other medical illnesses, from brain tumors through to serious infections. They can also be caused by intoxication with drugs. The diagnosis of schizophrenia is made when characteristic symptoms are present and no other cause can be discovered. The diagnosis is based not only on the symptoms present, but also on the impact that those symptoms have on an individual and the community. Generally, there is a need for symptoms to lead to suffering or problems in function for them to be considered a mental illness.

The symptoms of schizophrenia vary. They include delusions, hallucinations, problems with control of thought, social withdrawal, cognitive impairment, and depression. There are a number of other illnesses that have similar symptoms but not all the symptoms that are required for a diagnosis of schizophrenia. Over time, many people whose symptoms fall short of being diagnosable of schizophrenia eventually present with enough symptoms for a diagnosis to be made. Because of this some researchers feel it is better to consider schizophrenia and other psychoses as one group of illnesses. Of interest, others still, such as the past head of the National Institute of Mental Health in the USA, believe that diagnoses are not accurate for research and have suggested that looking at the cause of individual symptoms may be a better approach [13].

Schizophrenia and the other psychoses are considered a more severe form of mental illness because during acute presentations individuals may seem to have lost touch with reality. They may be hearing voices when no one is there; they may be responding to thoughts that have little clear basis in reality; and they may have difficulty knowing where the boundaries lie between themselves and other people. For instance, some people may think during a severe episode that other people can read their mind or place thoughts into their head. There is only 30% full symptomatic recovery and, for some, there is a gradual decline in their ability to advance themselves in the world. Many people with a diagnosis of schizophrenia do not work. This is as much because of stigma as the impact of the illness. On average, in high-income countries, the life expectancy of a person diagnosed with schizophrenia is decreased by 20 years because of co-morbidities such as smoking, poor diet, the impacts of medication to control symptoms on a person's metabolism, and suicide.

The treatment of schizophrenia and other psychoses includes medication, psychotherapy, family therapy, social interventions such as work and appropriate housing, and interventions to counter any cognitive decline, if there is any.

The treatments for psychoses are good, but even with excellent medical care the prognosis for many is not good. Interventions do not aim to cure psychoses; they aim to treat symptoms and support individuals. Long-term medication may help to prevent relapse, but there are side effects.

When treatment is less effective, prevention may be a better approach. The best prevention strategies are based on an understanding of the aetiology of an illness.

The idea that schizophrenia and other psychoses could be preventable may be surprising to some. This is, in part, because the

WHO's International Pilot Study of Schizophrenia in the 1970s suggested that the rates of schizophrenia were essentially the same across the world, which would indicate that significant differences in the social environment between countries had little impact on risk [14]. However, more recent attempts to investigate and collate incidence rates of schizophrenia using standard measures have reported significant differences between and within countries [15]. If you can identify the reasons for differences in rates of an illness between groups there is a possibility that you can find a strategy for prevention.

As with many chronic illnesses the causes are complex and work at many different levels. Recent advances in our understanding of the pathophysiology of psychoses such as schizophrenia have focused on the brain mechanisms that underlie particular symptoms in the search for improved pharmacological treatments. This may have inadvertently supported the perception that psychoses are 'brain diseases' and that the impact of social determinants may not be relevant. But the borders between the brain and the environment are being eroded by newer evidence on causation.

Balancing the development of our biological understandings there is a growing literature outlining the associations between a number of social or societal variables and the onset, course, and outcome of psychosis [16].

Rather than use these two sciences to better understand the aetiology, at times it seems like studies and the papers written from them have fueled an aetiological arms race, with biologists and social scientists building their arsenals of knowledge in the battle for superiority and, presumably, grant funding.

The understanding of the aetiology of schizophrenia and other psychoses may benefit from the approach in medicine, in general, where aetiological ideas have built on each other over time and the focus has been on the unique contribution of different types of risk and aetiological pathways rather than which is more important than the other.

The dichotomy between those who focus on the brain and those who focus on the environment produces conceptual difficulties because mental illness straddles both.

Biological risk factors

Biological theories of the development of schizophrenia are linked to the belief that the symptoms of schizophrenia are a consequence of a fault in the brain's neurotransmitter systems. An imbalance of specific neurotransmitters in specific brain regions leads to psychotic symptoms. There is a significant and compelling array of evidence to support the biological processes that are involved in psychosis. However, how the disruption of the neurotransmitter system comes about is less well delineated. There are many biological risk factors linked to the development of psychosis. I will not catalogue all the risk factors as they have been covered comprehensively elsewhere (see [17] and [18] for reviews).

Main biological risk factors such as identified by groups looking at seasonality, cannabis use, and obstetric complications have been at the level of demonstrating associations and to trying to identify what puts people or groups and increased risk. The theories of causation that they have spurned have been complex. They have included environmental factors, multiple other biological factors, and social factors.

Similarly, when associations have been identified between social factors and psychosis they have been linked to biological mechanisms when trying to determine possible causation.

The dichotomy between researchers who look at biological and those who look at social or psychological factors may be a fiction [17, 18].

Social risk factors

One of the main planks of the social theory studies in psychosis has been stress. Stress is a concept that everyone understands, but it is rarely properly described. Stress is a physiological response to a perception. When we encounter a threat our stress reaction kicks in and there are a number of acute changes that aim to improve the ability of the body to either think, fight, or run away. Our bodies are not developed to cope with the impacts of prolonged triggering of our physiological stress mechanisms and, over time, they may harm us. In addition, changes in the body to cope with what it thinks are continual threats may lead to issues. For instance, mobilization of stores to keep the blood sugar level up may harm the adrenal glands and be linked to an increased risk of diabetes. There are numerous other physical illnesses that are linked to continued stress, such as hypertension.

There is more detail to the vulnerability–stress model of mental illness [19, 20]. In general, it posits that genetic or developmental vulnerabilities interact with social adversity to influence a common pathway leading to stress-related effects that may culminate in psychosis. Genetic, biochemical, and neurological evidence support the link between stress and psychosis [21].

The biology of the stress response is that perceived stress activates the hypothalamic–pituitary–adrenal axis, which plays a pivotal role in governing our response to threat. The hypothalamus releases corticotropin-releasing hormone, which stimulates the secretion of adrenocorticotropic hormone from the pituitary gland into the bloodstream. In turn, adrenocorticotropic hormone stimulates the production and release of cortisol from the adrenal cortex, which binds to receptors across the brain and other organs in the body. The binding modulates brain function, immune responses, and cardiovascular function, as well as other processes important in the stress response [22].

However, if acquired vulnerabilities, such as genetic vulnerability, obstetric complications, or social adversity or cannabis misuse, are present the stress response may not work properly. Down-modulation of the response may be affected. The lack of down-modulation of the stress response may be linked to the development of psychosis. Vulnerabilities, such as a reduced size of the hippocampus in the brain, have been found in those at risk or whom have psychosis. The hippocampus makes sure that the stress response dampens down after it occurs [23].

In addition, pathways in the brain that are involved in the transmission of dopamine are sensitive to stress. This can lead to sensitization or an enhanced and persistent dopamine response in individuals with exposure to moderate levels of stress. People who live in stressful environments may be at particular risk of developing a psychotic illness [17, 24].

Whatever the cause of stress, the bottom line is that studies report that cumulative exposure to traumatic life events, or the number of life events experienced, is associated with an increased risk for psychosis [24], and the British National Psychiatric Morbidity Survey has reported that adverse life events are associated with subsequent psychotic experiences in the general population [25]. In addition to traumatic major life events, the accumulation of minor events or 'daily hassles' has also been linked to psychotic illness [20]. But it is not just the number of life events that is important. A life event such as bullying in childhood could lead to a chain of events because of reactions to that or changes in school or changes in self-esteem, which increase the chance of other stress-inducing environmental risk factors associated with psychosis.

The social model of causation argues that schizophrenia is the result of trauma or stress. The more social stress, the more impacts on neurotransmitter mechanisms, the higher the risk. But, in response to social adversity, there are often psychological processes that are triggered, either to decrease and normalize the perception of stress, or to make sense of it. Others suggest that stress may be linked to psychosis not through biological mechanisms, but through psychological ones.

Psychological risks and models

A more psychological model argues that adversity may lead to negative self-esteem or an increased chance that you will blame others for your situation. Being able to appraise situations and having a number of different ways of considering and understanding what is happening helps people to feel in control. Children develop social maps through interactions with their parents initially and then with others. Children in houses that are under strain may have less face-to-face time and may, on average, have fewer schema to help make decisions. Research shows that they may be less able to understand other people's intentions and to understand their agency. Partly because of this, social interactions provoke anxiety. Avoidance of anxiety-provoking situations in childhood can mean that the psychological mechanisms that are needed to deal with ambiguity are not well developed. When stress arises, the triggered coping style is more likely to be social withdrawal and suspicion of the actions of others. This increases the risk of developing paranoid ideation.

Literature outlining the association between childhood trauma and psychosis describes both psychological and neurobiological mechanisms, linking adverse experiences to psychosis [26]. These processes have neural correlates: sensitization of the mesolimbic dopamine system, which produces a heightened response to low-level stressors; changes in the immune system; and concomitant changes in the size and function of stress-related brain structures, such as the hippocampus and the amygdala.

These mechanisms also interact, as exemplified by the hypothesis that chronic exposure to social defeat may lead to sensitization of the mesolimbic dopaminergic system and increased risk of schizophrenia [27].

Physiologically and cognitively, exposure to early developmental stressors (e.g. childhood trauma) may act by sensitizing people to later adverse events, major or minor. Such exposures may increase the likelihood of adverse events, for instance, by shaping the capacity of individuals to form relationships [20]. Alternatively, they may interface with a person's attributional style—potentially making them more prone to psychotic thinking [28].

New thinking and new science

In industry, trade-offs are considered pivotal moments. The most successful manufacturers see trade-offs as an opportunity for innovation. Some argue that prior to the emergence of the Japanese car industry as a major exporter, world markets were dominated by a dichotomous model. The choice for many consumers was between high-cost, reliable cars and low-cost, less reliable cars. The industry trade-off was cost versus reliability. With significant investment in technology Japanese car manufacturers were able to sidestep this trade-off. They were able to produce low-cost, reliable cars. This gave them an entry into the market and their superior fuel efficiency meant that they became more popular during the 1970s' oil embargo. They now dominate the market.

Trade-offs are an opportunity for ingenuity and progress. The spurious trade-off between biological or social as the 'cause' of schizophrenia can be seen as an opportunity for improvement in our science and our thinking about aetiology. Researchers have already started to think differently and to move outside their specific field of exploration.

Social researchers are explaining their results using biological concepts, and biological researchers are trying to develop models of aetiology based on their understanding of social and environmental risks. Psychological theories have been shown to influence both biological and social causes.

A variety of findings in both the social and biological literature demonstrate that the two are linked and that maintaining a dichotomy between the two is increasingly difficult.

For instance, it is clear that the urban environment changes the exposure that a person or group has to biological risk factors. For example, there is some work that suggests that malnutrition *in utero* is linked to increased risk of psychosis in later life. Rates of malnutrition are increased in urban settings. Similarly, in many countries access to and use of cannabis is linked to place of residence.

More fundamental interactions between biological, environmental and social are found in the links between genetic predisposition and risk of illness. The vulnerability to developing schizophrenia in people with family members with the illness is influenced by urban residence. The increased risk of schizophrenia linked to being born or brought up in a city is mainly because of increased rates of schizophrenia in those who have familial risk. Studies have shown that the impact of urbanicity of psychotic symptoms is significantly greater in those who have a family history of psychosis and the impact of cities on rates and risk in this groups is increasing.

Genetic risk also potentiates other biological risks. When people are given the active ingredient in cannabis some develop psychotic symptoms, but most do not. The group that develop psychotic symptoms are overwhelmingly people with a family history of psychosis. Similarly, imaging studies have reported that the active ingredient in cannabis can have a direct toxic effect on the brain, leading to decreased brain volume. However, this toxic effect is only seen in people with a family history of schizophrenia. It is not seen in those without a family history [18].

Social factors also interact with each other. Social cohesion is linked to the rate of schizophrenia in an area. However, the impact of social cohesion on schizophrenia risk is only present in ethnic minority groups and those from lower socio-economic groups in studies that have reported so far.

These and other findings argue that the different risk factors may potentiate or decrease the impact of each other on overall risk. Different types of risk factors may interact and the actions of specific risk factors to increase the rates of illness may be dependent on other risk factors being present.

There is a complex web of causation, but there are different sciences at different levels—individual and ecological—involved.

Moreover, the biological literature (cannabis and seasonality), the psychological literature (development of concepts of self and schema), and the social (childhood social adversity) all point to the action of specific risk factors being exquisitely linked to specific time periods when the brain is maturing.

However, there is one factor that may not have been given enough prominence but which ushers in a new way of thinking. This is social context. Distress or problems with functioning, which are important facets of psychiatric diagnoses, are context related. They speak to an individual's interaction with society, their reflection of their own being, and their interaction with the environment.

To understand psychosis, it is important to understand these interactions.

One way of thinking about mental illness is that it can be considered a reflection of the biological and psychological mechanisms we use to adapt to the environment. The symptoms that we see and the behaviors or thoughts are the person trying to rise to challenges that are faced.

The psychological and social schema that we build to help us understand the world are there to maximize our ability to live in such a complex environment. Like our stress response these are adaptive mechanisms. Our response to social difficulties, life events, or everyday hassles is to use our psychological and social resources to be able better to understand the situation, predict what is going to happen, and be in control. We adapt our actions and thoughts based on our schema and so we minimize the risk to ourselves and maximize the benefit.

If our actions are in line with others, our adaptations to life's challenges are considered reasonable. If they are considered logical but unlawful, they are dealt with legally. But if they are considered illogical they may be dealt with by mental health professionals. In discussion with people with psychosis there is usually a reason for their actions. They are usually dealing with stressful situations or battling personal psychological issues that require action to decrease anxiety.

Whether these adaptations are considered illnesses or not depends on the differential acceptance by society to specific types of behaviors and thoughts. For instance, if you hear the voice of God in a charismatic church when you are looking to decrease your stress through worship of a higher being, that is not considered a symptom. But if you hear the voice of God while sitting in your office, and act on it, your co-workers may be troubled by it.

Context is enshrined in diagnoses and the building blocks of diagnosis—psychiatric symptoms. Diagnoses change over time. The ICD, DSM, and Chinese systems evolve with the social context and when they are too far out of step with social norms they tend to modify themselves. A recent debate has been about the changes in the diagnosis of depression during grief. Thirty years ago psychiatrists only diagnosed depression during a period of grief after 6 months. Depression before this time was considered a normal part of the process. Two decades ago guidance changed and if the symptoms were serious enough depression was diagnosed after 2 months. In DSM-5 the diagnosis of depression is possible 2 weeks into a period of grief [2].

Although there has been some consternation about this, and about what this means for us as a human race, pragmatists argue that people are expected to function 2 weeks after they have lost a loved on, and that most people can [4]. Allowing psychiatrists to diagnose and treat depression in the minority of people who are severely affected and cannot function 2 weeks after a bereavement aligns with societal expectations in some high-income countries. This would, of course, be viewed with horror by other cultures where there are clear expectations for defined periods of grief for relatives, almost all of which last longer than 2 weeks.

Similarly, with regard to symptoms, the definition of a delusion is not simply that a person has an unshakable thought that is not based on fact and is erroneous, but the thought needs to be outside the realm of normality for a person's social circle.

Our psychology is in a constant state of adaptation. Through the stress mechanism and through other neurotransmitter systems such as dopamine, our physiology is also adapting to maximize our ability to live in society.

However, there is a further complication; from a biological perspective, the brain not only helps us adapt to the environment, but it also develops in response to the environment. Some environmental factors promote healthy brain development and some impede it, but many have a variable impact depending on context. These can be considered intermediate social factors. Whether environmental events contribute to individual vulnerability or resiliency depends on many factors, including the previous history of socio-environmental exposures. Individuals who have been exposed to more positive socio-environmental influences, i.e. fewer social risk factors, tend to be more resilient. For these individuals, exposure to indeterminate social factors leads to the development of a more resilient coping style and they are more likely to be able to meet new challenges. However, if a person has been exposed to more negative social risk factors for mental illness, intermediate environmental factors are more likely to be experienced as burdensome, and this may further undermine the development of resilience.

These processes have neurodevelopmental parallels: both the structure and function of the brain are linked to environmental influences. van Os et al. have detailed the development of brain architecture, as well as neurocognition, affect regulation, and social cognition throughout childhood [18]. They reviewed the associations between specific factors in the social environment and neurocognitive development and linked problems in neurocognitive development during childhood to a later increased risk of schizophrenia [18].

If mental illnesses are disorders of adaptation, and the way the brain adapts is, in part, a response to social and environmental contexts, then mental illness lies in the interaction between brain and environment. The brain is married to the environment, and it is in that relationship that we see mental illnesses. Trying to understand the marriage by looking at only one partner is unlikely to give an accurate picture. Investigating one without the other resembles attempts to understand and repair a marriage without both parties present. It may give a distorted view of what is happening and may not offer the best basis for treatment.

This leads to a movement away from research that focuses entirely on biology or social factors toward investigations that focus on the interactions between the two, as well as the mechanisms underlying those interactions; this is a crucial development in the field [18].

From this it follows that we are less likely to find the causes of mental illness in the brain or in the social environment. We are more likely to find causes in the processes through which the brain adapts to the environment.

These processes can be considered not only at an individual level, but also at ecological and interactional levels. Because they are adaptations, we should consider them over time, but we should also consider how the ability to adapt may change over time.

Part of the new thinking of the causes of schizophrenia and other psychoses is to move towards investigation of neurogenesis, epigenetics, and inflammation. These are all dynamic ways in which the brain adapts itself to optimize the way the body reacts to the environment.

From complexity to utility

Using these understandings to produce interventions is still some way off. Self-regulation of adaptation through learning and other psychological processes are increasingly being seen as possible promising avenues for the treatment, if not cure, of some of the symptoms of schizophrenia. At a policy and ecological level the organization of our interpersonal safety net in response to the threats that make us stressed and the way we develop our communities and cities is likely to be a vital route to prevention.

I will use the four-dimensions model of causation to summarize our current understanding and to demonstrate the possible utility of our newer understanding of aetiology on the development of interventions. The four dimension approach includes biological, social, and psychological mechanisms at the individual level and also similar mechanisms at the ecological level. In addition to identifying interactions between individual and ecological levels it also recognizes interactions between risk factors within the different levels.

At an individual level our understanding is similar to that of heart disease in that there is an inherited risk, but whether one develops a heart attack or not depends on other risk, protective, and health-promoting factors that are encountered.

The risk of developing a psychosis for any individual depends on inherited vulnerabilities, but in addition rests on the balance of exposures to factors that either increase risk for illness or enhance mental health.

This chapter has detailed the genetic and other biological risk factors for schizophrenia and other psychoses. Social risk factors could include the use of certain drugs (especially cannabis), racial discrimination, and childhood experiences influencing development, such as bullying and psychological trauma, separation from parents, and other childhood adversities [29].

The number and severity of exposures, as well as their interactions, may all contribute to the risk of developing a psychotic illness. Previous work has shown that the greater the number of risk factors, the higher the risk of psychosis. Unfortunately, there has been less work on protective factors than risk factors.

At the ecological level, societal factors may change the amount and type of environmental exposures that a group is exposed to. This means they may change the risk profile for a whole population or increase the vulnerability of specific socially demarcated groups.

The model here is similar to that of diabetes, where changes in the availability and quality of certain types of food and cultural changes in activity with increasingly sedentary lifestyles have led to markedly increased rates of the illness.

Groups with similar individual-level risk profiles may have different rates of illness dependent on the ecological environment. In addition to factors like diet and exposure to infectious diseases, which influence early neurodevelopment, environmental risk factors that may contribute to the risk of psychosis include city birth and city living, social cohesion, social fragmentation, being a member of a minority group living in areas with low population densities of one's group, and migrants from countries that are predominantly black living in countries that are predominantly white.

Individual and ecological risks interact

For example, ecological factors may decrease the rates of illness by decreasing the impact of individual risk factors. The social safety net, for instance, may decrease the impact of certain life events on the risk of increasing the rate of schizophrenia at a population level and other ecological factors could interact with individual-level factors to increase risk. Social disorganization may decrease the capacity to cope with social risk factors, such as family discord or unemployment. There is some evidence that the impact of minority group membership on psychosis risk is linked to the density of that minority group in a geographical region or neighbourhood. The incidence of schizophrenia in minority groups is higher in those who live in areas where there are fewer other people from minority groups. However, institutional racism is likely to increase the impact of individual level racism on mental illness.

A further example would be cannabis use, and this demonstrates how interactions can produce a chain of events. Cannabis use may increase a person's risk of developing a psychotic illness. At an ecological level, the availability of cannabis in the community could increase the risk of cannabis use in the first place. Moreover, depending on social context, regular cannabis use may offer access to a subculture, or a different environment, characterized by an increase in daily hassles and life events, which increases the risk of exposure to other social factors associated with psychosis. Exposure to more life events and daily hassles may lead to higher levels of perceived stress and so increase cannabis use, thus further increasing the risk of psychosis. The link between individual and ecological processes in this example may trigger a chain of events resulting in further interactions among social risk factors.

Social factors also may alter biological risk in multiple ways. For example, socio-cultural factors at an ecological level, such as the trend toward older paternal age at conception, may change psychosis risk in offspring at a population level by increasing the rate of children with genetic vulnerability [30]. New evidence is rapidly emerging in this field. Binbay et al. [31], for instance, have reported that the association between familial liability to severe mental illness and the expression of illnesses within the psychotic spectrum is stronger in more deprived neighborhoods, in high unemployment neighbourhoods, and in neighbourhoods high in social control.

Further complexity is introduced by work on child brain development. This work has shown that the same exposure to an individual-level social determinant may have negative or positive impacts on the developing brain, depending on the individual's previous history of exposure to social determinants. If the balance of exposures has been negative, then an otherwise-neutral factor may be experienced as negative. Alternatively, if the balance of exposures has been positive, some challenges may actually enhance brain development [32]. Through this means, context may actually change the nature of an exposure, from positive to negative.

This also underlines the importance of 'time'; an individual's history and the possibility that the sequence of exposure may be important.

Time, is important in several other ways. First, sufficient exposure to an individual-level or ecological risk factor may only occur over time. Second, time may be needed for the interaction between individual and ecological risk factors to amplify. Third, there are sensitive periods in brain development during which exposure to certain risk factors may be more important. For instance, being born and brought up in a city is aetiologically more significant in schizophrenia than living in a city per se [33–35]. Other risk factors such as separation from parents may be more important in childhood than adult life. Fourth, there may be a delay in time between the exposure to a risk factor and the development of psychosis. For instance, the impact of maternal malnutrition on psychosis risk may only be evident when offspring reach early adulthood [36]. Last, the impact that a social factor has on an individual may be determined, in part, by the cumulative or profound effect of previous life experiences. These include the history of prior exposures linked to sensitization or resilience and the way that history may change our perception of our environment. A 10-year follow-up study on a population sample of 3021 people in Germany recently reported that early adversity may impact later expression of psychosis by increasing exposure to later adversity and/or by rendering individuals more sensitive to later adversity if these early experiences are severe [37].

It is exciting that there are mechanisms at an individual level such as neurogenesis, inflammation, and epigenetics that offer plausible explanations for how the social world gets under the skin to cause schizophrenia and other psychoses. Similarly, the psychological mechanisms for the production of psychosis offer avenues for treatment.

However, psychosis can ruin individuals and families. Acute psychosis is a dangerous condition that may lead to suicide and certainly can scar an individual's life and that of their family and friends. Minimizing the impact through effective treatment is one goal, but prevention is the one that I find more attractive.

Using our models of causation, we can think through possible intervention not just at the individual level, but also at the ecological and interactive levels. For example, we could use it to estimate whether decreasing access to cannabis, de-criminalizing it so that we de-link use from social harm, or whether we push hard for use after the age of 25 years would be the most efficient for protecting the public. We can investigate whether population-based measures would be best or whether we should target specific groups such as those with a family history of psychosis. We may want to investigate the links between the urban environment, the urban brain, and the risk of psychosis. Understanding how our environment programs our brain may be an important and vital area of research in the future, especially with the rise of the mega city in China, India, and Central and Southern America. We are set to transcend the nature or nurture debate with our understanding that for psychosis nature is nurture and our minds are a reflection of our adaptation to our environment.

These are exciting but early days in aetiological research into psychosis based on a multi-level understanding. We have not resolved the difficulty that schizophrenia and other psychoses are syndromes rather than specific illnesses, and so there may be many causes. But I believe that trying to understand the multiple possible pathways through which these psychoses are produced and allowing for a variety in mechanisms is useful. In some ways it forces us to consider what aetiology is rather than focusing on the aetiology of what.

The tension between the biological and the social led to a trade-off that has sparked ingenuity. Whether we use this to move to another level has yet to be seen, but all the elements are there for a revolution in our understanding of mental illness based on the work on the aetiology of psychosis. Simplifying this helps us understand what is going on and gives us a template on which to consider the possibility of interventions

References

1. World Health Organization. International Classification of Disease. Available at: http://www.who.int/classifications/icd/en/ (2015, accessed 26 December 2016).
2. American Psychiatric Association (APA). *Diagnostic and Statistical Manual of Mental Disorders.* 5th ed. Arlington, VA: American APA, 2015.
3. Wikipedia. Chinese Classification of Mental Disorders. Available at: https://en.wikipedia.org/wiki/Chinese_Classification_of_Mental_Disorders (accessed 8 February 2018).
4. McKenzie K. Mind Games. Available at: http://thewalrus.ca/mind-games/ (2013, accessed 25 December 2015).
5. Susser M, Susser E. Choosing a future for epidemiology: I. Eras and paradigms. *Am J Publ Health* 1996; 86: 668–73.
6. The John Snow Society. Welcome to the John Snow Society. Available at: http://www.johnsnowsociety.org/ (accessed 8 February 2018).
7. Mausner JS, Kramer S. *Mausner & Bahn Epidemiology: An Introductory Text.* Philadelphia, PA: W.B. Saunders Company, 1985.
8. Phelan, JC, Link BG, Tehranifar P. Social conditions as fundamental causes of health inequalities: theory, evidence, and policy implications. *J Health Soc Behav* 2010; 51: S28–S40.
9. Shah, Mizrahi R, McKenzie K. The four dimensions model for the social aetiology of psychosis *Br J Psychiatry* 2011; 199: 11–14.
10. Wikipedia. Causes of mental disorders. Available at: https://en.wikipedia.org/wiki/Causes_of_mental_disorders (accessed 8 February 2018).
11. Wikipedia. Causes of schizophrenia. Available at: https://en.wikipedia.org/wiki/Causes_of_schizophrenia (accessed 8 February 2018).
12. Insel TR. Rethinking How We Diagnose Psychosis. Available at: http://blogs.scientificamerican.com/mind-guest-blog/rethinking-how-we-diagnose-psychosis/ (accessed 8 February 2018).
13. Sartorius N, Shapiro R, Jablensky A. The international pilot study of schizophrenia. *Schizophr Bull* 1974; 1: 21–34.
14. McGrath J, Saha S, Chant D, Welham J. Schizophrenia: a concise overview of incidence, prevalence, and mortality. *Epidemiol Rev* 2008; 30: 67–76.
15. Morgan C, McKenzie K, Fearon P. *Society and Psychosis.* Cambridge: Cambridge University Press, 2008.
16. van Os J, Kapur S. Schizophrenia. *Lancet* 2009; 374: 635–645.
17. van Os J, Kenis G, Rutten B. Schizophrenia and the environment. *Nature* 2010; 468: 203–12.
18. Susser M, Susser E. Choosing a future for epidemiology: II. from black box to Chinese boxes and eco-epidemiology. *Am J Publ Health* 1996; 86: 674–7.
19. Nuechterlein KH, Dawson ME. A heuristic vulnerability/stress model of schizophrenic episodes. *Schizophr Bull* 1984; 10: 300–12.
20. Myin-Germeys I, van Os J. Adult adversity: do early environment and genotype create lasting vulnerabilities for adult social adversity in psychosis? In: Morgan C, McKenzie K, Fearon P (eds). *Society and Psychosis.* Cambridge: Cambridge University Press, 2008, pp. 127–42.
21. Jones SR, Fernyhough C. A new look at the neural diathesis–stress model of schizophrenia: the primacy of social-evaluative and uncontrollable situations. *Schizophr Bull* 2007; 33: 1171–7.
22. Walker E, Mittal V, Tessner K. Stress and the hypothalamic pituitary adrenal axis in the developmental course of schizophrenia. *Annu Rev Clin Psychol* 2008; 4: 189–216.

23. Fusar-Poli P, Perez J, Broome M, et al. Neurofunctional correlates of vulnerability to psychosis: a systematic review and meta-analysis. *Neurosci Biobehav Rev* 2007; 31: 465–84.

24. van Os J, Hanssen M, Bijl RV, Vollebergh W. Prevalence of psychotic disorder and community level of psychotic symptoms: an urban-rural comparison. *Arch Gen Psychiatry* 2001; 58: 663–8.

25. Johns LC, Cannon M, Singleton N, et al. Prevalence and correlates of self-reported psychotic symptoms in the British population. *Br J Psychiatry* 2004; 185: 298–305.

26. van Winkel R, van Nierop M, Myin-Germeys I, van Os J. Childhood trauma as a cause of psychosis: linking genes, psychology, and biology. *Can J Psychiatry* 2013; 58: 44–51.

27. Selten JP, Cantor-Graae E. Social defeat: risk factor for schizophrenia? *Br J Psychiatry* 2005; 187: 101–2.

28. Bentall RP, Kinderman P, Kaney S. The self, attributional processes and abnormal beliefs: towards a model of persecutory delusions. *Behav Res Ther* 1994; 32: 331–41.

29. Boydell J, van Os J, McKenzie K, Murray RM. The association of inequality with the incidence of schizophrenia—an ecological study. *Soc Psychiatry Psychiatr Epidemiol* 2004; 39: 597–9.

30. March D, Susser E. Invited commentary: taking the search for causes of schizophrenia to a different level. *Am J Epidemiol* 2006; 163: 979–81.

31. Binbay T, Drukker M, Alptekin K, et al. Evidence that the wider social environment moderates the association between familial liability and psychosis spectrum outcome. *Psychol Med* 2012;42: 2499–510.

32. Knudsen EI, Heckman JJ, Cameron JL, Shonkoff JP. Economic, neurobiological, and behavioral perspectives on building America's future workforce. *Proc Natl Acad Sci U S A* 2006; 103: 10155–62.

33. Lederbogen F, Kirsch P, Haddad L, et al. City living and urban upbringing affect neural social stress processing in humans. *Nature* 2011; 474: 498–501.

34. Marcelis M, Takei N, van Os J. Urbanization and risk for schizophrenia: does the effect operate before or around the time of illness onset? *Psychol Med* 1999; 29: 1197–203.

35. Pedersen CB, Mortensen PB. Evidence of a dose–response relationship between urbanicity during upbringing and schizophrenia risk. *Arch Gen Psychiatry* 2001; 58: 1039–46.

36. Susser E, St Calir D, He L. Latent effects of prenatal malnutrition on adult health the example of schizophrenia. *Ann NY Acad Sci* 2008; 1136: 185–92.

37. Lataster J, Myin-Germeys I, Lieb R, Wittchen HU, van Os J. Adversity and psychosis: a 10-year prospective study investigating synergism between early and recent adversity in psychosis. *Acta Psychiatr Scand* 2012; 125: 388–99.

CHAPTER 6

Genetic influences across the age span

Edward Shaw and Daniel J. Smith

Genetic influences on risk of developing mental illness

In the last few decades our understanding of social and psychological influences on population mental health has advanced significantly. This has been matched by more recent advances in the field of psychiatric genetic epidemiology, which is now delivering robust findings on the genetic architecture of several psychiatric disorders, as well as new insights on the importance of gene–environment interactions. In this chapter we will describe some examples of recent advances arising from psychiatric genetics research and consider the implications of this work from a global public mental health perspective.

Challenges in identifying genetic risk factors for mental illness

It is now established that many psychiatric disorders—including, for example, attention deficit hyperactivity disorder (ADHD), major depressive disorder (MDD), bipolar disorder (BD), schizophrenia and Alzheimer's disease (AD)—all have a strong heritable component (ranging from 35% to 80%) [1]. In this context 'heritability' is defined as the proportion of a disorder that can be attributed to genetic variation. As such, a positive family history is a major risk factor for most severe mental illnesses.

Further, we know that the genetic basis of most psychiatric disorders (in keeping with all complex human traits) is largely *polygenic* in nature, i.e. caused by the accumulation of a large number of genes each individually contributing only a small increase in risk. Although there are some examples of rare, highly penetrant genetic mutations that cause psychiatric syndromes, these represent only a very small proportion of the overall global burden of psychiatric disorders and are not considered in this chapter.

Some recent successes in the discovery of genetic variants that contribute to increased risk of psychiatric disorders are described in the following paragraphs, but it is important to contextualize these findings within the substantial challenges that exist when investigating the genetic basis of psychiatric disorders. Research in this area has moved from early family and adoption studies (which can identify estimates of heritability), through linkage studies within multiply-affected pedigrees (which can identify broad areas of the genome associated with disorder), to present-day large-scale genome-wide association studies (GWAS; which can identify specific loci or areas of the genome likely to contain disorder-associated gene variants). In the future, this work will be extended further by next-generation sequencing and advances in bioinformatics capabilities.

A major and longstanding issue with identifying genes for mental illness is that psychiatric diagnoses tend to be based on pragmatic consensus descriptions of clusters of symptoms and signs that do not necessarily map on to pathophysiological or brain mechanisms. As such, it has always been challenging to conduct genetic research using diagnostic categories, which, although reliable and clinically useful, are often internally heterogeneous and overlapping with each other. A good example of this is the current diagnosis of MDD, which covers a relatively wide range of discrete depression-related syndromes and shares considerable symptomatic overlap with BD, schizophrenia, and dementia. This difficulty was recognized recently by the suggestion that researchers should move towards investigating Research Domain Criteria (RDoC), which are dimensions of psychopathology (e.g. irritability, impulsivity, or anhedonia), rather than formal diagnostic groups [2]. The hope is that by targeting dimensions of psychopathology that cut across traditional diagnostic groups it will be possible to identify fundamental biological mechanisms. These new understandings can then be used to re-formulate diagnostic groupings so that they more closely relate to underlying aetiological and pathophysiological mechanisms. This work is underway within a number of research contexts, but it remains to be seen how it will move nosology and diagnosis forward in a practical sense. The challenge will be to demonstrate that the RDoC approach is both biologically valid and leads to an improvement in current clinical practice.

Another major challenge for psychiatric genetics has been the need for very large samples to conduct GWAS that are sufficiently powered to be able to detect the influence of multiple genes of small effect. In recent years the global collaboration of research groups within the Psychiatric Genetics Consortia has led to significant discoveries for conditions such as AD, schizophrenia, and BD [3, 4]. Technological advances, such as more efficient and cost-effective genotyping platforms and advanced bioinformatics infrastructures, have been fundamental in driving this field forward.

Although most of the research effort in recent years has focused on using GWAS, both copy number variations (which are large deletions or duplications in the genome) and the identification of rare variants are likely to contribute to our understanding of the overall genetic architecture of psychiatric disorders. Furthermore, as the cost of next-generation sequencing technologies decreases, it is likely that we will move beyond identifying areas of the genome that contain risk variants to describing the precise risk variants involved.

The contemporary challenge for the field of psychiatric genetics is how to translate these discoveries into advances in how we classify, diagnose, and treat a wide range of mental health problems, within the important context of complex interactions with multiple social, psychological cultural, and environmental risk factors.

Epigenetics

Epigenetics refers to modifications to DNA, such as DNA methylation and histone modification, which impact on the expression of genes without affecting the underlying genetic sequences. These epigenetic modifications, which can occur across the lifespan in response to a range of positive and negative environmental stimuli, are increasingly recognized as important in a range of psychiatric disorders. To date, most of the interest in psychiatric epigenetics research has focused on modifications to DNA that occur *in utero* or early in life, which then subsequently impact on increased risk for mental illness in adulthood. As such, epigenetic mechanisms represent an important bridge between underlying genetic vulnerability and dynamic environmental risk factors, such as exposure to stress or toxins *in utero*, or adverse childhood experiences. This is supported by recent work in schizophrenia, which has identified that epigenetic modifications may mediate the interaction between genetic and environmental risk factors (e.g. exposure to childhood trauma) to bring about aberrant neurodevelopment during adolescence and young adulthood [5].

Given the importance globally of issues such as poor nutrition during pregnancy, poverty, and early childhood adversity, it is likely that the study of epigenetic mechanisms will be increasingly important for understanding public mental health and developing new approaches to treatment.

Ethical considerations

The rapid pace of progress in psychiatric genomics raises several important ethical considerations. Inevitably, an oversimplified view of discovering genetic risk factors for mental illness may contribute to increased stigma against people with mental illness and could reignite concerns about eugenics and the potential for abuse of prenatal genetic testing. Similarly, there is a growing commercial interest in this area, which includes several companies now offering 'direct-to-consumer' genetic testing for conditions such as AD, autism, and schizophrenia. This is despite a scientific consensus that such tests are not yet sufficiently developed and tested to be clinically reliable. In the future, psychiatrists are likely to be called upon by patients and their families to provide advice and guidance on interpreting genetic test results [6]. The psychiatric genomics research community also has a responsibility to educate the public on issues relating to the pros and cons of genetic discoveries, as well as working more closely with the public, patients, and their families as fully engaged co-partners in future research. Another key issue is that an overemphasis within public mental health on genetic determinants of mental illness risks diverting attention

and resources away from important social, political, and cultural factors [7].

Genetic influences from childhood to old age: attention deficit hyperactivity disorder, schizophrenia, bipolar disorder, and Alzheimer's disease

The GWAS approach has led to improved understanding of genetic risk factors for a number of conditions. Here we summarize work on four 'exemplar' disorders, from childhood through adulthood to older age.

Attention deficit hyperactivity disorder

ADHD is a common disorder of childhood affecting 5.0–7.1% of children and 2.5–5.0% in adults worldwide [8]. Although the underlying mechanism is poorly understood, family and adoption studies suggest a strong genetic component. Environmental risk factors (e.g. low birthweight and delivery complications) are important, but genetic factors contribute a substantial risk, with most heritability estimates around 80% [9]. To date, progress by the global GWAS consortium for ADHD has been hindered by insufficient sample sizes, but this will improve with time. Case–control GWAS studies have not yet identified variants that are significant at the genome-wide level (i.e. with a P-value $< 5.0 \times 10^{-8}$), but a quantitative trait approach has identified several potential targets. A small number of candidate gene findings have been replicated and there has been some success in linking these to functional effects, for example *in vitro* and *in vivo* studies of the *DAT1* variable-number tandem repeat [9]. The high heritability estimates for ADHD suggest that multiple genes of small effect are likely to be discovered when case–control GWAS studies recruit sufficient sample sizes.

Schizophrenia

The most recently published GWAS of schizophrenia had over 36,000 cases and over 100,000 controls, and identified 108 areas of the genome with schizophrenia-associated variants [10]. Each of these loci had only a small impact on overall risk (with effect sizes typically in the region of 1.1–2.0), but subsequent analyses have confirmed that they contain genes that are expressed in the brain and involved with dopamine transmission, glutamate function, and immunity [10]. This has been a major advance for our understanding of the genetics of schizophrenia and has opened up a range of new areas of research and new potential therapeutic avenues.

Bipolar disorder

Within the next few months, a large GWAS of BD will be completed (making use of over 35,000 cases) and discoveries of multiple susceptibility loci containing genes for BD are expected to be published. To date, at least five novel risk genes for BD have been replicated within independent GWAS samples, including *TRANK1*, *ANK3*, *ODZ4*, *CACNA1C*, and *NCAN* [11, 12]. As with schizophrenia, such discoveries have the potential to open up new avenues of research, a good example of which relates to *CACNA1C*, which codes for a calcium channel receptor protein [13]. The discovery that aberrant calcium signalling plays a role in the pathophysiology of BD has important implications for the development of novel therapeutics, for example, raising the possibility that calcium channel antagonists (which are currently widely used as antihypertensive agents) might be usefully repurposed as novel treatments for BD.

Alzheimer's disease

AD is the predominant form of dementia (representing 50–75% of cases) and affects approximately 44 million people worldwide, with the number of cases expected to double by 2030 [14]. Pathologically, it is defined by severe neuronal loss, amyloid plaques, and neurofibrillary tangles of tau protein in the brain. Clinical manifestations include progressive deterioration of memory, cognitive function, and loss of independent living skills. The cost of caring for individuals with AD is considerable and as a consequence this is an area of priority for global public mental health.

Autosomal-dominant subtypes of AD account for only 1% of all cases, with three highly penetrant mutations in amyloid precursor protein, presenilin 1 and presenilin 2 [13]. Variants in apolipoprotein E, which is involved in lipid transport, neuronal growth, and the body's response to injury, were first identified in 1993, with some mutations elevating and some decreasing risk [15]. At least 21 AD-associated loci have now been identified in GWAS studies led by the International Genomics of Alzheimer's Disease Project, with odds ratios typically in the region of 1.1–2.0. This has led to suggestions of new pathophysiological pathways and GWAS findings have been functionally demonstrated in *Drosophila* (fruit fly) models of cognitive impairment [16]. So far, none of these developments has led to significant new treatment approaches, but there is currently a great deal of research investment in this area around the world, as evidenced by projects such as the multimillion-pound Dementia Platforms UK initiative (www.dementiasplatform.uk).

The public health significance of psychiatric genetics

Discoveries from psychiatric genetics research have the potential to improve global public health in a number of ways. A great deal of effort is currently underway to assess the usefulness of genetic risk factors as putative predictors of response to pharmacological treatments, most notably in the area of lithium treatment for BD, but also for a range of other psychiatric treatments and conditions. So far none of these pharmacogenomics studies has produced a test that is sufficiently specific to be of use in the clinic, but the pace of discoveries gives reason for optimism.

The polygenic nature of most psychiatric disorders and psychopathological traits means that it is now possible to construct 'polygenic risk scores' as a proxy for genetic loading for disorders such as schizophrenia and traits such as neuroticism. At the level of the individual, these scores will probably not be useful in terms of accurately predicting the development of clinical disorder from prodromal states, but they are likely to play an important future role in risk stratification and in estimations of clinical course and treatment outcomes. The use of these 'polygenic load' estimations, alongside the assessment of environmental exposures (e.g. adverse childhood experiences) might also be useful in stratifying patient populations, for example in terms of selecting the optimal combination of pharmacological and psychosocial interventions for a given individual.

Another area where genetic discoveries will play a role is psychiatric classification and diagnosis. As noted earlier, we know that there is considerable overlap in terms of genetic risk factors across traditional nosological boundaries. For example, many of the risk variants for schizophrenia have also been found to be risk variants for BD (and vice versa), telling us that nature does not conform to ICD or DSM definitions of disorder [17]. As the genetic architecture of psychiatric disorders and psychopathological traits becomes more fully understood, it is likely that this will lead to changes in how we classify psychiatric symptoms and signs. This will be a fundamental shift not only for the research community, but also for the way in which clinicians across the world approach the assessment and diagnosis of mental illness.

The precision-medicine approaches described earlier represent an approach to improving psychiatric outcomes by accounting for individual differences in genetic (and epigenetic) risk and environmental exposure. To date, most of the work in this area has focused on 'below-the-skin' genomic approaches. However, it should be noted that the full potential of precision medicine as it relates to mental health will not be fully realized unless such approaches are integrated with 'above-the-skin' considerations, which seek to describe and quantify the influence of economic circumstances, psychosocial barriers, social networks, cultural influences, healthcare organization, and policy- and political-level influences on mental health [18]. This clearly represents a major challenge for researchers and policymakers but will be necessary to make advances on a global scale.

Conclusions

After a long period of relatively slow progress, recent technological advances and the global cooperation of researchers and clinicians is now beginning to deliver real insights into the genetic architecture of most of the common psychiatric disorders. This progress is likely to lead to new approaches to classification, diagnosis, and treatment with far-reaching implications for the way in which mental health services are organized and delivered. The significance of this work is highlighted by the urgent need to fully integrate new discoveries in epigenetics and genetics within social, psychological, and cultural frameworks, in order to deliver robust improvements in mental health outcomes for a large number of individuals and their families globally.

References

1. Sullivan PF, Daly MJ, O'Donovan M. Genetic architectures of psychiatric disorders: the emerging picture and its implications. *Nat Rev Genet* 2012; 13: 537–51.
2. Cuthbert B, Insel T. Toward the future of psychiatric diagnosis: the seven pillars of RDoC. *BMC Med* 2013; 11: 126.
3. Cross-Disorder Group of the Psychiatric Genomics Consortium. Identification of risk loci with shared effects on five major psychiatric disorders: a genome-wide analysis. *Lancet* 2013; 381:1371–1379.
4. Cross-Disorder Group of the Psychiatric Genomics Consortium. Genetic relationship between five psychiatric disorders estimated from genome-wide SNPs. *Nat Genet* 2013; 45: 984–94.
5. Schmitt A, Martins-de-Souza D, Akbarian S, et al. Consensus paper of the WFSBP Task Force on Biological Markers: criteria for biomarkers and endophenotypes of schizophrenia, part III: molecular mechanisms. *World J Biol Psychiatry* 2017; 18: 330–56.

6. Appelbaum PS, Benston S. Anticipating the ethical challenges of psychiatric genetic testing. *Curr Psychiatry Rep* 2017; 19: 39.

7. Kong C, Dunn M, Parker M. Psychiatric genomics and mental health treatment: setting the ethical agenda. *Am J Bioethics* 2017; 17: 3–12.

8. Caye A, Swanson J, Thapar A, et al. Life Span Studies of ADHD—conceptual challenges and predictors of persistence and outcome. *Curr Psychiatry Rep* 2016; 18: 111.

9. Hawi Z, Cummins TDR, Tong J, et al. The molecular genetic architecture of attention deficit hyperactivity disorder. *Mol Psychiatry* 2015; 20: 289–97.

10. Schizophrenia Working Group of the Psychiatric Genomics Consortium. Biological insights from 108 schizophrenia-associated genetic loci. *Nature* 2014; 511: 421–7.

11. Goes FS. Genetics of bipolar disorder: recent update and future directions. *Psychiatr Clin North Am* 2016; 39: 139–55.

12. Craddock N, Sklar, P. Genetics of bipolar disorder. *Lancet* 2013; 381: 1654–62.

13. Green EK, Grozeva D, Jones I, et al. The bipolar disorder risk allele at *CACNA1C* also confers risk of recurrent major depression and of schizophrenia. *Mol Psychiatry* 2010; 15: 1016–22.

14. World Health Organization (WHO). *Dementia: A Public Health Priority.* Geneva: WHO, 2012.

15. Van Cauwenberghe C, Van Broeckhoven C, Sleegers K. The genetic landscape of Alzheimer disease: clinical implications and perspectives. *Genet Med* 2016; 18: 421–30.

16. Shulman JM, Chipendo P, Chibnik LB, et al. Functional screening of Alzheimer pathology genome-wide association signals in *Drosophila*. *Am J Hum Genet* 2011; 88: 232–8.

17. Craddock N, O'Donovan MC, Owen MJ. The genetics of schizophrenia and bipolar disorder: dissecting psychosis. *J Med Genet* 2005; 42: 193–204.

18. Gillman MW, Hammond RA. Precision treatment and precision prevention: Integrating "below and above the skin". *JAMA Pediatr* 2016; 170: 9–10.

CHAPTER 7

Public mental health and anthropology
An ecological approach

Joshua Moses and Rob Whitley

Introduction

Anthropology has contributed considerably to what we call public mental health, in ways both obvious and subtle. These contributions are sometimes divided into three broad approaches, namely (i) individual-level approaches, investigating mental health beliefs, behaviours, and illness narratives (sometimes known as 'phenomenology'); (ii) meso-level approaches, assessing the provision, nature, and practice of mental health care systems; and (iii) macro-level approaches, examining the mental health impact of societal structures, including political and economic structures (sometimes known as 'political economy'). In this chapter we will summarize and examine these three interrelated anthropological approaches to mental health. These three approaches are interrelated, with each affecting the other. Thus, we use the term ecological throughout, to emphasize the powerful bidirectional relationship between human experience and context.

In this chapter we emphasize the ecology of relationships among the macro-, meso-, and micro-levels, assessing research in each level. Indeed, one of the core strengths of anthropology is its ability to unify different spheres of influences. For example, a phenomenological-oriented study may focus on individuals' experience of a mental illness, such as depression. However, this experience will be interpreted by anthropologists as embedded in a structural context with an implicit understanding that individuals are created by the conditions under which they live. As such, anthropologists will deliberately assess the influence among macro, meso, and micro, implicitly acknowledging the relationship between the three.

Individual-level approaches

Anthropology has contributed much to the understanding of emotional distress in individuals. Arthur Kleinman is one of the key figures in medical anthropology over the last 40 years, contributing tremendously to a variety of subdisciplines, including his influential work on illness narratives [1]. In this work he suggests a distinction between illness and disease. Kleinman argues that illness refers to the everyday experience of patients, including impact on functional factors such as work and family. This is sometimes known as the 'illness experience'. Disease refers to the biological and medical details, or the ways that the medical world addresses and defines the patient's suffering. This emphasis on the non-clinical familial and social context has had an enduring impact on understandings of the patient in anthropology and psychiatry. This work, beginning in the 1970s, has highlighted a more holistic understanding of the patient, noting that healing is fostered by a plethora of factors outside of the conventional healthcare system.

Indeed, Thomas Csordas suggests that much literature on healing has focused on clearly demarcated benchmarks of recovery [2]. Instead, he argues that 'incremental healing', or small ways in which succour can be experienced, are better ways to understand relief from distress. He writes: 'What counts as change, as well as the degree to which that change is seen as significant by participants, cannot be taken for granted in comparative studies of therapeutic process' [2]. Particularly in cases where there is no clear or definitive resolution, defining 'minimal elements of efficacy' becomes important. According to Csordas, and many anthropologists working in mental health [3], the best way to come to understand this is through subtle ethnographic work that contextualizes healing processes in rich and complex experiences of day-to-day life—or what others call culture. He calls for interdisciplinary research and humanistic inquiry [2]:

> Medical anthropology and ethnopsychiatry pose fundamental problems of meaning upon which must be brought to bear theoretical as well as applied perspectives, comparative perspectives, comparative religion as well as medicine, and methods of understanding and interpretation as well as those of explanation and experiment (2: p. 57).

Another place where anthropological concepts have had widespread influence is in the development of cultural competence [4, 5]. Cultural competence has been defined as a set of skills and practices that lead to culturally appropriate services that respects patients' ethno-cultural beliefs, values, attitudes, and conventions [6]. Interest in cultural competence arose as healthcare research suggests large inequities in access to and quality of psychiatric care among ethno-racial groups, with non-white communities (and frequently those from lower-income groups) seeking care less and dropping out more [7, 8]. Cultural competence was posited as a concept that could help reduce these disparities by making services and treatment options more sensitive to ethno-cultural differences.

Meso-level: systems, policy, and advocacy

What we call here the 'anthropologist-as-advocate' tradition has a long history [9–11]. In the case of public mental health it can most clearly be seen in the work of anthropologists involved with social services and the recovery movement. Ethnographic methods are the hallmark of anthropology. This gives the discipline a uniquely intimate ability to understand those frequently left out of conversations about the provision and nature of mental health care.

Anthropologists have also found an important role in critiquing reductionist versions of biopsychiatry. Tanya Luhrmann's *Of Two Minds* outlines the transition from psychoanalytic and psychodynamic therapies to the ascendance of biopsychiatry in the 1970s and 1980s [12]. This far-ranging ethnography provides an example of how anthropologists can shed light on the processes of historical and organizational change, mapping how these changes create new institutional contexts and new forms of care.

Sue Estroff's *Making it Crazy* is another important example of how anthropologists illuminate daily lives of people in recovery [13]. This study illuminated the scantiness of follow-up supports and the concomitant struggles made by those attempting to survive in the community. Further examples include Paul Brodwin's *Everyday Ethics*, which asks 'what happens at the literal interface between frontline clinicians and individuals with severe psychiatric symptoms and profound social disenfranchisement' [14]? Again, what these ethnographies share is an attention to the moral components of care, the 'everyday ethics' of clinicians, and the lived experience of those living with mental illness.

Macro-level approaches: social structure and political economy

Those working with a structural and political economy framework see causes of distress as primarily rooted in inequalities and the social structures that are responsible for creating and maintaining them. A macro or structural/political-economy approach sees the locus of distress not primarily located in individual minds, but rather in how society itself is structured. In this view, the social arrangements created contexts that continually reproduce ill health.

Anthropologists have also collaborated on cross-national studies, which can contribute to a better understanding of social and cultural context. Among the most influential of such studies is the International Pilot Study of Schizophrenia, where a team of researchers, including anthropologists, compared the course and outcome of schizophrenia in nine countries, involving over 10,000 participants [15].

Key findings from this study—for example that recovery from schizophrenia appears to be better in developing countries [16]—have spawned in-depth case studies examining the role of factors such as spirituality, family dynamics, and stigma (or lack thereof) in influencing recovery [17, 18]. Such studies ensure that knowledge exchange between north and south is bidirectional. This can be mutually enriching, having important implications for policy in the developed, as much as the developing, world.

Again we see that anthropologists have provided critical cautionary evidence. By pointing towards the frequent misfit between 'Western' views and experiences of non-Western contexts, anthropologists have shown that public mental health must account for the day-to-day context of those living mental illness. Exporting programmes from resource-rich contexts to low-income contexts may, in fact, do more harm than good. As Neely Myers suggests [19], even concepts like 'empowerment', which seem, on the surface, to appear an unassailable good, may have unintended consequences. The author suggests that such policies may unintentionally increase stress for those recovering from schizophrenia without resources to be 'empowered'. Attending to local context, 'the better schizophrenia outcomes we have seen in developing countries for decades may decline in the push for one global fix-all for mental health' ([19].

Theresa O'Nell's important work on Flathead Indian depression initially focused on 'semantic networks' of experiences of loss and sadness among the Flathead [20]. She initially argued that *Diagnostic and Statistical Manual of Mental Disorder* understandings of depression pathologize the lived experience of suffering. Her interviews revealed that when asked about depression, those living on the reservation, who had 70–80% rates of depression, tended to speak about loneliness [20]. She argues that the depression is indicative of the large 'social pathologies' of colonialism. As with the postcolonial critiques mentioned earlier, the approach described here sees the causes of distress in large-scale historical forces of colonial and postcolonial domination. The avenues for succor, then, will not be found with increased provisions of mental health services, but rather in collective local efforts towards health and healing.

Climate change and emerging issues of public mental health

In a frequently cited passage, the influential polymath Gregory Bateson wrote [21]:

> You decide that you want to get rid of the by-products of human life and that Lake Erie will be a good place to put them. You forget that the eco-mental system called Lake Erie is a part of your wider eco-mental system—and that if Lake Erie is driven insane, its insanity is incorporated in the larger system of your thought and experience (21: p. 492).

Climate change pressures have increasingly given us the sense that the problems of the 'environment' are inseparable from human health [22–25]. Bateson's vision of ecology has a great deal to offer public mental health practitioners, who must begin to confront questions of these interrelations. How, for instance, might we begin to think of twinning the relationships of climate change to everyday experiences of anxiety? What are the subtle ways in which an analysis of multiple levels we have been discussing in this paper can inform responses to increasing climate pressures?

Recent work on climate change and mental well-being draws from a wide array of intellectual traditions. Environmental mourning, ecological anxiety, and climate melancholy offer interpretations of the quotidian shock associated with assimilating the reality of a rapidly warming climate and its present and future consequences [26–28]. Linking subjective experiences of chronic anxiety, despondency, and a seeming sense of hopelessness associated with environmental degradation, extinctions, and deforestation demand increased attention by those working in public mental health.

It appears much easier to avoid the idea that one's daily life is linked to an eco-social system that we are told is responsible for destruction of landscapes, the extinction of animals, and the possible future inhabitability of the planet by humans [29–33].

Jonathan Lear suggests that we require to work 'through the end of civilization' [34]. He applies a psychoanalytic lens to our collective sense of civilizational anxiety. Worth quoting at length, he writes [35]:

We live in a time of a heightened sense that civilizations are themselves vulnerable. Events around the world—terrorist attacks, violence social upheavals, and even natural catastrophes—have left us with an uncanny sense of menace. We seem to be aware of a shared vulnerability that we cannot quite name. I suspect that this feeling has provoked the widespread intolerance that we see around us today—from all points on the political spectrum. It is as though, without our insistence that our outlook is correct, the outlook itself might collapse. Perhaps if we could give a name to our shared sense of vulnerability, we could find better ways to live with it (35: p. 7).[1]

The implication of this shared vulnerability, along with collective anxiety, is one important area where anthropologists working in mental health can deepen our understanding of the affective or emotional components of climate change. Ethnographic methods are key for understanding the daily ways in which people navigate decisions and how they conceptualize futures, attachments to place, and community, which play important roles in supporting or hindering well-being.

Climate change encapsulates and intensifies many of the theoretical and practical challenges of public mental health. How do we distinguish between individual struggles that might be defined or diagnosed as mental health problems? How do we understand the relationship between politics and mental health? What role should mental health professions and systems have in determining care for widespread distress?

Unifying the approaches: anthropology, public mental health, and the case of indigenous suicide

The mental health response to indigenous suicide provides a particularly important example of how inequality and political economic factors play a critical role in producing and reproducing distress. Almost as disconcerting as suicide itself is the disconcerting nature of suicide research. Explanations are manifold, including genetics, epigenetic [36], psychoanalysis [37], political economy [38], and existentialism [39]. Yet there is a sense that while the data continue to pile up, and while more innovative studies are designed with ever-increasingly sophisticated statistical models, we have not got much closer to the causes of suicide or its prevention.

In the Arctic, the struggle to address suicide has a particularly dark and Sisyphean resonance. Vexing and painful for many, suicide rates in the Arctic as high as 20 times the national rates in the USA and Canada have been consistently documented [40–44].

As discussed, a vast body of psychiatric literature has articulated the cause of suicides, each leading to different kinds of interventions. Every intervention has an implied and/or explicit theory behind it. Some call for increased services, increased number of mental health professionals, or peer-support programs [45, 46]. Others suggest that psychiatric interventions are part of a colonial structure that reproduces the problems of suicide. Indigenous people, in this view, experience mental health interventions as a form of

violence [47–49]. A structural or political-economic (macro) perspective would look towards issues of housing, inequality, employment, and the politics of resource extraction and boom-and-bust economies. Ongoing housing shortages have been associated with lack of mobility, high levels of stress, and poor health.

A great deal of research has adopted a 'culturist' perspective [46, 50], using the culture concept as an explanatory framework for differences to explain high levels of suicide and other mental health outcomes. Here, the roots of suicide are seen as a loss of culture. The culture concept itself has been exported from anthropology as a way to identify in-group characteristics, and despite years of critique by anthropologists, the concept provides an important orienting framework for indigenous politics, as well many mental health researchers. The challenge is to understand the complexity of what culture is and how the concept at times functions to obscure political economic and structural causes of distress [51–53].

In a non-indigenous Western world, where a voluminous literature with a long history documents the psychological impacts of unemployment, underemployment and economic shifts more generally, the problems of aboriginal communities are framed in a very different way: as a problem of culture.

To focus on diagnostics, as seen earlier, is to miss the ongoing postcolonial, environmental and political-economic dynamics that play a determining role in the persistently high rates of suicide. Further, by using static versions of the culture concept and looking for solutions in versions of culture rooted in the past, rather than seeing culture as dynamically changing, the multi-level present-day causes are difficult to discern. An undue focus on culture obscures some of the key causes of distress: overcrowded and poor housing, environmental and social disruption caused by large-scale resource extraction, increasing climate disruption, and the enduring legacy of 'colonialism' and loss of livelihood [54, 55].

Importantly, a great deal has been written on the relationship between suicide and employment in the USA and Europe; however, much of the literature on aboriginal suicide maintains a focus on *culture*. The Marienthal study of 1931 [39] was one of the earliest detailed analysis of the impact of unemployment on mental health, and it still stands as an important contribution to understanding how communities weather the ups and downs of economic swings [40]. Or, in another context, the links between suicide and dispossession of farmers in India have clearly articulated relationships between livelihood, dispossession, and mental health [38]. Those working in public mental health have yet to fully apply such lessons to mental health issues among indigenous Arctic peoples.

Particularly because of the high costs of food, ammunition, fuel, and the equipment required to engage in subsistence activities, those interested in encouraging cultural activities should also be interested in wage employment. Public mental health research in indigenous communities would do well, for instance, to focus on young people's struggle to make a living and to forge identities in relationship to livelihoods that allow them to thrive [43]. Further, increased pressures of climate change are radically altering Arctic futures, changing the very possibility of human life in some communities. How might public mental health address the needs of communities who are being relocated and forced to search for new homes?

Lisa Stevenson's subtle and complex work on suicide in the Canadian Arctic eschews policy recommendations [49]. She

---

[1] Reproduced from Lear J, Radical Hope: Ethics in the Face of Cultural Devastation, Copyright (2008), with permission from Harvard University Press.

suggests a politics of care that places suicide in the context of on-going colonial violence and dispossession. In her view, psychiatric interventions are a continuation of the same colonial violence responsible for the suffering that has led to increased suicide rates. This work does not look towards the mental health system for solutions, nor does it offer a list of policy interventions. She suggests that there are different ways to define life, death, and mourning that elude the gaze of the settler colonial states. Stevenson points to a local politics of care informed by Inuit experience that finds that it does not readily fit the bureaucratic grid.

The case of the Arctic suicide struggle illustrates how different analytical lenses lead us to make different conclusions about the locus of distress and thus seek different policy, political, and clinical interventions. It also suggests that while carving up reality into discrete segments may be analytically necessary at times, it should be done with an acknowledgment that such divisions are provisional and artificial. It provides an example of complex socio-ecological problem, requiring a transdiscplinary, critical, and action-oriented approach. These are precisely the kinds of complex, confounding challenges a twenty-first-century public mental health professionals must engage with.

Conclusion

No single person can incorporate all of the perspectives discussed here in any one work or at all times. Understanding the three levels articulated in this chapter (the individual, the meso, and the macro) allows for a deeper understanding of the challenges of living in a world where we must simultaneously understand individual action and social forces that are frequently beyond our control. In other words, what appears to be an individual is, in fact, necessarily an instantiation of the social [21, 56–58].

A contemporary public mental health system informed by anthropology would focus on the conditions and contexts that are productive of health, wellness and well-being, and their unequal distribution, not solely on individuals. Given that government policies on all levels—from local to global governance—play a determining role, this is inherently a political task. There is simply no way around engaging with forces that reproduce inequality, and the environmental rupture that leads to precarity, as well as the loss livelihoods required for human well-being. The building of bridges among different traditions of thought, scales of analysis, and among disciplines is a critical enduring task.

References

1. Kleinman A. *The Illness Narratives: Suffering, Healing, And The Human Condition*. New York: Basic, 1989.
2. Csordas TJ. *Body/Meaning/Healing*. New York: Palgrave, 2002.
3. Desjarlais R. *Sensory Biographies*. Berkeley, CA: University of California Press, 2003.
4. Kirmayer LJ. Rethinking cultural competence. *Transcult Psychiatry* 2012; 49: 149–64.
5. Whitley R. Religious competence as cultural competence. *Transcult Psychiatry* 2012; 49: 245–60.
6. Bhui K, Warfa N, Edonya P, McKenzie K, Bhugra D. Cultural competence in mental health care: a review of model evaluations. *BMC Health Serv Res* 2007; 7: 1.
7. Desjarlais R, Eisenberg L, Good B, Kleinman A. *World Mental Health: Problems and Priorities in Low-Income Countries*: Oxford: Oxford University Press, 1996.
8. Vega WA. Higher stakes ahead for cultural competence. *Gen Hosp Psychiatry* 2005; 27: 446–50.
9. Hopper K. *Reckoning With Homelessness*. Ithaca, NY: Cornell University Press, 2002.
10. Tax S. Action Anthropology. *Curr Anthropol* 1975; 16: 514–17.
11. Scheper-Hughes N. The primacy of the ethical: propositions for a militant anthropology. *Curr Anthropol* 1995; 36: 409–40.
12. Luhrmann TM. *Of Two Minds: An Anthropologist Looks at American Psychiatry*. New York: Vintage, 2001.
13. Estroff SE. *Making it Crazy: Ethnography of Psychiatric Clients in an American Community*. Berkeley, CA: University of California Press, 1981.
14. Brodwin P. *Everyday Ethics: Voices From the Front Line of Community Psychiatry*. Berkeley, CA: University of California Press, 2013.
15. Hopper K, Harrison G, Janca A, Sartorius N (eds). *Recovery From Schizophrenia: An International Perspective: A Report From the WHO Collaborative Project, the International Study of Schizophrenia*. Oxford: Oxford University Press, 2007.
16. Leff J, Sartorius N, Jablensky A, Korten A, Ernberg G. The International Pilot Study of Schizophrenia: five-year follow-up findings. *Psychol Med* 1992; 22: 131.
17. Corin E, Thara R, Padmavati R. Shadows of culture in psychosis in south India: A methodological exploration and illustration. *Int Rev Psychiatry* 2005; 17: 75–81.
18. Halliburton M. Finding a fit: psychiatric pluralism in South India and its implications for WHO studies of mental disorder. *Transcult Psychiatry* 2004; 41: 80–98.
19. Myers NL. Culture. Stress and recovery from schizophrenia: lessons from the field for global mental health. *Cult Med Psychiatry* 2010; 34: 500–28.
20. O'Nell T. *Disciplined Hearts: History, Identity and Depression in an American Indian Community*. Berkeley, CA: University of California Press, 1996.
21. Bateson G. *Steps Towards an Ecology of Mind: Collected Essays in Anthropology, Psychiatry, Evolution, and Epistemology*. Chicago, IL: University of Chicago Press, 1972.
22. Berry HL, Bowen K, Kjellstrom T. Climate change and mental health: a causal pathways framework. *Int J Public Health* 2009; 55: 123–32.
23. Willox AC, Stephenson E, Allen J, et al. Examining relationships between climate change and mental health in the Circumpolar North. *Reg Environ Change* 2014; 15: 169–82.
24. Frumkin H, Hess J, Luber G, Malilay J, McGeehin M. Climate change: the public health response. *Am J Public Health* 2008; 98: 435–45.
25. Chivian E, Berstein A (eds) *Sustaining Life: How Human Health Depends on Biodiversity*. Oxford: Oxford University Press, 2008.
26. Robbins P, Moore SA. Ecological anxiety disorder: diagnosing the politics of the Anthropocene. *Cult Geogr* 2013; 20: 3–19.
27. Environment and/as Mourning. Digital Environmental Humanities. Available at: http://dig-eh.org/environment-andas-mourning/ (accessed 28 September 2016).
28. Scranton R. *Learning to Die in the Anthropocene: Reflections on the End of a Civilization*. San Francisco, CA: City Lights Publishers, 2015.
29. Doherty TJ, Clayton S. The psychological impacts of global climate change. *Am Psychol* 2011; 66: 265–76.
30. Macfarlane R. Generation Anthropocene: How humans have altered the planet for ever. Available at: http://www.theguardian.com/books/2016/apr/01/generation-anthropocene-altered-planet-for-ever (2016, accessed 9 April 2016).
31. McCright AM, Dunlap RE. Cool dudes: the denial of climate change among conservative white males in the United States. *Glob Environ Change* 2011; 21: 1163–72.
32. Palutikof JP, Boulter SL, Ash AJ, et al. *Climate Adaptation Futures*. Hoboken, NJ: John Wiley & Sons, 2013.
33. Maniates M. *Teaching for Turbulence*. Washington, DC: Island Press, 2013.

34. Lear J. Working through the end of civilization. *Int J Psychoanal* 2007; 88: 291–308.

35. Lear J. *Radical Hope: Ethics in the Face of Cultural Devastation.* Cambridge, MA: Harvard University Press, 2008.

36. McGowan PO, Sasaki A, D'Alessio AC, et al. Epigenetic regulation of the glucocorticoid receptor in human brain associates with childhood abuse. *Nat Neurosci* 2009; 12: 342–8.

37. Hillman J. *Suicide and the Soul.* Woodstock, CT: Spring, 1998.

38. Kennedy J, King L. The political economy of farmers' suicides in India: indebted cash-crop farmers with marginal landholdings explain state-level variation in suicide rates. *Glob Health* 2014; 10: 16.

39. Camus A. *The Myth of Sisyphus: And Other Essays.* Reissue ed. New York: Vintage, 1991.

40. Pollock NJ, Mulay S, Valcour J, Jong M. Suicide rates in aboriginal communities in Labrador, Canada. *Am J Public Health* 2016; 106: 1309–15.

41. Phippen JW. The Suicide Emergency Among Canada's First Nations. Available at: http://www.theatlantic.com/international/archive/2016/04/canada-suicide/477684/ (2016, accessed 28 September 2016).

42. Gone JP, Trimble JE. American Indian and Alaska Native mental health: diverse perspectives on enduring disparities. *Annu Rev Clin Psychol* 2012; 8: 131–60.

43. Wexler L, Hill R, Bertone-Johnson E, Fenaughty A. Correlates of Alaska native fatal and nonfatal suicidal behaviors 1990–2001. *Suicide Life Threat Behav* 2008; 38: 311–20.

44. Kirmayer LJ, Boothroyd LJ, Hodgins S. Attempted suicide among Inuit youth: psychological correlates and implications for prevention. *Can J Psychiatry* 1998; 43: 816–22.

45. Allen J, Mohatt G, Fok CCT, Henry D, People Awakening Team. Suicide prevention as a community development process: understanding circumpolar youth suicide prevention through community level outcomes. *Int J Circumpolar Health* 2009; 68: 274–91.

46. Chandler MJ, Lalonde C. Cultural continuity as a hedge against suicide in Canada's First Nations. *Transcult Psychiatry* 1998; 35: 191–219.

47. Kral MJ. Suicide and the internalization of culture: three questions. *Transcult Psychiatry* 1998; 35: 221–33.

48. Kral MJ. The weight on our shoulders is too much, and we are falling. *Med Anthropol Q* 2013; 27: 63–83.

49. Stevenson L. *Life Beside Itself: Imagining Care in the Canadian Arctic.* Berkeley, CA: University of California Press, 2014.

50. Hallett D, Chandler MJ, Lalonde CE. Aboriginal language knowledge and youth suicide. *Cogn Dev* 2007; 22: 392–9.

51. Dombrowski K. *Against Culture: Development, Politics, and Religion in Indian Alaska.* Lincoln, NE: University of Nebraska Press, 2001.

52. Dombrowski K. The white hand of capitalism and the end of indigenism as we know it. *Aust J Anthropol* 2010; 21: 129–40.

53. Dombrowski K, Khan B, Channell E, Moses J, McLean K, Misshula E. Kinship, family, and exchange in a Labrador Inuit community. *Arct Anthropol* 2013; 50: 89–104.

54. Ford JD, Pearce T, Duerden F, Furgal C, Smit B. Climate change policy responses for Canada's Inuit population: the importance of and opportunities for adaptation. *Glob Environ Change* 2010; 20: 177–91.

55. Willox AC, Stephenson E, Allen J, et al. Examining relationships between climate change and mental health in the Circumpolar North. *Reg Environ Change* 2014; 15: 169–82.

56. Jahoda M, Lazarsfeld PF, Zeisel H. *Marienthal; the sociography of an unemployed community.* Chicago, IL: Aldine, Atherton, 1971.

57. Hassan Z. *The Social Labs Revolution: A New Approach to Solving our Most Complex Challenges.* San Francisco, CA: Berrett-Koehler Publishers, 2014.

58. Appadurai A. *The Future as Cultural Fact: Essays on the Global Condition.* London: Verso, 2013.

CHAPTER 8

Social factors and mental health

Tom K. J. Craig

Prelude: diagnosis as a social construct

While the rest of this chapter will be concerned with how social conditions affect mental illness, it is worth noting at the outset that mental illness, especially when viewed categorically, can be thought of as a social construct, defined when a society (typically a sub-group of experts) labels certain behaviours as abnormal. Many of the symptoms of the phenomena so labelled exist on a continuum so that the point at which it is considered a disorder is rather arbitrary. Furthermore, many of the disorders have been described and categorized as they present in treatment centres that inevitably introduce further biases. For example, the marked apathy and withdrawal characteristic of the long-stay hospital patient was as much a reaction to the impoverished under-stimulating environment as it was to any inherent characteristic of the disorder that took the patient there in the first place. Of course, where the threshold is set and disorder declared may well determine which factors in the wider social environment seem to play a causal role.

Atheoretical observations

Many epidemiological surveys have documented associations between sociodemographic factors and mental ill health. For example, people with common mental disorders (CMDs) such as anxiety and depression are more likely to be female, aged between 35 and 54 years, separated or divorced, and of lower social class, living alone or as a single parent, unemployed, and with lower educational attainments. To these, for some conditions can be added migrant status, ethnicity, and residing in dense inner-urban settings, especially in downtrodden neighbourhoods with high levels of crime, illicit substance use and abundant graffiti.

Many of these factors are tightly intertwined. For example, poverty tends to go along with residence in economically deprived neighbourhoods that have higher crime rates than more affluent suburbs. More of the people living in these settings have lower educational attainments and more are economically inactive. Some disentangling of these effects can be attempted through statistical methods as in the Psychiatric Morbidity Survey, which found that lone mothers were twice as likely to have a CMD as other women but that this association was no longer significant after adjusting for social support and financial hardship [1]. Lone fathers, however, were also more likely to suffer from CMD than other fathers and this association remained even when age, income, debt, and social support were taken into account [2].

Living in dense urban areas crops up as a risk factor for both CMDs and major mental disorders such as schizophrenia and other psychoses. Here the association with urban density is remarkably consistent. Typically, meta-analyses across Europe show as much as a 70% higher incidence in urban versus rural areas [3], even when taking account of age, sex, genetic risk, social class, or ethnicity. It also seems that the length of exposure is important. Pedersen and Mortensen [4], in a study of Danish population registers, examined the association between risk of schizophrenia and the population density of the place of birth, and the place of residence before the age of 15 years. They found that at each age, the risk of schizophrenia increased with the extent of urbanization and, furthermore, that the risk increased with the length of residence in urbanized areas. People who lived in areas that had a higher density than 5 years earlier had an increased risk, whereas those living in a lower density than 5 years earlier had a decreased risk. According to these authors, if urbanization is causal, then it may account for as much as 30% of all cases of schizophrenia.

Some of these sociodemographic factors are more complex and difficult to get consensus on the best definition. A good example is that of ethnicity. In the UK, for example, people of Black Caribbean and African backgrounds have considerably elevated rates of first-episode psychosis than white British people of similar age and sex [5, 6], even though the rates of disorder in the home countries of these people do not differ from those found in white British people in the UK [7, 8]. Not surprisingly, these observations have been very controversial, but initial charges of bias and misdiagnosis have not been substantiated [9]. Earlier worries that the discrepancy might reflect under-enumeration of black minority people in the national census have also been largely put to rest and these findings keep getting repeated even when definitions of ethnic origin are more carefully considered. Evidence for similar findings comparing minority and majority ethnic groups crop up in studies in The Netherlands, Denmark, Sweden, Australia, and the USA [10], with the relative risk being particularly high in migrants from developing countries. While these studies suggest increased risk across different ethnic groups, the size of this risk varies so that in some studies, the risk appears to be much higher for some migrant groups than others [11].

It is apparent that just listing these associations is not taking us very far in terms of understanding why they arise, their causal direction (i.e. whether they explain or are explained by mental illness, or both) and what one might do about them in public health terms. One way to conceptualize what is involved is to view social factors operating a number of 'levels'. Firstly, there are general influences at a country or large regional level, such as the impact of income inequality between the richest and poorest of a society. Secondly, nested within these very global effects, are others operating at a neighbourhood level. These might include the quality of housing, crime rates, vandalism, and graffiti. Included, but at least partially independent of these neighbourhood effects are smaller networks involving work colleagues, friends, and family. Finally are individual person characteristics and experiences. The latter more individual detail may also be a meaningful consideration in an epidemiological/public health perspectiveinsofar as some experiences with profound health and well-being impacts (e.g. childhood maltreatment or domestic violence) are sufficiently common to be 'shared' across many individuals and so worthy of consideration for focused public health interventions. Two overarching theoretical models reflect conceptualization. Firstly, the *structural strain model* according to which the origins of mental disorder lie within the very structure and organization of society. Individuals develop mental illnesses because they fall foul of this structure and are excluded from participation. The model reflects the global and neighbourhood effects commented upon earlier, but, like them, only takes our understanding of mechanism a little distance. Secondly, the *social stress model* is to some extent an attempt to delve deeper to understand the components of social strain, expressed as environmental and social stressors, the effects of which are mediated by factors such as the individual's genetic make-up, personality, and available social support. These stressors include life events, ongoing difficulties, and problematical interpersonal relationships.

Structural strain models

Suicide

One of the earliest examples of an influential structural strain model was Emil Durkheim's concept of anomie (a state of normlessness and social disorganization) to explain the association between suicide and periods of rapid economic and social change [12]. In his view, all people needed to feel a sense of belonging to society, believing in it, and accepting the norms and rules of the community in return for support. In periods of rapid social change, many of the traditional structures are swept away or changed leaving the individual rudderless and divorced from those who more successfully negotiate change. This idea that suicide is linked in some way to poor social integration and a sense of alienation continues to feature in more recent theoretical models. Poor social integration is associated with increased risk of suicide even after taking account of employment and the presence of an established mood disorder [13]. Drilling down to the level of friends and family, and so to the lack of key social support, some experts suggest that what might be termed 'social comparison' is key. In this model, Mark Williams draws attention to the importance played by social rank in society pointing out that it is circumstances that reflect a defeat in life or a significant moral failure with consequent loss of face that is the real precipitant of suicide [14]. So being unemployed is more likely to result in depression and suicide when everyone else in the relevant social group has a job. In this model, it may not just be the loss of status that is important, but also the failure to attain it within what the individual would expect to be the 'norm' for their society. Associations at this level of abstraction are seldom straightforward. Suicide rates are not always found to fluctuate with rising and falling employment, and several longitudinal studies fail to find significant associations, especially for women [15]. Similarly, given the impact of migration (especially when enforced) on social

networks, it might be expected that suicide rates would increase. But some find increased rates only in subgroups, such as the elderly (> 75 years) [16], and yet others find migration to be protective; for example, one Dutch study found lower suicide rates in people suffering from psychotic conditions among migrants than in their Dutch counterparts [17].

Common mental disorder

Poverty is associated with mental ill health, found in all countries and societies, irrespective of their level of broad economic development [18]. However, it is not just absolute poverty that matters but rather the size of the gap between the haves and the have nots, so that some of the strongest associations are to be found in comparisons between the most affluent countries. Richard Wilkinson and Kate Pickett [19], in an analysis of survey data drawn from 12 countries in the 'developed' world, showed that there was a very strong linear association between the rates of mental illness and income inequality (the difference in income between the top and the bottom 20% of society) with a much higher percentage of the population suffering from mental ill health in the most unequal countries. The importance of this inequality goes beyond mental ill health, affecting diverse health indicators, including rates of obesity and diet-related health problems, illicit substance use and overall life expectancy, as well as a number of wider social indicators that themselves are indirectly associated with health outcomes. (e.g. educational attainment, teenage pregnancy, and delinquency)

Both social integration and income inequality can be represented at the neighbourhood level. Here, the concept of social capital is useful. Social capital can be conceptualized as the 'features of social life—networks, norms and trust—that enable participants to act together more effectively to pursue shared objectives' [20]. These social network relationships exist in two forms: 'bonding' and 'bridging' ties between people. Bonding ties are those that strengthen the cohesion of a social group and are characterized by features of mutual trust and loyalty. Positive aspects include caring for vulnerable members of the group, but there are also less desirable attributes, such as intolerance of outsiders. Bridging capital describes the links between diverse groups, of acquaintances, business partners, clubs, and so forth. This promotes social inclusion and is generally viewed as positive. Low social capital has been found to be associated with higher rates of CMD in adults and children [21, 22]. Although social capital is usually conceptualized as the total amount of resources in a society *potentially* available to an individual, the evidence for an association between social capital measured at this ecological level and mental health is inconsistent and weak at best [23].

Psychosis

As noted earlier, the association of psychosis and living in areas of high population density ('urbanicity') is one of the most robust associations of mental illness with social factors in psychiatry. Faris and Dunham, in a now classic early study, noted a disproportionate number of hospitalizations for schizophrenia came from the poorest areas of Chicago. The prevalence of schizophrenia declined progressively from a rate of over seven cases per 1000 adults in the central districts to below 2.5 per 1000 in the most affluent areas. This observation was replicated in many other North American and European contexts. They speculated that the stresses of living in poverty, in downtrodden neighbourhoods, and in relative social isolation were responsible for precipitating the illness, although the results of these studies can also be interpreted as evidence of social drift, where people in the prodromal stages of the illness find it increasingly difficult to sustain social ties and employment, and drift down the housing ladder [24], or at least stagnate, as the occupational level of the general population rises around them.

More recent research (also see Chapter 9) has tried to get behind these broad indicators by taking a closer look at the prevalence of some of the social conditions that might characterize inner city areas—poor built environment and socially fragmented neighbourhoods in which graffiti, delinquency, and crime are rife. For example, some studies have shown that the association between urbanicity and incidence of schizophrenia was fully explained when the level of social fragmentation and deprivation were taken into account in the statistical analysis [25]. Direct assessments of perceived social capital have produced rather more complicated results. Kirkbride et al. used postal questionnaires completed by residents of an area of South London to estimate neighbourhood levels of perceived social capital and related this to the incidence rates of schizophrenia from these areas [26]. They found a U-shaped relationship. Incidence rates were highest in areas with low social capital (incidence rate ratio 2.0), as well as in those where it was high (incidence rate ratio 2.5); this was independent of other neighbourhood characteristics including area deprivation. The authors conclude that areas of low social capital compound exposure to stress, whereas areas with high social capital may be problematic for those excluded for whatever reason

Structural strain models can also be called upon to throw some further light on the finding of higher incidence of psychotic disorders in some migrant populations as, for example, the recent studies showing that the risk of developing schizophrenia is correlated with ethnic density being highest in city areas where ethnic minorities make up the smallest proportion of the local population [27–29]. A similar observation was made in The Netherlands, where data from the Maastricht Mental Health Case Register found that people who were single had a higher risk of schizophrenia if they lived in areas where the majority of their neighbours lived with a partner [30]. Although intriguing, these results still do not provide us with an explanation of the mechanisms underlying a particular individual's response to these situations. It may be that being relatively isolated in areas of low ethnic density heightens the experience of exclusion and discrimination, or that being surrounded by people of a similar background is protective in some way.

Social stress theory

Measuring adversity

The findings at the level of social strain take us, at best, to the level of neighbourhood effects and imply unspecified stressors arising from these environments. But determining and measuring these individual level effects has proven challenging. Perhaps the biggest obstacle has been how to separate cause and effect. For practical reasons, most studies have to be retrospective with questions about prior stressors being asked of people who are already unwell. Early measures used checklists of common life events that ascribed arbitrary 'severities' that could be summed to provide an overall index. However, there are obvious problems with this approach, not least that some events may be recalled precisely because of the person's current mental state as they struggle to explain 'why me,

why now?' In addition, some experiences that are not experienced as very threatening at the time they occur may be elevated in severity when seen through the lens of current distress, others that occurred after onset recalled as having happened before, and others may plausibly be the result of behaviour that itself might be prodromal signs of illness. Most mental conditions are too infrequent at a population level to be able to use prospective designs to get round these problems—asking about events today will miss those happening closer to a future onset. Finally, not all stressors are discrete events, but include persisting adversity, such as poverty, poor-quality housing, and interpersonal relationship problems. One way forward through these methodological challenges was developed in the 1970s by George Brown and Tirril Harris for their epidemiological studies of depression [31]. They used a semi-structured interview (the Life Events and Difficulties Schedule; LEDS) based on careful cross-referencing of events with key calendar dates to identify details of possible stressors that met predetermined criteria for inclusion, distinguishing those that were logically independent of any influence the participant may have had from those that might have been the result of his/her actual behaviour as the result of incipient illness. The severity of the stressor was also rated by the investigator, taking into account the context in which it occurred. In this way, the severity of, say, the birth of a third child, would be seen to be much more threatening where the mother was a single parent, abandoned by her lover, and living in financial hardship than would a comparable birth in a woman in a stable and financially secure long-term relationship. This approach to measurement has been used in several studies a few of which are reviewed in the following subsections.

Common mental disorders

The first study to use the LEDS found that for both patients and community 'cases' of depression, one or more severely threatening events or difficulties preceded onset in 80% of depressed women but in only 30% of healthy women in the general population [31]. The essential findings have been replicated in many later studies internationally. The original concept of threat has undergone further refinement, with studies showing that stressors involving loss and humiliation are especially linked to depression, whereas 'danger' events are associated with anxiety, and the presence of two or more loss and danger events associated with mixed conditions where both depression and anxiety co-occur [32–34]. While most onsets of depression are preceded by one or more stressful experiences, only about a fifth of those who experience one of these stressors become depressed, suggesting that they operate against a background biological or psychosocial vulnerability. The relevant social vulnerability includes the lack of a close supportive relationship, particularly where this is manifest in a failure to deliver expected support at the time of the crisis [35]. But there are also more distal contributions to this vulnerability. Childhood maltreatment, defined as the presence of parental rejection, neglect, and physical or sexual abuse, is associated with depression in adulthood partly through the impact abuse can have on the individual's ability to form and maintain relationships across the lifespan. Childhood maltreatment is associated with early cohabitation and premarital pregnancy and with adult aversive partnerships that, in turn, are responsible for many of the severe events that immediately precede onset [36]. Childhood maltreatment may also play a role in maintaining depression [37].

Psychosis

The role of life events and difficulties in the onset of psychotic disorders is less well established. In part, this is because of the added difficulty of collecting this information in people where the onset is typically insidious with prodromal stages extending over many months making it difficult to date onset or distinguish events that might play an aetiological role from those that could be the result of behaviours associated with illness. A recent meta-analysis found just 16 studies published between 1968 and 2012 that met minimal criteria for research quality. Of these, 14 provided evidence for a causal link, but the majority of studies used checklist measures that did not take account of context or independence in the way described for depression [38]. The more robust studies include those carried out by George Brown and Jim Birley [39], who used an early version of the LEDS to examine the occurrence of life events prior to onset or relapse in a sample of hospitalized patients and a general population comparison. They found that independent events (i.e. those that could have no logical link to the psychotic condition or prodrome) occurred more frequently in the 3 weeks before the reported onset of the condition and speculated that the event stress triggered the onset of an essentially biologically determined disorder. Later studies have not replicated this 'triggering' effect as apparently causal associations have been found over the previous year and beyond [40–43]. Some later studies have confirmed the association when independent events are taken into account and there has been some effort to apply LEDS contextual measures of severity that suggest that 'intrusive' severe events may have a particularly strong impact. As is the case for depression, there is also evidence for a role for childhood experiences of abuse and neglect. Morgan and Fisher, in their comprehensive review, found average rates of childhood sexual abuse of 42% for females and 28% for males, far in excess of those reported by surveys of the general population [44]. Other meta-analyses have also noted these associations with emotional abuse [45], and the link is also observed in population-based studies of psychotic and psychotic-like experiences [46]. Studies in psychosis have yet to comprehensively unravel the pathways from such early abuse to later disorder, but the fact that such adversity is seen in the background of many people suffering from later mental ill health suggests that childhood is a particularly potent, albeit non-specific, causal factor.

While the aetiological role of stressful events in psychosis is uncertain, there is consistent evidence that the mundane stressors of family and everyday life can precipitate a relapse of established disorder. Studies have clearly shown increased risk of relapse among people with schizophrenia living in high expressed-emotion environments (characterized by expressions of criticism, hostility, and emotional over-involvement) [47]. This sensitivity has also been demonstrated by event sampling methods in which a mobile telephone or similar device is set to 'beep' at intervals throughout the day, at which point the participant records their thoughts, mood, and current context (where they are, what they are doing, and with whom). Studies have shown that people suffering from schizophrenia and first-degree relatives have a higher level of emotional reactivity to daily stress than do healthy controls and that symptoms vary in intensity according to the occurrence of minor hassles [48, 49]. In a recent study, sensitivity stress and an enhanced anticipation of threat were found to be associated with a sense of being an 'outsider' and of the environment being more personally meaningful (i.e. salient) in first-episode patients but not in healthy controls [50]. The study also found that these associations among patients were greatest in those who reported a history of childhood sexual abuse [51].

Social factors and the treatment pathway
Prevention

The evidence for the role of social factors in the aetiology of many mental disorders points to opportunities for prevention. Some strategies will involve broad efforts to benefit the population as a whole, whereas others are more focused on high-risk individuals. Of the two, it is the first that could deliver the greatest impact but could be the most difficult to deliver, not least because of resistance to the perceived interference of a 'nanny state' or resistance from vested interests. For example, the evidence may strongly suggest that societal change towards more equal societies would reduce the incidence of mental illness [19], but such change will be met with fierce resistance that will require considerable political will and unheralded cooperation across government and local authority departments that traditionally compete for resources, including health, education, housing, employment, justice, transport and leisure activities, the arts, and sport. In a smaller way, however, such change is sometimes achieved. For example, many urban regeneration programmes include an explicit target of improving conditions known to be linked to common mental disorders. One recent evaluation of a programme in Scotland showed sustained improvement in symptoms of common mental disorder that were linked not only to improvements in the fabric of buildings and their security, but also to opportunities for residents to choose kitchen and bathroom fittings, as well as increased employment opportunities in the locality [52].

One of the more specific areas where preventive intervention should bring considerable benefit is in childhood and parenting, including issues of child rearing and discipline. Conditions such as poor maternal nutrition, and alcohol and substance use during pregnancy, which are more frequent in some sectors of society, are obvious targets, with long-standing evidence that simple interventions can be beneficial [53]. Similarly, promoting a nurturing supportive relationship between parents and their children will have clear benefits, and several well-established programmes have been shown to be effective [54, 55]. Preventive programmes have also been used in schools with some success in terms of reducing conduct problems, antisocial behaviour, depression and impulsiveness while improving a range of social and emotional skills in the children [56, 57]. The most successful of these programmes work with the child, parents, and teachers to focus on improving social competence and behaviour, providing sessions that include home and classroom management of behaviour, problem-solving skills, and parenting skills, which all contribute to decreases in negative interactions and improved behaviours at home and at school. Interventions have also been developed to help children whose parents suffer from mental ill health in the hope that this may reduce transgenerational transfer of disorder. A recent meta-analysis found that the risk of developing a disorder in the offspring of mentally ill parents could be reduced by as much as 40% by these preventive interventions [58]. In another example of addressing childhood trauma, meta-analyses have demonstrated successful programmes for reducing bullying at school [59].

For adults, tackling pressures in the workplace is another area where preventive efforts could play a preventive role for CMD [60]. For the elderly, social isolation and loneliness are a major source of depression and simple social support and activity-based programmes have been shown to be effective in preventing depression [61]. For suicide, there is considerable evidence for the efficacy of broad-brush population level interventions such as restricting access to firearms and poisons [62]. Community-based, educational and practical interventions targeted on primary care have also been shown to be associated with reduce suicide rates in some studies [63], although specific interventions targeted at 'high-risk' individuals have been rather disappointing with few studies showing a clear benefit [64].

Health service access

Social factors also play an important role in determining whether, when, and how people will seek help for a mental health problem. Interestingly, while most studies find influences of sociodemographic factors on treatment seeking, the associations are not very consistent between studies especially when compared across different countries and times. For example, seeking medical help can be influenced by whether the sufferer takes an active problem-solving approach or tends to be passive and avoidant. The latter traits are said to be more prevalent among populations that traditionally have less social power and so explain some of the association between, say, ethnic minorities and low levels of help seeking. But these broad response styles will be heavily influenced by friends, family and tradition that encourages or delays consultation with official health care. One example of this is the different routes to specialist mental health care for first-episode psychosis in different ethnic groups in the UK. In the AESOP study, for example, people of black Caribbean and black African origins were far less likely to be arrive in psychiatric services via their general practitioner than were their white British contemporaries. Instead, they were more likely to come into care through presentations at the emergency departments of local hospitals or via the criminal justice system [65]. This has been attributed to the attitudes to mental disorder and psychiatric treatment within those communities, where severe mental illness is viewed as particularly shaming and the effects of treatment so awful that many patients and their families would prefer that the sufferer was labelled as 'bad' than 'mad'. This response to illness is also a response to what health care can offer and whether it, too, is seen as biased and institutionally racist. In response to these concerns, there have been some efforts to develop alternative services, as well as explicitly addressing shortcomings of mainstream services [66, 67].

The focus on social factors also serves as a good reminder of why people come for treatment and what should be the outcomes we seek to achieve. Typically, this has to go further than symptomatic improvement or reductions in distress because of the profound impact many mental health problems have on day-to-day function. Specialized interventions exist to improve housing outcomes [68], increase social networks [69], and return to employment [70], and

it is surprising and disappointing that few of these interventions make it out of research centres and into routine practice.

Conclusion

A consideration of the place of social factors should be at the heart of health care, whether accounted for as contributing to aetiology and so a target for prevention, as indicators of populations at risk of missing out on treatment, or, indeed, as themselves key outcomes of treatment.

References

1. Singleton N, Bumpstead R, O' Brien M, Lee A, Meltzer H. Psychiatric morbidity among adults living in private households 2000. *Int Rev Psychiatry* 2003; 15: 65–73.
2. Cooper C, Bebbington PE, Meltzer H, et al. Depression and common mental disorders in lone parents: results of the 2000 National Psychiatric Morbidity Survey. *Psychol Med* 2008; 38: 335–342.
3. Krabbendam L, van Os J. Schizophrenia and urbanicity: a major environmental influence—conditional on genetic risk. *Schizophr Bull* 2005; 31: 795–799.
4. Pedersen CD, Mortensen PB. Evidence of a dose-response relationship between urbanicity during upbringing and schizophrenia risk. *Arch Gen Psych* 2001; 58: 1039–1046.
5. Harrison G, Glazebrook C, Brewin J, et al. Increased incidence of psychotic disorders in migrants from the Caribbean to the United Kingdom. *Psychol Med* 1997; 27: 799–806.
6. Fearon P, Kirkbride JB, Morgan C, et al. Incidence in schizophrenia and other psychoses in ethnic minority groups: results from the MRC AESOP study. *Psychol Med* 2006; 36: 1541–1550.
7. Hickling FW, Rodgers-Johnson P. The incidence of first-contact schizophrenia in Jamaica. *Br J Psychiatry* 1995; 167: 193–196.
8. Mahy GE, Mallett R, Leff J, Bhugra D. First contact incidence of schizophrenia on Barbados. *Br J Psychiatry* 1999; 175: 28–33.
9. Hickling FW, McKenzie K, Mullen R, Murray RM. A Jamaican psychiatrist evaluates diagnoses at a London psychiatric hospital. *Br J Psychiatry* 1999; 175: 283–285.
10. Cantor-Graae E, Selten JP. Schizophrenia and migration: meta-analysis and review. *Am J Psychiatry* 2005; 162: 12–24.
11. Veling W, Selten, JP, Veen N, Laan W, Blom JD, Hoek HW. Incidence of schizophrenia among ethnic minorities in the Netherlands: a four-year first-contact study. *Schizophr Res* 2006; 86: 189–93.
12. Durkheim E. *Suicide*. Glencoe, IL: The Free Press, 1951.
13. Durbenstein PR, Conwell, Y, Connor KR, Eberly S, Evinger JS, Caine ED. Poor social integration and suicide: fact or artefact? A case-control study. *Psychol Med* 2004; 34: 1331–1337.
14. Williams M. *A Cry of Pain: Understanding Suicide and Self Harm*. Harmondsworth: Penguin, 1997.
15. Platt S, Hawton K. Suicidal behaviour and the labour market. In: Hawton K, van Heeringen K (eds). *The International Handbook of Suicide and Attempted Suicide*. Chichester: John Wiley and Sons, 2000, pp. 309–383.
16. Shah A, Lindesay J, Dennis M. Comparison of elderly suicide rates among migrants in England and Wales with their country of origin. *Int J Geriatr Psychiatry* 2009; 24: 292–299.
17. Termorshuizen F, Wierdsma AI, Visse, E, et al. Psychosis and suicide risk by ethnic origin and history of migration in the Netherlands. *Schizophr Res* 2012; 138: 268–273.
18. Patel V, Kleinman A. Poverty and common mental disorders in developing countries. *Bulletin of the World Health Organization* 2003; 81: 609–615.
19. Wilkinson R, Pickett K. *The Spirit Level: Why More Equal Societies Almost Always Do Better*. London: Allen Lane, 2009.

20. Putnam R. The strange disappearance of civic America. *American Prospect* 1996; 7: 34–48.
21. McCulloch A. Social environments and health: cross sectional national survey. *BMJ* 2001; 323: 208–209.
22. De Silva MJ, McKenzie K, Harpham T, Huttly SRA, Social capital and mental illness: a systematic review. *J Epidemiol Community Health* 2005; 59: 619–627.
23. McPherson K, Kerr S, McGee E, et al. The association between social capital and mental health and behavioural problems in children and adolescents: an integrative systematic review. *BMC Psychol* 2014; 2: 7.
24. Goldberg SM, Morrison SL. Schizophrenia and social class. *Br J Psychiatry* 1963; 109: 785–802.
25. Allardyce J, Gilmour H, Atkinson J Rapson T, Bishop J, McCreadie RG. Social fragmentation, deprivation and urbanicity: relation to first admission rates for psychoses. *Br J Psychiatry* 2005; 187: 401–406.
26. Kirkbride JB, Boydell J, Ploubidis GB, et al. Testing the association between the incidence of schizophrenia and social capital in an urban area. *Psychol Med* 2008; 38: 1083–1094.
27. Boydell J, van Os J, McKenzie K, et al. Incidence of schizophrenia in ethnic minorities in London: ecological study into interactions with environment. *BMJ* 2001; 323: 1336–1338.
28. Kirkbride JB, Morgan C, Fearon P, Dazzan P, Murray RM, Jones PB. Neighbourhood-evel effects on psychoses: re-examining the role of context. *Psychol Med* 2007; 37: 1413–1425.
29. Veling W, Susser E, van Os J Mackenbach JP, Selten JP, Hoek HW. Ethnic density of neighborhoods and incidence of psychotic disorders among immigrants. *Am J Psychiatry* 2008; 165: 66–73.
30. van Os J, Driessen G, Gunther N, Delespaul P Neighbourhood variation in incidence of schizophrenia. Evidence for person-environment interaction. *Br J Psychiatry* 2000; 176: 243–248.
31. Brown GW, Harris TO. *Social Origins of Depression: A Study of Psychiatric Disorder in Women.* London: Tavistock Press, 1978.
32. Finlay-Jones R, Brown G. Types of stressful life events and the onset of anxiety and depressive disorders. *Psychol Med* 1981; 11: 803–815.
33. Brown GW, Harris TO, Hepworth C. Loss, humiliation and entrapment among women developing depression: a patient and non-patient comparison. *Psychol Med* 1995; 25: 7–21.
34. Kendler KS, Hettema JM, Butera MA, Gardner CO, Prescott CA. Life event dimensions of loss, humiliation entrapment and danger in the prediction of onsets of major depression and generalized anxiety. *Arch Gen Psychiatry* 2003; 60: 789–796.
35. Brown GW, Andrews B, Harris T, Adler Z, Bridge L. Social support, self-esteem and depression. *Psychol Med* 1986; 16: 813–831.
36. Brown GW, Craig T, Harris TO, Handley RV, Harvey AL. Early maltreatment and adulthood cohabiting partnerships: a life-course study of adult chronic depression. *J Affect Dis* 2008; 110: 115–125.
37. Brown GW, Craig T, Harris TO. Parental maltreatment and proximal risk factors using the childhood Experience of Care and Abuse instrument: a life course study of adult chronic depression 5. *J Affect Dis* 2008; 110: 222–233.
38. Beards S, Gayer-Anderson C, Borges S, Dewey ME, Fisher HL. Morgan C. Life events and psychosis: a review and meta-analysis. *Schizophr Bull* 2013; 39: 740–747
39. Brown GW, Birley JL. Crises and life changes and the onset of schizophrenia. *J Health Soc Behav* 1968; 9: 203–214.
40. Faravelli C, Catena M, Scarpato A, Ricca V. Epidemiology of life events: life events and psychiatric disorders in the Sesto Fiorentino study. *Psychother Psychosom* 2007; 76: 361–368.
41. Lataster J, Myin-Germeys I, Lieb R, Wittchen HU, van Os J. Adversity and psychosis: a 10-year prospective study investigating synergism between early and recent adversity in psychosis. *Acta Psychiatr Scand* 2012; 125: 388–399.
42. Bebbington P, Wilkins S, Jones P, et al. Life events and psychosis. Initial results from the Camberwell Collaborative Psychosis Study. *Br J Psychiatry* 1993; 162: 72–79.
43. Raune D, Kuipers E, Bebbington P. Stressful and intrusive life events preceding first episode psychosis. *Epidemiol Psichiatr Soc* 2009; 18: 221–228.
44. Morgan C and Fisher H Environmental factors in schizophrenia: childhood trauma—a critical review. *Schizophr Bull* 2007; 33: 3–10.
45. Varese F, Smeets F, Drukker M, et al. Childhood adversities increase the risk of psychosis: a meta-analysis of patient-control, prospective- and cross-sectional cohort studies. *Schizophr Bull* 2012; 38, 661–671.
46. Janssen I, Krabbendam L, Bak M, Hanssen M, Vollebergh W, de Graaf R, van Os J. Childhood abuse as a risk factor for psychosis. *Acta Psychiatr Scand* 2004; 109: 38–45.
47. Barrowclough C, Hooley JM. Attributions and expressed emotion: a review. *Clin Psychol Rev* 2003; 23: 849–880.
48. Myin-Germeys I, van Os J, Schwartz JE, Stone AA, Delespaul PA. Emotional reactivity to daily life stress in psychosis. *Arch Gen Psychiatry* 2001; 58: 1137–1144.
49. Myin-Germeys I Delespaul P, van Os J. Behavioural sensitization to daily life stress in psychosis. *Psychol Med* 2005; 35: 733–741
50. Reininghaus U, Kempton MJ, Valmaggia L, et al. Stress sensitivity, aberrant salience and threat anticipation in early psychosis: an experience sampling study. *Schizophr Bull* 2016; 42: 712–722.
51. Reininghaus U, Gayer-Anderson C, Valmaggia L, et al. Psychological processes underlying the association between childhood trauma and psychosis in daily life: an experience sampling study. *Psychol Med* 2016; 46: 2799–2813.
52. Curl A, Keans A, Mason P, Egan M, Tannahill C, Ellaway A. Physical and mental health outcomes following housing improvements: evidence from the GoWell study. *J Epidemiol Community Health* 2015; 69: 12–19.
53. Windsor RA, Lowe JB, Perkins LL, et al. Health education for pregnant smokers: its behavioural impact and cost benefit. *Am J Public Health* 1993; 83: 201–206.
54. Webster-Stratton C, Reid MJ, Hammond M..Preventing conduct problems, promoting social competence: a parent and teacher training partnership in head start. *J Child Psychol Psychiat* 2001; 42: 943–952.
55. Olds DL. Prenatal and infancy home visiting by nurses: from randomized trials to community replication. *Prev Sci* 2002; 3: 1153–1172.
56. Weare K, Nind M. Mental health promotion and problem prevention in schools: what does the evidence say? *Health Promot Int* 2011; 26(Suppl. 1): 29–69.
57. Baker-Henningham H, Scott S, Jones K, Walker S. Reducing child conduct problems and promoting social skills in a middle income country: cluster randomised controlled trial. *Br J Psychiatry* 2012; 201: 101–108.
58. Siegenthaler E, Munder T, Egger M. Effect of preventive interventions in mentally ill parents on the mental health of the offspring: systematic review and meta-analysis. *J Am Acad Child Adolesc Psychiatry* 2012; 51: 8–17.
59. Vreeman RC, Carroll AE. A systematic review of school-based interventions to prevent bullying. *Arch Pediatr Adolesc Med* 2007; 161: 78–88.
60. Czabała C, Charzynska K, Mroziak B. Psychosocial interventions in workplace mental health promotion: an overview. *Health Promot Int* 2011; 26(Suppl. 1): i70–84.
61. Forsman AK, Nordmyr J, Wahlbeck K. Psychosocial interventions for the promotion of mental health and the prevention of depression among older adults. *Health Promot Int* 2011; 26(Suppl. 1): i85–107.
62. Yip PS, Caine E, Yousuf S, Chang SS, Wu KC, Chen YY. Means restriction for suicide prevention. *Lancet* 2012; 379: 2393–2399.
63. Hoven CW, Wasserman D, Wasserman C, Mandell DJ. Awareness in nine countries: a public health approach to suicide prevention. *Leg Med* 2009; 11(Suppl. 1): S13–S17.

64. Pitman A, Caine E. The role of the high risk approach in suicide prevention. *Br J Psychiatry* 2012; 201: 175–177.

65. Morgan C, Mallett R, Hutchinson G, et al. Pathways to care and ethnicity. 2. Source of referral and help-seeking. *Br J Psychiatry* 2005; 186: 290–296.

66. Bhugra D, Ayonrinde O, Butler G, Leese M, Thornicroft G. A randomized controlled trial of assertive outreach vs treatment as usual for black people with severe mental illness. *Epidemiol Psychiatr Sci* 2011; 20: 83–89.

67. Afuwape S, Craig TKJ, Harris T, et al. The Cares of Life Project (CoLP): an exploratory randomised controlled trial of a community-based intervention for black people with common mental disorder. *J Affective Disord* 2010; 127: 370–374.

68. Pleace N, Quilgars D. *Improving Health and Social Integration Through Housing First. A Review.* York: Centre for Housing Policy, 2013.

69. Pfeiffer PN, Heisler M, Piette JD, Rogers M, Valenstein M. Efficacy of peer support interventions for depression: a meta-analysis. *Gen Hosp Psychiatry* 2011; 33: 29–36.

70. Rinaldi M, Miller L, Perkins R. Implementing the Individual Placement and Support (IPS) approach for people with mental health conditions in England. *Int Rev Psychiatry* 2010; 22: 163–172.

CHAPTER 9

The epidemiological burden of major psychiatric disorders

Jennifer Dykxhoorn and James B. Kirkbride

Key definitions

Incidence: The number (frequency, rate, or proportion) of new health-related events in a defined population within a specified period of time [1].

Prevalence: The total number of individuals with a health-related event at a particular time/period in a defined population [1].

Point prevalence: The proportion of individuals with the condition at a specified point in time.

Period prevalence: The proportion of people with the condition at any point during a specified time period (e.g. annual **prevalence** or lifetime **prevalence**).

Measures of effect: Measures of effect summarize the strength of the relationship between an exposure and outcome, showing the amount of change a particular exposure has in the frequency or risk of the outcome [2, 3]. Measures of effect are used to compare the frequency of an outcome between two groups in relative or absolute terms [2]. Common relative effect measures include odds ratios and relative risks. Absolute effect measures include risk differences or 'number needed to treat.'

Measures of potential impact: Measures of potential impact are measures that estimate how much of the risk of a disease can be attributed to an exposure and, further, what quantifiable impact removing the exposure would have on the exposed group or the population. Measures of potential impact are necessary to translate epidemiological evidence into policy-relevant information [4]. Measures of impact assume a causal relationship between the exposure and the outcome [4]. Impact measures include attributable fraction among the exposed and attributable fraction for the population.

Attributable fraction (attributable proportion): The proportion of cases that can be attributed to a particular exposure. It is the proportion by which the risk would be reduced if the exposure would be eliminated. It can be estimated for exposed individuals (attributable fraction among the exposed) or for the whole population (attributable fraction for the population) [1].

Attributable fraction among the exposed: The proportion by which the **burden** of the outcome among the exposed would be reduced if the exposure were eliminated [1].

Attributable fraction for the population ('population attributable risk' or PAR): The proportion by which the **burden** of the outcome in the entire population would be reduced if the exposure were eliminated [1].

The burden of major psychiatric disorders

One striking feature of psychiatric disorders is that they are found in every human population worldwide. These disorders, which include depression and anxiety, schizophrenia, bipolar disorder, and autism spectrum disorders, contribute substantially to global burden of disease estimates. For example, in 2015, the aforementioned disorders were ranked in the top 21 of all disorders contributing to years lived with disability, with depression, anxiety, and schizophrenia ranked third, ninth, and twelfth, respectively [5]. Such severe morbidity is partly explained by the young age at onset for such disorders, which typically begin to emerge in childhood and adolescence, and may be associated with lifelong episodes of mental ill health. In turn, several mental health disorders are now associated with reduced life expectancy as a result of both excess suicide rates in people with mental health problems, as well as worse physical health, health care, and lifestyle choices. Most strikingly, people with schizophrenia may have a reduced life expectancy of between 10 and 25 years compared with the general population [6].

It is clear that this burden of psychiatric morbidity and mortality presents an imperative issue for public mental health. Beyond this, improving and ameliorating poor mental health will have a corresponding effect on physical health, well-being, and quality of life. But before we can move to such a point, we require a firm understanding of the burden of psychiatric disorders in the population. This is important for two reasons. Firstly, quantifying this burden—here, either in terms of *incidence* or *prevalence*—will allow mental health service planners, commissioners, and those designing interventions to improve psychiatric health, to make informed decisions about how to allocate finite resources most efficiently within a healthcare system. One such example from England is the development of a population-level prediction tool, which applies empirical epidemiological data on the risk of psychotic disorders to regional population demographics, providing accurate data about the annual *incidence* of schizophrenia and other psychoses in different communities [7]. Secondly, an understanding of any variance (or homogeneity) in *incidence* or *prevalence* of psychiatric disorders may inform or generate hypotheses about the possible causes of disorder.

In this chapter we provide an overview of the major epidemiological evidence describing the burden of three major psychiatric outcomes; common mental disorders (depression and anxiety), psychotic disorders (schizophrenia and other psychotic disorders), and suicide. Where major patterns of variation exist—by person or place—we also highlight these, with a special focus on the role of ethnicity and its implications for understanding the social and economic determinants of health. Because there is a substantial literature on these topics already, we have chosen to be selective rather than comprehensive in our treatment of the literature. We will refer to the major epidemiological studies conducted in psychiatric epidemiology over the past 30 years—typically in North America and Europe—as well as important systematic reviews and landmark studies. Finally, in this chapter, we briefly consider how this epidemiological data may inform possible interventions for public mental health.

Common mental disorders

A recent major systematic review of common mental disorders (CMD), which included both mood and anxiety disorders, placed the annual *prevalence* as 15.4% (95% confidence interval (CI) 12.8–18.6%) [8]. Remarkably, the pooled lifetime *prevalence* of disorders reported in this review rose to nearly one in three people (29.2%; 95% CI 25.9–32.6%). The annual *prevalence* of CMD appears to be almost twice as common in women than men, a pattern that holds for both mood (women: 7.3% (95% CI 6.5–8.1%); men: 4.0% (95% CI: 3.5–4.6%)) and anxiety disorders (women: 8.7% (95% CI 7.7–9.8%); men: 4.3% (95% CI 3.7–4.9%)). The same review found some global variation in these patterns, most notably with lower estimates from North and South East Asia, and Sub-Saharan Africa, and higher rates in English-speaking populations. It is unclear whether such differences reflect genuine ethnic, social, cultural variation in the manifestation of mental health symptomatology, or may arise for other reasons, including possible biases in the cultural sensitivity of diagnostic tools to detect mental health symptoms in different settings.

Epidemiological studies of CMD are most typically conducted using cross-sectional designs of the general population to estimate past symptomatology (i.e. in the past week, year, or lifetime) meeting diagnostic criteria for a disorder. While such studies may be somewhat prone to recall, they permit estimation of *prevalence* for a set of disorders, which may be under-reported in studies solely reliant on hospital records or routine databases, as many people meeting diagnostic criteria for CMD may never present to mental health services. *Incidence* studies of CMD are more rarely conducted, given this issue, and given that it may be particularly tricky to determine whether an episode of depression or anxiety is truly the first someone may have experienced. Furthermore, while CMDs are—vis-à-vis other psychiatric disorders—just that, relatively common, the absolute occurrence of episodes may be infrequent and require large sample sizes in order to provide precise *incidence* or *prevalence* estimates, or detect statistically robust differences in burden between different population subgroups. For these reasons, large, high-quality epidemiological studies of CMD are relatively infrequent.

Three of the largest and methodologically robust examples of their kind are the Epidemiologic Catchment Area (ECA) study [9], the National Comorbidity Surveys (NCS; I and II) [10]—both from the USA—and the Adult Psychiatric Morbidity Surveys (APMS) in the UK. The earliest of these three was the National Institute for Mental Health-funded ECA study, conducted in five sites to establish the 1-month and lifetime *prevalence* of psychiatric morbidity in the general population. The study represented a major advance in epidemiological enquiry of mental health disorders, using a standardized survey design across all five sites to establish the *prevalence* of mental health disorders according to validated diagnostic criteria (Diagnostic and Statistical Manual of Mental Disorders, third edition (DSM-III)), obtained from standardized diagnostic interviews. It is difficult to overestimate the magnitude of this advance; the ECA study—almost for the first time—sought to disaggregate 'global impairment' into specific, operationalized, and validated diagnostic categories. This approach recognized that differences in presentation may reflect underlying variation in aetiology, treatment, and care, in accordance with observations from other medical disciplines:

> We know from clinical information that persons with different mental disorders … have different demographic characteristics…family histories, life events, and neurobiologic correlates. They also have different responses to specific treatments. Such variations in correlates of other medical conditions are generally indicative of different diagnostic categories, etiologies, and need for care (Regier et al. 1984, pp.937-8 [9]).

Studies of specific psychiatric disorders required larger sample sizes, and this was recognized in the ECA study design, which sought to interview almost 20,000 people from its five sites. Subsequently, the study was able to provide precise estimates of the 1-month *prevalence* of all major psychiatric disorders in the adult population together (15.4%), as well as disorder-specific estimates [11]. The 1-month *prevalence* of affective disorders were higher in women (6.6%) than men (3.5%), a pattern that held for major depressive disorder, dysthymia, and anxiety disorders separately [12]. Further analysis of the ECA data has suggested that *prevalence* estimates of these disorders (most strongly for major depressive disorders and anxiety disorders) tended to be higher among people from lower socio-economic backgrounds, and those who were separated or divorced, although—like with any cross-sectional study—reverse causation (where the "outcome", mental disorders, actually causes the "exposure", lower socio-economic status) could explain such correlations. The study found little variation in CMDs by ethnicity, but both neighbourhood disadvantage and residential instability were associated with a higher 12-month *prevalence* of major depressive disorder [13].

Both the ECA study and the NCS study which followed a decade later, reported 12-month *prevalence* of any mental health disorders to be nearly one in three of the US population. Startlingly, both studies found that at least one in five of this group (rising to one in four in the NCS study) had not received treatment for their disorder, while half of those receiving treatment in the NCS study, did not meet DSM-III revised diagnostic criteria for a mental health disorder. Such studies are thus vital for taking the temperature of psychiatric morbidity in the population, as well as the level of untreated or over-treated need requiring redress through service reorganization. As mental health and well-being are not stochastically, or even solely genetically, determined, patterns of need at the population level will be influenced by changing sociodemographic, economic, and other (social or physical) environmental dynamics over time. Furthermore, patterns of care are also subject to changing social, economic, and political landscapes over time, and, as such, isolated measurements of a nation's mental health 'temperature' provided by single cross-sectional surveys may not detect broader climatic shifts in psychiatric morbidity over the longer term.

Such issues led the original authors of the NCS study to initiate a replication study (NCS-R) between 2001 and 2003, a decade after the first [10, 14]. While the NCS-R study found similar 12-month *prevalence* estimates of anxiety, mood, and substance abuse disorders to the earlier NCS study (of around one in three respondents), one major difference between the surveys was the increase in treatment for such disorders, rising from 24.3% to 40.4% of respondents with a diagnosable (DSM, fourth edition (DSM-IV)) mental health condition. Nonetheless, the majority of people who met criteria for psychiatric disorder in the year prior to each survey still received no treatment for their care, whereas there were substantial increases in treatment among people who did not meet criteria for a DSM-IV mental health disorder, or whose disorder was in the mild range. The authors noted various possible reasons for such changes, including more direct-to-consumer marketing strategies by the pharmaceutical industry (not permitted in other countries, including, e.g., the UK), better mental health awareness, increased insurance coverage, and better access to community services. Finally, the NCS-R highlighted the treatment gap between various groups; women, those aged between 35 and 54 years, and white groups (vis-à-vis non-Hispanic black and Hispanic populations) were more likely to receive treatment.

One further notable epidemiological study of CMD outside of the USA deserves attention; the APMS in the UK, a repeated cross-sectional household survey conducted over four successive waves in 1993 [15], 2000 [16], 2007 [17], and 2014 [18]. Compared with the US studies, the estimated 12-month *prevalence* of CMDs was lower in the UK, with around one in six people meeting diagnostic criteria in the last wave of the APMS study, albeit using a different diagnostic instrument (Clinical Interview Schedule–Revised). Nonetheless, trends between the US and UK surveys in treatment patterns exist. Like the ECA and NCS studies, the APMS surveys have found substantial levels of untreated mental health need in the community, with only one in three of the 2014 wave of the APMS reporting having sought treatment for their CMD [18]. As in the USA, treatment rates have risen over time, which the APMS authors attributed to greater use of psychotropic medications and psychological therapies. Finally, inequalities in receipt of treatment broadly echoed the findings of the NCS-R study, with older, female, and white participants all more likely to receive treatment for their mental health disorder.

Schizophrenia and other psychotic disorders

Cross-sectional surveys of psychotic disorders generally have more limited utility than cohort-based study designs. This arises for three primary reasons. Firstly, psychotic disorders occur less frequently than CMD (see previous section). Typically, the annual *prevalence* of schizophrenia has been estimated to be around four in 1000 [19], although heterogeneity may exist between populations. Therefore, cross-sectional surveys of psychotic disorders need to be very large to obtain precise *prevalence* estimates, and such studies tend to be less frequently conducted as a result. This reason alone, however, is insufficient to favour other designs over cross-sectional surveys, as the same, or even larger sample size requirements would apply

to, for example, cohort study designs. The second reason why cross-sectional surveys tend to be less frequently adopted to study schizophrenia and related psychotic disorders concerns the hunt for aetiological risk factors for psychosis, which has received substantial research attention. As cross-sectional surveys cannot establish direction of causation between a putative exposure and the outcome, they are of more limited use in this regard. Instead, cohort-based study designs often allow for temporal separation of exposure and outcome, to ensure the former precede the latter. This is important in mental health research, where patterns of exposure (e.g. by sociodemographic markers, deprivation, or urban living) may also mirror patterns of effect secondary to the onset of disorder (i.e. downward social drift following the onset of schizophrenia). The use of longitudinal designs, and focus on *incidence* (new cases) rather than *prevalence* (new and existing cases) minimizes (but may not altogether exclude) issues of reverse causality. In addition, in their seminal monograph on international variation in the *incidence* of schizophrenia (also discussed in more detail later) Jablensky et al. [20] also note that:

> [i]ncidence rates are better than *prevalence* rates [*sic*] for comparisons between different populations, because they are less affected by differential mortality, migration, and other demographic factors. The study of series of patients of recent onset is important also in view of the possibility that pathogenetic or triggering factors which are active in the period preceding the first manifestations of the disorder may cease to operate at later stages of its evolution (Jablensky et al. [20], pp. 43).

The final reason why cross-sectional surveys are less commonly used than cohort-based designs leverages a feature of psychotic disorders that differs notably from CMD: presentation to services. Because the onset of psychotic disorders is often marked by substantial, distressing, and overt symptomatology, including florid psychotic states, bizarre behaviour, social withdrawal, and cognitive impairment, people with psychotic disorder tend to present to mental health services at some point during their illness episode. That said, the duration of untreated psychosis may be long for some individuals [21], and is strongly associated with worse outcomes [22]. Thus, unlike CMDs—where a substantial proportion of people may be untreated (and undetected)—people with psychotic disorders are more routinely picked up in hospital records, healthcare registers, and other routine databases. As a result, while cohort-based study designs of the *incidence* of psychotic disorders may need to be extremely large, they can achieve such sample size requirements in a cost-efficient manner by leveraging use of reliable healthcare databases. In this section, we briefly review some selected major epidemiological studies of psychosis *incidence* in the past 30 years, and highlight the main findings from these studies.

A landmark study in the understanding of the epidemiology of schizophrenia and other psychotic disorders was the World Health Organization's (WHO) Determinants of Outcomes of Severe Mental Disorders study, colloquially known as the 'ten-country' study [20]. The study was conducted between 1978 and 1981 in 12 international settings in ten countries, designed to apply a systematic methodology to—amongst other aspects—the *incidence* of disorder. The study employed a robust case-finding approach to identify all new cases in defined catchment areas over a 2-year period, which met International Classification of Diseases, Ninth Revision (ICD-9) criteria for non-organic psychotic disorders. Importantly, the study established that schizophrenia could be reliably identified as a feature of all populations where it was studied, from Nigeria to India to Denmark to Japan. Furthermore, its manifestations across these settings were marked more by their similarities than their differences, suggesting broadly consistent cultural validity to the nosological entity defined in ICD-9 as 'schizophrenia'. *Incidence* data of sufficient epidemiological quality were eventually available from eight (including rural and urban Chandigarh as two separate sites) of the 12 centres, which were considered to have 'fairly complete coverage … of the various "helping agencies" that were likely to serve as first-contact sites for psychotic patients' [20]. Importantly, the study identified a two- to threefold variation in the *incidence* of narrowly and broadly defined schizophrenia, respectively, across these international settings. *Incidence* rates thus ranged from 7 to 14 per 100,000 for narrowly defined schizophrenia, and from 15 to 42 per 100,000 for its broadly defined counterpart, typically referred to today as schizophrenia spectrum disorders (SSD). Such variation may allude to important underlying risk factors for disorder (e.g. ethnicity, see 'How patterns of *incidence* and *prevalence* of mental health disorders vary by ethnicity'). Nonetheless, despite this apparent variation, and its potential importance for advancing our understanding of the causes of schizophrenia, an unfortunate legacy of the WHO 'ten-country' was a general misinterpretation of its principal findings (it should be noted, not by the original authors) that the study showed no international variation in risk. This dogma was solely based on the findings for narrowly defined schizophrenia, which were underpowered to detect a statistically significant variation in *incidence* (but not broadly defined schizophrenia, which showed statistically significant variation ($P < 0.05$)). The view that psychotic disorders were invariant to place effects dominated much of the psychiatric literature for the next 20 years, and was used to advance exploration of the possibility that schizophrenia was almost entirely genetic in origin [23, 24].

A series of important studies conducted since the WHO ten-country study [20] have added a strong evidence base to show that schizophrenia and other psychotic disorders vary by robust, replicable factors, including age (higher during late adolescence and the early 20s), sex (higher among men), ethnicity (higher among minority groups, see 'How patterns of *incidence* and *prevalence* of mental health disorders vary by ethnicity'), and place (higher in people exposed to more urban, deprived environments). For comprehensive systematic reviews on these topics, see McGrath et al. (all aspects) [25], Kirkbride et al. (all aspects) [26], March et al. (variation by place) [27], Bourque et al. (variation by migration and generation status) [28], and Cantor-Graae and Selten (variation by ethnicity and migration) [29]. One important example, conducted in the UK, was the Aetiology and Ethnicity in Schizophrenia and Other Psychoses (AESOP) study [30]. That study used a broadly comparable design to the WHO study, and sought to ascertain the *incidence* of first-episode psychotic disorders in community settings in three defined catchment areas in the UK, South East London, Nottinghamshire, and Bristol, comprising a mix of urban, suburban, and rural environments. In that study, Kirkbride et al. [30] found that the *incidence* of non-affective psychotic disorders varied from 13.9 in Nottinghamshire to 40.5 per 100,000 in South East London, consistent with international variance in rates observed by Jablensky et al. [20], albeit on a national scale. Register-based *incidence* studies using prospectively designed national cohorts have also provided valuable epidemiological evidence about the *incidence* of disorders, most notably from Sweden and Denmark

[31–33]. Linking entire population cohorts to hospital registers, such studies provide a powerful tool for the analysis of prospectively collected risk factors in relation to later mental health outcomes. Age-adjusted *incidence* rates of SSD from Sweden suggest that the rate in the background Swedish population is around 31 per 100,000 in women and 49 per 100,000 among men [31], reflecting known sex differences in the risk of psychotic disorders. *Incidence* rates of a similar or greater magnitude have been found for SSD in Danish registers [33], which were also able to estimate lifetime risk (similar to lifetime *prevalence*) at around 3.7% (similar for men and women).

Readers will note that the *incidence* and *prevalence* estimates obtained from these register-based cohort designs appear to be higher than comparable estimates of *incidence* from the first-contact studies described earlier (i.e. the WHO ten-country study, the AESOP study), or lifetime *prevalence* estimates from cross-sectional surveys. This pattern has been recently noted by Hogerzeil et al. [34, 35], using a dual first-contact and register-based design in the same population. Several reasons for this discrepancy may exist, but register-based designs may be more comprehensive in case identification, as 'hospital' registers will typically identify all people diagnosed with a disorder in a given healthcare system, including both in- and outpatient facilities. By comparison, first-contact designs, which rely on regular contact with a variety of secondary and tertiary care providers allied to mental health, may still be more likely to miss cases presenting to other parts of a healthcare system, unless these are also monitored. It is also possible that first-contact designs overestimate the population at risk (i.e. the denominator), because they typically take a static estimate of the population at risk at a single point in time (i.e. from a census or similar) and multiply this by the length of case ascertainment to approximate total person-years at risk [30]. This method thus ignores changes to the population at risk over time caused by entry to (owing to immigration, changes in birth and infant mortality rates) and exit from (emigration, adult mortality) the catchment area population. While such bias may be small over shorter periods of case ascertainment, they could be amplified over longer periods, or when coinciding with periods of rapid change in migration or mortality in the population. By contrast, via linkage to migration and death registers, register-based cohort studies can typically estimate the exact person-years at risk with a higher degree of precision. While these two reasons (better case finding and more precise denominator estimation) suggest that the higher rates observed in register-based cohort designs may be more reliable, we also note that first-contact designs can offer better validation of psychiatric diagnoses than register-based designs. First-contact studies, such as the WHO or AESOP studies, use standardized diagnostic assessments to validate any psychiatric diagnoses initially made in clinical settings to identify cases. By contrast, psychiatric case registers usually rely on clinical diagnoses made by mental health practitioners working in a variety of mental health settings, and may be more subject to inter-rater differences, and the vagaries of shifting diagnostic practices or sociocultural attitudes to mental health over time. While studies of register-based diagnoses for schizophrenia suggest they are valid for research purposes [36, 37], single-registry snapshots do not guarantee their validity for all psychotic (or psychiatric) disorders, or across all time periods, healthcare settings, or geographical locations. Allebeck (p. 390) suggests that these 'issues of validity and generalizability needs to be addressed for each specific study purpose' [38].

Suicide

Over 800,000 people die by suicide each year, making it an immense issue for global and public health. While we recognize the importance of understanding other suicidal outcomes, including suicidal thoughts, self-harm, and suicide attempts, we restrict this subsection to major studies of rates of completed suicide. Our focus here is, in part, because it represents the most severe suicidal outcome and, in part, because the available literature may be less subject to (although not free from [39]) under-reporting and detection biases than other suicidal outcomes. A larger literature on other important suicidal outcomes demonstrates how they contribute substantially to psychiatric morbidity in the general population, and particularly among young people [18, 40]. For *prevalence* examples, see the UK APMS (i.e. McManus et al. [18]), and the Australian population surveys [41], and for good reviews on this topic see Pitman et al. [40] and Evans et al. [42]).

Quantifying the overall burden of suicide is difficult, because rates vary by age, sex, ethnic group, and socio-economic position. Rates also vary cross-culturally and therefore by country, as well as over time. Nonetheless, since the 1960s and 1970s several studies, in several settings, have noted a decline in suicide among older people, with some more recent increases among young men, including in the UK, Japan, Australia, and New Zealand [43]. In the USA, although rates increased among young men between 1964 and 2013, the overall age pattern remains one of upward risk by age, with substantial peaks in men after 75 years of age. By contrast, rates for women are more uniform over age in the USA, as well as elsewhere [43]. Typically, suicide rates are about three times greater in men than women. This pattern is observed consistently in the UK, across all ages, where overall risks were estimated to be 16.6 in men and 5.4 in women per 100,000 of the population in 2015 [44]. Using the most recently available global estimates of suicide from WHO (2012) [45], age-standardized rates vary substantially worldwide, from fewer than 5 per 100,000 in much of North Africa, Southern Africa, Mexico, the Middle East, the Philippines, and Indonesia, to over 15 per 100,000 in parts of Russia and many countries in the former Soviet Bloc, East Africa, India, and Japan. For men, rates ranged from 0.6 per 100,000 in Saudi Arabia to 70.8 per 100,000 in Guyana; for women, rates ranged from 0.2 per 100,000 in Syria to 35.1 in the Democratic People's Republic of Korea [43]. Owing to these high rates, combined with large population bases, suicide in low- and middle-income countries are thought to account for around 75% of all suicides worldwide [45], making them a priority for global and public mental health.

Variations in suicide rates by person, place, and time are likely to occur for a variety of reasons, including changes in the availability of means, policy interventions, socio-economic factors, and other psychosocial stressors, as well as the influence of socio-cultural customs, values, and norms. The occurrence of some of these factors—most notably, availability of means and socio-economic stressors—may partially explain the higher rates of suicide observed in rural compared with urban populations [46–49], a pattern particularly pronounced amongst men [46, 47]. For example, higher suicide rates in rural parts of the USA, Canada, the UK, and Australia have been linked to the greater availability of firearms [47, 50–53], whereas pesticide poisonings have been observed to be more common in rural parts of Taiwan and South Korea [54, 55]. Socio-economic drivers of suicide rates are also important. There is accumulating evidence, for example, that economic recessions may impact on suicide rates through factors such as unemployment (see, e.g., Frasquihlo et al. [56]). In a further review of such evidence, the European Psychiatric Association [57] has suggested that various factors related to economic recession—including unemployment, indebtedness, precarious working conditions, inequality, housing security, and a loss of social cohesion (first noted in relation to suicide risk by Durkheim [58] in the nineteenth century)—are related to suicidal behaviours and a range of other mental health problems. Exposure to such factors is rarely distributed equitably throughout the population, and the authors suggest that certain high-risk groups, including working-age men and those of low socio-economic position, may bear a disproportionate burden of increased risk attributable to these effects, exacerbated during periods of economic recession. The European Psychiatric Association also noted that [57]:

> the existence of well-developed social protection and health services is also relevant. In this way, countries with a consolidated welfare state appears [sic] to be less exposed to adverse health outcomes related to economic decline (Martin-Carrasco et al. [57] pp. 105).

Nonetheless, they also note that the direction of causality in the association between suicide, economic hardship, and previous psychiatric morbidity has yet to be fully established. While further research is clearly required here, if true, such findings suggest that during periods of economic recession, policy-level decisions that seek to reduce government expenditure through cuts to mental health services may increase suicide deaths and other mental health problems. To combat the economic impact of recession on suicide and other areas of psychiatric morbidity, the European Psychiatric Association concludes by suggesting several areas of policy intervention, including initiatives that maintain income support, create jobs and more stable working environments, and tackle housing instability and structural inequalities present in society (for a detailed explanation of possible interventions see Martin-Carrasco et al. [57]). We note that many of the drivers of, and interventions against, increased suicide rates during periods of economic recession will also apply to subgroups of the population at all points in time. Given the heterogeneity in suicide rates between person and place over time, one area of policy intervention to provide appropriate treatment response and service provision for affected individuals and groups is accurate population surveillance, using consistent definitions of suicide and accurate recording via routine health observatories. Such accurate surveillance systems—although more challenging to implement in some settings—would allow early detection of emerging high risk groups for suicide, thus more effectively informing mental health service provision.

How patterns of *incidence* and *prevalence* of mental health disorders vary by ethnicity

The overall *incidence* and *prevalence* estimates highlighted in the first section may mask important heterogeneity within subgroups of the population. Closer investigation of groups that may be at increased risk is therefore important for public mental health and health service planning, and may also enrich our understanding of the aetiology of disorders. Ethnic variation in the *incidence* and *prevalence* of many health conditions has been widely documented [59], including psychiatric disorders. Early reports of high rates of hospitalization for schizophrenia, for example amongst Norwegians emigrating to the USA, date as far back as the 1920s [60]. Ethnic variation in mental illness was also identified in the aforementioned ECA study (see 'The burden of major psychiatric disorders'), which found that both the lifetime and 12-month *prevalence* of major mental disorders was higher among black respondents than those of white or Hispanic origin [61]. However, the study also noted that these ethnic groups tended to differ on important demographic characteristics (i.e. confounding), with black respondents more likely to be younger, poorer, and having less education than their white counterparts. In this section we briefly highlight the major epidemiological evidence describing any variation in the burden (*incidence* or *prevalence*) of CMD, psychotic disorders, and suicide by ethnicity and migration status.

Common mental disorders

Although a considerable literature exists on the overall *prevalence* of CMDs (see 'Common mental disorders'), until recently there has been little population-based investigation into ethnic variations in CMD [62]. Interestingly, the overall balance of evidence in regard to CMD does not provide consistent or conclusive evidence of ethnic variation.

Research from the USA initially suggested some ethnic variation in affective disorders existed. For example, the ECA study observed that rates of depression and dysthymia were higher in white and Hispanic groups than in black individuals [63]. However, this study did not find evidence for ethnic variation in bipolar disorder [63]. By contrast, the *prevalence* of depression across 23 countries in the European Social Survey was reported to be higher among ethnic minority groups (7.1%) than the majority-Caucasian population (5.9%) [64]. Meanwhile, research from another cross-sectional survey in England, known as EMPIRIC, noted some ethnic variation in the *prevalence* of CMD, although this was modest [62]. The APMS in England found that the higher CMD annual *prevalence* in ethnic minority groups was largely explained by sociodemographic confounders [65, 66]. In a meta-analysis on the relationship between mood disorders and migration, Swinnen and Selten concluded that, if anything, there was only a marginal increase in mood disorders amongst migrants overall (relative risk (RR) 1.38, 95% CI 1.17–1.62) [67].

Notwithstanding this mixed pattern, some authors have suggested that the experience of interpersonal racism and perceived racial discrimination in society are associated with CMD risk [68, 69]. UK-based research showed that the weekly *prevalence* of CMD increased significantly for Caribbean, Indian, Irish, and Pakistani ethnic groups who had experienced interpersonal racism compared with those reporting no harassment. This effect was particularly pronounced among ethnic minority women [68]. The study also found that the experience of employment-related discrimination increased the *prevalence* of CMD among many of these groups. Similarly, Bhui et al. found that CMD risk was highest among ethnic minorities who reported unfair treatment or racial insults [69]. This relationship was also demonstrated in the Netherlands, where perceived discrimination accounted for an estimated 25% of the depression risk for Turks and South-Asian Surinamese living in the Netherlands [70].

Variations in mental health service use by ethnicity for CMD have also been investigated. A detailed report using National Survey on Drug and Health Data revealed that access to care and quality of care varied according to ethnicity [71]. For example, white adults and those reporting mixed ethnicity were more likely to report using mental health services in the past year, to have a prescription for psychiatric medication, or to receive outpatient services than black adults [71]. Further research from the UK found that black and South Asian ethnic groups were less likely to have seen their doctor in the past year than white individuals, and even after controlling for symptom severity, black individuals were less likely to receive antidepressants than white individuals [65]. For people with depression in the past year in the USA, Latinos, Asians, and African Americans were less likely than non-Latino whites to have access to mental health treatment [72]. These minority groups were also less likely to have received adequate treatment for acute depressive episodes [72]. In general, ethnic minorities are less likely to receive care when they need it and are more likely to receive poor-quality care when they are treated [73]. These disparities in mental health care between ethnic groups could be driving ethnic differences in treated rates of mental health and mental illness, and, as such, public health policy must be developed to improve access to and quality of mental health care for ethnic minority groups.

Although the *prevalence* of CMD between different ethnic groups appears small, there is some evidence that first generation migrants (i.e. born abroad) may be at higher risk. For example, research from Sweden showed that migrants have increased CMD risk than native Swedes, although there was considerable between-group heterogeneity [74], with those from Finland and the Middle East at particularly elevated risk. Similarly, the Israel World Mental Health Survey found that the 12-month CMD *prevalence* was approximately double for migrants of North African or Asian origin than for European or American migrants, even after adjustment for socio-economic factors [75]. Other social determinants of health may underlie these differences, including the experience of structural or interpersonal discrimination. Furthermore, migration is often accompanied by a change in socio-economic position, and Das-Munshi et al. have proposed that downward intragenerational mobility (i.e. movement to a lower socio-economic position, including lower occupational or income status, during an individual's lifetime) is associated with international migration and increased vulnerability to CMD [76]. Other predisposing factors related to migration, including the economic circumstances in a migrant's country of origin, reasons for migration, and experiences in the host country may also play a role in differing CMD risk across migrant groups [77, 78].

Psychotic disorders

The elevated rates of psychotic disorders among ethnic minorities is one of the most replicated areas of psychiatric epidemiological research, providing clear and persuasive evidence that *incidence* rates are elevated in ethnic minority groups [79–81]. Some of the earliest evidence for this came from the seminal work of Ørnulv Ødegaard, who showed that migrant status was a risk factor for psychosis among Norwegians emigrating to Minnesota in the USA in the 1930s [60]. This finding has since been replicated, and extended to the descendants of migrants, in numerous settings [28, 29, 60,

82–87], including the UK [26, 88, 89], Sweden [90–92], Denmark [82, 84], the Netherlands [93], the USA [94], Canada [86, 95], and Israel [96]. The AESOP study in the UK found that ethnic minority groups were at increased risk for all psychotic disorders, with black Caribbean and African groups at highest risk [97]. A replication of this finding in a separate sample in East London found these excess *incidence* rates persisted after adjustment for socio-economic status [98]. A recent systematic review from England [26], where this issue has arguably been studied most often, suggests that the *incidence* of schizophrenia is around five times greater for people of black Caribbean (pooled RR 5.6, 95% CI 3.4–9.2) and African (pooled RR 4.7, 95% CI 3.3–6.8) backgrounds than white British people, with people from South Asian migrants (particularly Pakistani and Bangladeshi [98]) at around double the risk (pooled RR 2.4, 95% CI 1.3–4.5).

Research from the APMS study has shown that the *prevalence* of psychosis is also higher among black minority groups in the UK [66]. However, this study also suggested that the excess psychosis risk among some ethnic minority groups may be partly explained by socio-economic disadvantage [66], a finding only partially supported by comparable *incidence* studies.

The exact reasons for elevated risk of psychotic disorders among migrants and ethnic minority groups is still unknown (for good reviews of plausible hypotheses, see Bhugra [99], Fung et al. [100], and Morgan et al. [101]). The heterogeneity in risk between minority and migrant groups suggests that factors such as visible minority status, discrimination, or psychosocial adversity may be causally relevant to these differences. A meta-analysis found that the effect size was greater for migrants from developing versus developing countries (RR 3.3, 95% CI 2.8–3.9) [29]. One suggested explanation for higher rates among migrant groups is exposure to adversity in the country of origin, not limited to poverty, trauma, or political unrest. In support of this hypothesis, recent data from Hollander et al. demonstrated that refugees in Sweden are at even greater risk of schizophrenia than other non-refugee migrants from the same regions of origin [91]. Visible minority status may also contribute to ongoing adversities experienced by migrants and their descendants in their destination country following immigration [96, 102]. There are several other plausible mechanisms that may underpin these associations, including the suggestion that ethnic minority groups may be more likely to be misdiagnosed with a psychotic disorder than non-migrant groups. Although a body of indirect research does not support this idea (including the absence of differences in psychosis rates between people living in the Caribbean and the white British group in the UK [103–105], and similar symptomatic profiles by ethnicity at first presentation [106]), further research is required to examine all putative drivers of this public mental health tragedy [107].

Suicide

Despite the wide variation between countries in terms of overall suicide rates (see earlier 'Suicide' subsection), these aggregate estimates hide heterogeneity between groups within each country, including by ethnicity. In the UK, high rates of suicide have been demonstrated among black populations, as well as older South Asian women compared with the white British majority group [108]. Among past-year mental health service users, rates of suicide were lower among South Asians men but elevated for older South Asian women versus white individuals [109]. When stratified by age and sex, the research found that suicide rates were elevated among black Caribbean and black African men and women, as well as young women of South Asian origin [109]. In Sweden, suicide has been shown to be elevated among migrants and their children of Finnish (odds ratio (OR)$_{migrants}$ 1.4, OR$_{children\ of\ migrants}$ 1.7) or Western (including Norway, Denmark, Iceland, Germany, UK, USA, Canada) origin (OR$_{migrants}$ 1.2, OR$_{children\ of\ migrants}$ 1.7) [110].

Despite this variation, researchers since the 1920s have noted that suicide rates among immigrants were correlated with rates in their countries of origin [111]. This led researchers to hypothesize that migrants may 'import' their suicide risk [112, 113], as well as typical methods of suicide commonly found in their country of origin [113]. This evidence of the portability of suicide risk, coupled with evidence for the geographical differences in suicide rates between countries (see 'The burden of major psychiatric disorders') may strengthen genetic explanations of suicide risk, which posit that variation of rates between subgroups could be explained by genetic factors. Alternately, important socio-environmental factors that differ between the country of origin and host country may explain these findings [113]. Some studies have also suggested convergence of migrant suicide risk to the host country rate over time following immigration, perhaps owing to adopting new behavioural norms or sociocultural attitudes, which point to contextual and environmental risks for suicide [112, 114]. Others have suggested this may simply be explained by regression to the mean (the phenomenon where repeated measures vary non-systematically around the true mean, so unusually high or low measurements tend to be followed by measurements that are closer to the mean) [113, 115].

Globally, some of the highest rates of suicide are among Indigenous people in Australia, Canada, New Zealand, Greenland, and the USA [116, 117]. Estimates from Australia showed that the rates among Indigenous peoples was more than twice as high as those for non-Indigenous Australians [118]. For Inuit peoples, a group of Indigenous peoples in Canada, the suicide rate is 11 times higher than the Canadian average [119].

How the epidemiological burden of major psychiatric disorders translates into the potential for intervention

In section 'The burden of major psychiatric disorders' we provided an overview of the burden of major psychiatric disorders worldwide, and how these varied by the tenets of person and place. In the previous section, we gave greater detail on how these psychiatric disorders varied by migration and ethnicity, two factors along which there is considerable inequality in how the mental health burden is shared within populations. While a major goal of psychiatric epidemiology is to elucidate the underlying risk factors that cause these inequalities, it is also important to consider what impact the prevention of excesses risks may have on the global burden of psychiatric disorders. By doing so, psychiatric epidemiology can inform public mental health, policy interventions, and health service planning. In this section we consider, briefly, a thought experiment, by asking *if a risk factor for psychiatric disorder could be removed from the population, assuming causality, what proportion of cases could be prevented?* This question lies at the heart of the formula for the *population attributable risk* (PAR), which jointly considers the *measure of association* (i.e. a risk ratio), as well as the level (*prevalence*) of the exposure in the population [3]. Specifically, PAR estimates the reduction in *incidence* of an illness that would be achieved if the population was not exposed to the risk factor [3]. While PAR is useful for translating epidemiological risks into *measures of impact* for public health, it is based on a number of assumptions, including that a causal relationship between exposure and outcome exists, that removal of the exposure has a direct reduction on the outcome, and that the risk factor itself is modifiable (see Greenland and Rothman [3] and Rockhill et al. [120] for more coverage of these issues). Clearly, the latter is—depending on interpretation—both impossible and potentially troubling with respect to the issues of migration and ethnicity discussed in the previous section. This makes the search for the drivers of the increased risks for some migrant and ethnic minority groups an imperative issue for contemporary psychiatric epidemiology. If we can move closer to the identification of these risk factors, we can get a better handle on their public mental health impact. Nonetheless, PARs for the respective roles of migration and ethnicity in relation to psychiatric disorders (see later) may still be ideologically useful, as beacons for the potentially preventable burden of disorder in the population, if all underlying factors could be identified and prevented.

One challenge with applying research to public health interventions is that often the risk factors with the highest predictive power at the individual level (i.e. a large risk ratio) have a small population impact (i.e. because they are rare). Thus, epidemiological evidence that takes into account the magnitude of risk introduced by a risk factor, as well as the exposure patterns in the population is a powerful tool for public health intervention. Furthermore, PARs can be used to indicate the type of prevention strategies that may be most amenable to a given intervention. For example, as Geoffrey Rose made clear in his seminal 1984 lecture [121], population-level strategies may take priority over individual high-risk prevention approaches, when 'a large number of people at a small risk may give rise to more cases of disease than the small number who are at high risk'. This *prevention paradox* speaks to why the use of PAR can be important for public health interventions, as it provides a metric of which factors could result in the greatest potential impact.

Common mental disorders

Considering the wide range of risk factors for CMD, knowledge of PAR can potentially be used to help prioritize interventions and make informed use of limited public health resources. The multifactorial causes of CMD mean efforts to target high-risk individuals may be less effective from a public health perspective than population-based approaches. However, one major issue in designing such interventions is the level of unmet psychiatric need in the community which may never present to mental health services. Recognizing that previous episodes of depression and anxiety are one of the strongest predictors of future risk, the National Health Service in England launched a new model for treating psychological distress in the population in 2008, known as adult Improving Access to Psychological Therapies (IAPT). These services are designed to offer a stepped-care, evidence-based approach to treatment appropriate to the presenting psychological distress, including cognitive behavioural therapy and other treatments for which there is sufficient evidence as recommended by the National Institute for Health and Care Excellence [122].

These therapies are delivered by trained, accredited practitioners. Importantly, one major focus of IAPT provision is ease of access and use of the service. The national IAPT service model is designed to be highly accessible, with low barriers to entry (both self-referrals and referral via primary care are accepted), with services delivered by guided self-help, via telephone or in person, depending on the severity of the presenting symptoms. IAPT services also offer access to an employment adviser to reduce unemployment and lost work days, through both absenteeism and presenteeism. The IAPT intervention is designed to foster greater adherence to the intervention, be cost-effective (although whether it achieves this is unclear [123]), reduce stigma, and, most importantly, uses psychological approaches that have been shown to improve mental health outcomes for a larger proportion of society than would previously have had access to services [124, 125].

Elsewhere, other approaches to CMD prevention have identified targets for prevention. Research on adolescents in the USA, for example, has shown significant PARs across many areas, including interpersonal relationships (e.g. low family connectedness, including low understanding (PAR 31%), low attention (PAR 29%), and low paternal warmth (PAR 23%)); affect regulation and cognition (e.g. baseline depressed mood (PAR 39%)); delinquent/near-delinquent activities (e.g. early sexual relationships (PAR 41%)); and low levels of constructive community involvement conferred significant PAR to adolescent depression (e.g. not attending youth group (PAR 36%)) [126]. The PAR estimates from this study demonstrate that there are many risk factors from multiple domains that increase the risk of CMD. Further, this information can guide the focus of preventative interventions to areas such as family connectedness or constructive community engagement. Similarly, Goodman et al. [127] demonstrated that socio-economic factors contributed a significant PAR to adolescent depression: 40% and 26% for education and income, respectively [127]. If these socio-economic factors are causal, we would expect substantial reductions in the *incidence* of CMD if effective interventions were put in place to remove the damaging effect of these risk factors, including approaches highlighted in the WHO report on effective interventions and policy options for preventing mental disorders. The WHO has compiled a report highlighting the evidence for effective interventions and policy interventions on housing, education, or economic insecurity that have been shown to reduce the burden of CMD [128, 129].

Schizophrenia and other psychotic disorders

Both ethnic minority status and urbanicity have been identified as important risk factors for schizophrenia and other psychotic disorders, and the PAR for these two risk factors have been estimated in the UK [130]. In terms of ethnicity, the paper suggested that up to 22% of cases of psychotic disorders could be prevented if we were able to identify and remove all exposures that underlie the elevated risk of psychosis in ethnic minority populations. Furthermore, if it were possible to identify and remove all factors associated with the elevated risk among those living in urban environments, 27% of cases of non-affective psychosis could be prevented [130]. When considered together, the joint PAR for ethnicity and urbanicity in relation to non-affective psychosis was over 60% [130], reflecting possible synergistic effects between these two exposures. However, while these high PAR estimates suggest that urbanicity and ethnicity may be important targets for population strategies, the authors point out that it is the underlying drivers of risk that these markers represent which need to be identified, tested, and established as causal mechanisms for psychosis. Furthermore, any prevention strategy targeting a non-specific exposure such as 'urban living' is unlikely to be practical or cost-effective given the absolute *incidence* of psychotic disorders [130].

Suicide

The *prevention paradox* is clearly demonstrated in suicide prevention efforts. The robust association between psychiatric disorders and suicide has led many suicide prevention efforts to focus on individuals with mental illness, as they have high risk of suicide, despite the relatively low population *prevalence* of mental illnesses. By contrast, socio-economic factors, like education, income, social exclusion, or deprivation, are more distally associated with suicide risk, but because they are more commonly distributed in the population, efforts to make even small improvements in socio-economic conditions have the potential to substantially reduce suicide risk, if causal.

In their systematic review, Li et al. estimated the *population attributable risk* associated with psychotic disorders and socio-economic factors were of similar magnitude [131]. For example, the PAR in males for low educational achievement was 41% and low occupational status was 33%, whereas the PAR for affective disorders was 26% and substance use disorders was 9% [131]. Similar findings were also observed in females, suggesting that prevention strategies focusing on either would produce similar population-level effects on suicide [131]. This finding was replicated in Denmark using population registers, and the authors indicated the evidence highlights the need to combine suicide prevention programs that focused on both high risk groups (i.e. with mental illness), and on population interventions targeting unemployment and improving social cohesion [132].

Public mental health and variation in rates by ethnicity

In this chapter, we have paid particular attention to how the rates of schizophrenia and other psychotic disorders, CMD, and suicide vary by ethnicity, most notably for psychotic disorders. This issue has a particular public mental health challenge, given the inequality in risk faced by some ethnic minority groups. Ethnicity is not, of course, a modifiable risk factor, making it vital to consider why the health of minority populations is negatively influenced when thinking about putative intervention strategies to reduce harm. Mental health promotion and illness prevention efforts need to first identify the mechanisms that drive the increased rates in ethnic minority groups, and then find effective interventions to mitigate this risk. To use the well-known analogy in public health, we can design culturally sensitive and appropriate interventions that pull people out of the stream; however, it is important for us to consider what is causing so many to fall into the stream in the first place. There is an ethical imperative in public health to pay attention to large systemic shifts that are required to remove the excess burden of mental illnesses among ethnic minority populations. This requires cross-sectoral, intersectional efforts, as the reasons certain population groups are more likely to end up in the 'stream' of poor mental health have to do with systems of power, privilege, advantage, and systemic racism that are rooted in legacies of discrimination and disadvantage. The intersectionality lens is an important consideration as risks, like ethnic minority status, urban living, and low socio-economic status, tend to cluster, further exacerbating the increased risks. At minimum, 'preventive interventions must not directly affirm or contribute to inequality or injustice' [133]. However, an ethical approach insists that we go beyond this to actively promote equity and justice. While there does not seem to be any simple answers for how to address these systemic issues of power and injustice that may be contributing to increased risks of major psychiatric outcomes for marginalized populations, researchers and public health professionals need to continue to identify putative social and environmental determinants of mental health in order to build an evidence base around the potentially modifiable risk factors upon which we can intervene to improve population mental health.

References

1. Porta M (ed.). *A Dictionary of Epidemiology*. 6th ed. Oxford: Oxford University Press, 2016.
2. Tripepi G, Jager KJ, Dekker FW, Wanner C, Zoccali C. Measures of effect: relative risks, odds ratios, risk difference, and "number needed to treat." *Kidney Int* 2007; 72: 789–791.
3. Greenland S, Rothman KJ. Measures of effect and measures of association. In: Rothman KJ, Greenland S (eds). *Modern Epidemiology*. 2nd ed. Philadelphia, PA: Lippincott Willams and Wilkins, 1998, pp. 47–66.
4. Perez L, Künzli N. From measures of effects to measures of potential impact. *Int J Public Health* 2009; 54: 45–48.
5. Vos T, Allen C, Arora M, et al. Global, regional, and national incidence, prevalence, and years lived with disability for 310 diseases and injuries, 1990–2015: a systematic analysis for the Global Burden of Disease Study 2015. *Lancet* 2016; 388: 1545–1602.
6. Laursen TM, Munk-Olsen T, Vestergaard M. Life expectancy and cardiovascular mortality in persons with schizophrenia. *Curr Opin Psychiatry* 2012; 25: 83–88.
7. Kirkbride JB, Jackson D, Perez J, et al. A population-level prediction tool for the incidence of first-episode psychosis: translational epidemiology based on cross-sectional data. *BMJ Open* 2013; 3: 1–14.
8. Steel Z, Marnane C, Iranpour C, et al. The global prevalence of common mental disorders: a systematic review and meta-analysis 1980-2013. *Int J Epidemiol* 2014; 43: 476–493.
9. Regier DA, Myers JK, Kramer M, et al. The NIMH Epidemiologic Catchment Area program. Historical context, major objectives, and study population characteristics. *Arch Gen Psychiatry* 1984; 41: 934–941.
10. Kessler RC, Demler O, Frank RG, et al. Prevalence and treatment of mental disorders, 1990 to 2003. *N Engl J Med* 2005; 352: 2515–2523.
11. Regier DA, Boyd JH, Burke JD, Jr, et al. One-month prevalence of mental disorders in the United States. Based on five Epidemiologic Catchment Area sites. *Arch Gen Psychiatry* 1988; 45: 977–986.
12. Regier DA, Farmer ME, Rae DS, et al. One-month prevalence of mental disorders in the United States and sociodemographic characteristics: the Epidemiologic Catchment Area study. *Acta Psychiatr Scand* 1993; 88: 35–47.
13. Silver E, Mulvey EP, Swanson JW. Neighborhood structural characteristics and mental disorder: Faris and Dunham revisited. *Soc Sci Med* 2002; 55: 1457–1470.
14. Kessler RC, McGonagle KA, Zhao S, et al. Lifetime and 12-month prevalence of DSM-III-R psychiatric disorders in the United States. Results from the National Comorbidity Survey. *Arch Gen Psychiatry* 1994; 51: 8–19.

15. Jenkins R, Lewis G, Bebbington P, et al. The National Psychiatric Morbidity surveys of Great Britain—initial findings from the household survey. *Psychol Med* 1997; 27: 775–789.

16. Singleton N, Bumpstead R, O'Brien M, Lee A, Meltzer H. *Psychiatric Morbidity Among Adults Living in Private Households, 2000.* London: Her Majesty's Stationary Office, 2001.

17. McManus S, Meltzer H, Brugha T, Bebbington P, Jenkins R. *Adult Psychiatric Morbidity in England, 2007: Results of a Household Survey.* London: The NHS Information Centre for Health and Social Care, 2009.

18. McManus S, Bebbington PE, Jenkins R, Brugha T. Mental health and wellbeing in England: Adult Psychiatric Morbidity Survey 2014 Executive Summary. Available at: http://content.digital.nhs.uk/catalogue/PUB21748/apms-2014-exec-summary.pdf (2016, accessed 25 February 2018).

19. Saha S, Chant D, Welham J, McGrath J. A systematic review of the prevalence of schizophrenia. *PLOS MED* 2005; 2: e141.

20. Jablensky A, Sartorius N, Ernberg G, et al. Schizophrenia: manifestations, incidence and course in different cultures. A World Health Organization ten-country study. *Psychol Med* 1997; 20: 1–97.

21. Morgan C, Fearon P, Hutchinson G, et al. Duration of untreated psychosis and ethnicity in the AESOP first-onset psychosis study. *Psychol Med* 2006; 36: 239–247.

22. Melle I, Larsen TK, Haahr U, et al. Reducing the duration of untreated first-episode psychosis: effects on clinical presentation. *Arch Gen Psychiatry* 2004; 61: 143–150.

23. Crow TJ. Schizophrenia as the price that homo sapiens pays for language: a resolution of the central paradox in the origin of the species. *Brain Res Rev* 2000; 31: 118–129.

24. McGrath JJ. Myths and plain truths about schizophrenia epidemiology—the NAPE lecture 2004. *Acta Psychiatr Scand* 2005; 111:4–11.

25. McGrath J, Saha S, Welham J, El Saadi O, MacCauley C, Chant D. A systematic review of the incidence of schizophrenia: the distribution of rates and the influence of sex, urbanicity, migrant status and methodology. *BMC Med* 2004; 2: 1–22.

26. Kirkbride JB, Errazuriz A, Croudace TJ, et al. Incidence of schizophrenia and other psychoses in England, 1950-2009: A systematic review and meta-analyses. *PLOS ONE* 2012; 7: e31660.

27. March D, Hatch SL, Morgan C, et al. Psychosis and place. *Epidemiol Rev* 2008; 30: 84–100.

28. Bourque F, van der Ven E, Malla A. A meta-analysis of the risk for psychotic disorders among first- and second-generation immigrants. *Psychol Med* 2011; 41: 897–910.

29. Cantor-Graae E, Selten J-PP. Schizophrenia and migration: a meta-analysis and review. *Am J Psychiatry* 2005; 162: 12–24.

30. Kirkbride JB, Fearon P, Morgan C, et al. Heterogeneity in incidence rates of schizophrenia and other psychotic syndromes: findings from the 3-center AeSOP study. *Arch Gen Psychiatry* 2006; 63: 250–268.

31. Leao TS, Sundquist J, Frank G, Johansson LM, Johansson SE, Sundquist K. Incidence of schizophrenia or other psychoses in first- and second-generation immigrants: a national cohort study. *J Nerv Ment Dis* 2006; 194: 27–33.

32. Mortensen PB, Pedersen CB, Westergaard T, et al. Effects of family history and place and season of birth on the risk of schizophrenia. *N Engl J Med* 1999; 340: 603–608.

33. Pedersen CB, Mors O, Bertelsen A, et al. A comprehensive nationwide study of the incidence rate and lifetime risk for treated mental disorders. *JAMA Psychiatry* 2014; 71: 573–581.

34. Hogerzeil SJ, van Hemert AM, Rosendaal FR, Susser E, Hoek HW. Direct comparison of first-contact versus longitudinal register-based case finding in the same population: early evidence that the incidence of schizophrenia may be three times higher than commonly reported. *Psychol Med* 2014; 44: 3481–3490.

35. Hogerzeil SJ, van Hemert AM, Veling W, Hoek HW. Incidence of schizophrenia among migrants in the Netherlands: a direct comparison of first contact longitudinal register approaches. *Soc Psychiatry Psychiatr Epidemiol* 2017; 52: 147–154.

36. Dalman C, Broms J, Cullberg J, Allebeck P. Young cases of schizophrenia identified in a national inpatient register. *Soc Psychiatry Psychiatr Epidemiol* 2002; 37: 527–531.

37. Löffler W, Häfner H, Fätkenheuer B, et al. Validation of Danish case register diagnosis for schizophrenia. *Acta Psychiatr Scand* 1994; 90: 196–203.

38. Allebeck P. The use of population based registers in psychiatric research. *Acta Psychiatr Scand* 2009; 120: 386–391.

39. Claassen CA, Yip PS, Corcoran P, Bossarte RM, Lawrence BA, Currier GW. National suicide rates a century after Durkheim: do we know enough to estimate error? *Suicide Life Threat Behav* 2010; 40: 193–223.

40. Pitman A, Krysinska K, Osborn D, et al. Suicide in young men. Lancet 2012; 379: 2383–2392.

41. Fairweather-Schmidt AK, Anstey KJ. Prevalence of suicidal behaviours in two Australian general population surveys: methodological considerations when comparing across studies. *Soc Psychiatry Psychiatr Epidemiol* 2012; 47: 515–522.

42. Evans E, Hawton K, Rodham K, Deeks J. The prevalence of suicidal phenomena in adolescents: a systematic review of population-based studies. *Suicide Life Threat Behav* 2005; 35: 239–250.

43. Snowdon J, Phillips J, Zhong B, Yamauchi T, Chiu HFK, Conwell Y. Changes in age patterns of suicide in Australia, the United States, Japan and Hong Kong. *J Affect Disord* 2017; 211: 12–19.

44. Office for National Statistics. Suicides in the UK: 2015 registrations. Available at: https://www.ons.gov.uk/peoplepopulationandcommunity/birthsdeathsandmarriages/deaths/bulletins/suicidesintheunitedkingdom/2015registrations (2016, accessed 18 February 2018).

45. World Health Organization. Suicide data. Available at: http://www.who.int/mental_health/prevention/suicide/suicideprevent/en/ (2016, accessed 15 January 2017).

46. Yip PSF, Liu KY, Hu J, Song XM. Suicide rates in China during a decade of rapid social changes. *Soc Psychiatry Psychiatr Epidemiol* 2005; 40: 792–798.

47. Fontanella CA, Hiance-Steelesmith DL, Phillips GS, et al. Widening rural–urban disparities in youth suicides, United States, 1996–2010. *JAMA Pediatr* 2015; 169: 466.

48. Patel V, Ramasundarahettige C, Vijayakumar L, et al. Suicide mortality in India: a nationally representative survey. Lancet 2012; 379: 2343–2351.

49. Levin KA, Leyland AH. Urban/rural inequalities in suicide in Scotland, 1981–1999. *Soc Sci Med* 2005; 60: 2877–2890.

50. Ngamini Ngui A, Apparicio P, Moltchanova E, Vasiliadis H-M. Spatial analysis of suicide mortality in Québec: spatial clustering and area factor correlates. *Psychiatry Res* 2014; 220: 20–30.

51. Kapusta ND, Zorman A, Etzersdorfer E, Ponocny-Seliger E, Jandl-Jager E, Sonneck G. Rural–urban differences in Austrian suicides. *Soc Psychiatry Psychiatr Epidemiol* 2008; 43: 311–318.

52. Searles VB, Valley MA, Hedegaard H, Betz ME. Suicides in urban and rural counties in the United States, 2006–2008. *Crisis* 2014; 35: 18–26.

53. Qi X, Hu W, Page A, Tong S. Dynamic pattern of suicide in Australia, 1986–2005: a descriptive-analytic study. *BMJ Open* 2014; 4: e005311.

54. Chang SS, Sterne JA, Wheeler BW, Lu TH, Lin JJ, Gunnell D. Geography of suicide in Taiwan: spatial patterning and socioeconomic correlates. *Health Place* 2011; 17: 641–650.

55. Park B, Lester D. Rural and urban suicide in South Korea. *Psychol Rep.* 2012; 111: 495–497.

56. Frasquilho D, Matos MG, Salonna F, et al. Mental health outcomes in times of economic recession: a systematic literature review. *BMC Public Health* 2016; 16: 115.

57. Martin-Carrasco M, Evans-Lacko S, Dom G, et al. EPA guidance on mental health and economic crises in Europe. *Eur Arch Psychiatry Clin Neurosci* 2016; 266: 89–124.

58. Durkheim E, Spaulding JA, Simpson G. *Suicide: A Study in Sociology.* London: Routledge & Kegan Paul, 1952.

59. Nazroo JY. The structuring of ethnic inequalities in health: Economic position, racial discrimination, and racism. *Am J Public Health* 2003; 93: 277–284.

60. Ødegaard Ø. Emigration and insanity. *Acta Psychiatr Neurol* 1932; 4 (Suppl.): 1–206.

61. Robins L, Locke B, Regier D. An overview of psychiatric disorders in America. In: Robins LN, Regier DA (eds). *Psychiatric Disorders in America: The Epidemiologic Catchment Area Study*. Free Press: New York, 1991, pp. 228–267.

62. Weich S, Nazroo J, Sproston K, et al. Common mental disorders and ethnicity in England: the EMPIRIC study. *Psychol Med* 2004; 34: 1543–1551.

63. Weissman MM, Bruce ML, Leaf PJ, Florio LP, Holzer C, III. Affective disorders. In: Robins L, Regier DA (eds). *Psychiatric Disorders in America: The Epidemiologic Catchment Area Study*. Free Press: New York, 1991, pp. 53–80.

64. Missinne S, Bracke P. Depressive symptoms among immigrants and ethnic minorities: a population based study in 23 European countries. *Soc Psychiatry Psychiatr Epidemiol* 2012; 47: 97–109.

65. Cooper C, Spiers N, Livingston G, et al. Ethnic inequalities in the use of health services for common mental disorders in England. *Soc Psychiatry Psychiatr Epidemiol* 2013; 48: 685–692.

66. Brugha T, Jenkins R, Bebbington P, Meltzer H, Lewis G, Farrell M. Risk factors and the prevalence of neurosis and psychosis in ethnic groups in Great Britain. *Soc Psychiatry Psychiatr Epidemiol* 2004; 39: 939–946.

67. Swinnen SGHA, Selten JP. Mood disorders and migration: meta-analysis. *Br J Psychiatry* 2007; 190: 6–10.

68. Karlsen S, Nazroo JY, McKenzie K, Bhui K, Weich S. Racism, psychosis and common mental disorder among ethnic minority groups in England. *Psychol Med* 2005; 35: 1795–1803.

69. Bhui K, Stansfeld S, McKenzie K, Karlsen S, Nazroo J, Weich S. Racial/ethnic discrimination and common mental disorders among workers: findings from the EMPIRIC study of ethnic minority groups in the United Kingdom. *Am J Public Health* 2005; 95: 496–501.

70. Ikram UZ, Snijder MB, Fassaert TJL, Schene AH, Kunst AE, Stronks K. The contribution of perceived ethnic discrimination to the prevalence of depression. *Eur J Public Health* 2015; 25: 243–248.

71. Substance Abuse and Mental Health Services Administration(SAMHSA). *Racial/Ethnic Differences in Mental Health Service Use Among Adults*. HKHS Publication No. SMA-15-4906. Rockville, MD: SAMHSA, 2015.

72. Algeeria M, Chatterji P, Well SK, et al. Disparity in depression among racial and ethnic minority populations in the United States. *Psychiatr Serv* 2008; 59: 1264–1272.

73. McGuire T, Miranda J. Racial and ethnic disparities in mental health care: evidence and policy implications. *Health Aff (Millwood)* 2008; 27: 393–403.

74. Gilliver SC, Sundquist J, Li X, Sundquist K. Recent research on the mental health of immigrants to Sweden: a literature review. *Eur J Public Health* 2014; 24(Suppl. 1): 72–79.

75. Nakash O, Levav I, Gal G. Common mental disorders in immigrant and second-generation respondents: results from the Israel-based World Mental Health Survey. *Int J Soc Psychiatry* 2013; 59: 508–515.

76. Das-Munshi J, Leavey G, Stansfeld SA, Prince MJ. Migration, social mobility and common mental disorders: critical review of the literature and meta-analysis. *Ethn Health* 2012; 17: 17–53.

77. Lindert J, Ehrenstein OS von, Priebe S, Mielck A, Brähler E. Depression and anxiety in labor migrants and refugees—a systematic review and meta-analysis. *Soc Sci Med* 2009; 69: 246–257.

78. Porter M, Haslam N. Predisplacement and postdisplacement of refugees and internally displaced persons. *JAMA* 2005; 294: 610–612.

79. Schwartz RC, Blankenship DM. Racial disparities in psychotic disorder diagnosis: a review of empirical literature. *World J Psychiatry* 2014; 4: 133–140.

80. Kirkbride J, Errazuriz A, Croudace T, et al. *Systematic Review of the Incidence and Prevalence of Schizophrenia and Other Psychoses in England*. London: Department of Health Policy Research Programme, 2012.

81. King M, Coker E, Leavey G, Hoare A, Johnson-Sabine E. Incidence of psychotic illness in London: comparison of ethnic groups. *BMJ* 1994; 309: 1115–1119.

82. Cantor-Graae E, Pedersen CB. Full spectrum of psychiatric disorders related to foreign migration. *JAMA Psychiatry* 2013; 70: 427.

83. Cantor-Graae E, Pedersen CB. Risk of schizophrenia in second-generation immigrants: a Danish population-based cohort study. *Psychol Med* 2007; 37: 485–494.

84. Pedersen CB, Demontis D, Pedersen MS, et al. Risk of schizophrenia in relation to parental origin and genome-wide divergence. *Psychol Med* 2012; 42: 1515–1521.

85. Amad A, Guardia D, Salleron J, Thomas P, Roelandt JL, Vaiva G. Increased prevalence of psychotic disorders among third-generation migrants: Results from the French Mental Health in General Population survey. *Schizophr Res* 2013; 147: 193–195.

86. Kirkbride JB, Hollander AC. Migration and risk of psychosis in the Canadian context. *CMAJ* 2015; 187: 637–638.

87. Selten JP, Cantor-Graae E, Kahn RS. Migration and schizophrenia. *Curr Opin Psychiatry* 2007; 20: 111–115.

88. Coid JW, Kirkbride JB, Barker D, et al. Raised incidence rates of all psychoses among migrant groups: findings from the East London first episode psychosis study. *Arch Gen Psychiatry* 2008; 65: 1250–1258.

89. Tortelli A, Errazuriz A, Croudace T, et al. Schizophrenia and other psychotic disorders in caribbean-born migrants and their descendants in england: systematic review and meta-analysis of incidence rates, 1950–2013. *Soc Psychiatry Psychiatr Epidemiol* 2015; 50: 1039–1055.

90. Cantor-Graae E, Zolkowska K, McNeil TF. Increased risk of psychotic disorder among immigrants in Malmö: a 3-year first-contact study. *Psychol Med* 2005; 35: 1155–1163.

91. Hollander A-C, Dal H, Lewis G, Magnusson C, Kirkbride JB, Dalman C. Refugee migration and risk of schizophrenia and other non-affective psychoses: cohort study of 1.3 million people in Sweden. *BMJ* 2016; 352: i1030.

92. Zolkowska K, Cantor-Graae E, McNeil TF. Increased rates of psychosis among immigrants to Sweden: is migration a risk factor for psychosis? *Psychol Med* 2001; 31: 669–678.

93. Veling W. Ethnic minority position and risk for psychotic disorders. *Curr Opin Psychiatry* 2013; 26: 166–171.

94. Bresnahan M, Begg MD, Brown A, et al. Race and risk of schizophrenia in a US birth cohort: another example of health disparity? *Int J Epidemiol* 2007; 36: 751–758.

95. Smith GN, Boydell J, Murray RM, et al. The incidence of schizophrenia in European immigrants to Canada. *Schizophr Res* 2006; 87: 205–211.

96. Weiser M, Werbeloff N, Vishna T, et al. Elaboration on immigration and risk for schizophrenia. *Psychol Med* 2008; 38: 1113–1119.

97. Fearon P, Kirkbride JB, Morgan C, et al. Incidence of schizophrenia and other psychoses in ethnic minority groups: results from the MRC AESOP Study. *Psychol Med* 2006; 36: 1541–1550.

98. Kirkbride JB, Barker D, Cowden F, et al. Psychoses, ethnicity and socio-economic status. *Br J Psychiatry* 2008; 193: 18–24.

99. Bhugra D. Migration and schizophrenia. *Acta Psychiatr Scand* 2000; 102: 68–73.

100. Fung WLA, Jones PB, Bhugra D. Ethnicity and mental health: the example of schizophrenia and related psychoses in migrant populations in the Western world. *Psychiatry* 2009; 8: 335–341.

101. Morgan C, Charalambides M, Hutchinson G, Murray RM. Migration, ethnicity, and psychosis: toward a sociodevelopmental model. *Schizophr Bull* 2010; 36: 655–664.

102. Littlewood R, Lipsedge M. Migration, ethnicity and diagnosis. *Psychiatr Clin (Basel)* 1978; 11: 15–22.

103. Hickling FW, Rodgers-Johnson P. The incidence of first contact schizophrenia in Jamaica. *Br J Psychiatry* 1995; 167: 193–196.

104. Bhugra D, Hilwig M, Hossein B, et al. First-contact incidence rates of schizophrenia in Trinidad and one-year follow-up. *Br J Psychiatry* 1996; 169: 587–592.

105. Mahy GE, Mallett R, Leff J, Bhugra D. First-contact incidence rate of schizophrenia on Barbados. *Br J Psychiatry* 1999; 175: 28–33.

106. Demjaha A, Morgan K, Morgan C, et al. Combining dimensional and categorical representation of psychosis: the way forward for DSM-V and ICD-11? *Psychol Med* 2009; 39: 1943–1955.

107. Morgan C, Hutchinson G. The social determinants of psychosis in migrant and ethnic minority populations: a public health tragedy. *Psychol Med* 2009 (Epub ahead of print).

108. McKenzie K, Bhui K, Nanchahal K, Blizard B. Suicide rates in people of South Asian origin in England and Wales: 1993–2003. *Br J Psychiatry* 2008; 193: 406–409.

109. Bhui KS, McKenzie K. Rates and risk factors by ethnic group for suicides within a year of contact with mental health services in England and Wales. *Psychiatr Serv* 2008; 59: 414–420.

110. Hjern A, Allebeck P. Suicide in first- and second-generation immigrants in Sweden. A comparative study. *Soc Psychiatry Psychiatr Epidemiol* 2002; 37: 423–429.

111. Cavan R. *Suicide.* Chicago, IL: University of Chicago Press, 1928.

112. Spallek J, Reeske A, Norredam M, Nielsen SS, Lehnhardt J, Razum O. Suicide among immigrants in Europe—a systematic literature review. *Eur J Public Health* 2015; 25: 63–71.

113. Voracek M, Loibl LM. Consistency of immigrant and country-of-birth suicide rates: a meta-analysis. *Acta Psychiatr Scand* 2008; 118: 259–271.

114. Kliewer E. Immigrant suicide in Australia, Canada, England and Wales, and the United States. *J Aust Popul Assoc* 1991; 8: 111–128.

115. Barnett AG, van der Pols JC, Dobson AJ. Regression to the mean: what it is and how to deal with it. *Int J Epidemiol* 2005; 34: 215–220.

116. Leenaars A a, Echohawk M, Lester D, Leenaars L. What suicide among indigenous peoples: what does the international knowledge tell us? *Can J Native Stud* 2007; 2: 479–501.

117. McKenzie K, Serfaty M, Crawford M. Suicide in ethnic minority groups. *Br J Psychiatry* 2003; 183: 100–101.

118. Ferguson M, Baker A, Young S, Procter N. Understanding suicide among aboriginal communities. *Aust Nurs Midwifery J* 2016; 23: 36.

119. Crawford A. Inuit take action towards suicide prevention. *Lancet* 2016; 388: 1036–1038.

120. Rockhill B, Newman B, Weinberg C. Use and misuse of population attributable fractions. *Am J Public Health* 1998; 88: 15–19.

121. Rose G. Sick individuals and sick populations. *Int J Epidemiol* 1985; 14: 32–38.

122. Clark DM. Implementing NICE guidelines for the psychological treatment of depression and anxiety disorders: the IAPT experience. *Int Rev Psychiatry* 2011; 23: 318–327.

123. Mukuria C, Brazier J, Barkham M, et al. Cost-effectiveness of an Improving Access to Psychological Therapies service. *Br J Psychiatry* 2013; 202: 220–227.

124. Hammond GC, Croudace TJ, Radhakrishnan M, et al. Comparative effectiveness of cognitive therapies delivered face-to-face or over the telephone: an observational study using propensity methods. *PLOS ONE* 2012; 7: e42916.

125. Richards DA, Suckling R. Improving access to psychological therapies: phase IV prospective cohort study. *Br J Clin Psychol* 2009; 48: 377–396.

126. Booth KVP, Paunesku D, Msall M, Fogel J, Van Voorhees BW. Using population attributable risk to help target preventive interventions for adolescent depression. *Int J Adolesc Med Health* 2008; 20: 307–319.

127. Goodman E, Slap GB, Huang B. The public health impact of socioeconomic status on adolescent depression and obesity. *Am J Public Health* 2003; 93: 1844–1850.

128. Saxena S, Jané-Llopis E, Hosman C. Prevention of mental and behavioural disorders: implications for policy and practice. *World Psychiatry* 2006; 5: 5–14.

129. World Health Organization (WHO). *Prevention of Mental Disorders: Effective Interventions and Policy Options.* Geneva: WHO, 2004.

130. Kirkbride J, Coid JW, Morgan C, et al. Translating the epidemiology of psychosis into public mental health: evidence, challenges and future prospects. *J Public Ment Health* 2010; 9: 4–14.

131. Li Z, Page A, Martin G, Taylor R. Attributable risk of psychiatric and socio-economic factors for suicide from individual-level, population-based studies: a systematic review. *Soc Sci Med* 2011; 72: 608–616.

132. Qin P, Agerbo E, Mortensen PB. Suicide risk in relation to socioeconomic, demographic, psychiatric, and familial factors: a national register-based study of all suicides in Denmark, 1981–1997. *Am J Psychiatry* 2003; 160: 765–772.

133. Mrazek PJ, Haggerty RJ. *Reducing Risks for Mental Disorders: Frontiers for Preventive Intervention Research.* Washington, DC: National Academy Press, 1994.

CHAPTER 10

Critical epidemiology

Felix J. Rosenberg and Daniel Miranda

Introduction: what is health in critical epidemiology?

Prevailing texts consider epidemiology as a set of more or less complex and sophisticated tools for quantitative analysis of the distribution of specific diseases or health impairments according to predefined variables. It can also be referred to as a scientific discipline that aims to understand the complex interactions occurring during the health and disease process in populations, and, accordingly, orient the health systems at the various geographical levels to organize their public health plans and actions [1].

As a science (and not merely a tool) epidemiology is concerned with health as a *process* (and not a state or condition), a continuous and permanent movement across a subjective and abstract condition of *perfect health* and the various changing degrees of disease, illness, and/or sickness.

The idea of epidemiology as the study of 'health impairments' leads us to the concept of health as the *absence of disease*. Its frame of reference is what some authors consider the disease/illness/sickness complex [2]. According to the World Health Organization (WHO), 'Health is a state of complete physical, mental and social well-being and not merely the absence of disease or infirmity' [3]. This statement is crucial if we want to consider epidemiology as the science searching for explanations and proposals to reach the long desired dream of 'health for all', as established in 1977, by the World Health Assembly (WHA). Let us remember that WHA decided, on that occasion, that the main social target of governments and of the WHO should be the attainment by all the people of the world by the year 2000 of a level of health that would permit them to lead a 'socially and economically productive life' [4].

Naomar Almeida-Filho discusses quite extensively the issue of health and disease definitions, from the biological, semantic, anthropological, and philosophical points of view, trying to build what he calls a 'General Theory of Health', which, according to the author, is still to be built [2]. Juan Garay amends the WHO definition to include the concepts of equity and sustainability. He proposes that health is 'A state of well-being through the *adjustment* to physical, social and mental challenges in an *equitable and sustainable* way which enables the attainment of best feasible standards of health by all peoples' [5] (emphasis added).

The original people of the Andean civilizations interpret health as 'Sumak Kawsay', translated as 'good living', meaning in harmony with themselves, with their community, and with their social and natural environment. Diseases or other health impairments are not that important as long as they do not really interfere with that overall harmonic life. On the contrary, there cannot be good living just because of the absence of recognizable disease signals as long as the individual does not feel in harmony with his or her environment. The Constitution of Ecuador incorporates this concept of health, fully transforming the rights to health and the duties of the State [6]. This sense of health and disease or somehow similar meanings is still prevailing in many cultures other than the Anglo-Saxon-dominating world civilization.

For our purposes, we shall consider health as a multidimensional individual, cultural, social, and economic construction, and a human and social right that shall be equally enjoyed by all the people of the world, and (critical) epidemiology as the science of understanding and describing the distribution of health and of contributing to the achievement of this right.

Critical epidemiology is three times critical

1. Within an epistemological (philosophical) approach, critical epidemiology is critical of the prevailing and commonly used quantitative, clinical, or formal epidemiology. Despite full acknowledgement of the need to quantify health and disease objects and events, epidemiology should be considered as a science, having populations (and not individuals) as its major study object, and therefore a social science requiring social research methods, which also uses qualitative analysis as a significant operational tool. Epidemiology is about the dialectic relationship between individuals and populations where one builds and is reciprocally built by the other. It is critical to formal epidemiology, because the formal or causal approach to studying disease is phenomenological, i.e. it usually abstracts (segregates, separates) immediate cause–effect relationships from broader and very complex situations in which these relationships occur and which actually determine them.

2. We consider that the social structure is at the essence of the health and disease phenomena. Critical epidemiology will therefore necessarily criticize the class domination structure. Let us borrow a few words from Theresa's May first speech to the UK population after being appointed prime minister, on 13 July 2016: 'if you are born poor, you will die, on average, nine years earlier than others' [7]. This statement represents a very clear and synthetic structuralistic acknowledgment of critical epidemiology.

3. The third critical aspect of critical epidemiology is political. Criticism of the social class domination structure becomes a tool or instrument of political engagement and action for social transformation in order to reduce the social inequalities

as the determinant of health inequities. 'Critical epidemiology is critical because it looks after reality from a transformational perspective' [8].

The critics of epidemiological method: an epistemological debate

Epistemology is a branch of philosophy that studies the origin, nature, methods, rationality of beliefs, and limits of human knowledge [9].

Critical epidemiology is above all an epistemological issue. We essentially ask ourselves, what is the nature of knowing health and disease? Whose health and disease are we concerned about? How do we measure health and disease and what 'causes' diseases? Or, said in different terms, what 'determines' the health and disease process?

Since John Snow's brilliant deduction of the contamination of a water pump as the cause of the 1854 cholera outbreak in London [10], and Virchow considering social structure as the 'cause' of disease when studying—at about the same time—a typhus outbreak in Germany [11], much water has run under the bridge of epidemiological theory and methods.

Briefly, microbiological theories of a single cause—enhanced by the discoveries of Louis Pasteur and his disciples, and supported by Robert Koch's studies at the beginning of the twentieth century—were largely prevalent during the first half of the century.

Over the ensuing decades, Leavell and Clark's theory of the natural history of disease, and creation of the model of the ecologic triad, where *the host, the agent, and the environment* interact in complex ways to determine the outcome of specific diseases, was the basis of practically all prevailing epidemiological models.

This model is still solidly anchored in the cause–effect paradigm. The following statement, by the WHO, on prevention guidelines for mental health, based on the Leavell and Clark model, clearly demonstrates the strength of the paradigm, even 30 years after its first appearance:

The many causes of mental, neurological and psychosocial disorders are highly diverse in origin, effect, timing and mechanism. Complex multivariate social and health problems yield no simple and quick solution. Therefore, comprehensive but culturally-sensitive prevention plans must be tailored to a *specific cause and effect* [12] (emphasis added).

Sophisticated multivariate analysis were more recently proposed, including very diverse mathematical models, to explain and predict transmissible diseases. The rapid advance of biotechnology also led some researchers to propose the use of new paradigms in epidemiological approach and methods, such as the theory of non-linear complex systems able to analyse and synthesize adaptive organized complex systems [13].

Other multivariate models, including the use of the socio-economic status as a risk factor for non-communicable diseases, have also been proposed, but their approach is also cause and effect, not considering, for instance, the socio-historical trajectory of the studied population [14]. In order to explain the epidemiology of chronic non-transmissible diseases, Susser and Susser describe what they call the paradigm of the 'Black Boxes' [15], a not-well-known process mediating specific exposure factors to the outcome of chronic diseases, without any commitment with the definition of

their intermediate factors or even its pathogenesis. The theories of multivariate factors are still used to explain these not well known but empirically demonstrated relationships between exposure factors and diseases (lung cancer and tobacco being a clear example)

No matter how sophisticated they are, these models do not explain how these elements interact nor do they give a hint to what the mechanisms of the health and disease process in populations are. As stated by Pedro Luis Castellanos:

We observe today a paradox: despite the technical and technological development in the explosive field of epidemiology and epidemiological research production rocketing in the contemporary world, each time epidemiology contributes less to the understanding of health problems of populations and increasingly public health interventions tend to focus on interventions on individuals [16].

Are the social determinants of health and disease a new epistemological approach?

New disease patterns and advances in biotechnology led to a new paradigm, which some call the era of 'eco-epidemiology'. The model of 'Chinese boxes', integrating diverse systems that include molecular cause–effect relationships all the way through to very wide social system interactions, can represent this paradigm [15]. The epidemiological approach analyses determinants and outcomes in various organization levels. This, in turn, requires the establishment of a hierarchy between these organization levels and the concourse of the most different disciplines of science, able to incorporate mathematical models: biophysics, social sciences, and so on.

The contribution of social sciences is therefore necessary in order to understand the link between the individual hosting biological processes leading to disease and the social context in which that individual exists [17].

In order to approach this view, the WHO created, in March 2005, the Commission on Social Determinants of Health (CSDH) 'to support countries and global health partners in addressing the social factors leading to ill health and health inequities' [18]. For two years, the CSDH worked on the construction of a Conceptual Framework for Action on the Social Determinants of Health. An *eco-social perspective* is the theoretical basis involving epidemiological models to explain the determinants of health and disease [19]. Extensive literature review demonstrates and illuminates how social factors are related to biological elements generating health inequities within and between countries.

The final report of the CSDH focuses on the need for social justice; the existing evidence on the social determinants of health and, principally, on what actions are needed to face those social determinants and, consequently, to reduce health inequities [20]. Some of the epidemiological evidence presented includes the relationships of early education and nutrition; type of labour contracts and mental health; injuries related to existing preventive legislation; the global distribution of indicators of income and access to health services; education levels and life expectancy; infant mortality rates; and mother's education or family income. It also presents substantial information on the uneven distribution of income, public subsidies, and sex inequities, among others.

The report presents over 550 bibliographic citations, most of which include direct or indirect evidence of the role of social and economic factors determining health inequities. This solid construction led to the recognition of this issue, largely influencing the epidemiological framework, by the 62nd World Health Assembly, held in 2009 [21]. A very significant part of the conclusions of the CSDH is based on Marmot's review of health inequalities in England, which, in turn, presents a very long list of researchers who have now clearly proven the very strong relationship between the social, economic, and environmental determinants and the inequities in health [22].

It is important to highlight the CSDH's concept of social gradient of health among and within countries, which correlates average income and education levels (components of the so-called 'social capital') with life expectancy or other morbidity and mortality indexes. However, other authors use indicators of working-class power and welfare-state strength, available for 16 wealthy countries, to demonstrate that economic inequality and working-class power has a stronger association with health indicators than social capital. Health indicators analysed include life expectancy, self-rated health, low birthweight, and age- and cause-specific mortality [23].

The model of the multivariate social and economic determinants strengthens the discussion about health and health equity as a human right. The awareness of the political implications and difficulties in implementing actions towards health equity as a human right, the conceptual clarity and coherence of the arguments, the soundness of measurement methods, or the abundance of supporting data should become important resources for 'building societal consensus and arming advocates among and on behalf of the disenfranchised and marginalized'[24].

Assuming that social capital, i.e. average income, educational levels, and other social assets are valid variables to demonstrate the social and economic determinants of health and disease and, most particularly, of health inequities, some major questions arise: Is it possible to take real action on 'social determinants of health' under the theoretical epidemiological model adopted? Why are these so-called social and economic variables so uneven and unfair, even in the majority of the most developed countries? What is the role of public policies as an epidemiological variable in determining the health and disease process? Surprisingly, this latter variable is not considered in the above-mentioned analysis of social and economic determinants.

It should be noted that the large bibliographic investigation cited in this section does not make any substantial reference to the extensive work done on social medicine in Latin America since the second half of the last century, although a thorough description of its challenging theoretical and political role was published in *The Lancet* in 2001 [25].

Dialectics of concrete: health is a socio-historical construction

Some of the referenced Latin-American contributors to critical epidemiology, namely Laurell (Mexico), Breilh and Granda (Ecuador) and Almeida Filho (Brazil), among many others, are sources of inspiration when discussing antinomies and epistemological 'sutures' between the social–biological and the collective–individual contradictions within the field of social epidemiology [26].

Three major methodological issues challenge and contradict the formal logics prevalent in the positivist thinking that dominates the epidemiological sciences. In the first place, the relativity of choosing a limited set of causal relationships within an ecological process as an arbitrary process, as mentioned by Susser [1], demonstrates that

the supposed objectivity/'scientific evidence' of epidemiological associations between variables depends on the frame of reference subjectively chosen by the epidemiologist. The knowledge of *reality* is always a dialectic contradiction of man as object and subject of science.

A second relevant issue relates to the relativity of the direct or indirect association of the causal variables, depending on the research design. This is because the observed phenomena are not the reality itself. The dialectic concept of *concrete totality* is independent on the type or size of variables selected [27]. Whether we consider *environment* as the major vector of the health and disease process, or we search for *molecular biology* or even *subatomic particles* as the 'immediate causes', we shall still be talking of the phenomenological (apparent/measurable) sign of whatever stands behind: *the essence of the phenomenon we observe*. As in the Chinese boxes of Susser and Susser [15], the dialectics of concrete will realize that these apparently different levels are phenomena all representing the same essence. Causal/formal epidemiology will consider each of the boxes as isolated units instead of being an indivisible part of the whole, therefore *extracted/abstracted/isolated* from reality.

The logics of concrete establishes the dialectic relationships between *the proximate order* (which is the scope of interest of the traditional cause–effect epidemiology, i.e. the aetiological causation; studies on pathogenesis); *the near order* (ecological epidemiology; social, economic, and environmental multiple factors); and *the distant order* (the social structure organizing the space or territory where the health and disease process takes place) [28]. It also explains the double determination of the epidemiological process: *individual* (clinical epidemiology) and *collective* (social epidemiology). Both are one and indivisible. You cannot treat the one without the other.

Formal logics (the *logic of the form*, of the format of a given phenomenon) makes no sense out of its context. It becomes a mere abstraction. That is why it must be replaced by a *logic of the content* in which the formal logic is just one of its elements, a valid 'sketch' from the point of view of the formal plan, but uncertain and incomplete. The content is made by the interaction of subject (the thought) and object (to which the thought is applied), and this interaction is called the dialectic logic. When analysed separately, dialectics of form and of content remain empty because one explains the other. We can therefore state that, no matter what the level of organization we choose as the frame of reference (whether social or subatomic), there is no *absolute cause for any* phenomenon. There is a more or less proximal relationship. There may exist a 'conditioning' relation, and this relation is reciprocal in the concrete logics: the cause affects its effect and the effect affects its cause [28].

This is why the choice of a frame of reference for a cause–effect relationship in epidemiology is an arbitrary decision. No thought, no idea, and no reflection having an object and a content can be completely neutral. The so-called epidemiological *evidence* (the fetishism or the magic power of numbers) is restricted to measuring phenomena (i.e. risk rates) instead of considering the phenomenon as an expression of its essence, of *the thing itself* [27]. In order to understand the *thing itself* the observer has to know and reflect over the dialectic relationship between the essence and its manifest phenomena. How to approach this relationship is a subjective decision: this is what the dialectics of subject–object is about.

Karel Kosik explains that the dialectic thought must therefore destroy the pseudo-concrete vision of phenomenological evidence

[27]. This does not deny the existence or the objectivity of these phenomena, but it destroys its pretended independence demonstrating that they are always mediate causes; they derive from something else, from the *thing itself*. Destroying pseudo-concretion means that truth is not accessible once and for all, but it must be developed and realized. Knowledge is therefore not just contemplation, the immediate reflect of things. Man only really *knows* when he creates and understands the socio-human reality.

A quite simple demonstrative example of this epistemological understanding was applied by Steve Wing when analysing evidence of exposure disease in radiation epidemiology that does not consider the industries and social arrangements that produce these exposures [29]. Efforts to articulate an alternative epidemiology must consider the historical contexts of public health phenomena, Wing concludes.

When referring to the concrete totality (the essence or the thing itself), there is no possibility of thinking of any human phenomenon not related to a place (space) where this person lives, both individually and collectively. Therefore, the knowledge of this space is inherent to the knowledge of any process (as is the process of health and disease) linked to this person as an individual and as a member of his collectivity. People building the territory and the territory giving socio-historical sense to the human being can be called the dialectics of space [30] and will extensively be discussed in the next section.[1]

As clearly expressed by Milton Santos [30], 'actuality is a unit of universal and of particular: the latter appears as if it were separate, existing by itself, but it is sustained and maintained in the whole'. Citing Sartre (*Critique de La Raison Dialectique*, 1960, p. 139), '[...] the whole is entirely present in the part as its actual sense and destiny'

Critical epidemiology establishes the social structure as the determinant of health and disease

Although it might seem merely semantic, *social and economic determinants of health* is not equal to *social determination of health*. The paradigm of social and economical determinants of health maintains the epistemological approach of formal logics. When considering *distant, intermediate, and proximal* risk factors, combined for a multiple cause or multivariate determination of disease, the quantitative *description* of diverse phenomena prevails. You can hardly find any intellectual (thought) input to try to understand and recreate the socio-historic background responsible for that multiple causation, i.e. the dialectic relationship between the structural and historic essence and its expressions as phenomena. For instance, when income or education variables are associated with general health and disease indicators (i.e. life expectancy, etc.) or to specific pathologies (non-transmissible disease, etc.), there is generally no analysis of the historical process by which those social or economic differences were built, including the comparative study of the

state policies contributing to enhancing or softening these differences. It thus becomes difficult to correct. Do we correct health status (and health inequities) by universally increasing wages and providing universal education? How is it done? Are those actions feasible in the prevailing current national and global social structures? If we imagine that these social and economic inequalities cause health inequities in wealthy countries [23, 31], what can be said in the less-developed parts of the world and in view of the present trends of world capitalism increasing wealth concentration as never before [32, 33].

In order to answer these questions, a number of empirical research has been done, adopting Friedrich Engel's interpretations of health and disease based on historical and dialectic materialism [34]. Some authors even consider Engels as the 'father' of critical epidemiology [35, 36].

Jaime Breihl thinks that, historically and presently, the science of epidemiology is the expression of the power relations of a society [37]. In this line of thought, several Latin American researchers propose the category of *social class* as the major expression of the structural reality, historically determining the outcomes of the health and disease process in specific human and animal populations [26, 37–44].

Accordingly, epidemiology is a practical, empirical science that studies any element of the health and disease process in a given significant population in *a particular historical time*. Epidemiological research aims at building the characteristics of sanitary profiles according to the social reproduction profiles of the different social classes expressed as current productive agents, searching to critically understand the first (the health profiles) through the second (the social class in its daily practice) [45, 46].

Within this order of thinking, a close dialectic relationship was proposed between the concept of ecosystem (landscape epidemiology) and the social structure [47, 48]. The same dialectic relationship had been proposed earlier between the social and economic organization of specific forms of livestock production shaping those territories as the fundaments of veterinary epidemiology [49].

When specifically applied to epidemiological research in mental health, common disorders have been associated with socioeconomic characteristics (education and employment) [50]. However, José Sampaio, in his extensive and complex text, uses the social structure, social class, and sociocultural historical process to come nearer to the understanding of mental health as an object of epidemiology [36]. Carles Muntaner et al. also discuss socioeconomic position (SEP) and major mental disorders, concluding that measures of social class and socio-economic status are not empirically equivalent [51]. Reviewing 12 multi-level studies on SEP and mental health, they conclude that the area level of SEP deprivation (area of residence, neighbourhood, or city) is a stronger predictive indicator than the individual SEP condition. Studies showing that levels of income inequality rather than the low income itself affected rates of depression among low-income women in USA arrive at a similar conclusion [52].

Several authors discuss the challenge of using 'social class', an abstract concept, as an operational variable [41, 53, 54]. Trying to overcome the empiric difficulties of working with social class indicators, José Figueiredo uses Erik Wright's classification of social class strata based on productive assets to evaluate data of the Brazilian National Household Survey of 2008 [55–57]. Considering capital assets, access to information, and power ownership within

---

[1] For those who would like to deepen their knowledge and understanding of Dialect Materialism, we strongly recommend visiting the aforementioned references to Henri Lefevre, Karel Kosick, and Milton Santos.

occupational positions, he defines 15 class categories clustered in four major groups for Brazilian reality. Evaluating the distribution of individual self-rated health among those class categories, he shows accentuated discrepancies in the distribution of health chances across the Brazilian population capturing a pattern of social class associated health chances, which is independent of family income and education distribution.

Social classes are defined by the position they occupy in the capitalist production mode. The social structure as an abstract construction assumes concreteness in a territory. A geographical space is thus the dialectic relationship of the territory with its social organization. One could then assume that social class determines the health and disease outcome of a population in a given historical process mediated by its concrete exposure to biological and non-biological elements and mechanisms in a given space dialectically built by that social class.

This was the dominating theoretical ground for the forum: Social Class, Territory and Health, which took place in 2013 [58]. The Forum assumed the social class categories proposed by Figueiredo; the horizontal (socio-economic organization of the territory) and vertical (global vs local) dialectics of space [30], including its consequent discussion on the concepts of scaling in epidemiological research,[2] and the availability of health data at the required geographical scale in order to be able to develop a valid working proposal[3] for empirical research in critical epidemiology. Its conclusions are a relevant frame of reference to discuss the dialectic relationship between space and social class as the elementary category in scientific critical epidemiology [59].

Socially defined geographical clusters: a proposed key to developing methods in critical epidemiology

The epistemological debate in epidemiology is also present in health-related anthropology [60], as well as in geographical sciences, with its evident ideological and political implications.

Two major medical textbooks, both written in Brazil during the 1950s, fully express the general idea so far discussed in this chapter, integrating medical, epidemiological, anthropological, and geographical concepts—*The Geography of Hunger* by Josué de Castro, expert physician in nutrition [61]; and the *Social-Medical Essays*, by Samuel Pessoa, a physician specialized in parasitic diseases [62] —briefly, that *the social structure, derived from the hegemonic capitalist mode of production (the essence), determines a defined health and disease pattern, which expresses itself (the phenomena) in a particular territory built through a socio-historical process.*

According to formal logics, the territory is per se a study object, i.e. an epidemiological variable. On the contrary, critical geography considers it as the multiform scenario where the dialectic

interaction between the various human actions and the space occur [28, 30, 63–65]. The hegemonic mode of production is the real determinant of these interactions, understood as complex power-driven relations spatially expressed. It 'becomes concrete in a territorial base historically determined' [66].

For many authors, every cartographic representation is, potentially, a political instrument that throughout history has largely endorsed the vision of the territory as a space of *social and economic production*, along with the predominant quantitative and deterministic approach.

For instance, Rogerio Haesbaert reveals the point of rupture between what he calls the 'hegemonic paradigm', which considers land and territory as a basic functional resource and therefore a space of domination as opposed to the dialectic vision of territory [65]. According to the author, the etymology of the word *territory* gives historic support to its hegemonic comprehension, as its carries a double material and symbolic connotation. One relates to the political domination of land, inspiring *terror*, especially for those who cannot access or even enter the land (*térreo-territor*) and the other, on the contrary, inspires positive identification and effective appropriation for those who have the privilege of dominating it (*terra-territorium*). In full contradiction, the critical–dialectic perspective is fundamentally what the same author calls the 'Counter-hegemonic paradigm of the concept of space' (p. 54):

> … conceives the Territory above anything else as a lived space, densified through the multiple social and cultural relationships that turn the link society–land … a much denser tie, where men are not simply seen as subjects to be subjected to their milieu, but … composing their own milieu [sic] ([65], p.54).

The spatial perception of socio-sanitary vulnerabilities must move forward concomitantly with a political process of real territorial appropriation by those local actors in any way committed with social transformation. In order to reduce the *democratic deficit* present when formulating public policies for health, collective participation must condition new forms of spatial representations, generate cartograms circumscribed in scales 'closer' to the lived spaces, and, finally, target areas of social-sanitary interventions.

The need to construct a citizen-based cartography that considers the *lived space* as the starting point for the analysis and the proposal of intervention in the socio-sanitary reality is the leading concept in the development of an empirical methodology for research in critical epidemiology. Only a practice that considers the protagonist role of those who actually live the 'concreteness of the differences' can suggest or propose effective alternatives for reducing socio-sanitary inequities.

This concept leads to two major methodological implications within the framework of critical epidemiology: (i) the local expression of the global determination of the mode of production on the health and disease process; and (ii) the understanding of the socio-historical process continuously building and transforming the *lived space*, where the health and disease process expresses its specific patterns. In other words, critical epidemiology is about *space and time*.

The spatial representation of the sociocultural dimension of health

Nowadays, few people would disagree that the social and economic structure defines, globally speaking, health and disease indicators,

---

[2] The discussion refers to which is the most effective geographical scale to represent a dominant social class or class fraction and how to obtain valid population information not averaging various social classes.

[3] A valid working proposal means an epidemiological research methodology aimed at developing intervention proposals, which would effectively correct the determining elements of the adverse health and disease process in weakened social classes.

referring both to general demographic indicators, as well as to particular pathologies or general health impairments. However, all sorts of disease exposure elements (biological, environmental, social, economic, and cultural) will have a very different distribution in any single locality, even at the most reduced scales of analysis. This includes the subjective perception of the concept of health, as discussed earlier.

Santos synthesizes this dialogue between the concrete totality and the *relative particularities* of each territory (pp. 27–8): 'the space organized by men is like the other social structures, a subordinate–subordinating structure. And, like the other instances, space, although subject to the law of totality, has a certain autonomy …' [67]. In agreement with the relative singularity of the place, Nigel Thrift highlights the need for new spatial representations considering those territories where subjects do not *make* the places but *are* the places [68].

This approach forces us to reflect on the extent to which global health policies and guidelines should dogmatically be assumed and accepted as universal, considering that this practice, in fact, reproduces and enforces the hegemonic historically built export of subjectivities from the central countries towards the periphery. Even for operating purposes, the spectrum of intermediate categories of determination (biological, social, environmental) selected and established as a hierarchical criterion of health and well-being must be adapted and fit to the local realities.

As opposed to the implementation of global policies and guidelines (be it at international, regional, or national levels), critical epidemiology must prioritize *target areas*, geographical spaces where, because of their position within the social structure, human populations are exposed to all sorts of disease/illness/sickness conditioning elements. These populations, dialectically integrated to the geographical spaces where they live and relate to, can be designated as *clusters of destitution*. Because it is in these clusters where the social inequalities manifest themselves as health inequities, the construction of these socio-spatial diagnostics may drive to new strategies of support and intervention, to community mobilizing actions and to a new social positioning vis à vis what is 'strange' to the formal epistemological mainstream, i.e. the concrete reality.

The relevance of the historical accumulation process

Cycles of development and crises of the accumulation process are inherent to the capitalist production system [32, 33]. Consequently, the simultaneously articulating and disarticulating power of the productive links, migratory flows, and the whole modelling matrix of the geographical space are dynamic and historically fleeting.

This understanding seems to be fundamental when we consider the health and disease process intrinsically linked to the social structure determined by the mentioned mode of production. Critical epidemiology must be permanently concerned about the historical modifications of the simultaneous processes of capital, appropriating and leaving spaces where whole populations are conditioned to varying degrees of exposure and vulnerability to the most different elements conditioning disease and health impairments. In fact, these movements of capital, for example, are the real determinants of the occurrence of emerging and re-emerging diseases inasmuch as the transformations of the urban environment or rural landscapes deeply alter the social, economic, and biological elements of the respective ecosystems.

David Harvey refers to the dialectic relationship between the construction and deconstruction of capital reproduction as follows

(p. 150): 'capitalism makes an effort to create a social and physical landscape of its own image just to hide, break and even destroy that same landscape just on a following time instant. The internal contradictions of capitalism express themselves by incessantly forming and reforming the geographic landscapes' [63].

Therefore, critical epidemiology should implement a methodology of investigation and intervention that strongly considers the productive historical development of the chosen target areas instead of just working with present risk rates or any other artificially time-stabilized indicators.

Conclusion: a participative epidemiology will tackle the challenge of the Sustainable Development Goals

The epistemological exercise of systematically considering the dialectic relationship of essence and phenomenon and the methodological approach that effectively strengthens the protagonism of those actors who actually live the territorialities of inequalities are the keys to a truly critical epidemiology. This concept should prevent formal epidemiologists from falling into the methodological trap of quantification and super-valuing phenomenological 'evidence' that will finally be dissociated from the real cause or determination.

The essence of critical epidemiology is that the capitalist mode of production determines a social structure that is intrinsically unfair [33]. Inequality is inherent to capitalism [32]. Inequities are a consequence of its social structure. If the social structure is unfair, then its resulting health and disease process will also be unfair.

To move away from traditional epidemiological practices and to assume an 'epidemiology of action', two major strategies may be enforced:

1. Because epidemiology must shift its priorities from individual disease records to the practice of population health and well-being and from research cabinets to 'lived spaces', the social or public health agents working nearest to those lived spaces must appropriate epidemiological theory and practices. This means that epidemiology must become a major instrument for community (health) agents, equivalent staff, or voluntary agents working at primary health levels. We call this 'participative epidemiology'.

2. Because health is determined by the socio-historical development of 'lived spaces', the global approval of the Sustainable Development Goals, and their corresponding Agenda 2030, becomes a unique 'historical moment' to embrace these goals as an overall transformation process at the local levels of citizen organization [69]. The dialectics of concrete discussed here will probably completely shift the current concept and strategies of Health in All Policies [70], but this discussion is outwith the scope of this chapter.

References

1. Susser M. *Causal Thinking in the Health Sciences*. New York: Oxford University Press, 1973.
2. Almeida Filho N. For a General Theory of Health: preliminary epistemological and anthropological notes. *Cad Saúde Pública* 2001; 4: 753–799.
3. World Health Organization (WHO). Preamble to the Constitution of the World Health Organization. Official Records of the World Health

Organization. 1946; no. 2, p. 100. Available at: http://apps.who.int/iris/bitstream/10665/85573/1/Official_record2_eng.pdf (accessed 18 February 2018).

4. Mahler H. The meaning of Health for All by the year 2000. *Am J Public Health* 2016; 106: 36–38.

5. Garay J. Health equity: the key for transformational change. Available at: http://www.binasss.sa.cr/eng.pdf (accessed 15 August 2016).

6. Hermida C. Sumak Kawsay: Ecuador builds a new health paradigm. *MEDICC Rev* 2011; 13: 60.

7. May T. First speech as Prime Minister—BBC News. Available at: www.youtube.com/watch?v=FDyZ8trge2E (accessed 13 August 2016).

8. Breihl J. ¿Que critica la epidemiología crítica? *Boletín del Observatorio en Salud* 2009; 2: 18–28.

9. Webster's Universal College Dictionary. 'Epistemology'. New York: Gramercy Books, 1997.

10. UCLA Department of Epidemiology. John Snow. Available at: www.ph.ucla.edu/epi/snow.html (accessed 3 August 2016).

11. Silver G. Virchow, the heroic model in medicine: health policy by accolade. *Am J Public Health* 1987; 77: 82–88.

12. World Health Organization. Guidelines for the primary prevention of mental, neurological and psychosocial disorders. Available at: http://apps.who.int/iris/handle/10665/60992 (accessed 12 September 2016).

13. Bernardes MM. Epidemiologia e biotecnologia [Epidemiology and biotechnology]. In: Almeida Filho N, Barreto ML, Veras RP, Barata RB. (eds). *Teoria epidemiológica hoje: fundamentos, interfaces, tendências.* Rio de Janeiro: FIOCRUZ, 1998, pp. 165–184.

14. Hallal P, Clark VL, Assunção MC. et al. Socioeconomic trajectories from birth to adolescence and risk factors for non-communicable disease: prospective analyses. *J Adolesc Health* 2012; 51: S32–S37.

15. Susser M, Susser E. Um futuro para a epidemiologia [A future for epidemiology]. In: Almeida Filho N, Barreto ML, Veras RP, Barata R. (eds). *Teoria Epidemiológica Hoje: Fundamentos, Interfaces, Tendências.* Rio de Janeiro: FIOCRUZ, 1998, pp. 187–212.

16. Castellanos PL. O Ecológico na Epidemiologia [The ecologic in epidemiology]. In: Almeida Filho N, Barreto ML, Veras RP, Barata R. (eds). *Teoria Epidemiológica Hoje: Fundamentos, Interfaces, Tendências.* Rio de Janeiro: FIOCRUZ, 1998, pp. 129–147.

17. Germov J (ed.). Imagining health problems as social issues. In: *Second Opinion. An Introduction to Health Sociology,* 5th ed. Oxford: Oxford University Press, 2013, pp. 5–22.

18. World Health Organization. Comission on Social Determinants of Health, 2005–2008. Available at: http://www.who.int/social_determinants/thecommission/en/ (accessed 8 August 2016).

19. Krieger N. Theories for social epidemiology in the 21st century: an eco-social perspective. *Int J Epidemiol* 2001; 30: 668–677

20. Commission on Social Determinants of Health. *Closing the Gap in a Generation: Health Equity Through Action on the Social Determinants of Health. Final Report of the Commission on Social Determinants of Health.* Geneva: World Health Organization, 2008.

21. World Health Assembly. WHA62.14. Reducing health inequities through action on the social determinants of health. Available at: http://apps.who.int/gb/ebwha/pdf_files/A62/A62_R14-en.pdf (last accessed 10 August 2016).

22. Marmot M. Fair societies and healthy lives: the Marmot Review: strategic review of health inequalities in England post-2010. Available at: https://www.gov.uk/dfid-research-outputs/fair-society-healthy-lives-the-marmot-review-strategic-review-of-health-inequalities-in-england-post-2010 (accessed 18 February 2018).

23. Muntaner C, Lynch JW, Hillemeier M, et al. Economic Inequality, working class power, social capital, and cause-specific mortality in wealthy countries. *Int J Health Serv* 2002; 32: 629–656.

24. Braveman P. Social conditions, health equity, and human rights. *Health Hum Rights* 2010; 12: 31–48.

25. Waitzkin H, Iriart C, Estrada A, Lamadrid S. Social medicine in Latin America: productivity and dangers facing the major national groups. *Lancet* 2001; 358: 315–323.

26. Melo-Filho DA. Antinomies and epistemological 'sutures' between the social-biological and the collective-individual within the field of social epidemiology. *Rev Saúde Pública* 1996; 30: 383–391.

27. Kosik K. *Dialectics of the Concrete.* Berlin: Springer Science & Business Media, 1976.

28. Lefevre H. *Lógica Formal e Lógica Dialética [Formal Logic and Dialectic Logic].* 5th ed. Rio de Janeiro Civilização Brasileira, 1991.

29. Wing S. Limits of epidemiology. *Med Global Surviv* 1994; 1: 74–86.

30. Santos M. *A Natureza do Espaço [The Nature of Space].* 4th ed.. São Paulo: USP, 2006.

31. European Commission. Health inequalities in the EU—Final report of a consortium. Consortium lead: Sir Michael Marmot. Available at: https://ec.europa.eu/health/sites/health/files/social_determinants/docs/healthinequalitiesineu_2013_en.pdf (accessed 18 February 2018).

32. Piketti T. *Capital in the Twenty-First Century.* Cambridge, MA: The Belknap Press of Harvard University Press, 2014.

33. Harvey D. *The Limits to Capital.* Oxford: Basil Blackwell, 1982..

34. Engels F. *The Situation of the Working Class in England.* Moscow: Progress Publishers, 1973; São Paulo: Global, 1988.

35. Waitzkin H. The social origins of medicine: a forgotten history. *Int J Health Serv* 1981; 11: 77–103.

36. Sampaio JJ. *Epidemiologia da Imprecisão. Processo Saúde/Doença Mental Como Objeto da Epidemiologia [Epidemiology of Inaccuracy. Mental Health/Disease Process as Objetct of Epidemiology]* Rio de Janeiro" Editora FIOCRUZ, 1998.

37. Breilh J. Latin American critical ('Social') epidemiology: new settings for an old dream. *Int J Epidemiol* 2008; 37: 745–750.

38. Waitzkin H, Iriart C, Estrada A, Lamadrid S. Social medicine then and now: lessons from Latin America. *Am J Public Health* 2001; 91: 1592–1601.

39. Pereira Solla JS. Problems and limits in the utilization of the concept of social class in epidemiologic research: Cad. *Saúde Pública* 1996; 12: 207–216

40. Hernández LJ. Que critica la epidemiologia crítica: Una aproximación a la mirada de Naomar Almeida Filho (What does critical epidemiology criticize?). *Boletin del Observatorio em Salud* 2009; 2: 18–28.

41. Lombardi C, Bronfman M, Facchini L, et al. Operacionalização do conceito de classe social em estudos epidemiológicos [Turning the concept of social class operational in epidemiological studies]. *Rev Saude Publ* 1988; 22: 253–265.

42. Medeiros ARP, Larocca LM, Chaves LMM, Meier MJ, Wall ML. Epidemiology as a theoretical-methodological framework in the nurses' working process. *Rev Esc Enferm USP* 2012; 46: 1518–1522.

43. Rosenberg FJ. Estructura social y epidemiología veterinaria (Social structure and veterinary epidemiology). *Bol Centro Panam Fiebre Aftosa* 1986; 52: 1–24.

44. Aguilar MA, Roa IC, Kaffure LH, Ruiz LF, Sánchez G. Determinantes sociales de la salud: postura oficial y perspectivas críticas. [Social determinants of health: official stance and critical views]. *Rev Fac Nac Salud Públ* 2013; 31(Suppl. 1): S103–S110.

45. Breihl J. *Epidemiologia: Economia, Medicina y Política [Epidemiology: Economy, Medicine and Politics].* Dominican Republic: Colección SESPAS, 1980.

46. Breihl J, Granda E. *Investigación de la Salud en la Sociedad [Health Research in Society].* Quito: Centro de Estudios y Asesoría en Salud, 1980.

47. Pavlovsky E. *Natural Nidality of Transmissible Diseases.* Urbana, IL: University of Illinois Press, 1966.

48. Ferreira MU. Epidemiology and geography: the pathogenic complex of Max Sorre. *Cadernos Saúde Públ* 1991; 7: 301–309.

49. Obiaga JA, Rosenberg FJ, Astudillo VM, Goic R. Las características de la producción pecuaria como determinante de los ecosistemas de fiebre aftosa [Characteristics of livestock production as determinant of foot-and-mouth disease ecosystems]. *Bol Centro Panam Fiebre Aftosa* 1979; 33–42: 43–52.

50. Marín-León L. Social inequality and common mental disorders. *Rev Bras Psiquiatr* 2007; 29: 250–253.

51. Muntaner C, Eaton WW, Miech R, O'Campo P. Socioeconomic position and major mental disorders. *Epidemiol Rev* 2004; 26: 53–62.

52. Kahn RS, Wise PH, Kennedy BP, Kawachi, L. State income inequality, household income, and maternal mental and physical health: cross sectional national survey. *BMJ* 2000, 321: 1311–1315.

53. Barros MB. A utilização do conceito de classe social nos estudos dos perfis epidemiológicos: uma proposta [Using the concept of social class in studying epidemiologic profiles: a proposal]. *Rev Saúde Públ S Paulo* 1986; 20: 269–273.

54. Barata RB, Ribeiro MCS, da Silva ZP, Antunes JLF. Classe social: conceitos e esquemas operacionais em pesquisa em saúde [Social class: concepts and operationalization models in health research]. *Rev Saúde Públ* 2013; 47: 647–655.

55. Figueiredo JA. Class divisions and health chances in Brazil. *Int J Health Serv* 2011; 41: 691–709.

56. Wright E. *Class Counts: Comparative Studies in Class Analysis.* Cambridge: Cambridge University Press, 1997.

57. Wright E. *Foundations of a Neo-Marxist Class Analysis in: Approaches to Class Analysis.* Cambridge: Cambridge University Press, 2005.

58. Fiocruz/Palácio Itaboraí Fórum: Classes Sociais, Território e Saúde: Questões Metodológicas e Políticas (Social classes, Territory and Health: Methodologic and political issues). Available at http://www.forumitaborai.fiocruz.br/node/896 (accessed 18 February 2018).

59. Rosenberg Félix J. Clases sociales, territorio y salud: una propuesta para analizar e intervenir sobre la situación de salud a partir de su determinación social. [Social classes, territory and health: a proposal to analyze and intervene on the Health situation based on its social determination] *Biomédica* 2013; 33(Suppl. 2): 23–27.

60. Menendez EL. Antropologia médica e epidemiologia [Medical anthropology and epidemiology]. In: Alves PC and Rabelo MC (eds). *Antropologia da Saúde: Traçando Identidade e Explorando Fronteiras.* Rio de Janeiro: FIOCRUZ, 1998, pp. 71–93.

61. Castro J. *Geografia da fome [Geography of Hunger].* Rio de Janeiro: O Cruzeiro, 1946.

62. Pessoa S. *Ensaios Médicos Sociais [Socio-Medical Assays].* São Paulo: Cebes-Hucitec, 1978.

63. Harvey, D. *Spaces of Capital. Towards a Critical Geography.* Edinburgh: Edinburgh University Press, 2001.

64. Correa RL. *O Espaço Urbano [The Urban Space].* São Paulo: Ática, 1989.

65. Haesbaert R. *Viver no Limite: Território e Multi/Trans-territorialidade em Tempos de In-Segurança e Contenção [Living at the Limit: Territory and Multi/ Trans-territoriality in Times of Lack of Security and Contention].* Rio de Janeiro: Bertrand Brasil, 2014.

66. Santos M, Slaner S. Society and space: social formation as theory and method. *Antipode* 1977; 9: 5.

67. Santos M. *Por uma Geografia Nova.* São Paulo: HUCITEC, 1978.

68. Thrift N. Non-represental Theory: Space, Politics, Affect. Abingdon: Routledge, 1991.

69. United Nations Development Programme. Sustainable Development Goals. Available at: http://www.undp.org/content/undp/en/home/sdgoverview/post-2015-development-agenda.html (accessed 8 September 2016).

70. World Health Organization. Health in all policies training manual: 2016. Available at: http://who.int/social_determinants/publications/health-policies-manual/en/ (accessed 8 September 2016).

CHAPTER 11

Occupational epidemiology

Angelo d'Errico and Giuseppe Costa

Introduction

During the last 30 years, research on the mental health effects of occupational hazards has dramatically increased, in particular those related to exposure to psychosocial factors, usually grouped under the term 'workplace stress'. Stress at work has been implicated in the development of several health outcomes, for example cardiovascular diseases [1–3], autoimmune diseases [4], musculoskeletal disorders of the upper limb [5, 6], and the back [7].

Three main mental health outcomes have been studied in relation to workplace stress in the epidemiological literature: psychological well-being or psychological distress, depression, and burnout. The former has mainly been assessed via general health questionnaires, such as the Short Form (SF)-12 or the SF-36 [8], and the General Health Questionnaire (GHQ-12) [9]; depression via clinical diagnostic questionnaires, such as the Center for Epidemiologic Studies Depression Scale (CES-D) [10], the Composite International Diagnostic Interview (CIDI) [11] or the Beck Depression Inventory (BDI) [12]; and burnout mainly via the Maslach Burnout Inventory [13]. All these questionnaires have been used extensively for decades in the thematic literature and have been shown to have acceptable validity. Other outcomes investigated, as indicators of mental disorders, include physician-diagnosed psychiatric disorders, use of antidepressants or psychotropic medication, and disability pensions or sickness absence owing to depression or other mental disorders.

Exposure to psychosocial factors at work stems from characteristics of work organization, including temporal aspects of work, such as pace and shifts; features of the job content, such as repetitive work and lack of autonomy; unclear or conflicting tasks and demands; aspects related to the work group, such as social isolation and unequal workload; job supervision, including poor supervisor support and few possibilities of participating in the decision-making process; and exposure to offensive behaviour and discrimination [14].

In contrast to the measurement of exposure to physical or chemical hazards, the assessment of exposure to psychosocial hazards is commonly conducted using subjective methods, based on workers' self-reports. The use of objective methods, such as those based on workers' observations, focus groups, or the registration of tasks performed by the workers appears to be preferable to subjective information collected via questionnaires, as they are not influenced by subjects' health status [15, 16], and provide better identification of hazardous working conditions in order to prevent them [17]. Nevertheless, on one hand, there are problems regarding representativeness of the observation period with respect to tasks and activities actually performed by the workers over a long period, and, on the other hand, the theoretical construct of stress itself, which is a subjective experience, limits the utility of proposed objective evaluations of stressors. Cognitive appraisal of psychosocial factors, not accessible to external observers, appears necessary for stressors to exert their effects on health [18, 19].

An important problem in the interpretation of the results of epidemiological studies on the health effects of work stress is that they are obtained from studies with a cross-sectional design. These are potentially biased by a differential misclassification of the exposure based on recall bias, seeking meaning after the development of disease. This can result in an overestimate of the risk associated with the exposures. This bias is attributable to exposure overestimate by subjects affected by diseases [20], which may result in spurious associations between exposures and outcomes. For this reason, this chapter will focus mainly on the results of prospective studies, in which subjects affected by the disease under study at the beginning of the observation period are excluded from the analysis, or this is adjusted for its presence at the baseline interview.

Another relevant issue is adjustment for potential confounders, in particular socio-economic position and co-exposure to other work hazards. Regarding the former, its confounding effect relies on the fact that both the prevalence of exposure to adverse psychosocial factors, especially low control, and the occurrence of mental disorders generally are more frequent among less qualified workers [21–23]. Concerning potential confounding by co-exposure to other workplace hazards, psychosocial factors at work are often correlated with each other, as well as with ergonomic factors. Therefore, adjustment for these co-exposures is important to ascertain that the observed association actually relates to the exposure considered, instead of other variables unobserved or not included in the analysis. For example, this is particularly relevant for exposure to ergonomic factors, which are expected to correlate with psychosocial exposures, such as workload or time pressure, especially among manual workers, and may also be associated with the health outcomes examined [24].

Work stress models

Different definitions of workplace stress have been proposed over time, based on different schools of thought and theories: some, like the Michigan organizational stress model [25] or the 'effort–reward imbalance' model [26], are centred on the individual perception of the work environment, the organizational climate, and interpersonal relationships at work, whereas other theories are more focused on the assessment of objective job characteristics, rather than perceived stressors, like the demand–control model [27] or the action-theory model [28]. Accordingly, several models for the assessment of exposure to psychosocial factors at work have been created, together with many different questionnaires inspired by the different theories [29]. Historically, of these the most important are the Job Stress Survey [30], which focuses on high work pressure and lack of organizational support; the Occupational Stress Indicator [31] and the Work Environment Scale [32], intended to evaluate also aspects of the organizational climate; the Stress Scale, created by Spector and Jex [33], which emphasizes three main dimensions of stressors in work organizations: interpersonal conflicts, organizational ties, and workload; the 'Generic Job Stress Questionnaire', which measures in 13 questions exposure to just as many stress dimensions (workload, underuse of technical skills, work autonomy, psychological demand, work conflicts, responsibilites, etc.) [34].

In particular, two theoretical models, and the related measurement scales, have acquired popularity and have become widespread in the epidemiological literature in the last few decades: the 'demand–control' model, elaborated by Robert Karasek [27] and subsequently developed together with Töres Theorell [35], and the 'effort–reward imbalance' (ERI) model, proposed by Siegrist et al. [26].

Demand–control–support model

In the original model proposed by Karasek [27], the combination of exposure to psychological demand, defined as high work pressure combined with conflicting demands, and decision latitude, also named 'job control', would give rise to four types of job. High-strain jobs, i.e. jobs with high demand and low decision latitude, would be the most harmful in terms of negative effects on mental health because of exposure to high demand. This would not be moderated by sufficient resources of the worker, in terms of autonomy, variety of tasks and use of skills. The second type is that of the 'active' jobs, similarly characterized not only by high levels of demand, but also by high decision latitude, which buffers the deleterious effects of high demand. The third type includes jobs with low psychological demand and high decision latitude ('low-strain' jobs), which would be associated with the lowest risk of ill health, because the workers have limited challenges and enough resources to deal with these challenges. The last type if that of 'passive' jobs, characterized by both low levels of demand and decision latitude, which would lead to loss of motivation and atrophy of workers' skills but not to increased levels of psychological strain. The four job groups are obtainable by dividing the demand and the control scales at their median values, and in most studies the occurrence of health effects associated with exposure to high strain has been compared with that of the low-strain group or of the other three groups combined; however, in some the job-strain dimension was built as a continuous variable, obtained by dividing the value of the demand scale by that of the control one [36, 37]. In the demand–control model, the job control dimension is decomposable in two sub-dimensions, one related to autonomy in performing job duties (decision authority), and the other to possibility of using and developing technical skills at work (skill discretion). Karasek' model has been subsequently enriched by Johnson and Hall with the psychosocial dimension of 'social support', defined as support provided by colleagues and supervisors in performing job tasks [38]; according to this model, called 'iso-strain' or 'demand–control–support' (DCS), social support plays

a buffer role against the negative health consequences of high demand and low control. Although the type of social support at work considered by Johnson and Hall was limited to co-workers' support, in most subsequent studies the support of supervisors and of co-workers has been investigated separately [38, 39].

Since the first study by Karasek [27], who discovered from national survey data that a combination of low-decision latitude and high job demands was associated with mental strain, an impressive body of research has tested the model in empirical studies. In the earliest review on the subject, results from cross-sectional studies were supportive of an association of psychological distress with job strain or iso-strain, whereas those obtained from longitudinal studies gave almost no support to these associations; furthermore, the association between job strain and mental health was more consistent among males and manual workers [40].

Among longitudinal studies published until the end of the last century, several reported a significant increase in psychological distress, anxiety, or depression with regard to exposure to high demand [41–50], low control [42, 44, 45, 48, 49, 51], and low social support [42, 45, 46, 49, 51]; in contrast, only one study reported negative results for all these dimensions [52]. However, only a few of these studies gave support to the job-strain hypothesis [41, 47, 49].

A meta-analysis of 11 prospective studies of good methodological quality estimated significant excesses of 20–40% in the pooled risks of common mental disorders (neurotic and depressive disorders) for demand, control, and social support, whereas it was higher (around 80%) for job strain [53]. A high level of heterogeneity among risk estimates across studies was found for demand and, to a lesser extent, for social support; such a heterogeneity was likely due to differences in the accuracy of exclusion of cases or of adjustment for mental health at baseline, as studies showing the stronger associations were also those that did not exclude baseline cases or controlled only for sickness absence due to mental health problems, which may not account for milder psychiatric symptoms. For all the psychosocial exposures examined, stronger associations were found for men than for women, although results appeared more consistent for the latter.

Subsequently, two reviews on high-quality prospective studies focusing specifically on depression or depressive symptoms have confirmed that adverse exposure to stress, defined according to the demand–control model, was significantly associated with this outcome. In the review by Bonde [54], evaluating nine studies, relative risks (RR) of depression were significantly increased by 30% for high demand, by 20% for low job control, and by 44% for low social support; regarding job strain, risks estimates differed between the sexes, with an excess risk approaching twofold among men, but lower and less consistent among women. The other review [55], of seven studies, concluded that associations with depression were consistent for high demand and low social support, apparently stronger for co-worker support than for supervisor support, with a doubling of the RR for high demand and a 50% increase for low social support. Results regarding the relationship with job control were judged to be scarce and contradictory, whereas for job strain, three of five studies found a strong and significant association [56–58], and in another it was limited to men [59].

Later studies, with regard to job demands, showed a consistently increased risk of depression, ascertained through report of depressive symptoms or antidepressant medication [60–65], although in one study it was significant only among blue-collar workers [64] and in two only among men [59, 61]. Furthermore, a significant association with demand was observed in one study, where it was measured by objective ratings assigned to the jobs of a safety and hygiene manager [66], a characteristic that excludes the possibility of a spurious association due to differential misclassification of exposure by case status. However, the association with demand was not confirmed by other studies [67–69]. The job control and job strain dimensions were less consistently associated with depression: regarding the former, some studies were positive [62, 70–72] but were counterbalanced by many others with null results [60, 61, 63–67, 69, 73]; job strain was also only partially consistent across studies, although the majority displayed a significant association at least in one gender [60, 62, 71, 74–76]. Further support to the causal nature of the relationship between job strain and depression comes from a study that found an increased risk among subjects who changed exposure from low strain to high strain [57], as well as a dose–response effect found in three studies [45, 67, 75]. The relationship between social support and depression displays contradictory findings in the recent literature, especially when results were adjusted for potential confounders at baseline: a few studies found a significant relationship [60, 61, 67], but the majority were negative [65, 71, 73, 76, 77].

Regarding anxiety disorders, only a few studies have evaluated the association with work stress factors in prospective studies, with discordant findings. Among these, Stansfeld et al. [78] found that demand, control, job strain, and social support were all associated in the expected direction; Niedhammer and Chastang [73] reported a significant association with high demand but not with control or support; and Griffin et al. [79] found an association with low job control, although only among men, whereas in the study by Plaisier et al. [80] neither demand nor control were significantly associated. In a Swedish study, demand was found to significantly increase the risk of anxiety by 60%, but skill discretion and decision authority did not [81].

Effort–reward imbalance model

The 'ERI model identifies as the main stress determinant the imbalance between the effort sustained by workers in performing their job and the rewards provided by their work organization through three remuneration systems: money, esteem, and career opportunity (including job security). A prolonged experience of lack of reciprocity, in terms of high costs and low gains for the worker, would elicit negative emotions leading to an activation of the hypothalamic–pituitary–adrenal axis and of the sympathetic–adrenomedullary system, which would be responsible for the increased likelihood of developing physical and mental disorders [82]. Furthermore, according to this model a personality factor, named 'overcommitment', would increase workers' susceptibility to the health effects of ERI. Overcommitment, which characterizes part of the working population, has been defined as a person-specific characteristic reflecting an excessive involvement in work duties due to need for approval from others [83].

Also for the ERI model, the meta-analysis by Stansfeld and Candy [53] computed a pooled risk of common mental disorders similar to that of job strain (odds ratio 1.84), although this was estimated based on only two prospective studies [84, 85]. Another prospective study, the Whitehall II Study, not included in this review, found a positive association with mental health functioning in a large cohort of British civil servants [86]. Subsequent prospective studies have mostly confirmed the significant relationship of ERI with poor mental health, depression, use of antidepressant medications, or sickness absence for mental disorders [70, 74, 87–93]. A more recent review, evaluating the results of longitudinal cohort studies in 13 countries, estimated an almost twofold overall RR of depressive symptoms for US studies and an 80% increase for European studies, associated with exposure to ERI [89]; however, when controlled for health status at baseline the excess risk reduced to 50%, remaining significant only among European studies.

A recent study has also observed a significantly increased risk of disability pension for depression (hazard ratio 1.90) associated with high ERI, in a large cohort of Finnish public employees during a 9-year follow-up [94].

Other dimensions of work stress

Besides these two models, other dimensions of workplace stress have been proposed and tested in relation to health, among which emotional demand, organizational justice, work–family conflicts, job insecurity, and exposure to bullying, threat or violence appear the most promising. Furthermore, some temporal aspects of work, such as long working hours and shift work, have been considered as potential work stressors and many studies have evaluated their association with various health outcomes.

Emotional demand

Emotional demand has been defined by Arlie Hochschild [95] as the need to display certain emotional expressions in some jobs, implying a relationship with clients, pupils, or patients. Therefore, the construct of emotional demand refers to the quality of the interaction between workers and subjects outside the work organization, which is relevant especially in work settings such as education, health care, social work, and trading. Subsequent research has further characterized this psychosocial dimension, identifying four different components, including positive and negative emotions, sensitivity to clients' emotions, and emotional dissonance [96]; in particular, emotional dissonance, defined as the conflict between emotional spontaneous behaviour and the one workers are requested to display within the work organization [97], would be the main responsible factor for the mental health effects found in various studies.

Exposure to high emotional demand is diffused, with almost 30% of the employed population reporting exposure to it in the Danish Work Environment Survey, and about two-thirds of workers exposed in health care, education, and social services [98]. In the 2010 Eurofound Survey, 33% of men and 41% of women reported getting emotionally involved in their job always or most of the time (personal elaboration of the data).

High emotional demand has been found associated with several psychological outcomes, such as psychological distress [99, 100], depression [98, 101–103], and burnout [104–107]. A meta-analysis of the relationship between exposure to emotional demand and burnout estimated significantly increased meta-risks for both the emotional exhaustion and the depersonalization sub-dimensions [108]. In spite of most of the evidence relying on results from cross-sectional studies, which are more prone to several biases, as discussed above, a few authors have found these associations in prospective studies of good methodological quality, at least regarding psychological distress [99] and depression [98, 101].

Work–family conflicts

The dimension of work–family conflicts (WFC) refers to a condition in which the work and family domains interfere so much that one produces negative effects on the other [109]. The two main theories on which the construct of WFC is based are (i) the 'spillover' hypothesis, according to which alienation from the work sphere would be transferred to the sphere of the family [110]; and (ii) the 'role-strain' hypothesis, considering WFC as a conflict between the pressure exerted by different roles, which are somehow not compatible [109].

WFC are common in employed populations, as demonstrated by the 2010 Eurofound study, in which the prevalence was around 20% in the whole European Union but with a wide variability across countries and higher proportions of exposed workers in Southern European countries [111]. Heterogeneity in WFC among countries has been found to be mainly explained by differences in hours worked per week, work schedule regulations (in particular regarding schedule flexibility and the possibility of part-time work), and welfare typologies (indicator of availability of services for childcare, parental leave, social support of single parents, etc.) [111].

The presence of children in the household appears to be an important risk factor for WFC: it has been estimated that 40% of employed parents experience at some point in time a problematic work–family balance [112]. Moreover, occupations with frequent shift work have been reported to display a higher prevalence: in a survey of US nurses, 50% reported having experienced a WFC for more than 1 day per week during the previous 6 months [113]. In another US study, 16% of the general employed population reported suffering from WFC, with small sex, age, education, and marital status differences [114].

The most important work determinants of WFC, according to reviews by Byron [115] and Michel et al. [116], appear to be high workload, long working hours, role conflicts, poor social support from co-workers and supervisors, low autonomy, and task variety. Included among non-occupational determinants are family demands and associated factors, such as marital conflict and number of hours spent doing domestic work and taking care of children [115]. Frone et al. [117] first hypothesized that WFC was a mediation factor between some occupational exposures, such as excessive workload and long working hours, and health outcomes. In support of this theory, WFC have been found in a recent study to partly mediate the effect of exposure to ERI on mental disorders [118].

WFC has been repeatedly associated with the occurrence of mental symptoms or disorders, with RRs around 2 for anxiety or low mental well-being, in a range of 1.5–3.0 for depression, and threefold higher for burnout [111, 119–124]. However, in spite of the substantial body of research on the subject, most studies were cross-sectional, in which the direction of the effect was unclear, although a few longitudinal studies also reported significant associations between WFC and mental health, which were mainly similar in strength between the sexes [93, 120, 123]. A recent meta-analysis of longitudinal studies of WFC and psychological strain, including studies focusing on psychological distress, anxiety, depression, and emotional exhaustion, concluded that exposure to WFC was associated with a future risk of mental symptoms in the studies reviewed but with a small effect size [125].

Organizational justice

The term 'organizational justice' (OJ) refers to equity in rules and social norms governing enterprises, in particular in terms of resources and benefits distribution (distributive justice), of process and procedures (procedural justice), and of interpersonal relationships (relational justice, intended as respect of the management for workers' dignity) [126]. As for ERI, the construct of OJ stems from the social exchange theory, but it differs from the ERI concept in that it concerns workers' perception of fairness in their work organization at large, rather than that experienced only by themselves [127]. The health effects of OJ have been explained through the 'fairness heuristic theory', which proposes that workers' perception of procedural fairness would be a surrogate of management's trustworthiness when workers have scarce information on it, which would be protective for health because it would help workers to deal with situations of uncertainty [128].

Low OJ has been found associated with minor psychiatric disorders or psychological distress in various longitudinal studies conducted on different occupational cohorts, such as nurses and other hospital workers [129–131], British civil servants [132], as well as in the general employed population [133]. The most important review on the relationship with mental health evaluated the results of 11 prospective studies, concluding that both low procedural and relational justice increase the risk of mental disorders, and that these associations remained significant adjusting the analysis for exposure to work stress according to the DCS and the ERI models [134]. For relational justice, RRs among the exposed were in the range of 1.20–1.60 and they were almost all statistically significant; furthermore, in studies evaluating the effect of an improvement in relational justice, in both sexes there was a decreased risk of minor psychiatric morbidity, approximately by 25%, whereas the risk increased by 70–80% with a worsening of the exposure. Also with regard to procedural justice, the results of most studies were statistically significant, showing RRs of psychiatric morbidity, including depression, in the range of 1.4–1.9.

Job insecurity

According to data from the European Labour Force Surveys, workers hired on temporary contracts have increased by more than 25% from 1990 to 2007, making up 11.5–14.5% of the total workforce [135]. The recent economic crisis has accelerated this process, causing a higher diffusion of exposure to job insecurity among workers in the majority of European countries: workers in the 27 countries of European Union reporting being likely to lose their job in the next 6 months went up from 8.7% in 2007 to 13.2% in 2012 [136].

In the epidemiological literature, only since the 1970s has job insecurity been started to be considered a stress factor, with possible health effects. One of the first definitions of job insecurity is 'perceived powerlessness to maintain desired continuity in a threatened job situation' [137].

Therefore, its main features would be (i) the perception of the worker of a threat to work continuation; (ii) the importance for the worker of preserving his/her job; (iii) the feeling of not being able to do anything about the threat of losing the job; and (iv) the uncertainty about the possibility of losing the job.

Some categories of workers have been found more exposed to job insecurity, especially people with a low socio-economic position, women, migrants, ethnic minorities, and temporary workers [138].

Job insecurity, temporary work, and precarious work are characteristics that partly overlap. In particular, temporary work is a less specific surrogate indicator of job insecurity, as not all workers with temporary contracts are actually exposed to high insecurity. For example, in the 2010 European Working Condition Survey less than half of workers with temporary contracts reported being likely to lose their job in the next 6 months (41%), although this proportion decreased to 29% among workers with a permanent contract; as a consequence, differences in mental health observed between workers reporting or not reporting job insecurity were much stronger than those found between temporary and permanent workers [139]. Instead, the construct of precarious work has a wider scope, which also considers other adverse work characteristics, such as short-duration contracts, low level of negotiation with regard to working conditions, vulnerability to authoritarian treatment, low wages, few workplace legal rights and social security benefits, and powerlessness to exercise workplace rights [140].

Workers exposed to job insecurity have been found in many studies to be at higher risk of reporting low mental well-being [141, 142], as well as anxiety, depression, and burnout [65, 143–148], with 2–3-fold RRs associated with exposure.

The main literature reviews are concordant in stating that job insecurity is consistently associated with a lower level of mental well-being and an increased risk of anxiety, depression, and burnout [149–152]. An association with mental health has, in fact, also been found in longitudinal studies adjusting for health status at baseline or excluding diseased subjects [65, 153], features that limit the possibility of distortion of the risk estimates by selection bias or differential exposure misclassification, and in studies with a thorough adjustment for occupational and non-occupational potential confounders, especially other psychosocial factors in the workplace [65, 143, 153]. Furthermore, an increased risk was observed in longitudinal studies on companies undergoing downsizing, which examined the effect on health of the transition from a situation of high job security to one of low security [141, 154, 155]. Various groups of workers seem more susceptible to the health effects of job insecurity, in particular women [152], older workers [156, 157], and people employed in manual or low-status jobs [151, 152], likely because of their lower opportunities of finding a new job in case of dismissal. Welfare typology would be another important moderator of the health effects of job insecurity, according to a review showing that the association with mental health was modest or absent in Nordic countries (social-democratic welfare regime characterized by high levels of social protection) but present in other countries with different welfare regimes [152].

Bullying

The term 'workplace bullying' refers to a situation in which a person is repeatedly harassed at work, both directly, through abusive behaviour offending his/her personal dignity (insults, unsuitable remarks to the worker on how he/she carries out tasks, discrimination based on ethnic, religious, or political identity), or indirectly, by talking behind his/her back with colleagues or excluding the worker from social relationships or from information needed to perform the job correctly. In the 2010 Eurofound Survey, exposure to bullying at work in Europe was reported by 4% of workers, with small differences by sex [158], which is similar to figures reported by other authors [159, 160].

Nowadays, bullying is considered one of the most powerful stressors in the workplace, with potential impacts on both physical and psychological health, based on the results of several studies, which observed an increased risk of mental disorders associated with exposure to bullying or other forms of harassment, with risk mainly in a range of 1.2–3-fold [161–163]. A meta-analysis that evaluated the results of 14 prospective studies on the subject, mostly conducted in the Nordic countries, found that almost all of them observed a significant positive association with subsequent mental health problems (anxiety and depression) [164]. The results of this meta-analysis support a causal association, as in most studies the results were obtained from analyses adjusted for mental health at baseline, indicating that bullying was associated with new cases of mental disorders, and the likelihood of publication bias was considered low. The association was present both in studies conducted on the general employed population, as well as on specific occupational cohorts, indicating good generalizability of the results. It estimated a significant meta-odds ratio of 1.68 for exposure to bullying. This study also found that mental health problems increased significantly with the occurrence of subsequent bullying (meta-odds ratio 1.74), indicating the presence of a circular, self-reinforcing mechanism going from bullying to mental health and vice versa.

Among longitudinal studies conducted afterwards, most confirmed the association with mental health, anxiety, or depression in different working populations [165–168], except for one study where it disappeared after adjusting for baseline depressive symptoms [169].

Work hours

Both long working hours and shift work, especially night shifts, appear to increase the likelihood of developing different mental health outcomes, in particular depression and sleep disturbances.

It seems worth noting that the results of studies on shift work or long work hours are potentially affected by an important selection bias, i.e. the 'healthy worker survival effect', owing to the fact that workers with psychological problems tend, if possible, to move to daily work or to reduce overtime work. Therefore, studies with a cross-sectional design are likely affected by an attenuation bias, leading to an underestimate of the association between these exposures and the health outcomes investigated.

Long working hours

Long working hours are defined as working more than standard hours, which are widely different across countries. In Western, developed countries, standard working hours are generally 40 hours per week, but in many non-European countries, especially Asian ones, weekly hours are generally more than 40 and often in the range of 50–60 hours per week. The European Union Directive on work hours (2003/88/EC) has put the threshold at 48 weekly hours, which should not be exceeded, even considering overtime work. However, according to data from the European Survey on Working and Living Conditions 2010, 14.5% of men and 6.5% of women reported working beyond this limit (personal elaboration of the data).

There is a long-lasting debate over whether long working hours have an effect on mental health, which originated in early studies from the strong expectation of an association, in part contrasted by the modest strength of the associations observed and discordant results [170]. A main problem in the interpretation of these results is that the association between long work hours and mental health can potentially be confounded by other risk factors, such as demographic characteristics and workplace co-exposures, in particular demand [171]. According to the conceptual model proposed by the US National Institute for Occupational Safety and Health, long working hours would reduce time availability, as well as the ability of exploiting it to sleep, rest, or participate in family or leisure activities; moreover, they would expose workers to an excessive workload, reducing further their possibility of psycho-physical recovery. This would increase the likelihood of sleeping an insufficient number of hours and of developing sleep disturbances, fatigue, depression, physical symptoms, and changes in neurological, cognitive, and physiological functioning [172].

Several prospective studies have found an increased risk of developing anxiety or depression among workers exposed to long working hours or frequent overtime work [64, 173–176], although there are also some negative reports [177, 178]. Furthermore, in a Finnish study long hours significantly increased the risk of taking sleeping pills, but not antidepressants, and only among men; among women the RR was close to 1 [179]. Also, in a Korean study, a significant association with long working hours was found but only among subjects working more than 68 hours per week (RR 2.03) [180]. Some recent reviews support the existence of an association between long working hours and impaired mental health, although they highlight several methodological problems in the reviewed literature, which limit interpretation of the results, especially the wide variability in exposure definition, which makes uncertain which threshold value could be adopted to prevent mental problems [181, 182].

Shift work

In developed Western societies an increase in the diffusion of shift work occurred in the last few decades, which nowadays concerns about 20% of the employed population [183]. Work shift systems differ considerably in terms of shift duration, amount of night work, weekend work, shift start and end times, and length of shift cycle. In particular, night shifts and rotating shifts potentially interfere more with the circadian rhythms of individuals and with their family and social lives.

Despite earlier reviews on the relationship between shift work and mental health indicated a certain inconsistency of the association [184, 185], more recent ones suggest the presence of an increased risk of developing mental disorders, which, as for long working hours, seem to be mediated by fatigue, insufficient recovery periods, and poor work–family balance [186, 187].

Among longitudinal studies conducted in more recent years, several have found an increased risk of anxiety, depression, and poor mental health among shift workers [188–192]. In particular, a UK study observed a high risk of anxiety/depression in both men (RR 6.08) and women (RR 2.58) for having worked on night shift for at least 4 years [192]. In support of a causal relationship between shift work and mental health, a prospective study of Norwegian nurses observed that those moving from night to day work during a 2-year follow-up period showed decreased symptoms of anxiety and depression [193].

It has been suggested that the health effects of shift work are likely attributable to time schedule constraints, rather than to the shift work itself, based on the results of a Swedish study, which found an increased intention to leave the profession only among eldercare female workers with scarce influence on work [194]. A Cochrane review on efficacy of preventive interventions concluded that participation in programming work shifts improves mental health [195].

Conclusions

The evaluation of the literature on the effects on mental health of psychosocial factors at work indicates the presence of sound and consistent associations, likely of a causal nature, observed in many studies of good methodological quality, including in this definition longitudinal studies with at least adjustment for or exclusion of mental health cases at baseline, and adjustment for workplace co-exposure and socio-economic position. It is worth noting that, in the majority of the studies, exposure to psychosocial factors was measured only once in time, which would imply a non-differential misclassification of the exposure; in fact, exposure to these factors has a temporal variability that is not captured by a spot measurement, with the consequence of an underestimation of the associated risk estimates, especially in studies with a long follow-up. It is therefore likely that the strength of the association observed in many studies between the different hazards and the risk of mental disorders was actually lower than the true one.

The causal relationship between psychosocial factors and mental health is also supported by the reduction reported by several longitudinal studies in the incidence of mental disorders among workers who decreased their exposure in time. These findings also indicate that preventive interventions to decrease the level of exposure to psychosocial factors may be effective in reducing the burden of mental diseases in many work settings. The biological plausibility of the effects of these factors on mental health is supported by studies that observed an increase in the levels of cortisol and other hormones belonging to the hypothalamic–pituitary–adrenal axis [196] among subjects exposed to work stressors, as well as among people affected by depression [197, 198]. A summary evaluation on the consistency and the strength of association between the different workplace factors and mental health is presented in Table 11.1. Quantitative demands, job strain, ERI, organizational justice, job insecurity, and bullying appear to be the factors more consistently associated with this outcome, whereas the strength of association would be highest for job strain, ERI, WFC, and bullying.

Table 11.1 Summary evaluation of the association between exposure to workplace psychosocial hazards and risk of mental symptoms or disorders

Exposure	Consistency of the association	Strength of the association
Low control	+	+
High demand	++	+
High strain	++	++
High effort–reward imbalance	++	++
High emotional demand	+	+
High work–family conflicts	+	++
Low organizational justice	++	+
High job insecurity	++	+
Long working hours	+	+
Night work	+	+
Bullying	++	++

References

1. Bosma H, Peter R, Siegrist J, Marmot M. Two alternative job stress models and the risk of coronary heart disease. *Am J Publ Health* 1998; 88: 68–74.
2. Kuper H, Marmot M, Hemingway H. Systematic review of prospective cohort studies of psychosocial factors in the etiology and prognosis of coronary heart disease. *Semin Vasc Med* 2002; 2: 267–314.
3. Belkic KL, Landsbergis PA, Schnall PL, Baker D. Is job strain a major source of cardiovascular disease risk? *Scand J Work Environ Health* 2004; 30: 85–128.
4. Stojanovich L, Marisavljevich D. Stress as a trigger of autoimmune disease. *Autoimmun Rev* 2008; 7: 209–213.
5. Feuerstein M, Shaw WS, Nicholas RA, Huang GD. From confounders to suspected risk factors: psychosocial factors and work-related upper extremity disorders. *J Electromyogr Kinesiol* 2004; 14: 171–178.
6. Bernard BP. *Musculoskeletal Disorders and Workplace Factors: A Critical Review of Epidemiologic Evidence for Work-related Musculoskeletal Disorders of the Neck, Upper Extremity, and Low Back*. Cincinnati, OH: National Institute for Occupational Safety and Health, 1997.
7. National Research Council, Institute of Medicine. *Musculoskeletal Disorders and the Workplace: Low Back and Upper Extremities*. Washington, DC: National Academy Press, 2001.
8. Ware JE, Jr, Kosinski M, Keller SD. A 12-Item Short-Form Health Survey: construction of scales and preliminary tests of reliability and validity. *Med Care* 1996; 34: 220–233.
9. Goldberg DP, Williams P. *A User's Guide to the General Health Questionnaire*. Windsor: NFER-Nelson, 1978.
10. Radloff LS. The CES-D scale: a self-report depression scale for research in the general population. *Appl Psychol Meas* 1997; 1: 385–401.
11. Wittchen HU. Reliability and validity studies of the WHO—Composite International Diagnostic Interview (CIDI): a critical review. *J Psychiatric Res* 1994; 28: 57–84.
12. Johnson DA, Heather BB. The sensitivity of the Beck depression inventory to changes of symptomatology. *Br J Psychiatry* 1974; 125: 184–185.
13. Maslach C, Jackson SE. The measurement of experienced burnout. *J Occup Behav* 1981; 2: 99–113.
14. Kasl SV. Assessing health risk in the work setting. In: Schroeder H (ed.). *New Directions in Health Psychology Assessment*. Washington, DC: Hemisphere, 1991, pp. 95–125.
15. Kasl SV. Epidemiological contributions to the study of work stress. In: Cooper CL, Payne RL (eds). *Stress at Work*. New York: Wiley, 1978, pp. 3–38.
16. Kristensen TS. Job stress and cardiovascular disease: a theoretic critical review. *J Occup Health Psychol* 1996; 1: 246–260.
17. Frese M, Zapf D. Methodological issues in the study of work stress: objective vs. subjective measurement of work stress and the question of longitudinal studies. In: Cooper CL, Payne RL (eds). *Causes, Coping and Consequences of Stress at Work*. Chichester: Wiley, 1998, pp. 375–411.
18. Lazarus RS, Folkman S. Cognitive theories of stress and the issue of circularity. In: Appley ML, Trumbull R (eds). *Dynamics of Stress*. New York: Plenum, 1986, pp. 62–80.
19. Cox T, Rial-Gonzalez E. Risk management, psychosocial hazards and work stress. In: Rantanen J, Lehtinen S (eds). *Psychological Stress at Work*. Helsinki: Finnish Institute of Occupational Health, 2000.
20. de Lange AH, Taris TW, Kompier MA, Houtman IL, Bongers PM. 'The very best of the millennium': longitudinal research and the demand-control-(support) model. *J Occup Health Psychol* 2003; 8: 282–305.
21. Kosidou K, Dalman C, Lundberg M, Hallqvist J, Isacsson G, Magnusson C. Socioeconomic status and risk of psychological distress and depression in the Stockholm Public Health Cohort: a population-based study. *J Affect Disord* 2011; 134: 160–167.
22. Fryers T, Melzer D, Jenkins R. Social inequalities and the common mental disorders: a systematic review of the evidence. *Soc Psychiatry Psychiatr Epidemiol* 2003; **38**: 229–237.
23. Wiggins RD, Schofield P, Sacker A, Head J, Bartley M. Social position and minor psychiatric morbidity over time in the British Household Panel Survey 1991–1998. *J Epidemiol Commun Health*, 2004; 58: 779–787.
24. MacDonald LA, Karasek RA, Punnett L, Scharf T. Covariation between workplace physical and psychosocial stressors: evidence and implications for occupational health research and prevention. *Ergonomics* 2001; 44: 696–718.
25. Caplan R, Cobb S, French J, Harrison R. *Job Demands and Worker Health: Main Effects and Occupational Differences*. Washington, DC: National Institute for Occupational Safety and Health. 1975.
26. Siegrist J. Adverse health effects of high-effort/low-reward conditions. *J Occup Health Psychol* 1996; 1: 27–41.
27. Karasek RA. Job demands, job decision latitude and mental strain: implications for job redesign. *Adm Sci Q* 1979; 24: 285–308.
28. Frese M, Zapf D. Action as the core of work psychology: a German approach. In: Trinadis HC, Dunnette MD, Hough LM (eds.). *Handbook of Industrial and Organizational Psychology*, Vol. 4, 2nd ed. Palo Alto, CA: Consulting Psychologist Press, 1994, pp. 271–340.
29. Tabanelli MC, Depolo M, Cooke RM, et al. Available instruments for measurement of psychosocial factors in the work environment. *Int Arch Occup Environ Health* 2008; 82: 1–12.
30. Vagg PR, Spielberger CD. Occupational stress: measuring job pressure and organizational support in the workplace. *J Occup Health Psychol* 1998; 3: 294–305.
31. Cooper CL, Sloan SJ, Williams S. *Occupational Stress Indicator*. Windsor: Nfer-Nelson, 1988.
32. Moos RH, Insel PM. *Manual for Work Environment Scale*. Palo Alto, CA: Consulting, 1981.
33. Spector PE, Jex SM. Development of four self-report measures of job stressors and strain: interpersonal conflict at work scale, organizational constraints scale, quantitative workload inventory, and physical symptoms inventory. *J Occup Health Psychology* 1998; 3: 356.
34. Hurrell JJ, Murphy LR. Psychological job stress. In: Rom WM (ed.) *Environmental and Occupational Medicine*, 2nd ed. Boston, MA: Little, Brown & Company, 1992, p. 675.
35. Karasek R, Theorell T. *Healthy Work: Stress, Productivity and the Reconstruction of Working Life*. New York: Basic Books, 1990.
36. Landsbergis PA, Schnall PL, Warren K, Pickering TG, Schwarz JE. Association between ambulatory blood pressure and alternative formulations of job strain. *Scand J Work Environ Health* 1994; 20: 349–363.

37. Choi BK, Clays E, De Bacquer D, Karasek R. Socioeconomic status, job strain and common mental disorders—an ecological (occupational) approach. *Scand J Work Environ Health* 2008;Suppl. 6: 22–32.

38. Johnson JV, Hall EM. Job strain, work place social support, and cardiovascular disease: a cross-sectional study of a random sample of the Swedish working population. *Am J Publ Health* 1988; 78: 1336–1342.

39. LaRocco J, House J, French J. Social support, occupational stress and health. *J Health Soc Behav* 1980; 21: 202–218.

40. Van der Doef M, Maes S. The job demand-control (-support) model and psychological well-being: a review of 20 years of empirical research. *Work Stress* 1999; 13: 87–114.

41. Bromet EJ, Dew MA, Parkinson DK, Schulberg HC. Predictive effects of occupational and marital stress on the mental health of a male workforce. *J Organ Behav* 1988; 9: 1–13.

42. Parkes KR. Occupational stress among student nurses: a natural experiment. *J Appl Psychol* 1982; 67: 784.

43. Kawakami N, Haratani T, Araki S. Effects of perceived job stress on depressive symptoms in blue collar workers of an electrical factory in Japan. *Scand J Work Environ Health* 1992; 18: 195–200.

44. Barnett RC, Brennan RT. Change in job conditions, change in psychological distress, and gender: a longitudinal study of dual-earner couples. *J Organ Behav* 1997; 18: 253–274.

45. Bourbonnais R, Comeau M, Vézina M. Job strain and evolution of mental health among nurses. *J Occup Health Psychol* 1999; 4: 95–107.

46. Daniels K, Guppy A. Occupational stress, social support, job control, and psychological well-being. *Hum Relat* 1994; 47: 1523–1544.

47. Niedhammer I, Goldberg M, Leclerc A, Bugel I, David S. Psychosocial factors at work and subsequent depressive symptoms in the Gazel cohort. *Scand J Work Environ Health* 1998; 24: 197–205.

48. Stansfeld SA, Fuhrer R, Shipley MJ, Marmot MG. Work characteristics predict psychiatric disorder: prospective results from the Whitehall II Study. *Occup Environ Med* 1999; 56: 302–307.

49. Cheng Y, Kawachi I, Coakley EH, Schwartz J, Colditz G. Association between psychosocial work characteristics and health functioning in American women: prospective study. *BMJ* 2000; 320: 1432–1436.

50. Parkes KR. Locus of control as moderator: an explanation for additive versus interactive findings in the demand-discretion model of work stress? *Br J Psychol* 1991; 82: 291–312.

51. Johnson JV, Hall EM, Ford DE, et al. The psychosocial work environment of physicians. The impact of demands and resources on job dissatisfaction and psychiatric distress in a longitudinal study of Johns Hopkins Medical School graduates. *J Occup Environ Med* 1995; 37: 1151–1159.

52. Steptoe A, Wardle J, Lipsey Z, et al. A longitudinal study of work load and variations in psychological well-being, cortisol, smoking, and alcohol consumption. *Ann Behav Med* 1998; 20: 84–91.

53. Stansfeld SA, Candy B. Psychosocial work environment and mental health--a meta-analytic review. *Scand J Work Environ Health* 2006; 32: 443–462.

54. Bonde JP. Psychosocial factors at work and risk of depression: a systematic review of the epidemiological evidence. *Occup Environ Med* 2008; 65: 438–445.

55. Netterstrom B, Conrad N, Bech P, et al. The relation between work-related psychosocial factors and the development of depression. *Epidemiol Rev* 2008; 30: 118–132.

56. Shields M. Stress and depression in the employed population. *Health Rep* 2006; 17: 11–29.

57. de Lange AH, Taris TW, Kompier MA, Houtman IL, Bongers PM. Effects of stable and changing demand-control histories on worker health. *Scand J Work Environ Health* 2002; 28: 94–108.

58. Wang J. Perceived work stress and major depressive episodes in a population of employed Canadians over 18 years old. *J Nerv Ment Dis* 2004; 192: 160–163.

59. Virtanen M, Honkonen T, Kivimaki M, et al. Work stress, mental health and antidepressant medication findings from the Health 2000 Study. *J Affect Disord* 2007; 98: 189–197.

60. Theorell T, Hammarström A, Gustafsson PE, Magnusson-Hanson L, Janlert U, Westerlund H. Job strain and depressive symptoms in men and women: a prospective study of the working population in Sweden. *J Epidemiol Commun Health* 2014; 68: 78–82.

61. Thielen K, Nygaard E, Rugulies R, Diderichsen F. Job stress and the use of antidepressant medicine: a 3.5-year follow-up study among Danish employees. *Occup Environ Med* 2011; 68: 205–210.

62. Wahrendorf M, Blane D, Bartley M, Dragano N, Siegrist J. Working conditions in mid-life and mental health in older ages. *Adv Life Course Res* 2013; 18: 16–25.

63. Endo M, Muto T, Haruyama Y, Yuhara M, Sairenchi T, Kato R. Risk factors of recurrent sickness absence due to depression: a two-year cohort study among Japanese employees. *Int Arch Occup Environ Health* 2015; 88: 75–83.

64. d'Errico A, Cardano M, Landriscina T, et al. Workplace stress and prescription of antidepressant medications: a prospective study on a sample of Italian workers. *Int Arch Occup Environ Health* 2011; 84: 413–424.

65. Andrea H, Bültmann U, van Amelsvoort LG, Kant Y. The incidence of anxiety and depression among employees--the role of psychosocial work characteristics. *Depress Anxiety* 2009; 26: 1040–1048.

66. DeSanto Iennaco J, Cullen MR, Cantley L, Slade MD, Fiellin M, Kasl SV. Effects of externally rated job demand and control on depression diagnosis claims in an industrial cohort. *Am J Epidemiol* 2010; 171: 303–311.

67. Bonde JP, Munch-Hansen T, Wieclaw J, Westergaard-Nielsen N, Agerbo E. Psychosocial work environment and antidepressant medication: a prospective color study. *BMC Public Health* 2009; 9: 262.

68. Ylipaavalniemi J, Kivimaki M, Elovainio M, Virtanen M, Keltikangas-Jarvinen L, Vahtera J. Psychosocial work characteristics and incidence of newly diagnosed depression: a prospective cohort study of three different models. *Soc Sci Med* 2005; 61: 111–122.

69. Fandiño-Losada A, Forsell Y, Lundberg I. Demands, skill discretion, decision authority and social climate at work as determinants of major depression in a 3-year follow-up study. *Int Arch Occup Environ Health* 2013; 86: 591–605.

70. Lunau T, Wahrendorf M, Dragano N, Siegrist J. Work stress and depressive symptoms in older employees: impact of national labour and social policies. *BMC Public Health* 2013; 13: 1086.

71. Clumeck N, Kempenaers C, Godin I, et al. Working conditions predict incidence of long-term spells of sick leave due to depression: results from the Belstress I prospective study. *J Epidemiol Commun Health* 2009; 63: 286–292.

72. Inoue A, Kawakami N, Haratani T, et al. Job stressors and long-term sick leave due to depressive disorders among Japanese male employees: findings from the Japan Work Stress and Health Cohort study. *J Epidemiol Commun Health* 2010; 64: 229–35.

73. Niedhammer I, Chastang JF. Psychosocial work factors and first depressive episode: retrospective results from the French national SIP survey. *Int Arch Occup Environ Health* 2015; 88: 835–847.

74. Wang J, Smailes E, Sareen J, Schmitz N, Fick G, Patten S. Three job-related stress models and depression: a population-based study. *Soc Psychiatry Psychiatr Epidemiol* 2012; 47: 185–193.

75. Clays E, De Bacquer D, Leynen F, Kornitzer M, Kittel F, De Backer G. Job stress and depression symptoms in middle-aged workers--prospective results from the Belstress study. *Scand J Work Environ Health* 2007; 33: 252–259.

76. Stansfeld SA, Shipley MJ, Head J, Fuhrer R. Repeated job strain and the risk of depression: longitudinal analyses from the Whitehall II study. *Am J Publ Health* 2012; 102: 2360–2366.

77. Lassalle M, Chastang JF, Niedhammer I. Working conditions and psychotropic drug use: cross-sectional and prospective results from the French national SIP study. *J Psychiatr Res* 2015; 63: 50–57.

78. Stansfeld SA, Clark C, Caldwell T, Rodgers B, Power C. Psychosocial work characteristics and anxiety and depressive disorders in midlife: the effects of prior psychological distress. *Occup Environ Med* 2008; 65: 634–642.

79. Griffin JM, Fuhrer R, Stansfeld SA, Marmot M. The importance of low control at work and home on depression and anxiety: do these effects vary by gender and social class? *Soc Sci Med* 2002; 54: 783–798.

80. Plaisier I, de Bruijn JG, de Graaf R, ten Have M, Beekman AT, Penninx BW. The contribution of working conditions and social support to the onset of depressive and anxiety disorders among male and female employees. *Soc Sci Med* 2007; 64: 401–410.

81. Liu B, Lavebratt C, Nordqvist T, et al. Working conditions, serotonin transporter gene polymorphism (5-HTTLPR) and anxiety disorders: a prospective cohort study. *J Affect Disord* 2013; 151: 652–659.

82. Weiner H. *Perturbing the Organism: The Biology of Stressful Experience.* Chicago, IL: University of Chicago Press, 1992.

83. Siegrist J, Starke D, Chandola T, et al. The measurement of effort-reward imbalance at work: European comparisons. *Soc Sci Med* 2004; 58: 1483–1499.

84. Stansfeld SA, Bosma H, Hemingway H, Marmot MG. Psychosocial work characteristics and social support as predictors of SF-36 health functioning: the Whitehall II study. *Psychosom Med* 1998; 60: 247–255.

85. Godin I, Kittel F, Coppieters Y, Siegrist J. A prospective study of cumulative job stress in relation to mental health. *BMC Publ Health* 2005; 5: 67.

86. Kuper H, Singh-Manoux A, Siegrist J, Marmot M. When reciprocity fails: effort-reward imbalance in relation to coronary heart disease and health functioning within the Whitehall II study. *Occup Environ Med* 2002; 59: 777–784.

87. Kivimäki M, Vahtera J, Elovainio M, Virtanen M, Siegrist J. Effort-reward imbalance, procedural injustice and relational injustice as psychosocial predictors of health: complementary or redundant models? *Occup Environ Med* 2007; 64: 659–665.

88. Ndjaboué R, Brisson C, Vézina M, Blanchette C, Bourbonnais R. Effort–reward imbalance and medically certified absence for mental health problems: a prospective study of white-collar workers. *Occup Environ Med* 2014; 71: 40–47.

89. Siegrist J, Lunau T, Wahrendorf M, Dragano N. Depressive symptoms and psychosocial stress at work among older employees in three continents. *Global Health* 2012; 8: 27.

90. Li J, Weigl M, Glaser J, Petru R, Siegrist J, Angerer P. Changes in psychosocial work environment and depressive symptoms: a prospective study in junior physicians. *Am J Ind Med* 2013; 56: 1414–1422.

91. Lamy S, De Gaudemaris R, Lepage B, et al. The organizational work factors' effect on mental health among hospital workers is mediated by perceived effort-reward imbalance: result of a longitudinal study. *J Occup Environ Med* 2013; 55: 809–816.

92. Rugulies R, Aust B, Madsen IE, Burr H, Siegrist J, Bültmann U. Adverse psychosocial working conditions and risk of severe depressive symptoms. Do effects differ by occupational grade? *Eur J Publ Health* 2013; 23: 415–420.

93. Peter R, March S, du Prel JB. Are status inconsistency, work stress and work-family conflict associated with depressive symptoms? Testing prospective evidence in the lidA study. *Soc Sci Med* 2016; 151: 100–109.

94. Juvani A, Oksanen T, Salo P, et al. Effort-reward imbalance as a risk factor for disability pension: the Finnish Public Sector Study. *Scand J Work Environ Health* 2014; 40: 266–277.

95. Hochschild AR. *The Managed Heart: Commercialization of Human Feelings.* Berkeley, CA: University of California Press.

96. Zapf D, Vogt C, Seifert C, Mertini H, Isic A. Emotion work as a source of stress: the concept and development of an instrument. *Eur J Work Organ Psychol* 1999; 8: 371–400.

97. Middleton DR. Emotional style: the cultural ordering of emotions. *Ethos* 1989; 17: 187–201.

98. Madsen IE, Diderichsen F, Burr H, Rugulies R. Person-related work and incident use of antidepressants: relations and mediating factors from the Danish work environment cohort study. *Scand J Work Environ Health* 2010; 36: 435–444.

99. Bültmann U, Kant IJ, Van den Brandt PA, Kasl SV. Psychosocial work characteristics as risk factors for the onset of fatigue and psychological distress: prospective results from the Maastricht Cohort Study. *Psychol Med* 2002; 32: 333–345.

100. Burr H, Albertsen K, Rugulies R, Hannerz H. Do dimensions from the Copenhagen Psychosocial Questionnaire predict vitality and mental health over and above the job strain and effort-reward imbalance models? *Scand J Publ Health*, 2010; 38(3 Suppl.): 59–68.

101. Muntaner C, Van Dussen DJ, Li Y, Zimmerman S, Chung H, Benach J. Work organization, economic inequality, and depression among nursing assistants: a multilevel modeling approach. *Psychol Rep* 2006; 98: 585–601.

102. Wieclaw J, Agerbo E, Mortensen PB, Burr H, Tuchsen F, Bonde JP. Psychosocial working conditions and the risk of depression and anxiety disorders in the Danish workforce. *BMC Publ Health* 2008; 8: 280.

103. Andrea H, Bültmann U, Beurskens AJ, Swaen GM, van Schayck CP, Kant IJ. Anxiety and depression in the working population using the HAD Scale--psychometrics, prevalence and relationships with psychosocial work characteristics. *Soc Psychiatry Psychiatr Epidemiol* 2004; 39: 637–646.

104. Zapf D. Emotion work and psychological well-being: A review of the literature and some conceptual considerations. *Hum Resource Manag Rev* 2002; 12: 237–268.

105. Bakker AB, Demerouti E, Verbeke W. Using the job demands-resources model to predict burnout and performance. *Hum Resource Manag* 2004; 43: 83–104.

106. Morris JA, Feldman DC. Managing emotions in the workplace. *JMI* 1997; 257–274.

107. Abraham R. Emotional dissonance in organizations: antecedents, consequences, and moderators. *Gen Soc Gen Psychol Monogr* 1998; 124: 229.

108. Bono JE, Vey MA. Toward understanding emotional management at work: a quantitative review of emotional labor research. In: Ashkanasy N, Hartel C (eds). *Understanding Emotions in Organizational Behavior.* Mahwah, NJ: Erlbaum, 2004, pp. 212–233.

109. Greenhaus JH, Beutell NJ. Sources of conflict between work and family roles. *Acad Manag Rev* 1985; 10: 76–88.

110. Kabanoff B, O'Brien G. Work and leisure: a task attributes analysis. *J Appl Psychol* 1980; 65: 596–609.

111. Lunau T, Bambra C, Eikemo TA, van der Wel KA, Dragano N. A balancing act? Work-life balance, health and well-being in European welfare states. *Eur J Publ Health* 2014; 24: 422–427.

112. Galinsky E, Bond JT, Friedman DE. *Highlights: The National Study of the Changing Workforce.* New York: Families and Work Institute, 1993.

113. Grzywacz JG, Frone MR, Brewer CS, Kovner CT. Quantifying work-family conflict among registered nurses. *Res Nurs Health* 2006; 29: 414–426.

114. Alterman T, Luckhaupt SE, Dahlhamer JM, Ward BW, Calvert GM. Job insecurity, work-family imbalance, and hostile work environment: prevalence data from the 2010 National Health Interview Survey. *Am J Ind Med* 2013; 56: 660–669.

115. Byron K. A meta-analytic review of work–family conflict and its antecedents. *J Vocat Behav* 2005; 67: 169–198.

116. Michel JS, Kotrba LM, Mitchelson JK, Clark MA, Baltes BB. Antecedents of work–family conflict: a meta-analytic review. *J Organ Behav* 2011; 32: 689–725.

117. Frone MR, Russell M, Cooper ML. Antecedents and outcomes of work-family conflict: testing a model of the work-family interface. *J Appl Psychol* 1992; 77: 65.

118. du Prel JB, Peter R. Work-family conflict as a mediator in the association between work stress and depressive symptoms: cross-sectional evidence from the German lidA-cohort study. *Int Arch Occup Environ Health* 2015; 88: 359–368.

119. Obidoa C, Reeves D, Warren N, Reisine S, Cherniack M. Depression and work family conflict among corrections officers. *J Occup Environ Med* 2011; 53: 1294–1301.

120. Leineweber C, Baltzer M, Magnusson-Hanson LL, Westerlund H. Work-family conflict and health in Swedish working women and

men: a 2-year prospective analysis (the SLOSH study). *Eur J Publ Health* 2013; 23: 710–716.

121. Frone MR. Work–family conflict and employee psychiatric disorders: the national comorbidity survey. *J Appl Psychol* 2000; 85: 888.

122. Wang Y, Chang Y, Fu J, Wang L. Work-family conflict and burnout among Chinese female nurses: the mediating effect of psychological capital. *BMC Publ Health* 2012; 12: 915.

123. Magnusson-Hanson L, Leineweber C, Chungkham HS, Westerlund H. Work-home interference and its prospective relation to major depression and treatment with antidepressants. *Scand J Work Environ Health* 2014; 40: 66–73.

124. Nistor K, Nistor A, Ádám S, Szabó A, Konkolÿ Thege B, Stauder A. [The relationship of work-related psychosocial risk factors with depressive symptoms among Hungarian workers: preliminary results of the Hungarian Work Stress Survey]. *Orvosi Hetilap* 2015; 156: 439–448 (article in Hungarian).

125. Nohe C, Meier LL, Sonntag K, Michel A. The chicken or the egg? A meta-analysis of panel studies of the relationship between work-family conflict and strain. *J Appl Psychol* 2015; 100: 522–536.

126. Elovainio M, Heponiemi T, Sinervo T, Magnavita N. Organizational justice and health; review of evidence. *G Ital Med Lav Ergon* 2010; 32(3 Suppl. B): B5–B9.

127. Adams JS. Inequity in social exchange. *Adv Exp Soc Psychol* 1965; 2: 267–299.

128. Van den Bos K, Wilke HA, Lind EA. When do we need procedural fairness? The role of trust in authority. *J Pers Soc Psychol* 1998; 75: 1449.

129. Elovainio M, Kivimäki M, Vahtera J. Organizational justice: evidence of a new psychosocial predictor of health. *Am J Publ Health* 2002; 92: 105–108.

130. Kivimäki M, Elovainio M, Vahtera J, Virtanen M, Stansfeld SA. Association between organizational inequity and incidence of psychiatric disorders in female employees. *Psychol Med* 2003; 33: 319–326.

131. Kivimäki M, Elovainio M, Vahtera J, Ferrie JE. Organisational justice and health of employees: prospective cohort study. *Occup Environ Med* 2003; 60: 27–33.

132. Ferrie JE, Head J, Shipley MJ, Vahtera J, Marmot MG, Kivimäki M. Injustice at work and incidence of psychiatric morbidity: the Whitehall II study. *Occup Environ Med* 2006; 63: 443–450.

133. Ybema JF, van den Bos K. Effects of organizational justice on depressive symptoms and sickness absence: a longitudinal perspective. *Soc Sci Med* 2010; 70: 1609–1617.

134. Ndjaboué R, Brisson C, Vézina M. Organisational justice and mental health: a systematic review of prospective studies. *Occup Environ Med* 2012; 69: 694–700.

135. Eurostat. *Health and Safety at Work in Europe (1999-2007). A Statistical Portrait.* Luxembourg: Publications Office of the European Union, 2010.

136. Eurofound. *Impact of the Crisis on Working Conditions in Europe.* Luxembourg: Office for Official Publications of the European Commission, 2013.

137. Greenhalgh L, Rosenblatt Z. Job insecurity: toward conceptual clarity. *Acad Manag Rev* 1984; 3: 438–448.

138. Landsbergis PA, Grzywacz JG, LaMontagne AD. Work organization, job insecurity, and occupational health disparities. *Am J Ind Med* 2014; 57: 495–515.

139. Eurofound. *Health and Well-being at Work: A Report Based on the Fifth European Working Conditions Survey.* Luxembourg: Office for Official Publications of the European Commission, 2012.

140. Vives A, Amable M, Ferrer M, et al. The Employment Precariousness Scale (EPRES): psychometric properties of a new tool for epidemiological studies among waged and salaried workers. *Occup Environ Med* 2010; 67: 548–555.

141. Swaen GM, Bültmann U, Kant I, van Amelsvoort LG. Effects of job insecurity from a workplace closure threat on fatigue and psychological distress. *J Occup Environ Med* 2004; 46: 443–449.

142. Lau B, Knardahl S. Perceived job insecurity, job predictability, personality, and health. *J Occup Environ Med* 2008; 50: 172–181.

143. D'Souza RM, Strazdins L, Lim LL, Broom DH, Rodgers B. Work and health in a contemporary society: demands, control, and insecurity. *J Epidemiol Commun Health* 2003; 57: 849–854.

144. Boya FO, Demiral Y, Ergör A, Akvardar Y, De Witte H. Effects of perceived job insecurity on perceived anxiety and depression in nurses. *IND Health* 2008; 46: 613–619.

145. Edimansyah BA, Rusli BN, Naing L, Mohamed Rusli BA, Winn T, Tengku Mohamed Ariff BR. Self-perceived depression, anxiety, stress and their relationships with psychosocial job factors in male automotive assembly workers. *IND Health* 2008; 46: 90–100.

146. Burgard SA, Brand JE, House JS. Perceived job insecurity and worker health in the United States. *Soc Sci Med* 2009; 69: 777–785.

147. Rugulies R, Bültmann U, Aust B, Burr H. Psychosocial work environment and incidence of severe depressive symptoms: prospective findings from a 5-year follow-up of the Danish work environment cohort study. *Am J Epidemiol* 2006; 163: 877–887.

148. Norlund S, Reuterwall C, Höög J, Lindahl B, Janlert U, Birgander LS. Burnout, working conditions and gender--results from the northern Sweden MONICA Study. *BMC Publ Health* 2010; 10: 326.

149. De Witte H. Job insecurity: review of the international literature on definitions, prevalence, antecedents and consequences. *Eur J Work Organ Psychol* 1999; 8: 155–177.

150. Quinlan M, Mayhew C, Bohle P. The global expansion of precarious employment, work disorganisation and occupational health: a review of recent research. *Int J Health Serv* 2001; 31: 335–414.

151. Sverke M, Hellgren J, Näswall K. No security: a meta-analysis and review of job insecurity and its consequences. *J Occup Health Psychol* 2002; 7: 242–264.

152. Kim IH, Muntaner C, Vahid Shahidi F, Vives A, Vanroelen C, Benach J. Welfare states, flexible employment, and health: a critical review. *Health Policy* 2012; 104: 99–127.

153. Hellgren J, Sverke M, Isaksson K. A twodimensional approach to job insecurity: Consequences for employee attitudes and well-being. *Eur J Work Organ Psychol* 1999; 8: 179–195.

154. Kivimäki M, Vahtera J, Pentti J, Ferrie JE. Factors underlying the effect of organisational downsizing on health of employees: longitudinal cohort study. *BMJ* 2000; 320: 971–975.

155. Ferrie JE, Shipley MJ, Stansfeld SA, Marmot MG. Effects of chronic job insecurity and change in job security on self reported health, minor psychiatric morbidity, physiological measures, and health related behaviours in British civil servants: the Whitehall II study. *J Epidemiol Commun Health* 2002; 56: 450–454.

156. Vahtera J, Kivimäki M, Pentti J. Effect of organisational downsizing on health of employees. *Lancet* 1997; 350: 1124–1128.

157. Cheng Y, Chen IS, Chen CJ, Burr H, Hasselhorn HM. The influence of age on the distribution of self-rated health, burnout and their associations with psychosocial work conditions. *J Psychosom Rese* 2013; 74: 213–220.

158. Ardito C, d'Errico A, Leombruni R. Exposure to psychosocial factors at work and mental well-being in Europe. *Med Lav* 2014; 105: 85–99.

159. Einarsen S, Skogstad A. Prevalence and risk groups of bullying and harassment at work. *Eur J Work Organ Psychol* 1996; 5: 185–202.

160. Kivimäki M, Virtanen M, Vartia M, Elovainio M, Vahtera J, Keltikangas-Järvinen L. Workplace bullying and the risk of cardiovascular disease and depression. *Occup Environ Med* 2003; 60: 779–783.

161. Lahelma E, Lallukka T, Laaksonen M, Saastamoinen P, Rahkonen O. Workplace bullying and common mental disorders: a follow-up study. *J Epidemiol Commun Health* 2012; 66: e3.

162. Lallukka T, Haukka J, Partonen T, Rahkonen O, Lahelma E. Workplace bullying and subsequent psychotropic medication: a cohort study with register linkages. *BMJ Open* 2012; 2: pii: e001660.

163. Rugulies R, Madsen IE, Hjarsbech PU, et al. Bullying at work and onset of a major depressive episode among Danish female eldercare workers. *Scand J Work Environ Health*, 2012; 38: 218–227.

164. Nielsen MB, Magerøy N, Gjerstad J, Einarsen S. Workplace bullying and subsequent health problems. *Tidsskr Nor Laegeforen* 2014; 134: 1233–1238.

165. Bonde JP, Gullander M, Hansen ÅM, et al. Health correlates of workplace bullying: a 3-wave prospective follow-up study. *Scand J Work Environ Health* 2016; 42: 17–25.

166. Rodríguez-Muñoz A, Moreno-Jiménez B, Sanz-Vergel AI. Reciprocal relations between workplace bullying, anxiety, and vigor: a two-wave longitudinal study. *Anxiety Stress Coping* 2015; 28: 514–530.

167. Gullander M, Hogh A, Hansen ÅM, et al. Exposure to workplace bullying and risk of depression. *J Occup Environ Med* 2014; 56: 1258–1265.

168. Loerbroks A, Weigl M, Li J, Glaser J, Degen C, Angerer P. Workplace bullying and depressive symptoms: a prospective study among junior physicians in Germany. *J Psychosom Res* 2015; 78: 168–172.

169. Hogh A, Conway PM, Grynderup MB, et al. Negative acts at work as potential bullying behavior and depression: examining the direction of the association in a 2-year follow-up study. *J Occup Environ Med* 2016; 58: e72–e79.

170. Sparks K, Cooper C, Fried Y, Shirom A. The effects of hours of work on health: a meta-analytic review. *J Occup Organ Psychol* 1997; 70: 391–408.

171. Spurgeon A, Harrington JM, Cooper CL. Health and safety problems associated with long working hours: a review of the current position. *Occup Environ Med* 1997; 54: 367–375.

172. Caruso CC, Bushnell T, Eggerth D, et al. Long working hours, safety, and health: toward a National Research Agenda. *Am J Ind Med* 2006; 49: 930–942.

173. Shields M. Long working hours and health. *Health Rep* 1999; 11: 33–48.

174. Virtanen M, Ferrie JE, Singh-Manoux A, et al. Long working hours and symptoms of anxiety and depression: a 5-year follow-up of the Whitehall II study. *Psychol Med* 2011; 41: 2485–2494.

175. Amagasa T, Nakayama T. Relationship between long working hours and depression: a 3-year longitudinal study of clerical workers. *J Occup Environ Med* 2013; 55: 863–872.

176. Kleiner S, Schunck R, Schömann K. Different contexts, different effects? Work time and mental health in the United States and Germany. *J Health Soc Behav* 2015; 56: 98–113.

177. Michelsen H, Bildt C. Psychosocial conditions on and off the job and psychological ill health: depressive symptoms, impaired psychological wellbeing, heavy consumption of alcohol. *Occup Environ Med* 2003; 60: 489–496.

178. Varma A, Marott JL, Stoltenberg CD, Wieclaw J, Kolstad HA, Bonde JP. With long hours of work, might depression then lurk? A nationwide prospective follow-up study among Danish senior medical consultants. *Scand J Work Environ Health* 2012; 38: 418–426.

179. Laaksonen M, Lallukka T, Lahelma E, Partonen T. Working conditions and psychotropic medication: a prospective cohort study. *Soc Psychiatry Psychiatr Epidemiol* 2012; 47: 663–670.

180. Kim W, Park EC, Lee TH, Kim TH. Effect of working hours and precarious employment on depressive symptoms in South Korean employees: a longitudinal study. *Occup Environ Med* 2016; 73: 816–822.

181. Bae SH, Fabry D. Assessing the relationships between nurse work hours/overtime and nurse and patient outcomes: systematic literature review. *Nurs Outlook* 2014; 62: 138–156.

182. Bannai A, Tamakoshi A. The association between long working hours and health: a systematic review of epidemiological evidence. *Scand J Work Environ Health* 2014; 40: 5–18.

183. Kantermann T, Juda M, Vetter C, Roenneberg T. Shift-work research: Where do we stand, where should we go? *Sleep Biol Rhythms* 2010; 8: 95–105.

184. Rutenfranz J, Colquhoun WP, Knauth P, Ghata JN. Biomedical and psychosocial aspects of shift work. A review. *Scand J Work Environ Health* 1977; 3: 165–182.

185. Harrington JM. Shift work and health—a critical review of the literature on working hours. *Ann Acad Med Singapore* 1994; 23: 699–705.

186. Tucker P, Knowles SR. Review of studies that have used the Standard Shiftwork Index: evidence for the underlying model of shiftwork and health. *Appl Ergon* 2008; 39: 550–564.

187. Sancini A, Ciarrocca M, Capozzella A, et al. Lavoro a turni e notturno e salute mentale. *G Ital Med Lav Ergon* 2012; 34: 76–84.

188. Kaneko SY, Maeda T, Sasaki A, et al. Effect of shift work on mental state of factory workers. *Fukushima J Med Sci* 2004; 50: 1–9.

189. Arimura M, Imai M, Okawa M, Fujimura T, Yamada N. Sleep, mental health status, and medical errors among hospital nurses in Japan. *IND Health* 2010; 48: 811–817.

190. Selvi Y, Özdemir PG, Özdemir O, Aydın A, Beşiroğlu L. Influence of night shift work on psychologic state and quality of life in health workers. *Dusunen Adam* 2010; 23: 238–243.

191. Driesen K, Jansen NW, van Amelsvoort LG, Kant I. The mutual relationship between shift work and depressive complaints—a prospective cohort study. *Scand J Work Environ Health* 2011; 37: 402–410.

192. Bara AC, Arber S. Working shifts and mental health—findings from the British Household Panel Survey (1995–2005). *Scand J Work Environ Health* 2009; 35: 361–367.

193. Thun E, Le Hellard S, Osland T, et al. Circadian clock genes, insomnia, sleepiness and shift work disorder. *J Sleep Research* 2014; 23: 251–251.

194. Nabe-Nielsen K, Kecklund G, Ingre M, Skotte J, Diderichsen F, Garde AH. The importance of individual preferences when evaluating the associations between working hours and indicators of health and well-being. *Appl Ergon* 2010; 41: 779–786.

195. Joyce K, Pabayo R, Critchley JA, Bambra C. Flexible working conditions and their effects on employee health and wellbeing. *Cochrane Database Syst Rev* 2012; 2: CD008009.

196. Chida Y, Steptoe A. Cortisol awakening response and psychosocial factors: a systematic review and meta-analysis. *Biol Psychol* 2009; 80: 265–278.

197. Deuschle M, Schweiger U, Weber B, et al. Diurnal activity and pulsatility of the hypothalamus-pituitary-adrenal system in male depressed patients and healthy controls. *J Clin Endocrinol Metab* 1997; 82: 234–238.

198. Carroll BJ, Cassidy F, Naftolowitz D, et al. Pathophysiology of hypercortisolism in depression. *Acta Psychiatr Scand Suppl* 2007; 433: 90–103.

CHAPTER 12

Public mental health and occupational health

Katie Blissard Barnes and Max Henderson

Introduction

Public mental health is concerned with the mental health of the general population, including both the prevention of mental illness and broader promotion of good mental health and well-being [1]. Poor mental health affects up to one in four of the population, most of whom are in work [2–4]. Using the workplace as a focus for public mental health may bring benefits to the employer and the employee, and has the potential to reach a large proportion of the wider population. Managing the potential risks posed by work and supporting those with psychiatric disorders to enter and remain in work can have positive business impacts. Preventing mental illness can reduce absenteeism, thereby boosting productivity and improving wider economic performance [5, 6]. Promoting good-quality work can be perceived as one way of achieving improved public mental health [7].

Occupational health

Occupational medicine is a medical specialty that focuses on the interface between health and work [8]. Multidisciplinary occupational health (OH) teams work to keep people healthy at work. They provide advice to employers and employees about all aspects of the working environment, including the psychosocial work environment, in order to prevent injury and ill health. They help identify injury and ill health when it arises in the workplace or interferes with occupational function. They assist the employer and the employee in making decisions about fitness to work, and many assist employees in accessing appropriate therapeutic interventions, although very few provide treatment themselves. They do, however, liaise with other specialists and general practitioners to devise and implement strategies to rehabilitate and return to work those who have been off sick.

OH professionals have a responsibility to both employer and employee. The responsibility to the employee is delivered at both the individual and the group level; group level ranges from small teams to multinational organizations. In the UK, the Health and Safety at Work Act (1974) provides a framework within which employers must manage the health of employees [9].

Public mental health and occupational health

OH practitioners and OH services focus not only on individuals, but also on the workplace and the organization. Depending on the organization they may influence aspects of physical safety, systems of work, and employee emotional and psychological health. This dual role provides an opportunity for OH teams and professionals to affect the health of the population, whether that is the population employed by the organization, the population local to the organization, or the population made up of the organization's customers.

Historically, OH has been more concerned with physical risks, such as heat, noise, dust, and chemicals. As work has changed so the risks have changed. In many countries heavy manufacturing has been replaced by service industries. Workplaces have changed, work has changed, and workers have changed. There is a growing appreciation that symptom-based conditions, including, although not exclusively, psychiatric disorders, represent a greater risk than conditions where a clear cause could be identified in the physical environment [10]. This has required a shift in approach, with perhaps an even greater recognition that both 'exposures' and 'outcomes' must be understood at the population and group level. Employee mental health is now an important business issue owing to the acknowledgement of the effect it can have on the functioning of a business.

Mental health at work

Mental illness is under-recognized and still highly stigmatized [11–14]. Many employees do not disclose their psychiatric disorder to their employer [15]. A history of a psychiatric disorder can have an impact at multiple stages of the employment process. People with psychiatric disorders may not apply for jobs, either for fear their history will be held against them, or because they themselves believe they are not up to the job—so-called self-stigmatization [16–18]. Sadly, the perception that having a mental health disorder reduced your risk of employment used to be true, with over a third of employers stating they would not employ someone with a mental health disorder [11, 19]. Once in work, similar influences impact on access to training or promotion [20].

Deciding whether or not to disclose, to whom, and when can be a big decision. Those who decide not to disclose a history of psychiatric disorder run a number of risks [13, 21], not least that then accessing appropriate help should the need arise becomes more difficult. Brohan et al. [22] have described in detail the range of positive and negative influences on the decision-making process. Their study suggests that employer understanding of mental health—a vital component in any disclosure decision—has been slow to evolve. Limited by understanding of mental health issues, people still do not seek help for mental health problems as early as with a physical health problem [22, 23]. Henderson et al. [24] have developed and trialed a tool to help employees make the decision about disclosure. Early results—admittedly on small numbers—showed reduced decisional conflict in those using the CORAL tool [25].

In the UK the Disability Discrimination Act 1995 made it an offence to treat someone differently on the basis of a disability [26]. The definition of disability used in the Act, with a focus on the ability to perform normal day-to-day activities, allowed a number of psychiatric disorders to be included. The Disability Discrimination Act 1995 was incorporated into the Equality Act in 2010 [27, 28]. Legislation is a public statement about the values held by society, and the drafting of disability legislation to include psychiatric illness has been a major step forward. Under the terms of the Act employers are required to make 'reasonable' adjustments to the jobs of employees who are 'qualifying persons'. While raising awareness and providing a structure are positive, legislative solutions remain limited by the fact that the onus is on the disabled person to show that they are, indeed, a 'qualifying person' and then to persuade the court that a proposed adjustment is 'reasonable'.

OH is in a unique position to start and, indeed, encourage conversations and openness about mental health and ill health in the workplace. Providing a safe place to disclose mental ill health can then facilitate a better awareness of psychiatric disorders by employers and all employees, and lead to better support structures being adopted. The dual responsibility of OH to employer and employee can also allow OH to impact both at an individual clinical level and at a population level. The approach to stigma is one example. OH can interact with individual employees and individual line managers to educate and challenge preconceived ideas about psychiatric illness, including self-stigma. The role that a number of OH professionals and services have in shaping organizational culture can have a wider population-level impact on reducing stigmatizing responses to those with psychiatric disorders.

Work and the social determinants of health

While biological medicine is advancing rapidly there is also a growing recognition of the wider social determinants of health. A range of reports, at the national and international level, have highlighted the key role of social circumstances in influencing general health and well-being [29–32]. High-quality, safe working conditions promote positive health outcomes, including mental health outcomes; poor working environments, low wages, and insecure employment can all contribute to poor health [31, 32].

With hours needing to link with the global economy for many jobs, and the expanding 24/7 lifestyle, more and more people are working shift work, with hours into and across the night [33]. This is true in medicine and is now becoming commonplace for other roles such as finance, retail, and transport. Working nights, and long stretches of days, including weekends, can be exhausting and can impact on day-to-day routines of eating and sleeping. It can contribute to social isolation. There is a small but growing literature linking night working and common mental disorders (CMD) [34, 35].

Health inequalities

'Health inequalities' refers to variation in the health and the determinants of health between different groups and populations. These inequalities are seen in many aspects of public mental health.

Those in the most deprived areas suffer the most with psychiatric disorders and are at risk of a slower recovery from mental illness [5, 36]. Poor mental health can be seen as both an exposure and an outcome in this context. Mental illness can lead directly or indirectly, for example via worsening of a physical illness, to an employee exiting employment. This, in turn, can lead to greater poverty. Those already some distance from the labour market, often the least well educated, with poorer housing, have a high prevalence of psychiatric disorders, which, in turn, holds them down at the bottom of society [37]. Any service provision that helps reduce the development of ill health at work, secures early identification of ill health at work, helps keep employees in work or at least close to work despite being ill, and assists a successful and sustainable return to work for those who have been absent as a result of illness can act as a counterweight to the negative relationship between poor mental health and poor occupational function.

Inverse care law

The inverse care law, first described by Tudor Hart, observes that those who need good health care the most are often the least likely to receive it [38]. Initially described in primary care, it can also be recognized in employment and OH. Those in the least secure jobs, on low pay, and in the lowest-quality working conditions would seem the most likely to benefit from robust OH support. This could be to ensure their safety, to minimize absence, or to facilitate a sustainable and successful return to work after illness. In the UK, however, occupational medicine provision is patchy and limited. Large organizations, and much of the public sector, are most likely to have access to high-quality OH services [39], perhaps in 70%. It is often much more readily available to employees higher up in an organization than those at the bottom. However, in the UK more people are employed by small- and medium-sized employers, leaving over 60% of the UK workforce without specialist occupational medicine. Primary care works hard to fill in, and is better trained than ever, but still most general practitioners will have little or no specialist training on occupational medicine.

Physical–mental health interface

Long-term conditions and common mental disorders

Long-term conditions (LTCs) include diseases that cannot currently be cured, such as heart disease, diabetes, and chronic obstructive pulmonary disease [40]. LTCs are common and expensive, with almost a third of the UK population having at least one and as much as 70% of the National Health Service (NHS) budget being spent on them [40]. The number with more than one LTC is also set to increase over the coming years, putting more strain on healthcare systems. In addition, LTCs carry a significantly higher risk of mental health problems compared with those who do not have an LTC, with almost double the numbers of CMDs with just one LTC [41]. The converse is also true with those suffering from CMD being more likely to have a LTC [3, 42]. Patients with both conditions are likely to struggle more to recover from physical health problems, or manage their LTC, i.e. comorbid LTCs and CMDs lead to poor health outcomes and quality of life [41].

The role of employment and occupational health

Public health is both mental and physical; public mental health cannot exist in isolation. Strategies need to take into account the relationship between mental and physical health. Similarly, OH deals with both physical and mental health problems, alone and in combination presenting in the workplace. The role of the OH professional, and the position of OH within an organization are not always clear to employees. Some may be reluctant to either attend or to disclose some aspects of their medical history for fear of it being passed to management.

This is a particular issue with mental illness. Employees may be more comfortable with a physical diagnosis, or a less precise term such as 'stress', where there is a problem outside them that has been 'done to' them. Many still see mental illness as evidence of personal failure. Mental and physical comorbidity is an even greater challenge as the mental health component may be missed or under-appreciated by both patient and clinician. An 'either mental or physical' mindset can be seen in sickness absence records, including the UK Fit Note record, where often only a single diagnosis is recorded. OH practitioners need to have a low threshold for considering that a mental disorder may be part of the presentation. There is little evidence to recommend a formal 'screening' process, but rather the development of a mindset and a recognition that psychiatric disorder is common yet may not announce itself. OH can assist stigma reduction by creating an environment where disclosure is as easy and as non-threatening as possible.

Risk to health from work

Work is usually beneficial to health, including mental health [43, 44]. Beyond just providing an income, it gives people a sense of purpose, a structure to the day or week, a sense of achievement, and the opportunity to interact with others [43]. Poor mental health is strongly associated with unemployment [45, 46]. OH has an important role in helping those with mental heath problems stay in, or close to, work.

Not all work is good for you. 'Work is good for your health' has been updated to 'Good work is good for your health'. Poor-quality work may be worse for your health than no job at all [7]. Features that define poor-quality work include long hours, antisocial shift patterns, low pay, and job insecurity [29, 47]. Some suggest that having a poor job is as bad as being unemployed [47]. A number of groups are over-represented in the population employed in low-quality employment. These include those with lower educational attainment, those with a history of contact with the criminal justice system, and those with a history of difficulties with drugs or alcohol. People in these groups are also more likely to suffer with mental health problems. In addition, they may find even these jobs hard to sustain—the low-pay no-pay cycle [48]. This can precipitate worsening of that individuals' mental health.

The remit of OH is the health of a particular group of employees, but public mental health is concerned with the wider population. They may not be as far apart as might initially be thought, however. Every employee has a social network, a community to which they belong, friends, and family. Adverse effects of mental illness on occupational function and job retention can negatively impact on these social circles. The impact of decisions taken by OH is felt more widely than the workplace.

How to make bad work good?

The stigma associated with mental illness can prevent people seeking help, which, in turn, means individuals suffer their mental illness without support [22]. This can lead to absence from work and either leaving entirely or a slow process of return to work. Reducing stigma makes up a huge barrier to public mental health and is equally important within businesses.

The psychosocial work environment

Efforts to understand how the psychosocial work environment can impact on employee mental health have resulted in at least three models, each with a body of supporting evidence. It is important to understand what factors within work contribute to poor mental health to therefore overcome it. There are three models that have been developed that outline the different risks to mental health from work. These are job strain [49, 50], effort–reward imbalance [51], and organizational justice [52, 53].

Job strain model

The job strain model, also known as the job demand–control model contrasts the demands placed on an employee with their ability to control their work. High job strain is the combination of high demands and low control/decision latitude. A number of adverse health and employment outcomes have been associated with job strain, including cardiovascular disease [54], CMD [55], greater sickness absence [56], and ill-health retirement [57, 58]. More recently, it has been suggested that support at work can mitigate some of the effects of job strain. This may be support from fellow colleagues or management, with the support mechanisms acting as a buffer when the demand may be high or control low [59–62].

These factors are consistent across different jobs and populations, suggesting this is not just relevant for individual businesses and employers, but a wider public mental health issue. OH physicians can play a key role here to not only work with individuals, but also at an organization-wide level to educate all on coping strategies, improving communication, increasing control within their role, and so on. This can positively affect individuals and the organization [6, 59–61, 63].

Effort-reward imbalance model

The effort–reward imbalance model was proposed by Johannes Siegrist [51]. Here, the efforts expended by an individual employee are contrasted with the rewards received by the employee. Both effort and reward are defined. Notably, reward is understood far more broadly than simply financial rewards. Siegrist suggested that a combination of high effort but low reward led to adverse outcomes and a substantial literature now supports this. Effort–reward imbalance is associated with increased risk of poor mental health, mainly depression and anxiety [64], both short-term and long-term sickness absence [65], and an increased risk of cardiovascular disease [66].

This is not to say that jobs should have a low demand in order to make work a more positive experience, but mediating this so that expected effort is not unattainable and that receiving an element of reward for that hard work done is important. This can be achieved in many ways, but often these can be simple strategies that OH physicians can work with employers to incorporate into their business structure.

What this model did differently to that of Robert Karasek's, is to consider the role of overcommitment, a personality characteristic of the individual that would act as a catalyst towards poor mental health in the situation of high effort, low reward [67]. This is an area OH can explore with individuals, so that improving employees mental health does not just become the responsibility of the employer.

Organizational justice model

Organizational justice concerns the extent to which an employee perceives the way he is treated by his employers to be fair [68]. Different types of justice are described, and although correlated, each type has an independent association with a range of occupational outcomes, in particular sickness absence [53].

Low perceived organizational justice is causally related to poor mental health, and this can be applied to men and woman and across a range of occupations and employers [52]. 'Procedural justice', the say employees have over changes in the workplace, had a much larger effect on those higher paid and more skilled jobs. Procedural injustice has been shown to have a stronger impact on mental health than 'relational injustice', i.e. how you believe you are treated by supervisors. Organizational justice models contain an element of interpersonal relationships missing from the other models of the psychosocial work environment [53].

Irrespective of the model, there are two critical points of intervention for improving mental health in the workplace—to reduce the primary causes of mental ill health, and to better enable employees and employers to identify and treat it when it does arise. Supporting and involving all members in discussion about adapting an organization increases the sense of control and organizational justice. This involvement in decision-making can reduce the negative impact of work on mental health and help to reduce stigma.

Preventative strategies need to sit alongside plans for early recognition when mental illness does occur. Models of the psychosocial work environment provide a blueprint for creating more mentally health workplaces where, for example, support is easily available for employees in difficulty [6, 22]. This is discussed more fully in the next subsection. Sometimes, avoiding risks for fear of poor mental health is not possible, but improving resilience and coping strategies might help. One study found that an outreach programme to identify those with depression and offer treatment early, rather than once they were already absent from work gained a positive outcome in terms of being financially beneficial and keeping employees in work [69, 70].

Health and Safety Executive 'Management Standards'

The body responsible for the enforcement of health, safety, and welfare legislation in the UK is the Health and Safety Executive (HSE), created by the 1974 Health and Safety at Work Act [9]. In response to concerns about the rise in 'stress at work' and, in particular, its economic impact, the HSE established the 'Management Standards' [71]. These cover what the HSE regards as the 'primary causes' of 'stress at work'—demands, control, support, relationships, role, and change. The HSE recommends organizations use a risk-management approach and suggest incorporating the HSE Management Standards Indicator Tool, a 35-part questionnaire, to generate data from employees. The Management Standards set out 'States to Be Achieved' across the six areas, namely that 85% of employees in an organization report that they are able to, for example, 'deal with the demands of their job'.

The HSE Management Standards lean heavily on Karasek's job strain model, and were established before research emerged questioning its simple adoption [72, 73]. 'Stress' is difficult to define

and the Management Standards uses 'the adverse reaction people have to excessive pressure or other types of demand placed upon them'. This is problematic as not only is it somewhat circular, but it just moves the problem of definition onto what is an 'adverse reaction': how can one be sure that the 'adverse reaction' is associated with the 'excessive pressure' and, indeed, how does one tell if pressure is 'excessive'?

That a statutory body such as the HSE has taken such a keen interest in occupational mental health is of great significance to both occupational medicine and to public mental health. The clear implication that Health and Safety at Work includes mental, as well as physical health is important, and represents an early example of so-called parity of esteem. The generation and utilization of the Management Standards has a number of limitations, however, arising, in part, from a perceived need to instrumentalize what is a rather nuanced phenomenon. By attaching a scoring approach the 'equivalence' of each standard is implied, and suggesting a cut-off where these data generate a binary position 'acceptable' versus 'not acceptable' seems an oversimplification. No recognition is given to the possible role of factors relating to the individual (background, history, etc.) on the alleged causal pathway between exposure ('excessive pressure') and outcome ('stress') [73–75]. The intersection between 'stress' and frank ill health is not addressed at all

Risk to work from poor health

Mental illness results in the greatest burden of disease in the UK [42]. The World Health Organization has identified that mental illness accounts for the biggest cause of lost disability-adjusted life years [76]. Worldwide the amount of money spent on mental illness was US\$2.5 trillion and this is predicted to rise by 2030 to US\$6 trillion [76]. It is believed the total cost of poor mental health in the UK is over £100 billion [39, 77]. This includes days of productivity lost via sick days, the cost of reduced efficiency of staff suffering from mental health problems, and the cost of care for these individuals. Sick days alone contribute to over 10 million days lost due to CMD such as depression [3, 42], with up to three times the risk of unemployment if you have a mental disorder [78].

Risk to whom?

The impact of poor mental health on work can be felt at a number of levels. Employee health is a major focus for employers, in part because it can impact on the bottom line in terms of profit and growth [3, 79]. It can also be felt more widely in its effects on colleagues and managers. In safety-critical businesses, such as the airline industry or health care, there are potentially greater impacts.

Risk to the business

Poor staff mental health can have both financial and non-financial impacts on business. Adverse financial impacts arise from the cost of sick pay, ill-health retirement, staff recruitment and replacement costs, and lower productivity. Lower productivity costs can emerge whether staff go on sick leave or not. The cost to UK businesses from reduced productivity and sickness absence has been estimated as £26 billion [39]. The most recent 2016 Green Paper in the UK states that 1.7 million people of working age have a mental health problem and are not in work. This lack of employment is not only detrimental financially and psychologically to the individuals, but also represents a loss of valuable skills and labour for businesses.

This is being increasingly recognized by key government and NHS leaders, in particular [5]. The better workplace leaders understand the implications of poor mental health in work, the easier it will be to involve them in changes.

As a clinical medical specialty, occupational medicine has a role in the assessment of individual employees. In many organizations, notably larger organizations, occupational medicine may have the ability to influence policies and guidelines, and through these organizational culture, in line with a public mental health agenda. In many instances the case will need to be made on purely economic grounds, but there are increasing examples of organizations who view their position on staff health, including mental health, as part of their wider corporate responsibility agenda. By definition, large organizations employ large numbers of people, meaning the impact of measures taken here can be significant. These benefits to the organization are not wholly distinct from the financial benefits. Organizations that develop a culture of high engagement and well-being, where employees feel able to be open about the difficulties the face, either work- or non-work-related, will attract higher-calibre job applicants, retain them longer, and allow them to be more productive.

Presenteeism is the phenomenon where sick employees remain in work but are less productive [80–82]. They can be more difficult to identify and therefore to help [3, 83]. Presenteeism is strongly associated with psychiatric illness, in part because mental disorders are 'invisible' and because there can be such a stigma associated with disclosure. It can be very expensive, costing, in some reports, more than absenteeism [84].

The current Green Paper [39], published in the autumn of 2016 by the UK government, outlines a new approach to provide continued support to those individuals who were unemployed, once they have found employment. This will provide further support, including financial to those on a low income, aiming to keep people in work, further benefiting the employer. The approach specifically recognizes the role that OH can play.

Risk to the customer

The adverse impact of mental illness on employee function brings additional difficulties for safety-critical industries. Two obvious examples are the aviation industry and health care. Notable cases such as the 'German Wings' incident, where a pilot with a history of psychiatric illness deliberately flew his plane into the side of a mountain, in an apparent suicide, have focused attention on how the concept of fitness to fly is defined and assessed, and by whom [85]. Should anyone with a history of mental illness be allowed to fly, and if so whom? In such situations the challenges of psychiatry, such as the lack of objective tests like blood tests or scans, are amplified, making the role of the occupational physician especially difficult. A strict regulatory framework is placed around the certification of pilots, for example in the UK by the Civil Aviation Authority. As ever, these regulations are only ever as good as their weakest link, often the human tasked with applying them.

Health care, too, is subject to tight regulation—in the UK the General Medical Council regulates doctors, and the Nursing and Midwifery Council regulates nurses and midwives, for example. Mental illness can impair the way a healthcare professional works within their team, or impact on crucial decisions they may make. While this may have catastrophic consequences for patients, modern health care is delivered by teams, often multidisciplinary teams, in part to minimize the impact of any single individual. Again, occupational medicine has a crucial role in assessing and advising on the fitness to work of healthcare professionals. Here, though, they face an additional complication, that of working with the doctor-patient.

Doctors have high rates of mental illness, high rates of drug and alcohol misuse [86], and a reputation for being difficult patients to manage if they seek help at all [87]. Doctoring doctors brings issues of seniority, confidentiality, trust, and honesty, especially if the doctor-patient believes the treating doctor may prevent them working. However, doctors deserve the same quality of health care as the rest of the population and must be managed within whatever disability discrimination legislation applies in their country [88, 89]. And patients need doctors to be well and at work to care for them! Large numbers of people are employed in health care in many countries; occupational medicine provided to this sector of the workforce has a substantial double opportunity to progress the public mental health agenda by influencing the health and well-being of the workforce, and the populations they care for.

Conclusion

One of the key roles of the OH team and OH practitioner is the work that is done with the individual employee-patient. On the surface this has a limited interface with the wider public mental health agenda. But work and the workplace are so focal to public mental health that a high-quality OH interaction can have a positive public mental health impact. Improving the mental health of one employee or improving their ability to manage their mental ill health in the workplace, and therefore keep them in work, has benefits beyond that individual. A culture of a mentally healthy workplace can develop: colleagues with similar difficulties notice and are more prepared to disclose mental health problems and employers' fears of an employee with a mental illness are assuaged. The individual stays in work, benefiting their family and their children have a parent in work rather than on benefits. The employee produces, and pays tax, both of which benefit the wider economy. The dual responsibility of OH to employer and employee provides an unrivalled platform for this work.

OH is more often found in large organizations than small- and medium-sized enterprises. While this means many employees miss out, those within bigger organizations can benefit from work done by OH without ever coming into direct contact. The workplace is an ideal place to deliver improvements in public mental health, and OH is the main channel into the workplace with regard to health. Encouraging organizations, from line managers up to board level to engage with the public mental health agenda is a worthwhile challenge for OH. Using the increasing evidence base available, although moving beyond the stale 'stress' approach exemplified by the HSE Management Standards, OH can deliver benefits at the individual organization and population level. This must be fundamentally good for OH, too.

References

1. Faculty of Public Health. Why public mental health matters. Available at: http://www.fph.org.uk/why_public_mental_health_matters (2010, accessed 13 September 2016).

2. NHS Digital. Adult Psychiatric Morbidity in England – 2007, Results of a household survey. Available at: http://digital.nhs.uk/catalogue/PUB02931 (2007, accessed 20 February 2018).

3. Sainsbury Centre for Mental Health (SCMH). *Mental Health at Work: Developing the Business Case (Policy Paper 8)*. London: SCMH, 2007.

4. World Health Organization (WHO). *The World Health Report 2001—Mental Health: New Understanding, New Hope*. Geneva: WHO, 2001.

5. NHS Confederation. *Public Mental Health and Wellbeing—The Local Perspective*. London: NHS, 2011.

6. LaMontagne AD, Martin A, Page KM, et al. Workplace mental health: developing an integrated intervention approach. *BMC Psychiatry* 2014; 14: 131.

7. Butterworth P, Leach LS, Strazdins L, Olesen SC, Rodgers B, Broom DH. The psychosocial quality of work determines whether employment has benefits for mental health: results from a longitudinal national household panel survey. *Occup Environ Med* 2011; 68: 806–812.

8. Palmer KT, Brown I, Hobson J (eds). *Fitness for Work: The Medical Aspects*. London: Oxford University Press, 2013.

9. Health and Safety Executive. Health and Safety at Work etc Act 1974. Available at: http://www.hse.gov.uk/legislation/hswa.htm (accessed 20 February 2018).

10. Henderson M, Holland-Elliott K, Hotopf M, Wessely S. Liaison psychiatry and occupational health. *Occup Med (Lond)* 2001; 51: 479–481.

11. Bunt K, Shury J, Vivian D. *Recruiting Benefit Claimants: A Qualitative Study of Employers who Recruited Benefit Claimants (Research Report No. 150)*. London: Department for Work and Pensions, 2001.

12. McGrath B. *Mental Health, The Last Workplace Taboo*. London: Shaw Trust, 2010.

13. Royal College of Psychiatrists. *Mental Health and Work*. London: The Stationery Office, 2008.

14. Stuart H. Mental illness and employment discrimination. *Curr Opin Psychiatry* 2006; 19: 522–526.

15. National Health Service. NHS Health and Well-being. Final Report. Available at: http://webarchive.nationalarchives.gov.uk/20130107105354/http://www.dh.gov.uk/prod_consum_dh/groups/dh_digitalassets/documents/digitalasset/dh_108907.pdf (2008, accessed 17 October 2016).

16. Corrigan PW, Rao D. On the self-stigma of mental illness: stages, disclosure, and strategies for change. *Can J Psychiatry* 2012; 57: 464–469.

17. Corrigan PW, Larson JE, Rusch N. Self-stigma and the 'why try' effect: impact on life goals and evidence-based practices. *World Psychiatry* 2009; 8: 75–81.

18. Corrigan PW, Watson AC. Understanding the impact of stigma on people with mental illness. *World Psychiatry* 2002; 1: 16–20.

19. Manning C, White P, Attitudes of employers to the mentally ill. *Psychiatr Bull* 1995; 19: 541–543.

20. Michalak EE, Yatham LN, Maxwell V, Hale S, Lam RW. The impact of bipolar disorder upon work functioning: a qualitative analysis. *Bipolar Disord* 2007; 9: 126–143.

21. MacDonald-Wilson KL, Russinova Z, Rogers ES, et al. Disclosure of mental health disabilities in the workplace. In: Schultz IZ Rogers ES (eds). *Handbook of Work Accommodation and Retention in Mental Health*. New York: Springer, 2010, pp. 191–217.

22. Brohan E, Henderson C, Wheat K, et al. Systematic review of beliefs, behaviours and influencing factors associated with disclosure of a mental health problem in the workplace. *BMC Psychiatry* 2012; 12: 11.

23. Corrigan P. How stigma interferes with mental health care. *Am Psychol* 2004; 59: 614–625.

24. Henderson C, Brohan E, Clement S, et al. A decision aid to assist decisions on disclosure of mental health status to an employer: protocol for the CORAL exploratory randomised controlled trial. *BMC Psychiatry* 2012; 12: 133.

25. Henderson C, Brohan E, Clement S, et al. Decision aid on disclosure of mental health status to an employer: feasibility and outcomes of a randomised controlled trial. *Br J Psychiatry* 2013; 203: 350–357.

26. Act of Parliament. Disability Discrimination Act 1995. Available at: http://www.legislation.gov.uk/ukpga/1995/50/contents (accessed 20 February 2018).

27. Act of Parliament. Equality Act 2010. Available at: http://www.legislation.gov.uk/ukpga/2010/15/pdfs/ukpga_20100015_en.pdf (accessed 20 February 2018).

28. Lockwood G, Henderson C, Thornicroft G. The Equality Act 2010 and mental health. *Br J Psychiatry* 2012; 200: 182–183.

29. Commission on Social Determinants of Health. *Closing the Gap in a Generation: Health Equity Through Action on the Social Determinants of Health. Final Report of the Commission on Social Determinants of Health*. Geneva: World Health Organization, 2008.

30. Marmot M, Goldblatt P, Allen J, et al. *Fair Society Healthy Lives (The Marmot Review)*. Available at: http://www.instituteofhealthequity.org/resources-reports/fair-society-healthy-lives-the-marmot-review (accessed 20 February 2018).

31. Organisation for Economic Co-operation and Development (OECD). *Transforming Disability Into Ability: Policies to Promote Work and Income Security for Disabled People*. Paris: OECD, 2003.

32. Bartley M, Ferie J, Montgomery S. Health and labour market disadvantage: unemployment, nonemployment and job insecurity. In: Marmot M, Wilkinson RG (eds). *Social Determinants of Health*. Oxford: Oxford University Press, 2006, pp. 78–96.

33. TUC. Number of people working night shifts up by more than 250,000 since 2011, new TUC analysis reveals. Available at: https://www.tuc.org.uk/economic-issues/industrial-issues/workplace-issues/number-people-working-night-shifts-more-250000 (2016, accessed 14 December 2016).

34. Jaradat YM, Nielsen MB, Kristensen P, Bast-Pettersen. Shift work, mental distress and job satisfaction among Palestinian nurses. *Occup Med (Lond)* 2017; 67: 71–74.

35. Norder G, Roelen CAM, Bültmann U, van der Klink JJL. Shift work and mental health sickness absence: a 10-year observational cohort study among male production workers. *Scand J Work Environ Health* 2015; 41: 413–416.

36. Fryers T, Melzer D, Jenkins R, Brugha T. The distribution of the common mental disorders: social inequalities in Europe. *Clin Pract Epidemiol Mental Health* 2005; 1: 14.

37. Siegrist J, Benach J, McKnight A, Goldblatt P, Muntaner C. *Employment Arrangements, Work Conditions and Health Inequalities. Report on New Evidence on Health Inequality Reduction, Produced by Task Group 2 for the Strategic Review of Health Inequalities Post-2010*. London: UCL Institute of Health Equity, 2010.

38. Tudor Hart J. The inverse care law. *Lancet* 1971; 1: 405–412.

39. Department for Work and Pensions (DWP). *Improving Lives. The Work, Health and Disability Green Paper*. London: DWP, 2016.

40. Department of Health (DoH). *Long Term Conditions Compendium of Information*. Leeds: DoH, 2012.

41. Naylor C, Parsonage M, McDaid D, Knapp M, Fossey M, Galea A. Long-term conditions and mental health: The cost of co-morbidities. Available at: https://www.kingsfund.org.uk/sites/default/files/field/field_publication_file/long-term-conditions-mental-health-cost-comorbidities-naylor-feb12.pdf (2012, accessed 20 February 2018).

42. Royal College of Psychiatrists (RCP). *No Health Without Public Mental Health; The Case for Action*. London: RCP, 2010.

43. Waddell G, Burton A. *Is Work Good for Your Health and Well-being?* London: The Stationery Office, 2006.

44. National Institute for Health and Care Excellence (NICE). *Promoting Mental Wellbeing at Work: Full Guidance*. NICE: London, 2009.

45. Yoo KB, Park EC, Jang SY, et al. Association between employment status change and depression in Korean adults. *BMJ Open* 2016; 6: e008570.

46. McGee RE, Thompson NJ. Unemployment and depression among emerging adults in 12 states, Behavioral Risk Factor Surveillance System, 2010. *Prev Chronic Dis* 2015; 12: E38.

47. Ervasti J, Vahtera J, Virtanen P, et al. Is temporary employment a risk factor for work disability due to depressive disorders and delayed return to work? The Finnish Public Sector Study. *Scand J Work Environ Health* 2014; 40: 343–352.

48. Bambra C. *Work, Worklessness, and the Political Economy of Health.* Oxford: Oxford University Press, 2011.

49. Karasek R. Job demands, job decision latitude, and mental strain: implications for job redesign. *Adm Sci Q* 1979; 24: 285–307.

50. Karasek R, Theorell T. *Healthy Work. Stress, Productivity, and the Reconstruction of the Working Life.* New York: Basic Books, 1990.

51. Siegrist J. Adverse health effects of high-effort/low-reward conditions. *J Occup Health Psychol* 1996; 1: 27–41.

52. Kivimäki M, et al. Organisational justice and health of employees: prospective cohort study. *Occup Environ Med* 2003; 60: 27–33.

53. Ndjaboue R, Brisson C, Vezina M. Organisational justice and mental health: a systematic review of prospective studies. *Occup Environ Med* 2012; 69: 694–700.

54. Kuper H, Marmot M. Job strain, job demands, decision latitude, and risk of coronary heart disease within the Whitehall II study. *J Epidemiol Community Health* 2003; 57: 147–153.

55. Stansfeld SA, Fuhrer R, Shipley MJ, Marmot MG. Work characteristics predict psychiatric disorder: prospective results from the Whitehall II Study. *Occup Environ Med* 1999; 56: 302–307.

56. North FM, Syme SL, Feeney A, Shipley M, Marmot M. Psychosocial work environment and sickness absence among British civil servants: the Whitehall II study. *Am J Public Health* 1996; 86: 332–340.

57. Laine S, et al. Job strain as a predictor of disability pension: the Finnish Public Sector Study. *J Epidemiol Community Health* 2009; 63: 24–30.

58. Mäntyniemi A, Oksanen T, Salo P, et al. Job strain and the risk of disability pension due to musculoskeletal disorders, depression or coronary heart disease: a prospective cohort study of 69,842 employees. *Occup Environ Med* 2012; 69: 574–581.

59. Michie S, Williams S. Reducing work related psychological ill health and sickness absence: a systematic literature review. *Occup Environ Med* 2003; 60: 3–9.

60. Bambra C, Egan M, Thomas S, Petticrew M, Whitehead M. The psychosocial and health effects of workplace reorganisation. 2. A systematic review of task restructuring interventions. *J Epidemiol Community Health* 2007; 61: 1028–1037.

61. Egan M, Bambra C, Thomas S, Petticrew M, Whitehead M, Thomson H. The psychosocial and health effects of workplace reorganisation. 1. A systematic review of organisational-level interventions that aim to increase employee control. *J Epidemiol Community Health* 2007; 61: 945–954.

62. Häusser J, Mojzisch A, Niesel M, Shculz-Hardt S. Ten years on: a review of research on job demand-control (-support) model and psychological well being. *Work Stress* 2010; 24: 1–35.

63. Lamontagne AD, Keegel T, Louie AM, Ostry A, Landsbergis PA. A systematic review of the job-stress intervention evaluation literature, 1990–2005. *Int J Occup Environ Health* 2007; 13: 268–280.

64. Ndjaboué R, Brisson C, Vézina M, Blanchette C, Bourbonnais R. Effort–reward imbalance and medically certified absence for mental health problems: a prospective study of white-collar workers. *Occup Environ Med* 2014; 71: 40–47.

65. Head J, Kivimäki M, Siegrist J, et al. Effort-reward imbalance and relational injustice at work predict sickness absence: the Whitehall II study. *J Psychosom Res* 2007; 63: 433–440.

66. Peter R, Siegrist J. Chronic psychosocial stress at work and cardiovascular disease: the role of effort-reward imbalance. *Int J Law Psychiatry* 1999; 22: 441–449.

67. Siegrist J, Li J. Associations of extrinsic and intrinsic components of work stress with health: a systematic review of evidence on the effort-reward imbalance model. *Int J Environ Res Public Health* 2016; 13: 432.

68. Elovainio M, Kivimaki M, Vahtera J. Organizational justice: evidence of a new psychosocial predictor of health. *Am J Public Health* 2002; 92: 105–108.

69. Wang PS, Simon GE, Avorn J, et al. Telephone screening, outreach, and care management for depressed workers and impact on clinical and work productivity outcomes: a randomized controlled trial. *JAMA* 2007; 298: 1401–1411.

70. Hill D, Lucy D, Tyers C, James L. *What Works at Work.* London: Institute of Employment Studies, 2007.

71. Health and Safety Executive (HSE). *Tackling Stress: The Management Standards Approach.* London: HSE, 2005.

72. Henderson M, Harvey SB, Overland S, Mykletun A, Hotopf M. Work and common psychiatric disorders. *J R Soc Med* 2011; 104: 198–207.

73. Henderson M, Clark C, Stansfeld S, Hotopf M. A lifecourse approach to long-term sickness absence—a cohort study. *PLOS ONE* 2012; 7: e36645.

74. Henderson M, Richards M, Stansfel S, Hotopf M. The association between childhood cognitive ability and adult long-term sickness absence in three British birth cohorts: a cohort study. *BMJ Open* 2012; 2(2).

75. Henderson M, Stansfeld S, Hotopf M. Self-rated health and later receipt of work-related benefits: evidence from the 1970 British Cohort Study. *Psychol Med* 2013; 43: 1755–1762.

76. World Health Organization (WHO). The global economic burden of noncommunicable diseases. Available at: http://apps.who.int/medicinedocs/en/d/Js18806en/ (2011, last accessed 20 February 2018).

77. Centre for Mental Health (CMH). *The Economic and Social Costs of Mental Health Problems in 2009/10.* London: CMH, 2010.

78. Melzer D, Fryers T, Jenkins R (eds). *Maudsley Monograph 44: Social Inequalities and the Distribution of Common Mental Disorders.* Hove: Psychology Press, 2004.

79. National Institute for Health and Care Excellence (NICE). *Promoting Mental Wellbeing at Work: Full Guidance PH22.* NICE: London, 2009.

80. Schultz AB, Edington DW. Employee health and presenteeism: a systematic review. *J Occup Rehabil* 2007; 17: 547–579.

81. Dew K, Keefe V, Small K. 'Choosing' to work when sick: workplace presenteeism. *Soc Sci Med* 2005; 60: 2273–2282.

82. Bergström G, Bodin L, Hagberg J, Aronsson G, Josephson M. Sickness presenteeism today, sickness absenteeism tomorrow? A prospective study on sickness presenteeism and future sickness absenteeism. *J Occup Environ Med* 2009; 51: 629–638.

83. National Institute for Health and Care Excellence (NICE). *Promoting Physical Activity in the Workplace: Full Guidance.* London: NICE, 2008.

84. Black C. *Working for a Healthier Tomorrow.* London: The Stationery Office, 2008.

85. Henderson M. Germanwings: Should there be screening for mental illness at work? Available at: http://www.bbc.co.uk/news/health-32735801 (2015, accessed 20 February 2018).

86. Murray RM. Characteristics and prognosis of alcoholic doctors. *Br Med J* 1976; 2: 1537–1539.

87. Brooks SK, Gerada C, Chalder T. Review of literature on the mental health of doctors: are specialist services needed? *J Ment Health* 2011; 20: 146–156.

88. Department of Health (DoH). *Mental Health and Ill Health in Doctors.* London: DoH, 2008.

89. Department of Health (DoH). *Good Doctors, Safer Patients: Proposals to Strengthen the System to Assure and Improve the Performance of Doctors and to Protect the Safety of Patients.* London: DoH, 2006.

CHAPTER 13

Health equity

Hideki Hashimoto and Norito Kawakami

Introduction

Achievement of health equity is a pivotal goal of healthcare systems [1]. However, the underlying philosophical definition of health equity is ambiguous, which complicates the formulation of policies and targets, and precludes effective implementation of the concept. This chapter has three objectives. Firstly, it seeks to review the existing literature to demonstrate the heterogeneity of the concept of health equity, and will review what is needed for health equity to be achieved in the context of the ethical basis referred to, such as libertarianism, utilitarianism, Kantian liberalism, and capability theory. Secondly, it will discuss the importance of mental health in the achievement of health equity, with reference to existing reviews of public mental health, and will examine the influence of social stigma and subsequent social exclusion as a barrier to achieving health equity. Finally, it will discuss the policy agenda to achieve health equity in the context of public mental health. The chapter refers to the concept of 'social determinants of health' to inform the formulation of a range of policies to achieve health equity.

Equity and equality

The most widely cited definition of 'health equity' is that proposed by Margaret Whitehead in her influential 1992 paper, namely that a lack of health equity is a condition where differences in health exist that 'are not only unnecessary and avoidable but, in addition, are considered unfair and unjust' [2]. Since then, however, the terms 'equity' and 'equality' have been used ambiguously and interchangeably too often, and the meaning of 'equity' varies across the literature.

For example, the United States Healthy People programme defines health equity as the 'attainment of the highest level of health for all people' [3]. In contrast, the World Health Organization (WHO) extends Whitehead's argument to define health equity as 'the absence of avoidable or remediable differences among groups of people … therefore involves more than inequality with respect to health determinants, access to the resources needed to improve and maintain health or health outcomes' [4]. In the latter context, inequity implies the existence of social injustice, and achievement of health equity requires moral discussion, whereas 'inequality' is a more value-neutral term and is taken semantically to equate with 'disparity'.

Equity is the absence of avoidable or remediable differences among groups of people, whether those groups are defined socially,

economically, demographically, or geographically. *Health inequities* therefore involve more than inequality with respect to health determinants, access to the resources needed to improve and maintain health or health outcomes. They also entail a failure to avoid or overcome inequalities that infringe on fairness and human rights norms.

Reducing health inequities is important because health is a fundamental human right and its progressive realization will eliminate inequalities that result from differences in health status (such as disease or disability) in the opportunity to enjoy life and pursue one's life plans.

A characteristic common to groups that experience health inequities—such as poor or marginalized persons, racial and ethnic minorities, and women—is lack of political, social or economic power. Thus, to be effective and sustainable, interventions that aim to redress inequities must typically go beyond remedying a particular health inequality and also help empower the group in question through systemic changes, such as law reform or changes in economic or social relationships.[1]

Others argue that inequity is a difference in the opportunities or means to achieve health, whereas inequality is a difference in ends, or health as a final outcome of concerns (e.g. Pan-American Health Organization). Equity therefore requires that all individuals in a population have equal opportunities to achieve health, whereas equality concerns whether consequences are equal. In this context, the differences between equity and equality reflect differences in appropriate targets for policy interventions to close gaps.

Disparities in consequential health outcomes will arise from several sources, including differences in availability of baseline resources and opportunities. Some may be less modifiable and may be distributed randomly, such as genetic properties and subsequent physical or cognitive capacities. Others are more susceptible to non-random selection due to socio-economic, cultural (e.g. caste), demographic (e.g. race or ethnicity), and political factors. Finally, given equal availability of baseline resources and opportunities, outcomes could still differ according to an individual's commitment to achieving goals, as well as by external influences such as accidents, economic shocks, conflict, and natural disasters.

Some differences in health outcomes can therefore be attributed to random chance, systemic selection by social structures, and individual commitment. There is a wide consensus that differences caused by systemic social selection beyond an individual's control are 'unfair', and should be alleviated by distributional justice

---

[1] Reproduced from Health Systems Topics: Equity, with permission from the World Health Organization. Available at http://www.who.int/healthsystems/topics/equity/en/

[5]. Differences arising solely from individual commitment and voluntary choice are attributed to individual responsibility, and interventions cannot (or should not) be made. However, individual commitment is often shaped by factors other than an individual's free will, such as the availability of resources, future projection, and sense of control, which are further influenced by social selection and subsequent resource availability. Thus, it may not be possible to attribute health outcome differences separately to social, individual, and chance attributes. This leads to the moral debate on how to achieve 'fairness' in equity.

Ethical basis for 'health equity'

What equity means depends on which ethical basis is referred to. As Amartya Sen elegantly stated, equity achieved under one school of ethical theory may be inequity under another [6]. This highlights the importance of understanding the contributions of different schools of ethical theory to the health equity debate.

Utilitarianism

Utilitarianism seeks for the maximization of social utility; an individual's utility is counted as one and no more than one, and any individual's welfare is treated equally. Utilitarianism weighs consequences regardless of the nature of interests, original positions, or conditions. Resource allocation is to be determined when the marginal utility gain derived from the obtained consequence of one (or one group) equals the marginal loss of others, so that no additional net gain is achievable in a society. Because it is concerned with consequences and ignores processes, utilitarianism is often criticized as lacking justice. In the health equity context, utilitarianism would seek to maximize the sum of 'quality adjusted life years', or a utility-weighted life year in the society [7]. As those with chronic conditions tend to have a lower chance of recovering their health status for a given investment, utilitarianism will assign a lower priority to investment for those with chronic conditions. As such, a utilitarian approach may not well address inequalities in opportunities to achieve health [8].

Libertarianism

Libertarianism takes the most value in self-governance, or an individual's right to determine her/his own destiny without external interference. If self-governance is equally secured, the outcomes that an individual could achieve are determined by her/his own commitment and responsibility. Differences in initial conditions leading to differences in outcomes do not induce a moral claim in the libertarian context. Those with impaired life chances, for example those with permanent disability and reduced opportunities to participate in the formal workforce, would be left to fend for themselves with or without informal care or support from family or charity. Redistribution through taxation to help those in need is against libertarian ethics, because the government institution coerces individuals into paying for somebody else. Thus, some criticize libertarianism for generating inequality in health outcomes [8].

Kantian liberalism

Kantian liberalism, also known as Rawlsian ethics, claims that differences in outcome caused by factors beyond an individual's control should be compensated, and further claims the 'min-max'

rule, namely that the least advantaged should be provided with the greatest possible opportunity. The concept is based on liberalism, in that individuals should be responsible for their own acts and decisions. Kantian liberalism claims that factors such as sex, race, ethnicity, socio-economic position, political minority status, and inherited physical or cognitive capacities are all beyond an individual's voluntary choice, and the baseline disadvantage due to these factors should be compensated for by 'equal-footing'. The concept thus seeks equal opportunities for individuals with different original positions.

Kantian liberalism is often criticized for presuming that individuals with capacity will fully commit to social activities, and precludes those with permanent physical or psychiatric disability [9]. For example, individual capacity to translate a given resource or opportunity into a health outcome would vary, and those with permanent disability would need larger investment to achieve the same level of health as those without the condition. How to 'fairly' compensate for differences in capacity is not explicitly discussed in this ethical claim.

Capability approach

The capability approach has been proposed by Sen as a means of achieving equity beyond utilitarianism-based welfarism and liberalism ethics [6]. Sen argued that utility-based welfarism simply focuses on what is achieved, and does not consider how choices are made. If an individual makes a choice, but only from a limited set of alternatives, it should not be considered to equate to the same choice made from a broader, richer range of alternatives. Sen claims that fairness should be sought not only in realized well-being, but also in the freedom and potential to choose alternative statuses of well-being, or different kinds of living.

Sen further argued that liberalism narrowly focuses on opportunities, and fails to consider what is actually or potentially achieved. He introduced the concept of 'functionings', or 'beings and doings', as the ultimate ends to constitute a valuable living. For example, 'being healthy' is a type of functioning. Then, he claimed that individuals should be free to realize their own goals with the 'capability' to achieve valuable functionings. The capability approach requires a set of valuable functionings to be achievable, and freedom of choice to act for one's own value to be equally distributed for fairness to be achieved. In this approach, health equity means more than equal achievement of health status or equal access to health resources, as Sen commented:

> (Health equity) includes concerns about achievement of health and the capability to achieve good health, not just the distribution of health care, but it also includes the fairness of processes and thus must attach importance to non-discrimination in the delivery of healthcare [10].

The concept of capability was recently applied to health by Jennifer Ruger [11], who defined 'health capabilities' as 'the conditions affecting health and one's ability to make health choices to achieve optimal health under given genetic, social, political, and economical environment', and provided a list of factors affecting capabilities composed of internal factors (e.g. health literacy, self-efficacy, and health values) and external factors (e.g. social norms, social networks, economic and political power, and access to health care).

The capability approach explicitly incorporates the difference in individual capacity to translate a given investment to well-being (e.g. inherited cognitive capacity, and permanent physical and mental health conditions). The approach argues that instead of realized outcomes and resource investment, equity should be sought in the degree of functioning potentially realized, or the capabilities. This may explain why the concept has high affinity with the conceptual model of what makes 'disability'.

The International Classification of Functioning, Disability and Health, released by the WHO in 2001, sought to integrate medical and social models of disability, and took into account individual and environmental factors that influence functioning, disability, and quality of life [12, 13]. Some argue that the model has a considerable conceptual overlap with the capability approach, in that it also treats functioning as a realization of valuable social inclusion that is affected by personal and environmental conditions [14].

In summary, different ethical schools view health equity differently. In the context of public mental health, the capability approach seems to be the most promising ethical basis for equity, as mental health is a consequence, as well as a target, of public health policy. However, the capability approach can be criticized for being too broad and being resistant to standardization or operationalization for measurement and evaluation, giving rise to challenges when translating health equity into public mental health policy-making and action. To use the health equity concept based on the capability approach effectively, sharing a working definition and goals to be realized should be carefully and transparently discussed by stakeholders.

Why and how equity matters in public mental health discussion

Good mental health is a resource that enables an individual to fully realize their value in life. Accumulated evidence consistently indicates that those who experience social and economic hardship, including sex and ethnic status, are at higher risk of poor mental well-being and developing mental ill health [15–20]. Poor mental well-being and mental ill health further preclude fair access to quality health care [21–23], and a broader range of social, economic, and other resources to achieve full social participation [24, 25]. Consequent social exclusion further leads to higher risks of developing mental ill health [26, 27].

As such, when addressing equity in public mental health, mental health should be regarded not merely as a consequence or a cause of inequity, but as an important medium that reciprocally links social structure and individual well-being. In other words, mental health, as well as physical health, is a key target to break a vicious cycle linking ill health and socio-economic disadvantage (Fig. 13.1) [18].

Socio-economic inequity in mental health within and between countries

There are many known risk factors for the development of mental ill health, ranging from genetic and biological factors to social environments in high-income countries [15, 16] and middle-to-low-income countries [17]. Depression has been most rigorously studied; the results provide convincing evidence that educational attainment of individuals and their parents, and sex-determined status such as marital disadvantage, within-family power imbalance, and related domestic violence are significant risk factors for depression. There is also reasonable evidence that low economic status has a role to play [18].

Low educational attainment may lead to higher chance of being exposed to social stress, and may also be related to low mental health literacy that precludes adequate coping with stress and timely seeking of self-help and professional help [28]. Self-efficacy and lack of control often accompany socio-economic hardship, and all are associated with depression [26, 27]. Some studies also suggest that immigrant populations are more susceptible to mental

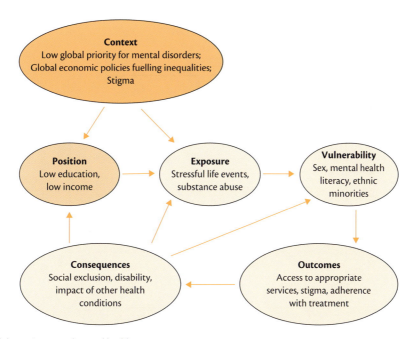

Fig. 13.1 Vicious cycle of social determinants and mental health.

Source: Reproduced from Patel, V, Lund C, Hatheril, S, et al., Mental disorders: Equity and social determinants. In: E. Blas & A.S. Kurup (Eds.), Equity, Social Determinants and Public Health Programmes, pp. 115–134, Copyright (2010), with permission from the World Health Organization

ill health because of acculturation and perceived discrimination [29], and the association is further intensified by low educational background [30].

The risk factors for depression are not randomly distributed, but are systematically shaped by social structures such as social class, and are over-represented in socio-economically and culturally vulnerable populations reflected in the socio-economic gradients of mental ill health within a society [18].

From the macroscopic point of view, there are some national-level factors that affect population-level trends in mental ill health prevalence. A classic study by Emile Durkheim found differences in suicide rates between countries with different religion-related norms about social control [31], although the methodology and interpretation was criticized. Most recent economic studies have found consistent relationships between the incidence of suicide and economic growth [32, 33]. However, the impact of the 2008 global economic shock was differentially presented in the suicide rate across countries [34, 35], suggesting there are population-level moderators affecting economic impact on the risk of mental ill health and subsequent suicide behaviour, such as national policy regarding workers' compensation and social security (Fig. 13.2).

Examples of population-level determinants of mental health can also be found from international studies of aged populations. The Survey of Health, Ageing and Retirement in Europe (SHARE) is a transnational panel study of middle-aged and older populations following the US Health and Retirement Study [36, 37]. Depression was measured using the Euro-D scale to translate the results of different measurement batteries used between countries into a comparable score. The survey found commonality, as well as differences, across countries in risk factors for depression. Not being married and living alone were consistently found to correlate with depression status across countries. The report also confirmed that female sex was related to higher odds of being depressed, although there was a significant country–sex interaction; the correlation was stronger in Southern European countries. Equivalent household income was not consistently related to depression prevalence across countries, although an association between low income and depression was observed in Northern European countries, which reflected the findings of a sister study in Japan [38]. Although European panel data found that older age is associated with depression prevalence, the Japanese counterpart study did not find a clear correlation with age. A possible explanation is that elderly Japanese

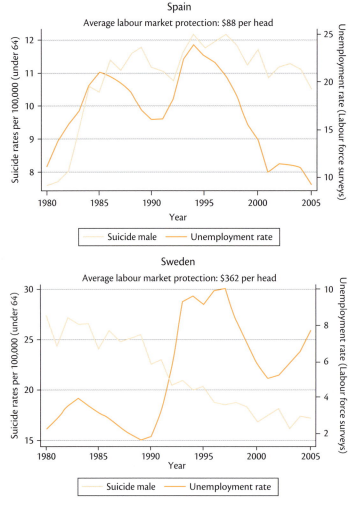

Fig. 13.2 Body economics by Stuckler.

people face fewer financial risks for healthcare co-payment thanks to a reduced co-payment rate for those aged over 75 years under public universal coverage, which exhibited a protective effect for mental health status [39]. These transnational variations strongly suggest that important structural mediators work to influence associations between depression and individual socio-economic status.

Life course perspective in public mental health

Exposure to risk factors for mental ill health are accumulative over an individual's life, starting in the very early developmental stage, including the prenatal period. Childhood adversity, ranging from maltreatment of any type (e.g. physical, emotional, and sexual), neglect by carers, parental maladjustment (e.g. parental mental ill health conditions, including substance abuse), and the experience of domestic violence, all damage emotional, behavioural, and psychological development, and lead to higher risks of mental ill health in adulthood [40–43]. Again, these conditions are disproportionally distributed in socio-economically vulnerable populations.

Some studies have reported that the early onset of mental disorders is associated with significantly reduced household income in later life [44, 45]. However, the impact was found only in high- and upper-middle-income countries and not in low- or lower-middle-income countries [24]. In addition, mental disorders further trigger job discrimination, and there is increasing awareness of the economic costs incurred by mental disorders and subsequent lost productivity [25].

Mental ill health, discrimination, and socio-economic disadvantages are intertwined to reproduce disadvantage and inequity in mental health, which can be transferred intergenerationally [20]. Thus, the life course perspective indicates that earlier intervention in the life course is most important, and that interventions at different stages of the life course through different institutions are required. It further indicates that interventional activities in different stages should be integrated in consistent health policy.

Stigma and healthcare access

Discrimination and subsequent social exclusion are critical themes in the discussion of public mental health. Discrimination evokes the perception of stigma to those with mental ill health conditions. Perceived stigma forces people with mental illness to react 'to avoid the label of mental illness' [22]. Perceived stigma damages self-esteem and is itself a risk factor for depression. More seriously, perceived stigma discourages people with mental illness to seek timely and appropriate healthcare attention [22, 23]. Discouraging access to quality care further widens disparities in mental health, especially among those with lower education and who are socially isolated [21].

Social determinants of health and health equity in public mental health

It is not sufficient to provide equal access to quality mental health care to achieve equity in public mental health. Health equity is not only about the equal distribution of health status, but also about the equal distribution of functionings and freedom to choose alternative functionings, as the capability approach stipulates. As this review has so far confirmed, public mental health is strongly determined by social, economic, cultural, and even political factors (e.g. in the cases of humanitarian crisis during wartime and political turmoil). Thus, it is logical to argue that equal distribution of social determinants of mental health to prevent, treat, and compensate for the burden of mental ill health is required to achieve public mental health equity [5]. For this purpose, health policy and a range of social, economic, and welfare policies should be implemented in a coordinated fashion [18, 20, 46].

Allen et al. [20] have extended the discussion initiated by the WHO's Commission on Social Determinants of Health into the public mental health context to propose four principles for the 'social determinants of health' approach. The first is 'proportionate universalism', meaning that a policy should target the whole population, with a calibrated focus on those with greater needs and vulnerabilities. The second is the trans-sector approach to realize effective coordination of social, economic, and health policies that can be accountable for health impact. The third is the importance of early intervention. Finally, the review also highlighted the interdependency of mental and physical health and emphasized that public mental health policy should be given higher priority with intensified allocation of financial, medical, and human resources, with a long-term vision and effective combination of global and local actions.

The Faculty of Public Health and the Mental Health Foundation in the UK recently issued a comprehensive policy advocacy report to achieve public mental health equity [46]. The report called for the reform of current biomedical models of mental health to take into account the social context of mental ill health and the cumulative impacts of discrimination, poverty, and exclusion. It also argued that 'a fairer society with a better distribution of opportunities' should be realized through increasing mental health literacy in the community to reduce stigma and discrimination.

A comprehensive review and policy proposal by the WHO also listed a table of policy targets ranging from economic development, education, labour, housing, welfare, and drug and alcohol policies (Table 13.1) [18], with special emphasis on targeting early adolescence and social intervention to reduce stigma.

Despite enthusiasm for the 'social determinants of health' approach to achieve public mental health equity, currently available evidence mainly supports the effectiveness of provision of quality mental health care and income support to those with mental ill health, whereas there is limited support for the effectiveness of policies to tackle social determinants of mental health [18]. The relative lack of supportive evidence for this approach may not be because of a lack of effectiveness of such policies in practice, but rather because of limited implementation of the policy so far. Indeed, there are several challenges to implement the approach into real-world practice. The most important challenge is the current lack of political awareness of the approach that has reduced the priority given to public mental health policy [47]. It is also methodologically challenging to evaluate the effectiveness of 'social determinants of health' policy in an experiment to evaluate its impact precisely and accurately.

It requires political, academic, and civic commitment to achieve health equity in public mental health. It will be a substantial

Table 13.1 Interventions for mental disorders targeting socio-economic context and differential vulnerability with indicators

Interventions targeting	Indicators
Socio-economic context and position	
Mental health policy, legislation and service infrastructure coordinate service provision	Presence, date, development, and content of policies, legislation and plans
Alcohol and drug policies to reduce substance-related disorders	
Economic policies promo«ing financialsecurity of populations, funding for key services	
Labour policies promoting employment and protection against stress	
Welfare policies protecting the disabled, sick and unemployed	
Education poilcies that provide quality basic education and cater for special needs	
Differential exposure	
Providing safe home and community environments for children	Child abuse rates, conviction of child abusers
Prevention of injury,violence and crime	Statistics on injury, violence and crime, improved community safety
Provision of adequate housing	Housing backlog, % of population homeless
Relocation of people with mental disorders to less adverse neighbourhood	Access to employment and economic opportunities
Improved antenatal and obstetric care	Infant and maternal mortality rates
Employment creation and skills development	Employment rate, skill levels, available training programmes
Differential vulnerability	
Early childhood development programmes targeting impoverished populations, mother–infant interventions, parent training	Number of parents/children in receipt of programme, longitudinal indicators of child health and development
Depression prevention programmes	Number of target population receiving programmes, mental health outcomes
Targeted screening programmes, e.g. following head injury	Detection and treatment rates
Provision of adequate nutrition	Rates of malnutrition and micronutrient deficiency
Antidiscrimination programmes targeting racism, gender discrimination, stereotyping	Social attitudes to and service utilization by age, gender, ethnicity
Access to financial facilities for poor	Households receiving microcredit and savings schemes

Source: Reproduced from Patel V, Lund C, Hatheril S, et al., Mental disorders: equity and social determinants. In: E. Blas & A.S. Kurup (Eds.), Equity, Social Determinants and Public Health Programmes, pp. 115–134, Copyright (2010), with permission from the World Health Organization.

challenge to reach a social consensus on how to achieve a fairer society on the basis of a shared ethical basis in the society.

References

1. Institute of Medicine. *Guidance for the National Healthcare Disparities Report. Committee on Guidance for Designing a National Healthcare Disparities Report.* Washington DC, National Academy Press.
2. Whitehead M. The concepts and principles of equity in health. International *J Health Serv* 1992; 22: 429–445.
3. Department of Health and Human Services, US. Healthy People 2020. Available at https://www.healthypeople.gov/2020/about/foundation-health-measures/Disparities (2010, accessed 20 February 2018).
4. World Health Organization. Equity. Available at http://www.who.int/healthsystems/topics/equity/en/ (accessed 1 March 2017).
5. Braveman P, Gruskin S. Defining equity in health. *J Epidemiol Commun Health* 2003; 57: 254–258.
6. Sen A. *Inequality Re-examined.* Cambridge, MA: Harvard University Press, 1992.
7. Anand S, Hanson K. Disability-adjusted life years; a critical review. In: Anand S, Peter F, Sen A (eds). *Public Health, Ethics, and Equity.* Oxford: Oxford University Press, 2004, pp. 183–200.
8. Marmot M. Social causes of social inequalities in health. In: Anand S, Peter F, Sen A (eds). *Public Health, Ethics, and Equity.* Oxford: Oxford University Press, 2004, pp. 37–62.
9. Cureton A. A Rawlsian perspective on justice for the disabled. Essays Philos 2009; 9: Article 4.
10. Sen A. Why health equity? In: Anand S, Peter F, Sen A (eds). *Public Health, Ethics, and Equity.* Oxford: Oxford University Press, 2004, pp. 21–34.

11. Ruger JP. Health capability; conceptualization and operationalization. *Am J Public Health* 2010; 100: 41–49.
12. World Health Organization (WHO). *International Classification of Functioning Disability, and Health*. WHO: Geneva, 2001.
13. Ustun TB, Chatterji S, Bickenbach JE, Kostanjsek N, Schneider M. International Classification of Functioning, Disability and Health: a new tool for understanding disability and health. *Disabil Rehabil* 2003; 25: 565–571.
14. Mitra S. The capability approach and disability. *J Disabil Policy Stud* 2006; 16: 236–247
15. Melzer D, Fryers T, Jenkins R, Brugha T, McWilliams B. Social position and the common mental disorders with disability: estimates from the National Psychiatric Survey of Great Britain. *Soc Psychiatry Psychiatr Epidemiol* 2003; 38: 238–243.
16. Fryers T, Melzer D, Jenkins R, Brugha T. The distribution of the common mental disorders; Social inequalities in Europe. *Clin Pract Epidemiol Mental Health* 2005; 1: 14.
17. Lund C, Breen A, Flisher A, et al. Poverty and common mental disorders in low and middle income countries; a systematic review. *Soc Sci Med* 2010; 71: 517–528.
18. Patel V, Lund C, Hatheril S, et al. Mental disorders: equity and social determinants. In: Blas E, Kurup AS (eds). *Equity, Social Determinants and Public Health Programmes*. Geneva: World Health Organization, 2010, pp. 115–134.
19. Department of Health. No Health Without Mental Health; a cross-Government mental health outcomes strategy of people of all ages. Available at: https://www.gov.uk/government/publications/no-health-without-mental-health-a-cross-government-mental-health-outcomes-strategy-for-people-of-all-ages-a-call-to-action (2011, accessed 20 February 2018).
20. Allen J, Balfour R, Bell R, Marmot M. Social determinants of mental health. *Int Rev Psychiatry* 2014; 26: 392–407.
21. Wang PS, Aguilar-Gaxiola S, Alonso J, et al. Use of mental health services for anxiety, mood, and substance disorders in 17 countries in the WHO World Mental Health Surveys. *Lancet* 2007; 370: 841–850.
22. Corrigan P. How Stigma interferes with mental health care. *Am Psychol* 2004; 59: 614–625.
23. Sirey JA, Bruce ML, Alexopoulos GS, et al. Perceived stigma as a predictor of treatment discontinuation in younger and older outpatients with depression. *Am J Psychiatry* 2001; 158: 479–481.
24. Kawakami N, Abdulghani EA, Alonso J, et al. Early-life mental disorders and adult household income in the World Mental Health Surveys. *Biol Psychiatry* 2012; 72: 228–237.
25. Stuart H. Employment equity and mental disability. *Curr Opin Psychiatry* 2007; 20: 486–490.
26. Dalgard OS. Social inequalities in mental health in Norway: possible explanatory factors. *Int J Equity Health* 2008; 7: 27.
27. Anaf J, Baum F, Newman L, Ziersch A, Jolley G. The interplay between structure and agency in shaping the mental health consequences of job loss. *BMC Public Health* 2013; 13: 110.
28. Jorm AF. Mental health literacy: public knowledge and beliefs about mental disorders. *Br J Psychiatry* 2000; 177: 396–401.
29. Torres L, Driscoll MW, Voell M. Discrimination, acculturation, acculturative stress, and Latino psychological distress: a moderated mediational model. *Cultur Divers Ethnic Minor Psychol* 2012; 18: 17–25.
30. Asakura T, Gee GC, Nakayama K, Niwa S. Returning to the 'homeland':work-related ethnic discrimination and the health of Japanese Brazilians in Japan. *Am J Public Health* 2008; 98: 743–750.
31. Durkheim E. Suicide—a study in sociology (originally published in 1897 in French, *Le Suicide*). New York: The Free Press, 1951.
32. Ruhm C. Are recessions good for your health? *Q J Econ* 2000; 115: 617–650.
33. Ruhm C. Recessions, Healthy No More? National Bureau of Economic Research Working Paper 19287. Available at: http://www.nber.org/papers/w19287 (2013, accessed 20 February 2018).
34. Stuckler D, Basu S, Suhrcke M, Coutts A, McKee M. The public health effect of economic crises and alternative policy responses in Europe: An empirical analysis. *Lancet* 2009; 374: 315–323.
35. Stuckler D, Basu S, Suhrcke M, Coutts A, McKee M. Effects of the 2008 recession on health: a first look at European data. *Lancet* 2011; 378: 124–125.
36. Dewey ME, Prince MJ. Mental Health. In: Borsch-Supan A, Brugiavini A, Jurges H, Mackenbach J, Siegrist J, Weber G (eds). *Health, Ageing and Retirement in Europe. First results from the Survey of Health, Ageing and Retirement in Europe*. Mannheim: Mannheim Research Institute for the Economics of Aging, 2005, pp. 108–117.
37. Grundy E, van Campen C, Deeg D, et al. Task group on older people. Health inequalities and the health divide among older people in the WHO European Region. Copenhagen: World Health Organization Regional Office for Europe, 2013.
38. Ichimura H, Hashimoto H, Shimizutani S. First report of Japanese Study of Aging and Retirement. RIETI Working Paper Series. Available at: https://www.rieti.go.jp/en/projects/jstar/ (2008, accessed 20 February 2018).
39. Nishi A, McWilliams JM, Noguchi H, et al. Health benefits from reduced patient cost sharing in Japan. *Bull World Health Organ* 2012; 90: 426–35A,
40. Green JG, Berglund P, Gruber MJ, et al. Childhood adversities and adult psychopathology in the National Comorbidity Survey Replication (NCS-R) I: associations with first onset of DSMIV disorders. *Arch Gen Psychiatry* 2010; 67: 113e23.
41. Kessler RC, McLaughlin KA, Green et al. Childhood adversities and adult psychopathology in the WHO Mental Health Surveys. *Br J Psychiatry* 2010; 197: 378–385.
42. Fryers T, Brugha T. Childhood determinants of adult psychiatric disorder. *Clin Pract Epidemiol Ment Health* 2013; 9: 1–50.
43. Fujiwara T, Kawakami N, World Mental Health Japan Survey Group. Association of childhood adversities with the first onset of mental disorders in Japan; Results from the World Mental Health Japan Survey Group. *J Psychiatr Res* 2011; 45: 481–487.
44. Smith JP, Smith GC. Long-term economic costs of psychological problems during childhood. *Soc Sci Med* 2010; 71: 110–115.
45. Gibb SJ, Fergusson DM, Horwood LJ. Burden of psychiatric disorder in young adulthood and life outcomes at age 30. *Br J Psychiatry* 2010; 197: 122–127.
46. Faculty of Public Health and Mental Health Foundation. *Better Mental Health for All: A Public Health Approach to Mental Health Improvement*. London: Faculty of Public Health and Mental Health Foundation.
47. Campion J, Coombes C. Bhaduri N. Mental health coverage in needs assessments and associated opportunities. *J Public Health (Oxf)* 2017; 39: 813–820.

SECTION II

Evidence

CHAPTER 14

Social capital and mental health

Kwame McKenzie

Introduction

Understanding the factors that prevent illness or promote health is fundamental to the practice of public health medicine and should be fundamental to psychiatry.

The fact that the rates of illness are different within and between groups offers a lens to identify causes from which to develop interventions that could decrease disparities [1]. To this end, public health agencies across the world have been considering what factors are linked to health and what policy initiatives could mitigate any negative impacts. One example is the Public Health Agency of Canada, which has identified 12 key determinants of health (Box 14.1) [2].

As would be expected given the web of causation, many of these factors are interrelated [3]. But it is of note that social factors are far more numerous than biological or physical determinants. This reflects the often-quoted finding that the differential risk of illness is mostly related to exposure to the social determinants of health [2]. These social determinants are the conditions in which people are born, grow, live, work, and age. A better understanding of the social determinants could improve our ability to prevent and fight disease [4].

Most reputable public health bodies agree with the World Health Organization that understanding of and action on the social determinants of health are crucial to recognizing our potential to improve health and decrease inequities in health [1, 5].

Significant progress has been made in understanding and measuring many of the social determinants, including a growing knowledge of the impact of income, income inequality, early childhood development, education, and personal health practices, such as diet and exercise, on health [1]. However, understanding and changing factors considered to reflect 'the social environment' has proved tricky [6].

This is, in part, because of the difficulty in understanding the different facets of the social environment that could be considered important for health. It is easier to investigate income and social support than it is to understand and change the fabric of society and the way communities are set up [7].

The impact of the social environment or, more precisely, the structure of society on psychological health has been the subject of debate and research in mental health for over 100 years. Emile Durkheim's theories on suicide from the 1890s are notable, and Robert Faris and Warren Dunham argued in the 1930s that the level of 'disorganization' within a neighbourhood was a factor that could explain differential rates of mental disorder within the city of Chicago [8, 9]. More recently, work on the aetiology of psychosis has

investigated factors such as the concentration of ethnic minorities in an area and facets of city living that could impact on illness risk [10, 11].

But over the last 20–30 years another way of conceptualizing the social world. Social capital has captured the imagination of researchers and policymakers [1, 12–16]. Some have even considered it to be a pivotal idea in social policy and health. They have argued that it is particularly important to psychiatry because of the clear theoretical links between aspects of social capital and the causes of mental health problems, and because some of the impacts of social capital on physical health are through psychological processes [13, 14, 17].

What is social capital?

Social capital is a theory that attempts to describe features of the fabric of society. It identifies factors in populations such as the level of civic participation, social networks, and levels of trust because such forces shape the quality and quantity of social interactions and the institutions that underpin society. It is a complex multi-component concept that aims to help us better understand the world that we live in and has been used to produce better social policy [12, 13].

Like many concepts in the social space, social capital cannot be simply considered as a single continuous variable. It is difficult to consider areas or people as having high or low social capital. This is, in part, because social capital is multifaceted. In some ways it would be more correct to talk about the different types of social capital that a person, group, or area has rather than their total social capital. Different mental health problems could be linked to different aspects of social capital in different ways. These links may be direct or through other physical, environmental, and societal mechanisms [7, 13].

In his study of the impact of community centres on health, Lyda Hanifan is probably the first person to have described social capital in modern literature [18]. However, many cite Jane Jacobs as the first person to make an explicit reference to the term social capital [14, 19]. Jacobs states:

> Underlying any float of population must be a continuity of people who have forged neighbourhood networks. These networks are a city's irreplaceable social capital [19].

Since the 1960s many theorists have attempted to better refine the term. Although it is difficult to find an agreed definition of social capital, most theories consider trust, networks, and norms to be the main components. But rather than focusing on definitions, it is

Box 14.1 Determinants of health

Income and social status
Social support networks
Education and literacy
Employment and working conditions
Social environments
Physical environments
Personal health practices and coping skills
Healthy child development
Biology and genetic endowment
Health services
Gender
Culture

Source: Data from Public Health Agency of Canada, What determines health?, Available at http://www.phac-aspc.gc.ca/ph-sp/determinants/index-eng.php

more important to consider the different features of social capital as a multidimensional concept.

We can consider social capital to have at least four dimensions:

individual/ecological;

cognitive/structural;

bonding/bridging;

vertical/horizontal.

Individual/ecological social capital

The sociologist Pierre Bourdieu's view of social capital may be considered to reflect an assumption that it is a property of an individual [15]. In summary, his view is that a person's individual's social relationships and knowledge allow access to resources (e.g. health care and education), and these relationships define their social capital [15]. Social capital lies in access to existing and well-researched factors that influence health, such as social support and social networks, rather than in those networks or supports per se. Other researchers who analyse social capital at the individual level include trust, a sense of belonging, and civic engagement as measures of social capital [20–22].

An alternative approach is to consider social capital as ecological. This is in line with Jane Jacobs' view that social capital is a property of an area [6, 23, 24]. Those who follow this conceptualization see social capital as being embodied in relationships between individuals, between groups, and between groups and abstract bodies such as the state. One of the more commonly used ecological definitions of social capital originates from the political scientist Robert Putnam [12]. This definition arose out of empirical work on the performance of regional government in Italy and consists of five principal characteristics:

1. Community networks, voluntary, state, personal networks and density.

2. Civic engagement, participation, and use of civic networks.

3. Local civic identity-sense of belonging, solidarity, and equality with local community members.

4. Reciprocity and norms of cooperation, a sense of obligation to help others, and confidence in return of assistance.

5. Trust levels in the community.

Structural and cognitive social capital

Structural social capital describes the relationships, networks, associations, and institutions that link people and groups together. They can thus be measured numerically or through an analysis of linkages or network density. For instance, the number of church groups, local societies, Sunday league football teams, or volunteer groups in an area and the percentage of people who participate may be considered a measure of structural social capital. Some consider an individual correlate to be an individual's level of participation in groups outside the work environment. It can also be considered as the development and existence of a social safety net and collective investments in human capital such as education and accessible health care [6, 12, 17, 21].

Cognitive social capital consists of values, norms, reciprocity, altruism, and civic responsibility, sometimes called 'collective moral resources'. Some have measured this by performing surveys of the level of trust in neighbours and civic identity and comparing rates of trust in one area to another. At an individual level one could measure perceptions of community like a sense of belonging or trust [7, 13, 17, 25].

Bonding and bridging social capital

Social capital can be considered as bridging (inclusive) or bonding (exclusive). Bonding social capital is inward focused and characterized by homogeneity, strong norms, loyalty, and exclusivity. It is intra-group and relies on strong ties. It can be thought of as the type of social capital that a family unit has or that which is found in small, close-knit migrant groups who need mutual support [14, 16, 12, 25, 26].

Bridging social capital is outward-focused and links different groups in society. The ties between people are weaker and some would consider bridging social capital to be more fragile. An individual's social networks reflect their bridging social capital [13, 17].

Bonding social capital can have positive impacts such as increasing social supports available to people but can also have a negative effect on society. For example, organized crime groups like the Mafia are often depicted as being closely bonded. In contrast, bridging social capital is generally considered to be a positive thing. It acts as a sociological superglue binding groups in the community together and so can facilitate common action [14].

Horizontal and vertical social capital

A final dimension on which social capital can be split is horizontal and vertical. Horizontal social capital describes social capital between people in similar strata of society and vertical social capital describes social capital that provides integration between people in different strata of society.

Essentially, horizontal social capital can be considered to include the bonding social capital, bridging social capital, cognitive, and structural social capital that is confined to particular social strata. An example would be bonding social capital within a wealthy family and bridging social capital through exclusive clubs (which link them to similarly rich families) together with all their structural and cognitive correlates.

Vertical social capital can be seen as the degree of integration of groups within a hierarchical society that allows it to influence policy and access justice and resources from those in power. It can be seen as a type of bridging social capital with structural components referring to the organizational integrity, penetration, and effectiveness of the state and cognitive elements reflecting group identity [16].

Measuring social capital

There are many different tools available to measure social capital [17, 27]. Although tools are available, many have not been validated and few capture all the dimensions of social capital. It is easier to produce tools to measure individual social capital than measuring it at an ecological level. In fact, studies trying to work ecologically often rely on measuring the individual's perception of society and then aggregating individual perceptions to group or area levels. It is unclear how valid this is. It could be argued that instead of questionnaires that rely on the sum of individual perception, other, observational, measures of societal structure are more precise. The number of civic associations have been used, as have measures of community effectiveness, and indicators of trust such as whether local petrol stations demand pre-payment before motorists fill their tanks or whether stores allow credit.

But it could also be argued that the sum of individual perceptions in an area or group are more important for community building and the psychological health of the community than actual structures in society.

There are, of course, the fundamental questions that come with measuring context, such as whether community is geographical, and how to deal with dispersed communities or Internet-linked groups. The assumption that communities are generally place-based may be erroneous and this issue needs further attention. Some sociologists have claimed that modern society is characterized by constant change, with individuals constantly constructing and reconstructing their sense of self [28, 29]. This is made possible by the range of choices and 'lifestyles' available in the modern world and leads to a semi-permanent state of dislocation and instability. Place as a factor in the perception of security is considered to have diminished rapidly, owing to a combination of globalization, technology, postmodernism, and infra-structural developments. The present is marked by greater heterogeneity in terms of demography, behaviour, and lifestyle. It is vastly different from the world of self-contained homogenous and stable neighbourhoods that characterized earlier traditional eras. In this social milieu, non-spatial communities may dwarf the neighbourhood community in importance for individuals.

An example from the literature better explains the issue

'... a refugee living in a stable neighbourhood of a large city may find support in the city wide refugee community from the same country far more important than the neighbourhood community. Many faith groups find their faith community more important than their residential community especially if they are in the minority in their geographic area. Socially excluded groups such as those suffering from mental illness may link with each other through support groups which are increasingly based on telephone lines and the internet. It is an open question as to whether the concepts of social capital developed for spatial communities are applicable in

non-spatial communities and what kind of impact it has on community members' [13].[1]

But these concerns need to be balanced by the fact that for most people geographically based associative behaviour is important. People are likely to continue to belong to a number of different communities, both geographically and non-spatially. The balance may differ through one's life, will be different for different groups, and these may have different impacts on specific health conditions. For example, relatively immobile groups such as children and the elderly may be more affected by neighbourhood social capital than groups who have high relative mobility. It must also be borne in mind that area-based government and health services are likely to find area-based policy easier to promote.

Published reviews of the association between social capital and mental illness

Despite its perceived importance there have been few good reviews of social capital and mental illness [14, 17, 27, 30, 31].

That being said, there have been reviews in children's health, adult mental illness, in general, common mental disorders (CMD), and mental health in old age. The general conclusion from these is that there is an association between higher levels of some types of social capital and a lower risk of mental health problems [14, 17, 27, 30, 31].

One of the first published attempts to review the association between social capital and mental illness in the peer-reviewed literature was undertaken in 2005 [14]. This narrative review traced the historical development of the concept of social capital and then examined the relationship between social capital and depression and anxiety, and then psychoses. The study concluded that despite its promise there is a lack of strong evidence supporting the hypothesis that social capital protects mental health.

But the most quoted review is that that of De Silva et al. [17]. They systematically reviewed quantitative studies examining the association between social capital and mental illness. Twenty-one studies met the inclusion criteria for the review. Fourteen measured social capital at the individual level and seven at an ecological level. At an individual level higher rates of cognitive social capital were associated with lower rates of CMD and child mental illness. There was also evidence that combined measures of social capital were associated with lower rates of CMD. The impact of ecological social capital on health was difficult to assess because of the diverse nature of the seven studies that were included. The review concluded that individual and ecological social capital may measure different aspects of the social environment.

A further review by Ehsan and De Silva [27] focused specifically on CMD. They systematically reviewed peer-reviewed published quantitative studies examining the direct association between social capital and CMD and attempted to investigate the association between different types of social capital and CMD. They included 39 studies: 31 cross-sectional and eight cohort studies. These studies included 39 effect estimates for individual level cognitive, 31 for individual level structural, nine for ecological level cognitive, and 11 for ecological level structural social capital. They report that individual cognitive social capital is protective against developing CMD. Ecological cognitive social capital is also associated with reduced risk of CMD, but they add the caveat that studies were cross-sectional. For structural social capital there was overall no association at either the individual or ecological levels. However, 'Two cross-sectional studies found that in low-income settings, a mother's participation in civic activities is associated with an increased risk of common mental disorder'. They concluded that there was sufficient evidence to design and evaluate individual and ecological cognitive social capital interventions to promote mental well-being and prevent CMD.

The initial finding of an association between childhood mental health problems and social capital was followed up in a review by McPherson et al. [31]. They undertook an integrative systematic review of the international research findings on the role and impact of family and community social capital on mental health/behavioural problems in children and adolescents to provide a consolidated evidence base to inform future research and policy development. A meta-analysis/meta-synthesis was not undertaken Because of the heterogeneity in study design and outcomes, and the results were presented in narrative form. The review included 55 studies. The majority were cross-sectional surveys and were conducted in North America ($n = 33$); seven were conducted in the UK. Samples ranged in size from 29 to 98,340. They reported that family and community social capital are associated with mental health/behavioural problems in children and adolescents. Positive parent–child relations, extended family support, social support networks, religiosity, neighbourhood, and school quality appear to be particularly important for good mental health. Their conclusion was that social capital generated and mobilized at the family and community level can influence mental health/problem behaviour outcomes in young people.

Nyqvist et al.'s systematic review aimed to explore the relationship between social capital and mental well-being in older people [30]. They found 11 studies that met the inclusion criteria. All the studies found positive associations between types of social capital and aspects of mental well-being. However, the types of social capital linked with mental well-being varied. It was unclear whether this reflected the lack of a 'gold standard' in the measurement of social capital or mental well-being. Despite this the authors concluded that family and friends at the micro-level may be the key factors in generating social capital and well-being in older people.

Is there a causal relationship between social capital and mental illness?

Social capital is a complex, multifactorial concept. Mental illness is another complex variable and the different illnesses within this broad church have different causation [6]. Given these facts, a general theory of the mechanisms through which social capital may impact rates of mental illness should be considered with caution. Notwithstanding this caveat, two linked questions have dominated the debate on social capital and mental health:

1. Can social capital prevent or cause mental illness?

2. Does the level or type of social capital have an impact on the rate of mental illness?

Causation

In answer to the first question, before an exposure can be considered to a possible cause there are a number of issues that need to be considered. These can be reduced to four tests.

1. First, there needs to be an association or correlation between the exposure and the illness. The reviews presented in the previous section confirm that there is an association between aspects of social capital and types of mental illness or well-being—although these vary from review to review.

2. Second, there needs to be a temporal sequence of events. The proposed cause has to come before the disease. This is often problematic in medicine and especially in mental illness because many disorders have a long lag time between exposure and the development of problems [32]. Longitudinal research investigating social capital and mental health is methodologically challenging, expensive, and, not surprisingly, rare or inconclusive [17, 27].

3. Third, there needs to be no other explanatory variable that affects both the cause and the outcome, which could explain the association. Causation theories in mental illness get into difficulty here. Most mental illnesses are complex, multifactorial problems where there are a number of other possible explanatory variables. This is partly because many illnesses are caused by a number of factors acting directly on a person or their social and behavioural environment, which increase or decrease risk. It is also because aetiological factors in many illnesses act indirectly through complex intervening mechanisms to produce their effects [32].

Given this complexity, most epidemiological studies in mental illness do not attempt to demonstrate the cause of an illness, but to identify risk or preventative factors or other factors that may help predict an illness or its outcome. The aim is not to find a single cause but to work out what proportion of the rate of an illness or risk of an illness can be explained by its association with the 'causative' variable [32].

Social capital is another complex variable. It is difficult to conceptualize and measurement is still in its infancy. Epidemiological research into social capital to date has rarely attempted to answer the question whether social capital causes mental illness, rather whether social capital is associated with mental illness and the size of the association.

4. The fourth test for causality is that there needs to be a plausible mechanism by which the exposure can lead to the illness. Or, in other words, how could differing rates of social capital lead to mental illness? Here there is little evidence, although the disaggregation of social capital into its constituent parts could offer a lens through which this could be considered. And, although it is reasonable to conclude that the strong associations between aspects of social capital and different mental illnesses and mental health problems would not satisfy the test of causation, the face validity of some of the speculative mechanisms that have been used to explain the associations have caught the imagination of policymakers. They have also led some researchers to call for the development of interventions to increase social capital to improve rates of mental illness [27].

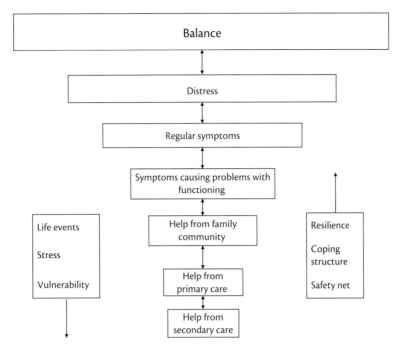

Fig. 14.1 A simplified pathways diagram for the development of mental illness.

What mechanisms could explain reported associations between social capital and mental illness?

The risk of mental illness is associated with biological, psychological, and social factors. These factors may be risk factors for illness or protective factors that build resilience to illness. Biological, psychological, and social factors interact at an individual level to change their risk of developing an illness and at a group level to change the environment in which the individual lives and the rate of illness.

Biological factors include the genetic endowment of an individual or group. Psychological factors such as the way a person reacts to stress or their proneness to addiction can also be seen at a group level with particular cultural or subcultural groups having different strengths and vulnerabilities because of specific ways they react to social stress.

Some argue that the risk of mental illness is linked to the total of risk factors and protective factors acting on a person or group over time. Others argue that there are sensitive periods in which specific factors may have a significant impact on mental health. It is most likely that both are true and a combination of risks, protective factors, and the timing of exposure to these forces over time explain variations in mental illness.

The impact of different factors may be considered in four dimensions, individual factors, ecological factors, the interaction between individual and ecological factors, and time [33].

There is an added level of complexity. For mental illnesses with clear biological aetiologies, such as purely genetic illnesses, some could argue that no level of social or societal risk factors will be important. This would be of more concern if they were the majority rather than the vast minority of mental illnesses. Indeed it is arguable whether there is really any illness which is completely biological in its aetiology.

A simplified pathways diagram for the development of mental illness is displayed in Fig. 14.1. This ignores the multi-level causation and puts both individual and ecological factors on the same plane. There are factors that promote wellness and those which drive the development of mental health problems. As an individual moves from balance through different levels of distress, they tend to call of individual, as well as social, factors to try to promote restitution. They continue to move down the pathway if the impact of forces promoting mental illness are greater than the forces promoting mental wellness. They move back towards balance when the forces promoting wellness have a greater action than those promoting illness.

Many factors have been linked with the development of mental health problems (Box 14.2). The exposure to risk factors is not only linked to the individual, but also the society they live in. The likelihood of encountering a risk factor, as well as having the supports to overcome it, are linked to the social environment, as well as your personal risk of exposure and access to services or supports. Many of the factors that have been shown to be linked to the risk of mental health problems are also linked to the presence of social capital.

The possible mechanisms through which social capital is considered to have an impact on the rates of mental illness have rarely been empirically researched, but there are some hypotheses [13, 34].

Cognitive and structural social capital

The ties that link communities may also facilitate the development of trust. Association membership and civic trust are highly correlated. Per capita group membership, for instance in the USA, has been shown to be inversely correlated with age-adjusted all-cause mortality [35]. Density of civic association membership is similarly a predictor of deaths from coronary heart disease, malignant neoplasms, and infant mortality [7, 34].

Box 14.2 Factors linked with the development of mental health problems

Some individual risk factors for mental illness:

- low birthweight;
- parents with a mental illness;
- physical illness;
- substance misuse;
- lower educational and employment level;
- low-autonomy workplace;
- urban birth and residence;
- life events (e.g. victim of violence).

Some individual protective factors for mental illness:

- social support;
- education/higher social position;
- marriage—for men;
- autonomy at work.

Some factors that increase rates of mental illness in a community:

- disorganization;
- unpredictable;
- low trust, high anxiety, high vigilance;
- high migration;
- high crime;
- low safety net provision;

Community risk-lowering factors:

- cohesive/predictable;
- low crime rates;
- low income inequality;
- high safety net provision;
- high investment in human capital.

Levels of distrust are significantly correlated with age-adjusted mortality rates.

Apart from the potentially injurious effects and anxiety produced by having to continually reassess your environment in a low trust community, higher levels of physical illness lead to higher levels of mental illness as people try to cope psychologically.

The provision of health services and levels of education in an area may be linked to the level of investment in human capital—higher investment could be expected in areas with high trust and high levels of social cohesiveness. Health service provision would be expected to influence the prevalence of mental illness.

From a different perspective, but with the same outcome, the level of social capital may influence government performance, such as the government's capacity to develop and implement policy.

Social capital could affect this capacity by, for example, affecting support for re-distributive policies or for universal healthcare insurance, both of which could represent core government objectives.

A government operating in a jurisdiction with a low level of social capital may lack electoral support for such interventions and so could not proceed with them (at least not without significant political risk) [36].

Areas with low levels of investment in infrastructure may accentuate disability and impairment for instance by poor maintenance of streets and transport systems. There is evidence that disability and impairment, especially in older people, is a direct risk factor for the aetiology and maintenance of depression [37].

Moreover, social disorganization, defined as the 'inability of a community structure to realize the common values of its residents and maintain effective social controls', correlates with rates of suicide and crime [38].

Poorer informal community surveillance and non-enforcement of conventional norms (by both the authorities and the civil population) could lead to increased rates of crime. With regard to the origins of crime and residents of cohesive communities may be better able to control the youth behaviours that set the context for gang violence [7].

Lower levels of informal community control have been associated with increased rates of various forms of 'deviancy'. Health norms such as avoiding drugs of misuse and teenage pregnancy are less well enforced. Because of this one would expect higher levels of addiction, teenage pregnancy, and involvement with the criminal justice system. These are all risk factors for mental illness. In addition, higher rates of substance misuse and teenage pregnancy would predict increased rates of fetal abnormalities and lower-birthweight babies. Low-birthweight babies and those with abnormalities are at an increased risk of mental illness when they grow up. Moreover, the mothers of children with abnormalities are also at increased risk of suffering from postnatal mental illness. The model would therefore predict that lower levels of social capital lead to a cascade that increases the rate mental illness.

Income inequality is recognized by many to be a social cancer—leading to the undermining and disintegration of many factors developed for the social good. The rise of income inequality across high-income countries has been indentified as an important factor in health. There has been a long-standing discussion about the mechanisms through which income inequality leads to differences in health. Some have argued that income inequality undermines social capital and this leads to poorer investment in the social space and so produces a more toxic environment. While others have argued that changes in cognitive social capital are required for increasing income inequality to be acceptable. Simply put, for a society to go from being more equal to allowing gross inflation of incomes for a few while others are struggling would require a change in the ideals and norms of a community. It is of note that the world GINI coefficient—a measure of inequality—is higher in 2015 than it was in 1820. Recently, Putnam has presented data demonstrating that social changes pointing to a decrease in collectivism pre-date the rise of income inequality in the USA. This supports the argument that changes in cognitive social capital pre-date changes in income inequality.

Bonding and bridging social capital and mental health

Civic associations and groups glue society together. They offer a number of different access points so that individuals and families can be involved in society and meet each other. These allow the development of civic identity and enhance social status. They offer social support, pathways to identify resources, and opportunities for employment and social connection.

The weak social ties created by voluntary associations socially cohere communities

Weak social ties prevent individuals from becoming isolated and encourage active engagement within the community. They can decrease fear and anxiety and help make society more predictable. They also offer places where conflicts can be understood and managed. The skills acquired through being involved in civil society are important both on a horizontal level and vertically when negotiating with organizations. Moreover, being able to identify and articulate the needs of a constituency is a persuasive political position. Communities with high levels of bridging social capital may not only manage conflict better, but the skills developed may also allow them to apply pressure to government to obtain resources. These communities would be considered to have high social efficacy. Areas with higher levels of social efficacy may be better at protecting their structural social capital, such as social and health services. They may be more able to organize to fight budget cuts such as the closure of a school or a hospital. They may be more able to unite to form pressure groups that produce appropriate social organizations that can easily be accessed. In times of crisis, for instance during war or drought, they are more able to unite to protect and support their residents.

Communities with higher levels of bonding and bridging social capital produce better environments in which their populations live, and grow. Through these mechanisms the cumulative impacts of bonding and bridging social capital may decrease the risk of mental health problems.

Areas low in bonding and bridging social capital may have fractured social relations. A relative absence of societal safety nets could be considered likely due to low levels of willingness to invest. These areas would be less able to offer the types of social support, which could act as a buffer so preventing the progression of life's challenges into mental illness. Similarly, they may be less able to provide support, which may aid restitution, to family and carers of those with a mental illness.

The ties between individuals in areas are also used to transmit knowledge. In areas with higher levels of bonding and bridging social capital communication is easier. Positive health messages may be easier to promote.

Variations in the availability of psychosocial resources at the community level may help to explain the anomalous finding that socially isolated individuals residing in more cohesive communities do not appear to suffer the same ill health consequences as those living in less cohesive communities [7].

However, it would be wrong to think that social capital will necessarily be good for mental health. Highly bonded communities may have little tolerance for people with psychological difficulties. Rather than help them they may seek to exclude them. They may promote negative health norms and may be burdensome on individuals [6, 14].

Vertical and horizontal social capital and mental illness

Conceptualization of the possible impacts of bonding and bridging social capital tend to consider its impacts at a horizontal level. We consider access to resources such as social support or psychological support at a family, friend, or neighbourhood level. We tend to think about access to the social safety net such as mental health services or local homecare for seniors. Accessing care is facilitated by good bridging social capital—as this increases awareness of services and support, knowledge that other people may have had the same problems, and can decrease anxiety in seeking help. Thick social supports from bonded families can help individuals through difficult times.

However, vertical aspects of social capital also need to be considered [13, 14]. The availability of the social safety net and, more fundamentally, local investment in factors linked to the development of thriving, resilient individuals, such as high-quality accessible daycare in early years, good education, access to green space, and other extracurricula activities that help develop social brain and access to higher education and jobs, depends on local areas being able to access resources. For more marginalized communities this depends on how well they are linked to parts of society that may have more money and influence government decisions [34].

Areas low in social efficacy may be more politically marginalized. Add to this lower vertical social capital in a society and it is not hard to imagine that it may be difficult for such communities to produce an adequate safety net itself, to accrue sufficient support for investment in human capital (e.g. a high level of education for all) and to encourage wider Government to develop relevant policies that will help develop a good social infrastructure. The social environment, social safety net, and educational resources in the community will be lower. This would decrease the ability of the community to support people who are getting into difficulty back towards a state of psychological balance. Hence, as a community, rates of mental health problems could be considered likely to increase. The fabric of the lives of people in more marginalized areas depends on how well vertically integrated a society is. Or, in other words, it depends on that community's vertical social capital. Horizontal social capital can help people and communities help themselves, but the scope and impact of their ability to help themselves depends on the resource that is available in a community [13, 14].

Conclusion

Social capital is many things to many people. Its appeal seems to be in its face validity and the possibility that it may help us to better understand complex social processes. Its problems lie in the fact that it is conceptualized as a complex variable which could be linked to many different mechanisms that change the risk of mental illness. Given the multi-level nature of social capital it is better considered as a plural. A person or an area may have different types of social capital than one overall level of social capital. By disaggregating the concept it may be possible to better understand the associations between social capital and mental illness.

References

1. World Health Organization (WHO). *World Health Report 2002. Reducing Risks, Promoting Health Lives*. Geneva: WHO, 2002.
2. Public Health Agency of Canada. What Determines Health. Available at: http://www.phac-aspc.gc.ca/ph-sp/determinants/index-eng.php (accessed 21 February 2018).
3. Krieger N Epidemiology and the web of causation: has anyone seen the spider? *Soc Sci Med* 1994; 39: 887–903.

4. Marmot M, Wilkinson R. *Social Determinants of Health.* Oxford: Oxford University Press, 2005.

5. Braveman P, Ergerter S, Williams D. Social determinants of health coming of age. *Annu Rev Public Health* 2011; 32: 381–398.

6. McKenzie K, Whitley R, Weich S. Social capital and mental illness. *The Br J Psychiatry* 2002; 181: 280–283.

7. Berkman L, Kawachi I. *Social Cohesion, Social Capital, and Health. Social Epidemiology.* New York, Oxford: Oxford University Press, 2000.

8. Durkheim E. *Suicide.* New York: Free Press, 1951.

9. Faris REL, Dunham HW. *Mental Disorders in Urban Areas.* Chicago, IL: University of Chicago Press, 1939.

10. Morgan C, Fearon P, McKenzie K. *Society and Psychosis.* London: Cambridge University Press, 2008.

11. Drukker M, Buka SA, Kaplan C, McKenzie K, Van Os J. Social capital and young adolescents' perceived health in different sociocultural settings. *Soc Sci Med* 2005; 611: 185–198.

12. Putnam R. *Making Democracy Work: Civic Traditions in Modern Italy.* Princeton, NJ: Princeton University Press, 1993.

13. McKenzie K, Harpham T. *Social Capital and Mental Health.* London: Jessica Kingsley Publishers, 2006.

14. Whitley R, McKenzie K. Social capital and psychiatry: review of the literature. *Harv Rev Psychiatr* 2005; 13: 71–84.

15. Bourdieu P. The forms of social capital. In: Richardson G (ed.) *The Handbook of Theory and Research for the Sociology of Education..* New York: Greenwood Press , 1986, pp. 241–258.

16. Woolcock M. Social capital and economic development: toward a theoretical synthesis and policy framework. *Theory Soc* 1998; 27: 151–208.

17. De Silva M, McKenzie K, Harpham T, Huttly S. Social capital and mental illness: a systematic review. *J Epidemiol Community Health* 2005; 59: 619–627.

18. Hanifan L. *The Community Centre Boston.* Boston, MA: Silver Burdett, 1920.

19. Jacobs J. *The Death and Life of Great American Cities.* London: Penguin, 1961.

20. Weber MP Huxley PJ. Measuring access to social capital the reliability and validity of the resource generator and its association with common mental disorder. *Soc Sci Med* 2007; 65: 481–492.

21. Weber MP. Access to social capital and the course of depression. PhD thesis. Available at: http://martinwebber.net/wp-content/uploads/2012/02/webber-phd-thesis.pdf (accessed 21 February 2018).

22. De silva M, Harpham T, Tuan T, Bartolini R. Penny M, Huttly S. Psychometric and cognitive validation of a social capital measuring tool in Peru and Vietnam *Soc Sci Med* 2006; 62: 941–953.

23. Kawachi I, Kim D, Coutts A, Subramanian SV. Commentary: Reconciling the three accounts of social capital. *Int J Epidemiol* 2004; 33: 682–690.

24. Inter-university Consortium for Political and Social Research. Project on Human Development in Chicago Neighborhoods. Available at: https://www.icpsr.umich.edu/icpsrweb/PHDCN/about.jsp (accessed 21 February 2018).

25. Putnam R. Bowling alone: America's declining social capital. *Journal of Democracy* 1995; 6: 65–78.

26. Woolcock M, Narayan D. Social capital: implications for development theory, research, and policy (English). Available at: http://documents.worldbank.org/curated/en/961231468336675195/Social-capital-implications-for-development-theory-research-and-policy (accessed 21 February 2018).

27. Ehsan AM, De Silva MJ. Social capital and common mental disorder: a systematic review. *J Epidemiol Community Health* 2015; 69: 1021–1028.

28. Giddens A. *Modernity and Self-identity.* Cambridge: Polity Press, 1991.

29. Cohen S, Wills TA. Stress, social support and the buffering hypothesis. *Psychol Bull* 1985; 98: 310–357.

30. Nyqvist F, Forsman AK, Giuntoli G, Cattan M. Social capital as a resource for mental well-being in older people: a systematic review. *Aging Ment Health* 2013; 17: 394–410.

31. McPherson KE, Kerr S, McGee E, et al. The association between social capital and mental health and behavioural problems in children and adolescents: an integrative systematic review *BMC Psychol* 2014; 2: 7.

32. Gelder M, Mayou R, Cowen P. *Shorter Oxford Textbook of Psychiatry Part 1.* Oxford, New York: Oxford University Press, 2004.

33. Shah J, Mizrahi R, McKenzie K. The Four dimensions model for the social aetiology of psychosis. *Br J Psychiatry*, 2011; 199: 11–14.

34. Cullen M, Whiteford H. *The Interrelations of Social Capital with Health and Mental Health. National Mental Health Strategy.* Canberra: Commonwealth Department of Health and Aged Care, 2001.

35. Kawachi I, Kennedy BP, Lochner K, et al. Social capital, income inequality, and mortality. *Am J Public Health* 1997; 87: 1491–1498.

36. Lavis J, Stoddart G. Social Cohesion and Health. *McMaster University Centre for Health Economics and Policy Analysis Working Paper Series,* 99–09, 1999.

37. Prince M, Harwood RH, Blizard RA, Thomas A, Mann AH. Impairment, disability and handicap as risk factors for depression in old age. The Gospel Oak Project V. *Psychol Med* 1997; 27: 311–321.

38. Sampson R, Groves W. Community structure and crime: testing social-disorganization theory. *Am J Sociol* 1989; 94: 774–802.

CHAPTER 15

Policy challenges
Well-being as a priority in public mental health

Felicia A. Huppert and Kai Ruggeri

Introduction

There has been a sustained struggle within the public health community to accept and integrate scientifically viable evidence on mental well-being into policy and practice. Although the term well-being is commonly used to include physical wellness, economic prosperity, and sometimes social relationships, in this chapter we confine the use of the term well-being to mental well-being, and regard this as synonymous with positive mental health. Regrettably, the term well-being is frequently used as a euphemism for mental illness or ill-being; however, we use the term in its literal meaning, namely being well.

In this chapter, we confront the reluctance of some members of the psychiatry and public health communities to take well-being seriously. To do so, we examine unresolved issues, such as how precisely to define and measure well-being in its true sense, as well as how to address doubts and barriers to accepting the value and public health benefits of improving the well-being of a population.

To provide a background to understanding these issues, we begin with a very brief history of well-being. After summarizing evidence for the psychological and social benefits of well-being interventions, we outline the health economic case for the financial benefits of promoting well-being in the population. Finally, we draw conclusions about the current state of our knowledge, and argue that despite some remaining limitations, there are compelling reasons to recognize and even prioritize well-being as a goal for public policy, and to introduce programmes that promote well-being into policy and practice.

We should bear in mind that well-being science is a relatively new endeavour [1], and like any important new field of science, it needs to be cultivated through constructive criticism of its methods and findings. Simply dismissing the entire enterprise because its methods have not yet been perfected is counterproductive.

A very brief history of well-being

Happiness and well-being are concepts that have been used for thousands of years to describe how well life is going, but it is only in the last few decades that they have attracted serious empirical research. Philosophers and religious thinkers from many traditions have debated the meaning of happiness and well-being, and their significance in our lives [2]. Within the Western tradition, these debates can be traced back to the ancient Greek philosophers, where one school of thought espoused the hedonic view, defining happiness as leading a pleasurable life, whereas the opposing, eudaimonic view espoused by Aristotle, defined happiness as leading a meaningful and virtuous life, not merely fulfilling one's desires. Two centuries before this, Buddhism taught that genuine well-being came about not through pleasurable experiences—external or internal—but through the cultivation of mental balance leading to wisdom and compassion [3].

Like the eudaimonic and Buddhist perspectives in which happiness was more than individual pleasure, early economic theory adopted the utilitarian ethics that emerged from the eighteenth-century Enlightenment, which regarded the moral worth or 'utility' of an action as the totality of happiness it produced. According to this view, the aim of policy should be to provide 'the greatest happiness for the greatest number' [4–6], and that 'whatever the form or constitution of government may be, it ought to have no other object than the general happiness' [7]. To this end, John Sinclair [8], a Scottish statistician, identified the need for 'An inquiry into the state of a country for the purposes of ascertaining the quantum of happiness enjoyed by its inhabitants and the means of its future improvement', but there is no definition of the 'quantum of happiness' in the account, and no prescription for applying the findings of the account in a way that would increase this quantum.

As happiness was evidently hard to measure, generations of economists settled for a proxy measure, namely the satisfaction of preferences or desires, of which consumption was a key indicator. However, some leading economists, most notably Richard Layard [9] and Joseph Stiglitz, Amartya Sen, and Jean-Paul Fitoussi [10] have challenged the traditional emphasis on preferences and consumption. They argue that we need to return to a utilitarian view of economics, as growing wealth and consumption do not lead to the experience of life going well, which is an increasingly shared view among economists and psychologists [11].

From the mid-twentieth century, psychologists began to take an interest in positive aspects of well-being, rather than focusing on disorder and dysfunction. Some, like Marie Jahoda [12], Carl Rogers [13] and Abraham Maslow [14] used a eudaimonic perspective, characterizing very good mental health in terms of being fully functional as individuals and in relationships. Later scholars who also took a eudaimonic perspective include Carol Ryff [15], Alan Waterman [16] and Edward Deci and Richard Ryan [17]. However, Gregory Ashby and colleagues [18], Ed Diener [19],

Barbara Fredrickson [20], and Daniel Kahneman and colleagues [21] have adopted a hedonic view, regarding positive emotions as the defining feature of well-being.

The historical and philosophical context of the various theories of well-being has influenced the way different scholars define and measure well-being, and their approach to improving well-being, as we describe in later sections.

Why well-being matters

Health and well-being are desirable states for individuals and are good for society. As we have seen, generations of philosophers and religious scholars have argued that well-being is the ultimate good, so it follows that well-being should be promoted and nurtured. However, the promotion and nurturing of well-being requires not only a commitment to its central importance in our lives, but also the expenditure of financial and other resources. This is why the instrumental benefits of high levels of well-being are frequently cited to persuade politicians and policymakers that the levels of expenditure required are fully justified.

What is the evidence that well-being leads to improvements in more readily quantifiable areas of our lives? A vast body of cross-sectional data, as well as longitudinal data, shows that higher levels of subjective well-being[1] are associated with many desirable characteristics, such as better learning and educational attainment, greater productivity at work, better relationships, more pro-social behaviour, and better health and life expectancy [1, 22]. This relationship is illustrated in Fig. 15.1.

As cross-sectional data shed no light on the direction of causality, we consider here only the evidence from longitudinal and experimental studies. There is compelling evidence from prospective longitudinal studies of normal and clinical populations that various measures of subjective aspects of well-being (e.g. positive affect, optimism, self-esteem) predict later physical health and longevity, controlling for baseline health and socioeconomic status [23–25]. A higher level of well-being increases resistance to developing illness (as seen in experimental studies of the effects of nasal introduction of the common cold virus [26]) and provides a protective role in the course of physical illness [27]. Mechanisms may include the effects of subjective well-being on reducing the stress response and improving immune function [28, 29].

Subjective well-being early in life has also been shown to reduce the risk of mental disorder.

To our knowledge only one study has specifically addressed this issue. Participants in the nationally representative British 1946 birth cohort study were rated by teachers on their positive mood and behaviour in their early teens, and assessed on a range of outcomes several decades later. Controlling for sociodemographic factors, cognitive function, and personality, high ratings by teachers were associated with a 62% reduction in the risk of a mental health problem later in life [30]. Other good outcomes later in life

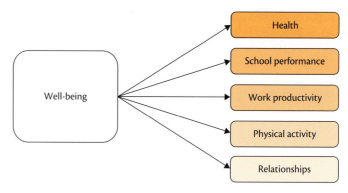

Fig. 15.1 Conceptual model of how well-being is typically considered as having impacts on other outcomes.

associated with high levels of subjective well-being in childhood include higher satisfaction with work, a high frequency of contact with friends or family, engagement in social activities, and pro-social behaviour [30, 31].

Overall, this growing evidence for the positive consequences and impacts of well-being lends increasing weight to the merit of intervening to enhance well-being, whether through individual or group interventions, or at the social level through public policy.

Although the wide range of instrumental benefits of well-being are frequently cited as the reason for its importance, we reiterate that the instrumental benefits are not the main reason why well-being is important. They are merely a by-product or dividend of a high level of well-being. The real reason well-being matters is that well-being is an end in itself—an ultimate good.

Defining mental health and well-being

One of the biggest challenges in the field is that there is no agreed definition of well-being. This is true even when we disregard the confusing euphemistic use of the term well-being (or mental health) to mean mental disorders. (A striking illustration of euphemism is the peculiar use of the term 'mental health prevention'. Why would anyone wish to prevent mental health?)

One approach to defining well-being is called 'objective list theory', whereby an expert lists the objective conditions deemed necessary for individuals to experience well-being. Some influential bodies such as the Organisation for Economic Co-operation and Development (OECD) [32] and the UK Office for National Statistics (ONS) [33] define well-being primarily in objective terms: the combination of factors such as health, education, income, quality of housing, and quality of relationships. This approach confuses contextual aspects of well-being with well-being itself, and downplays the centrality of people's lived experience, i.e. their subjective well-being. There can be no doubt that many people whose lives can be considered as fortunate by objective criteria may be deeply unhappy, unfulfilled, isolated, and perceive their functioning to be impaired. In contrast, there are many people whose objective circumstances may be poor, who nevertheless lead happy and fulfilled lives. Although individual and population well-being is influenced by objective circumstances, at its core, well-being is a subjective state—it is how well a person perceives their life to be going.

---

1 Note that this refers generally to measures of psychological well-being and mental health, which are inherently subjective, not the narrow framework of 'subjective well-being' (SWB), which is defined as life satisfaction, high levels of pleasant affect, and low levels of unpleasant affect.

Even when we put aside definitions that focus on objective circumstances that may be related to well-being and consider only definitions that are concerned with subjective aspects of well-being or the behaviours that characterize it, there is as yet no agreement on how broadly or narrowly such experience should be defined. For instance, the World Health Organization (WHO) definition of mental health describes it as 'a state of well-being in which every individual realizes his or her own potential, can cope with the normal stresses of life, can work productively and fruitfully, and is able to make a contribution to her or his community' [34]. This definition focuses on some aspects of high level functioning, but it is not clear how this list of components was derived.

As outlined in the brief history section, some scholars regard positive emotion such as happiness as a sufficient definition of well-being (hedonic perspective [9, 21, 35]), whereas others insist that the essence of well-being is perceived functional ability, sense of meaning, and positive relationships (eudaimonic perspective [15, 17]). Still others define well-being as the combination of feeling good and functioning well, believing that both are necessary for the experience of well-being [36–38]. This lack of a cohesive, consensus-driven, and widely applied definition has undoubtedly slowed progress in both scientific work on well-being and general appreciation for its value among the medical community. However, this is not a sufficient basis for withholding efforts to establish well-being as a primary outcome of interest rather than simply the reduction of disease across populations [39]. On the contrary, this is where progress originates.

Moving forward

What is the way forward in developing a consensus on the definition of well-being or positive mental health? To begin with, there needs to be agreement that mental health is multidimensional, and cannot be defined in terms of a single construct such as happiness or life satisfaction. However, to date, most lists of well-being dimensions are based either on the author's theoretical background or personal preferences (e.g. Ryff based her list on psychodynamic theory and developmental psychology), and as theories and preferences vary, it is unlikely that there would be agreement on this basis. But perhaps a more systematic approach to identifying the relevant dimensions may gain more traction. For example, a systematic approach based on the nature of the relationship between mental health and mental illness might have a greater chance of gaining widespread acceptance.

One such attempt has been made by Huppert and So [36], based on the idea that positive mental health lies at the opposite end of a continuum to mental illness as represented by the common mental disorders (CMD; depression and generalized anxiety). These disorders are common both in the sense that they are highly prevalent in the population, and that they may afflict any member of the population at some point in their life. Acknowledging that there are internationally recognized criteria and lists of symptoms for the diagnosis of these CMD (Diagnostic and Statistical Manual of Mental Disorders, International Classification of Diseases), these investigators systematically defined the opposite of each symptom. For example, they suggest that the opposite of the *loss* of interest and pleasure is *being* interested and engaged, and the opposite of the sense of hopelessness that characterizes major depressive episodes is being optimistic. Using this systematic approach, they identified 10 dimensions that appear to define the positive end of the mental health spectrum. These are: sense of competence, emotional stability, engagement, sense of meaning, optimism, positive emotions, positive relationships, resilience, self-esteem, and vitality. There is considerable overlap between these dimensions and the dimensions specified in other lists. These include Martin Seligman's PERMA (positive emotion, engagement, relationships, meaning, accomplishment) or Ryff's six dimensions of psychological well-being (autonomy, environmental mastery, personal growth, positive relationships, purpose in life, self-acceptance). However, the systematic way in which the 10 dimensions of Huppert and So were derived perhaps puts them on a more solid footing. Future psychometric and longitudinal research will establish the extent to which these 10 dimensions are independent of one another. But at this relatively early stage in the science of well-being, it may be useful to accept these as a provisional list, and measure all of these dimensions wherever possible when undertaking a mental health/well-being survey.

Measuring mental health and well-being

Innumerable studies that purport to measure well-being use scales that are designed to measure symptoms of mental illness or distress. Even if an individual does not endorse a single symptom on such a scale, we cannot conclude that they have a high level of subjective well-being—all we can conclude is that they do not have symptoms of disorder. In order to measure positive well-being, we need questions that ask about positive experiences. It is entirely possible for an individual to endorse neither symptoms nor positive experiences. It is the extent of endorsement of positive experiences that indicates the level of subjective well-being. Therefore, questions designed to measure well-being need to be positively worded, i.e. the content of the question needs to be about positive features.

Some measures of distress or disorder include questions about positive feelings or functioning. A good example is the General Health Questionnaire [40], most versions of which have equal numbers of negatively and positively focused items. It has been shown that insights into well-being, its determinants and impacts, can be achieved by comparing responses to the positive and negative items [41]. For example, although the literature, based largely on measures of symptomatology, suggests that depressive symptoms are associated with adverse events such as unemployment and mortality, Huppert and Whittington [41] have shown that these are better predicted by the absence of positive features than by the presence of depressive symptoms. In other words, adverse outcomes may be better predicted by a low level of well-being than by the presence of mental disorder. Such a finding has profound implications for policy and practice [42], suggesting that the promotion of well-being may be at least as important as the treatment and prevention of disorder.

Perhaps the best example of the misalignment between measures of mental health and mental illness comes from the five-item WHO Well-Being Index (WHO-5), which was first published in 1998 and has since been used globally, becoming the focus of systematic reviews, policies, and major international strategies [43]. Although the measure itself has been constructed as an instrument to assess psychological well-being, and all five questions concern positive feelings and functioning, much of the literature on it has focused on its application as a screening tool for depression. This further builds arguments that measuring positive features may offer more insight into mental illness than measuring negative features, and this ironic application is another illustration of the interchangeable use of the terms mental health and mental illness. Given this mindset, it is unsurprising that there is confusion about how to measure mental health as distinct from mental illness.

If we accept that subjective well-being can only be measured using questions about positive features, we now discuss what are the most widely used measures, and how effectively they measure subjective well-being or positive mental health. By far the most commonly used metric for population well-being is life satisfaction, usually assessed by a single question. In many cases, this is the primary or even sole measure of well-being, resulting in a single mean applied to a particular group with further analyses to identify determinants and covariates. However, while there is already debate around the value of life satisfaction as a measure of well-being [44], it is very evidently *not* a measure of mental health. Equating a general evaluation of life—which integrates current attitudes, future expectations, and past experiences in a dynamic and ever-changing way—to well-being has impeded research, as such a measure is both extremely difficult to interpret and clearly an inadequate proxy for mental health.

A single-item measure of happiness is also widely used in population studies to assess subjective well-being. Usually it is asked about a person's general level of happiness, but in some recent applications it assesses the momentary or recent experience of happiness. The ONS in the UK now routinely asks 'How happy were you yesterday?' Even if it can be argued that this is an adequate way to assess subjective well-being, either in its general or momentary/recent formulation, it is clearly an inadequate proxy for evaluating mental health.

Mental health, like mental illness is multidimensional, and an acceptable measure of mental health needs to assess the relevant dimensions. There are a number of widely used multidimensional measures of well-being/mental health, and although the universal adoption of a single measure is not a requirement for scientific progress (for instance, there are numerous scales measuring depression and anxiety) there should be agreement on which dimensions need to be measured. Unfortunately, this is not the case in relation to measures of well-being. For example, Ryff's Scales of Psychological Well-being measure six dimensions of well-being, based on psychodynamic theory and developmental psychology: autonomy, environmental mastery, personal growth, positive relationships, purpose in life, and self-acceptance. For Deci and Ryan [17] the key dimensions are autonomy, competence, and relatedness, which they describe as basic psychological needs, whereas Seligman's list comprises PERMA (positive emotions, engagement, relationships, meaning, and accomplishment) [38]. The corresponding scales can be used to yield a total score, as well as information about each of these dimensions.

In a pragmatic rather than theory-driven exercise, some national and international bodies undertake population surveys. These include the OECD's 'How's Life?' survey [32] and ONS surveys [33] using a combination of questions, which include life satisfaction to measure a person's global evaluation of well-being, recent feelings of happiness and anxiety to measure mood, and a question about sense of meaning as an indicator of eudaimonic well-being. In two other widely used measures (Warwick-Edinburgh Mental Well-being Scale [45]; Flourishing Scale [46]) each scale incorporates several dimensions of well-being, but only a total score is derived rather than scores on each individual dimension. Nevertheless, because these measures are simple, in terms of face validity as well as scoring, and because they provide a single number, they have had a significant impact on public capacity to relate to the concept of mental well-being.

As described in the 'Definition' section, the only multidimensional approach that is solidly and explicitly rooted in the mental health/illness literature is that of Huppert and So [36]. Defining positive mental health (also known as well-being or flourishing) as the opposite of the CMD (depression, generalized anxiety) they identified 10 dimensions of well-being, and suggested that all needed to be measured in order to capture fully the construct of positive mental health. Using a set of 10 indicator items, one for each dimension, which had been administered in the European Social Survey, they developed a method of both combining the items to measure overall well-being, and examining the separate profiles of the 10 dimensions to gain an understanding of how these profiles varied across population subgroups and nations [36, 47].

This approach is invaluable for policymakers, as it identifies where strengths and weaknesses lie, and, accordingly, which dimensions need to be targeted for particular groups. Although the framework used in these studies is very promising, there is not yet a corresponding, psychometrically validated scale that includes multiple items to measure accurately each of the 10 dimensions. Research on the development of such a scale is almost completed, and should go some way towards allaying concerns about whether we have a high-quality, appropriate scale for measuring positive mental health that is suitable for policy [42].

When evaluating findings from studies of well-being, we always need to bear in mind how exactly well-being was conceptualized in the particular investigation, and how exactly it was measured, as this can greatly influence the interpretation and implications of the findings. A useful step towards greater rigour would be for publishers, editors, and reviewers to insist on authors being very precise in how the term well-being is being used.

Evidence for the effectiveness of interventions to improve well-being

One of the key questions following discussion on measurement and terminology is simply, 'How do we do anything about it?' There is a rapidly growing body of research using a variety of programmes across different population groups and contexts to enhance well-being; that is, where well-being (measured in a variety of ways) is the main outcome, or at least one of the primary outcomes. While this is not the most developed aspect of the field, the quality of the research is also improving, going from basic pre-post study designs to randomized, controlled trials, some with active control groups.

There is also a growing number of systematic reviews and meta-analyses of interventions to enhance well-being, including the impressive series of reviews from the international DataPrev project [48]. However, caution must be urged in taking these publications at face value, as many publications that purport to provide evidence of improved well-being are conducted on small samples, often with narrow inclusion criteria, and, in fact, use outcomes that demonstrate symptom reduction rather than improvements on well-being measures. As such, this may be seen as the next challenge in *public* mental health regarding well-being, although recent insights are encouraging.

Many of the intervention programmes provide behavioural training such as teaching the skills that are known to be associated with high levels of well-being. One set of programmes is derived from positive psychology and coaching psychology, which use goal-oriented and solution-focused approaches, and targets skills such as resilience, gratitude, positive affect, and character building [49–53]. Another set of programmes emanates from the mindfulness literature, and targets skills such as attention and awareness, emotion regulation, curiosity, non-judgement, and self-kindness [54–57]. There is also growing interest in mindfulness and compassion-based programmes and growing evidence of their benefits both for individual and relational well-being [58].

Physical exercise programmes have also been linked to psychological well-being. While the extensive research in this area is almost exclusively focused on association studies, there is some evidence of a causal relationship between physical activity interventions and psychological well-being, as seen in experimental trials which show that moderate exercise increases positive affect and self-esteem [59, 60].

While most of these well-being interventions use group-based training, some are one-to-one, and an increasing number are self-help programs, including an escalating number of web-based programs or apps, disturbingly few of which have been properly evaluated. One notable exception is the study by Powell et al [61]. They undertook a randomized, controlled trial using a web-based intervention teaching cognitive behavioural principles in a general population sample. Well-being, assessed by the Warwick-Edinburgh Mental Well-Being Scale (WEMWBS)[45], was measured at baseline, after 6 weeks of training, and again 6 weeks later. Significant improvements were found at both 6 and 12 weeks in the intervention group compared with the control group. Web-based interventions and e-learning clearly have the potential to reach large sectors of the population at low cost, although improvements in their design are needed to avoid the high rates of failure to complete the programme.

Other interventions to enhance well-being focus on changing the context or the environment, rather than individual skills training. Examples are changing a school's ethos, changing workplace structures or practices, or encouraging social connection among older people to reduce isolation. A growing number of studies examine the effect on psychological well-being of making changes to the urban or the natural environment [62–66].

A recent review of the effectiveness of interventions to enhance well-being at different stages in the life course has been undertaken by Kristian Wahlbeck [67]. Results are grouped according to the different contexts in which the intervention was provided—parenting and early years, schools, workplaces, and for older people. Most of the programmes described in the following paragraph are universal, and some clinicians and policymakers are sceptical about the benefit of this approach, preferring to target interventions to those with the greatest need. However, one of the most important findings from a public mental health perspective is that these universal programmes have their greatest effect on those with the greatest need. A further advantage of these universal programmes is that they normalize the intervention procedure and thereby avoid stigma.

Parenting interventions, including early parent–child interaction and approaches to fostering positive behaviours are regarded as an important target for mental health promotion. Promoting a nurturing early interaction between parents and children increases the child's resilience in the face of adverse life events and promotes lifelong mental health and well-being. Parenting programmes also improve the well-being of parents and the relationship between parents, which would likely further increase the well-being of the child. Intervention approaches include one-to-one training, programmes targeted at families where children are showing early signs of mental health problems, and universal programmes delivered to all parents in schools, community settings, antenatal classes, or via the Internet [68, 69]. Programmes that use trained home visitors to strengthen parent–child interaction and provide counselling have been shown to be effective when delivered by trained nurses in developed countries [70], or by trained laywomen in developing countries [71]. Such programmes have been found to improve maternal sensitivity, to reduce criticism and harsh upbringing, and to improve child attachment.

Mental health promotion in schools has grown rapidly in recent decades, and there are many good research studies [72–75]. Interventions focus on teaching students skills such as resilience, behaviour regulation, social skills, and mindfulness, as well as teacher education, peer support, or a whole-school approach, including work on school leadership and ethos. While many studies show beneficial impacts on the reduction of depressive symptoms and problem behaviours, many also show increases in well-being and behaviours conducive to well-being, such as social and emotional skills, increased problem-solving ability, cooperation, empathy, and a positive and realistic self-concept.

The workplace is an important setting for mental health promotion in the adult population. Psycho-social interventions, including skills training, relaxation, and structuring employment to create good working conditions have all been shown to bring well-being benefits to the individual (e.g. mental health improvement, stress reduction, increased job satisfaction) and to social relationships and performance in the workplace [76–79]. There are also completed and ongoing studies of the effects of interventions to improve well-being or decrease stress in very specific settings, such as in prisons [80, 81], and among military personnel [82, 83].

Psychosocial interventions that aim to increase the social connectedness of older people have been shown to improve psychological well-being and reduce feelings of loneliness. A review and meta-analysis has shown that social activities among older people significantly improve positive mental health, life satisfaction, and quality of life, and reduce depressive symptoms when compared with no intervention [84, 85].

While the aforementioned studies provide ample evidence that well-being interventions can be effective, they are often brief (days or weeks) so they may have only short-term benefits, although little research has been done on duration of effect. Maybe like some medications that are taken for life, well-being interventions need to be repeated regularly. Or, like exercise, the skills that have been learned need to be practised regularly. Detailed investigation of such issues will inform policy and identify best practice.

As sample sizes and study quality continue to improve, it will become possible to address the time-honoured question: 'Which interventions work best for whom, for which outcomes, and for how long?' For instance, if we compare different forms of skills training, some people may respond better to meditation-based learning, whereas others may respond better to the more cognitive, goal-focused skills training offered by typical positive psychology interventions. Or perhaps the best results might arise from learning several different approaches to enhancing well-being, and the effects of programme length and programme order on well-being outcomes could be investigated.

In addition, as was described earlier, there are two main approaches to improving well-being—programmes designed to change individual attitudes and behaviours, and programmes designed to change the context or environment. Little is known about the relative benefits of change at the individual level versus the contextual level. Further research is needed to establish whether providing opportunities for people to learn and cultivate the skills of well-being may be more or less effective than changing the context in which people live or work. It may be that learning the skills that underpin well-being will enable people to experience greater well-being across diverse areas of their life, whereas changes in specific contexts (e.g. school or workplace) may be needed to support and sustain individual change. A new generation of public health field trials will yield answers to these questions, providing a firm evidence base for promoting the most effective public mental health policies and programmes.

The financial case for improving well-being

McDaid and Cooper state [86]: 'It is not enough to know what factors contribute to wellbeing, we then need to carefully evaluate the cost-effectiveness of actions to promote better wellbeing in society' (p. 5). While well-being is itself the ultimate outcome, there may be concerns that financial investment toward study and intervention may take away from other areas of public mental health and psychiatry. However, there are a number of examples demonstrating that investment in improving mental health yields major returns, which should relieve such concerns.

The DataPrev project reviewed 47 studies of varying quality, which looked either at promotion of mental health and well-being and/or primary prevention of poor mental health. It concluded that there were significant economic benefits from investing in improving well-being [87]. One example is an estimated annual cost saving of 30% when mental health promotion programmes are administered in the workplace. This study also estimated the benefit to cost ratio of positive parenting interventions, reporting a range from 1.26:1 to 28.42:1. Additionally, Knapp et al. [88] have undertaken some analyses of the cost-effectiveness of a multi-component well-being intervention in a workplace setting, and calculated an annual return on investment of 9 to 1. Such approaches are critical given the finite resources available for population mental health programmes [89].

If economic gain must be visible to invest in the promotion of mental health and well-being, what would be the implication if this return was not shown? In other words, if improved mental health meant greater financial costs than returns, or if improved population well-being coincided with decreasing gross domestic product, what do we choose as a society to prioritize? Such considerations may be, on some level, directly related to the 'controversy' of well-being within all policy.

Integrating well-being into public mental health policy

Probably the biggest barrier among clinicians to accepting the importance of well-being is the persistence of the medical model, in which there are just two states: disease and normality. Medical training emphasizes that diseases need to be understood, treated, and prevented, and clinicians often regard this to be enough to produce health. Yet, since 1948, the WHO has made it clear that 'health is more than the absence of disease or infirmity'. Furthermore, patients do not regard it as enough to be relieved of their symptoms; what they want is to be restored to a fully functional state where they can enjoy life to the full [90]. Recovery from mental illness has been defined as the process of building a meaningful and satisfying life, as defined by the person themselves, which has been shown to include finding and maintaining hope, re-establishment of a positive identity, building a meaningful life, and taking responsibility and control [91, 92]. Patient-centred medical care therefore needs to recognize the key role of well-being in the recovery process.

Another barrier to accepting the importance of studying and promoting well-being is the problem of limited resources. The argument is that if the limited resources available are spent on improvement of well-being, this takes away from resources for treatment (and possibly prevention) of mental disorder. This is a fair concern, because even improving population well-being will not eliminate mental disorders. As long as major underfunding continues in the mental health sector, we will need to ensure adequate resources for treatment and prevention because of the extremely damaging effect that mental disorders have on individuals and those around them. Clearly, as has been cogently argued by Layard [93], the mental health sector needs a much larger slice of the pie that represents how health funds are allocated between physical and mental health/illness. In order to decide what percentage of the (augmented) mental health budget should go to the promotion of well-being, we need to understand more about the extent of population shift following interventions that promote or increase well-being.

Perhaps the most convincing way to demonstrate the impoverishment of the medical model and the value of promoting positive well-being is to provide evidence that by improving the average level of well-being in the population, we can reduce the burden of CMD. Evidence might include reducing the severity or duration of a disorder, or, better still, lowering the probability of a disorder occurring. Various lines of evidence suggest that this may, indeed, be the case. In this chapter we have already shown a high level of well-being early in life produces a large reduction in the likelihood of a mental disorder later in life [30], adjusting for baseline socioeconomic factors, cognitive function, and personality. Further, the majority of well-being interventions described in an earlier section have been shown to decrease depression, anxiety, and stress, as well as increasing psychological well-being [49, 50, 51, 55, 56]. At present, however, the intervention studies have been undertaken on relatively small groups, and what is needed is a large-scale demonstration that a well-being intervention can both shift the population curve towards well-being, and reduce the prevalence of CMD. In other words, we seek evidence at the population level that is congruent with the Rose hypothesis [94].

According to this model, the prevalence of any common health condition is directly related to the population mean of the underlying risk factors. The key insight from this model is that the most effective way to reduce the prevalence of a common disorder is to shift the mean of the population in a positive direction. The effectiveness of this approach has been demonstrated in diverse conditions such as alcohol abuse and heart disease [95, 96]. The question we address here is whether the model applies to mental illness and mental health. To answer this question, we must ask if CMD fulfil certain criteria. We need to establish first whether the prevalence of CMD is related to the average level of well-being in the population. The answer is yes. A study by Anderson, Huppert, and Rose [97] showed a close relationship between mean scores on a measure of mental health and the prevalence of clinically significant disorder in subgroups of the population. Secondly, we need to establish whether there is a reduction in CMD if the population mean shifts in a positive direction. Again, the answer is yes. In a 7-year longitudinal study of a representative population sample, Huppert and Whittington [41] confirmed that a small positive shift in the population mean on a measure of mental health was associated with a large reduction in the prevalence of CMD. They found a 6% reduction in clinically significant mental disorder for every 1-point increase on their measure of mental health, and this compared favourably with their Rose model prediction of a 7% decrease. The study was an observational one, but had it been an intervention study, a 6% decrease in population mental disorder would represent not only huge cost benefits, but also a very substantial reduction in personal suffering and its subsequent impact on families and the wider community. A similar association has been reported more recently in a study of adolescents [98].

What remains to be established is whether a well-being *intervention* can decrease the prevalence of CMD in the population by shifting the population mean towards higher well-being. We urge researchers who are undertaking large-scale well-being interventions to test this model of population shift.

The road ahead

Although there is as yet no agreement on a single definition or best measure of well-being, and more research is required on whether and how the population curve shifts following well-being interventions, it is very encouraging that there is almost universal agreement among governments and international organizations about the importance of subjective well-being. For example, the WHO advocates that there should be 'health in all policies', including 'mental health in all policies', in a manner that integrates the work across sectors to improve population health and health equity [99, 100]. This ambition is founded upon the insistence that 'there is no health without mental health', first advocated in 1999 by the Finnish National Research and Development Centre for Welfare and Health (STAKES), when Finland held the Presidency of the European Union [101]. This perspective was subsequently embraced in 2003 by the New York City Department of Health and Mental Hygiene [102], and in 2011 in the English Mental Health Strategy [103], entitled 'No Health Without Mental Health'. Finally, the US Centers for Disease Control and Mental Health Europe endorse the specific need to 'promote positive mental health and wellbeing in all policies' [104, 105].

In an economic context, one example of the commitment to well-being is the Millennium Development Goals (MDGs), which

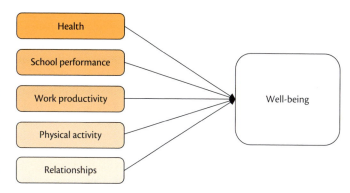

Fig. 15.2 Making well-being the outcome of interest.

were established by the United Nations in 2000 and replaced by the Sustainable Development Goals (SDGs) in 2015. In the MDGs, there was no mention of mental health nor was there any scientific approach to understanding or improving well-being. In response to the growing evidence, the SDGs have as the third goal: 'Ensure healthy lives and promote well-being for all at all ages' [106].

David McDaid [107] highlights that well-being has, indeed, become a major commitment for governments globally, but this is of little use unless research on well-being is actually used to inform policy and practice. As demonstrated in the previous section, there seems to be sufficient evidence to initiate policy field trials and policy experiments implementing what is already known from subjective well-being research. Asking why this change has not already taken place, the distinguished economist John Helliwell argues that the relatively slow progress from accumulating evidence to changes in policies and practices is partly due to the human predilection to adhere to old ways despite the arrival of contradictory evidence [108]. This pervasive effect is hard to dislodge because decision-makers are generally unaware of their subconscious biases in favour of evidence supporting the view they already hold. Helliwell concludes that if taking SWB[2] more seriously has the potential to increase quality of life while reducing pressures on available resources, there should be a stronger commitment to broadening the range of policy alternatives to include those with a strong chance of improving SWB.

Critically, however, the most significant implication for policy—which will have direct ramifications for research on the topic—will be the shift in thinking about well-being as an outcome as opposed to a mechanism by which other outcomes are achieved. This is depicted in Fig. 15.2, which simply but crucially alters the paradigm described earlier and visualized in Fig. 15.1. This implies that for valid and sustained impacts to be recognized within public mental health, well-being must not be treated as a footnote or superficially recognized policy outcome. Instead, it should be on a par with other impacts sought within a given policy, or even as the pinnacle impact of all policy, with relevant underlying initiatives resourced appropriately to achieve desired effects.

---

[2] In this context, we refer specifically to the defined construct 'subjective well-being', typically written as SWB, which necessarily includes measures of life satisfaction, high levels of pleasant affect, and low levels of unpleasant affect. It is important to note this narrow but critical distinction to avoid any confusion in semantics or constructs.

Conclusion

Regardless of where anyone sits on views of well-being, it remains important: if you believe treatment is most important, then well-being is critical in recovery; if you believe prevention is important, well-being can reduce risks of illness; if you believe well-being is ultimately what everyone wants from life, then it should be *the* target and indicator of ultimate interest.

Encouragingly, narratives around well-being as a matter of public interest have evolved. In the past, well-being was not considered a priority for public policy. However, as poorly defined approaches have been replaced by improved understanding and terminology, there is now extensive debate on how to best measure well-being on a global level. We have gone from a focus on interventions to alleviate symptoms to interventions to reduce the risk of illness to interventions to optimize flourishing. In short, we have come a long way: What needs to happen next?

If we genuinely care about good public mental health, the most critical thing is that we have appropriate definitions for well-being, although it is not mandatory to have only one. These must in turn emphasise that it is the positive end of the mental health spectrum and that it is multidimensional. These must become the way we measure well-being as *the* outcome of interest for public mental health (and all policies), by whatever name is deemed most accurate.

As has been argued, such progress is only possible with sufficient investment in understanding well-being, its underlying factors, and how interventions do (or do not) improve it across populations. There is no implication that doing this—certainly not from the authors—requires forsaking investment in the treatment of mental illness or the prevention of disease. On the contrary, to overcome the controversial discussion of well-being, there must be appreciation for the entire spectrum of mental health with appropriate investment made at each stage.

Once this whole-population perspective is in place, the focus can shift toward discussions of the best interventions to facilitate the highest well-being for the largest number of people. Doing this will establish well-being as the ultimate aim of policy within and beyond mental health programmes, and not simply as a footnote in major public programmes. It will ultimately promote positive outcomes for most individuals within a population, putting well-being ahead of focusing on incomes, illness, or other objective indications of how life is going. Instead, it will recognize what is most important to populations and thereby promote systematic attempts to facilitate improvement on those dimensions in a meaningful and sustainable way.

References

1. Huppert FA. The state of wellbeing science: concepts, measures, interventions, and policies. *Wellbeing* 2014; 6: 1–49.
2. Schoch R. *The Secrets of Happiness: Three Thousand Years of Searching for the Good Life.* New York: Simon and Schuster, 2006.
3. Wallace BA, Shapiro SL. Mental balance and well-being: building bridges between Buddhism and Western psychology. *Am Psychol* 2006; 61: 690.
4. Bentham J. *The Principles of Morals and Legislation.* London: Printed for T. Payne, 1789 (republished in 1988 by Prometheus Books, New York).
5. Mill JS. *Utilitarianism.* London: Parker, Son and Bourn, 1863.
6. Priestley J. *An Essay on the First Principles of Government; and on the Nature of Political, Civil, and Religious Liberty.* London: History of Economic Thought Books, 1768.
7. Paine T. *Rights of Man.* London: J.S. Jordan, 1791.
8. Sinclair J. *Statistical Account of Scotland, vol. 2.* Edinburgh: Creech, 1792.
9. Layard R. *Happiness: Lessons From a New Science.* London: Penguin, 2011.
10. Stiglitz JE, Sen A, Fitoussi JP. Report by the Stiglitz Commission on the Measurement of Economic Performance and Social Progress. New York: United Nations, 2009.
11. Kahneman D, Deaton A. High income improves evaluation of life but not emotional well-being. *Proc Natl Acad Sci* 2010; 107: 16489–16493.
12. Jahoda M. Current concepts of positive mental health. *J Occup Environ Med* 1959; 1: 565.
13. Rogers CR. The concept of the fully functioning person. *Psychotherapy* 1963; 1: 17.
14. Maslow AH. *Toward a Psychology of Being.* New York: Van Nostrand, 1962.
15. Ryff CD. Happiness is everything, or is it? Explorations on the meaning of psychological well-being. *J Person Soc Psychol* 1989; 57: 1069.
16. Waterman AS. Two conceptions of happiness: contrasts of personal expressiveness (eudaimonia) and hedonic enjoyment. *J Person Soc Psychol* 1993; 64: 678.
17. Deci EL, Ryan RM. *Intrinsic Motivation and Self-determination in Human Behavior.* New York: Plenum, 1985.
18. Ashby FG, Isen AM, Turken AU. A neuropsychological theory of positive affect and its influence on cognition. *Psychol Rev* 1999; 106: 529.
19. Diener E. Subjective well-being. *Psychol Bull* 1984; 95: 542–575.
20. Fredrickson BL. What good are positive emotions? *Rev Gen Psychol* 1998; 2: 300.
21. Kahneman D, Diener E, Schwarz N (eds). *Well-being: Foundations of Hedonic Psychology.* New York: Russell Sage Foundation, 1999.
22. Dolan P, Peasgood T, White M. Do we really know what makes us happy? A review of the economic literature on the factors associated with subjective well-being. *J Econ Psychol* 2008; 29: 94–122.
23. Dolan P, Peasgood T, White M. Do we really know what makes us happy? A review of the economic literature on the factors associated with subjective well-being. *J Econ Psychol* 2008; 29: 94–122.
24. Danner DD, Snowdon DA, Friesen WV. Positive emotions in early life and longevity: findings from the nun study. *J Person Soc Psychol* 2001; 80: 804.
25. Diener E, Chan MY. Happy people live longer: subjective well-being contributes to health and longevity. *Appl Psychol* 2011; 3: 1–43.
26. Cohen S, Doyle WJ, Turner RB, Alper CM, Skoner DP. Emotional style and susceptibility to the common cold. *Psychosom Med* 2003; 65: 652–657.
27. Lamers SM, Bolier L, Westerhof GJ, Smit F, Bohlmeijer ET. The impact of emotional well-being on long-term recovery and survival in physical illness: a meta-analysis. *J Behav Med* 2012; 35: 538–547.
28. Fredrickson BL, Mancuso RA, Branigan C, Tugade MM. The undoing effect of positive emotions. *Motiv Emot* 2000; 24: 237–258.
29. Davidson RJ, Kabat-Zinn J, Schumacher J, et al. Alterations in brain and immune function produced by mindfulness meditation. *Psychosom Med* 2003; 65: 564–570.
30. Richards M, Huppert FA. Do positive children become positive adults? Evidence from a longitudinal birth cohort study. *J Pos Psychol* 2011; 6: 75–87.
31. Olsson CA, McGee R, Nada-Raja S, Williams SM. A 32-year longitudinal study of child and adolescent pathways to well-being in adulthood. *J Happiness Stud* 2013; 14: 1069–1083.
32. Organisation for Economic Co-operation and Development (OECD). *How's Life? 2015: Measuring Well-being.* Paris: OECD Publishing, 2015.
33. Office of National Statistics (ONS). *Personal Well-being in the UK: Jan to Dec 2016.* London: Office of National Statistics, 2017.

34. World Health Organization (WHO). *The World Health Report 2001: Mental Health: New Understanding, New Hope*. Geneva: WHO, 2001.

35. Fredrickson B. *Positivity*. New York: Harmony, 2009.

36. Huppert FA, So TT. Flourishing across Europe: application of a new conceptual framework for defining well-being. *Soc Indic Res* 2013; 110: 837–861.

37. Keyes CL. Promoting a life worth living: human development from the vantage points of mental illness and mental health. In: Lerner RM, Jacobs F, Wertlieb D (eds). *Handbook of Applied Developmental Science: Promoting Positive Child, Adolescent, and Family Development Through Research, Policies, and Programs*. Thousand Oaks, CA: SAGE, 2003, pp. 257–274.

38. Seligman ME. *Flourish: A Visionary New Understanding of Happiness and Well-being*. New York: Simon and Schuster, 2012.

39. Stewart-Brown S, Middleton J, Ashton J. Responses to the Chief Medical Officer's report 2013. *Lancet* 2015; 385: 2576.

40. Goldberg D, Williams P, Williams P. *A User's Guide to the General Health Questionnaire*. Windsor: NFER-Nelson, 1988.

41. Huppert FA, Whittington JE. Evidence for the independence of positive and negative well-being: Implications for quality of life assessment. *Br J Health Psychol* 2003; 8: 107–122.

42. Farver-Vestergaard I, Ruggeri K. Setting national policy agendas in light of the Denmark results for well-being. *JAMA Psychiatry* 2017; 74: 8.

43. Topp CW, Østergaard SD, Søndergaard S, Bech P. The WHO-5 Well-Being Index: a systematic review of the literature. *Psychother Psychosom* 2015; 84:167–176.

44. Krueger AB, Schkade DA. The reliability of subjective well-being measures. *J Public Econ* 2008; 92: 1833–1845.

45. Tennant R, Hiller L, Fishwick R, et al. The Warwick-Edinburgh mental well-being scale (WEMWBS): development and UK validation. *Health Qual Life Outcomes* 2007; 5: 63.

46. Diener E, Wirtz D, Tov W, et al. New well-being measures: short scales to assess flourishing and positive and negative feelings. *Soc Indic Res* 2010; 97: 143–156.

47. Ruggeri K, Garcia Garzon E, Maguire A, Huppert FA. Comprehensive psychological wellbeing. In: Harrison E, Quick A, Abdallah S (eds). *Looking Through the Wellbeing Kaleidoscope*. London: New Economics Foundation, 2016, pp. 10–29.

48. Cooper C. Special supplement on mental health promotion. *Health Promot Int* 2011; 26 (1).

49. Bolier L, Haverman M, Westerhof GJ, Riper H, Smit F, Bohlmeijer E. Positive psychology interventions: a meta-analysis of randomized controlled studies. *BMC Public Health* 2013; 13: 119.

50. Gander F, Proyer RT, Ruch W, Wyss T. Strength-based positive interventions: Further evidence for their potential in enhancing well-being and alleviating depression. *J Happiness Stud* 2013; 14: 1241–1259.

51. Sin NL, Lyubomirsky S. Enhancing well-being and alleviating depressive symptoms with positive psychology interventions: a practice-friendly meta-analysis. *J Clin Psychol* 2009; 65: 467–487.

52. Weiss LA, Westerhof GJ, Bohlmeijer ET. Can we increase psychological well-being? The effects of interventions on psychological well-being: a meta-analysis of randomized controlled trials. *PLOS ONE* 2016; 11: e0158092.

53. Wood AM, Froh JJ, Geraghty AW. Gratitude and well-being: a review and theoretical integration. *Clin Psychol Rev* 2010; 30: 890–905.

54. Creswell JD. Mindfulness interventions. *Annu Rev Psychol* 2017; 68: 491–516.

55. Keng SL, Smoski MJ, Robins CJ. Effects of mindfulness on psychological health: A review of empirical studies. *Clin Psychol Rev* 2011; 31: 1041–1056.

56. Kuyken W, Weare K, Ukoumunne OC, et al. Effectiveness of the mindfulness in schools programme: non-randomised controlled feasibility study. *Br J Psychiatry* 2013; 203: 126–131.

57. Sedlmeier P, Eberth J, Schwarz M, Zimmermann D, Haarig F, Jaeger S, Kunze S. The psychological effects of meditation: a meta-analysis. *Psychol Bull* 2012; 138: 1139.

58. Huppert FA. Living life well: the role of mindfulness and compassion. In: Forgas J, Baumeister R (eds) *The Social Psychology of Living Well*. London: Psychology Press, 2017.

59. Biddle SJ, Mutrie N. *Psychology of Physical Activity: Determinants, Well-being and Interventions*. London: Routledge, 2007.

60. Spence JC, McGannon KR, Poon P. The effect of exercise on global self-esteem: a quantitative review. *J Sport Exercise Psy* 2005; 27: 311–334.

61. Powell J, Hamborg T, Stallard N, et al. Effectiveness of a web-based cognitive-behavioral tool to improve mental well-being in the general population: randomized controlled trial. *J Med Internet Res* 2013; 15: e2.

62. Anderson J, Ruggeri K, Steemers K, Huppert F. Lively social space, well-being activity, and urban design findings from a low-cost community-led public space intervention. *Environ Behav* 2017; 49: 685–716.

63. Björk J, Albin M, Grahn P, et al. Recreational values of the natural environment in relation to neighbourhood satisfaction, physical activity, obesity and wellbeing. *J Epidemiol Commun Health* 2008; 62: e2.

64. Bowler DE, Buyung-Ali LM, Knight TM, Pullin AS. A systematic review of evidence for the added benefits to health of exposure to natural environments. *BMC Public Health* 2010; 10: 456.

65. Gidlow CJ, Jones MV, Hurst G, et al. Where to put your best foot forward: psycho-physiological responses to walking in natural and urban environments. *J Environ Psychol* 2016; 45: 22–29.

66. Hartig T, Mang M, Evans GW. Restorative effects of natural environment experiences. *Environ Behav* 1991; 23: 3–26.

67. Wahlbeck K. Public mental health: the time is ripe for translation of evidence into practice. *World Psychiatry* 2015; 14: 36–42.

68. Stewart-Brown S. Parenting interventions to promote wellbeing and prevent mental disorder. In: Huppert FA, Cooper CL (eds). *Interventions and Policies to Enhance Well-being*. Oxford: Wiley-Blackwell, 2014, pp. 53–91.

69. Stewart-Brown SL, Schrader-Mcmillan A. Parenting for mental health: what does the evidence say we need to do? Report of Workpackage 2 of the DataPrev project. *Health Promot Int* 2011; 26(suppl. 1): i10–28.

70. Olds DL. Prenatal and infancy home visiting by nurses: from randomized trials to community replication. *Prev Sci* 2002; 3: 153–172.

71. Cooper PJ, Tomlinson M, Swartz L, et al. Improving quality of mother–infant relationship and infant attachment in socioeconomically deprived community in South Africa: randomised controlled trial. *BMJ* 2009; 338: b974.

72. Adi Y, Killoran A, Janmohamed K, Stewart-Brown S. Systematic review of the effectiveness of interventions to promote mental wellbeing in children in primary education. Report 1: Universal approaches: non-violence related outcomes https://www.ncbi.nlm.nih.gov/pubmedhealth/PMH0024581/ (2007, accessed 21 February 2018).

73. Durlak JA, Weissberg RP, Dymnicki AB, Taylor RD, Schellinger KB. The impact of enhancing students' social and emotional learning: A meta-analysis of school-based universal interventions. *Child Dev* 2011; 82: 405–432.

74. Weare K, Nind M. Promoting mental health and wellbeing in schools. In: Huppert FA, Cooper CL (eds) *Interventions and Policies to Enhance Well-being*. Oxford: Wiley-Blackwell, 2014, pp. 93–140.

75. Weare K. Mindfulness in education. In: West MA (ed.) *The Psychology of Meditation: Research and Practice*. Oxford: Oxford University Press, 2016, pp. 259–281.

76. Czabala C, Charzynska K. A systematic review of mental health promotion in the workplace. In: Huppert F, Cooper CL (eds). *Interventions and Policies to Enhance Wellbeing*, vol. 6. Chichester: Wiley-Blackwell, 2014, pp. 221–276..

77. Czabała C, Charzyńska K, Mroziak B. Psychosocial interventions in workplace mental health promotion: an overview. *Health Promot Int* 2011; 26(Suppl 1.): i70–i84.

78. Good DJ, Lyddy CJ, Glomb TM, et al. Contemplating mindfulness at work: an integrative review. *J Manag* 2016; 42: 114–142.

79. Robertson IT, Cooper CL, Sarkar M, Curran T. Resilience training in the workplace from 2003 to 2014: a systematic review. *J Occup Organ Psychol* 2015; 88: 533–562.

80. Auty KM, Cope A, Liebling A. A systematic review and meta-analysis of yoga and mindfulness meditation in prison: effects on psychological well-being and behavioural functioning. *Int J Offender Ther Comp Criminol* 2017; 61: 689–710.

81. Dunn JM. Benefits of mindfulness meditation in a corrections setting. Available at: https://www.upaya.org/uploads/pdfs/DunnB enefitsofMeditationinCorrectionsSettingrev7110.pdf (accessed 21 February 2018).

82. Harms PD, Herian M, Krasikova DV, Vanhove AJ, Lester PB. The Comprehensive Soldier and Family Fitness Program Evaluation. Report #4: Evaluation of Resilience Training and Mental and Behavioral Health Outcomes. Available at: https://digitalcommons.unl.edu/cgi/viewcontent.cgi?referer=https://www.google.co.uk/&httpsredir=1&article=1009&context=pdharms (2013, accessed 21 February 2018).

83. Stanley EA, Schaldach JM, Kiyonaga A, Jha AP. Mindfulness-based mind fitness training: A case study of a high-stress predeployment military cohort. *Cogn Behav Pract* 2011; 18: 566–576.

84. Forsman AK, Nordmyr J, Wahlbeck K. Psychosocial interventions for the promotion of mental health and the prevention of depression among older adults. *Health Promot Int* 2011; 26(Suppl. 1): i85–i107.

85. Forsman AK, Stengard E, Wahlbeck K. Enhancing mental health and mental wellbeing in older people. In: Huppert FA, Cooper CL (eds). *Interventions and Policies to Enhance Well-being*. Oxford: Wiley-Blackwell, 2014, pp. 331–354.

86. McDaid D, Cooper CL. Introduction. In: McDaid D, Cooper CL (eds). *The Economics of Wellbeing*, Vol. 5. Oxford: Wiley Blackwell, 2014, pp. 1–9.

87. McDaid D, Park AL. Investing in mental health and well-being: findings from the DataPrev project. *Health Promot Int* 2011; 26(Suppl. 1): i108–i139.

88. Knapp M, McDaid D, Personage M. *Mental Health Promotion and Mental Illness Prevention: The Economic Case*. London: Department of Health, 2011.

89. Luyten J, Naci H, Knapp M. Economic evaluation of mental health interventions: an introduction to cost-utility analysis. *Evid Based Ment Health* 2016; 19: 49–53.

90. Oades L, Deane F, Crowe T, Lambert WG, Kavanagh D, Lloyd C. Collaborative recovery: an integrative model for working with individuals who experience chronic and recurring mental illness. Australa Psychiatry 2005; 13: 279–284.

91. Andresen R, Oades L, Caputi P. The experience of recovery from schizophrenia: towards an empirically validated stage model. *Aust N Z J Psychiatry* 2003; 37: 586–594.

92. Shepherd G, Boardman J, Slade M. *Making Recovery a Reality*. London: Sainsbury Centre for Mental Health, 2008.

93. Layard R. *A New Priority for Mental Health*. London: Centre for Economic Performance, London School of Economics, 2015.

94. Rose G. *Rose's Strategy of Preventive Medicine*. Oxford: Oxford University Press, 1992.

95. Colhoun H, Ben-Shlomo Y, Dong W, Bost L, Marmot M. Ecological analysis of collectivity of alcohol consumption in England: importance of average drinker. *BMJ* 1997; 314: 1164.

96. Puska P, Vartiainen E, Tuomilehto J, Salomaa V, Nissinen A. Changes in premature deaths in Finland: successful long-term prevention of cardiovascular diseases. *Bull World Health Organ* 1998; 76: 419.

97. Anderson J, Huppert F, Rose G. Normality, deviance and minor psychiatric morbidity in the community. *Psychol Med* 1993; 23: 475–485.

98. Goodman A, Goodman R. Population mean scores predict child mental disorder rates: validating SDQ prevalence estimators in Britain. *J Child Psychol Psychiatry* 2011; 52: 100–108.

99. World Health Organization. Health in all policies. Available at: http://www.healthpromotion2013.org/health-promotion/health-in-all-policies (2013, accessed 21 February 2018).

100. European Union. Joint Action on Mental Health and Well-being: Mental Health in all Policies. Available at: http://www.mentalhealthandwellbeing.eu/assets/docs/publications/MHiAP%20Final.pdf (2015, accessed 21 February 2018).

101. Finnish National Research and Development Centre for Welfare and Health (STAKES). *Framework for Promoting Mental Health in Europe*. Hamina: Ministry for Social Affairs and Health.

102. New York City Department of Health and Mental Hygiene. There is no health without mental health. Available at: http://www1.nyc.gov/site/doh/data/data-sets/community-health-survey.page (2003, accessed 21 February 2018).

103. Department of Health (DoH). *No Health Without Mental Health. A Cross-government Mental Health Outcomes Strategy for People of All Ages*. London: DoH.

104. Kottke TE, Stiefel M, Pronk NP. 'Well-being in all policies': promoting cross-sectoral collaboration to improve people's lives. *Prev Chron Dis* 2016; 13: E52.

105. Mental Health Europe. Activity Report 2016. Available at: https://mhe-sme.org/wp-content/uploads/2017/08/MHE-Activity-Report-2016.pdf (2016, accessed 21 February 2018).

106. United Nations. (Sustainable Development Goals. Available at: http://www.undp.org/content/undp/en/home/sustainable-development-goals.html (2016, accessed 21 February 2018).

107. McDaid D. Making use of evidence from wellbeing research in policy and practice. In: McDaid D, Cooper CL (eds). *The Economics of Wellbeing*. Oxford: Wiley-Blackwell, 2014, pp. 285–297.

108. Helliwell J. How can subjective wellbeing be improved? In: Huppert FA, Cooper CL (eds). *Interventions and Policies to Enhance Well-being*. Oxford: Wiley-Blackwell, 2014, pp. 611–631.

CHAPTER 16

Unemployment and mental health

Mel Bartley

A concern with the effect of unemployment on mental health in the community was the rationale for one of the first excursions of psychiatry and psychology into public health. In 1930 the great economic depression had hit the Austrian town of Marienthal [1, 2]. A wish to understand and mitigate effects on psychological well-being led a team, headed by Marie Jahoda and Paul Lazasfeld, to go and live in the town, mixing with the population to monitor the ways in which people were affected by the closure of the town's textile factory. This was a path-breaking study in many ways [3]. Perhaps most striking is the way in which the investigators 'embedded' themselves in the community. They used what would now be called 'mixed methods' of survey, interviews, and participant observation. They recruited community members into the study team. They even provided some services such as a sewing class and lessons on household budgeting. Their primary finding was that the unemployed, over time, sank into a state of apathy and helplessness. Income deprivation was the most obvious reason for this. But people no longer seemed to have the energy to partake even in activities that cost nothing. Fewer books were borrowed from the free library, people no longer read newspapers nor, in a time and place of strong political discussion, did they participate in political activity. At this time there were few validated scales of psychological well-being of the kind that we now have. Interestingly, however, this meant that the Marienthal study focused more on what was going on in the community and its families; their approach was more holistic than most present-day studies.

As willingly admitted by Jahoda, one shortcoming of the Marienthal study was its methodology. Nowadays, the small sample and the close involvement of the investigators would be regarded as a threat to the validity of the results. Arguments about method have continued to haunt research on unemployment and health from that day to this. This has been particularly true of research on unemployment and physical health or mortality [4, 5]. But claims that unemployment is harmful to mental health have also come in for a fair bit of criticism. In both cases, however, the upside of the sceptical reception of the work in some circles has been the close attention paid to methods, and the use of more advanced techniques, which has benefited the fields of social psychiatry and social epidemiology considerably.

Trends in the labour market

We are now 86 years and three more major recessions beyond the time of the Marienthal study. Fig. 16.1 shows how unemployment has increased in each of these: 1980–86, 1992–94 and 2008–14.

In that time, research has become far more sophisticated and data have improved beyond recognition. We have moved from community studies to ecological studies tracing correlations over time in national trends of, for example, unemployment and psychiatric hospital admission [6] to cross-sectional studies using representative samples [7–10] to longitudinal studies of individuals passing through changing economic circumstances [11]. But change in society is now threatening the ability of research to keep up. The recession of 2008 in the UK, for example, although the worst since 1930, did not result in such a major increase in unemployment, as can be seen from Fig. 16.1 [12, 13]. Fig. 16.2 shows how while the unemployment rate fell back to pre-crisis levels by late 2014, the proportion working part time who wanted full-time work remained well above its pre-crisis level.

In Fig. 16.2, the dotted lines represent the long-term average for unemployment, the proportion working part time because they could not find full-time work, and a combination of these two, termed the 'underemployment' rate. So, whereas the unemployment rate had, by 2015, fallen below its long-term average, the proportion wanting full-time work who could only find part-time work remained high above it. Taken together, this 'underemployment' rate was therefore still above its pre-crisis average 9 years later.

The whole of the labour market is now changing. Companies are able to employ people on short-term and zero-hours contracts. The trend for the number of stable jobs for people with sub-degree-level education to fall, which started in the 1980s [14], has continued. Since 2007, the total number of jobs increased, but during that period the increase was entirely accounted for by full- and part-time self-employed and part-time employees. This is not to say there is no longer plenty of 'unskilled' work to be done in industrial economies. On the contrary, the ageing population and the increasing levels of employment among women have created a high level of demand for care work, which is regarded as non-skilled and tends to be low paid. But in the opinion of some economic historians, the phenomenon of the post-war 'full employment' economy with stable jobs paying a living wage for all (men at least), regardless of education, was temporary. We shall not see its like again. And this means a major reassessment of the relationship between work, unemployment, and mental health [15].

The 'new service economy' contains fewer stable jobs, and these are jobs that require interpersonal skills rather than craft skills and physical resilience. Even among those with craft skills, such as carpentry and plumbing, many more workers are self-employed than

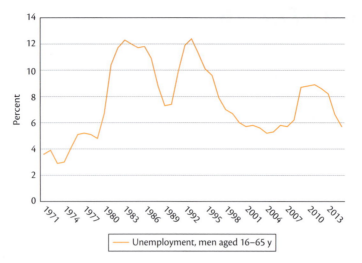

Fig. 16.1 Trends in unemployment.

Source: Data from Office for National Statistics, Labour Force Survey, Copyright (2016).

employed in large-scale workplaces. The disciplines of timekeeping and work organization fall far more onto the individual rather than a central management, as does the task of communicating with customers. Lower-educated men, and those with poorer social and communication skills, have been particularly hard hit by this aspect of labour market change. Just taking one example that is so simple and obvious as to be almost totally overlooked: regional accents. I am not sure how relevant this would be outside of the UK. The most famous story of stage and film that dramatizes the need for a certain type of speech in order to succeed socially, *My Fair Lady*, is set in England. But the world-leading sociologist Pierre Bourdieu wrote of the importance of accent for success in the top educational institutions of France [16], and there has been similar research on accent as a source of stigma in working-class Paris [17] China [18],

and cities all over the world adopting the 'new service economy' [19]. One of the major barriers to employment in newer sectors, such as tele-sales and call centres, which form an ever higher proportion of non-graduate employment, is the difficulty of understanding different accents that are associated with social status, region, ethnicity, or other potentially stigmatizing characteristics [20]. In this way, an aspect of the personal 'habitus' (to use Bourdieu's sociological term), which would have been totally irrelevant or even have given access to supportive social networks in the 1970s, has become a disadvantage in the hunt for jobs More generally, an economy dominated by service occupations will have fewer roles for those with lower levels of communication skills of all types. This also means that mild psychological problems, such as high-functioning autism or problems with anger management, take

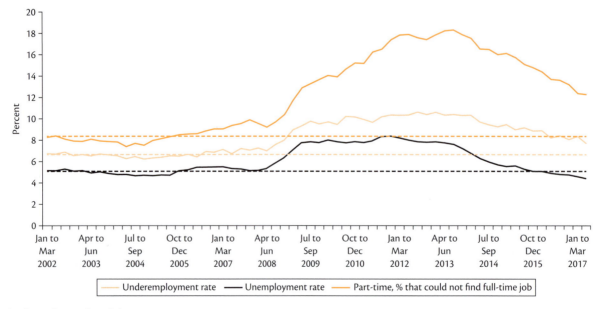

Fig. 16.2 'Underemployment' trends from 2002 to 2017.

Reproduced from Drake N, Monahan E, Suresh N, et al., Economic review: October 2017, Copyright (2017), Office for National Statistics, reproduced under the Open Government Licence v3.0, Available at https://www.ons.gov.uk/economy/nationalaccounts/uksectoraccounts/articles/economicreview/october2017

on a far higher importance. Instead of being a source of structure and stability in the life of people already dealing with psychosocial issues of various kinds, the workplace is closed to those who may most benefit from it [21].

Two facts have emerged from the research. The first thing we now know that was not understood in the recessions of the 1980s and 1990s is that not just any job protects mental health. It is as bad to have a 'poor job' as to have none [22]. Although stable jobs may have been a source of emotional stabilization, the kinds of jobs now available to many people without higher education (and, indeed, to many who have been to university) seem to constitute a hazard to psychological health. The second is that one cannot understand the relationship between unemployment and mental health outside the life course framework. The more sophisticated the research became, the clearer these facts became.

Social distribution of unemployment

Research on the health consequences of unemployment disappeared more or less completely after the end of the Second World War. Given the acceptance of the definition of 'full employment' to mean full employment for men only (there was no consideration of women), there seemed no need for further scientific inquiry. A leading British authority on unemployment was told in the 1970s that his work would be 'of historical interest only' (R.A. Sinfield, personal communication).

Important advances in understanding of labour markets took place during this period, however, that were to influence research on unemployment and health in the major recession that shortly followed. Most important among these advances was the realization that unemployment is not randomly distributed throughout the working population. Far from it. In 1975 the epidemiologist Jerry Morris, in his book *Uses of Epidemiology*, extended his earlier work with Richard Titmuss. In their 1944 paper, on the 'poverty complex', the tendency of low income, job insecurity, and poor housing to be clustered in certain geographical areas and to be experienced by the same groups of people [23]. They admitted the difficulties involved in separating out the effects of any single aspect of this complex from the others. Then, in the 1970s ,the work of Adrian Sinfield [24], Jon Stern [25], and others showed that a small proportion of all workers experienced the great majority of days spent without a job.

This 'labour market segmentation' was the reason for the failure of the British welfare system to cope with the financial consequences of unemployment, even outside of recessions. Social insurance was one of the founding principles of the Beveridge welfare state. At times of financial sufficiency, workers paid into an insurance fund (National Insurance) so that at times of inability to work they could receive as of right a replacement income. This was intended to be the same for everyone, across the social scale. Unlike taxation, it did not redistribute income between rich and poor, but rather within the life course of the same person it shifted some income from the good times to the bad times. In this way the reformers hoped to ensure that unemployment benefit was not stigmatized as 'charity'. National Assistance (as opposed to National Insurance) was the fallback safety net available when the insurance benefit ran out, and this was (and still is, although the names of all these benefits change rapidly) funded from general taxation (for a fuller explanation of these terms see [26]). Even at times of high employment,

those who were most at risk of job loss tended to be those with the least stable work histories and, accordingly, the least likely to have fully paid up social insurance. As a result, a large proportion of unemployed people required payments from the 'safety net' social assistance scheme. This more stigmatized source of income would be expected to have a more detrimental effect on psychological well-being. However, it took quite a long time until the implications of labour market segmentation for the relationship between unemployment and mental health to be fully understood.

The recession of the 1980s not only temporarily increased unemployment, but also introduced what was perhaps the first of the major changes to the British post-Second World War labour market. This was the massive increase in economic inactivity. Those who are economically inactive are not 'unemployed', i.e. those who are not actively looking for work at all. The 'rate' of unemployment is calculated by dividing the numbers of unemployed (judged in several different ways, but the easiest to understand is simply the count of those receiving unemployment benefit) by the number of workers plus jobseekers. So the economically inactive do not enter the calculation of the unemployment rate at all [26]. The work of Beatty and Fothergill has shown that increasingly during the 1980s and 1990s people unable to find work were encouraged by employment advisers to declare themselves as 'permanently sick' in order to reduce the headline unemployment figure [27, 28]. Fig. 16.3 compares the unemployment and inactivity rates of men in working age. The series only starts in 1975 as before that economic inactivity in men was very low.

Before the late 1970s the vast majority of economically inactive people were women looking after the home and family. They were financially dependent on the income of their husbands. Men who were regarded as inactive owing to ill health (the great majority) were (and still are) dependent on the 'social assistance' type of tax-funded benefit. The two most common diagnoses in these men are musculoskeletal conditions and psychiatric conditions (see Fig. 16.4). Since 2010 governments have radically changed policy towards making the receipt of sickness and disability benefit more strongly conditional on attempts to find work. Such policy changes

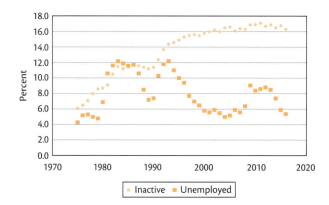

Fig. 16.3 Economic inactivity in working-age men.
Source: data from Office for National Statistics, Labour Force Survey: Unemployment rate: UK: Male: Aged 16-64: %: SA, Copyright (2014), Available at https://www.ons.gov.uk/employmentandlabourmarket/peoplenotinwork/unemployment/timeseries/ybtj/lms; Office for National Statistics, Labour Force Survey: Economic inactivity rate: UK: Male: Aged 16-64: %: SA, Copyright (2014). Available at https://www.ons.gov.uk/employmentandlabourmarket/peoplenotinwork/economicinactivity/timeseries/ybtm/lms

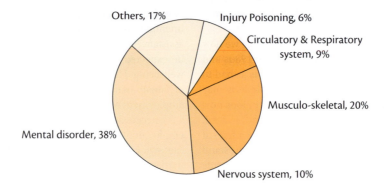

Fig. 16.4 Reasons for claiming incapacity benefits.
Source: Reproduced from Layard R, Mental Health: Britain's biggest social problem?, Copyright (2005), with permission from Richard Layard.

should throw into sharp relief the question of the relationship be-tween unemployment and mental health. At the present time, there appears to be little research on the effects of the new policies on mental health at the population level, or in the groups of un-employed or 'inactive'.

Early studies of the 1980s' recession

In some ways it is paradoxical that damage to mental health from unemployment is seen as a problem at all. During the increase in unemployment that started in the 1980s in the UK and in the 1990s in many other European nations, employers did not, in fact, see 'full employment' as a desirable state of affairs. It was believed that economies, to run efficiently, needed not to undershoot the 'non-accelerating inflation rate of unemployment', or NAIRU. The economists' famous 'Phillips curve' seems to show that as un-employment rises, the rate of increase in wages falls. The argu-ment went like this: when the demand for labour is too high (too little unemployment), workers will be able to demand higher and higher wages. Employers will then increase prices to compensate, which will be countered by workers with yet further demands for wage increases. The inflation of the late 1970s was widely blamed on this. It is believed that a certain level of unemployment, the NAIRU, was necessary in order to stop this happening. In add-ition, many believed that at times of low unemployment, workers had too much power in the workplace and threatened the 'right to manage' of their employers, leading to inefficiency and low productivity. Thus, the idea of the threat of unemployment as a discipline on workers is not exactly consistent with a concern for the mental health of the unemployed. Unemployment will need to be an unpleasant experience. But were there unintended costs of the experience of unemployment, costs that would have to be absorbed elsewhere in the criminal justice or health systems? These questions began to be raised in the late 1970s by an American aca-demic whose work had considerable influence in the UK and the rest of Europe [29].

As unemployment increased in the late 1970s and early 1980s, some commentators were pointing out that there was an even greater increase in long-term unemployment (a result of the way in which unemployment is distributed in a working population, as discussed earlier). Even if policymakers were willing to impose a

certain amount of short-term misery on workers in order to have low inflation and a 'flexible' labour market, the health consequences of so many people spending a year or more out of work seemed to need further thought.

These doubts were increased by the publication in the USA in 1976 of a paper 'Estimating the social costs of national eco-nomic policy: implications for mental and physical health, and criminal aggression' by Harvey Brenner [29], claiming that high unemployment had effects outside of the purely economic. In an earlier paper, Brenner had shown a tendency of psychiatric hospital admissions to vary alongside trends in unemployment. Brenner's work was promoted in the UK by practitioners of public health (at that time called 'Community Medicine') [30]. The (then) Department of Health and Social Security (DHSS) initiated in 1977 a cohort study of the unemployed [31], not to study mental health, but to estimate the influence of the amount of benefits on the duration and frequency of unemployment spells. Because of Brenner's work, at the third sweep of this study a few questions on health were included. These were intended to focus on any damage by long-term unemployment: the idea was to compare those who had remained unemployed during the whole of the study with those who found work again. The conclusion of the study was that there was nothing especially harmful about long-term unemployment.

However, in the interim a subsample of the DHSS cohort study had been interviewed by the psychiatrist Len Fagin and his colleague Martin Little. They used a more clinical approach, and were restricted, partly by the rules of the Government Survey Control Unit, to 22 families. Fagin concluded that [32]:

...the loss of a job can set in motion psychological changes which in some male breadwinners result in clinical depression, with feelings of...self-blame...loss of self-esteem...suicidal thoughts...and an increased use of tobacco or alcohol (p. 115).

And it was clear from their rich account of these families' experiences that the lack of money and time structure had a severe impact on both mood in the unemployed men and on their family relationships. In fact, this work presented a rather grim picture of the extent to which family harmony depended on having money to buy things and to justify the dominant role of the male breadwinner. In this respect, Fagin and Little's work stands in the tradition of community psychiatry and psychology of the Marienthal study, which emphasizes the relationship of economic change to social relationships rather than focusing purely on the 'mental health' of individuals. Like Lazarsfeld [1], Fagin theorized job loss as a form of bereavement, followed by successive stages of shock, pessimism when attempts to find a job fail, active distress, and, finally, fatalism in which (as in Marienthal) the unemployed become passive and withdrawn, living in a narrow world.

Brenner and Fagin's papers stimulated a great deal of publicity. Government concerns resulted in new studies being funded: unemployment was now no longer 'of historical interest only'. Some of these studies attempted to replicate Brenner's time series of national unemployment, suicide, and psychiatric hospital admissions. But these kinds of data are rare and often difficult to interpret. Other, more manageable data could be collected at a smaller scale by interviews and surveys of individuals, comparing the employed and unemployed. These studies attempted to square the circle created by the contradictory findings of the earliest work, using larger samples than were available to Fagin and Little [33].

A lot of the most influential research on unemployment and mental health during the recession of the1980s was done at the University of Sheffield's Social and Applied Psychology Unit under the leadership of Peter Warr. During the 1980s his group carried out a large number of studies to investigate the ways in which unemployment might exert its impact on mental health [10, 34, 35]. These suggested that life satisfaction was reduced amongst the unemployed, whereas negative affect, strain, anxiety, and mood disturbance serious enough to suggest clinical depression, as measured on the General Health Questionnaire (GHQ), were increased. Warr summed up the results in terms of a 'vitamin theory' of benefits of work for mental health, which include physical and mental activity, use of skills, decision latitude, interpersonal contact, social status, and 'traction'—a reason to go on through the day and from one day to the next. In different demographic groups (sex, age, social class, education) the various 'vitamins' were found to have different levels of importance [36].

Another prominent body of work during the 1980s was that of the Medical Research Council's Unit for Epidemiological Studies in Psychiatry led by Norman Kreitman. This began with a unique study of parasuicide by Platt and Kreitman made possible by the Unit's close link with the Edinburgh Regional Poisoning Treatment Centre, which received over 90% of all cases of self-poisoning and self-injury requiring hospital admission in the city [37]. As a result, admissions could be used as a reasonably valid numerator for studying time trends and area differences in suicide and parasuicide in the region. This study had three main findings. The first was that as unemployment increased in Edinburgh, so did the incidence of parasuicide. The authors admitted that this was an 'ecological correlation' only, unable even to say if it had been unemployed people committing parasuicide. However, their individual-level analysis showed a fairly steady relative risk of parasuicide in the unemployed of around 10 to 1 over the whole time period. And hidden within this figure was the fact that in those unemployed for over a year, the excess risk was twice as high as in those unemployed for less than a year [37].

Although the subsequent recessions of the 1990s and 2008–14 have not stimulated the same volume of research on unemployment and mental health, a steady trickle of new papers appeared. Paul and Moser carried out a comprehensive systematic review of all these [38]. It concluded that:

> … the health level of unemployed persons is [about] half a standard deviation below the health level of employed persons. This effect is a rather broad one, since it can be detected on a large range of mental health indicators (mixed symptoms of distress, depression, anxiety, psychosomatic symptoms, subjective well-being, and self-esteem). The effect … is equivalent to an increase in the rates of persons with psychological problems with potential clinical severity from 16% to 34% ([38] pp. 277–8).[1]

Paul and Moser also confirmed, to a large extent, the findings of the Sheffield studies on the different relationships of unemployment to mental health in different age, sex, and regional groups.

This comprehensive and careful review does admit, however, that meta-analytic methods cannot ensure against all of the problems that arise when claiming a causal effect.

The problem of causality: longitudinal studies

Studies of unemployment and health have always been accompanied by lively debates around causality. In 1944, Morris and Titmuss, in their discussion of physical health in areas hard hit by the recession of the 1930s in the UK, wrote of the 'poverty complex', the tendency of low income, job insecurity, and poor housing to be clustered in certain geographical areas and to be experienced by the same groups of people. They admitted the difficulties involved in separating out the effects of any single aspect of this complex from the others, but nevertheless felt that: 'We are not … absolved from the attempt to break up the poverty complex and assess the role of the different component elements' [23].

It would not be plausible to attribute the rise of two million in the number of claimants of unemployment benefit in the UK that took place between 1979–86, 1990–93, and 2008–12 to an increasing prevalence of either physical or psychological illness (see Fig. 16.1 and 16.2). In that sense, 'health' cannot possibly 'cause unemployment'. As Townsend [39] has expressed it: 'personal characteristics are clearly subsidiary in any explanation of expansions or contractions of the labour force, or of its subdivisions, into more or less secure groups' (p. 646). However, the existing evidence does indicate that it is the less physically and mentally fit who remain unemployed [5, 40]. It also appears that considerations of health may be significant in the loss of, and failure to regain, work, even when redundancy or unemployment is not explicitly stated by respondents to be a consequence of illness. One method that has been used to try and correct for this possibility is the so-called 'factory closure study'. This considered only people who became unemployed when their whole workplace was closed. The argument was that unemployment in this case is 'exogenous' to the individual. The results have been mixed, with some showing little association

---

[1] Reproduced from *Journal of Vocational Behavior*, 74(3), Paul KI, Moser K, Unemployment impairs mental health: Meta-analyses, pp. 264–82, Copyright (2009), with permission from Elsevier.

between job loss and health [41, 42], and others showing quite a strong one [43–45].

Selection as an explanation of any observed relationship between unemployment and psychological distress can take two forms. In 'direct selection', the presence of a psychological illness is the cause of either job loss or failure to regain employment or both. In 'indirect selection', as conventionally understood, there is a third characteristic, such as a personality trait, which confounds the relationship between unemployment and psychological ill health by 'causing' both states. In the 1980s there were no longitudinal studies suitable to test for these phenomena. Platt and Kreitman appealed to the large size (10 times in those unemployed for less than a year and 18 times in those unemployed for over a year) of the excess risk of parasuicide in unemployed persons [37]. In their own words: 'Such a relation is of course in line with the hypothesis that unemployment is a cause of parasuicide, though other interpretations are (just) possible'.But research had to await the maturing of, for example, the British Birth Cohorts and British Household Panel Study (BHPS) to go further into the question of causality.

The first longitudinal insights into the relationship between unemployment and mental health to emerge from a British Birth Cohort appeared in 1999. This study included men only, owing to the difficulty of defining unemployment in women of this cohort. But all had been followed-up from birth to the age of 33 years, which they attained in 1991, having passed through the high-unemployment period of the 1980s. It was possible to define their employment status in every month from the age of 16 to 32 years and so to distinguish between the total amount of time spent unemployed and the recency of any experience of unemployment. A degree of direct and indirect selection was confirmed, in that behavioural maladjustment in childhood, disadvantaged social class in childhood, and slow growth were all found to be related to the amount of unemployment a cohort member was to experience during the 1980s recession [46].

It was also possible to explore the possibility of a causal relationship of unemployment to psychological ill health by controlling for measures of psychological well-being both at the age of 11 years, i.e. before entry to the labour market, and at 23 years of age at the time of a rapid increase in unemployment. The definition of psychological ill health was narrow and specific: medical consultation for any of a range of psychological symptoms. Because respondents to the survey gave the dates of their medical consultation, the relatively new method of survival analysis with time-varying coordinates ('Cox regression') could be used. The relationship of psychological ill health to total months of unemployment was explained away in terms of the confounding variables (prior psychological problems, class at birth, and education), thus supporting the idea that there is a complex of adversities involved rather than a simple relationship to unemployment, even in the long term. However, unemployment in the year prior to onset remained significant in the face of full adjustment. In addition, both accumulated and recent unemployment were more strongly related to the onset of psychological distress symptoms when those showing signs of distress at the age of 23 years were excluded from the analysis [47]. This paper therefore hinted at a more complex relationship than merely selection or causation, of a kind that had not been possible to observe in the research done 10 years earlier.

Longitudinal data emerged from the BHPS, which began in 1991 and re-surveyed a representative sample of 5000 households every year through the recession of the 1990s. Using data from 1991 and 1992, Weich and Lewis found that the main damage of unemployment to mental health (measured each year by the GHQ) was in making it less likely that people who already had high (bad) scores in 1991 would recover by the following year. It was, in this study, poverty rather than employment status that had the clearest impact on mental health. This supported their contention that poverty is the most important mediator of the mental health effects of unemployment [48]. However, with only 12 months of data they had no opportunity to test for selection.

A more rigorous test was undertaken by Winkelmann and Winkelmann [49], who applied an econometric approach to data from the German SocioEconomic Panel study and aimed to use repeated measurements to address the problem of selection in relating unemployment to 'life satisfaction'. They had no measure of mental health per se, but their methodological approach showed the way that future studies would develop. They describe the selection problem as follows:

> Assume … that inherently dissatisfied persons are more likely to be laid off; in a cross-section study, this effect would be falsely interpreted as an effect of unemployment on satisfaction. Second, the presence of unobserved common determinants of satisfaction and unemployment may lead to a spurious correlation, or omitted variable bias. Health is one such factor that is commonly difficult to measure correctly. With repeated observations for the same individuals, it becomes possible to control for unobserved, but time-invariant, individual specific effects that are correlated with unemployment [49].[2]

They approached their research question by first pooling all the data (the 'person-years') so that each individual contributed 6 years of data, during which time they might be employed or unemployed and satisfied or dissatisfied. To test strictly for a causal relationship between unemployment and dissatisfaction, they took only data from those people who had changed their employment status at some point between 1984 and 1990. In effect, these people were being used as their own controls; it could be assumed that their unobserved personal characteristics that might bias the relationship between employment status and life satisfaction were held constant (this is known as a 'fixed effect'). With this method, they showed that life satisfaction dropped sharply after job loss, even after allowing for the fact that those who went on to become unemployed did have slightly lower life satisfaction to begin with. In further analysis they showed that decreasing income was likely to be an important reason for the change.

Thomas et al. [50] were able to use more sweeps of the BHPS, from 1991 to 1998. They found that transitions out of employment into any non-employed state were accompanied by deterioration in mental health, measured with the GHQ, in both men and women. They were also able to take possible selection into account by adding a score on the GHQ and a variable indicating ill health prior to the transition. Even after these adjustments, those becoming unemployed were twice as likely to be 'GHQ cases' as those remaining in employment.

---

[2] Reproduced from Economica, 65(257), Winkelmann L, Winkelmann R, Why Are the Unemployed So Unhappy? Evidence from Panel Data, pp. 1–15, Copyright (1998), with permission from John Wiley and Sons.

By the late 2000s, however, questions still remained over the causal status of the relationship between unemployment and any kind of health. Although the link to psychological health had always been less controversial than that to physical morbidity and mortality, researchers were not unanimous.

In 2012, Steele et al. [51] commented that:

> Studies investigating the relationship between individuals' health and changes in employment status over the life course may provide stronger evidence for a causal link, especially where regular repeated measurements are available for a long follow-up period.

As with other forms of social and economic disadvantage, the maturing of longitudinal studies such as the British Birth Cohorts and the BHPS threw new light on how unemployment might fit into the life course. Flint et al. [11] used 16 years of annual data to examine the associations of both unemployment and insecure work with mental health measured according to the GHQ. Like Winkelman and Winkelman [49], Flint et al. used a multi-level model that compared the mental health of each individual who experienced any unemployment each time they were unemployed with when they were employed over the 17 years of observation. On average, the individual's GHQ score was elevated by 2.2 units at a time of unemployment compared with a time of secure employment. Taking into account possible confounding variables such as education, age, income, type of housing (social vs private), physical health, and drug or alcohol problems varied little to change the size of this relationship.

Steele et al. [51] used slightly more years of observation from the BHPS and a more sophisticated method to examine the role of selection even more carefully. Similarly to Flint et al. [11], they found that, on average, a person scored an extra 2.52 GHQ points (about half a standard deviation) when unemployed rather than employed. In order to rule out 'direct health selection', they adjusted the relationship of employment status to GHQ for each person's GHQ score in the previous year. This made little difference, reducing the increase in score from 2.52 to 2.45 (a 3% reduction). But the innovation of this study was the method used to take indirect selection into account. This technique, a multi-level multi-process model, allowed for the possibility that the same people might have a propensity to become both anxious or depressed and unemployed over their lives. The method does not allow anything to be inferred about why such a propensity might exist. But taking it into account did reduce the estimated worsening of the GHQ score relative to employment from 2.45 to 2.23 (over 11% reduction). In the words of Steele et al. [51], 'men whose unmeasured characteristics placed them at above-average levels of anxiety and depression tended also to have above-average chances of being out of employment' (p. 708).

Fig. 16.5 shows one simple example of the way in which life course influences may produce this kind of 'indirect selection' effect. In male participants in the 1958 British Birth Cohort, those with moderate levels of behavioural maladjustment as long ago as age 7 years have double the risk of unemployment and three times the risk of permanent sickness by the age of 50 years when compared with those with normal adjustment. The risk of permanent sickness is increased by an even greater amount. A similar graph could be shown for childhood poverty. We do not yet have studies of the extent to which childhood material (poverty, parental unemployment) and psychological (parental conflict, divorce) might, indeed,

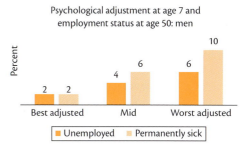

Psychological adjustment at age 7 and employment status at age 50: men

Fig. 16.5 Life course influences on risk of unemployment or economic inactivity at 50 years of age.
Source: Data from Centre for Longitudinal Studies, National Child Development Study (1958 Birth Cohort), Copyright (1958), Economic and Social Research Council.

amount to a 'life-course poverty complex', to paraphrase the words of Morris and Titmuss.

Implications of labour market change

Flint and colleagues also addressed the issue of the changes in the labour market. They take to task much of the earlier research for failing to address job insecurity, and the possibility that a lot of apparent economic inactivity may, in fact, be hidden unemployment. In the words of Flint et al. [11]: 'A limitation of much of the research in this field has been an overemphasis on unemployment and employment, a false dichotomy which fails to capture the various ways in which individuals engage with the formal labour market'. Accordingly, they calculate the worsening of GHQ score of 1.1 points (out of a range of 1–12) in those moving from secure to insecure employment robust to adjustment for many confounding variables. Once again it is possible that a similar unobserved individual propensity could account for some of the association between moving into insecure work and mental health that was found by Steele et al. [51] for unemployment. But this work remains to be done.

However, as it is not possible for an epidemic of mental illness to account for an increase in unemployment at the national or regional level, nor for increases in job insecurity or deterioration in job quality. We have seen in Fig. 16.2 that although the numbers of employed people in the British economy continued to rise after only a short decline after the crisis of 2008, this rise was almost entirely accounted for by 'non-typical' jobs: temporary, part-time, and self-employment. Hellgren and Sverke [52] conducted a sophisticated longitudinal analysis to investigate the extent to which mental health may itself be a cause of movement from more to less secure employment, finding a far greater effect the other way around: deterioration in job conditions leading to worse mental health. Virtanen et al. [53] investigated the relationship between temporary employment in a systematic review. They found that temporary workers were not only less likely to have sickness absence (for reasons that may seem rather obvious), but also tended to have worse mental health than comparable permanent workers. There is a tendency for workers who are displaced during economic downturns to find themselves in less secure and less-well-paid jobs, even when they do return to work [54]. De Witte et al. [55] reviewed more recent longitudinal evidence, finding once again a strong case for a harmful effect of job insecurity.

Benach et al. [56] have highlighted the emergence of 'precarious work' as a major concern for public health research going forward. In their excellent narrative review, they link the newer flexible types of work contract with the issues surrounding management control of workers that were outlined at the beginning of this chapter. In a review paper, Macassa [57] found few studies, but those that existed appear to extend the evidence of the risks of temporary employment into other types of precarity.

As with the threat of unemployment, but perhaps even more effectively, temporary work and the 'zero-hours contracts' put workers in a weak position to bargain for better conditions or higher wages. The rapid increase in these types of work arrangements following the downturn of 2008, illustrated for the UK in Fig. 16.2, must have played a role in the failure of real wages to increase over this period despite the appearance of an increase in 'employment'.

Conclusion

As has so often been the case, the task of public health when assessing the extent of any health effects of unemployment and employment precarity addresses the consequences of social change for the individual and community. Historically, there have been many economic shifts that prove to be double-edged swords. Industrial urbanization massively increased the productivity of societies and had the potential to raise living standards. Many of the task of mitigating epidemics, pollution, and abrupt declines in the availability of jobs over the business cycles fell to public health. In nineteenth-century London, for example, it was well known that the urban population did not reproduce itself owing to very high infant mortality from infectious disease and the rapid wearing-out of adult workers by factory and home conditions. Strangely enough there is a current parallel to this 150-year-old example at the present time. Increasingly we hear of labour shortages, of the need to recruit workers from other nations. Not just because of shortages of specific technical skills, but also it seems even of normal social skills, in other words, mental health. As shown in Fig. 16.3, the rate of economic inactivity (people not even well enough to search for work) almost tripled between the mid-1970s and 2010. And Fig. 16.4 shows that almost 40% of inactive people of working age suffer from psychological ill health. It seems that stable employment was, indeed, providing 'vitamins', as envisaged by Warr [36]. But the health effects of such vitamins are not simply lost during a spell of unemployment and then regained easily. For some people they are needed to develop psychological capacity throughout life. Public mental health, enriched by new information on mental health and employment conditions over the life course, can develop its ability to understand these processes. In doing so it will not only contribute to the relief of suffering, but also to solving urgent economic problems.

References

1. Lazarsfeld P. An unemployed village. *J Person* 1932; **33**: 147–151.
2. Jahoda M, Lazarsfeld P, Ziesel H. *The Sociography of an Unemployed Community: Marienthal*. London: Tavistock, 1972.
3. Fryer D. Editorial: introduction to Marienthal and beyond. *J Occup Organ Psychol* 1992; 65: 257–268.
4. Lundin A, Lundberg I, Hallsten L, Ottosson J, Hemmingsson T. Unemployment and mortality—a longitudinal prospective study on selection and causation in 49321 Swedish middle-aged men. *J Epidemiol Community Health* 2010; 64: 22–28.
5. Böckerman P, Ilmakunnas P. Unemployment and self-assessed health: evidence from panel data. *Health Econ* 2009; 18: 161–179.
6. Brenner H. *Estimating the Social Costs of National Economic Policy: Implications for Mental and Physical Health, and Criminal Aggression*. Washington, DC: US Government Printing Office, 1976.
7. Daniel WW, Stilgoe E. *Where Are They Now? A Follow-up Study of the Unemployed*. London: Political and Economic Planning, 1978.
8. Warr P. A study of psychological well-being. *Br J Psychol* 1978; 69: 111–121.
9. Moylan S, Davies R. The disadvantages of the unemployed. *Employment Gazette* 1980; 88: 830–832.
10. Banks MH, Jackson PR. Unemployment and risk of minor psychiatric disorder in young people: cross-sectional and longitudinal evidence. *Psychol Med* 1982; 12: 789–798.
11. Flint E, Bartley M, Shelton N, Sacker A. Do labour market status transitions predict changes in psychological well-being? *J Epidemiol Community Health* 2013; 67: 796–802.
12. Gregg P, Wadsworth J. Employment in the 2008–2009 recession. *Labour Gazette* 2010; 4: 37–43.
13. Bell DNF, Blanchflower DG. UK unemployment in the Great Recession. *Natl Inst Econ Rev* 2010; 214: R3–R25.
14. Nickell S, Bell B. The collapse in demand for the unskilled and unemployment across the OECD. *Oxf Rev Econ Policy* 1995; 11: 40–62.
15. Bambra C. *Work, Worklessness, and the Political Economy of Health*. Oxford: Oxford University Press, 2011.
16. Bourdieu P. *Distinction*. London: Routledge, 1984.
17. Stewart CM. On the socio-indexicality of a Parisian French intonation contour. *J Fr Lang Stud* 2012; 22: 251.
18. Wong FKD, Chang YL, He XS. Correlates of psychological wellbeing of children of migrant workers in Shanghai, China. *Soc Psychiatry Psychiatr Epidemiol* 2009; 44: 815–824.
19. Hall P. The end of the city? *City* 2003; 7: 141–152.
20. Dovidio JF, Gluszek A, John MS, Ditlmann, R, Lagunes P. Understanding bias toward Latinos: discrimination, dimensions of difference,and experience of exclusion. *J Soc Issues* 2010; 66: 59–78.
21. Bartley M, Ferrie J, Montgomery S. Health and labour market disadvantage: unemployment, non-employment, and job insecurity. In: Marmot M, Wilkinson R. (eds). *Social Determinants of Health*, 2nd ed. Oxford: Oxford University Press, 2005, pp. 78–96.
22. Butterworth P, Leach LS, McManus S, Stansfeld SA. Common mental disorders, unemployment and psychosocial job quality: is a poor job better than no job at all? *Psychol Med* 2013; **43**: 1763–1772.
23. Morris JN, Titmuss R. Health and social change: recent history of rheumatic heart disease. *Med Off* 1944; 69–71, 77–79, 85–87.
24. Sinfield RA. *What Unemployment Means*. Oxford: Martin Robertson, 1981.
25. Stern J. Who bears the burden of unemployment? In: Beckerman W (ed.). *Slow Growth in Britain*. Oxford: Clarendon, 1979, pp. 134–145.
26. Bartley M, Ferrie J. Glossary: unemployment, job insecurity, and health. *J Epidemiol Community Health* 2001; 55: 776–781.
27. Beatty C, Fothergill S, Macmillan R. A theory of employment, unemployment and sickness. *Reg Stud* 2000; 34: 617–630.
28. Beatty C, Fothergill S. The diversion from 'unemployment' to 'sickness' across British regions and districts. *Reg Stud* 2005; 39: 837–854.
29. Brenner MH, Mooney A. Unemployment and health in the context of economic-change. *Soc Sci Med* 1983; 17: 1125–1138.
30. Draper P, Dennis J, Griffiths J, Partridge J, Popa J. Micro-processors, macro-economic policy, and public health. *Lancet* 1979; 313: 373–375.
31. Department of Health and Social Security (DHSS). *Cohort Study of Long Term Unemployed Men, 1978*. London: DHSS, 1982.
32. Fagin L, Little M. *The Forsaken Families*. London: Penguin, 1985.
33. Banks M, Ullah P. *Youth Unemployment: Social and Psychological Perspectives: Department of Employment Research Paper No. 61*. London: HMSO, 1987.
34. Warr PB. Job loss, unemployment and psychological well-being. In: Ilen V, van de Vliert F (eds). *Role Transitions*. New York: Plenum Press, 1984, pp. 55–67.

35. Warr PB. Twelve questions about unemployment and health. In: Roberts B, Finnegan R, Gallie D (eds). *New Approaches to Economic Life*. Manchester: Manchester University Press, 1985, pp. 92–114.

36. Warr P. A conceptual framework for the study of work and mental health. *Work Stress* 1994; 8: 84–97.

37. Platt S, Kreitman N. Trends in parasuicide and unemployment among men in Edinburgh, 1968–82. *BMJ* 1984; 289: 1029–1032.

38. Paul KI, Moser K. Unemployment impairs mental health: Meta-analyses. *J Vocat Behav* 2009; 74: 264–282.

39. Townsend P. *Poverty in the UK*. Harmondsworth: Penguin, 1979.

40. Butterworth P, Leach LS, Pirkis J, Kelaher M. Poor mental health influences risk and duration of unemployment: a prospective study. *Soc Psychiatry Psychiatr Epidemiol* 2012; 47: 1013–1021.

41. Martikainen P, Maki N, Janti M. The effects of unemployment on mortality following workplace downsizing and workplace closure: a register-based follow-up study of Finnish men and women during economic boom and recession. *Am J Epidemiol* 2007; 165: 1070–1075.

42. Strully KW. Job loss and health in the US labour market. *Demography* 2009; 46: 221–246.

43. Beale N, Nethercott S. Job-loss and family morbidity: a study of a factory closure. *J R Coll Gen Pract* 1985; 35: 510–514.

44. Kuhn A, Lalive R, Zweimüller J. The public health costs of job loss. *J Health Econ* 2009; 28: 1099–1115.

45. Salm M. Does job loss cause ill health? *Health Econ* 2009; 18: 1075–1089.

46. Montgomery SM, Bartley MJ, Cook DG, Wadsworth ME. Health and social precursors of unemployment in young men in Great Britain. *J Epidemiol Community Health* 1996; 50: 415–422.

47. Montgomery SM, Cook DG, Bartley MJ, Wadsworth ME. Unemployment pre-dates symptoms of depression and anxiety resulting in medical consultation in young men. *Int J Epidemiol* 1999; 28: 95–100.

48. Weich S, Lewis G. Poverty, unemployment, and common mental disorders: population based cohort study. *BMJ* 1998; 317: 115–119.

49. Winkelmann L, Winkelmann R. Why are the unemployed so unhappy? Evidence from panel data. *Economica* 1998; 65: 1–15.

50. Thomas C, Benzeval M, Stansfeld SA. Employment transitions and mental health: an analysis from the British household panel survey. *J Epidemiol Community Health* 2005; 59: 243–249.

51. Steele F, French R, Bartley M. Adjusting for selection bias in longitudinal analyses using simultaneous equations modeling: the relationship between employment transitions and mental health. *Epidemiology* 2013; 24): 703–711.

52. Hellgren J, Sverke M. Does job insecurity lead to impaired well-being or vice versa? Estimation of cross-lagged effects using latent variable modelling. *J Organ Behav* 2003; 24: 215–236.

53. Virtanen M, Kivimäki M, Joensuu M, Virtanen P, Elovainio M, Vahtera J. Temporary employment and health: a review. *Int J Epidemiol* 2005; 34: 610–622.

54. Brand JE. The far-reaching impactof job loss and unemployment. *Annu Rev Sociol* 2015; 41: 359–375.

55. De Witte H, Pienaar J, De Cuyper N. Review of 30 years of longitudinal studies on the association between job insecurity and health and well-being: is there causal evidence? *Aust Psychol* 2016; 51: 18–31.

56. Benach J, Vives A, Amable M, Vanroelen C, Tarafa G, Muntaner C. Precarious employment: understanding an emerging social determinant of health. *Annu Rev Public Health* 2014; 35: 229–253.

57. Macassa G. Precarious employment and health outcomes in Sweden: a systematic review. *J Publ Health Epidemiol* 2016; 8: 169–174.

CHAPTER 17

Housing and mental health

Tom K. J. Craig and Jed Boardman

Introduction

The quality of our living environment has been a key concern for public health since its inception. Attempts to tackle the onset and spread of infectious diseases in the nineteenth century identified poor housing, poor sanitation, and overcrowding as significant causes of ill health. The rapid urbanization that took place in the 1800s resulted in overcrowding in the cities and towns and a profusion of poorly built and inadequate housing. These conditions were described by public health campaigners such as Edwin Chadwick and Charles Booth, and by authors such as Charles Dickens and Elizabeth Gaskell. Friedrich Engels, in his account of *the Condition of the Working Classes in England in 1844*, noted [1]:

> … the disgusting state of the working class districts…. which is chiefly attributable to their unpaved streets, irregular architecture, numerous courts and alleys, and total lack of the most ordinary means of cleanliness, all taken together is explanation enough of the excessive mortality in those unhappy abodes of filthy misery ([1] p. 39).

Today, such conditions may have all but disappeared in the UK, but remain in the favelas, shanty towns, displaced peoples camps, and other dwellings in the towns and cities of many low-income countries. Even in the UK, much poor-quality housing persisted into the twentieth century, with slum clearances being a commonly used strategy of urban regeneration and health improvement.

Maintaining the quality of housing remains an important part of public health. In this chapter we will examine the relationship between housing and mental health and the importance of good-quality housing for the population and housing support for people with long-term mental health problems.

What is housing?

The average adult in developed countries spends as much as 80–90% of their day in buildings of one kind or another, most of this in the home. Looked at in this way it is not difficult to see why housing has direct implications for our health and well-being. The house (or dwelling) provides a physical structure in which to shelter from the elements and other external forces. As such, it needs to have a sound structure and be free from hazards. It gives us a place to sleep, to store and prepare food, and to look after our personal hygiene. Moreover, it provides the social, cultural, and economic structures that we call a 'home'. A refuge, a place to for privacy, security, quiet, relaxation, and for social exchange with family, friends, and others. It is also a place to bring up our children. But our house and home exist in wider local environment, the neighbourhood, and the community. This gives us access to local services and facilities, green spaces, and to our social networks and a sense of social cohesion. The quality of this local environment has an impact on the quality of our house, home, and health, and, as the Engels quote implies, to the possible hazards of poor sanitation, environmental pollution and decay, crime, and violence.

Housing, physical health, and hazards

There are strong links between the quality of housing and physical disorders, in particular infectious diseases, chronic diseases and injuries [2, 3]. Children and older adults may be particularly at risk [4]. Housing may present many hazards that have direct and indirect effects on our health, such as poor sanitation (e.g. lack of safe drinking water, ineffective waste disposal); cold, damp, and mouldy conditions; exposure to toxic substances (e.g. smoke, lead, radon); and fire and injury hazards. A list of these hazards that form part of the Housing Health and Safety Rating System (HHSRS) used in England are shown in Box 17.1.

Jaakkola et al. [5], in an important report for the World Health Organization, noted that damp and mouldy conditions across European households ranged from 5% to 20% in colder countries (e.g. Scandinavia) to up to 29% of homes in the UK. Based on a meta-analysis of data from 45 European countries, they estimated 50 asthma-related disability-adjusted life years per 100,000 children related to exposure to damp dwellings and up to 83 deaths per year to mould exposure. Similarly, as many as 70% excess winter deaths from cardiovascular disease and 33% from respiratory disease in the elderly can be attributed to excessive exposure to low indoor temperatures that, in turn, result from inefficient or inadequate indoor heating and insulation [5]. To these can be added the excess morbidity and mortality associated with poor indoor air quality, be that from tobacco smoke, inadequate ventilation of wood burning, carbon monoxide poisoning from old and faulty gas appliances, or even increased cancer prevalence associated with exposure to radon gas from geological sources.

Housing and mental health

There are fewer studies examining the association between housing and mental health than for physical health. These are mainly cross-sectional surveys and have all taken a very broad approach to the assessment of mental disorder, focusing mainly on common conditions of anxiety and depression often assessed by screening measures rather than more comprehensive diagnostic assessment. The factors these studies show to be related to mental health are summarized in Box 17.2.

Box 17.1 Hazards to health

Physiological hazards

Accident hazards
Damp or mould
Excessive cold
Excessive heat
Asbestos and MMF (manufactured mineral fibres) biocides
Carbon monoxide and fuel combustion products
Lead
Radiation (e.g. radon)
Uncombusted fuel gas
Volatile organic compounds

Accident hazards

Falls associated with bathrooms
Falls on the level
Falls associated with stairs and steps
Falls between levels
Poor electrical wiring
Fire risks
Hot surfaces and materials
Collision and entrapment risks
Explosion risk
Poor position and operability of amenities
Risk of structural collapse and falling elements

Psychological hazards

Overcrowding
Entry by intruders
Poor lighting
Excess noise

Infection hazards

Poor domestic hygiene and/or pests
Poor facilities for food safety
Poor sanitation and drainage
Poor water supply for domestic purposes

Source: Data from the Office of the Deputy Prime Minister, Housing Health and Safety Rating System: Operating Guidance. Housing Act 2004: Guidance about inspections and assessment of hazards given under Section 9, Copyright (2006), Crown copyright.

Box 17.2 Housing factors associated with poor mental health

Poor-quality housing

- State of housing (e.g. presence of damp, cold, mould) associated with poor mental health [6–11].
- Structural deficiencies in housing associated with use of tranquilizers and psychological symptoms [12].
- Insufficient daylight—associated with increased symptoms of depression [7].
- Move to better-quality housing (or improvements to existing housing) linked with reduction of psychological symptoms [13, 14].

Overcrowding and neighbourhood noise

- In adults—associated with depression, increase in psychological symptoms, accidental and violent death (including suicide) [6–8, 15].
- In children—increases in irritability, tension, aggression, lower levels of interaction with other children, poor educational attainment and adjustment [8].

Multiple occupancy and temporary accommodation

- In adults—increased depressive symptoms, domestic violence, alcoholism, family stress, relationship breakdown [8].
- In children—delayed development, poor educational attainment, irritability, temper tantrums, disturbed [8].
- People living in temporary bed and breakfast accommodation are 2.5 times more likely to experience poor mental health than people housed in permanent accommodation in the same area [16].

Tenure and control over housing

- Lack of control over the internal environment and choice of housing—associated with poor mental health [8].

Housing type

- High-rise housing—associated with poorer mental health in adults, high rates of physician visits for mental health problems, behavioural problems in children, and restricted play opportunities [6, 7, 17–19].
- People living in houses rather than flats tend to have better mental health [20].
- Multi-dwelling housing is associated with poor mental health [17, 19].
- Deck-access flats—associated with increased levels of diagnosed depression [21].

Quality of neighbourhood

Poor mental health associated with physical aspects of the environment (e.g. presence of derelict buildings, lack of green space),

In summary, the key factors affecting mental health include building quality, multi-family occupancy, and the impact of living in high-rise buildings. In Europe, for example, according to one recent review, 7% of the population are exposed to severe housing deprivation, defined as overcrowding and one or more of problems with leaking roofs, no indoor toilet, or bath/shower. Around a half of all accommodation is multi-family and an average of 15% of housing is in buildings of four or more stories [24]. As might be expected, there is a wide variation in these figures between countries and also the significance afforded to each by local politicians and housing experts. But, regardless of this variation, there is near universal recognition that poor quality and the disparity in quality between the poorest and richest in society is a significant contributor

dissatisfaction with access to green spaces, and community facilities; fear of crime and feeling unsafe to go out in the day; and limited opportunities for social participation [6, 7, 21–23].

- ◆ Higher levels of mental well-being associated with:
  - ◆ living in an area perceived to have attractive buildings;
  - ◆ living in an attractive, quiet, peaceful environment;
  - ◆ perceiving the area to have a good internal reputation;
  - ◆ being satisfied with the house and landlord;
  - ◆ feeling that both home and neighbourhood contribute to a sense of well-being (Bond et al. [20]).

to unhappiness and to mental and physical ill health affecting, especially, vulnerable population groups such as migrants and people with disabilities, including severe mental illness.

Lack of housing: homelessness

Of course, if inadequate housing is bad for health there is no surprise that homelessness is also associated with a high risk of both physical and mental illness. Getting hold of accurate numbers of homeless people is difficult because some counts include both people sleeping 'rough' on the streets, as well as those in direct-access hostels and in temporary or other unstable housing. Nevertheless, the numbers seem to be on the rise in England, rough sleeping up by as much as 55% between 2010 and 2014 and a parallel rise in annual statutory 'homelessness acceptances' (an official administrative record of local government), much of which can be attributed to rising numbers of homeless people (and families) from the private-rent sector [25]. Studies in Western countries have repeatedly found higher rates of physical and mental illness among homeless populations versus the general population, although there is considerable variation between different surveys. So, for example, one meta-analysis found substance use disorders (alcohol and drug dependency) to be the most commonly recorded, but rates of psychosis were also markedly elevated from 3% to 42% versus just 1% in the general population, and rates of depression were as high as 49% versus around 7% in the general population [26]. Many of these problems co-occur with physical illness, including both infectious causes (including HIV) and non-communicable conditions, of which cardiovascular disease is the most prevalent. Not surprisingly, mortality is substantially higher than in the general population, with the excess risk being most notable among younger people [27]. Unfortunately, many studies also demonstrate inefficient and poorly coordinated services that fail to integrate medical and social care.

Interpreting the link between housing and health

That there is an association between the quality of housing and health is well established, but the relationship is a complex one, not least because the concept of 'housing' includes aspects of the physical structure of the building, the infrastructure of the neighbourhood, and the economic and social structure of the wider community; all of these, in turn, interact with each other and the unique social, economic, and cultural components of the individual household. In addition, it may be difficult to separate confounding factors such as income, deprivation, and social position, which are also strongly linked to mental health and housing. Poor housing design and decrepit fabric cause or contribute to household accidents, including fatalities that in some European countries exceed deaths due to road traffic accidents. Indeed, it is usual for risk factors for poor health to converge, so that houses in poorer neighbourhoods are likely to be inadequately insulated and heated, encouraging the growth of mould that, in turn, is associated with respiratory disease. Lack of access to recreational outdoor space contributes to rising levels of sedentary behaviour and onwards to obesity and to related health problems.

The quality of the built environment is also firmly associated with mental well-being. Living in decrepit housing is fraught with hassles and stress. Poor-quality housing tends to go along with environmental problems of damp and mould indoors, and multiple occupancy typically in high-rise buildings (which have additional problems of restricted access to green space and noisy neighbours) and with neighbourhood problems, including rapacious landlords, vandalism, graffiti, and crime all contributing to the chronic stress that can be a cause of depression and other common mental disorders (CMD). Finally, where one lives is also a powerful indicator of social standing and so is linked to feelings of inadequacy and stigmatization.

Given the entanglement of housing, the wider environment, and poverty, it is very difficult to say with certainty what aspects of housing are most associated with ill health. Research has therefore tended to prioritize some characteristics over others. For example, an interesting early study of the general practice records of 558 families of British servicemen living in either high- or low-rise accommodation found that general practitioner consultation rates were far higher for the high-rise dwellers than for those living on the ground floor. The most common complaint was respiratory, but the rate of consultations for mental and psychoneurotic consultations was 36.1 per 1000 residents in high-rise accommodation versus 17.4 per 100,000 in low-rise accommodation. The author comments that these probably underestimate the true rate and that many of the other conditions may well have had co-morbid mental ill health that went unrecorded. Although these conditions had multiple causes, many of the women in the high rise attributed problems to boredom, inadequate outdoor space, and lack of communication with their neighbours [19]. Problems of greater subjective social isolation and loneliness have been reported in other comparisons of high- versus low-rise accommodation [28, 29].

The association between the wider aspects of the built environment and CMD was explored as part of an evaluation of an urban regeneration programme. Prior to the start of the regeneration programme, two electoral wards were identified (one scheduled for regeneration and the other selected on the basis of similar housing and sociodemographic characteristics but not scheduled for regeneration). A built environment survey was carried out in order to identify discrete housing areas in which each was homogenous in terms of the character of the housing. A total of 1300 households and within these up to two residents were selected for inclusion using random probability sampling. Each respondent provided sociodemographic details and completed a measure of depression. There was a strong and significant association between depression score and living in a property with predominantly deck access, abundant graffiti, few private gardens, and shared recreational space, these associations persisting even after taking account of socio-economic status, floor or residence, and reported structural problems such as damp or infestations in the home [21].

Another way to explore the association is to examine what happens after renovations or relocations to better facilities. There are a handful of relevant studies. In one study, for example, 56 residents of public housing who had requested a housing transfer on medical grounds of mental ill health, were randomly allocated to priority re-housing or a waiting list. Of the 28 allocated to the priority group, 23 had moved by the end of the study, as had six of the non-priority group. Mental state was assessed at baseline, after moving and at the 12-month follow-up. Participants who moved reported significant reductions in symptom scores for anxiety and depression compared with those who did not [13]. Similarly encouraging reports in early studies suggest some benefit from improving housing quality, but all suffer from defects in randomization or mental state assessment or both, making it very difficult to generalize [11, 14, 30, 31]. A more recent example of the presumed benefits of renovation is reported by Angela Curl et al. [32]. The study used a quasi-experimental design to evaluate the impact on physical and mental health of four types of housing improvement—central heating, secure front doors, fabric works (i.e. repairs to roofs, balconies, stonework, etc.), and fitting new kitchens and bathrooms, all offered as part of a renovation programme in Glasgow, UK. They studied the impact of these renovations on the lives of 1933 residents though data collected in three cross-sectional surveys carried out approximately 2 years apart in which health outcomes (physical and mental) were assessed. Outcomes between those who had properties renovated between baseline and the second survey or between the second and third survey were compared with those who remained on the waiting list for housing improvements. The analysis explored associations with any housing improvement and then separately for each of the four types of renovation. There was an overall improvement in mental health associated with the renovation programme over time. Improvements to the fabric of the housing were associated with better mental and physical health; improvements to security and to kitchens and bathrooms were associated with better mental health, but, interestingly, the positive benefits of greater front door security was only seen in the first year and not thereafter, whereas the benefits of new kitchens and bathrooms were sustained, possibly reflecting the greater personal investment in the design of these, where, unlike the other changes, residents had a choice over colours and layout.

Unfortunately, the positive findings from these studies are balanced by almost as many where no significant association is seen or even where the association is reversed. Large-scale urban regeneration projects where improved housing is a major goal, are also accompanied by many other interventions that are likely to benefit health—better leisure facilities, initiatives to tackle unemployment, and others to improve uptake of welfare benefits. The upshot of this confounding is that the majority of studies fail to find statistically significant benefit [31, 33–35]. A recent Cochrane review of 33 housing improvement initiatives found that only two showed clear gains in overall health following interventions to improve heating/warmth, and four reported some non-significant improvements in general physical health following rehousing or refurbishment [36]. This Cochrane review, in keeping with other earlier reviews (e.g. [31]) notes that many of the studies

suffered from serious methodological shortcomings, including small sample sizes, lack of experimental design, short follow-up, and a lack of good information on baseline health status. The interventions themselves are multifaceted but only studied in overview so it is not possible to disentangle what aspects matter most. As the authors of the Glasgow study say [32], there is a question about how big an effect on health can be realistically disentangled from all the other impacts, including random events thrown up by the highly unstable, impoverished communities that these renovation programmes target or, indeed, from wider positives, such as improved employment opportunities. In the Glasgow study, for example, gaining employment was more likely after renovation and associated with both physical and mental health gains that were at least as great as any association with that resulting from the housing improvement.

The costs of unsatisfactory housing

In England, the HHSRS hazard ratings form part of the definition of a 'Decent Home', which is one that meets all of the following criteria:

- is free from category 1 hazards (the most serious hazard score), as assessed by the HHSRS;
- is in a reasonable state of repair;
- has reasonably modern facilities and services;
- provides a reasonable degree of thermal comfort.

This definition has been, since 2006, in the annual English Housing Survey, a national survey of people's housing circumstances and the condition and energy efficiency of housing in England. In 2014, 20% of dwellings (4.6 million homes) failed to meet the Decent Homes standard. This is a reduction of 3.1 million homes since 2006, when 35% of homes failed to meet the standard. Privately rented accommodation is more likely to fail to meet the standard than socially rented (29% vs 14%). Nineteen per cent of owner-occupied homes failed to meet the Decent Homes standard in 2014.

Using data from the 2011 English Housing Survey, Nicol et al. [37] estimated the treatment costs to the National Health Service (NHS) of people living in accommodation with HHSRS category 1 hazards (the poorest 15% of housing stock in England) to be £1.4 billion per annum (extrapolated to £2.0 billion for homes with other significant HRSRS hazards). These estimates are similar to those of the cost burden to the NHS of smoking and alcohol [38]. Furthermore, the analysis estimated that if £10 billion was now spent to improve all of the 3.5 million 'poor' homes in England, this would save the NHS £1.4 billion in first year treatment costs. It is suggested that such an investment would pay for itself in just over 7 years and then continue to accrue benefits into the future.

Housing and severe mental illness

Studies of severe mental disorders such as schizophrenia and other psychoses have also demonstrated associations with impoverished environments. In what is now a classic study, Robert Faris and Warren Dunham [39] found that the highest rates for treated schizophrenia occurred in the slum areas of the city and declined progressively as their survey progressed towards the more affluent areas. This observation has been replicated many times and in many countries around the world. One plausible explanation for the association is that prodromal impairments affecting functional ability, including the ability to hold down employment, leads the individual to drift towards low-income accommodation. The alternative to this social-drift hypothesis is that the stresses and strains of living in these environments play a causal role. As we have said earlier, there is no doubt that being poor and having to live in a downtrodden neighbourhood with high levels of vandalism, graffiti, and unruly behaviour and crime is stressful. And there is also abundant evidence for an association between exposure to stressful circumstances and psychosis [40]. In addition to evidence linking environment, including housing quality, to psychosis is the evidence of a greater risk of having these conditions with increasing population density and the observation that risk is increased the longer one spends in these environments [41, 42]. To this can be added the intriguing observation that, in these urban areas, risk seems greatest for minority populations. So, for example, the increased incidence of psychosis among black people and ethnic minorities in cities across Europe that some research suggests may be highest for those minorities residing in neighbourhoods where they are in the greatest minority [43–45].

Regardless of whether the association is best explained by drift or causal models, it is also clear that, once established, schizophrenia and other severe mental disorders have a profound impact on a person's everyday ability to maintain the environment, finances, and myriad tasks that go along with housing tenure. The result is that most people with these conditions need support of one kind or another from family and the state. Until the middle of the last century, the preferred state provision for severe and persistent mental disorder was the hospital asylum. These large institutions became unpopular partly because of humanitarian concerns about the institutional environment and the quality of care they provided. Perhaps the most significant influence was economic as it became evident that welfare reforms, including the introduction of health insurance, enabled disabled people to live more cheaply outside institutions [46]. The result was a dramatic reduction in the number of long-stay beds in parts of Europe and North America. In England, for example, the number of beds reduced from over 150,000 in 1955 to fewer than 3000 by 2010. The residents of these asylums were discharged to a variety of supported community settings, including 'hospital hostels' with 24-hour staffing, and group homes with varying levels of residential and visiting support. Research showed that this deinstitutionalization in England was not associated with any significant worsening in mental health or social behaviour, no increase in homelessness, and was preferred by the patients, who were seen to make greater use of community facilities [47, 48]. Other countries around the world have also moved towards replacing the hospital asylum with community-based care. Trieste in Italy probably comes closest to what was provided in England. Here, some buildings of the old asylum were converted into group homes for people with the highest needs, but the majority of patients were cared for either in their own homes or with visiting support to range of apartments across the city. In North America, the process was more abrupt and welfare support and sheltered housing less well developed, resulting in homelessness reaching epidemic proportions in some cities and the criminal justice system rapidly becoming the alternative asylum [49]. These problems became so difficult to resolve that even today there are professional voices calling for the return of the hospital asylum [50]. While few in Europe would go so far as to call for the re-introduction of the asylum, there are, nevertheless, concerns

that deinstitutionalization has not proceeded as far or as smoothly as envisaged. Surveys carried out across countries in Europe noted that while the numbers of hospital beds declined, there was a parallel increase of beds in forensic units, residential nursing and group homes, and in prison, amounting, it was said, to evidence of trans-institutionalization as the people who would otherwise be cared for in a hospital are now found in prisons, private hospitals, and residential care homes [51].

Supported accommodation for severe mental illness: research evidence

The model of housing provision and support for people with severe mental illness has changed considerably from the early hospital closure programmes that offered discharged patients lifelong tenancies in staffed group homes. Today the emphasis is on helping people to live as independently as possible, ultimately to the point where they can manage their accommodation without assistance. Ideally, support is tailored to the individual's needs and provided collaboratively with the recipient. The result is an elaborate matrix of housing types and of support. At one extreme are people in mainstream housing who require minimal support, perhaps managing some aspect of their tenancy, and at the other extreme are those residing in 24-hour staffed accommodation with meals, medication, and domestic cleaning provided every day. Between these two extremes is accommodation provided with varying levels of support from mental health workers who work with the explicit aim of helping the resident acquire the skills to be able to move through gradual steps towards greater independence. But although this move-on-to-independence model of rehabilitation has near-universal acceptance, there is, in fact, very little by way of quality randomized controlled evaluations of the different schemes, which is surprising given their cost [52], although perhaps understandable given the conviction of many clinicians, managers, and, indeed, patients that the graduated approach is less risky. As a result, research in the post-deinstitutionalization era is largely confined to simple surveys and qualitative evaluations. Early surveys across different kinds of housing in England found few differences in the characteristics of residents in the different schemes and considerable variation in the support offered [53]. A recent nationwide survey in England attempted to investigate differences in the quality of care, costs, and experiences of residents across the spectrum of supported care. A total of 619 residents were recruited from 22 residential care, 35 supported housing, and 30 floating outreach services, and face-to-face interviews were carried out with service managers, staff, and residents. As expected, residents in residential care and supported housing had more severe mental health problems than those in floating outreach and this was reflected in the gradient of costs with residential care the most and floating outreach the least expensive. Satisfaction with care was similar across services. Interestingly, quality of life was higher in settings with more support possibly because of the challenges faced by people struggling with the greater demands of independent living [54].

Recent reviews show that most residents report a moderate degree of satisfaction with their supported housing, although most would prefer independent living with visiting support rather than having staff on site [55, 56]. Quite a lot is known from qualitative studies of the characteristics of this supported housing that are valued by residents. These findings are summarized in Box 17.3.

Box 17.3 Qualitative studies: characteristics of successful supported housing

Choice and flexibility

♦ Active participation in decisions about housing [55].

♦ Provided with choice, autonomy, and control over living environment [55, 57].

♦ Having goals and choices in everyday life [58].

♦ Increased competence and better self-confidence [59].

♦ Increased independence, improved sense of well-being [60].

♦ Coherence, stability, security, and flexibility [61].

Quality of relationships between residents and staff

♦ Dignity, trust, respect, and choice [55].

♦ Person-centred, individualized approach [55].

♦ Supportive atmosphere and good relationship with staff [62].

♦ Community spirit, having someone to attach to [63].

♦ Good-quality supportive relations [64].

♦ Good case worker, having someone who understands [57, 65].

♦ Continued access to a support worker and long-term case management [55].

Provision of a range of supports

♦ Support with independent living, preventing and managing crises, pursuing work and education, maintaining social connections and physical and mental health [55].

♦ Structured programming (if too rigid, this proved unsatisfactory for residents) [62].

♦ Engaging in an activity [66].

Tenancy and environment

♦ Maintaining tenure over time [64].

♦ Place of rest [63].

♦ Security and privacy [67].

♦ Choice of residential area and accommodation [67].

♦ Neighbourhood fit: matching needs and goals of residents to the environment best suited to them, e.g. close to community resources and social connections, stable neighbourhoods with lower crime rates [55].

♦ More diverse a neighbourhood may be more accepting [55].

♦ Integrated with mainstream housing—thus 'anonymous' and neighbours unaware of their mental health problems [55].

Or

♦ Clustered housing—benefit from the support of peers [55, 68].

In North America, early re-housing models were similar to those described earlier, with a progression from emergency shelters towards own tenancy by way of intermediate supported housing and rehabilitation focused on daily living skills. But in the mid-1990s, some experts argued that this stepwise model could be replaced by more or less immediate access to permanent, independent housing and only then introducing whatever support the individual needed in order to maintain the tenancy. Early trials of this approach in New York showed that as many as 80% of homeless people placed in these 'Housing First' schemes were stable over a 2-year period versus just 30% of those following the more traditional rehabilitation approach, with 78% of the housing first clients continuously housed over a 4-year period [69, 70].

A larger programme in five Canadian cities has recently been reported [71, 72]. It involved 2148 people with mental health problems who were randomly placed in one of three groups: two Housing First groups who received either Assertive Community Treatment (ACT) or Intensive Case Management (ICM), and a control group who had access to existing housing and support services in their local area. The three groups of people were followed-up over a 2-year period. As with the US studies, housing stability was high, with 62% of the Housing First groups remaining housed over the 2-year period versus 31% of the control group. Housing stability was almost identical in those offered ACT or ICM. There was also some evidence that Housing First services were cost-effective for people with the highest level of need. One possible criticism of large-scale randomized controlled trials is the very uneven quality of treatment as usual comparison services. A later analysis focused on a high-need subsample in Toronto where there was already a robust housing pathway and related support service, including well-established assertive community treatment teams, community mental health centres with a focus on homelessness and access to 7000 supported housing placements. The high-risk sample randomized to Housing First or treatment as usual comprised people with diagnosis of psychosis or bipolar disorder, who met one of four criteria: hospitalization at least twice in one year in the previous 5 years; or had problems with substance dependency or a recent arrest or incarceration. The Housing First group spent more time stably housed than those in the treatment as usual group, and taking account of baseline scores, showed significantly superior community functioning and quality of life with fewer arrests. There were no differences between groups in substance use or health service contacts [73].

By and large, the most striking benefit of these Housing First programmes lies in housing stability—a key outcome for formerly homeless people, especially those with lengthy or multiple episodes of homelessness. Other effects or mental health status, engagement with care and wider improvements in social function are modest, although some studies have shown benefit [74]. No large-scale evaluations of Housing First have been reported outside North America, but the smaller studies in Europe have also found high rates of housing retention [75, 76].

Conclusion

The quality of the built environment and that of local neighbourhoods has been universally recognized to play a crucial role in the health and well-being of the population. Adequate housing, defined in terms of legal security of tenure; availability of services, materials, facilities, and infrastructure; affordability; habitability; accessibility; location; and cultural adequacy has been recognized by the United Nations as a basic human right [77]. Its importance is not confined to a causal agent in people's ill health, but also as an important means of supporting and maintaining health in people with disabilities and long-term conditions, including those with mental health problems. Adequate housing not only provides the means to maintain health, but also a setting where support can be provided to people with mental health problems and is essential to the provision of community-based care [78]. The provision of good-quality housing also has the capacity to reduce health, social service, and societal costs [79, 80]. To improve and maintain population health it is essential that there is greater integration of government institutions that control housing policy with those who coordinate health and social policies. In addition, there is a burning need for providers of housing services to be better integrated with providers and commissioners of health and social services [81]. The provision of quality housing is by its very nature a health intervention.

References

1. Engels F. *The Condition of the Working Class in England*. New York, London: Allen & Unwin, 1952.
2. Krieger J, Higgins DL. Housing and health: time again for public health action. *Am J Public Health* 2002; 92: 758–768.
3. Braubach M, Jacobs DE, Ormandy D. *Environmental Burden of Disease Associated With Inadequate Housing*. Geneva: World Health Organization, 2011.
4. Barnes M, Cullinane C, Scott S, Silvester H. *People Living in Bad Housing—Numbers and Health Impacts*. London: NatCen Social Research, 2013.
5. Jaakkola M, Haverinen-Saughnessy U, Douwes J, Nevalainen A. Indoor dampness and mould problems in homes and asthma onset in children. In: Braubach M, Jacobs DE, Ormandy D (eds). *Environmental Burden of Disease Associated With Inadequate Housing*. Geneva: World Health Organization, 2011, pp. 5–31.
6. Guite HF, Clark C, Ackrill G. The impact of the physical and urban environment on mental well-being. *Public Health* 2006; 120: 1117–1126.
7. Evans GW. The built environment and mental health. *Bull N Y Acad Med* 2003; 80: 536–555.
8. Page A. Poor housing and mental health in the United Kingdom: changing the focus for intervention. *Int J Environ Health Res* 2002; 1: 31–40.
9. Hopton J, Hunt S. The health effects of improvements to housing: a longitudinal study. *Hous Stud* 1996; 11: 271–286.
10. Hunt SM, McKenna SP. The impact of housing quality on mental and physical health. *Hous Rev* 1992; 41: 47–49.
11. Gifford R, LaCombe C. Children's socioemotional health and housing quality. *J Hous Built Environ* 2006; 21: 177–189.
12. Duvall D, Booth A. The housing environment and women's health. *J Health Soc Behav* 1978; 19: 410–417.
13. Elton PJ, Packer JM. A prospective randomized trial of the value of rehousing on ground of mental illness. *J Chronic Dis* 1986; 39: 221–227.
14. Halpern D *Mental Health and the Built Environment*. London: Taylor & Francis, 1995.
15. Gabe J, Williams P. Women, housing and mental health. Int J Health Serv 1987; 17: 667–79.
16. National Housing Federation. *Housing and Mental Health*. London: National Housing Federation, 1999.
17. Evans GW, Wells NM, Moch A. Housing and mental health: a review of the evidence and a methodological and conceptual critique. *J Soc Issues* 2003; 59: 475–500.
18. Saegert S. Environment and children's mental health: residential density and low income children. In: Baum A, Singer JE (eds). *Handbook of Psychology and Health*, vol. II. Hillsdale NJ: Erlbaum, 1982, pp. 247–271.
19. Fanning DM. Families in flats. *BMJ* 1967; 4: 382–386.
20. Bond L, Kearns A, Mason P, Tannahill C, Egan E, Whitely E. Exploring the relationships between housing, neighbourhoods and mental wellbeing for residents of deprived areas. *BMC Public Health* 2012; 12: 48.
21. Weich S, Blanchard M, Prince M, Burton E, Erens B, Sproston K. Mental health and the built environment: cross-sectional survey of individual and contextual risk factors for depression. *Br J Psychiatry* 2002; 180: 428–433.
22. Ellaway A, Macintyre S, Kearns A. Perceptions of place and health in socially contrasting neighbourhoods. *Urban Stud* 2001, 38: 2299–2316.
23. Araya R, Dunstan F, Playle R, Thomas H, Palmer S, Lewis G. Perceptions of social capital and the built environment and mental health. *Soc Sci Med* 2006; 62: 3072–3083.
24. Evans GW. Housing and mental health. In: Braubach M, Jacobs DE, Ormandy D. (eds). *Environmental Burden of Disease Associated With Inadequate Housing*. Geneva: World Health Organization, 2011, pp. 173–177.
25. Fitzpatrick S, Pawson H, Bramley G, Wilcox S, Watts B. The homeless monitor: England 2016. Available at: https://www.crisis.org.uk/media/236829/the_homelessness_monitor_england_2016_es.pdf (2016, accessed 12 November 2016).
26. Fazel S, Khosla V, Doll H, Geddes J. The prevalence of mental disorders among the homeless in western countries: systematic review and meta-regression analysis. *PLOS Med* 2008; 5: e225.
27. Fazel S, Geddes J, Kushel M. The health of homeless people in high income countries: descriptive epidemiology, health consequences and clinical and policy recommendations. *Lancet* 2014; 384: 1529–1540.
28. McCarthy D, Saegert S. Residential density, social overload, and social withdrawal. *Hum Ecol* 1976; 6: 253–272.
29. Wilcox BL Holahan CJ. Social ecology of the megadorm in university student housing. *J Educ Psychol* 1976; 68: 453–458.
30. Evans GW, Wells NM, Chan HY, Saltzman H. Housing quality and mental health. *J Consult Clin Psychol* 2000; 68: 526–530.
31. Thomson H, Petticrew M, Morrison D. Health effects of housing improvement: systematic review of intervention studies. *BMJ* 2001; 323: 187–190.
32. Curl A, Keans A, Mason P, Egan M, Tannahill C, Ellaway A. Housing improvements: evidence from the Go Well study. *J Epidemiol Community Health* 2015; 69: 12–19.
33. Barton A, Basham M, Foy C, Buckingham K, Somerville M. The Watcombe Housing Study: the short term effect of improving housing conditions on the health of residents. *J Epidemiol Community Health* 2007; 61: 771–777.
34. Kearns A, Whitley E, Mason P, Petticrew M, Hoy C. Material and meaningful homes: mental health impacts and psychosocial benefits of rehousing to new dwellings. *Int J Public Health* 2011; 56: 597–607.
35. Thomas R, Evans S, Huxley P, Gately C, Rogers A. Housing improvement and self-reported mental distress among council estate residents. *Soc Sci Med* 2005; 60: 2773–2783.
36. Thomson H, Thomas S, Sellstrom E, Petticrew M. Housing improvements for health and associated socio-economic outcomes. *Cochrane Database Syst Rev* 2013; 28: CD008657.
37. Nicol S, Roys M, Garrett H. *The Cost of Poor Housing to the NHS. Briefing Paper*. Watford: Building Research Establishment (BRE) Trust, 2015.
38. Scarborough P, Bhatnagar P, Wickramasinghe KK, Allender S, Foster C, Rayner M. The economic burden of ill health due to diet, physical inactivity, smoking, alcohol and obesity in the UK: an update to 2006/07 NHS costs. *J Public Health* 2011; 33: 527–535.

39. Faris REL, Dunham HW *Mental Disorders in Urban Areas: An Ecological Study of Schizophrenia and Other Psychoses.* Chicago, IL: University of Chicago Press, 1939.

40. Beards S, Gayer-Anderson C, Borges S, Dewey ME, Fisher HL, Morgan C. Life events and psychosis: a review and meta-analysis. *Schizophr Bull* 2013; 39: 740–747.

41. Krabbendam L, van Os J. Schizophrenia and urbanicity: a major environmental influence—conditional on genetic risk. *Schizophr Bull* 2005; 31: 795–799.

42. Pedersen CD, Mortensen PB. Evidence of a dose-response relationship between urbanicity during upbringing and schizophrenia risk. *Arch Gen Psych* 2001; 58: 1039–1046.

43. Cantor-Graae E, Selten JP. Schizophrenia and migration: meta-analysis and review. *Am J Psychiatry* 2005; 162: 12–24.

44. Boydell J, van Os J, McKenzie K, et al. Incidence of schizophrenia in ethnic minorities in London: ecological study into interactions with environment. *BMJ* 2001; 323: 1336–1338.

45. Kirkbride JB, Morgan C, Fearon P, Dazzan P, Murray RM, Jones PB. -level effects on psychoses: re-examining the role of context. *Psychol Med* 2007; 37: 1413–1425.

46. Scull A. *Decarceration: Community Treatment and the Deviant. A Radical View,* 2nd ed. Cambridge: Polity Press, 1984.

47. Leff J. *Care in the Community. Illusion or Reality?* Chichester: Wiley, 1997.

48. Leff J, Trieman N. Long stay patients discharged from psychiatric hospitals. Social and clinical outcomes after five years in the community. TAPS Project 46. *Br J Psychiatry* 2000; 176: 217–223.

49. Warner R. *Recovery From Schizophrenia: Psychiatry and the Political Economy.* London: Routledge & Kegan Paul, 1985.

50. Sitsi DA, Segal AG, Emanuel EJ. Improving long-term psychiatric care: bring back the asylum. *JAMA* 2015; 313: 243–244.

51. Priebe S, Badesconyi A, Fioritti A, et al. Reinstitutionalisation in mental health care: comparison of data on service provision from six European countries. *BMJ* 2005; 330: 123–126.

52. Chilvers R, Macdonald G, Hayes A. Supported housing for people with severe mental disorders. *Cochrane Database Syst Rev* 2006; 4: CD000453.

53. Priebe S, Saidi M, Want A, Mangalore R, Knapp M. Housing services for people with mental disorders in England: patient characteristics, care provision and costs. *Soc Psychiatry Psychiatr Epidemiol* 2009; 44: 805–814.

54. Killaspy H, Priebe S, Bremner S, et al. Quality of life, autonomy satisfaction, and costs associated with mental health supported accommodation services in England: a national survey. *Lancet Psychiatry* 2016; 3: 1129–1137.

55. Kirsh B, Gewurtz R, Bakewell R, Singer B, Badsha M, Giles N. *Critical Characteristics of Supported Housing: Findings From the Literature, Residents and Service Providers.* Toronto: Wellesley Institute, 2009.

56. Gonzalez MT, Andvig E. Experiences of tenants with serious mental illness regarding housing support and contextual issues: a meta-synthesis. *Issues Ment Health Nurs* 2015; 36: 971–988.

57. Andvig E, Hummelvoll JK. From struggling to survive to a life based on values and choices: first-person experiences of participating in a Norwegian Housing First project. *Nord J Soc Res* 2015; 6: 167–183.

58. Petersen KL, Hounsgaard BT, Nielsen CV. User involvement in mental health rehabilitation: a struggle for self-determination and recognition. *Scand J Occup Ther* 2012; 19: 59–67.

59. Pejlert A, Asplund K, Norberg A. Towards recovery: living in a home-like setting after the move from a hospital ward. *J Clin Nurse* 1999; 8: 663–673.

60. Nelson G, Clarke J, Febbraro A, Hatzipantelis M. A narrative approach to the evaluation of supportive housing: stories of homeless people who have experienced serious mental illness. *Psychiatr Rehabil J* 2005; 29: 98–104.

61. Carpenter-Song E, Hipolito MM, Whitley R. 'Right here is an oasis': How 'recovery communities' contribute to recovery for people with serious mental illnesses. *Psychiatr Rehabil J* 2012; 35: 435–440.

62. Goering P, Sylph J, Foster R, Boyles S, Babiak T. Supportive housing: a consumer evaluation study. *Int J Soc Psychiatry* 1992; 38: 107–119.

63. Bengtsson-Tops A, Ericsson U, Ehliasson K. Living in supportive housing for people with serious mental illness: a paradoxical everyday life. *Int J Ment Health Nurs* 2014; 23: 409–418.

64. Browne G, Courtney M. Housing, social support and people with schizophrenia: a grounded theory study. *Issues Ment Health Nurs* 2005; 26: 311–326.

65. Browne G, Hemsley M, StJohn W. Consumer perspectives on recovery: a focus on housing following discharge from hospital. *Int J Ment Health Nurs* 2008; 17: 402–409.

66. Lindstrom M, Sjostrom S, Lindberg M. Stories of rediscovering agency: home-based occupational therapy for people with severe psychiatric disability. *Qual Health Res* 2013; 23: 728–740.

67. Brolin R, Rask M, Syren S, Baigi A, Brunt DA. Satisfaction with housing and housing support for people with psychiatric disabilities. *Issues Ment Health Nurs* 2015; 36: 21–28.

68. Bowpitt G, Jepson M. Stability versus progress: finding an effective model of supported housing for formerly homeless people with mental health needs. Available at: http://irep.ntu.ac.uk/id/eprint/23617 (2007, accessed 12 November 2016).

69. Tsemberis S. *Housing First: The Pathways Model to End Homelessness for People With Mental Illness and Addiction.* Center City, MN: Hazelden, 2010.

70. Stefancic A, Tsemberis S. Housing First for long-term shelter dwellers with psychiatric disabilities in a suburban county: a four-year outcome study of housing access and retention. *J Prim Prev* 2007; 28: 265–279.

71. Goering P, Veldhuizen S, Watson A, et al. *National At Home/ Chez Soi Final Report.* Calgary, AB: Mental Health Commission of Canada, 2014.

72. Aubry T, Nelson G, Tsemberis S. Housing First for people with severe mental illness who are homeless: a review of the research and findings from the At Home/Chez soi demonstration project. *Can J Psychiatry* 2015; 60: 467–474.

73. O'Campo P, Stergiopoulos V, Nir P, et al. How did a housing first intervention improve health and social outcomes among homeless adults with mental health illness in Toronto? Two year outcomes from a randomised trial. *BMJ Open* 2016: 6: e010581.

74. Pleace N, Quilgars D. *Improving Health and Social Integration Through Housing First. A Review.* York: Centre for Housing Policy, 2013.

75. Busch-Geertsema, V. Housing First Europe—results of a European social experimentation project. *European Journal of Homelessness* 2014; 8: 13–18. Available at: http://www.feantsaresearch.org/download/article-01_8-13977658399374625612.pdf (accessed 5 March 2018).

76. Bretherton J, Pleace N. *Housing First in England. An Evaluation of Nine Services.* York: Centre for Housing Policy, 2015.

77. United Nations. The Right to Adequate Housing. Available at: https://www.un.org/ruleoflaw/files/FactSheet21en.pdf (1991, accessed 22 February 2018).

78. Boardman J. *More Than shelter. Supported Accommodation and Mental Health.* London: Centre for Mental Health, 2016.

79. Buck D, Simpson M, Ross S. *The Economics of Housing and Health. The Role of Housing Associations.* London: King's Fund, 2016.

80. The National Housing Federation. *Developing a Business Case for Health—What Does Good Look Like?* London: National Housing Federation, 2016.

81. National Housing Federation. *Common Cause Consulting Mental Health & Housing. Housing on the Pathway to Recovery.* London: HACT, 2016.

CHAPTER 18

Social class and mental health
The impact of international recession and austerity

M. Harvey Brenner

Introduction

The Great Depression of the 1930s gave rise to the first US studies of the ecological relation between lower social class and proportionately higher levels of mental disorder [1]. These findings were replicated by epidemiological methods at the individual level following the Second World War and thereafter throughout the twentieth and early twenty-first centuries. Interpretation of the dynamics of these findings involving exposure to economic instability, unemployment, and downward social mobility were advanced with time series data especially showing that the Great Depression had precipitated the highest levels of hospitalized mental disorder and suicide in the twentieth century [2]. Did the Great Recession of 2007–09 and its aftermath of government austerity, job insecurity, and poverty replay the Great Depression experience in elevating the rates of mental disorder and suicide? Were these relations intensified by the widening social class differences due to technological change and globalization? In general, do losses of employment and income increase the population rate of mental disorder and are lower social classes most vulnerable to these economic crises?

The current international literature on psychological disorder and suicide do show significantly elevated rates in conjunction with unemployment increases during the Great Recession and with its timing over 2007–09. US studies additionally indicate that mental disorder and suicide increased in relation to the housing and mortgage crises. Yet, almost entirely lacking were studies of the health effects of the Great Recession using gross domestic product (GDP) as a major economic indicator of the recession. This is the case despite the fact that GDP represents the principal indicator used by economists to specify the dating and magnitude of recessions. However, it can be seen with recent models that GDP declines have been a major source of increase in suicide, as well as total mortality during the Great Recession and the accompanying government austerity. The somewhat more popular indicator of economic recession is the unemployment rate, which has been traditionally linked to nationally elevated suicide rates and, during and since the Great Recession, to elevated psychological morbidity.

These findings, in conjunction with the current literature, are the background of a multistage sequence of circular relations that is developed as a paradigm in this chapter. This circularity involves relations among social class, stress-related mental disorder, national economic changes, and overall population health.

This chapter discusses the impact of the Great Recession and austerity measures on global mental health in the context of social class differences. Lower social class status puts populations at higher risk for experiencing mental stressors and provides fewer resources to cope with them. Lower social class also often involves subcultural coping styles, and normative patterns, that include multiple behavioral risks to health (e.g. smoking, high-calorie food consumption, alcohol abuse, low risk aversiveness, social withdrawal, violence, opioid and illegal drug use).

Social classes themselves, however, represent and serve to categorize the industrial and occupational structures of societies as they go through the evolutionary process of economic development. With long-term economic growth, the real income, educational and occupational-skill levels of the lower social classes are substantially enhanced, and long-term mental and physical health, as well as longevity, are usually improved. Thus, the principal impact of the Great Recession—via GDP decline and unemployment increase—on mental health (e.g. depression, anxiety, and suicide) can be observed. However, while the evolutionary factors of economic development are largely beneficial for mental and physical health, there are also damaging implications for mental health that are consequences of population ageing.

Longer-lived populations of the post-industrialized societies are subject to the 'epidemiological transition'. In this transition, infectious diseases are replaced as the dominant sources of illness and mortality by the chronic diseases, that endure throughout much of life, and are subject to the risks related to alcohol, tobacco, overweight, reduced physical activity, altered social relations, and environmental toxins. These long-term illnesses and sources of mortality (e.g. cancer, tuberculosis, HIV) then become important risks to depression and especially suicide.

In this chapter the literature on the Great Recession and austerity policies as they have influenced mental health outcomes are critically examined. Key studies have involved the individual-level impact of unemployment and the effects of business organization downsizing on the mental health of job losers, as well as survivors. There is evidence of a reciprocal effect whereby previously poor mental health, which is far more prevalent in low social classes (and interacts with poor physical health), influences the likelihood of both job loss in recessions, and, subsequently, income decline and further deterioration of mental health. By integrating previous and recent literatures, the principal population risks to damaged mental health are brought together in models predicting global suicide rates as a consequence of the Great Recession and austerity policies taking into account the added physical health risks posed by social class differences and by the economic crisis.

The models are grounded on national income (GDP per capita) as a source of increasing household economic resources (and thus poverty reduction), increased sophistication of technology, which elevates the scientific-informational basis of employment, and investment in education—which makes it possible for populations to absorb higher levels of technology through elevated job skills—thus advancing productivity. The GDP can be understood as a continuous variable that is the leading source of overall economic development. As such, GDP also subsumes those elements of economic development that are unequally distributed throughout the social class structure. With this in mind, it is clear that, since at least the 1980s, the benefits of economic growth have inordinately gone to the higher social classes, especially emphasizing those occupations and industries with the highest levels of income, education, and occupational skill levels. Continuation of the expanded social class disparities in income and wealth, in the aftermath of the Great Recession, portends increasing health disparities, especially involving psychological morbidities and their sequelae.

Significance of social class for psychiatric epidemiology

Social class represents the status of a person with respect to cognitive, economic, social, and emotional resources required to adapt to the physical and human environment. The extent of those resources underlie both the vulnerability, and the capacity of the person to successfully respond, to psychological and physical stressors.

The modern epidemiological literature tends to focus on three metrics of social class, often using the term 'socio-economic status'. These are income, educational, and occupation levels. The metrics are used as convenient and extremely practical means of linking specific attributes of social class to health measures by statistical methods. However, these broad statistical approaches occasionally leave the reader with the view that social class consists *only* of the three metrics. The concept of 'social class' goes beyond socioeconomic status as often measured in epidemiological studies. Social class includes authority-power in the workplace hierarchy; the distinction between ownership, management, and 'worker' status; the intergenerational continuity of wealth and poverty, the industrial basis of occupational differences in work content; the regional economic maintenance of socio-economic and ethnic patterns of working life; and national differences in standards of living based on residential, economic, technological-cultural, and political development. Therefore, it is important to take into account work organization, industry, economic region, national-cultural distinctions, and political party orientation in considering social class from global and historical perspectives.

Ecological span of social class

In general, the distinction between measures of socio-economic status and the more general construct of social class, is revealed in the 'spread effects' of parent to child continuity of class status [3, 4], as discussed in the previous section. Beyond family continuity are the regionally based patterns of industrial development. Thus, we observe in Europe and North America that there are regions traditionally specialized in different types of manufacturing, agriculture, and services, including the professions of finance, retailing, the restaurant industry, and tourism. Individuals born into those regional-industrial ecological niches are likely to obtain employment in them, given the traditions of family and culture, unless beset by major recessions, industrial decline, technological change, or globalization. In those cases, they will tend to migrate from these areas and disrupt the continuity of social class values, attitudes, and work.

In addition, there has now emerged an epidemiological literature that examines the effect of social class on mental and physical health where neighborhood is the unit of analysis. This form of geospatial analysis of health problems is especially discerning because the different social classes are typically dispersed in relatively homogenous neighborhoods according to the economic necessities of residence and transportation.

Ethnicity and social class

Ethnicity often further subdivides the social classes, generally placing those of lower social status at predominantly lower class levels. This frequently occurs because of cultural discrimination that limits specific ethnic groups in their access to, for example, educational opportunities, particular types and levels of employment, residential areas, health care, criminal justice, and political participation. Beyond physiologically or culturally based ethnicity, recently arrived generations of immigrants are often subject to discrimination, which limits entry into the social classes most relevant to their educational and job skills. These discriminatory practices tend to expand lower social class population segments by intensifying downward social mobility. This is exemplified by the historical pattern of development of the US social class system, based on successive waves of immigration since the colonial period [5, 6]. Upward social mobility and integration of immigrant groups is enhanced under conditions of long-term economic growth, the provision of employment opportunities, and investment in education.

Social class, economic crises, and mental illness before the Great Recession

Following A.B. Hollingshead's development of the two-factor index of social class for use with US populations, Hollingshead (sociologist) and Frederick Redlich (psychiatrist) produced the original epidemiological study, at the individual level, of treated mental disorder in New Haven, Connecticut [7]. Their classic finding is that psychiatric disorders, in general, and both depressive illness and schizophrenia, were found in greater prevalence at increasingly low levels of social class. The basic interpretation was that mental disorders partly result from early and mid-life crises or stressors that were more common in lower social class subcultures wherein resources to cope adequately with these stressors were less available as they depended on income, education, and contacts at both social and professional levels. It also did not escape these authors that genetic factors or early-life deprivations or traumas could provide a template of predisposing factors upon which later stressors could precipitate psychiatric symptoms or longer-term disorders.

Two major epidemiological studies of populations not in treatment further supported the New Haven findings of substantially higher mental illness rates at lower social class levels in Nova Scotia and New York City [8, 9]. The inverse relation between social class and mental disorder has been confirmed throughout the twentieth and twenty-first centuries, and is a basic component of the 'social gradient' of health [10]. Much of this relation has continued to be interpreted within the framework of stress theory [11]. From the 1970s to the 1990s, psychosocial stress interpretations of both psychological and physical illness gained considerable momentum following the discoveries of Walter Cannon in the 1920s of the 'fight or flight' syndrome [12], and identification of the 'general adaptation syndrome' by Hans Selye [13, 14]. Within this tradition, the first widely used stress scales were developed in 1967 [15], and have been used in various forms that elucidate the inverse social class and mental illness relation [16–20].

In accordance with a stress-based interpretation of the social class–mental illness findings, a second line of research, involving economic change and business cycles at the aggregate level, was introduced in 1973 [2]. This study found that economic recessions, and especially vulnerability to employment losses, were substantially responsible for mental hospitalization in New York State from 1841 to 1967. Since publication of the New York State findings [2], a series of studies covering the twentieth and early twenty-first centuries has shown that mortality involving stress-related diagnoses—especially cardiovascular disease, cirrhosis of the liver, suicide, and homicide—declined in relation to GDP growth and increased in conjunction with higher unemployment rates [21–27]. The theoretical perspective is that national and regional economic change—the principal source of social change—is a fundamental factor that underlies both long-term social well-being—and, under economically unstable circumstances, societal distress. When economic growth is not sustained and employment declines, increases in these stress-related causes of death tend to be elevated over at least a 1–6-year period. Furthermore, an extensive literature focused on unemployment has shown consistent relations to deterioration in mental health measures [28–31]. Finally, at the individual level, epidemiological studies have consistently confirmed positive relations among unemployment and stress-related illnesses, including cardiovascular diseases [32–37].

Over the remainder of the twentieth century, an econometric and epidemiological literature concentrating on mental disorder, suicide, and alcohol abuse continued to demonstrate damage to mental health in relation to elevated unemployment rates [28, 29, 38]. This research has been further supported by a substantial literature, at the individual level, on the impact of unemployment on physical health levels [30, 32–34], with an emphasis on stress-related cardiovascular illness.

Recent literature: impact of the Great Recession on mental health psychiatric disturbance

In this section evidence of the influence of the Great Recession on a number of mental health indicators is outlined, including psychiatric disturbance, suicide, and alcohol and drug abuse. This is a burgeoning topic in the social sciences, psychiatric, and economic literature, which is rapidly expanding and already contains literature reviews, including both theoretical interpretations and practical policy implications [31, 39–41]. The studies identified in the following paragraphs are restricted to quantitative mental health correlates of the Great Recession.

European studies at the individual level demonstrate that loss of job or income during the Great Recession increased the risk of psychiatric disturbance. The countries that were the sources of these studies include Greece [42, 43], Spain [44–46], Sweden [47], and France, Hungary, Sweden, and the UK [48]. In addition, findings were published from Hong Kong and Australia [49, 50].

There is also a noticeable gap, in much of the European literature, between the number of persons affected by psychiatric disorders and those treated appropriately during the Great Recession due to multiple factors, including austerity [39]. Aggregate-level cross-sectional studies in Europe indicate moderate implications for psychiatric disturbance in the Great Recession largely confined to males [51, 52], and specifically in Spain and the UK [46, 53, 54]. These findings were reinforced when diagnosed psychiatric disorders were examined.

US studies appear to show somewhat stronger effects of the Great Recession on psychiatric disturbance. Individual-level studies indicate that unemployment or loss of economic resources represent a highly significant set of risks to symptoms of mental disorder [55–57]. Findings from aggregate population studies, based on national survey data, also emphasized elevated psychological disturbance during the Great Recession. African Americans appear to have experienced more pronounced symptoms of mental disorder [58].

The housing crisis, igniting much of the Great Recession in the USA, stimulated a substantial literature on implications for psychological disorders. Rigorously conducted analyses covering individuals, neighbourhoods, and counties consistently showed increases in psychological disorder based on foreclosures and housing wealth decline [59, 60]. Several of the more prominent studies were at the individual level [61–63] and at the county and neighbourhood levels [64–66].

Suicide

Suicide rates were substantially elevated in much of the industrialized world in relation to unemployment and timing of the Great Recession. Indeed, more recent research shows that unemployment has been a primary factor responsible for reattempt at suicide [67]. These represent perhaps the most valid and reliable findings of elevated disturbance of mental health in the recession as they are based on a conservative estimate of depressive symptomatology eventuating in the most severe outcome. These relationships were detailed for industrialized countries, Europe [52, 68], and especially Western Europe [69], and a broad range of high-income countries, including the USA [70–75]. Elevated trends for suicidality were also found to be significantly related to unemployment and timing of the Great Recession in Western Europe [69], Greece [76–78], Finland [79], Italy [80, 81], Spain [82, 83], Sweden [84], the UK [85], Iceland [86], New Zealand [87], Korea [88], Japan [89], and the USA [90, 91].

More specialized studies of the impact of the recessional housing and foreclosure crisis similarly showed evidence of heightened suicide rates [92, 93]. The overall debt crisis was also pronounced in

European countries, which were studied extensively. Indebtedness was a risk factor during the European Recession for both mental disorder and elevated suicide rates [94–98].

Alcohol abuse

Alcohol consumption per capita during the Great Recession has shown declines in the general population. This is consistent with a pattern in which lower incomes would reduce consumption in restaurants and social gatherings. It is not clear whether this reduction of alcohol consumption promotes better or worse health in the general population. On the assumption that average population consumption of alcohol is moderate, there is considerable evidence that such ingestion significantly reduces the risk of heart disease [99]. However, there is a tradition in public health that links high rates of population alcohol consumption to increased mortality due to liver cirrhosis and related illnesses. At the individual level of analysis in both European countries and the USA the Great Recession appears to have resulted in higher pathological consumption—i.e. 'binge drinking'— in the USA [100–105], European Union (EU) [106], Iceland [107], Italy [108], and the UK [109]. This is consistent with stress-related alcohol consumption being used as a moderator of anxiety and depression.

Drug abuse

Evidence during the Great Recession points to an unequivocal increase in drug abuse rates—especially of illicit drugs—particularly among those who have experienced loss of employment or income, or are anxious about that possibility. This is consistent with traditional findings that lower social class populations, especially vulnerable to drug abuse on the grounds of economic hardship, are generally at higher risk for drug abuse [110], and is demonstrated specifically in Australia [111], France [112], Iceland [113], Italy [114], Portugal [115], and the USA [116, 117]. The higher drug addiction prevalence among lower socio-economic groups increases both their risk of economic loss during the recession and the intensified use of drugs to mitigate subsequent psychological morbidity.

Limitations of the current literature

The most important gap in the current literature involves the almost total absence of studies that utilize GDP, as a principal measure of recession, in studies that estimate the mental or physical health impact of the Great Recession [118]. Currently, the most frequently cited evidence of the health effects of the Great Recession relies on the unemployment rate at the aggregate level and on the individual-level experience of unemployment, debt, or consequences of the US housing crisis. However, the GDP is a necessary component of this evidence because it is the traditional indicator used by economists to specify the dates and magnitude of recession [118]. More specifically, according to the National Bureau of Economic Research Dating Committee: 'A recession is a significant decline in economic activity spread across the economy, lasting more than a few months, normally visible in real GDP, real income, employment, industrial production and wholesale-retail sales' [119].

In addition, the standard objection, among labour economists, to using the unemployment rate as the entire measure of recession is that it only involves persons who lost employment and are currently seeking work—thus eliminating those who gave up looking for work. Among the labour statistics that could be used to estimate more precisely the mental health impact of job loss are the long-term unemployment rate, the rate of underemployment, and the share of the population (or age 25–54 years) not employed.

Moreover, the general view is that examining the contemporaneous, or short-term, relation between recessional unemployment and psychological morbidity or suicide will omit most of the relation—which is medium-to-long-term [120–123]—i.e. over at least 5–10 years [21, 25]. The issue here is that there are not only long-duration effects of unemployment—influencing reduced wages, poverty, labour force withdrawal, and psychological and physical disability. Overall, poverty levels both in the European Great Recession and the US crisis resulted in more pronounced indications of mental disorder [41, 121–123]. Indeed, if economic crisis occurs relatively early in life, the cumulative effect of ensuing multiple stresses could be distributed over the life course. This would be the case especially where unemployment results in decreased family economic status to a lower social class level. Nevertheless, hardly any health studies of the Great Recession attempt to go beyond a short-term estimate.

Equally important, to understand mental health implications of the international recession of 2007–09 and its aftermath, analyses of psychological morbidity, such as suicide, including a global sample involving developing countries, would be needed.

Further, with respect to estimating the impact of economic changes on psychological morbidity or mortality, epidemiological methodology requires controls for the most important risk or benefit factors that relate to health deterioration. This not only includes addiction, violence, and environmental risks, but benefits including healthcare expenditures and educational attainment. Such controls have thus far been largely absent from studies of health effects of the Great Recession.

The circularity trap: mental morbidity, social class, and economic crisis

In outlining the literature on the impact of social class on mental health, reference was made to the relation between social class and physical well-being, both in terms of illness and mortality. Part of the rationale for emphasizing physical illness and mortality is that these measures of harm are important risk factors to subsequent mental morbidity. This constitutes one mechanism whereby social class is linked to mental health, i.e. through the multiple mediating factors represented by stressful life events that result in diminished physical well-being.

Among the top-10 stressful life events identified in the 'social readjustment rating scale' are those involving (i) harm to health, (ii) damage to family relations, and (iii) loss of employment or retirement [15]. The next 10 most stressful events also include damage to health (two items) and five items relating to economic hardship (i.e. business readjustment, changes in financial state, change to different line of work, major mortgage). The two additional major stressors are foreclosures of mortgage or loan, and changes in responsibilities at work. The incidence of damage to health and life expectancy, the most salient stressors, are classically shown to be inversely related to social class level, known as the 'social gradient' or 'health gradient', as is mental illness prevalence [10]. Epidemiological studies at the individual level of analysis have also uniformly shown that unemployment is consistently related to deteriorating health, mortality and poor mental health [28–30].

Thus, the epidemiological literature underlies the foundational observation that lower social classes bear the heaviest burden of physical and mental health problems. These health problems, in turn, should also be seen as stressors with future implications for decreased capacity for work. Diminished work capacity often results in poor work performance with implications for career damage or complete loss of employment.

The relations between mental health, on the one hand, and the combined effects of social class, the Great Recession, and government austerity, on the other, can be seen in a circular pattern of causation (see Fig. 18.1). In this circular sequence, a *first stage* is introduced involving traditional lower social class preponderance of mental illness prior to the Great Recession, exacerbated by technological change and globalization, and engendering a higher prevalence of physical illness and mortality. Stress theory informs us that those mental and physical disorders are themselves stressors, as they can considerably diminish social (and especially work) functioning and are sources of stigma, which often diminish social status. Psychological and physical disorders are frequently linked as much somatic illness—especially cardiovascular disease—is influenced by mental stress. Thus, even among the fully employed, lower social class position can be understood as a stressor, incorporating lower social status, fewer cognitive and material resources, vulnerability to crises, and lower access to social capital [124].

In a second stage, the Great Recession disproportionately damaged the employment, income, wealth, and inequality positions of the lower social classes, partly resulting from relatively low education and initially higher illness levels.

The effect of the Great Recession on economic inequality has been studied intensely in the USA, which was the source of the international economic crisis. In the USA, the lowest social class groups fell into a smaller share of income during 2007–09, largely due to job losses [125]. The most important differential in loss among social class groups involved wealth, where the bottom 90% of the income groups suffered the greatest losses in wealth,

in addition to disposable income losses, which might make them vulnerable to persistent future earnings decline [126]. In general, all groups lost wealth during the Great Recession, but the declines were greatest for the least advantaged [127]. Thus, the impact of the Great Recession, especially where high unemployment was involved, increased mental and physical illness levels not only owing to absolute losses, but also probably owing to an expansion of social class inequalities.

However, adding further to the circularity of the relations among social class, illness, and the recession, there is extensive economic opinion that high levels of income inequality substantially influenced the occurrence of both the Great Depression and the Great Recession, and the high level of inequality may be part of the *root* cause of the Great Recession [128]. Furthermore, recent economic opinion suggests that the secular growth in income inequality is a major threat to long-term economic growth [129–132].

In a *third stage*, one observes that the recessional and austerity losers of employment and income have a difficult time finding new employment if they are lacking intermediate-to-high-level work skills or educational qualifications. In those cases, particularly after middle age, even if new employment is secured, it is generally at a lower level of income and job status [133, 134]. This situation will be most pronounced if the recessional loss occurs in industries with declining employment, such as manufacturing, and if, as has recently been the case, there is a trend of rising income inequality interacting with a major recession, such as in 2007–09. This third stage serves to maintain the intergenerational divisions of the social class structure, owing to very minimal upward mobility among the lower social classes.

In a *fourth stage*, and, ultimately, the effects of the Great Recession on mental health are largely maintained as a result of the continued expansion of economic inequality and the maintenance of historically high poverty rates. The circularity of this sequence is maintained under conditions of slow economic growth and the hollowing out of the middle classes, largely due to loss of manufacturing employment and increases in low-wage services employment. The consequences are that much of the 'working class' now becomes the working poor, characterized by having less than a

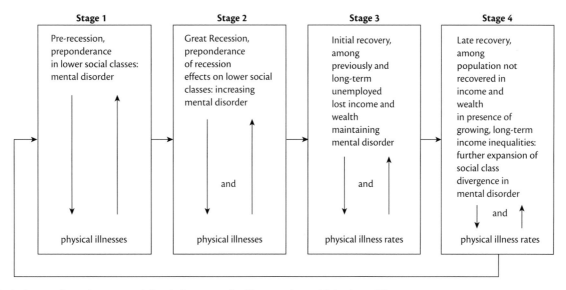

Fig. 18.1 Circular impact of recession on mental disorder in context of stable or growing social class inequalities.

tertiary education. This slow restructuring of the social class configuration involves limited upward mobility of the lower social classes and the intensification of the inverse relation of social class status to mental illness. Further, in this *fourth stage*, we see the continued elevation of social stressors resulting from the sustained decline in the social status, resources, and social capital among those who did not recover (or recovered minimally) in the aftermath of the recession. These post-recession stressors, in turn, perpetuate new and interacting mental and physical health problems. The circular model specifies further that these health issues continue to suppress the capacity for highly productive work—especially among the lower social class populations. These conditions return our analysis to *stage one*.

The stability of this feedback loop can be broken by greatly improved economic growth, social welfare, and educational investment. But, in the face of slow economic growth, government austerity, diminution of manufacturing employment, precarious work, and long-term increases in income inequality, the continuity of this adverse feedback loop seems more likely.

Adding to this problem of circularity among low social class, recession and poor mental health is a standard phenomenon that can be referred to as the 'spread effect'. Thus, it is often a problem to identify which individuals, within a family experiencing recessional job loss, will actually be subject to damaged mental or psychophysiological health. In the most traditional case, a head of household may lose employment or income, and subsequently experience personal isolation and status loss. However, the effect of those losses and isolation then is dispersed among the other family members—be they a spouse, child, or elderly parent. The internal disruption commonly known to occur within family life emanates from this singular loss of employment—even though the ultimate harm to mental or physical health may be found in infants, young adults, husbands or wives, and the elderly, who depend on the principal household earner for their economic and social status.

Impact of the Great Recession and diminished economic growth on suicide: multivariate analyses

A multivariate predictive model of worldwide suicide rates can be used as a means of understanding the international distribution of life-threatening clinical depression. This model updates, internationally, an earlier multivariate suicide model covering industrialized societies [68]. The importance of focusing on depression is that it is the leading cause of disability worldwide and is the fourth leading contributor to the burden of disease [135]. But depression itself is difficult to measure on a population basis, given variation in symptomatology and diagnoses across different world cultures and international distinctions in technical psychiatric approaches. Therefore, suicide is used in this chapter as one measure of the international distribution and trends in clinical depression. Depression, further, has traditionally been linked to suicide [136]. Ironically, even when depression is treated pharmacologically, there is increased risk to suicide from drug therapy [137].

Suicide is probably the best-known cause of death to be found related to economic recessions. But few multivariate studies have pointed to this relation during the Great Recession of 2007–09. An increase in the suicide rate has been documented during and following the interval of the Great Recession [70, 138]. Fully

quantitative, multivariate epidemiological, and econometric models using the standard recessional indices of GDP decline and unemployment increases, and controlling for relevant confounders, in world and industrialized country samples, are presented in this chapter.

The epidemiology of suicide involves the diagnoses of affective disorders—especially depression, feelings of hopelessness, helplessness and worthlessness, and risks of socio-economic disadvantage—especially unemployment, homelessness, economic dependence; contact with police or justice system; relationship disruption or loss; and substance use/abuse [139]. This epidemiological background draws attention to the relations, across world societies, between the recessional variables of GDP decline and increased unemployment—specifically during the Great Recession of 2007–09. The multivariate models attempt to explain variation in the age-adjusted suicide rate for 165 countries over the years 2000–13 in a pooled cross-sectional time series regression analysis. Tables 18.1 and 18.2 show the predictability of the overall model components.

Table 18.1 Relationships between worldwide recessional indicators, gross domestic product (GDP) per capita (average last 5 years), and the unemployment rate (without lag) to age-adjusted global suicide rates for 165 countries, controlling for education, behavioural, and environmental risk factors, and diagnosis-specific mortality and illness rates associated with suicide

Suicide (ICD-10 codes X60–X84) age-adjusted death rate per 100,000 of total overall population

Predictor	Overall R^2: 0.69		
	Coefficient		95% CI
GDP per capita PPP (average last 5 years)	−0.15	***	−0.17 to −0.13
Education index (range 0–100)	−0.02	**	−0.03 to 0.00
Unemployment rate (%) in total population age 15+ years	0.05	***	0.02 to 0.07
CO_2 emissions in grams per capita and year (average last 20 years)	0.32	***	0.26 to 0.37
Total neoplasms, age-standardized death rate per 100,000	0.03	***	0.02 to 0.04
Alcohol and drug use disorders, age-standardized death rate per 100,000	0.14	***	0.10 to 0.18
Unintentional injuries, age-standardized death rate per 100,000	0.17	***	0.15 to 0.19
Homicides, age-standardized death rate per 100,000	0.12	***	0.09 to 0.15
HIV prevalence, age standardized per 100,000 of total population	0.001	***	0.001 to 0.001
Constant	0.72		−0.89 to 2.33

Note: One hundred and sixty-five countries of the world, 1995–2013. Regression results are adjusted with regional dummy variables for (i) Eastern and Western Africa; (ii) Eastern Asia; (iii) Republic of Korea and Japan; (iv) Russia, Ukraine, Belarus, and Kazakhstan; (v) Bosnia, Croatia, Montenegro, Serbia, and Slovenia. ICD-10: International Classification of Diseases, 10th Edition; CI: confidence interval; PPP: purchasing power parity.

*, **, and *** denote statistical significance of the estimated coefficient at the 10%, 5%, and 1% confidence levels, respectively.

Table 18.2 Relations between worldwide recessional indicators, gross domestic product (GDP) per capita (average last 5 years), and the unemployment rate (average last 5 years) to age-adjusted global suicide rates for 165 countries, controlling for education, behavioural, and environmental risk factors, and diagnosis-specific mortality and illness rates associated with suicide

Suicide (ICD-10 codes X60–X84) age-adjusted death rate per 100,000 of total overall population

Predictor	Overall R^2: 0.69		
	Coefficient		95% CI
GDP per capita PPP (average last 5 years)	−0.14	***	−0.16 to −0.12
Education index (range 0–100)	−0.02	**	−0.03 to −0.01
Unemployment rate (%) in total population age 15+ years (average last 5 years)	0.09	***	0.06 to 0.12
CO_2 emission in grams per capita and year (average last 20 years)	0.33	***	0.27 to 0.38
Total neoplasms, age-standardized death rate per 100,000	0.03	***	0.02 to 0.04
Alcohol and drug use disorders, age-standardized death rate per 100,000	0.13	***	0.09 to 0.18
Unintentional injuries, age-standardized death rate per 100,000	0.17	***	0.14 to 0.19
Homicides, age-standardized death rate per 100,000	0.12	***	0.09 to 0.15
HIV prevalence, age standardized per 100,000 of total population	0.001	***	0.001 to 0.001
Constant	0.20		−1.42 to 1.82

Note: One hundred and sixty-five countries of the world, 1995–2013. Regression results are adjusted with regional dummy variables for (i) Eastern and Western Africa; (ii) Eastern Asia; (iii) Republic of Korea and Japan; (iv) Russia, Ukraine, Belarus, and Kazakhstan; (v) Former Yugoslavia. ICD-10: International Classification of Diseases, 10th Edition; CI = confidence interval; PPP: purchasing power parity.

*, **, and *** denote statistical significance of the estimated coefficient at the 10%, 5%, and 1% confidence levels, respectively.

In the world model, the key recessional variable is GDP, as a decline over two-quarters in GDP growth is usually understood to indicate minimally the presence of recession [118]. The GDP, as the central measure of economic development, is also the basis of upward mobility, i.e. the extent to which a population can, on average, advance in its social class status, based on the development of new occupations in the 'knowledge' economy and the diminution of manufacturing and agricultural employment contingent on technological change. But the more popular indictor in journalistic writing and epidemiological measurement involves a sharp elevation of the unemployment rate followed by a substantial decline, usually within a year. The presence of national GDP decline and unemployment increase generally indicates substantial elevation of poverty rates and underemployment, i.e. employment involving shorter hours, reduced wages, and jobs requiring lower skill levels—and a decrease in labour force participation for those who have given up searching for new employment.

The consequences of the austerity are also incorporated in the longer-term effects of the recession, especially diminished or slow growth in GDP, and include the effects of government policies in minimizing government spending.

The relation between the unemployment and suicide rates can be seen at lags from 0 to 5 years. The 0-year lag shows the significant contemporaneous relation of unemployment to suicide. But the lagged effect of unemployment over a 5-year period is especially intense. It takes into account that the suicide rate has been continually elevated over the Great Recession and smaller subsequent recessions experienced by several countries, especially in Europe, in the aftermath of the austerity and continued economic decline (see Table 18.1). The cumulative relation of unemployment rates to suicide rates can be measured over the full 0–5-year average of the unemployment rate during the 6-year period as the predictor of suicide (see Table 18.2). A similar Recessional effect is observed when the relation of GDP to suicide is measured over a 0–5-year interval (see Tables 18.1 and 18.2).

Control for confounders in the Great Recession–suicide relation

These multivariate suicide models take account of the fact that various other external causes of death than suicide are frequently based on underlying emotions, such as depression and anxiety, which give rise to and often predict suicide (alcohol abuse, drug abuse, unintentional injuries). The related causes of death are therefore under control in the suicide model. In fact, frequently these causes of death on official certificates will be used to mask actual suicide, which is stigmatized (and is often proscribed by religion or law) in some societies. Furthermore, under control are causes of illness and death that are often risk factors for depression and suicide (e.g. cancers and tuberculosis). These sources of illness can be especially debilitating, particularly when inadequately treated, or result in loss of employment, and therefore act as major sources of stress. Additionally, mortality resulting from these frequent causes of death become prominent stressors as in the death of spouse or close relation. However, all of these causes of death are themselves made more likely in the face of losses of income and employment and are found in substantially greater frequency in lower socio-economic groups. Thus, when estimates are made of the impact of the recession and government austerity on suicide, health factors that are closely associated with depression and suicide are placed under control (see Tables 18.2 and 18.3). At the same time, abundant literature indicates that the recession, unemployment, and austerity are risks to these same diagnoses of morbidity and mortality.

The sustained relation of GDP declines and unemployment increases to suicide over 0–5 years can also be found among the advanced industrialized countries of the Organisation for Economic Co-operation and Development (OECD) where suicide, and clinical depression, in general, would be measured more accurately (according to Diagnostic and Statistical Manual of Mental Disorders criteria) and with less cultural variability (see Table 18.3). These findings, covering the OECD countries' suicide rates, are similar to those for stress-related cardiovascular mortality rates in EU countries that also increased in relation to GDP declines and higher unemployment during the Great Recession [140].

Table 18.3 Relation between industrialized country (Organisation for Economic Co-operation and Development; OECD) recessional indicators, gross domestic product (GDP) per capita (average last 5 years), and the unemployment rate (average 5 years) to age-adjusted total suicide rates for 35 countries, controlling for education, environmental risk factors, and diagnosis-specific mortality rates associated with suicide

Suicide (ICD-10 codes X60–X84) age-adjusted death rate per 100,000 of total overall population

Predictor	Overall R^2: 0.70		
	Coefficient		95% CI
GDP per capita PPP in '000 (average last 5 years)	−0.13	***	−0.18 to −0.07
Education index (range o0–100)	−0.11	***	−0.16 to −0.06
Unemployment rate (%) in total population age 15+ years (average last 5 years)	0.14	***	0.08 to 0.21
CO_2 emission in grams per capita and year (average last 20 years)	0.15	**	0.03 to 0.27
Total neoplasm, age-standardized death rate per 100,000	0.05	***	0.03 to 0.06
Transport injuries, age-standardized death rate per 100,000	0.12	***	0.04 to 0.20
Other unintentional injuries,[†] age-standardized death rate per 100,000	0.48	***	0.41 to 0.55
Homicides, age-standardized death rate per 100,000	0.57	***	0.41 to 0.73
Constant	10.52	***	4.68 to 16.37

Note: Thirty-five OECD countries, 1995–2013. Regression results are adjusted with regional dummy variables for (i) Chile and Mexico; (ii) Greece and Turkey; (iii) Republic of Korea and Japan. ICD-10: International Classification of Diseases, 10th Edition; CI = confidence interval; PPP: purchasing power parity.

*, **, and *** denote statistical significance of the estimated coefficient at the 10%, 5%, and 1% confidence levels, respectively. [†]Other unintentional injuries: unintentional injuries excluding transport accidents

Estimate of the impact of the austerity on health

The austerity policies essentially involved reduced government spending and increased taxation, with the combined effect of slowing economic growth, maintaining elevated unemployment rates, and increasing income inequality [141, 142]. Considering the consequences of reduction of government expenditures, it is clear that specific decreases in expenditures for health care—as a proportion of GDP, in industrialized countries of the OECD—has occurred, on average, over 1995–2013. Government expenditure on health as a percentage of national income is inversely related to the age-adjusted mortality rate (see Table 18.4). In this model, level of educational attainment is used to infer the long-term implications of government expenditures on education, as a critical investment in health and economic growth; it is strongly inversely related to overall mortality rates. Under control in the predictive model are variables expressing mortality due to alcohol and drug abuse, violence, traffic accidents, other unintentional accidents,

Table 18.4 Relationship between industrialized country (Organisation for Economic Co-operation and Development; OECD) recessional indicators, gross domestic product (GDP) per capita (average last 5 years), and the unemployment rate (without lag) to age-adjusted total mortality rates for 35 countries, controlling for education, environmental risk factors, and diagnosis-specific mortality rates associated with suicide

Total age-adjusted death rate per 100,000 of total overall population

Predictor	Overall R^2: 0.75		
	Coefficient		95% CI
GDP per capita PPP in '000 (average last 10 years)	−7.53	***	−8.62 to −6.44
Total expenditure on health as % of GDP	−12.77	***	−16.46 to −9.09
Education index (range 0–100)	−4.75	***	−5.73 to −3.77
Unemployment rate (%) in total population age 15+ years	1.03	**	0.08 to 1.97
CO_2 emission in grams per capita and year (average last 20 years)	3.90	***	1.82 to 5.98
Smoking prevalence (%) in total population age 15+ years	0.88		−0.41 to 2.17
Fertility rate per 100,000 of female population aged 10–14 years	2.22	***	1.88 to 2.56
Obesity prevalence per 10,000 in total population age 20+ years, lag 5 years	4.81	***	2.98 to 6.64
Tuberculosis prevalence, age-standardized, per 100,000 of total population, lag 1 year	3.88	***	3.27 to 4.49
Constant	971.10	***	854.54 to 1087.67

Note: Thirty-five OECD countries, 1995–2014. Regression results are adjusted with one regional dummy variable for Chile, Mexico, Turkey, and Republic of Korea. CI: confidence interval; PPP: purchasing power parity.

*, **, and *** denote statistical significance of the estimated coefficient at the 10%, 5%, and 1% confidence levels, respectively.

intense physical illness, and mortality (malignancies and tuberculosis) (see Tables 18.1 and 18.2). The conclusion is that the austerity in important government expenditures had, overall, a damaging effect on industrialized country life expectancy. In addition, overall mortality, which also increased in relation to the Great Recession (see Table 18.4), being a known risk for clinical depression in family members and other close relations, is likely to have further influenced the suicide rate in several countries.

Unemployment and labour force participation in US suicide prediction

It can be seen that suicide rate increases have been related to recessions in 19 of the 23 recessions since 1900, and especially in the

Great Depression and the Great Recession (Fig. 18.2a). However, in the USA, suicide increased sharply during and after the Great Recession, despite the fact that the unemployment rate immediately and continually declined following that recession. This may be because the US unemployment rate was no longer sufficient to describe the loss of labour force participation due to discouraged workers giving up on seeking new employment. Thus, while the US suicide rate is very well predicted by high unemployment in the Great Depression, and several subsequent recessions, it loses some of its predictive precision, starting in the 1990s. In the 2007–09 recession and its aftermath, decline in the labour force participation rate is the far superior predictor of elevated suicide rates (see Fig. 18.2a, b).

Suicide and the circularity trap: empirical models

The multivariate suicide models as sources of statistical explanation focus on the main themes of this chapter, namely the linkage of social class, the Great Recession, and financial austerity, as they have influenced worldwide and industrialized country suicide rates. These suicide models can be understood as a sequence of circular relations among the variables, taking into account both mental and physical health indices. More specifically, it can be seen (see Table 18.1) that the primary predictors of suicide include mortality due to alcohol, drug abuse, unintentional injuries, violence, HIV infection, and, especially, malignancies.

In a first stage (see Fig. 18.1) one can view the mutual relations between suicide and both mortality due to unintentional injuries and malignancies. Unintentional injuries include automobile traffic, falls, drug overdoses, and poisoning. It is possible that a substantial proportion of these are self-destructive in nature or actual suicides not technically classified as such due to stigma or other restraints in reporting. As these are also causes (i.e. diagnostically) of mortality, these deaths themselves are major stressors and risks to the depression and potential suicide of loved ones. HIV and malignancies are unusually debilitating illnesses and are substantial risks to suicide [143]. Similarly, deaths attributable to HIV and cancer are themselves stressors potentially influencing depression and suicide in loved ones. It is also apparent from the literature that alcohol, drug abuse, and violence represent high risks of depression and suicide, and that deaths due to these societal harms are sufficient stressors to be risks for depression and suicide in closely related persons. It is clear that all of these causes of death (depression, alcohol abuse, drug abuse, unintentional injuries, malignancies, and HIV infection) are inversely related to social class status along the lines of the health gradient and that this gradient expands and increases in influence under conditions of greater inequality of income and wealth [144].

In stage two (see Fig. 18.1), it can be observed that the damaging effect of the Great Recession is strongest in the lowest social class groups, with the highest prevailing rates of mental and physical illness. In stage two one can calculate the damaging effect of the Great Recession on suicide—most particularly through the impact of heightened unemployment rates and declining national income, and the subsequent influence of the austerity regime on maintaining or enlarging these economic shocks and their effects on poverty. It is also known, epidemiologically, as is estimated in this suicide model, that alcohol, drug use, violence, unintended

injuries, malignancies, and HIV infection are associated with suicide [143], partly because of their common link to lower class prevalence and to unemployment and income loss. HIV prevalence and cancer mortality are epidemiologically linked to lower income and employment loss partly through the comparatively deficient access of lower class populations to health care [145, 146].

The effect of the losses of employment and income further increase the economic and stress burden on the society as a whole, but especially on the middle and very lowest social classes, where unemployment has been highest. The Great Recession produced the largest earnings inequality among industrialized country populations (where data have been observable), especially in countries that saw large increases in unemployment between 2007 and 2009.

Stage 3 (see Fig. 18.1) involves the recovery phase of the Great Recession after 2009. Despite the technical language of 'recovery', however, the USA and other industrialized countries, including those of the EU, saw the rate of poverty maintained and usually increased, as a result of their strong linkage to the high, sustained, unemployment rates. Following recessions, the unemployed who subsequently do find new employment re-enter the workforce at lower social class status and lower wages, which are maintained during the remainder of their careers [134]. Nevertheless, there has been a post-Recession increase in long-term unemployment and substantial reduction in the labour force among discouraged job seekers. It is also found, in conjunction with austerity measures, that the post-Recession economies continued to stall and elevate income inequalities [147].

Additional literature reveals that the business downsizing that was heavily intensified during the Great Recession not only led to increased mental health problems stemming from unemployment, but also elevated levels of depression and anxiety, even among those who remained employed in downsized firms [47, 48]. In the case of the world suicide model, an optimal lag averaging over 5 years for both national income and unemployment can be observed. This appears to reflect at least a medium-term impact of the Great Recession on suicide. However, even among the wealthiest industrialized countries of the OECD, the principal impact of unemployment on the suicide rate occurs within 12 months but extends for at least 5 years (see Table 18.3).

In stage 4 (see Fig. 18.1), as shown in the aftermath of the Great Recession, we continue to see increases in the poverty rate and in the unemployment rate as well, especially in EU countries. In both North America and the EU, income and wealth inequality have continued to increase [129, 147]. The social class differentials in mental illness continue to grow as re-employment increases at lower social class levels. This returns the circular sequence to its origins in stage one, where the economy is not yet in another recessional phase.

Implications: mental health and reconstitution of the social classes

General improvements in mortality related to mental and somatic health are associated with long-term, sustainable, economic development. Secular economic growth, in turn, depends on improved productivity, which is substantially based on scientific and technological innovation. But the 'creative destruction' brought by innovation simultaneously reduces employment in the superseded occupations.

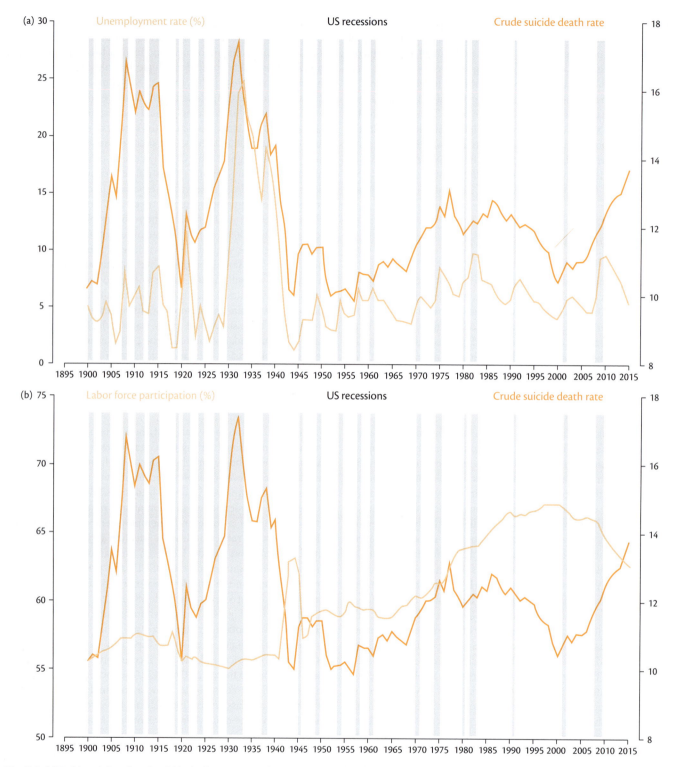

Fig. 18.2 (a) Positive relation of crude suicide death rate to unemployment rate over time, 1900–2015. Unemployment and suicide rate typically increase during recessions (shaded). Since 1980 the precise positive relation has diminished somewhat but remains highly significant. (b) Inverse relation of crude suicide death rate to labour force participation rate over time 1900–2015. The inverse relation has been relatively weak, but significant, before and during the Great Depression of the 1930s, but has become stronger after 1940 and is highly predictable since 1980.

Note: Shaded areas show recessions in the USA, 1900–2015.

This implies that unless new employment in innovative industries, at equivalent wage levels, quickly replaces obsolescent occupations, there will be a net long-term economic loss to the displaced workers and their mental and physical health. This is what has happened to lower-skilled occupational classes as a result of secular decline in manufacturing employment across much of the industrialized world. It has resulted from technological change and the movement of manufacturing jobs to Asia and Central America in the accelerated pattern of globalization [148].

In the current generation, this has now left us with a partly reconstructed social class system. The traditional 'working class' representing manufacturing and manual labour has been disappearing and its remnants are no longer a 'middle class'. This reconstituted class structure should be seen against the backdrop of the Great Recession and its subsequent policy responses involving decline in government spending on health and social protection, i.e. the 'austerity'. Additionally, many economists suggest that a post-Recession, longer-term decline in the rate of economic growth has prevented a return to the middle class-wage jobs that characterized much of the twentieth century.

Looming larger in the macroeconomic background is the very long-term increase in economic inequality that has been seen in nearly all industrialized societies' reconstitution of the 'middle class' [149]. Evidence provided by major economic organizations and independent authorities points to further decline in the rate of economic growth if economic inequality persists in accordance with its current trend [147]. This would mean that the enlarging income-wealth gap between the highest social classes and all others would tend to expand the differences in our current class structure and their implications for disparities in mental illness rates.

Alleviating the circular progression of psychological morbidity over the twenty-first century will require policies that foster sustainable economic growth and reduced economic inequality, especially through education and training oriented toward the lower-skilled social classes. But social protection, including unemployment insurance and retraining—referred to as active labour market policies—will also be essential to maintenance and enlargement of the skilled labour force. Equally crucial, however, will be further access to and sophistication of health care for mental disorders. In the present environment, this especially includes alcohol, drug abuse, opioid addiction, and violence.

References

1. Faris RE, Dunham HW. *Mental Disorders in Urban Areas: An Ecological Study of Schizophrenia and Other Psychoses*. Chicago, IL and London: The University of Chicago Press, 1939.
2. Brenner MH. *Mental Illness and the Economy*. Cambridge, MA: Harvard University Press, 1973.
3. Rothstein R. *Class and Schools: Using Social, Economic and Educational Reform to Close the Black–White Achievement Gap*. New York: Teachers College, Columbia University, 2004.
4. Erola J, Jalonen S, Lehti H. Parental education, class and income over early life course and children's achievement. *Res Soc Stratif Mobil* 2016; 44: 33–43.
5. Warner WL, Lunt PS. *The Social Life of a Modern Community*. New Haven, CT: Yale University Press, 1941.
6. Warner WL, Meeker M, Eells KL. *Social Class in America; A Manual of Procedure for the Measurement of Social Status*. Oxford: Science Research Associates, 1949.
7. Hollingshead AB, Redlich FC. *Social Class and Mental Illness: A Community Study*. New York: John Wiley, 1958.
8. Leighton AH. *My Name is Legion: Foundations for a Theory of Man in Relation to Culture*. New York: Basic Books, 1959.
9. Srole L, Langner TS, Michael ST, Opler MK, Rennie TA. *Mental Health in the Metropolis: The Midtown Manhattan Study*. New York: Blakiston Division, McGraw-Hill, 1962.
10. Kelly MP, Doohan E. The social determinants of health. In: Merson MH, Black RE, Mills AJ (eds). *Global Health: Diseases, Programs, Systems and Policies*, 3rd ed. Burlington, MA: Jones & Bartlett Learning, 2012, 75–114.
11. Baum A, Garofalo JP, Yali A. Socioeconomic status and chronic stress: does stress account for SES effects on health? *Ann N Y Acad Sci* 1999; 896: 131–144.
12. Cannon WB. *Bodily Changes in Pain, Hunger, Fear and Rage: An Account of Recent Researches Into the Function of Emotional Excitement*. New York: D. Appleton and Co., 1929.
13. Selye H. A syndrome produced by diverse nocuous agents. *Nature* 1936; 138: 32.
14. Selye H. The general adaptation syndrome and the diseases of adaptation 1. *J Clin Endocrinol Metab* 1946; 6: 117–230.
15. Holmes TH, Rahe RH. The social readjustment rating scale. *J Psychosom Res* 1967; 11: 213–218.
16. Kessler RC. Stress, social status, and psychological distress. *J Health Soc Behav* 1979; 20: 259–272.
17. Paykel ES, Myers JK, Dienelt MN, Klerman GL, Lindenthal JJ, Pepper MP. Life events and depression: a controlled study. *Arch Gen Psychiatry* 1969; 21: 753–760.
18. Myers JK, Lindenthal JJ, Pepper MP, Ostrander DR. Life events and mental status: a longitudinal study. *J Health Soc Behav* 1972; 13: 398–406.
19. Thoits PA. On merging identity theory and stress research. *Soc Psychol Q* 1991; 54: 101–112.
20. Dohrenwend BS, Dohrenwend BP. *Stressful Life Events: Their Nature and Effects*. New York: John Wiley & Sons, 1974.
21. Brenner MH. *Estimating the Social Costs of National Economic Policy: Implications for Mental and Physical Health, and Criminal Aggression: A Study Prepared for the use of the Joint Economic Committee, Congress of the United States*. Washington, DC: US Government Printing Office, 1976.
22. Brenner MH. Mortality and the national economy: a review, and the experience of England and Wales, 1936–76. *Lancet* 1979; 314: 568–573.
23. Brenner MH, Swank RT. Homicide and economic change: recent analyses of the Joint Economic Committee Report of 1984. *J Quant Criminol* 1986; 2: 81–103.
24. Brenner MH, Mooney A. Unemployment and health in the context of economic change. *Soc Sci Med* 1983; 17: 1125–1138.
25. Brenner MH. *Estimating the Effects of Economic Change on National Health and Social Well-being: A Study*. Washington, DC: US Government Printing Office, 1984.
26. Brenner MH. Economic change, alcohol consumption and heart disease mortality in nine industrialized countries. *Soc Sci Med* 1987; 25: 119–132.
27. Brenner MH. Commentary: Economic growth is the basis of mortality rate decline in the 20th century—experience of the United States 1901–2000. *Int J Epidemiol* 2005; 34: 1214–1221.
28. Catalano R, Goldman-Mellor S, Saxton K, et al. The health effects of economic decline. *Annu Rev Publ Health* 2011; 32: 431–450.
29. Dooley D, Catalano R, Wilson G. Depression and unemployment: panel findings from the Epidemiologic Catchment Area study. *Am J Community Psychol* 1994; 22: 745–765.
30. Kasl SV, Jones BA, The impact of job loss and retirement on health. In: Berkman LF, Kawachi I (eds). *Social Epidemiology*. Oxford: Oxford University Press, 2000, pp. 118–136.
31. Zivin K, Paczkowski M, Galea S. Economic downturns and population mental health: research findings, gaps, challenges and priorities. *Psychol Med* 2011; 41: 1343–1348.
32. Gallo WT, Bradley EH, Falba TA, et al. Involuntary job loss as a risk factor for subsequent myocardial infarction and stroke: findings from the Health and Retirement Survey. *Am J Ind Med* 2004; 45: 408–416.
33. Noelke C, Avendano M. Who suffers during recessions? Economic downturns, job loss, and cardiovascular disease in older Americans. *Am J Epidemiol* 2015; 182: 873–882.
34. Dupre ME, George LK, Liu G, Peterson ED. The cumulative effect of unemployment on risks for acute myocardial infarction. *Arch Intern Med* 2012; 172: 1731–1737.
35. Zagożdżon P, Parszuto J, Wrotkowska M, Dydjow-Bendek D. Effect of unemployment on cardiovascular risk factors and mental health. *Occup Med* 2014; 64: 436–441.

36. Janlert U, Asplund K, Weinehall L. Unemployment and cardiovascular risk indicators data from the MONICA survey in Northern Sweden. *Scand J Publ Health* 1992; 20: 14–18.

37. Naimi AI, Paquet C, Gauvin L, Daniel M. Associations between area-level unemployment, body mass index, and risk factors for cardiovascular disease in an urban area. *Int J Environ Res Publ Health* 2009; 6: 3082–3096.

38. Dooley D, Catalano R, Rook K, Serxner S. Economic stress and suicide: multilevel analyses. *Suicide Life Threat Behav* 1989; 19: 321–332.

39. Martin-Carrasco M, Evans-Lacko S, Dom G, et al. EPA guidance on mental health and economic crises in Europe. *Eur Arch Psychiatry Clin Neurosci* 2016; 266: 89–124.

40. Margerison-Zilko C, Goldman-Mellor S, Falconi A, Downing J. Health impacts of the Great Recession: a critical review. *Curr Epidemiol Rep* 2016; 3: 81–91.

41. World Health Organization. Impact of economic crises on mental health. Available at: www.euro.who.int/__data/assets/pdf_file/0008/134999/e94837.pdf (2011, accessed 23 December 2016).

42. Drydakis N. The effect of unemployment on self-reported health and mental health in Greece from 2008 to 2013: a longitudinal study before and during the financial crisis. *Soc Sci Med* 2015; 128: 43–51.

43. Economou M, Madianos M, Peppou LE, Patelakis A, Stefanis CN. Major depression in the era of economic crisis: a replication of a cross-sectional study across Greece. *J Affect Disord* 2013; 145: 308–314.

44. Urbanos-Garrido RM, Lopez-Valcarcel BG. The influence of the economic crisis on the association between unemployment and health: an empirical analysis for Spain. *Eur J Health Econ* 2015; 16: 175–184.

45. Gili M, Roca M, Basu S, McKee M, Stuckler D. The mental health risks of economic crisis in Spain: evidence from primary care centres, 2006 and 2010. *Eur J Publ Health* 2013; 23: 103–108.

46. Bartoll X, Palència L, Malmusi D, Suhrcke M, Borrell C. The evolution of mental health in Spain during the economic crisis. *Eur J Publ Health* 2014; 24: 415–418.

47. Andreeva E, Hanson LL, Westerlund H, Theorell T, Brenner MH. Depressive symptoms as a cause and effect of job loss in men and women: evidence in the context of organisational downsizing from the Swedish Longitudinal Occupational Survey of Health. *BMC Public Health* 2015; 15: 1045.

48. Brenner MH, Andreeva E, Theorell T, et al. Organizational downsizing and depressive symptoms in the European recession: the experience of workers in France, Hungary, Sweden and the United Kingdom. *PLOS ONE* 2014; 9: e97063.

49. Lee S, Guo WJ, Tsang A, et al. Evidence for the 2008 economic crisis exacerbating depression in Hong Kong. *J Affect Disord* 2010; 126: 125–133.

50. Sargent-Cox K, Butterworth P, Anstey KJ. The global financial crisis and psychological health in a sample of Australian older adults: a longitudinal study. *Soc Sci Med* 2011; 73: 1105–1112.

51. Buffel V, van de Straat V, Bracke P. Employment status and mental health care use in times of economic contraction: a repeated cross-sectional study in Europe, using a three-level model. *Int J Equity Health* 2015; 14: 29.

52. Reeves A, McKee M, Gunnell D, et al. Economic shocks, resilience, and male suicides in the Great Recession: cross-national analysis of 20 EU countries. *Eur J Public Health* 2015; 25: 404–409.

53. Astell-Burt T, Feng X. Health and the 2008 economic recession: evidence from the United Kingdom. *PLOS ONE* 2013; 8: e56674.

54. Katikireddi SV, Niedzwiedz CL, Popham F. Trends in population mental health before and after the 2008 recession: a repeat cross-sectional analysis of the 1991–2010 Health Surveys of England. *BMJ Open* 2012; 2: e001790.

55. Hyclak TJ, Meyerhoefer CD, Taylor LW. Older Americans' health and the Great Recession. *Rev Econ Househ* 2015; 13: 413–436.

56. Riumallo-Herl C, Basu S, Stuckler D, Courtin E, Avendano M. Job loss, wealth and depression during the Great Recession in the USA and Europe. *Int J Epidemiol* 2014; 43: 1508–1517.

57. McInerney M, Mellor JM, Nicholas LH. Recession depression: mental health effects of the 2008 stock market crash. *J Health Econ* 2013; 32: 1090–1104.

58. Lo CC, Cheng TC. Race, unemployment rate, and chronic mental illness: a 15-year trend analysis. *Soc Psychiatry Psychiatr Epidemiol* 2014; 49: 1119–1128.

59. Tsai AC. Home foreclosure, health, and mental health: a systematic review of individual, aggregate, and contextual associations. *PLOS ONE* 2015; 10: e0123182.

60. Downing J. The health effects of the foreclosure crisis and unaffordable housing: A systematic review and explanation of evidence. *Soc Sci Med* 2016; 162: 88–96.

61. Yilmazer T, Babiarz P, Liu F. The impact of diminished housing wealth on health in the United States: evidence from the Great Recession. *Soc Sci Med* 2015; 130: 234–241.

62. Burgard SA, Seefeldt KS, Zelner S. Housing instability and health: findings from the Michigan Recession and Recovery Study. *Soc Sci Med* 2012; 75: 2215–2224.

63. Osypuk TL, Caldwell CH, Platt RW, Misra DP. The consequences of foreclosure for depressive symptomatology. *Ann Epidemiol* 2012; 22: 379–387.

64. Houle JN. Mental health in the foreclosure crisis. *Soc Sci Med* 2014; 118: 1–8.

65. McLaughlin KA, Nandi A, Keyes KM, et al. Home foreclosure and risk of psychiatric morbidity during the recent financial crisis. *Psychol Med* 2012; 42: 1441–1448.

66. Cagney KA, Browning CR, Iveniuk J, English N. The onset of depression during the great recession: foreclosure and older adult mental health. *Am J Public Health* 2014; 104: 498–505.

67. Mendez-Bustos P, de Leon-Martinez V, Miret M, Baca-Garcia E, Lopez-Castroman J. Suicide reattempters: a systematic review. *Harvard Rev Psychiatry* 2013; 21: 281–295.

68. Brenner MH. Profound unhappiness in the international recession: the case of suicide in industrialized countries. In: Klein LR, Dalko V, Wang MH (eds). *Regulating Competition in Stock Markets: Antitrust Measures to Promote Fairness and Transparency Through Investor Protection and Crisis Prevention*. Hoboken, NJ: John Wiley & Sons, 2012, pp. 27–44.

69. Laanani M, Ghosn W, Jougla E, Rey G. Impact of unemployment variations on suicide mortality in Western European countries (2000–2010). *J Epidemiol Community Health* 2015; 69: 103–109.

70. Reeves A, McKee M, Stuckler D. Economic suicides in the great recession in Europe and North America. *Br J Psychiatry* 2014; 205: 246–247.

71. Phillips JA, Nugent CN. Suicide and the Great Recession of 2007–2009: the role of economic factors in the 50 US states. *Soc Sci Med* 2014; 116: 22–31.

72. Gemmill A, Falconi A, Karasek D, Hartig T, Anderson E, Catalano R. Do macroeconomic contractions induce or 'harvest' suicides? A test of competing hypotheses. *J Epidemiol Community Health* 2015; 69: 1071–1076.

73. Norström T, Grönqvist H. The Great Recession, unemployment and suicide. *J Epidemiol Community Health* 2015; 69: 110–116.

74. Corcoran P, Griffin E, Arensman E, Fitzgerald AP, Perry IJ. Impact of the economic recession and subsequent austerity on suicide and self-harm in Ireland: An interrupted time series analysis. *Int J Epidemiol* 2015; 44: 969–977.

75. Barr B, Taylor-Robinson D, Scott-Samuel A, McKee M, Stuckler D. Suicides associated with the 2008–10 economic recession in England: time trend analysis. *BMJ* 2012; 345: e5142.

76. Branas CC, Kastanaki AE, Michalodimitrakis M, et al. The impact of economic austerity and prosperity events on suicide in Greece: a 30-year interrupted time-series analysis. *BMJ Open* 2015; 5: e005619.

77. Fountoulakis KN, Savopoulos C, Siamouli M, et al. Trends in suicidality amid the economic crisis in Greece. *Eur Arch Psychiatry Clin Neurosci* 2013; 263: 441–444.

78. Economou M, Angelopoulos E, Peppou LE, Souliotis K, Stefanis C. Suicidal ideation and suicide attempts in Greece during the economic crisis: an update. *World Psychiatry* 2016; 15: 83–84.

79. Mäki N, Martikainen P. A register-based study on excess suicide mortality among unemployed men and women during different levels of unemployment in Finland. *J Epidemiol Community Health* 2012; 66: 302–307.

80. De Vogli R, Marmot M, Stuckler D. Excess suicides and attempted suicides in Italy attributable to the great recession. *J Epidemiol Community Health* 2013; 67: 378–379.

81. De Vogli R, Vieno A, Lenzi M. Mortality due to mental and behavioral disorders associated with the Great Recession (2008–10) in Italy: a time trend analysis. *Eur J Public Health* 2014; 24: 419–421.

82. Miret M, Caballero FF, Huerta-Ramírez R, et al. Factors associated with suicidal ideation and attempts in Spain for different age groups. Prevalence before and after the onset of the economic crisis. *J Affect Disord* 2014; 163: 1–9.

83. Bernal JA, Gasparrini A, Artundo CM, McKee M. The effect of the late 2000s financial crisis on suicides in Spain: an interrupted time-series analysis. *Eur J Public Health* 2013; 23: 732–736.

84. Garcy AM, Vågerö D. Unemployment and suicide during and after a deep recession: a longitudinal study of 3.4 million Swedish men and women. *Am J Public Health* 2013; 103: 1031–1038.

85. Saurina C, Bragulat B, Saez M, López-Casasnovas G. A conditional model for estimating the increase in suicides associated with the 2008–2010 economic recession in England. *J Epidemiol Community Health* 2013 67: 779–787.

86. Oskarsson H, Bjarnadottir S. Suicides and the economic crisis: the Icelandic experience. *Eur Psychiatry* 2013; 28: 1.

87. Goldman-Mellor SJ, Caspi A, Harrington H, et al. Suicide attempt in young people: a signal for long-term health care and social needs. *JAMA Psychiatry* 2014; 71: 119–127.

88. Chan CH, Caine ED, You S, Fu KW, Chang SS, Yip PS. Suicide rates among working-age adults in South Korea before and after the 2008 economic crisis. *J Epidemiol Community Health* 2014; 68: 246–252.

89. Koo J, Cox WM. An economic interpretation of suicide cycles in Japan. *Contemp Econ Policy* 2008; 26: 162–174.

90. Harper S, Charters TJ, Strumpf EC, Galea S, Nandi A. Economic downturns and suicide mortality in the USA, 1980–2010: observational study. *Int J Epidemiol* 2015; 44: 956–966.

91. Nandi A, Prescott MR, Cerdá M, Vlahov D, Tardiff KJ, Galea S. Economic conditions and suicide rates in New York City. *Am J Epidemiol* 2012; 175: 527–535.

92. Fowler KA, Gladden RM, Vagi KJ, Barnes J, Frazier L. Increase in suicides associated with home eviction and foreclosure during the US housing crisis: findings from 16 national violent death reporting system states, 2005–2010. *Am J Public Health* 2015; 105: 311–316.

93. Houle JN, Light MT. The home foreclosure crisis and rising suicide rates, 2005 to 2010. *Am J Public Health* 2014; 104: 1073–1079.

94. Meltzer H, Bebbington P, Brugha T, Farrell M, Jenkins R. The relationship between personal debt and specific common mental disorders. *Eur J Public Health* 2013; 23: 108–113.

95. Sweet E, Nandi A, Adam EK, McDade TW. The high price of debt: household financial debt and its impact on mental and physical health. *Soc Sci Med* 2013; 91: 94–100.

96. Jenkins R, Bebbington P, Brugha T, et al. Mental disorder in people with debt in the general population. *Public Health Med* 2009; 6: 88–92.

97. Meltzer H, Bebbington P, Brugha T, Jenkins R, McManus S, Dennis MS. Personal debt and suicidal ideation. *Psychol Med* 2011; 41: 771–778.

98. Richardson T, Elliott P, Roberts R. The relationship between personal unsecured debt and mental and physical health: a systematic review and meta-analysis. *Clin Psychol Rev* 2013; 33: 1148–1162.

99. Rimm EB, Klatsky A, Grobbee D, Stampfer MJ. Review of moderate alcohol consumption and reduced risk of coronary heart disease: is the effect due to beer, wine, or spirits? *BMJ* 1996; 312: 731–736.

100. Kaplan MS, Huguet N, Caetano R, Giesbrecht N, Kerr WC, McFarland BH. Economic contraction, alcohol intoxication and suicide: analysis of the National Violent Death Reporting System. *Inj Prev* 2015; 21: 35–41.

101. Dávalos ME, Fang H, French MT. Easing the pain of an economic downturn: macroeconomic conditions and excessive alcohol consumption. *Health Econ* 2012; 21: 1318–1335.

102. Mulia N, Zemore SE, Murphy R, Liu H, Catalano R. Economic loss and alcohol consumption and problems during the 2008 to 2009 US recession. *Alcoholism* 2014; 38: 1026–1034.

103. Vijayasiri G, Richman JA, Rospenda KM. The Great Recession, somatic symptomatology and alcohol use and abuse. *Addict Behav* 2012; 37: 1019–1024.

104. Zemore SE, Karriker-Jaffe KJ, Mulia N. Temporal trends and changing racial/ethnic disparities in alcohol problems: results from the 2000 to 2010 National Alcohol Surveys. *J Addict Res Ther* 2014; 4: 160.

105. Richman JA, Rospenda KM, Johnson TP, et al. Drinking in the age of the great recession. *J Addict Dis* 2012; 31: 158–172.

106. Dom G, Samochowiec J, Evans-Lacko S, Wahlbeck K, Van Hal G, McDaid D. The impact of the 2008 economic crisis on substance use patterns in the countries of the European Union. *Int J Environ Res Public Health* 2016; 13: 122.

107. Ásgeirsdóttir TL, Corman H, Noonan K, Ólafsdóttir Þ, Reichman NE. Was the economic crisis of 2008 good for Icelanders? Impact on health behaviors. *Econ Hum Biol* 2014; 13: 1–9.

108. Mattei G, Ferrari S, Pingani L, Rigatelli M. Short-term effects of the 2008 Great Recession on the health of the Italian population: an ecological study. *Soc Psychiatry Psychiatr Epidemiol* 2014; 49: 851–858.

109. Harhay MO, Bor J, Basu S, et al. Differential impact of the economic recession on alcohol use among white British adults, 2004–2010. *Eur J Public Health* 2014; 24: 410–415.

110. Storti CC, De Grauwe P, Sabadash A, Montanari L. Unemployment and drug treatment. *Int J Drug Policy* 2011; 22: 366–373.

111. Chalmers J, Ritter A. The business cycle and drug use in Australia: evidence from repeated cross-sections of individual level data. *Int J Drug Policy* 2011; 22: 341–352.

112. Lakhdar CB, Bastianic T. Economic constraint and modes of consumption of addictive goods. *Int J Drug Policy* 2011; 22: 360–365.

113. Almarsdóttir AB, Karlsdóttir ÁD, Gumundsson A, Halldórsson M, Gizurarson S. Did the fall of the Icelandic banks affect psychotropic drug use in the population? *Pharmacoepidemiol Drug Saf* 2011; 20: 87–88.

114. Zuccato E, Castiglioni S, Tettamanti M, et al. Changes in illicit drug consumption patterns in 2009 detected by wastewater analysis. *Drug Alcohol Depend* 2011; 118: 464–469.

115. Furtado C. The effect of the financial crisis in the use of psychotropics drugs in Portugal. *Pharmacoepidemiol Drug Saf* 2013; 22: 422–423.

116. Compton WM, Gfroerer J, Conway KP, Finger MS. Unemployment and substance outcomes in the United States 2002–2010. *Drug Alcohol Depend* 2014; 142: 350–353.

117. Arkes J. Recessions and the participation of youth in the selling and use of illicit drugs. *Int J Drug Policy* 2011; 22: 335–340.

118. National Bureau of Economic Research. Business Cycle Dating Committee, National Bureau of Economic Research. Available at: http://www.nber.org/cycles/sept2010.html (2010, accessed 12 December 2016).

119. National Bureau of Economic Research. US Business Cycles Expansions and Contractions. Available at: http://www.nber.org/cycles.html (2010, accessed 15 January 2017).

120. Mather M. Effects of the Great Recession on Older Americans' Health and Well-being. Available at: http://www.prb.org/Publications/Reports/2015/todays-research-aging-great-recession.aspx (2015, accessed 23 February 2018).

121. Reeves A, McKee M, Stuckler D. Economic suicides in the great recession in Europe and North America. *Br J Psychiatry* 2014; 205: 246–247.

122. Danziger S, Chavez K, Cumberworth E. *Poverty and the Great Recession.* Stanford, CA: Stanford Center on Poverty and Inequality, 2012.

123. Gutman A, Failing Economy, Failing Health. Available at: https://www.hsph.harvard.edu/magazine/magazine_article/failing-economy-failing-health/ (2014, accessed 15 December 2016).

124. Kawachi I, Kennedy BP, Lochner K, Prothrow-Stith D. Social capital, income inequality, and mortality. *Am J Public Health* 1997; 87: 1491–1498.

125. Smeeding T. Income Wealth and Debt and the Great Recession. Available at: https://web.stanford.edu/group/recessiontrends/cgi-bin/web/sites/all/themes/barron/pdf/IncomeWealthDebt_fact_sheet.pdf (2012, accessed 20 October 2016).

126. Perri F. Inequality, Recessions and Recoveries. Available at: https://www.minneapolisfed.org/publications/the-region/inequality-recessions-and-recoveries (2013, accessed 15 December 2016).

127. Pfeffer FT, Danziger S, Schoeni RF. Wealth disparities before and after the Great Recession. *Ann Am Acad Polit Sci* 2013; 650: 98–123.

128. Report by the U.S. Congress Joint Economic Committee. Income Inequality and the Great Recession. Available at: http://www.jec.senate.gov/public/_cache/files/91975589-257c-403b-8093-8f3b584a088c/income-inequality-brief-fall-2010-cmb-and-ces.pdf (2010, accessed 5 December 2016).

129. Aghion P, Caroli E, García-Peñalosa C. Inequality and Economic Growth: The Perspective of the New Growth Theories. Available at: http://nrs.harvard.edu/urn-3:HUL.InstRepos:12502063 (1999, accessed 23 January 2017).

130. Cingano F. Trends in Income Inequality and its Impact on Economic Growth. Available at: http://www.oecd-ilibrary.org/social-issues-migration-health/trends-in-income-inequality-and-its-impact-on-economic-growth_5jxrjncwxv6j-en (2014, accessed 23 February 2018).

131. Dabla-Norris E, Kochhar K, Suphaphilphat N., Tsounta E. Causes and Consequences of Income Inequality: A Global Perspective. Available at: https://www.imf.org/external/pubs/ft/sdn/2015/sdn1513.pdf (2015, accessed 12 October 2016).

132. Stiglitz JE. Inequality and economic growth. *Political Q* 2015; 86: 134–155.

133. Greenstone M, Looney A. Unemployment and Earning Losses: A Look at Long-Term Impacts of the Great Recession on American Workers. Available at: https://www.brookings.edu/blog/jobs/2011/11/04/unemployment-and-earnings-losses-a-look-at-long-term-impacts-of-the-great-recession-on-american-workers/ (2011, accessed 10 December 2016).

134. Faber H. Job Loss in the Great Recession: Historical Perspective from the Displaced Workers Survey, 1984–2010. Available at: http://www.nber.org/papers/w17040 (2011, accessed 6 October 2016).

135. World Health Organization. Depression. Available at: http://www.who.int/mediacentre/factsheets/fs369/en/ (2016, accessed 23 February 2018).

136. Oquendo MA, Galfalvy H, Russo S, et al. Prospective study of clinical predictors of suicidal acts after a major depressive episode in patients with major depressive disorder or bipolar disorder. *Am J Psychiatry* 2004; 161: 1433–1441.

137. Nelson JC, Spyker DA, Morbidity and mortality associated with medications used in the treatment of depression: an analysis of cases reported to U.S. Poison Control Centers, 2000–2014. *Am J Psychiatry* 2017; 174: 438–450.

138. Reeves A, Stuckler D, McKee M, Gunnell D, Chang SS, Basu S. Increase in state suicide rates in the USA during economic recession. *Lancet* 2012; 380: 1813–1814.

139. European Commission. Actions against depression. Available at: http://ec.europa.eu/health/ph_determinants/life_style/mental/docs/depression_en.pdf (2004, accessed 23 February 2018).

140. Brenner MH. Impact of unemployment on heart disease and stroke mortality in European Union countries. Available at: http://ec.europa.eu/social/main.jsp?catId=738&langId=en&pubId=7909&furtherPubs=yes (2016, accessed 23 February 2018).

141. Stuckler D, Basu S. *The Body Economic Why Austerity Kills. Philadelphia*. PA: Basic Books, 2013.

142. Fazi T. How Austerity Has Crippled The European Economy–In Numbers. Available at: https://www.socialeurope.eu/2016/03/austerity-crippled-european-economy-numbers/ (2016, accessed 23 February 2018).

143. Cholera R, Pence BW, Bengtson AM, et al. Mind the gap: gaps in antidepressant treatment, treatment adjustments, and outcomes among patients in routine HIV care in a multisite U.S. clinical cohort. *PLOS ONE* 2017; 12: e0166435.

144. Wilkinson RG, Marmot M. *Social Determinants of Health*, 2nd ed. Oxford: Oxford University Press, 2006.

145. Gonzalez JS, Batchelder AW, Psaros C, Safren SA. Depression and HIV/AIDS treatment nonadherence: a review and meta-analysis. *J Acquir Immune Syndr* 2011; 58: 181–187.

146. Nakash O, Levav I, Aguilar-Gaxiola S, et al. Comorbidity of common mental disorders with cancer and their treatment gap: findings from the World Mental Health Surveys. *Psychooncology* 2014; 23: 40–51.

147. Joint Economic Committee Congress of the United States on the 2016 Economic Report of the President. Available at: http://www.jec.senate.gov/public/_cache/files/0db793da-5e90-4f9d-ad9e-487f28652c7a/3-2-2016-joint-economic-report-w-minority-views-final.pdf (2016, accessed 23 February 2018).

148. Autor DH, Dorn D, Hanson GH. The China shock: learning from labor-market adjustment to large changes in trade. *Annu Rev Econ* 2016; 8: 205–240.

149. Stiglitz JE. *The Price of Inequality: How Today's Divided Society Endangers Our Future*, 1st ed. New York: WW Norton, 2012.

CHAPTER 19

The social determinants of mental health

Kamaldeep Bhui

Introduction

Public health is defined by the UK's Faculty of Public Health as 'the science and art of promoting and protecting health and well being, preventing ill-health and prolonging life through the organised efforts of society'. This approach locates the causes of ill health and the remedial actions in society, at the level of populations outside, although inclusive, of formal health services. It is well established that healthy societies include strong interpersonal relationships that are supportive, offer protections and opportunities, and contribute to social fabric through forming trusting relationships; society works towards improving material conditions, and levels of activity that provide purpose and meaning, as well as physical fitness. Personal agency and collective contributions to society contribute to one's own sense of purpose and agency (and therefore empowerment) in the collective effort, and personal well-being is thus maximized. Public health interventions are intended to be population based, and span across sectors, in partnership with the public healthcare agencies, local government, transport hubs, law enforcement, housing agencies, schools, and those responsible for green space and clean air. Public health approaches seek to take all private and public measures to prevent disease, promote health and prolong life among the population as a whole [1]. The public health approach aims to reduce the burden of disease through population-level interventions. This can involve changes to legislation, for example banning smoking in public places to reduce the hazards of secondary smoking [2], or some targeted approaches, for example cross-government suicide prevention strategy [3].

What are the social determinants of poor mental health?

The social determinants of ill health have been highlighted in the UK since the early 1980s, with the publication of the Black Report [4]. Despite the clear links between social inequalities and causes of sickness and consequent shortened and blighted lives, little progress has been made [5, 6]. Different policies and idioms of action have been seen over the decades, with the most recent being alignment of action with Millennium Development Goals, and, in the UK, acknowledgement of the need to promote positive actions to minimize disabilities and offer opportunities for all [7].

Over 90% of our health is determined by lifetime physical, behavioural, social, and environmental factors rather than the consequences of healthcare services. Relevent factors include poor nutrition, excessive alcohol use, smoking nicotine-based tobacco and illegal drug use, poor levels of physical inactivity, traumas such as adverse childhood experiences and violence, poor education, food insecurity, poor housing quality, unemployment, and discrimination [8, 9]. Experiences of adversity are also gendered, and specific adversities are evident in childhood and at times of war and conflict [10–12]. Solutions include school-based programmes for children, as well as actions to ensure a fairer society emerges in which all people have chances for education and success, and are protected from adversity [12, 13]. There are significant opportunities to ensure preventive actions are provided in a timely way, to realize maximum health and economic gains over the life course [14]; yet these have been rather undermined owing to the need for immediate resources with significant delay in realizing such gains, which is rather inconvenient for governments making the investment as they cannot demonstrate success within their term of office.

Social determinants of inequalities remain of great importance for health consequences. For example, Michael Marmot's recent work highlights how almost all health indices in the population are subject to the influence of structural disadvantage [15, 16]. For example, mothers living in mixed- or high- rather than low-status neighbourhoods have a 65% lower risk of having no friends in the neighbourhood and a 41% lower risk of depression or anxiety [17]. Large income differences have damaging health and social consequences, and in most countries social inequality is increasing [18]. Income inequality appears to produce social stratification for critical periods of development in the life course, especially in children, and so could explain between-country differences in income and inter-country differences in health status as a function of social stratification [19]. So health-risk behaviours, smoking, exercise, educational progression, and drug and alcohol use are all targeted as behavioural and lifestyle causes of ill health, but these are patterned by social status and poverty.

However, intervention requires that we understand mechanisms to intervene in society, the real world, not in a laboratory or in an artificial setting of a carefully orchestrated trial with restrictive criteria for who does and does not enter the trial, so limiting applicability of trials in the real world. This includes not only health professionals and agencies, but interventions around the political economy and structure in society, including sources of power imbalance.

The 2016 report of Bramley et al. [20] on poverty and its impacts on health concludes that:

◆ health care accounts for the largest portion of additional public spending associated with poverty (approximately £29 billion per year);

◆ healthcare use and costs are strongly related to immediate and historical poverty;

◆ around a quarter of all spending in acute hospital care together with spend in primary care can be attributed to greater use of these services by people in poverty.

The evidence suggests poverty and other social determinants of poor physical and mental health are driven by the circumstances into which people are born, grow up, live, work, and grow old. These circumstances are, in turn, shaped by a wider set of forces such as economics, social policies, and politics. As social determinants are modifiable, influence health outcomes many years later, and might be the most effective targets for preventive interventions, they need action alongside structural interventions to break the intergenerational cycles of inequality [21].

Brain, mind, and body in a social context

One of the unhelpful distinctions made in scientific discourse is the notion that mind and body are somehow separate entities and that they exist in isolation from one another; that medical or physical diseases are not the same as mental or psychiatric diseases, as these lack a measureable pathophysiology. The assumption here is that social and psychological markers are insufficient as a basis of defining illness and disease, and only biomarkers legitimize the existence of illness, the sick role, and need for health intervention. At the same time, the social experience and construction of illness and wellness for accepted medical diseases/disorders with biomarkers are neglected.

Although the Royal College of Psychiatrists' campaign on 'parity of esteem' appears to challenge stigma and frank discrimination against mental disorders, it also reflects societal failures to address interactions between medical disease/illnesses and the social nexus in which these arise, through interaction with biology. This is the case for both physical conditions and psychiatric conditions. Depression shows a 2–3-fold risk of both heart disease and cancer, and there is reverse causality of a similar magnitude [22, 23].

Explanations for why these co-morbidities occur and what we should do to prevent them invoke notions of greater total disease burden that arises in the context of poor environments with material and social disadvantages. Failed efforts to address these multiple disadvantages are captured in the term 'wicked diseases', where the causes are multiple, persistent, and forever changing and the solutions have also to be equally 'wicked' [24]. Merrill Singer coined the term 'syndemic' as a useful way of thinking about, measuring and treating multiple social causes and diseases that are connected through interactive social and biological vulnerabilities [25]. For example, this approach has been applied in gay and bisexual men and Hispanic people with HIV, and exposures to violence and discrimination [26, 27]. The 'expression' of a particular disease

depends on the precise individual biological, social, and psychological expressions of vulnerabilities and coping. A clustering of illnesses is shaped by geographical spaces in which material deprivation also clusters, providing a potent mixture of an unequal, unhealthy, and substantially less resilient or successful locale.

This perspective emphasizes that health and illness are social, as well as medical, issues. Smoking, obesity, and road traffic accidents cause obvious medical issues such as chronic obstructive pulmonary disease, heart disease/diabetes, and trauma, respectively. Individually, the medical problems caused by these behaviours all have established evidence based treatment regimes. Conversely, the individual choice to indulge in certain behaviours and the social environment that permits these choices remain an underutilized pathway of reducing harmful behaviour. That is, the way that the social contingencies within which an individual chooses to act could be targeted to change influences on individual decisions.

This requires measuring intersectional impacts and contextual determinants of risk factors associated with different life stages, by gender and ethnic group, income, employment, and for children in care, ethnic and migrant populations, offenders, homeless people and those with unstable housing, and people who identify themselves as lesbian, gay, bisexual, and transgender [28–33]. These groups share exclusion, a lack of social and political agency, and experiences of stigma and discrimination (see Chapter 52).

Tackling inequity

Economic inequality continues to drive different patterns of socio-economic disadvantage, poor health, and premature mortality [13]. Economically, wealth is linked to health, with increased debt resulting in more mental disorder [34]. Suicides in England are rising and the prominent explanation is of financial crisis, unemployment, social isolation, and a breakdown in coping and social support [35]. Living in a safe environment free from discrimination and violence improves mental health [36], but interventions to improve social capital need funding models that work across sectors [37]. Reducing inequality is arguably a matter of fairness and social justice as a core value of society, however, there is a cost. Difficulties remain in targeting the poorest in society in order to reduce inequality, with those better off often benefitting proportionally more [38]. Proportionate universalism has been recommended by the World Health Organization [39], but applying this in practice creates tensions between preventive population interventions and those focused on the most unwell. Social factors are often included in treatment packages. However, this individual-level intervention overlooks the systemic and structures sources of ill health and tackling social determinants can not be successful unless focused at the broader societal and health economic, and the structures and processes by which people flourish, develop social capital, ward of misfortune and poor health and by which they collective take action to remove structural and institutional sources of injustice and inequality. Within this context, greater personal responsibility to manage ill health must work alongside more active engagement and interventions within industries responsible for food, alcohol, and smoking, and agencies with influence over green space and leisure, the psychosocial work environment, and the management of exposures to adversity, conflict, war, and trauma.

References

1. Kindig DA. Understanding Population Health Terminology. *Milbank Q* 2007; 85: 139–161.

2. Myers DN, He J. Cardiovascular effect of bans on smoking in public places. *J Am Coll Cardiol* 2009; 54: 1249–1255.

3. HM Government. Preventing suicide in England: a cross-government outcomes strategy to save lives. Available at: https://www.gov.uk/government/uploads/system/uploads/attachment_data/file/430720/Preventing-Suicide-.pdf (2012, accessed 25 February 2018). .

4. Gray AM. Inequalities in health. The Black Report: a summary and comment. *Int J Health Serv* 1982; 12: 349–80.

5. Smith GD, Bartley M, Blane D. The Black report on socioeconomic inequalities in health 10 years on. *BMJ* 1990; 301: 373–377.

6. Sim F, Mackie P. Health inequalities: the Black Report after 25 years. *Public Health* 2006; 120: 185–186.

7. Battams S. Editorial: Public mental health policy, mental health promotion, and interventions which focus on the social determinants of mental health. *Front Public Health* 2016; 4: 285.

8. Sederer LI. The social determinants of mental health. *Psychiatr Serv* 2016; 67: 234–235.

9. Alexander K. Social determinants of methadone in pregnancy: violence, social capital, and mental health. *Issues Ment Health Nurs* 2013; 34: 747–751.

10. Stewart DE. Social determinants of women's mental health. *J Psychosom Res* 2007; 63: 223–224.

11. Kohrt BA, Jordans MJ, Tol WA, et al. Social ecology of child soldiers: child, family, and community determinants of mental health, psychosocial well-being, and reintegration in Nepal. *Transcult Psychiatry* 2010; 47: 727–753.

12. Yearwood EL. The social determinants of health and mental health: global foundations for improving child and family mental health. *J Child Adolesc Psychiatr Nurs* 2010; 23: 196–197.

13. Marmot MA, Goldblatt J, Boyce P, McNeish T, Grady D, Geddes M. I. Fair Society, Healthy Lives. Strategic Review of Health Inequalities in England post-2010. Available at: http://www.parliament.uk/documents/fair-society-healthy-lives-full-report.pdf (accessed 25 February 2018).

14. Campion J, Bhugra D, Bailey S, Marmot M. Inequality and mental disorders: opportunities for action. *Lancet* 2013; 382: 183–184.

15. Marmot M, Bell R. Social inequalities in health: a proper concern of epidemiology. *Ann Epidemiol* 2016; 26: 238–240.

16. Marmot M. Social determinants of health inequalities. *Lancet* 2005; 365: 1099–1104.

17. Albor C, Uphoff EP, Stafford M, Ballas D, Wilkinson RG, Pickett KE. The effects of socioeconomic incongruity in the neighbourhood on social support, self-esteem and mental health in England. *Soc Sci Med* 2014; 111: 1–9.

18. Pickett KE, Wilkinson RG. Income inequality and health: a causal review. *Soc Sci Med* 2015; 128: 316–326.

19. Wilkinson R, Pickett K. The problems of relative deprivation: why some societies do better than others. *Soc Sci Med* 2007; 65: 13.

20. Bramley G, Hirsch D, Littlewood M, Watkins D. Counting the cost of UK poverty. Available at: https://www.jrf.org.uk/report/counting-cost-uk-poverty (2016, accessed 25 February 2018).

21. Marmot M. Health in an unequal world. *Lancet* 2006; 368: 2081–2094.

22. Jiang W, Krishnan RR, O'Connor CM. Depression and heart disease: evidence of a link, and its therapeutic implications. *CNS Drugs* 2002; 16: 111–127.

23. Charlson FJ, Stapelberg NJ, Baxter AJ, Whiteford HA. Should global burden of disease estimates include depression as a risk factor for coronary heart disease? *BMC Med* 2011; 9: 47.

24. Petticrew M, Tugwell P, Welch V, et al. Better evidence about wicked issues in tackling health inequities. *J Public Health (Oxf)* 2009; 31: 453–456.

25. Singer M. Pathogen-pathogen interaction: a syndemic model of complex biosocial processes in disease. *Virulence* 2010; 1: 10–18.

26. Egan JE, Frye V, Kurtz SP, et al. Migration, neighborhoods, and networks: approaches to understanding how urban environmental conditions affect syndemic adverse health outcomes among gay, bisexual and other men who have sex with men. *AIDS Behav* 2011; 15(Suppl. 1): S35–S50.

27. Gonzalez-Guarda RM, Florom-Smith AL, Thomas T. A syndemic model of substance abuse, intimate partner violence, HIV infection, and mental health among Hispanics. *Public Health Nurs* 2011; 28: 366–378.

28. Ghavami N, Katsiaficas D, Rogers LO. Toward an intersectional approach in developmental science: the role of race, gender, sexual orientation, and immigrant status. *Adv Child Dev Behav* 2016; 50: 31–73.

29. Vinnerljung B, Hjern A, Lindblad F. Suicide attempts and severe psychiatric morbidity among former child welfare clients—a national cohort study. *J Child Psychol Psychiatry* 2006; 47: 723–733.

30. Bhui K MK. Suicide rates in people of South Asian origin in England and Wales 1993–2003. *Br J Psychiatry* 2008; 193: 406–409.

31. Eynan R, Langley J, Tolomiczenko G, et al. The association between homlessness and suicidal ideation and behaviours: results of a cross-sectional survey. *Suicide Life Threat Behav* 2011; 32: 418–427.

32. Fazel S, Yu, R. Psychotic disorders and repeat offending: systematic review and meta-analysis. *Schizophr Bulle* 2011; 37: 800–810.

33. Chakraborty Aea. Mental health of the non-heterosexual population of England. *Br J Psychiatry* 2011; 198: 143–148.

34. Jenkins Rea. Debt, income and mental disorder in the general population. *Psychol Med* 2008; 38: 1485–1493.

35. Barr B, Taylor-Robinson D, Scott-Samuel A, McKee M, Stuckler D. Suicides associated with the 2008-2010 economic recession in England: time trend analysis. *BMJ* 2012; 345: e5142.

36. Lindert JL, I. *Violence and Mental Health—Its Manifold Faces*. Berlin: Springer, 2015.

37. De Silva MJ, McKenzie K, Harpham T, Huttly SR. Social capital and mental illness: a systematic review. *J Epidemiol Community Health* 2005; 59: 619–627.

38. Barat LM, Palmer N, Basu S, Worrall E, Hanson K, Mills A. Do malaria control interventions reach the poor? A view through the equity lens. *Am J Trop Med Hyg* 2004; 71: 174–178.

39. World Health Organization. Social determinants of mental health. Available at: http://www.who.int/mental_health/publications/gulbenkian_paper_social_determinants_of_mental_health/en/ (accessed 25 February 2018).

CHAPTER 20

Social determinants in low-income countries

Syed Masud Ahmed and Mohammad Didar Hossain

Introduction: mental health scenario in low-income countries

The global population is living longer, thanks to the spectacular development of curative medicine [1], but with more morbidities and disabilities, of which mental health disorders constitute an important component. According to Global Burden of Diseases 2013 study, of the top-10 diseases major depressive disorder (MDD) ranked third in 1990 but second in 2013 [2]. Besides developed regions of the world, interestingly, MDD also ranked second in South Asia, North Africa, and the Middle East, and first in Sub-Saharan Africa. Globally, mental and substance abuse disorders together accounted for 21% of the years lived with disability versus 28.5% in 2010 [2]. Gender divide in mental disorders was also prominent, with MDD and anxiety being more common among women. Since the publication of World Health Report 2001 [3], mental health disorders is increasingly being recognized as an important public health problem. To address this, an action plan has been prepared based on available evidence related to vulnerabilities and risk factors for the disadvantaged population [4].

There is a lack of regular, up-to-date, and comprehensive population-based data on the mental health situation in the low-income countries of Asia and Africa. Moreover, in most instances, data from low- and middle-income countries are combined in different studies and reports. Whatever data are available, from local or national levels, a dismal scenario is presented. For example, a recent systematic review of the mental health situation in Bangladesh found the prevalence of mental disorders to be high (6.5–31.0% in adults and 13.4–22.9% in children) but largely under-recognized and under-reported owing to stigma associated with mental health illnesses [5]. A systematic review of published literature in Pakistan found the prevalence of anxiety and depressive disorders to be 34% [6]. In another systematic review of community-based epidemiological studies in India, the prevalence of mental disorders was found to be 190–200 per 1000 of the population, or around 20% of the population [7]. Other studies from India found the prevalence of mental disorders to vary from as low as < 5% in the general population to 9.4% in children and adolescents to as high as 26.7% among the elderly [8]. Data from a nationally representative sample in Nepal revealed the prevalence of anxiety and depression to be 16.1% and 4.2%, respectively, and anxiety–depression co-morbidity to be 5.9% [9].

In sub-Saharan Africa, a systematic review of published literature on childhood mental health disorders found the prevalence of any psychological disorder to be around 14.5% (among those aged ≤16 years) [10]. Another study from the same region, found the prevalence of depression symptoms and major depression among HIV-positive individuals on antiretroviral therapy to be quite high (31.2% and 18%, respectively) [11]. In a nationally representative epidemiological survey from South Africa, the most common mental health disorders were found to be agoraphobia (4.8%), MDD (4.9%), and alcohol abuse or dependence (4.5%) [12]. In Zimbabwe, common mental disorders (CMD) and depression were quite high in its high HIV/AIDS-prevalent population [13]. In the Yoruba-speaking population of Nigeria, the lifetime prevalence of anxiety disorder was found to be 5.7%, MDD was found to be 3.3%, and the prevalence of alcohol abuse to be 2.8% [14]. Mental health disorders are common among Moroccans: the prevalence of anxiety disorder was found to be 37% and that of major depression to be 26.5% [15]. A household survey in five regions of Egypt found mental health disorders prevalence of 16.9% among the population surveyed [16]. Of these, anxiety disorders was found to have a prevalence of 4.8%, depression disorders of 6.4%, and combined prevalence of 4.7%.

Social determinants of mental health in low-income countries

According to the World Health Organization, mental health is 'a state of well-being in which every individual realizes his or her own potential, can cope with the normal stresses of life, can work productively and fruitfully, and is able to make a contribution to her or his community.' As is evident from the previous section, mental health disorders are also becoming an increasingly important public health problem in low-income countries, thanks to the fallouts from the very competitive globalized economy, as well as the sociopolitcal instability that is a spin-off of the former. The magnitude of the problem is reflected in the call for 'the promotion, protection and restoration' of mental health so that we can 'think, emote, interact with each other, earn a living and enjoy life' [17].

Besides biological and psychological factors, various social, economic, and environmental factors ('conditions in which people are born, grow, live, work, and age') also come into play to determine mental health status, together called the 'social determinant of mental health'. These determinants act throughout the life cycle starting from *in utero* to old age: 'beginning before birth and progressing into early childhood, older childhood and adolescence, during family building and working ages, and through to older age' [17]. These determinants or risk factors for disorder(s) of mental health include poverty and exclusion, education, gender and violence, employment status, work and living environment, and social capital. A poor socio-economic and education status, being female, being in low-paid irregular employment or unemployment/hidden unemployment, having an unhealthy working and living environment with air, water, soil, and sound pollution, and having non-genial relationships and poor social capital make a perfect recipe for poor mental health.

Poverty, exclusion, education, and mental health

In low- and middle-income countries (LAMICs), poverty and exclusion are intimately associated with common mental health disorders, such as anxiety and depression. Poverty results in economic deprivation, income inequalities, and poor levels of education, and thus a low probability of gainful employment and a high probability of indebtedness [18], ultimately leading to mental disorders. Gainful employment and indebtedness are part of a vicious cycle: poverty perpetuates mental disorders and the latter interferes with engagement in productive activities and income-earning, therefore exacerbating poverty. Also, in LAMICs, between 40% and 50% of mental health care costs are borne out of pocket, which further impoverishes the individual and the family [19].

The prevalence of mental disorders usually follows a social gradient: compared with others, the poor and the disadvantaged groups suffer disproportionately from mental disorders and the adverse consequences [20]. But the strength of the association between poverty and mental health disorders varies according to which particular dimension of poverty is measured [18]. Again, others argue that it is not the level of poverty, but changes in life circumstances, such as onset of severe illness (e.g. cancer), that has a greater impact on mental health [21]. Still others think it to be due to measurement errors [22]. The significant role of poverty in initiating/perpetuating/precipitating mental health disorders is well established in small-scale studies from low-income Asian countries like Bangladesh [5], India [23, 24], Pakistan [6, 25], and Indonesia [26], and countries in Sub-Saharan Africa, such as Kenya [27], and Zambia, Ghana, and Uganda [28].

Education is important for mental health in low-income countries as a lack of education may be a proxy for lack of opportunity or low socio-economic status [29]. Like poverty, this inverse relationship between education level and mental disorders is found to be strong in studies from LAMICs in South Asia and Latin America [29, 30], comparable with what has been observed in high-income European countries [31, 32].

Unemployment and mental health

Unemployment is both a consequence and a cause of illness, including mental illness [33]. Unemployment leads to deterioration of both physical and mental health including suicide [34], and long-term unemployment causes a higher burden of mental illnesses than short-term unemployment, with the burden of illness increasing with the duration of unemployment [33]. It has been found that unemployment leaves a long-term 'scarring effect' on the mental health of the individual [35]. A meta-analysis of 237 cross-sectional and 87 longitudinal studies found the prevalence of psychological problems to be higher (34%) among the unemployed than the employed (16%) [36], which was also found by Lund et al. [19] in a systematic review of 115 studies. This deleterious effect of unemployment on mental health is especially prominent in countries with a low level of economic development, including the absence of an appropriate safety net for the unemployed [36]. The effect of unemployment on mental health status, for example stress level is mediated by factors such as subsequent income loss and poverty, and stigma and social isolation [37].

Work environment and mental health

Work or engagement in gainful activities can be beneficial for an individual's overall well-being, including mental well-being, especially if the work environment is favourable and the supervision is good. It is also identified with providing one with sense of purpose and social identity, and opportunities for personal development, which, again, is crucial for mental well-being [38]. In an organizational environment, issues such as 'overwork, lack of clear instructions, unrealistic deadlines, lack of decision-making, job insecurity, isolated working conditions, surveillance, and inadequate child-care arrangements' produce job stress, and consequent CMD and reduced productivity, especially in low-income settings [39, 40].

Living environment and mental health

A healthy environment and living arrangement is essential for better health, including mental health [41]. External environment may determine exposure to various physical, biological, or chemical pollutants, producing health effects such as accidents/injury (direct) and bronchial asthma from air pollution (indirect) [42]. Housing or built environment has effects on mental health, either directly (e.g. increasing psychological distress) or indirectly (e.g. altering psychosocial processes with known mental health affects), through elevating the stress level and its consequences [43]. This is especially important for poor and disadvantaged people in urban slums (resulting from massive rural–urban migration and rapid urbanization in low-income countries) [44, 45].

Gender, violence, and mental health

Women's experiences of social, economic, and environmental factors are different from those of men, including the level of stress of everyday life, and, as such, they tend to have higher levels of CMD (e.g. depression) than men [46], at every level of household income [47]. Also, society's negative attitude towards mental disorders, i.e. stigma [48], is more dominant in the case of women, which interferes with their connectivity with society at large [49, 50].

Violence against women and children and its consequences, including mental disorders, is an important public health problem in LAMICs [51]. This is especially true for a specific from of violence: intimate partner violence [52]. Depression during pregnancy, both ante- and postnatally, is very common in women in low-income countries and affects infant and child growth and nutritional status [53]. Violence/intimate partner violence has been implicated for all forms of mental disorders (anxiety, depression, suicide attempts, and post-traumatic stress disorder) in low-income countries like Bangladesh [54], Rwanda [55], Ghana [56], and India [57].

Social capital and mental health

Social capital plays a significant role in people's health and well-being in resource-poor settings, for example in LAMICs [58]. It works both as a source of health information in times of need and also as a safety net in the absence of formal financial resources [59]. However, much less importance is given to the study of social capital as an important determinant of health (including mental health) in low-income countries. There is an inverse relationship between levels of social capital and occurrence of CMD in times of peace and disaster [60, 61]. The individual level of social capital (e.g. level of trust and harmony in society) in women and men has been shown to be inversely associated with CMD in diverse low-income settings, such as Peru, Ethiopia, Vietnam, and Andhra Pradesh of India [62], Bangladesh [63], and Vietnam [64]. Besides self-health, the social capital of women is also related to child nutritional status in low-income countries [65].

Conclusions

CMD such as anxiety and depression are relatively common among the populations of low-income countries in South Asia and Sub-Saharan Africa. CMD are proportionately more prevalent among women in these countries owing to the women's vulnerable and precarious position in society. Social attitude towards CMD also complicates the situation and hinders access to care, especially for women. Other marginalized populations such as ethnic and religious minorities also have a greater preponderance of CMD compared with others.

Beside biological and psychological factors, various socio-economic and environmental factors also play a significant role in precipitating/initiating CMD, throughout the life cycle. This is especially true in the case of women, owing to the patriarchal nature of societies across low-income countries. Significant social determinants influencing mental health and well-being include poverty and exclusion; illiteracy/semi-literacy; unemployment/underemployment; unhygienic work and living environment; gender, stigma, and violence; and relationships and network, for example social capital. The association is not always straightforward: sometimes, the social determinants act in a vicious circle like poverty and CMD, which, in turn, is exacerbated in situations of low level of education and unemployment.

However, for people of low-income countries, poverty is all pervasive and affects physical, as well as mental, health in various ways. Any attempt to ameliorate mental illnesses calls for attention to be paid to these important social determinants and take appropriate measures to overcome adverse conditions.

References

1. Nolte E, Mckee M. Does health care save lives? Avoidable mortality revisited. Available at: http://www.nuffieldtrust.org.uk/sites/files/nuffield/publication/does-healthcare-save-lives-mar04.pdf (2004, accessed 26 February 2018).
2. Vos T, Barber RM, Bell B, et al. Global, regional, and national incidence, prevalence, and years lived with disability for 301 acute and chronic diseases and injuries in 188 countries, 1990–2013: a systematic analysis for the Global Burden of Disease Study 2013. *Lancet* 2015; 386: 743–800.
3. World Health Organization (WHO). *The World Health Report 2001: Mental Health: New Understanding, New Hope.* Geneva: WHO, 2001.
4. World Health Organization (WHO). *Mental Health Action Plan 2013–2020.* Geneva: WHO, 2013.
5. Hossain MD, Ahmed HU, Chowdhury WA, Niessen LW, Alam DS. Mental disorders in Bangladesh: a systematic review. *BMC Psychiatry* 2014; 14: 216.
6. Mirza I, Jenkins R. Risk factors, prevalence, and treatment of anxiety and depressive disorders in Pakistan: systematic review. *BMJ* 2004; 328: 794.
7. Math SB, Srinivasaraju R. Indian psychiatric epidemiological studies: learning from the past. *Indian J Psychiatry* 2010; 52(Suppl. S3): 95–103.
8. VenkatashivaReddy B, Gupta A, Lohiya A, Kharya P. Mental health issues and challenges in India: a review. *Int If Sci Res Publ* 2013; 3: 1–3.
9. Risal A, Manandhar K, Linde M, Steiner TJ, Holen A. Anxiety and depression in Nepal: prevalence, comorbidity and associations. *BMC Psychiatry* 2016; 16: 102.
10. Cortina MA, Sodha A, Fazel M, Ramchandani PG. Prevalence of child mental health problems in Sub-Saharan Africa: a systematic review. *Arch PediatrAdolesc Med* 2012; 166: 276–281.
11. Nakimuli-Mpungu E, Bass JK, Alexandre P, et al. Depression, alcohol use and adherence to antiretroviral therapy in sub-Saharan Africa: a systematic review. *AIDS Behav* 2012; 16: 2101–2118.
12. Williams DR, Herman A, Stein DJ, et al. Twelve-month mental disorders in South Africa: prevalence, service use and demographic correlates in the population-based South African Stress and Health Study. *Psychol Med* 2008; 38: 211–220.
13. Chibanda D, Cowan F, Gibson L, Weiss HA, Lund C. Prevalence and correlates of probable common mental disorders in a population with high prevalence of HIV in Zimbabwe. *BMC Psychiatry* 2016; 16: 55.
14. Gureje O, Lasebikan VO, Kola L, Makanjuola VA. Lifetime and 12-month prevalence of mental disorders in the Nigerian Survey of Mental Health and Well-Being. *Br J Psychiatry* 2006; 188: 465–471.
15. Kadri N, Agoub M, Assouab F, et al. Moroccan national study on prevalence of mental disorders: a community-based epidemiological study. *Acta Psychiatr Scand* 2010; 121: 71–74.
16. Ghanem M, Gadallah M, Meky FA, Mourad S, El-Kholy G. National Survey of Prevalence of Mental Disorders in Egypt: preliminary survey. *East Mediterr Health J* 2009; 15; 65–75.
17. World Health Organization (WHO). *Social Determinants of Mental Health.* Geneva: WHO, 2014.
18. Patel V. Mental health in low- and middle-income countries. *Br Med Bull* 2007; 81/82: 81–96.
19. Lund C, Breen A, Flisher AJ, et al. Poverty and common mental disorders in low and middle income countries: a systematic review. *Soc Sci Med* 2010; 71: 517–528.
20. Allen J, Balfour R, Bell R, Marmot M. Social determinants of mental health. *Int Rev Psychiatry* 2014; 26: 392–407.
21. Das J, Do QT, Friedman J, McKenzie D, Scott K. Mental health and poverty in developing countries: revisiting the relationship. *Soc Sci Med* 2007; 65: 467–480.
22. Corrigall J, Lund C, Patel V, Plagerson S, Funk MK. Poverty and mental illness: fact or fiction? A commentary on Das, Do, Friedman, McKenzie & Scott (65:3, 2007, 467–480). *Soc Sci Med* 2008; 66: 2061–2063.
23. Poongothai S, Pradeepa R, Ganesan A, Mohan V. Prevalence of depression in a large urban South Indian population—the Chennai Urban Rural Epidemiology Study (Cures – 70). *PLOS ONE* 2009; 4: e7185.
24. Malik MK, Jacob KS. Psychological morbidity among co-residents of older people in rural South India: prevalence and risk factors. *Int J Soc Psychiatry* 2015; 61: 183–187.

25. Husain N, Gater R, Tomenson B, Creed F. Social factors associated with chronic depression among a population-based sample of women in rural Pakistan. *Soc Psychiatry Psychiatr Epidemiol* 2004; 39: 618–624.

26. Tampubolon G, Hanandita W. Poverty and mental health in Indonesia. *Soc Sci Med* 2014; 106: 20–27.

27. Jenkins R, Njenga F, Okonji M, et al. Prevalence of common mental disorders in a rural district of Kenya, and socio-demographic risk factors. *Int J Environ Res Public Health* 2012; 9: 1810–1819.

28. Flisher AJ, Lund C, Funk M, et al. Mental health policy development and implementation in four African countries. *J Health Psychol* 2007; 12: 505–516.

29. Araya R, Lewis G, Rojas G, Fritsch R. Education and income: which is more important for mental health? *J Epidemiol Community Health* 2003; 57: 501–505.

30. Cheng HG, Shidhaye R, Charlson F, et al. Social correlates of mental, neurological, and substance use disorders in China and India: a review. *Lancet Psychiatry* 2016; 3: 882–899.

31. Sironi M. Education and mental health in Europe: School attainment as a mean to fight depression. *Int J Ment Health* 2012; 41: 79–105.

32. Alonso J, Angermeyer MC, Bernert S, et al. Prevalence of mental disorders in Europe: results from the European Study of the Epidemiology of Mental Disorders (ESEMeD) project. *Acta Psychiatr Scand* 2004; 109: 21–27.

33. Herbig B, Dragano N, Angerer P. Health in the long-term unemployed. *Dtsch Arztebl Int* 2013; 110: 413–419.

34. Wanberg CR. The individual experience of unemployment. *Annu Rev Psychol* 2012; 63: 369–396.

35. Daly M, Delaney L. The scarring effect of unemployment throughout adulthood on psychological distress at age 50: Estimates controlling for early adulthood distress and childhood psychological factors. *Soc Sci Med* 2013; 80: 19–23.

36. Paul KI, Moser K. Unemployment impairs mental health: Meta-analyses. *J Vocat Behav* 2009; 74: 264–282.

37. Bartley M. Unemployment and ill health: understanding the relationship. *J Epidemiol Community Health* 1994; 48: 333–337.

38. Harvey SB, Joyce S, Tan L, et al. Developing a mentally healthy workplace: a review of the literature. Available at: https://www.headsup.org.au/docs/default-source/resources/developing-a-mentally-healthy-workplace_final-november-2014.pdf?sfvrsn=8 (2014, accessed 26 February 2018).

39. Harnois G, Gabriel P, World Health Organization, International Labour Organisation. Mental Health and Work: Impact, Issues and Good Practices. Available at: http://digitalcommons.ilr.cornell.edu/cgi/viewcontent.cgi?article=1223&context=gladnetcollect (2000, accessed 26 February 2018).

40. Chopra P. Mental health and the workplace: issues for developing countries. *Int J Ment Health Syst* 2009; 3: 4.

41. Krieger J, Higgins DL. Housing and health: time again for public health action. *Am J Public Health* 2002; 92: 758–768.

42. Australian Institute of Health and Welfare. Health and the environment: a compilation of evidence. Cat. no. PHE 136. Available at: http://www.aihw.gov.au/WorkArea/DownloadAsset.aspx?id=10737418532 (2011, accessed 26 February 2018).

43. Evans GW. The built environment and mental health. *J Urban Health* 2003; 80: 536–555.

44. Gee GC, Payne-Sturges DC. Environmental health disparities: a framework integrating psychosocial and environmental concepts. *Environ Health Perspect* 2004; 112: 1645–1653.

45. Vlahov D, Freudenberg N, Proietti F, et al. Urban as a determinant of health. *J Urban Health* 2007; 84: 16–26.

46. Trivedi JK, Mishra M, Kendurkar A. Depression among women in the South-Asian region: the underlying issues. *J Affect Disord* 2007; 102: 219–225.

47. Allen J, Balfour R, Bell R, Marmot M. Social determinants of mental health. *Int Rev Psychiatry* 2014; 26: 392–407.

48. Rusch N, Angermeyer MC, Corrigan PW. Mental illness stugma: concepts, consequences, and initiatives to reduce stigma. *Eur Psychiatry* 2005; 20: 529–539.

49. Corrigan PW, Watson AC. Understanding the impact of stigma on people with mental illness. *World Psychiatry* 2002; 1: 16–20.

50. World Health Organization (WHO). *Women's Mental Health: An Evidence Based Review.* Available at: http://apps.who.int/iris/bitstream/10665/66539/1/WHO_MSD_MDP_00.1.pdf (2000, accessed 28 February 2018).

51. Ribeiro WS, Andreoli SB, Ferri CP, Prince M, Mari JJ. Exposure to violence and mental health problems in low and middle-income countries: a literature review. *Rev Bras Psiquiatr* 2009; 31(Suppl. II): S49–S57.

52. Dillon G, Hussain R, Loxton D, Rahman S. Mental and physical health and intimate partner violence against women: a review of the literature. *Int J Fam Med* 2013: 313909.

53. Fisher J, de Mello MC, Patel V, et al. Prevalence and determinants of common perinatal mental disorders in women in low-and lower-middle-income countries: a systematic review. *Bull World Health Organ* 2012; 90: 139–149G.

54. Nasreen HE, Kabir ZN, Forsell Y, Edhborg M. Low birth weight in offspring of women with depressive and anxiety symptoms during pregnancy: results from a population based study in Bangladesh. *BMC Public Health* 2010; 10: 515.

55. Umubyeyi A, Mogren I, Ntaganira J, Krantz G. Intimate partner violence and its contribution to mental disorders in men and women in the post genocide Rwanda: findings from a population based study. *BMC Psychiatry* 2014; 14: 315.

56. Sipsma H, Ofori-Atta A, Canavan M, Osei-Akoto I, Udry C, Bradley EH. Poor mental health in Ghana: who is at risk? *BMC Public Health* 2013; 13: 288.

57. Kumar s, Jeyaseelan l, Suresh S, Ahuja RC. Domestic violence and its mental health correlates in Indian women. *Br J Psychiatry* 2005; 187: 62–67.

58. Perkins JM, Subramanian SV, Christakis NA. Social networks and health: a systematic review of sociocentric network studies in low- and middle-income countries. *Soc Sci Med* 2015; 125: 60–78.

59. Chuang Y, Schechter L. Social networks in developing countries. *Annu Rev Resour Econ* 2015; 7: 451–472.

60. Kawachi I, Berkman LF. Social ties and mental health. *J Urban Health* 2001; 78: 458–467.

61. Wind TR, Fordham M, Komproe IH. Social capital and post-disaster mental health. *Glob Health Action* 2011; 4: 6351.

62. De Silva MJ, Huttly SR, Harpham T, Kenward MG. Social capital and mental health: A comparative analysis of four low income countries. *Soc Sci Med* 2007; 64: 5–20.

63. Islam MS, Alam MS. Social capital and mental health: results from a cross-sectional study in Bangladesh. *Asian Soc Sci* 2014; 10: 118–225.

64. Thuy NTM, Berry HL. Social capital and mental health among mothers in Vietnam who have children with disabilities. *Glob Health Action* 2013; 6: 18886.

65. De Silva MJ, Harpham T. Maternal social capital and child nutritional status in four developing countries. *Health Place* 2007; 13: 341–355.

CHAPTER 21

Mental and physical health

Mike McHugh

Introduction: mental health and physical health are inextricably linked

This chapter aims to bring together theory and practice in linking physical and mental health through exploration of the biopsychosocial model of health and illness. It will investigate mechanisms for enhancing both mental health (and well-being) and physical health using a population health approach.

René Descartes (1637) may have been wrong in playing down the physical dimensions of living when he said 'I think therefore I am'. Instead, mental health and physical health are fully integrated and co-dependent. The mind and body are intrinsically linked on a physiological level.

Until the 1990s, a biomedical model dominated Western thinking about both physical health and mental health [1]. This model predominately focused on illness and its genetic and biological causes, and largely overlooked developmental, social (relational, systematic, and structural), and environmental determinants of health. This approach generated solutions that were largely pharmaceutical and technological. Without question this delivered immense advances for health in general. Nevertheless, this paradigm is now being superseded by the biopsychosocial model, which expands the theory of health and illness as originating from a combination of *biological* factors (e.g. genes), *psychological* factors (e.g. behaviour, lifestyle, stress, and health beliefs), and *social* conditions (e.g. cultural influences, family relationships, and social support) [2].

Links between physical and mental illnesses

The increased risks of poor physical health and premature death experienced by people with mental illness [3], and the increased risk of poor mental health among people with physical health problems [4], are now widely accepted and understood.

Physical ill health has been shown to be as detrimental to mental health as much as poor mental health contributes to poor physical health [5]. People with chronic diseases are at increased risk of poor mental health, particularly depression and anxiety—around 30% of people with a long-term physical health condition also have a mental health problem [4]. In some cases, depression appears to result from specific biological effects of chronic illness. For example, malnourishment in infants can increase the risks of cognitive and motor deficits, and heart disease and cancer can increase the risk of depression [6].

Meanwhile, mental ill health has been clearly shown to have a negative association with physical health. A particular concern relates to the health needs of people with serious mental illness as they experience poorer health and die earlier than average. People with serious mental illness now have the same life expectancy as the general population had in the 1950s, this equates currently to between 8 and 15 years lower than expected [7].

Mental health and well-being

This chapter will investigate the links between mental health and well-being. We know that improving mental well-being appears to protect against developing mental illness [8, 9] *and* to improve significantly physical health, and reduce morbidity and mortality [10, 11].

Promoting mental health and well-being and preventing mental health problems should be key elements of every public health strategy because mental health and well-being influence all other health outcomes.

This chapter will explore the underlying risk factors for mental and physical illness, as well as the factors that increase mental well-being and thereby improve mental and physical health. It will also consider the links between mental health and physical health and behaviour. Finally, some of the physiological systems through which this interaction plays out will be examined as a means of better understanding the main pathways through which a person's mental and physical health and functioning mutually influence each other against a wider background of interacting social and environmental influences.

Parity of esteem

'Parity of esteem' is the label being used by those calling for mental health to be given equal priority to physical health. The term is used primarily in England, and is not well understood outside the UK. The Royal College of Psychiatrists proposed that parity of esteem should be defined as 'valuing mental health equally with physical health'. The usefulness of the term is contested, although there is consensus that mental health services are underfunded in comparison with physical health services. 'Parity of esteem' means that a person's physical and mental health needs are understood to be of equal importance, and treated as such. In reality, it is impossible to separate our physical and mental health from one another, although many of us—health professionals and public alike—can still see them as very separate.

Although the discourse around parity of esteem currently focuses on addressing the critically important issue of poor health and life expectancy of people with serious mental health problems, the debate needs to broaden into challenging all aspects of disparity enshrined in how society and policymakers view mental and physical health from prevention through to treatment. Linking mental health so closely to physical health raises challenges, and it is important that calls for mental health parity are not too reductive or narrow, as mental health is not just the responsibility of the health and social care system.

Definitions and concepts of mental health and well-being and physical health: basic principles

Over time there have been many changing terminologies used to describe the realities of mental health, well-being, and mental illness [12]. They encompass positive health, health problems, illness, and disorders. Different communities of interest have preferences for different terms and it has been challenging to reach a consensus.

It is important to agree a common vocabulary if we are to understand the links between physical and mental health. Language is crucial in communicating with the wide range of professionals, patients, carers, and members of the public outside medicine and the health service with whom public health staff work every day.

Health 'is a state of complete physical, mental and social well-being and not merely the absence of disease or infirmity' [13]. It could be argued that good physical health arises when the body functions optimally and in keeping with how it is designed.

Mental health 'is a state of well-being in which every individual realizes his or her own potential, can cope with the normal stresses of life, can work productively and fruitfully, and is able to make a contribution to her or his community' [14]. The emphasis on positive health is crucial here. 'Mental health' is increasingly used to describe a spectrum from mental well-being or positive mental health through to mental health problems, conditions, illnesses, and disorders.

Mental well-being, as used in this chapter, encompasses the positive end of mental health covering both the hedonic (feeling good) and eudemonic components (functioning well). Feeling good is subjective and embraces happiness, life satisfaction [15], and other positive affective states. Functioning well encompasses the components of psychological well-being (self-acceptance, personal growth, positive relations with others, autonomy, purpose in life, and environmental mastery) [16].

The term *well-being* is often used synonymously with mental well-being, partly, perhaps, to counterbalance prevailing trends to focus on physical well-being. 'Well-being' is relatively new as an academic field. There are also conceptual and measurement issues, which mean that the available evidence for effective and specifically defined well-being interventions in the field of public mental health is in its infancy compared with evidence from more established scientific disciplines.

Mental and *social well-being* are inextricably linked in both cause and effect, and social well-being is positively linked to good health. Good relationships with others—partners, family, and friends, and to a lesser extent more formal social groups—reduces the risk of mortality [17]. More recent work reinforces the impact of the social context on health in confirming that neighbourhood social capital is linked to improved health [18, 19].

Mental capital encompasses a person's cognitive and emotional resources. It includes their cognitive ability, how flexible and efficient they are at learning, and their 'emotional intelligence', such as their social skills and resilience in the face of stress. It determines how well an individual is able to contribute effectively to society, and also to experience a high personal quality of life [20].

Positive mental health, as described by George Vaillant [21], examines a number of models of positive mental health states and the empirical evidence or conceptualization that supports them. *Positive psychology* relates to concepts such as optimism and 'authentic happiness', as explored by Martin Seligman [22], and is based on the idea that if people are taught to be resilient and optimistic they will be less likely to suffer from depression and they will lead happier, more productive lives. Building on human strengths can be seen as building psychological 'muscles' before problems occur [23].

Resilience means 'being able to cope with the normal stress of life' and 'bounce back from problems'. This is an important component of many definitions of mental well-being and mental health, with great relevance for the prevention of mental health problems [24]. It is not a fixed attribute but a balance between the mechanisms and processes of protection and vulnerability [25].

Another important concept includes mental health as *social and emotional* intelligence [26], which highlights the importance of being able to recognize and respond appropriately to the emotions of the self and others.

Common risk factors for mental health/illness and physical health/illness

There are common determinants shared between physical health, mental health, and illness, and these are the starting point for approaches to prevention and improvements in health in its widest sense. The factors that promote and protect mental health and well-being, and those that are associated with the risk of poor mental health are widely understood to be differentially distributed: influenced by aspects of social identity, including gender, ethnicity, sexual orientation and age, and by the experience of disability [27].

Social and economic conditions impact on both physical and mental health throughout life, with the result that, for example, if you are poorer you are more likely to experience worse physical and mental health and to die younger. This association between poverty and mental and physical disorders appears to be universal, occurring in all societies, irrespective of their levels of development [28].

Poverty and disadvantage may impact on physical health by affecting mental health, by the experience of disadvantage and exclusion mediated through feelings of hopelessness, anxiety, and powerlessness, which lead to physical health consequences [27, 29].

Fig. 21.1 summarizes these multiple and mutually reinforcing influences [27].

Specific risk factors for both poor mental and physical health also include low control at work and poor social support, both of which have important influences on physical health (e.g. cardiovascular morbidity) and psychological health (e.g. depression) [29]. Factors such as insecurity and hopelessness, rapid social change, and the risks of violence and physical ill health may also explain this greater vulnerability [30, 31].

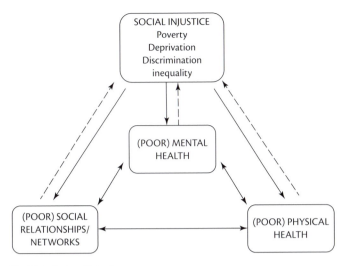

Fig. 21.1 Cycles of injustice.
Source: Reproduced from Scottish Development Centre for Mental Health, National Programme for Improving Mental Health and Well-Being: Addressing Mental Health Inequalities in Scotland - equal minds, Copyright (2005), Crown Copyright

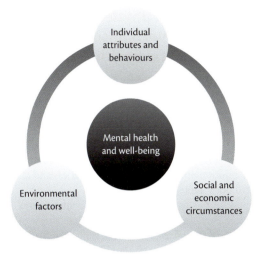

Fig. 21.2 What influences mental health and mental well-being.
Source: Reproduced from Risks to Mental Health: An overview of vulnerabilities and risk factors, Copyright (2012), with permission from World Health Organization.

Mental well-being and its relationship to mental and physical health: underlying risk and protective factors for mental health, mental well-being, mental illness, and therefore physical illness

Determinants of mental health and well-being overlap and include not only individual attributes such as the ability to manage one's thoughts, emotions, behaviours, and interactions with others, but also social, cultural, economic, political, and environmental factors such as national policies, social protection, living standards, working conditions, and community social supports. Fig. 21.2 illustrates the factors that influence mental well-being and therefore mental health.

The relationship between 'health' and 'well-being' appears to have two-way causality, i.e. good health improves well-being and good well-being improves health [32].

The benefits of good mental well-being are broad, deep-reaching, and societal. They include children who learn easily and are able to fulfil their full potential as members of society; people who are better able to manage life events and traumas; people who live in a way that supports their own and others' health, who can manage their health issues and provide compassionate support for relatives and friends when they are vulnerable; employees who are creative, adaptable, resilient, and productive; and people who age well [33, 34].

Emerging evidence suggests that improving mental well-being can contribute substantially to improving physical health and to reducing morbidity and mortality [10, 11]. Affective, eudemonic, and evaluative well-being all predict future subjective health, suggesting that impaired well-being is not just a product of poor health, but it is also systematically associated with the development of poor health [35].

Negative affective styles such as anxiety and hostility have been shown to predict increased risk for illness and mortality [36, 37].

Subjective well-being is also predictive of mortality across a number of health conditions, including depression, anxiety, coronary heart disease, and cancer [38].

Social relationships, social well-being, and mental well-being

Good social relations combined with positive attitudes to self, environmental mastery, and the positive relationships with others underpin resilience and are essential components of mental well-being [39].

Loneliness has a significant detrimental effect on people's health and well-being. The influence of social relationships on the risk of death are comparable to other established mortality risk factors such as smoking and alcohol consumption, and actually exceed the influence of physical activity and obesity [39]. There is some evidence to suggest the reductions in all-cause mortality associated with high levels of well-being are partially or completely mediated by social networks [40].

To summarize: in an integrated and evidence-based model of health, mental health (including emotions and thought patterns) and well-being have emerged as a key determinant of overall health (see Fig. 21.3).

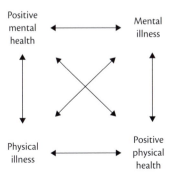

Fig. 21.3 Mental and physical health: a holistic view.
Source: Reproduced from Promoting Mental Health: Concepts, Emerging Evidence, Practice, Copyright (2005), with permission from World Health Organization.

Understanding the physiological and neuroendocrine mechanisms that link physical and mental health

Life course

We are beginning to understand the molecular mechanisms by which early experience confers lasting changes in health and behaviour. Fifty per cent of mental health problems are established by the age of 14 years and 75% by the age of 24 years [41]. It is therefore critical to understand how early life events influence life-long patterns of emotionality and stress responsiveness and alter the rate of brain and body ageing.

The hippocampus, amygdala, and prefrontal cortex undergo stress-induced structural remodelling, which alters behavioural and physiological responses. It has been suggested that chronic elevation of stress hormones particularly at critical times of bonding and attachment has deleterious effects on the developing central nervous system, and this includes increasing the risk for major depressive disorder [42]. Cross-fostering experiments have shown that maternal behaviour rather than genetic and biological maternal traits largely determine adult behaviour [43].

Ultimately, mental and physical health and functioning mutually interact through physiological systems, such as neuroendocrine and immune functioning. There is evidence that happiness is linked to the physiological processes that affect health and high levels of well-being directly affect good health through these pathways [38]. Anxious and depressed moods initiate a cascade of adverse changes in endocrine and immune functioning and increase susceptibility to a range of physical illnesses, for example development of the common cold [44], and delayed wound healing [45].

Stress involves two-way communication between the brain and the cardiovascular, immune, and other systems via neural and endocrine mechanisms. The brain is a target of stress because it determines what is threatening. Stress and stress hormones produce both adaptive and maladaptive effects on the brain throughout the life course and the brain also generates the physiological and behavioral responses that can be either adaptive or damaging. Stress biology illuminates the mechanisms by which emotional distress exacerbates susceptibility to physical illness. How people feel (stressed, depressed, isolated, scared, excluded) has a direct effect on both the immune and cardiovascular systems.

Beyond the 'flight-or-fight' response to acute stress, there are events in daily life that produce a type of chronic stress and lead over time to wear and tear on the body ('allostatic load'). Mental health is linked to physiological processes in the body mammalian (fight and flight) and the more phylogenically ancient (freeze) stress responses [46].

The autonomic nervous system is integrally linked to emotional states and regulates cardiovascular, respiratory, digestive, repair, and defence functions of the body at a subconscious level and so has a profound effect on resilience and susceptibility to disease. This is an important underlying mechanism to explain why cohort studies looking at different aspects of mental health demonstrate a survival advantage in those with good mental well-being [11]. The strong gradient in health described earlier in the chapter may result from relative deprivation working as a catalyst for a range of negative emotional and cognitive responses to inequity, which then mediate their impacts through the neuroendocrine systems.

The role of the immune system as an important physiological mediator underlying the relationship between positive emotions, health, and survival is also suggested [47], in that well-being predicts better immune functioning in older adults—this has been found both in healthy adults and clinical samples, and is independent of poor health [48].

Social isolation is not only a risk factor for depression, but also increases the risk of coronary disease and mortality, probably through influences on blood pressure, and endocrine and immune responses [49, 50].

We also know that positive relationships which are a key component of mental well-being, are protective against loneliness and death [39], and whereas the precise mechanisms are yet to be elucidated it is very likely that the physiological processes described earlier—the adoption of healthy lifestyles, the proactive management of long-term disease, and the relative influence of wider determinants—all play a part.

As an adjunct to pharmaceutical therapy, social and behavioural interventions such as regular physical activity and social support reduce the chronic stress burden and benefit brain and body health and resilience [51].

Fig. 21.4 summarizes how these physiological and neuroendocrine phenomena shape and directly impact on risk factors for illness and on behaviour.

Links between mental health/well-being, physical health, and behaviour

One of the main pathways through which a person's mental and physical health and functioning mutually influence each other is through behaviour. The health behaviour of an individual is highly dependent on that person's mental health [52].

The term 'health behaviour' covers a range of activities, such as eating sensibly, getting regular exercise and adequate sleep, avoiding

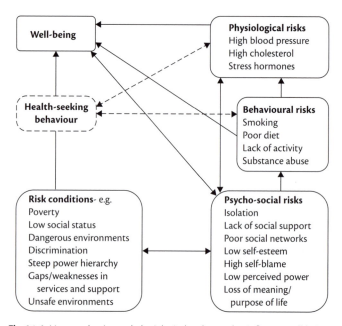

Fig. 21.4 Neuroendocrine and physiological pathways that influence well-being.
Source: Reproduced courtesy of Chris Bentley.

smoking and illicit drugs, engaging in safe sexual practices, wearing safety belts in vehicles, and adhering to medical therapies.

Positive aspects of behaviour

Indirect links exist between 'happiness' and healthy lifestyles. People with high levels of well-being are more likely to have healthier lifestyles. For instance, students at college with higher life satisfaction have demonstrated a higher propensity to exercise and eat healthier food, as well as being a healthier weight [53].

Mental well-being and resilience are protective factors for physical health, partly through reducing the prevalence of risky behaviours such as heavy drinking, illegal drug use, smoking, and unhealthy food choices, which are often used as coping and management mechanisms in the absence of other support [54].

Diet

There is a complex relationship between mental health and diet. We know that improvement in quality of diet leads to higher levels of good mental health in adolescents [55]. Healthy foods, particularly emphasizing fruit and vegetable consumption—up to eight portions a day—can positively affect mental, as well as physical, health [56, 57].

Physical exercise: the miracle cure?

There is strong evidence that increased physical activity improves the well-being of people in general and older people in particular. Therefore, engaging in physical activity is paramount to ageing well [58]. Being physically active is inextricably linked to independent living and other factors such as social support, both of which are also crucial aspects for well-being in older adults. Regular physical activity is also linked to improvements in immune function and resistance to illness [48].

Levels of physical activity can also impact on mental well-being in terms of mood, stress, self-esteem, anxiety, dementia, and depression [59].

Exercise for preventing depression

Physical activity has been shown to reduce depression risk [60]. Exercise is moderately more effective than no therapy for reducing symptoms of depression [61], and is similar in effectiveness to antidepressants and to psychological therapies. Current National Institute for Health and Care Excellence guidance recommends the use of structured physical activity in the treatment of depression [62].

Two 45-minute exercise sessions a week are suggested as a minimum, but the evidence around the optimum level is unclear. Benefits may be additionally increased by access to green space and associated increased activity levels [63].

Exercise in dementia

There is some evidence that exercise programmes can improve the ability of people with dementia to perform daily activities, although there is no evidence of benefit from exercise on cognition, psychological symptoms, and depression [64].

Negative aspects of behaviour

People with mental health problems are more likely to smoke, be overweight, have disrupted education, be unemployed, take time off work, fall into poverty, and find themselves in the criminal justice system [65]. Mental health problems in childhood predict the adoption of unhealthy lifestyles in adolescence [65].

Unhealthy lifestyles can be a response to stress, which plays a part in the course of many chronic diseases, and whereas other factors like social norms, availability, price, and legality are important opportunities for regulation, a key reason most people find it difficult to change their lifestyle for the better is because the lifestyle assuages emotional distress. For example, eating carbohydrates increases serotonin levels, which may boost mood [54].

Obesity

There are bi-directional associations between mental health problems and obesity. Obese people have been found to have a 55% increased risk of developing depression over time, whereas depressed persons have a 58% increased risk of becoming obese [66]. Women appear to be at greater risk of obesity and common mental health disorders than men [67].

There are various theories to explain why obesity might lead to poor mental health in adults, for example increased medical problems and mobility restrictions associated with obesity, which can have a direct impact on psychological well-being, and can lead to depression, eating disorders, distorted body image, and low self-esteem [68]. A combination of the biological impact of increased stress alongside poor adherence to weight-loss programmes, binge eating, negative thoughts, and reduced social support may make it difficult for a depressed person to avoid weight gain [69].

Intervention strategies to tackle obesity should consider both the physical and mental health of patients. Care providers should monitor the weight of depressive patients and, similarly, in overweight or obese patients, mood should be monitored. This awareness could lead to prevention, early detection, and co-treatment for people at risk, ultimately reducing the burden of both conditions. Current research in this area is limited and there is an urgent need for evaluations of weight-management interventions, both in terms of weight loss and psychological benefits.

Other lifestyle approaches

At present, health services in supporting people with mental illness tend to address mental health issues independently from services to address unhealthy lifestyles. Lifestyle-change programmes could be more successful if they fully consider the individual's underlying mental health and psychological state [70].

Smoking

Smoking is detrimental to well-being in older adults. Current smokers were significantly more depressed than ex-smokers or those who had never smoked (26% vs 13% and 15%, respectively) [35]. Smaller differences were seen for enjoyment of life, eudemonic well-being, and life satisfaction.

Stop smoking

There is also a correlation between smoking cessation and gains in mental health and subjective well-being, as well as lower levels of anxiety and depression [71].

Alcohol

The associations between alcohol and drug misuse and health are well documented [72]. Although the research is limited, moderate alcohol consumption has potential benefits [73], and is part of normal social interactions for many people and, in turn, has an important positive influence on well-being.

Where alcohol consumption is at harmful levels, brief interventions led by nurses delivered in a primary care setting have been found effective in lowering the consumption of alcohol. A wide range of physiological and pharmacological interventions have been shown to be effective in supporting people to overcome alcohol dependence and addiction [74].

Summary of interventions to improve mental health, well-being, and physical health

Public health practitioners and governments alike now have extensive information on risk and protective factors for mental and physical health and well-being. This knowledge can be used to develop and implement actions to prevent mental and physical disorders from developing and to protect and promote mental and physical health at all stages of life. It is important to take a life-course approach as early stages of life present a particularly important opportunity to promote mental health and prevent mental disorders. There are two main areas of focus in order to develop sustainable population approaches:

1. Reduce risk factors for mental and physical illness.

2. Strengthen mental health, well-being, and therefore physical health.

Public health practitioners can effect positive change by combing four broadly overlapping areas of public health practice: leadership, partnership, advocacy, and measuring change.

- As *leader*: directly using resources to commission and implement programmes.

- As *partner*: working in partnership to understand the health impact of other departments' and partner's policies; can include joint strategies, commissioning, and sharing of resources, including budgets.

- As *advocate*: when not in a position to have any direct control over an issue or policy, a key role is to champion and advocate for change, tackling mental health inequalities, stigma, and discrimination.

- As *evaluator*: adopt an evidence-based approach in all of the programmes/activities to commission, including addressing gaps in the evidence base.

There is a continuum between health and illness [75], as described by Geoffrey Rose, who proposed that where a health issue is continuously distributed in the population, the mean predicts the proportion of the population with a diagnosable illness.

This has been demonstrated to be true for both child and adult populations with regard to common mental disorders (CMD; depression and anxiety in adults, and emotional and behavioural problems in children). It follows, at least for CMD, that if it can be demonstrated than an intervention offered at a universal level improves the mean mental health in a universal population, that the intervention will reduce the level of diagnosable illness in the population.

The Rose hypothesis has apparently not yet been demonstrated as either true or false for severe and enduring mental illness. However, the ubiquity of CMD and their substantial cost to the economy are sufficient justification for universal approaches, regardless of the effect on severe and enduring mental illness.

Population-wide approaches involve reducing the average levels of the population's risk and also strengthening average levels of mental health and well-being, while not overlooking the importance of intervening intensively for those few at the highest level of risk.

Reducing shared risk factors for mental and physical illness

Public health practitioners have an important role in tackling and influencing the broader social and economic conditions and determinants that impact on both physical and mental health and well-being as described earlier. We must also fully support people to address unhealthy lifestyles, including diet, exercise, smoking, alcohol, substance misuse, and sexual health, as this is also an important opportunity to reduce the burden of both mental and physical illness.

Promoting 'mental well-being' to prevent mental illness (and therefore physical illness)

As discussed earlier, there is a strong evidence base for investing in the promotion of mental health and well-being and the prevention of mental health problems as an integral part of improving physical health. Equally, taking a proactive approach to tackling the mental health and well-being needs of those with chronic physical illnesses remains an important goal if we are to enhance and improve overall health at a population level.

Protection and promotion of mental well-being, including early intervention and prevention, improves quality of life, life expectancy, educational achievement, productivity and economic outcomes, and reduces violence, antisocial behaviour, and crime.

Good evidence exists for a range of public mental health interventions across the life course that could be commissioned to promote mental well-being, encourage a healthy lifestyle, and thereby prevent chronic disease and mental illness [76]. These can work in conjunction with other public health interventions focused on behaviour change and risk factor reduction to improve physical health.

Specific interventions to improve wellbeing: what works

Policy interventions may not directly target well-being; however, these interventions may still affect well-being as an outcome:

- learning;

- work;

- environment;

- social inclusion, activity, and relationships;

- parenting and early-years interventions.

Learning

Children's well-being can be improved by supporting school readiness [77], as implemented through:

◆ strengthening the home learning environment;

◆ preschool and early child education programmes to promote early language acquisition and literacy;

◆ high-quality preschool education programmes to improve education, social interactions, and school readiness.

Adult well-being

Taking part in informal learning has also been found to improve older people's levels of well-being. There is some qualitative literature to suggest that for older people both the social aspect of learning and the intrinsic value placed on learning were key incentives for older people to participate [78].

Work

The relationship between work and well-being has a two-way causality [32].

A number of work-related interventions have been found to be effective in enhancing people's levels of well-being [79].

Environment

The physical and psycho-social environments have been shown to be key factors in people's well-being. Interventions to improve housing can improve health outcomes, as well as changing people's perceptions across a range of factors such as crime and safety [80]. Neighbourhood improvements also increase mental well-being [81].

Active Travel Town Schemes have been found to enhance the levels of non-car travel. Reducing the amount of traffic and its speed has been found to increase levels of play and social activity and quality of life [82].

Social inclusion, activity, and relationships

Social networks are important tools in building people's resilience. Taking part in social activities, and having good relationships and strong social networks are all shown to be good for people's levels of well-being. Older people have been found to have higher levels of resilience when provided with a high level of social support both before and during adverse circumstances [83].

Social prescriptions link patients in primary care with non-medical support in the community. They have been found to improve mental health outcomes, improve community well-being, and lower social exclusion [84]. Befriending has been found to have benefits in terms of tackling depression and to be cost-effective. Community navigators have also been found effective in helping older people in terms of tackling isolation and improving well-being.

For young people, friends, support networks, social roles that are valued, and foster a positive perspective on the local area have been found to help reduce the likelihood of emotional and behavioural problems, as well as the severity of these problems [83].

Parenting and early-years interventions

Early-years interventions can raise the levels of well-being of children and young people [77, 85]. Preschool interventions have been

found to be the most cost-effective, but school-age interventions have also been found to be effective.

Foresight Report

The Foresight Report identified the well-being equivalent of 'five fruit and vegetables a day' [20]. The suggestions for individual action to enhance well-being, based on an extensive review of the evidence are shown in Box 21.1.

Conclusions

The biopsychosocial model of health helps draw together the theoretical origins and forces that bring physical and mental health (and disease) closer together. This model expands on earlier theories in describing health and illness as originating from a combination of *biological* factors, for example genes, *psychological* factors (e.g. behaviour, lifestyle, stress, and health beliefs), and *social* conditions (e.g. cultural influences, family relationships, and social support).

It is now more useful to frame health as an integrated totality, one that includes our overlapping physiological functioning, our

---

Box 21.1 Foresight Report

'Five ways to wellbeing'

◆ *Connect* … With the people around you. With family, friends, colleagues and neighbours. At home, work, school or in your local community. Think of these as the cornerstones of your life and invest time in developing them. Building these connections will support and enrich you every day.

◆ *Be active* … Go for a walk or run. Step outside. Cycle. Play a game. Garden, Dance. Exercising makes you feel good. Most importantly, discover a physical activity you enjoy and that suits your level of mobility and fitness.

◆ *Take notice* … Be curious. Catch sight of the beautiful. Remark on the unusual. Notice the changing seasons. Savour the moment, whether you are walking to work, eating lunch or talking to friends. Be aware of the world around you and what you are feeling. Reflecting on your experiences will help you appreciate what matters to you.

◆ *Keep learning* … Try something new. Rediscover an old interest. Sign up for that course. Take on a different responsibility at work. Fix a bike. Learn to play an instrument or how to cook your favourite food. Set a challenge you enjoy achieving. Learning new things will make you more confident as well as being fun.

◆ *Give* … Do something nice for a friend, or a stranger. Thank someone. Smile. Volunteer your time. Join a community group. Look out, as well as in. Seeing yourself, and your happiness, as linked to the wider community can be incredibly rewarding and creates connections with the people around you.

Source: Reproduced from Government Office for Science, Mental Capital and Wellbeing: Making the most of ourselves in the 21st century. Executive Summary, Copyright (2008), Crown copyright.

mental and spiritual processes, and our behaviour. We can begin to explore the separation and joining of mental and physical health not in terms of actual, distinct, underlying differences, but as tools for understanding the whole, and as a mechanism for introducing measures and changes that positively impact on both mental and physical health at a population level.

The evidence base is growing, that by strengthening mental health and well-being we not only reduce the risk of mental illness, but in so doing we enhance population health in its widest sense. Equally, improving physical health has a significantly positive influence on population mental health.

The concomitant reduction in the burdens of both mental and physical disease is of growing importance and concern to policymakers and the wider public. We must build on our expanding knowledge and evidence base to implement wider strategies and interventions that truly draw physical and mental health together as a mutually dependent, integrated whole. In many respects this journey is just beginning.

References

1. Mehta N. Mind-body dualism: a critique from a health perspective. *Mens Sana Monogr* 2011; 9: 202–209.
2. Engel GL. The need for a new medical model: a challenge for biomedicine. *Science* 1977; 196: 129–136.
3. De Hert M, Correll CU, Bobes J, et al. Physical illness in patients with severe mental disorders. I. Prevalence, impact of medications and disparities in health care. *World Psychiatry* 2011; 10: 52–77.
4. Naylor C, Parsonage M, McDaid D, Knapp M, Fossy M, Galea A. Long-term conditions and mental health: the cost of co-morbidities. Available at: https://www.kingsfund.org.uk/sites/files/kf/field/field_publication_file/long-term-conditions-mental-health-cost-comorbidities-naylor-feb12.pdf (2012, accessed 26 February 2018).
5. Herrman H, Jané-Llopis E. Mental health promotion in public health. The evidence of mental health promotion effectiveness: strategies for action. Available at: http://www.gencat.cat/salut/imhpa/Du32/html/en/dir1663/Dd12975/iuhpe_special_edition_no2.pdf (2005, accessed 26 February 2018).
6. Patel V, Woodward A, Feigin V, Quah SR, Heggenhougen K. *Mental and Neurological Public Health: A Global Perspective.* Boston, MA: Academic Press, 2010.
7. Chang CK, Hayes RD, Perera G, et al., Life expectancy at birth for people with serious mental illness and other major disorders from a secondary mental health care case register in London. *PLOS ONE* 2011; 6: e19590.
8. Lyubormirsky S, Sheldon KM, Schkade D. Pursuing happiness: the architecture of sustainable change. *Rev Gen Psychol* 2005; 9: 111–131.
9. Keyes CLM, Dhingra SS, Simoes EJ. Change in level of positive mental health as a predictor of future risk of mental illness. *Am J Public Health* 2010; 100: 2366–2371.
10. NHS Information Centre. Health Survey for England – 2010. Respiratory Health: Chapter 7. Available at: https://digital.nhs.uk/catalogue/PUB03023 (accessed 7 March 2018).
11. Chida Y, Steptoe A. Positive psychological wellbeing and mortality: a quantitative review of prospective observational studies. *Psychosom Med* 2008; 70: 741–756.
12. Hornsby J. Longworth G. (eds). *Reading Philosophy of Language.* Chichester: Wiley, 2005.
13. World Health Organization. Constitution of WHO: principles. Available at: http://www.who.int/about/mission/en/ (accessed 26 February 2018).
14. World Health Organization. Mental health: a state of well-being. Available at: http://www.who.int/features/factfiles/mental_health/en/ (accessed 26 February 2018).
15. Diener E, Suh EM, Lucas RE, Smith HL. Subjective well-being: three decades of progress. *Psychol Bull* 1999; 125: 276–302.
16. Ryff CD. Happiness is everything, or is it? Explorations on the meaning of psychological well-being. *J Pers Soc Psychol* 1989; 57: 1069.
17. Berkman LF, Syme SL. Social networks, host resistance and mortality: a nine-year follow up study of Alameda County residents. *Am J Epidemiol* 1979; 109: 186–204.
18. Berkman LF, Kawachi I (eds). *Social Epidemiology.* Oxford: Oxford University Press, 2000.
19. Tampubolon G, Subramanian SV, Kawachi I. Neighbourhood social capital and individual self-rated health in Wales. *Health Econ* 2013; 22: 14–21.
20. Government Office for Science. Mental Capital and Wellbeing: Making the most of ourselves in the 21st century. Available at: https://www.gov.uk/government/uploads/system/uploads/attachment_data/file/292450/mental-capital-wellbeing-report.pdf (2008, accessed 26 February 2018).
21. Vaillant GE. Positive mental health: Is there a cross-cultural definition? *World Psychiatry* 2012; 11: 93–99.
22. Seligman MEP. *Authentic Happiness: Using the New Positive Psychology to Realize Your Potential for Lasting Fulfillment.* New York: Free Press, 2002
23. Boniwell I, Ryan L. *Personal Well-Being Lessons For Secondary Schools: Positive Psychology in Action for 11 to 14 year olds.* Oxford: Oxford University Press, 2012.
24. Mental Health Foundation. Better Mental Health For All: A public health approach to mental health improvement. Available at: http://www.fph.org.uk/uploads/Better%20Mental%20Health%20For%20All%20FINAL%20low%20res.pdf (2016, accessed 26 February 2018).
25. World Health Organization. Mental Health Action Plan 2013–2020. Available at: http://apps.who.int/iris/bitstream/10665/89966/1/9789241506021_eng.pdf?ua=1 (2013, accessed 26 February 2018).
26. Vaillant GE, Davis JT. Social/emotional intelligence and midlife resilience in schoolboys with low tested intelligence, *Am J Orthopsychiatry* 2000; 70: 215–222.
27. Scottish Government Report: *National Programme for Improving Mental Health and Well-Being: Addressing Mental Health Inequalities in Scotland—equal minds*, published, 2005, Available at http://www.gov.scot/Publications/2005/11/04145113/51151 *(part 6)*
28. CSDH. *Closing the Gap in a Generation: Health Equity Through Action on the Social Determinants of Health. Final Report of the Commission on Social Determinants of Health.* Geneva: WHO, 2008
29. Wilkinson R, Marmot M (eds). Social Determinants of Health: The solid facts. Available at: http://www.euro.who.int/__data/assets/pdf_file/0005/98438/e81384.pdf (2003, accessed 26 February 2018).
30. Kopp MS, Skrabski A, Szedmák S. Psychosocial risk factors, inequality and self-rated morbidity in a changing society. *Soc Sci Med* 2000; 51: 1351–1361.
31. Patel V, Kleinman A. Poverty and common mental disorders in developing countries. *Bull World Health Organ* 2003; 81:609–615.
32. De Neve JE, Diener T, Xuereb C. The objective benefits of subjective wellbeing. In: Helliwell J, Layard R, Sachs J (eds). *World Happiness Report 2013.* New York: UN Sustainable Development Solutions Network, 2013.
33. Herrman HS, Saxena S, Moodie R (eds). Promoting Mental Health: Concepts, Emerging Evidence, Practice. Available at: http://www.who.int/mental_health/evidence/MH_Promotion_Book.pdf (2005, accessed 26 February 2018).
34. Knapp M, Ardino V, Brimblecombe N, et al. Youth Mental Health: New Economic Evidence. Available at: http://www.pssru.ac.uk/archive/pdf/5160.pdf (2016, accessed 26 February 2018).
35. Steptoe A, Demakakos P, de Oliverira C (eds). The psychological wellbeing and health functioning of older people in England. In: *The Dynamics of Ageing: Evidence from the ENGLISH LONGITUDINAL STUDY OF AGEING 2002–10.* London: Institute for Fiscal Studies, 2012, pp. 98–182.

36. Nabi H, Kivimaki M, De Vogli R, Marmot MG, Singh-Manoux A. Positive and negative affect and risk of coronary heart disease: Whitehall II prospective cohort study. *BMJ* 2008; 337: a118.

37. Cohen S Pressman SD. Positive affect and health. *Curr Dir Psychol Sci* 2006; 15: 122–125.

38. Diener E, Chan MY. Happy people live longer: subjective wellbeing contributes to health and longevity. *Appl Psychol* 2011; 3: 1–43.

39. Holt-Lunstad J, Smith TB, Layton JB. Social relationships and mortality risk: a meta-analytic review. *PLOS Med* 2010; 7: P11.

40. Xu J, Roberts RE. The power of positive emotions: it's a matter of life or death—subjective wellbeing and longevity over 28 years in a general population. *Health Psychol* 2010; 29: 9–19.

41. Kessler RC, Berglund P, Demler O, Jin R, Merikangas KR, Walters EE. Lifetime prevalence and age-of-onset distributions of DSM-IV disorders in the National Comorbidity Survey replication. *Arch Gen Psychiatry* 2005; 62: 593–602.

42. National Research Council (US) and Institute of Medicine (US) Committee on Depression, Parenting Practices, and the Healthy Development of Children; England MJ, Sim LJ (eds). *Depression in Parents, Parenting, and Children: Opportunities to Improve Identification, Treatment, and Prevention.* Washington, DC: National Academies Press, 2009.. Available at: https://www.ncbi.nlm.nih.gov/books/NBK215119/ (accessed 26 February 2018).

43. Francis D, Diorio J, Liu D, Meaney MJ. Nongenomic trasmission across generations of maternal behavior and stress responses in the rats. *Science* 1999; 286: 1155–1158.

44. Cohen S, Tyrrell DAJ, Smith AP. Psychological stress and susceptibility to the common cold. *N Engl J Med* 1991; 325: 606–612.

45. Kielcot-Glaser JK, Page GG, Marucha PT, MacCallum RC, Glaser R. Psychological influences on surgical recovery: perspectives from psychoneuroimmunology. *Am Psychol* 1999; 53: 120–128.

46. Porges SW. *The Polyvagal Theory: Neurophysiological Foundations of Emotions, Attachment, Communication and Self regulation.* New York: WW Norton, 2011.

47. Marsland AL, Pressman SD, Cohen SD. Positive affect and immune function. In: Ader R (ed.). *Psychoneuroimmunoloy*, 4th ed., Vol. 2. San Diego, CA: Elsevier, 2007, pp. 761–779.

48. Friedman EM. Wellbeing, ageing and immunity. In: Segerstrom SC (ed.) *The Oxford Handbook of Psychoneuroimmunology.* New York: Oxford University Press, 2012, pp. 37–60.

49. House JS, Landis KR, Umberson D. Social relationships and health. *Science* 1998; 241: 540–545.

50. Kaplan GA, Salonen JT, Cohen RD, Brand RJ, Syme SL, Puska P. Social connections and mortality from all causes and from cardiovascular disease: prospective evidence from eastern Finland. *Am J Epidemiol* 1988; 128: 370–380.

51. McEwen BS. Physiology and neurobiology of stress and adaptation: central role of the brain. *Physiol Rev* 2007; 87: 873–904.

52. World Health Organization. The world health report 2001 - Mental Health: New Understanding, New Hope. Available at: http://www.who.int/whr/2001/en/ (2001, accessed 26 February 2018).

53. Lustig R. *Fat Chance—The Bitter Truth About Sugar.* London: Fourth Estate, 2013.

54. Pettay RS. *Health Behaviors and Life Satisfaction in College Students.* Doctoral Dissertation, Kansas State University, 2008.

55. O'Neil A, Quirk SE, Housden S, et al. Relationship between diet and mental health in children and adolescents: a systematic review. *Am J Public Health* 2014; 104: e31–e42.

56. Brown JS, Learmonth AM, Mackereth CJ. *Promoting Public Mental Health and Well-being; Principles Into Practice.* London: Jessica Kingsley Publishers, 2015.

57. Knifton L, Quinn N. *Public Mental Health: Global Perspectives.* London: Open University Press, 2013.

58. Department of Health. A Compendium of Factsheets: Wellbeing Across the Lifecourse. Ageing Well. Available at: https://www.gov.uk/government/uploads/system/uploads/attachment_data/file/277584/Ageing_Well.pdf (accessed 12 March 2018).

59. Cattan M, Tilford S. *Mental Health Promotion: A Lifespan Approach.* London: Open University Press, 2006.

60. Warburton DER, Nicol CW, Bredin SSD. Health benefits of physical activity: the evidence. *CMAJ* 2006; 174: 801–809.

61. Cooney GM, Dwan K, Greig CA, et al. Exercise for depression. *Cochrane Database Syst Rev* 2013; 9:: CD004366.

62. Joint Commissioning Panel for Mental Health. Guidance for commissioning public health services. Available at: www.jcpmh.info (2013, accessed 26 February 2018).

63. Ward Thompson C, Roe J, Aspinall P, Mitchell R, Clow A, Miller D. More green space is linked to less stress in deprived communities: evidence from salivary cortisol patterns. *Landscape Urban Plan* 2012; 105: 221–229.

64. Forbes D, Forbes SC, Blake CM, Thiessen EJ, Forbes S. Exercise programs for people with dementia. *Cochrane Database Syst Rev* 2015; 4: CD006489.

65. Royal College of Psychiatrists. No health without public mental health. The case for action. Position Statement PS4. Available at: http://www.rcpsych.ac.uk/pdf/Position%20Statement%204%20website.pdf (2010, accessed 26 February 2018).

66. Luppino FS, de Wit LM, Bouvy PF, et al. Overweight, obesity, and depression: a systematic review and meta-analysis of longitudinal studies. *Arch Gen Psychiatry* 2010; 67: 220–229.

67. McCarty CA, Kosterman R, Mason WA, et al. Longitudinal associations among depression, obesity and alcohol use disorders in young adulthood. *Gen Hosp Psychiatry* 2009; 31: 442–450.

68. Ivbijaro GO. Mental health and chronic physical illnesses: the need for continued and integrated care—World Mental Health Day 2010. *Ment Health Fam Med* 2010; 7: 127.

69. Markowitz S, Friedman MA, Arent SM. Understanding the relation between obesity and depression: causal mechanisms and implications for treatment. *Clin Psychol* 2008; 15: 1–20.

70. NHS Confederation. From illness to wellness archiving efficiencies improving outcomes. Available at: http://www.nhsconfed.org/~/media/Confederation/Files/Publications/Documents/illness_to_wellness_241011.pdf (2011, accessed 26 February 2018).

71. Public Health England. Smokefree mental health services in England: Implementation document for providers of mental health services. Available at: https://www.gov.uk/government/uploads/system/uploads/attachment_data/file/509262/SF_MH_services_in_England__Guidance_for_Providers.pdf (accessed 12 March 2018).

72. Crawford V. *Co-Existing Problems of Mental Disorder and Substance Misuse ('Dual Diagnosis'): A Review of Relevant Literature. Final Report to the Department of Health.* London: Royal College of Psychiatrists' Research and Training Unit, 2001.

73. Goldberg IJ, Mosca L, Piano MR, Fisher EA. AHA Science Advisory: Wine and your heart: a science advisory for healthcare professionals from the Nutrition Committee, Council on Epidemiology and Prevention, and Council on Cardiovascular Nursing of the American Heart Association. *Circulation* 2001; 103: 472–475.

74. Public Health England. The Public Health Burden of Alcohol and the Effectiveness and Cost-Effectiveness of Alcohol Controll Policies: An evidence review. Available at: https://www.gov.uk/government/uploads/system/uploads/attachment_data/file/583047/alcohol_public_health_burden_evidence_review.pdf (accessed 12 March 2018).

75. Rose G. Sick individuals and sick populations. *Int J Epidemiol* 2001; 30: 427–432.

76. Campion J, Fitch C. Guidance for commissioning public mental health services. Available at: http://www.jcpmh.info/wp-content/uploads/jcpmh-publicmentalhealth-guide.pdf (2012, accessed 26 February 2018).

77. Mayor of London. Evidence base for a Healthy Early Years Programme in London. Available at: https://www.london.gov.uk/sites/default/files/evidence_base_for_a_healthy_early_years_programme_in_london_jan_2016.pdf (accessed 12 March 2018).

78. Jenkins A, Mostafa T. *BIS Research Paper Number 92. Learning and Wellbeing Trajectories Among Older Adults in England.* London: Department of Business, Innovation and Skills, 2012.

79. Department of Health. A Compendium of Factsheets: Wellbeing Across the Lifecourse: What works to improve wellbeing. Available at: https://www.gov.uk/government/uploads/system/uploads/attachment_data/file/277593/What_works_to_improve_wellbeing.pdf (accessed 12 March 2018).

80. Thomson H, Petticrew M, Morrison D. Health effects of housing improvement: systematic review of intervention studies. *BMJ* 2011; 323: 187–190.

81. Clark C, Candy B, Stansfield S. *A Systematic Review on the Effect of the Built and Physical Environment on Mental Health.* London: Centre for Psychiatry, Wolfson Institute of Preventive Medicine, Queen Mary's School of Medicine and Dentistry, University of London.

82. Hart J. No Friends? Blame the Traffic . . . . Available at: https://onthelevelblog.wordpress.com/2008/09/19/no-friends-blame-the-traffic/ (2008, accessed 26 February 2018).

83. Cooke A, Friedli L, Coggins T, et al. *Mental Wellbeing Impact Assessment: A Toolkit for Wellbeing*, 3rd ed. London: National MWIA Collaborative, 2011.

84. Friedli L, Watson S. *Social Prescribing for Mental Health*. Leeds and York: Northern Centre for Mental Health, 2004.

85. National Institute for Health and Care Excellence. Social and emotional wellbeing: early years. Available at: https://www.nice.org.uk/guidance/ph40/chapter/1-Recommendations#whose-health-will-benefit (2012, accessed 26 February 2018).

CHAPTER 22

Clinical outcome assessment in mental health

Skye P. Barbic and Stefan J. Cano

Introduction

For more than 30,000 years, there has been evidence of humans using measurement to quantify variables of interest. For example, ancient peoples use notched pieces of wood or bone called 'tally sticks' to record numbers. In the twelfth century, tally sticks were adopted by the Exchequer of England as the measurement tool for collecting the King's taxes [1], and were used across England and many Commonwealth countries as a 'language of assessment' until 1826 [2].

The rationale for quantification in society has evolved significantly in the last two centuries—especially in the health sciences. In the mid-nineteenth century, Florence Nightingale used data to demonstrate how basic sanitation and hygiene standards led to decreased mortality of soldiers wounded in the Crimean War [3]. In the early twentieth century, Ernest Amory Codman introduced the concept of 'End Result Cards', to track patient data including demographics, diagnoses, treatments, and outcomes [4]. Codman also formed 'the Committee for Hospital Standardization', at the Massachusetts General Hospital, the first known committee focused on systematically identifying and tracking patient outcomes to improve the care of current and future patients. He wrote:

> We believe it is the duty of every hospital to establish a follow-up system, so that as far as possible, the result of every case will be available at all times for investigation by members of the staff, the trustees, or administration, or by other authorized investigators or statisticians [5].

Rigorous measurement approaches and quality standards benefit both the patient and key stakeholders, including clinicians, families, policymakers, and researchers.

The concept of clinical outcome assessment (COA) and data collection is rooted in the simple and yet important realization that health is a continuum. The goal of health assessment is to generate data that characterizes where a person is at on the continuum, where they are going, and how they can get there. As a result, COA is a vital form of communication. As with human language, it involves a cognitive ability to learn and convey information from one person to another. The ways in which information is conveyed in health has wide-reaching impacts on clinical decision-making, health care costs, and research.

'If you cannot measure it, you cannot improve it'.

So said Lord Kelvin, who is credited with the Kelvin thermodynamic measurement scale. In 1848, Kelvin argued for the need for a temperature scale with a null point (absolute zero) and a unit increment (degree Celsius). The Kelvin has been widely accepted as a unit and language for quantifying temperature. Temperature, as a variable of interest, is an outcome that most of us take advantage of. Despite not being directly observable, individuals across the globe have developed systematic methods for quantifying and communicating this outcome. In parallel, in mental health, most outcomes are also not directly observable. With one in four people around the world affected by mental disorders at some point in their lives, quantifying mental health outcomes robustly and systematically—just as temperature is quantified—is of critical importance [6].

What is clinical outcome assessment?

COA is the process of gathering empirical data to estimate or evaluate the nature, health quality, or ability of a person. As clinicians and researchers, we must systematically collect and use data, both to estimate where an individual is on a health continuum, and also to inform we how evaluate programmes or make treatment decisions with patients and their families. In the field of mental health, the challenge is to estimate outcomes in a precise, comparable, and reproducible manner. COA is essential in supporting advances in care in nearly all areas of mental health practice and research. COA can serve as a platform from which new and existing interventions can be built upon, easily evaluated, and shared. Nevertheless, before determining how to measure clinical outcomes in mental health, we must first understand the term 'measurement' at a nuanced level.

What is measurement?

Measurement is a process that involves description and quantification [7]. The science of measurement is pursued in the field of metrology. Metrology has been essential for establishing a common language of internationally accepted units of measurement and realizing these units in practice. Historically, assessment tools were developed to measure physical qualities such as weight, height, distance, and temperature. In 1795, France called for a harmonization of units to create an understanding of outcomes measured in any field of science, medicine, and technology. This led to the creation of the decimal-based metric system and eventually, over 200 years later, the International System of Units (SI). In 2017, the SI system is used by nearly every country across the globe to inform economic, health, industry, energy, and environmental decisions. The impact of metrology on international trade is perhaps the easiest to conceptualize [2]. Market success depends on an agreed upon system of measurement and symmetry between buyers and sellers, just as it was in the twelfth century with the use of tally sticks for taxation calculations [2]. In mental health, the impact of service provision and evidence-based practice also requires an agreed-upon system of measurement and symmetry between stakeholders.

Identifying outcomes for clinical assessment in mental health

The range of outcomes to consider in mental health is vast. However, in a 2017 review of studies describing the development of nearly 200 COAs, only 11% actually asked patients which outcomes are worth measuring [8]. The practice of asking patients to identify and prioritize outcomes has been described as 'surprisingly rare' [9]. As Coulter notes, consulting key stakeholders, particularly patients and families, about health outcomes is essential to:

> Highlight(ing) issues such as the ability to live well despite their health condition, minimising dependency and treatment burden, participating in meaningful activities, reducing stigma, avoiding loneliness, and having a sense of control over their daily life [9].

These outcomes are important to patients and are increasingly identified in the literature as critical to predicting long-term outcomes and quality of life [10].

In mental health, the philosophy of assessment and treatment has shifted dramatically. Moving from a focus on purely medical-somatic care, the centre has shifted towards patient- and family-centred care that emphasizes a person's capacity to live a full and meaningful life [10, 11]. In Western countries, mental health organizations face increasing pressure to articulate how their interventions and outcomes fit within a recovery-oriented framework [12–14]. This has added increased debate about the need to collect data relevant to patient goals to inform quality of care. To date, a core set of clinical assessments to measure both medical-somatic and functional outcomes in mental health has not been agreed upon. In order to optimize the mental health to our communities, clinicians, researchers, policymakers, and other key stakeholders must set standards for measuring the full range of outcomes important to patients.

Challenges to standardized clinical outcome assessment in mental health

Measuring physical characteristics in medicine is based on rigorous principles of quantity, number, and exactitude, to meet the criteria of objective measurement [14, 15]. For example, measurements of heart rate, oxygen saturation, and respiratory rate can all be compared against a standard unit to establish quantitative differences that represent numerical magnitudes on an equal-interval scale [15]. In psychiatry and other mental health fields, measuring attributes and personal characteristics such as emotions, attitudes, and perceptions can be more challenging. These attributes cannot be observed directly and can only be inferred subjectively by the use of rating scales to query attitudes, thoughts, and behaviors believed to reflect the underlying construct [14–16]. An

attribute that cannot be directly observed, but that must rather be inferred from other, observed variables, is called a *latent variable*. The method of obtaining the information needed to quantify latent variables is often in the form of a *rating scale*.

What is a rating scale?

Rating scales can be used to quantify mental health outcomes, which, in turn, can be used to inform fundamental decisions in clinical practice, health policy, and treatment trials [16–20]. In the USA, nearly one-quarter of all drug labels include information about treatment benefits based on patient rating scales [20]. Recently, methodological standards for the development and use of rating scales in clinical trials have been developed [21–23]. These standards have important implications for all areas of medicine, notably psychiatry and other field of mental health where outcomes are commonly latent.

How to choose clinical outcome assessments in practice and research

COAs must be fit for purpose. Perhaps the most common phrase used in any peer-reviewed research article is 'the assessment was selected because it was deemed reliable and valid'. Consideration for the implications of this phase are necessary. What does it mean for a COA to be *reliable* and *valid*?

Reliability is the extent to which measurement is error free [24, 25]. Reliability is thus an overall measure of consistency of a COA [25]. A COA has high reliability if it produces similar results under consistent conditions, such as across time or across contexts of use. Reliability is typically measured using reliability coefficients with scores that range from 0.00 (high error) and 1.00 (no error) [25]. Common types of reliability are described in Table 22.1.

A commonly accepted rule for reliability is shown in Table 22.2.

Intuitively, a stakeholder would hope for high reliability of a COA. However, as shown in Table 22.1, clinicians and researchers must interpret the trustworthiness of a measure deemed 'reliable' with caution, considering from all angles the consistency or stability of the measure [26].

Validity is the extent to which a COA measures what it purports to measure [27]. The way in which the term is commonly used is guided by Cronbach and Meehl's classic article entitled 'Construct validity in psychological tests' [27]. These are described in Table 22.3.

In mental health, specifically psychiatry, controversy with assessing the validity of diagnostic categories has been strongly debated. In this context, these terms are often used beyond the purposes of COA [30]. For example, *content validity* can be used to describe symptoms and diagnostic criteria; *criterion validity*—specifically *predictive validity*—may refer mainly to diagnostic stability over time; and *discriminant validity* may be used to describe the delimitation of one disorder from another. Kendell and Jablensky [29] emphasize the importance of considering all types of validity and distinguishing validity and utility. In order to be useful, COAs must be fit for purpose to measure what they purport to measure (valid) and inform clinical decision-making (utility).

Stenner et al. [30] describe validity as the 'story' about what it means to move up a variable of interest. Not only should stakeholders consider the content of a COA, but also the underlying

Table 22.1 Types of reliability tests commonly described to qualify clinical outcome assessments

Type	Purpose
Test–retest	Assesses the degree to which test scores are consistent from one test administration to the next. Measurements are gathered from a single rater who uses the same methods or instruments and the same testing conditions.
Inter-rater	Assesses the degree of agreement between two or more raters in their appraisals.
Intra-rater	Assesses the degree of agreement of a rater over time.
Inter-method	Assesses the degree to which test scores are consistent when there is a variation in the methods or instruments used.
Parallel-form (also called equivalent forms reliability)	Uses one set of questions divided into two equivalent sets ('forms'), where both sets contain questions that measure the same construct, knowledge or skill. The two sets of questions are given to the same sample of people within a short period of time and an estimate of reliability is calculated from the two sets.
Internal consistency	Assesses the consistency of results across items within a test to assess whether several items that propose to measure the same construct produce similar scores. It is typically measured using Cronbach's alpha [25].

Source: Reproduced from Psychometrika, 16(3), Cronbach LJ, Coefficient alpha and the internal structure of tests, pp. 297–334, Copyright (1951), with permission from Springer.

Table 22.2 Common rule for reliability.

Cronbach alpha (α)	Internal consistency
$\alpha \geq 0.9$	Excellent
$0.9 > \alpha \geq 0.8$	Good
$0.8 > \alpha \geq 0.7$	Acceptable
$0.7 > \alpha \geq 0.6$	Questionable
$0.6 > \alpha \geq 0.5$	Poor
$0.5 > \alpha$	Unacceptable

Source: Reproduced from Kelley TL, Interpretation of educational measurements, Copyright (1927), World Book Company

validity of its measurement structure. This approach ensures that outcomes are meaningful and develops a language of assessment, which is critical for translating outcomes into purpose. This common language in mental health can be used to compare performance metrics of clinical services to evidence-based guidelines or standards, as well as create meaningful conversations between key stakeholders. The item hierarchy of a commonly used screening questionnaire for trauma can be seen later in Fig. 22.2. Items on the measurement continuum of interest are located from easiest (low stress) to hardest (high stress). In this example, a person's location on the measurement continuum can be directly mapped to

the item(s) in this location. This allows stakeholders to validate the total score and interpret it meaningfully based on a theoretical and measurement model.

Beyond reliability and validity, mental health stakeholders should reflect on a series questions when considering COA.

What is the context of use?

The first step in considering a COA is to describe clearly the health condition under investigation. In identifying the context of use, a clinician or researcher should describe the severity, onset, co-morbidities, and phenotypes of the disease or chronic health condition. Moreover, mental health stakeholders must understand their target population: mapping out key demographic characteristics will be critical when making decisions about selecting the most sensitive and culturally appropriate COA. This understanding will ensure that the stakeholder is clear about how their context of use or clinical population compares to the studies in which the COA was developed and tested.

What is the rationale for assessment in this context of use?

Increasingly strong evidence suggests that the therapeutic targeting of conventionally measured outcomes—anatomy, pathophysiology, service utilization, and symptoms—may not necessarily translate into outcomes that are valued to the patient and their families. While these conventional outcomes are unquestionably important,

Table 22.3 Common types of validity commonly described in clinical outcome assessment.

Type	Purpose
Face	To estimate whether a test appears to measure a certain criterion.
Construct	To estimate the degree to which a test measures what it claims, or purports, to be measuring.
Content	Describe whether the assessment content covers a representative sample of the construct under investigation. This is described in a non-statistical manner and relies on evidence from experts or key stakeholders.
Criterion	Consider whether scores on an instrument agree with a definitive 'gold standard' measurement of the same theme. Can be divided into (1) concurrent and (2) predictive validity.

Source: Data from American Psychological Association, Standards for educational & psychological tests, Copyright (1974); Am J Psychiatry, 160(1), Kendell R, Jablensky A, Distinguishing between the validity and utility of psychiatric diagnoses, pp. 4-12, Copyright (2003), American Psychiatric Association.

they are not the only variables that have a strong rationale for inclusion in a COA. The intent of assessment in psychiatry and mental health optimally includes clinical and patient-valued outcomes as well.

What type of clinical outcome assessment is needed?

Bombardier and Tugwell [31] provide three purposes for measuring health: (i) diagnostic, (ii) prognostic, and (iii) evaluative. *Diagnostic* tools include measures that can identify the nature or cause of some phenomenon under investigation. The most commonly used diagnostic tool used in psychiatry is the *Diagnostic and Statistical Manual of Mental Disorders* (DSM). In its current, fifth version, the DSM-V is used by health professionals and other stakeholders such as forensic and legal specialists to diagnose and classify mental disorders. The intention of diagnostic tools is to facilitate an objective assessment of symptom presentations through the use of concise and explicit criteria. Clinicians and researchers use *prognostic* COAs to predict how an outcome will develop. Often, prognostic assessments include screening tools, such as the Patient Health Questionnaire-9 to screen for behavioural health symptoms. Another example is the use of blood tests to screen for conditions that may necessitate prescribing certain medications over others (e.g. blood, heart, thyroid, and kidney conditions). Finally, mental health stakeholders use *evaluative* measures to quantify the change in a person over time. As mentioned previously, many variables in psychiatry are latent and are measured indirectly by how they manifest in a population. Therefore, methods to transform the manifestations of these latent variables into clinically meaning numbers that can be taken as measurements and compared across time are needed [17, 31].

What considerations are needed for using rating scales in clinical outcome assessment?

Two types of rating scales are commonly used to measure latent variables in psychiatry: single-item scales (e.g. Global Assessment of Functioning (GAF) [32]) and multiple-item scales (e.g. Centre for Epidemiologic Scale for Depression [33], Beck Depression Inventory [34], Hamilton Anxiety Rating Scale [35]). Each type of scale has advantages and disadvantages.

Single-item rating scales

Single-item scales are easy to use and generate scores that can be easily communicated to patients (e.g. most psychiatrists can recognize that someone with a GAF score of 10 has low function and is at persistent risk of hurting themselves or others). However, single-item scales are scientifically weak because they have poor reliability, poor validity, and poor responsiveness [17, 36, 37]. The poor reliability is due to the random error associated with substantial random error, and adequately high levels of reproducibility are difficult to achieve [17, 37]. Poor validity arises because it is difficult to represent a complex construct such as function with a single question [37, 38]. For example, in measuring 'function' using the GAF (see Fig. 22.1), the descriptions of several categories are challenging to disentangle and score. For instance, categories at the upper end of the scale encompass different levels of function (social, occupational, and school), symptomology, response to stress,

and engagement in meaningful interpersonal relationships. DSM-V editors have recently concluded that the GAF is too subjective of a measurement instrument, and consequently they have not included it in the DSM-V [39, 40].

Single-item scales are also limited in that they do not consider a person's frame of reference [17]. An example of this is using a commonly used quality-of-life item: 'Rate your own health state today'. This item is ambiguous because it does not provide the frame of reference for interpretation. Different people may bring different frames of reference when answering this question, thereby making comparisons across individuals or groups difficult.

The limited responsiveness of single-item scales is due to the division of wide variables into only a few levels. For example, for the complex construct 'function', the single-item rating scale represents different levels of the continuum by dividing the continuum into 10 thick bands (Fig. 22.1). This thick-band division makes it difficult both to localize people precisely on the continuum, and to interpret their score in a clinically meaningful way. Therefore, single-item rating scales have limited reliability. This limitation has been previously well established empirically and discussed at length in the literature [41–45]. Nonetheless, researchers and clinicians continue to use single-item scales in clinical trials and practice [46–50].

Multiple-item rating scales

Hobart et al. [17] note that 'multiple item scales comprise of a set of items, each of which has two or more ordered response categories that are assigned sequential integer scores'. For clinical or research purposes, items are typically added together to produce a total score—also called the raw, summed, or scale score. Hobart et al. [17] suggest that the use of multiple-item rating scales has two fundamental requirements: (i) evidence that the values produced are actually rigorous measurements and not just numbers; and (ii) evidence that the items measure the variable of interest that they are intended to measure.

Multiple item scales are commonly used in mental health. In multiple item scales, scores from each item are combined to give a total score. This practice may seem clinically sensible: combining multiple items reduces random error, and therefore enhances scale reliability. Use of multiple items allows for constructs to be captured comprehensively and broken down into their component parts. This ability to break down captured information is especially important in mental health clinical practice and research, given the complex nature of many of the outcomes that are measured [51, 52]. For example, the 'function' outcome described previously could be captured on a multiple-item rating scale through items that are divided into sub-domains that qualify the construct. Thus, validity, responsiveness, and precision are improved because their continuum is divided into more parts. Unlike single-item scales, the theoretical advantages of multiple-item scales in mental health and are supported by empirical evidence [51–55].

Although multiple-items scales are scientifically strong, the scores they produce are less clinically actionable. For example, what does a score of 15 mean in a depression scale that ranges from 0 to 60? How does that same score of 15 compare with the total scores generated by the over 300 other existing depression scales? Interpretation of these scores can be challenging for research purposes and can present problems when communicating results to patients, families, and other health professionals.

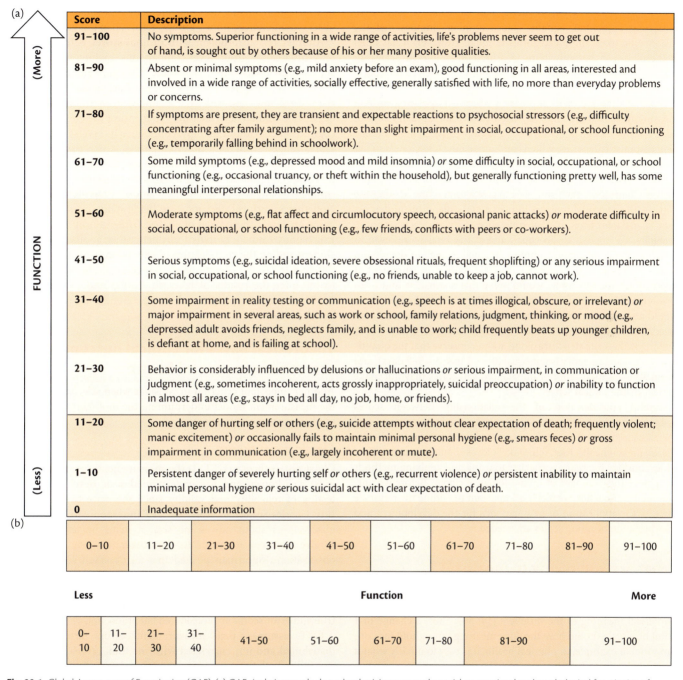

Fig. 22.1 Global Assessment of Functioning (GAF). (a) GAF single-item scale that asks physicians to rate the social, occupational, and psychological functioning of adults. The GAF comprises of 10 ordered categories that are, by convention, assigned sequential integer scores (0–100). (b) The 'function' continuum. Each scoring category represents a range on the function continuum, with a point of transition between the 10 equally spaced categories. Each category is assumed to be equally spaced. However, as shown in this example with 700 young adults with mental illness, the scoring categories are not equally spaced. As a result, the stakeholders are unable to locate the points of transition accurately relative to each other. As a result, the ranges of function are not the same for each category.

Source: Reproduced from Appl Psychol Meas, 1(3), Radloff LS, The CES-D Scale: a self-report depression scale for research in the general population, pp. 385-401, Copyright (1977), with permission from SAGE Publications.

Ordered scores are not scientific measurements

Four types of scales are commonly used to elicit health information: *nominal, ordinal, interval,* and *ratio.* In mental health, the majority of scales are comprised of questions with *ordinal* response categories. An ordinal scale orders the category response options,

but unlike interval scales, it does not define the magnitude of the interval between the categories [31]. Ordinal scales have an obvious hierarchy to the scoring; however, the spacing between response options is not necessarily equal [17, 31]. For example, for an item such as 'How would you rate your health today?', a typical response option structure may be 'poor'/'fair'/'good'/'very good'/'excellent'. Each response category is typically assigned numerical values (e.g. 1, 2, 3, 4, 5), so that a total score can be generated. Assigning sequential, equally spaced numbers implies that the distance between these categories is equal. However, it has been well established that only items measured on an *interval* scale—in which the units are equally spaced—should be added to produce a total score [3, 4, 37].

Another example of multiple-item scales extrapolating ordinal measurement is the commonly used Centre for Epidemiological Scale for Depression (CES-D) [33]. The CES-D has 20 items in four item response categories, which summarize how often a person felt a certain way over the last week. Response categories include 0 (< 1 day), 1 (1–2 days), 2 (3–4 days), and 3 (5–7 days). The response category figures are then summed to give a total score. Scoring the items with sequential integers implies equal differences in depression at the item level, in that differences between each response category are implied to be equal, and at the total score level, in which a change of 1 point implies an equal change in depression across the range of the scale. So, is a total score a measurement of depression? The 'no' lobby would argue that a constant unit is an absolute requirement for measurement [7], whereas the 'yes' lobby would argue that ordinal scores are weaker forms of measurement or adequately approximate interval level measurement [55]. Yet in looking at the scale structure alone, we can observe that the quantification of each category is not equal (0 = < 1 day; 3 = 5–7 days), and so justifying a total score of imbalanced categories may not make perfect mathematical sense.

Careful consideration of the relationship between scores assigned to item response categories and generated by scales and the measurements they imply is required. When reading state-of-the art mental health research, stakeholders should, whenever possible, consider the best approaches to using and applying methods to achieve this standard of methodological rigour. Before we outline such approaches, we feel it is important to outline the rationale for why the application of new methods for the development and interpretation of rating scales are needed.

What are you trying to measure?

Information generated from rating scales is most meaningful if statistical analysis does not alter the unit of measurement or the numerical meaning of the numbers [14, 56]. Thus, a change in 1 point on a scale should have the same meaning throughout the continuum. For example, in physical health, it is easy to qualify what it means to have a weight increase of 10 kg or lbs. Such an easy interpretation is not often possible for ordinal scales, in which a change or difference in 1 point can be variable across the continuum (see Fig. 22.2).

When measuring mental health outcomes such as mood, cognition, and function, mental health stakeholders face an ambiguous task when attempting to qualify the meaning of a 1-point change throughout the measurement continuum [56, 57]. This ambiguity both makes it difficult to describe the changes observed and also complicates how total scores can be used to infer relationships between other health outcomes. As a result, quantifying meaningful linear relationships using ordinal rating scales is unlikely. In fact, the relationship is S-shaped (Fig. 22.3). Empirical studies show that a 1-point change in an ordinal score can vary up to 15-fold across the scale range, and the variation is scale dependent [58–61]. This variability has obvious and serious implications for clinical trials,

in which fundamental decisions are being made based on overall observed differences among groups, rather than individuals.

Another related problem with ordinal scores is that they are only suitable for group-level comparisons, making comparisons across individuals often impossible. Comparisons can only be made at the group level because the confidence intervals around the ordinal score are wide. For example, in recent studies using depression and anxiety measures to measure the effectiveness of cognitive–behavioural therapy, confidence intervals around total scores ranged from ±4.0 to ±10.5 points, which equates to 33–40% of their respective total score ranges [62–64]. Consequently, there are limitations for how clinical trials can legitimately compare changes and differences among individuals [17, 65]. Nonetheless, critical decisions are being made on these group-based analyses. These types of analyses only inform the extent to which one treatment in statistically better than another treatment. Understanding the complexities of why an individual undergoes different levels and directions of change would be advantageous to interpret the results of research studies and to inform the quality of care for people with complex and long-term mental health problems.

Theoretical bases for clinical outcome assessment in mental health

Another important criterion to consider when selecting a COA is the measurement model underpinning the tool. Three commonly used measurement models exist.

Classical test theory

Classical test theory (CTT) is the measurement theory that is the most well-known and has underpinned scale development and testing of reliability and validity since the early twentieth century. Charles Spearman proposed CTT in response to his repeated observations about how some sets of items he tested seemed to give more consistent results than other sets [66]. From these observations, Spearman posited that an observed score 'O' was composed of a true score 'T' and an error score 'E'. CTT proposes that there is a linear model linking O to the sum of T and E, such that: $O = T + E$. Only the observed score 'O' is observable, and the true and error scores are considered latent [66, 67].

CTT assumes that measurement errors are randomly distributed and not correlated with the total score. Further, for any individual, the measurement error associated with one scale is not correlated with the true score or measurement error of another scale. Error may be the result of many different influences that can affect an individual at any moment during the testing, and so clinicians and researchers must consider these influences. For example, an individual may have just lost their housing, or may have just won the lottery. The influence may be both negative and positive and can cause a range of error around the true score [67].

Errors can also be described as *systematic* or *random*. A *systematic error* refers to a characteristic of the test or the testing situation that will affect all measurements equally [67]. The systematic error may occur if a test repeatedly measures something other than what the test was intended to measure [55]. The impact of this error may influence all testing candidates equally. CTT assumes that systematic error does not take place. Thus, stakeholders must carefully

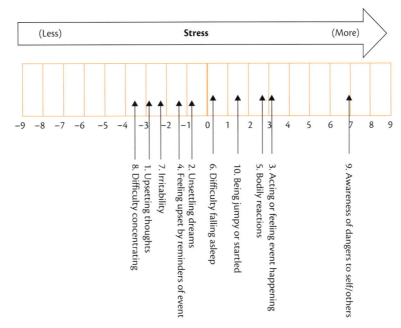

Fig. 22.2 How items on a measurement continuum can tell a clinical story. This is an example of the Trauma Screen Questionnaire (TSQ) filled in by adults who experience mental illness and marginalization in an urban community. The TSQ is a 10-item screening assessment for stress. Each item is scored as 0 or 1. Items are summed to produce a total score that ranges from '0' (all responses 'no') to '10' (all responses 'yes'). This figure shows the distribution of the items along the continuum of the concept of interest. This can be seen as the story of items how a person, on average, moves up the concept of interest. For example, a person is likely to endorse item #8 (difficulty concentrating) most strongly first as an early indicator of stress. As the person moves up the continuum (more stress), he/she is more likely to endorse the next set of items (#1, #7 … #9). In this example, item #9 is the most 'difficult' item. A person who endorses this item has a high probability for also endorsing the items that came before it. The hierarchy of items can inform the story of where a person is at on the continuum. This can be advantageous for clinical decision-making, research purposes, or for developing a language between stakeholders.

consider their context of use and testing process to ensure that systematic errors are minimized. This may include standardizing the ways in which assessment takes place: the day, time, assessment location, and rater, for instance.

Random error in COA is associated with unknown or unpredictable changes in the assessment. In mental health, random error is common and can be minimized by taking more frequent measures of an outcome. An example of random error is patient

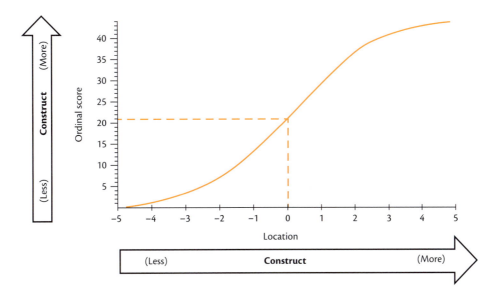

Fig. 22.3 Example of how total scores often do not have a linear relationship with a person's ability estimate. This is an example of a sample of patients with mental illness who completed all items on a 10-item questionnaire. Each item is scored 0–4, for a total scoring range of 0–40. The figure shows that the total score on the questionnaire (vertical axis) can be mapped to the unique estimate of ability of the person (horizontal axis). The shape of the curve is generally sigmoid shaped. Thus, the precise relationship between total scores and person estimates depends on the items on the test. In this example, a person who scores 21 falls approximately in the middle of the distribution.

or rater fatigue or illness. The error may produce an estimate that is different from the true underlying value. In mental health care, many important decisions may rely on the outcome generated from COAs. Thus, minimizing random error through frequent assessment and averaging observations can help to minimize the impact of these values.

One critique of CTT is that it is sample dependent. In measuring outcomes, ideally a COA is free of measurement error or bias. As an analogy: when measuring weight, a bathroom scale does not care whether the person on the scale is male or female, old or young, well rested or fatigued. The value produced is independent of these characteristics; it does not vary. *Invariance* is the term often used to describe the property of remaining unchanged regardless of changes in the conditions of measurement. Fortunately, new psychometric approaches to measurement development and testing can provide valuable information about invariance.

Item response theory

Item response theory (IRT), also known as latent trait theory, is a statistical modelling paradigm that is used to find mathematical models that explain data [68]. IRT is commonly used for the design, analysis, and scoring of rating scales in health to quantify latent outcomes. IRT emerged as a measurement theory during the 1950s and 1960s, and became more widely used in the late 1970s and 1980s as information technology introduced software that made computations feasible. IRT tests the relationship between patients' performances on a test item and an overall measure of the ability that item was designed to measure. IRT can produce several *statistical models* to represent the characteristics of the items in a test and the test-takers themselves.

One key feature of IRT is that it does not assume each item is equally difficult. This distinguishes the approach from CTT, where it is assumed that all items are replications of each other and can be added equally to produce a total score.

The IRT includes three key assumptions [69]. Firstly, the trait under investigation is *unidimensional*; that is, a COA should measure only one underlying trait. Secondly, *local dependence* of items must be met. Local dependence requires that (i) the chance of one item being used is not related to another item or items on the assessment; and (ii) the response to an item is the person's independent decision, separate from any external influence or group [70]. Finally, the third assumption is that the response of a person to an item can be modelled and described by an *item response function* (IRF). The IRF, described more comprehensively elsewhere [71, 72], posits the probability that a person with a given ability will endorse an item a certain way. For example, consider a set of items ordered from low (easiest) to high (hardest). Persons with lower ability have less of a chance to endorse the more difficult items, whereas people with high ability are very likely to endorse difficult items. To use a rough example: if a person can successfully run 5 km, it is likely that they can also run 1, 2, 3, and 4 km distances (although this example incorporates dependence). However, if the person is unable to complete 6 km—a more difficult item—the probability of them completing longer distances at that point in time is lower. The IRF also comes with a set of parameters that help to determine the exact probability—in this case, the exact probability of the person being able to complete a 6-km run based on their failed attempt to run further than 5 km. The IRF's parameters can include factors such as gender and age. This information can be important for tailoring

coaching and training. In mental health, it can also be helpful to use IRT output to generate information about a person's ability and the level of support (item difficulty) that they may need to improve their health.

Rasch measurement theory

The Rasch model, named after the Danish mathematician Georg Rasch (1901–80), is also widely used in health outcome measurement to transform ordinal response categories onto a linear scale with interval-like properties. Rasch measurement theory (RMT) is an experimental psychometric paradigm used to examine the extent to which the observed rating scale data fit the assumption of an underlying hierarchical construct [73, 74]. Compared with IRT, RMT uses a priori hypotheses about the ordering of the items and how they cover the latent concept of interest from low to high. RMT is based on a logit transformation of the probability of response to a particular item. An item that 50% of respondents pass or endorse has a logit of 0 [73, 75]. A scale that defines the full spectrum of a construct will range from –4 to + 4 logits, corresponding to ± 4 standard deviations defining the full range of a standard normal distribution.

Similarly to IRT, people at the low end of the logit scale are described to have less ability, whereas people at the high end have more ability. Correspondingly, items at the low end are easy to pass or endorse, whereas items at the high end are difficult to pass or endorse [76, 77]. A range of parameters arising from the Rasch analysis can be used to judge misfit and the resultant extent to which scoring and summing is defensible in the data collected according to the Rasch model [78]. This ability to judge and defend scoring and summation is a particular strength for researchers and clinicians working in mental health.

The routine use of COA that meet RMT criteria provides an opportunity to help drive how health care is organized, delivered, and funded [79–81]. Mental health stakeholders are increasingly using RMT tools because they can enable a common language between patients, clinicians, researchers, and other involved parties. This common outcome language in mental health can be used to compare performance metrics of clinical services to evidence-based guidelines or standards.

Conclusions

COAs measure key aspects of disease burden in medicine. In addition, they can provide a rich profile about where a person is at, where they are going, and what level of support is needed to reach a target or end point. Careful attention is needed to develop, test, select, administer, and interpret information generated from these tools. The fundamental challenge with assessment in mental health is that many of these outcomes cannot be measured directly, which, in turn, challenges how data can be used to inform new levels of healthcare efficiency and quality. However, with the availability of new methods, the routine use of COA in mental health now provides an opportunity to help drive how health care is organized and delivered.

In this chapter, we outlined several recommendations for maximizing the contributions of assessment in research and practice. Clinical insight, consideration of patient and family needs, and robust measurement provide opportunities to ensure that the right patient receives the right intervention at the right time. By focusing on patient priorities and improving patient outcomes, mental health stakeholders—from clinicians and researchers up to hospital administrators, policymakers, and politicians—can optimize healthcare systems and practices. As we work towards the aim of having a mental health system with agreed-upon assessments and units, it is critical for all stakeholders to use theoretically driven data to improve healthcare systems and practices.

Thus, Ernest Amory Codman was far ahead of his time when, in the early 1900s, he began tracking data to improve patient outcomes. It would have been a wonder to have both he and the forerunners of measurement theory side by side. Fortunately, their efforts and methods have been well documented. The importance of their ideas, incorporated with modern-day methods of assessment administration, cannot be overemphasized. Advances in measurement science can improve healthcare systems and practices by bringing innovative approaches to the point of care. Increased understanding of the evolution of measurement in mental health is needed to ensure greater quality, accountability, and accessibility of care.

References

1. Maddox T. *The History and Antiquities of the Exchequer of the Kings of England, in Two Periods: To wit, From the Norman Conquest, to the End of the Reign of K. John; and From the End of the Reign of K. John, to the End of the Reign of K. Edward II.* Vol T. London: Printed for W. Owen, 1711.
2. Baxter TW. Early accounting, the tally and the checkerboard. *Account Hist J* 1989; 16: 43–83.
3. Chun J, Bafford AC. History and background of quality measurement. *Clin Colon Rectal Surg* 2014; 27: 5–9.
4. Mallon B. *Ernest Amory Codman: The End Result of a Life in Medicine.* Philadelphia, PA: WB Saunders, 2000.
5. Codman EA, Chipman WW, Clark JW, Kanavel AB, Mayo WJ. Standardization of hospitals: report of the committee appointed by the Clinical Congress of Surgery of America. *Trans Clin Con Surg North America* 1913; 4: 2–8.
6. World Health Organization. Mental disorders. Available at: http://www.who.int/mediacentre/factsheets/fs396/en/ (2016, accessed 31 March 2017).
7. Michell J. Measurement: a beginner's guide. *J Appl Meas* 2003; 4: 298–308.
8. Wiering B, de Boer D, Delnoij D. Patient involvement in the development of patient-reported outcome measures: a scoping review. *Health Expect* 2017; 20: 11–23.
9. Coulter A. Measuring what matters to patients. *BMJ* 2017; 356: j816.
10. Anthony WA. Recovery from mental illness: the guiding vision of the mental health service system in the 1990's. *Psychosoc Rehabil J.* 1993; 16: 11–23.
11. Kidd SA, McKenzie KJ, Virdee G. Mental health reform at a systems level: widening the lens on recovery-oriented care. *Can J Psychiatry* 2014; 59: 243–249.
12. Kidd SA, George L, O'Connell M, et al. Fidelity and recovery orientation in Assertive Community Treatment. *Community Ment Health J* 2010; 46: 342–350.
13. Slade M, Amering M, Farkas M, et al. Uses and abuses of recovery: implementing recovery-oriented practices in mental health systems. *World Psychiatry* 2014; 13: 1–12.
14. Bezruczko N. *Rasch Measurement in Health Sciences.* Maple Grove, MN: JAM Press, 2005.
15. Tesio L. Measuring behaviors and perceptions: Rasch analysis as a tool for rehabilitation research. *J Rehabil Med* 2003; 35: 105–115.
16. Cano SJ, Barrrett LE, Zajicek JP, Hobart JC. Beyond the reach of traditional analyses: using Rasch to evaluate the DASH in people with multiple sclerosis. *Mult Scler J* 2011; 17: 214–222.
17. Hobart JC, Cano SJ, Zajicek JP, Thompson AA. Rating scales as outcome measures for clinical trials in neurology: problems, solutions, and recommendations. *Lancet Neurol* 2007; 6: 1094–1105.
18. Gnanasakthy A, Mordin M, Clark M, DeMuro C, Fehnel S, Copley-Merriman C. A review of patient-reported outcome labels in the United States: 2006 to 2010. *Value Health* 2012; 15: 437–442.
19. Brundage M, Blazeby J, Revicki D, et al. Patient-reported outcomes in randomized clinical trials: development of ISOQOL reporting standards. *Qual Life Res* 2013; 22: 1161–1175.
20. Patrick D, Burke LB, Gwaltney CJ, et al. Content validity—establishing and reporting the evidence in newly developed patient-reported outcomes (PRO) instruments for medical product evaluation: ISPOR PRO good research practices task force report: part 2—assessing respondent understanding. *Value Health* 2011; 14: 978–988.
21. Patrick DL, Burke LB, Gwaltney CJ, et al. Content validity—establishing and reporting the evidence in newly developed patient-reported outcomes (PRO) instruments for medical product evaluation: ISPOR PRO good research practices task force report: part 1—eliciting concepts for a new PRO instrument. *Value Health* 2011; 14: 967–977.
22. United States Department of Health and Human Services. *Guidance for Industry: Patient Reported Measures: Use in Medical Product Development to Support Labeling Claims.* Rockville, MD: Food and Drug Administation, 2009.
23. Department of Health. *Guidance on the Routine Collection of Patient Reported Outcome Measures (PROMs).* London: Department of Health, 2009.
24. de Vet HCW, Terwee CB, Mokkink LB, Knol DL. *Measurement in Medicine: A Practical Guide.* Cambridge: Cambridge University Press, 2011.
25. Cronbach LJ. Coefficient alpha and the internal structure of tests. *Psychometrika* 1951; 16: 297–334.
26. Kelley TL. *Interpretation of Educational Measurements.* Yonkers, NY: World Book Company, 1927.
27. Cronbach LJ, Meehl PE. Construct validity in psychological tests. *Psychol Bull* 1955; 52: 281–302.
28. American Psychological Association (APA). *Standards for Educational and Psychological Tests.* Washington, DC: APA, 1974.
29. Kendell R, Jablensky A. Distinguishing between the validity and utility of psychiatric diagnoses. *Am J Psychiatry* 2003; 160: 4–12.
30. Stenner AJ, Fisher WP, Jr, Stone MH, Burdick DS. Causal Rasch models. *Front Psychol* 2013; 4: 536.
31. Bombardier C, Tugwell PA. Methodological framework to develop and select indices for clinical trials: statistical and judgmental approaches. *J Rheumatol* 1982; 9: 753–757.
32. Hall RC. Global assessment of functioning. A modified scale. *Psychosomatics* 1995; 36: 267–275.
33. Radloff LS. The CES-D Scale: a self-report depression scale for research in the general population. *Appl Psychol Meas* 1977; 7: 385–401.
34. Beck AT, Ward CH, Mendelson M, Mock J, Erbaugh J. An inventory for measuring depression. *Arch Gen Psychiatry* 1961; 4: 561–571.
35. Hamilton M. The assessment of anxiety states. *Br J Med Psychol* 1959; 32: 50–55.
36. Grootenboer EM, Giltay EJ, van der Lem R, van Veen T, van der Wee NJ, Zitman FG. Reliability and validity of the Global Assessment of Functioning Scale in clinical outpatients with depressive disorders. *J Eval Clin Pract* 2012; 12: 502–507.
37. Nunnally J, Bernstein I. *Psychometric Theory*, 3rd ed. New York: McGraw-Hill, 1994.
38. Manning W, Newhouse J, Ware JE, Jr. The status of health in demand estimation: or beyond excellent, good, fair, and poor. In: Fuchs V (ed.). *Economic Aspects of Health.* Chicago, IL: Univeristy of Chicago Press, 1982, pp. 143–184.
39. American Psychiatric Association (APA). *Diagnostic and Statistical Manual of Mental Disorders*, 5th ed. Arlington, VA: APA, 2013.
40. Haas BM, Bergstrom E, Jamous A, Bennie A. The inter rater reliability of the original and of the modified Ashworth scale for the assessment

of spasticity in patients with spinal cord injury. *Spinal Cord* 1996; 34: 560–564.

41. Hobart J, Freeman J, Thompson A. Kurtzke scales revisited: the application of psychometric methods to clinical intuition. *Brain* 2000; 123: 1027–1040.

42. Blackburn M, van Vliet P, Mockett SP. Reliability of measurements obtained with the modified Ashworth scale in the lower extremities of people with stroke. *Phys Ther* 2002; 82: 25–34.

43. Clopton N, Dutton J, Featherston T, Grigsby A, Mobley J, Melvin J. Interrater and intrarater reliability of the Modified Ashworth Scale in children with hypertonia. *Pediatr Phys Ther* 2005; 17: 268–274.

44. Wilson JT, Hareendran A, Hendry A, Potter J, Bone I, Muir KW. Reliability of the modified Rankin Scale across multiple raters: benefits of a structured interview. *Stroke* 2005; 36: 777–781.

45. McFarlane WR, Levin B, Travis L, et al. Clinical and functional outcomes after 2 years in the early detection and intervention for the prevention of psychosis multisite effectiveness trial. *Schizophr Bull* 2015; 41: 30–43.

46. Chaudhry M, Maqsood A, Diab-Agha S, Rosenberg J. Nicardipine-induced acute hepatitis in an intensive care unit patient. *Am J Ther* 2009; 16: 71–73.

47. Vaney C, Heinzel-Gutenbrunner M, Jobin P, et al. Efficacy, safety and tolerability of an orally administered cannabis extract in the treatment of spasticity in patients with multiple sclerosis: a randomized, double-blind, placebo-controlled, crossover study. *Mult Scler* 2004; 10: 417–424.

48. Cameron JI, Cheung AM, Streiner D, Coyte PC, Stewart DE. Stroke survivor depressive symptoms are associated with family caregiver depression during the first 2 years poststroke. *Stroke* 2011; 42: 302–306.

49. Uyttenboogaart M, Luijckx GJ, Vroomen PC, Stewart RE, De Keyser J. Measuring disability in stroke: relationship between the modified Rankin scale and the Barthel index. *J Neurol* 2007; 254: 1113–1117.

50. Bird VJ, Le Boutillier C, Leamy M, Williams J, Bradstreet S, Slade M. Evaluating the feasibility of complex interventions in mental health services: standardised measure and reporting guidelines. *Br J Psychiatry* 2014; 204: 316–321.

51. Hung CI, Wang SJ, Yao YC, Yang CH. The cut-off points of the Depression and Somatic Symptoms Scale and the Hospital Anxiety and Depression Scale in detecting non-full remission and a current major depressive episode. *Int J Psychiatry Clin Pract* 2012; 16: 33–40.

52. Ambrosini PJ, Metz C, Bianchi MD, Rabinovich H, Undie A. Concurrent validity and psychometric properties of the Beck Depression Inventory in outpatient adolescents. *J Am Acad Child Adolesc Psychiatry* 1991; 30: 51–57.

53. Andresen R, Caputi P, Oades L. Stages of recovery instrument: development of a measure of recovery from serious mental illness. *Aust N Z J Psychiatry* 2006; 40: 972–980.

54. Bridges JF, Slawik L, Schmeding A, Reimer J, Naber D, Kuhnigk O. A test of concordance between patient and psychiatrist valuations of multiple treatment goals for schizophrenia. *Health Expect* 2013; 16: 164–176.

55. Nunnally JC. *Psychometric Theory*, 1st ed. New York: McGraw-Hill, 1967.

56. Wright BD, Linacre JM. Observations are always ordinal; measurements, however, must be interval. *Arch Phys Med Rehabil* 1989; 70: 857–860.

57. Hedeker D. Methods for multilevel ordinal data in prevention research. *Prev Sci* 2015; 16: 997–1006.

58. Wright BD. A history pf social science and measurement. *Educ Meas* 1997; 52: 33–52.

59. Kersten P, White PJ, Tennant A. Is the pain visual analogue scale linear and responsive to change? An exploration using Rasch analysis. *PLOS ONE* 2014; 9: e99485.

60. Katzenschlager R, Schrag A, Evans A, et al. Quantifying the impact of dyskinesias in PD: the PDYS-26: a patient-based outcome measure. *Neurology* 2007; 69: 555–563.

61. Sargent-Cox KA, Anstey KJ, Luszcz MA. Patterns of longitudinal change in older adults' self-rated health: the effect of the point of reference. *Health Psychol* 2010; 29: 143–152.

62. Hedman E, Axelsson E, Gorling A, et al. Internet-delivered exposure-based cognitive-behavioural therapy and behavioural stress management for severe health anxiety: randomised controlled trial. *Br J Psychiatry* 2014; 205: 307–314.

63. Wiles N, Thomas L, Abel A, et al. Clinical effectiveness and cost-effectiveness of cognitive behavioural therapy as an adjunct to pharmacotherapy for treatment-resistant depression in primary care: the CoBalT randomised controlled trial. *Health Technol Assess* 2014; 18: 1–167.

64. Wiles N, Thomas L, Abel A, et al. Cognitive behavioural therapy as an adjunct to pharmacotherapy for primary care based patients with treatment resistant depression: results of the CoBalT randomised controlled trial. *Lancet* 2013; 381: 375–384.

65. McHorney CA, Tarlov AR. Individual-patient monitoring in clinical practice: are available health status surveys adequate? *Qual Life Res* 1995; 4: 293–307.

66. Traub R. Classical test theory in historical perspective. *Educ Meas* 1997; 16: 8–14.

67. Streiner D, Norman G. *Health Measurement Scales: A Practical Guide to Their Development and Use*, 3rd ed. Oxford: Oxford University Press, 2007.

68. Frost MH, Reeve BB, Liepa AM, Stauffer JW, Hays RD, Mayo/FDA Patient-reported outcome consensus meeting group. What is sufficient evidence for the reliability and validity of patient-reported outcome measures? *Value Health* 2007; 10(Suppl. 2): S94–S105.

69. Lord F. A theory of test scores. *Psychometr Monogr* 1952; 7: 84.

70. Lord F. The relation of the reliability of multiple-choice tests to the distribution of item difficulties. *Psychometrika* 1952; 17: 181–194.

71. Cook KF, Teal CR, Bjorner JB, et al. IRT health outcomes data analysis project: an overview and summary. *Qual Life Res* 2007; 16(Suppl. 1): 121–132.

72. Lord FM. *Applications of Item Response Theory to Practical Testing Problems*. Hillsdale, NJ: Lawrence Erlbaum Associates, 1980.

73. Rasch G. *Probabilistic Models for Some Intelligence and Attainment Tests*. Copenhagen: Danish Institute for Education Research, 1980.

74. Hobart JC, Cano SJ, Posner H, et al. Putting the Alzheimer's cognitive test to the test II: Rasch Measurement Theory. *Alzheimers Dement* 2013; 9(1 Suppl.): S10–S20.

75. Rasch G. On general laws and the meaning of measurement in psychology. In: *Proceedings of the Fourth Berkeley Symposium in Mathematical Statistics and Probability, IV*. Berkeley, CA: University of California Press, 1961, pp. 321–334.

76. Andrich D. Rating scales and Rasch measurement. *Expert Rev Pharmacoecon Outcomes Res* 2011; 11: 571–585.

77. Andrich D. *Rasch Models for Measurement*. Beverly Hills, CA: SAGE, 1988.

78. Andrich D, Sheridan B, Luo G. RUMM 2030. 4.0 for windows (upgrade 4600.0109). Perth, WA: RUMM laboratory Pty Ltd, 1997–2010.

79. Reeve BB, Wyrwich KW, Wu AW, et al. ISOQOL recommends minimum standards for patient-reported outcome measures used in patient-centered outcomes and comparative effectiveness research. *Qual Life Res* 2013; 22: 1889–1905.

80. Ahmed S, Berzon RA, Revicki DA, et al. The use of patient-reported outcomes (PRO) within comparative effectiveness research: implications for clinical practice and health care policy. *Med Care* 2012; 50: 1060–1070.

81. Kirwan JR, Bartlett SJ, Beaton DE, et al. Updating the OMERACT filter: implications for patient-reported outcomes. *J Rheumatol* 2014; 41: 1011–1015.

CHAPTER 23

Environmental contaminants and mental health
The chemicalization of life as a matter of violation of the right to health and renewal of the 'disease industry'

Paulo Amarante and Eduardo Torre

Introduction

Contemporary society faces a major global dilemma: food insecurity and environmental contamination due to a predatory development model that began in the post-war period, which has produced an unsustainable and poisoned society. The predatory model of post-industrial capitalism had its start linked to central factors such as chemical-dependent agriculture, social medicalization, and the nutrition transition, associated with the perverse mercantilization of natural resources. The expansion of large-scale monocultures using agrochemicals and pesticides, pharmaceutical industry and medical technification, and additivated industrial food are consequences of these interconnected factors. This process is institutionally and legally permitted, and it has been producing multiple violations of human rights and deepening various forms of intoxication and illnesses: it is the model known as the chemicalization of life.

In this sense, one of the major discussions is post-war agriculture and its contemporary configuration, especially the teratogenic effects, violation of human rights, and environmental injustice [1–7].

After the Second World War there was a global change in agriculture, which is today commonly referred to as the 'green revolution', with the introduction of chemical inputs to the production of food and in the extensive monoculture controlled by large transnational corporations. This change in agriculture leads to production processes dependent on the use of 'agricultural defensives', mechanization, and massive production, resulting in soil depletion and contamination of water resources and living beings.

The consequences of this process are severe illnesses, the loss of rights and vulnerability of disadvantaged social groups, and exacerbated environmental contamination. In this context, it becomes evident that the right to health presents a condition of extreme contradiction and is often reduced to the discussion on the access to health services. It is also evident that the result of this process is sanitary and environmental injustice, and the precariousness of rural and urban living conditions.

On the one hand, studies in the area of collective health have gained strength and are instrumental in social movements and political struggles facing interests linked to the model of the chemicalization of life and agrointoxication of society; on the other hand, there appears to be a need to broaden the investigation and even the thematization on the relation between mental health and the effects and consequences of environmental contaminants, agrochemicals, and food additives. The studies on the relations between polyintoxication and the chemicalization of life and the various forms of mental illness need funding.

This means that the use and consumption of agrochemicals and food additives, associated with very diverse factors of environmental contamination and social insalubrity, such as the innumerable overlapping forms of pollution, exposure to risks and stress, food insecurity or malnutrition, and many factors of social insecurity and precarious living conditions, lead to complex combinations of conditions that are related to many diseases or health insults. Some examples are hypertension, diabetes, infarction, stroke, obesity, child and adult allergies, depression, sexual impotence, suicide, cancer, reproductive infertility, and there are even studies and indications of a relation to autism and attention deficit hyperactivity disorder. Surely these are complex and multifaceted diseases to which it is not possible to associate only one factor; but in all of them one finds many cases in which it is possible to state that these are prevailing or vastly relevant factors. As in the perverse triad in young men suffering from and being victimized by the sequence sexual impotence–depression–suicide, it was believed that those were isolated cases, but they are being revealed as systematically repetitive, in worrisome and under-reported conditions occurring in developed countries, as well as in developing and peripheral countries [8–14].

This extremely important field of studies seeks to discuss the relations between environmental contaminants and mental health, leading to the problematization of the effects of mental illnesses in the population resulting from food insecurity and environmental injustice arising from what one could denominate 'industry of multiple intoxications' or 'industry of poisoning'. In the same way, it is possible to refer to the 'industry of disease' as linked to the interests concerning the mercantilization of suffering and the privatization of health.

In other words, what is configured is the institutionalization of multiple intoxication engendering violations to the right to health and the right to food, with severe impacts on physical and mental health, as well as on social and cultural rights and the protection of life.

Mental health and agrochemicals: the emblematic case of the 'perverse triad' of impotence, depression, and suicide

It is crucial for the field of collective health to face the issue of food and nutrition security, and the violations of the right to health and food, including the effects of food insecurity on health and the environment. In this debate, much evidence and many documented problems have been presented relating the multiple impacts from the industrial and agrointoxicated food model to the mental and physical health of workers and society in general. Thus, it is possible to affirm the need to question the legality and feasibility of this model from the point of view of the right to health as a fundamental right in democratic societies [15, 16]; and this leads to verifying that the model of chemical-dependent agriculture has been producing multiple forms of intoxication and deep precariousness of living conditions in rural and urban areas [17–-19].

In this context stands out a perverse triad that has been present on the international scene and demands urgent and further research and debates: the perverse triad of sexual impotence, depression, and suicide, which has been repeatedly occurring among rural workers who use agrochemicals.

The impacts from agrochemical intoxication on health are well known, but in this case there is a domino effect, with biopsychosocial consequences, as the use of agrochemicals by workers, even with the wearing of personal protective equipment, has triggered sexual impotence and depression as conditions that are directly associated with intensive exposure. Suicide has also been observed as a consequence of chemical intoxication, whether acute and intense, or as a consequence of depression from intoxication, associated with marital crisis and economic insecurity, and in some cases associated with threats and pressures undergone by workers.

The use of certain agrochemicals is directly related to high suicide rates among agricultural workers in several countries because it directly affects the central nervous system (CNS), triggering psychiatric disorders, including anxiety, irritability, insomnia or sleep disorders, depression, and suicide, often caused by the voluntary ingestion of the same poison used on crops [8, 10].

Neurological and behavioural alterations have been confirmed in relation to acute or subacute intoxication with dramatic consequences, as in a pioneer study of the repercussions of the use of organophosphate agrochemicals in tobacco cultivation in Brazil, causing neurological disorders, symptoms of Parkinson disease, and suicide among agricultural workers [20], as well as other studies with similar results [8, 21].

Mental health, human rights, and environmental justice: the debate in the field of collective health

Several researchers have been pointing to the need for the thematization and integration of studies on the relations between environmental contamination and chemical intoxication with impacts on mental health.

The effects of exposure to pesticides on neurobehavioural and cognitive development are associated with neurotoxicity among adolescent and adult workers, as well as among the non-working population, including children. This association has been investigated in various forms, including the assessment of experimental data for 'developmental neurotoxicity' from pesticides. The majority of neurotoxic compounds are included in organophosphates and carbamates, pyrethroids, and organochlorines, among others, which interfere in the normal development of the CNS. Studies assess not only the potential toxicity of pesticides on children, but also the effects during the gestational period, with a special focus on developmental neurotoxicity.

Preventing neurotoxic diseases related to pesticides depends on investigation in order to provide guidance to intervention policies for the protection of human health, with an emphasis on examining potential long-term effects since pre-adolescence, childhood, or prenatal exposure.

Studies on developmental neurotoxicity show the challenges in understanding the effects of exposure to pesticides on health across the lifespan, i.e. in the various stages of the life course, and especially important is the evidence on neurobehavioural deficits and attention deficit hyperactivity disorder (ADHD) in children, as well as neurobehavioural changes in adolescents who work with organophosphate pesticides [22].

High levels of exposure, including poisoning, result in high levels of multiple damage, with agricultural contamination and neuropsychiatric sequelae, including the use of pesticides as a cause of suicide. Poisoning from pesticides alters the brain and leads to an increase of anxiety and depression. Exposure to organophosphate pesticides causes depression, impulsivity, and mood disorders, which explains the increased association between exposure to organophosphates and suicide.

In developed countries, high levels of neurobehavioural deficits have been found in children exposed to pesticides in the prenatal period. Also, ADHD has been found in the USA among children aged 8–15 years, associated with urinary metabolites of organophosphate pesticides. Besides, studies have been conducted on the impact of the exposure to pesticides in adolescents who work during the period of poison application. In other countries, there is also evidence of similar phenomena in the association of suicide and depression with exposure to organophosphates among agricultural workers [22].

Adverse results in pregnancy/procreation among women working in Colombian floriculture, exposed to pesticides and other risk factors, were investigated with regard to their association with spontaneous abortion, premature birth, and congenial malformation [23]. In Ecuador, an investigation was conducted on neurobehavioural development in children potentially exposed to pesticides and environmental contamination in the flower industry owing to the proximity of rural communities to large agricultural industries, and found impairment of fine and gross motor skills and problem-solving skills [24]. But there are results that still cause controversy. The approach of biomedical and experimental research, prevalent in toxicological and clinical studies, has a reductionist character and contrasts with systemic, sociological and transdisciplinary analyses, in relation to broader and critically deeper research protocols that include the consideration of environmental causes.

One of the most worrisome issues in investigations worldwide is the relationship between autism and agricultural pesticides; they highlight the urgent need to integrate data sources for surveillance and research, as in the Centers for Disease Control and Prevention's Environmental Public Health Tracking Program. The large convergence of data on birth, social services, and agriculture has allowed researchers to relate environmental exposure to agricultural pesticides and autism spectrum disorders (ASD) in children. The study focused on autism in children and its association with their mothers' residence during pregnancy and at the time of birth near well-defined agricultural fields with pesticide applications, including the commonly used dicofol and endosulfan, in the production of cotton, fruit, vegetables, beans, and nuts in the region of California's Central Valley [25, 26].

Respiratory diseases have been associated with environments with concentrations of polycyclic aromatic hydrocarbons (PAHs), a type of air pollutant, confirming that chemical contaminants are a problem of great importance to preschool children, the same way as fine particles (PM2.5) represent a risk to very young children. PAHs and PM2.5 are primarily formed from the combustion of products from petroleum, charcoal, wood, tobacco, garbage, and fat, among other substances. The production of polychlorinated biphenyls (PCBs) has similar effects; PCBs were widely used in electrical transformers, plastics, and other products, and production of them has been banned in the USA since the 1970s. However, virtually all US citizens present measurable levels of PCBs because their compounds persist in the environment and are accumulated in organisms (bioaccumulation) [26]. Epidemiological studies have associated prenatal exposure to PCBs with impaired neurodevelopment in children and babies; in studies with animals, prenatal exposure caused a decrease in the levels of thyroid hormones, such as thyroxine, which are essential for neurodevelopment. The rupture of the thyroid system is one of the pathways via which PCBs can cause damage, but the endocrine disruptors have been studied in a much broader way and this is only one of the most robustly proven effects on human health. Dozens of environmental chemicals were found in the blood samples of 285 pregnant women in a cohort study from Salinas Valley, California, including 34 congeners of PCBs, which have at least 209 congeners. In the same source, reference is made to the use of dichlorodiphenyltrichloroethane since the 1960s, with evidence of its association with breast cancer in women, and cancer, in general [26].

Another important study regarding the findings of environmental causes of ASD and neurodevelopmental disabilities (NDD) has been conducted at the School of Medicine at Mount Sinai in New York along with the National Institute of Environmental Health Services. Genetic research has always received attention and funding, but despite the hereditary component often present in ASD and in other NDD, this research should be complemented by environmental studies for the investigation of causes of NDD. The great sensibility of the developing human brain regarding toxic elements, especially during the embryonic and fetal stages, considered as 'windows of vulnerability', indicates the need to study the environmental causes of ASD and other NDD. With follow-up of the mother and child over time, researchers have been conducting prospective studies to discover the aetiological association between prenatal exposure and NDD. In the same way, an association of ASD with drugs used in the first trimester of pregnancy, such as thalidomide, misoprostol, and valproic acid, and also with rubella infection, has been discovered [27].

An association was made between autistic behaviours and prenatal exposure to organophosphate chlorpyrifos insecticide, and also between cognition loss, dyslexia, and ADHD with exposure to lead, methylmercury, organophosphate insecticides, organochlorine insecticides, endocrine disruptors, phthalates, arsenic, manganese, PAHs, bisphenol A, brominated flame retardants, and perfluorinated compounds, among many others. Toxic chemical elements cause damage to the developing human brain and also through direct toxicity and interactions with the genome. This means that a significant part of neurobehavioural disorders is directly caused by toxic environmental exposure, and an even greater part is caused by interactions between environmental factors, defined in a broad way, and inherited susceptibilities. The mechanisms of gene–environment interactions are related to epigenetic changes in gene expression, caused by toxic chemical elements, resulting in the impaired DNA methylation [27]. Considering that in the last 50 years over 80,000 new synthetic chemical substances have been developed, and that a least 3000 are produced in large amounts and present a great potential risk for human exposure, pregnant women and children are at risk of greater impact. At least 200 of these substances, mostly via consumption, are found in the blood of the entire North-American population. The consequences for child health and pregnancy are not completely known. A large number of the total chemical substances have not yet received the minimum assessment for their toxicity potential and only one-quarter have been tested for their toxicity potential during the early development of life.

In the same direction, several studies have investigated environmental causes of ASD and learning disabilities, from chemical products and mixtures widely distributed in the environment that are suspected of causing developmental neurotoxicity and many other effects [27–34].

Perhaps the most important is that of Stephanie Seneff of the Massachusetts Institute of Technology (MIT), which indicates a probable association between the use of agrochemicals and cases of child autism, related specifically to the use of glyphosate [35]. Predictions are that from 2025 onwards half of children born in the USA will be diagnosed with ASD. Seneff, too, does not consider autism as a neurological disorder arising only from genetics, but also from environmental factors, especially exposure to Monsanto Roundup® herbicide (glyphosate) and to a cocktail of heavy metals, including aluminium [36–39].

Seneff has been on the receiving end of pressure from the pharmaceutical industry and industrial agriculture against the dissemination of her research, which combines data processing with biological and toxicological studies. Aluminium and glyphosate, specifically, interrupt the functioning of the pineal gland (melatonin sulphate), in direct relation to autism. Glyphosate also interferes in important pathways of the absorption of amino acids in the gastro-intestinal system, destroying the intestinal flora, which is essential to health and responsible for the immune system, with harmful effects and precocious ageing. The harm caused by glyphosate to the intestine also causes impairment in the normal excretion of aluminium, which accumulates especially in the pineal gland, thus causing brain damage. Glyphosate forms an encasement over the aluminium, preventing its absorption by the organism and so the aluminium remains in tissues and its accumulation causes a chain reaction of problems. Furthermore, autistic children who had their regular diets, containing agrochemicals and neurotoxins, substituted with organic foods have shown improvements in speech patterns and in social and cognitive skills, with visible changes in just a few weeks.

Within a period of 5 years, the level of ASD in the USA increased from 1 in 150 to 1 in 50, and there is also an assumption that studies on environmental causes will point to similar associations for other diseases, such as Parkinson's and Alzheimer's, which were practically unheard of 50 years ago. Within only 10 years, the use of Roundup® in farms in the USA increased by over 80% and currently over 80,000 tons are used on transgenic corn, soya, and other crops, with unprecedented poisoning.

A final consideration on a crucial issue: since the 1980s and 1990s, cancer has been associated with pollution, exposure to contamination from toxic substances, and intoxication from agrochemicals; however, nowadays there is consensus that one of the causes of the vertiginous increase in the number of cancer cases in the last decades is the use and consumption of agrochemicals and multiple exposures to environmental contaminants [8, 40–43].

In Argentina, a tragic condition has been documented of an exponential increase in cancer cases, malformation of babies, and neonatal death, way above levels reported in historical records and levels registered in other countries. In 2010, the Argentinian media announced that agrochemicals had tripled cancer cases and quadrupled the number of babies born with malformations [8].

Institutionalized agrointoxication and the effects on human health: the case of Brazil

Brazil is the world largest consumer of agrochemical products since 2010 in terms of quantity and types, with proven use of products that are not legally permitted, and even among those permitted in the country many have been banned in several others. Brazil has a permissive legislation regarding the list of agrochemicals with commercial authorization and a low capacity for surveillance and regulation of this sector, which generates over US$5 billion net profit per year. This implies contamination of ecosystems, water, and air, with severe consequences to health in rural and urban areas. Although the *Conselho Nacional de Segurança Alimentar e Nutricional* (CONSEA; National Council for Food and Nutrition Security) has been active in putting pressure on the national administration in several ways, governmental control on agrochemicals, both by registration of permitted substances and banning those that are forbidden, must advance tremendously, because even the *Agência Nacional de Vigilância Sanitária* (ANVISA; National Agency for Sanitary Surveillance) has many difficulties to undertake this necessary control [9].

Thus, Brazil appears as the most agrointoxicated country on the planet, having little protection against agribusiness lobbies. Despite the fact that Brazilian environmental legislation is considered to be very advanced, there is a model of development based on commodities and extensive use of land for monocultures directed to the export of raw materials, resulting in the expulsion of traditional communities and vulnerable populations from territories under the speculation of the agribusiness. The greatest driving forces of this model have been transgenic soya, corn, and eucalyptus for the production of cellulose and feedstock, among others [9].

Therefore, the current situation may be defined as institutionalized agrointoxication, jeopardizing the quality of food and water for human consumption, with an obvious violation of the right to adequate food and nutrition that should be guaranteed according to Constitutional Amendment 64/2010; to be highlighted is the practice of biocides pulverization, which contaminates large areas beyond the territory of application, with severe impacts on the biodiversity of extensive regions, and this includes the contamination of rainwater [9].

Regarding the field of mental health, phenomena have been described such as the presence of agrochemicals in breast milk and impairments in child development [9]. In the state of Mato Grosso, a study of breast milk contamination by agrochemicals, conducted by Wanderley Pignati and Danielly Cristina Palma (see [9]), had a great impact on the national media because it denounced an extremely severe condition; as a consequence, they suffered threats and pressures, engendering the debate in the field of collective health in Brazil about the creation of mechanisms to protect scientists threatened by groups with commercial and industrial interests in the agribusiness [9].

Several researchers have been investigating multiple exposure to agrochemicals and pollutants as the cause of cancer and mutagenicity; reproductive infertility; child allergies; depression; child cognitive deficit and hyperactivity; neurological, respiratory, cardiological and lung disorders; immunological and endocrine systems disorders; panic syndrome; sexual impotence; and suicide in Brazil and other countries, with an important contribution to the development of knowledge on this theme [1, 2, 9, 17–19, 44–47].

In Brazil, there are currently several methods of resistance to the agrointoxication process gathered in an active and acknowledged social movement: the *Campanha Permanente Contra o Agrotóxico e Pela Vida* (Permanent Campaign Against Agrochemicals and For Life) [40], conducted by dozens of signatory institutions, standing out as one of the most important movements for food and nutrition security in the world (www.contraosagrotoxicos.org). This movement has promoted five editions of National Conferences on Food and Nutrition Security (CESAN). Since 2010, these conferences have been crucial moments in the defence of the right to food, with stages of mobilization at municipal and state levels that have strengthened the debate on civil society and grassroots movements, for the social control over the policies for the sector [48].

Other highlights of the movement in Brazil are the protagonism of *Grupo de Trabalho Saúde e Ambiente* (Work Group Health and Environment) of *Associação Brasileira de Saúde Coletiva* (ABRASCO; Brazilian Association of Collective Health); the creation of *Rede Brasileira de Justiça Ambiental* (RBJA; Brazilian Network for Environmental Justice); the launching of *Mapa de Conflitos envolvendo Injustiça Ambiental e Saúde no Brasil* (Map of Conflicts Involving Environmental Injustice and Health in Brazil) [18, 49]; and the launching of the documentary films *O Veneno está na Mesa* (The Poison is on the Table, 2011) and *Brasil Orgânico* (Organic Brazil, 2013). Following the biggest environmental disaster in the country's history, which occurred in November 2015 with the bursting of a mining dam in the state of Minas Gerais operated by Samarco, the *Caravana Territorial da Bacia do Rio Doce* (Territory Caravan through Rio Doce Basin), which gathered researchers and activists together in April 2016, travelled over 600 km in the area and saw innumerable effects of severe mental and physical suffering, social vulnerability, and emergency conditions for many of the urban populations throughout the basin; destruction/extermination of flora and fauna; and contamination from mineral residues in the entire hydrographic complex [50].

The 'green revolution' and the paradigm of chemicalization of life: from agrointoxication to social medicalization

A deep change in agriculture and cultivation patterns occurred as a result of the fact that the chemical weapons industry was reoriented in the post-war period, especially from the 1970s onwards, to the production of the so-called 'agricultural defensives'. This represented a market renewal, resulting in the introduction of agrochemicals and pesticides associated with the monopoly of seeds. Creole seeds (non-transgenic), which had always been mostly in the possession of and available to small-scale agricultural producers, have gradually been substituted by genetically modified seeds, patented by transnational corporations responsible for this change. Ironically called the 'green revolution', this change was officially announced as modernization and great technological and productive advances, in substitution of family and small-scale agriculture. Thus, a new production paradigm arises: the agrointoxicated agriculture [9].

Transgenic seeds and 'agricultural defensive' are inseparable, i.e. the transgenic seed has been genetically modified in order to bear the use of agricultural poison, killing pests (and any other living being), and keeping large-scale crops. Therefore, agricultural producers, in general, have been held hostage by being obliged to buy the 'package' of modified seed/defensive to be able to produce and fight pests.

The first important 'agricultural defensive' used in the green revolution was Roundup® (glyphosate), associated with the genetically modified Bt corn seed, created by Monsanto from 'Agent Orange', which was used by the US military force during the Vietnam War to eliminate forest cover and be able to attack the Viet Cong troops that hid in the forests. The reorientation of the chemical industry of war, with a chemical weapon transformed into an agricultural defensive, allowed for a new era of agricultural production and food and environmental poisoning due to the intensive and large-scale production in monocultures. Social and environmental injustices produced by this model have great impact on rural and urban populations and on health and the environment [9].

A final, timely issue of little visibility, although extremely severe, also using Brazil as an example, is the use of industrial residues in the production of micronutrients for agriculture in order to minimize costs and maximize profits. This is a clear violation of international agreements on the environment and of fully consolidated principles of human health and constitutional rights. The interests of the steel and metal industry led to pressure by national and international firms on the State to legalize so-called 'hazardous waste' for agribusiness. However, ANVISA has proven, by means of the *Programa de Análise de Resíduos de Agrotóxicos* (PARA; Program of Agrochemical Residues Analysis) and data systems, the damage to

human health and the expansion of food insecurity in case the use of dangerous residues in agriculture is permitted [9].

The model of industrial food associated with the use of agrochemicals is maintained by interests that have promoted several ways of pressurizing and influencing to prompt institutions to legalize this type of business in Brazil—the use of industrial residue in agriculture—and while this does not happen, illegal use has been documented for decades. The illegal import of toxic residues from countries such as USA, Canada, Mexico, Spain, Holland, and England occurs in contravention of the Basel Convention (1989) on the Control of Transboundary Movements of Hazardous Wastes and their Disposal, and also of the Brazilian environmental legislation, as well as the *Receita Federal* (Internal Revenue Service), which has been making apprehensions in large Brazilian ports since the 1980.

For chemical-dependent agriculture, it is necessary to correct soil deficiencies using several products, because poisoned soils become depleted soils, and micronutrients from natural minerals (e.g. boron, cobalt, copper, iron, manganese, molybdenum, nickel, and zinc) are important for this correction. But the fact is that since the end of the 1970s micronutrient fertilizer industries became interested in low-cost raw material and started to make illegal use of hazardous industrial waste [9].

Since the 1980s investigations have demonstrated that hazardous industrial waste contains other inorganic and organic chemical elements and compounds (arsenic, mercury, lead, cadmium, chromium, organochlorines, furans, dioxins) that are not metabolized by plants. Besides being extremely toxic, these compounds accumulate in food, soil, and water, with severe risks and impairments, and causing irreversible damage in some cases [9].

It is important to highlight the effects of ingestion or progressive intoxication from heavy metals on the human CNS and behaviour, which can engender neurological damage and induce syndromes related to dementia, as well as irritability, agitation, cognitive deficit, and aggressiveness, as has been investigated in recent decades [9, 51].

Another relevant aspect to observe is that industrial interests seek to complete the contaminant cycle by having industrial waste transformed into feedstock for poisoned agriculture, ignoring all ethical and legal limits.

Yet, completing the cycle of programmed poisoning and the chemicalization of life does not end at this point. One of the most important key points in the discussion of the relationships between environmental contaminants and mental health is the fact that the same corporations that created and maintain the model of agrointoxicated agriculture are often those that produce medicines. In other words, the agrochemical and pharmaceutical industries are deeply connected: BASF, Bayer, Novartis, Monsanto, and Syngenta are chemical companies that produce agricultural defensives and, at least partially, medicines and pharmaceutical feedstock. This is not a casual phenomenon; interests linked to agrochemicals are associated with the same interests that induce the expansion of social medicalization—those linked to the paradigm of the chemicalization of life. Profits from oncological and psychiatric drugs, for example, are very high.

In particular, psychotropic drugs are of interest to the pharmaceutical industry, related to the dissemination within society of an amplified psychopathological view linked to the diagnostic hyperinflation and the dissemination of the *Diagnostic and Statistical Manual of Mental Disorders,* and the expansion of psychiatric diagnoses. Therefore, related to this is the consequent massive use of generations of antidepressants, antipsychotics, and anticonvulsants, previously more restricted to institutionalized patients, and nowadays functioning as a panacea for mental suffering stimulated by the phantasy of the 'magic pill'. This process may also be described as social medicalization or the medicalization of everyday life, or even the pathologization of behaviours [52–56].

The mercantilization of mental suffering is linked to the production of knowledge and policies by the pharmaceutical and psychiatric industry that aims to produce more hospitalization, more procedures and examinations, and the continuous and uninterrupted use of drugs, with the consequent effect of chronic chemical dependence and the development of tolerance: exactly the same as in chemical-dependent agriculture, in which increasing amounts of poison are needed to produce the same effects, because pests develop resistance. Equally, the same phenomenon refers to the indiscriminate use of antibiotics and the expansion of super bacteria as one of the most severe emergent aspects of medical iatrogenesis.

This allopathic biomedical and psychiatric paradigm is centred on the individual and on the disease, rather than on the promotion of health. It is based on examinations and procedures of high technological density, has institutionalizing characteristics, and has increasing costs. Thus, it is not capable of effectively producing health.

This leads to the 'epidemics' of psychotropic drug prescriptions for all types of behaviour considered deviant or unacceptable, and to the pathologization of daily life. For this reason, there is a debate in the field of mental health about the interest of the psychiatric industry in reinforcing the role of disease—the idea of the incurability of mental disorder; the idea of chronification and interminable treatment [54].

The 'triple load of diseases' and the demographic, epidemiologic and nutrition transition: the social production of disease and the industrial food model

Morbidity and mortality patterns have presented great changes in the last few decades, as well as living and health conditions of populations; this issue has been studied in collective health by way of the concept of demographic and epidemiological transition. This concept explains why changes in the pattern of disease distribution have occurred, related to historical and social changes, and associated with urban and lifestyle changes since the 1970s, such as increased life expectancy, ageing of the population, a decrease in the female fertility rate, and the increase in non-communicable chronic diseases, among other factors, which impact the distribution of diseases within the population.

However, a new phenomenon is being observed that makes the sanitary context even more complex, named the 'triple transition' or the 'triple burden of diseases' [57]. This means that besides demographic transition (changes in living conditions and lifestyle) and epidemiological transition (overlapping of chronic degenerative diseases with re-emerging infectious diseases and mother–child health problems related to social inequality and vulnerability), there is a nutrition transition (changes in the forms of production and consumption of food), causing multiple impacts.

Demographic and epidemiological changes are due to intricate and multifaceted factors. However, some changes have been introduced by interests of the capital, for example with agrointoxicated agriculture there is a precariousness of life and work in rural areas, followed by an increase of rural exodus to cities and consequent 'favelization' growth. And there is a crucial change in the society's dietary model with a process of food massification—the concept of fast food—and the consumption of industrialized food with innumerous additives and excessive salt, sugar, and fat.

It is obvious that the model of industrialized food is directly linked to the 'epidemics' of hypertension and diabetes, as well as obesity. Studies have also been proving that in the organism there is a cumulative effect from chemical substances, such as additives and agrochemicals, which is related to the vertiginous increase in cancer and child cancer cases, and in diseases and damage associated with food. The morbidity and mortality profiles composed of the three major causes of death and illness (infarction, cardiovascular and metabolic diseases, and cancer, among other causes of illness, such as depression and obesity) have inexorably been associated with nutrition transition in developed countries, as well as in developing and peripheral countries.

It can be considered that nutrition transition, as a crucial component of morbidity and mortality profiles, has not only been socially produced from economic and industrial interests, but it has also introduced an industrial and agrointoxicated dietary model that is highly disease-producing. Thus, it results from a food model that causes diseases, in the same way that agrointoxication of society and environment results from agribusiness; in this sense, these models, as components of the paradigm of chemicalization of life constitute some of the major contemporary forms of renewal of the 'disease industry'.

In the last few decades there has been a deep change in the population's diet that causes concern to regulatory agencies and the scientific community owing to the substitution of natural food by processed food, resulting in an impoverished diet. This contributes to the occurrence of chronic non-communicable diseases, especially circulatory system diseases, diabetes, and neoplasia, with a multifactorial aetiology associated with factors such as inadequate diet, obesity, dyslipidaemia, addiction to tobacco/nicotine, and insufficient physical activity [58].

Finally, the issue of food additives constitutes another example of the monopoly of food by the interests that violate the right to health. Furthermore, the technology used by the food industry to extend the shelf life of products has been questioned regarding the safety of food additives, especially dyes and flavour enhancers. The adverse and cumulative effects of food additives do not permit justification of the use of acceptable daily intake parameters, criteria accepted by World Health Organization, especially owing to the impact of additive consumption on child health [58]. In the same way, regulation of the use of agrochemicals follows parameters of 'maximum levels permitted' following a similar logic.

Food sovereignty and agroecology: from the chemicalization of life to a new paradigm in mental and environmental health

In the context of generalized agrointoxication, a food model that causes illness, and the medicalization of the society, there are several trends of thought on health and food that are being produced, drawing on researchers and investigations in varied fields of study.

One of the most important themes on health and food and nutrition security in relation to human rights is the debate on food sovereignty of countries, because it is in the domain of transnational corporations that control the seeds and the agrochemical market.

The Nyéléni Declaration on Food Sovereignty (28 February 2007) from the Forum for Food Sovereignty, one of the most important documents on this issue [59], defines food sovereignty as 'the right of peoples to healthy and culturally appropriate food produced through ecologically sound and sustainable methods, and their right to define their own food and agriculture systems'. It proposes that food security be guaranteed above the interests of markets and corporations, ensuring the right to use and manage land, territories, and biodiversity, and implying new social relations free of oppression and inequalities.

Regarding the field of mental health, the analysis of its relation to human rights and environmental justice is important for a new vision of mental suffering and the processes of becoming psychically ill and psychosocially vulnerable. It is necessary to broaden the point of view, being attentive not to be captured by technicism and objectivation of the subjects, which prevail in the traditional psychiatric intervention.

In view of the issues discussed in this chapter, there is nowadays a worldwide mobilization around agroecology and the production of organic food that seeks the eradication of the agrochemical industry, associated with the struggle for rights and strengthening of social movements, against the institutionalized poisoning maintained by the strong interests of agribusiness [60].

Finally, there are some very important documentary films on the current scenario that we would like to highlight: *Food Matters* (USA, 2008); *Super Size Me* (USA, 2004); *A Carne é Fraca* (*The Flesh is Weak*; Brazil, 2005); *The Future of Food* (USA, 2004); and *The World According to Monsanto* (France, 2007).

Conclusions

The paradigm of the chemicalization of life, supported by the pillars of chemical-dependent agriculture, social medicalization, and nutrition transition, points to a renewal of the contemporary forms of the disease industry, producing social and environmental injustice, severe social and environmental damages, and violation of the right to health and the right to food, endangering democracies and the achievements of social movements in the last decades. But the production of knowledge and the articulation of struggles and activists in different spheres involving multiple actors and institutions have been giving rise to new possibilities and ways to face this industry of disease and death that is the paradigm of chemicalization of life.

In other words, when linking the problems in the fields of mental health, human rights, and environmental justice, the transdisciplinary debate points, primarily, in the direction of surpassing the various forms of environmental contamination and surpassing the model of chemical-dependent agriculture and its unfolding, as crucial in the struggle for food and nutrition security, in the sense of avoiding the processes of becoming physically and mentally ill, for the consolidation of the rights to health and food.

Therefore, setting up research and integration networks in the production of knowledge is not only urgent, but is also an ethical and political imperative for the actors in the field of collective health, mental health, and environmental health in defense of human rights and the right to life.

References

1. Porto MF, Finamore R. Riscos, saúde e justiça ambiental: o protagonismo das populações atingidas na produção de conhecimento. *Cien Saude Colet* 2012; 17: 493–501.
2. Porto MF, Soares WL. Modelo de desenvolvimento, agrotóxicos e saúde: um panorama da realidade agrícola brasileira e propostas para uma agenda de pesquisa inovadora. *Rev Bras Saude Ocup* 2012; 37: 17–31.
3. Ziegler J. *Destruição em Massa: Geopolítica da Fome*. São Paulo: Cortez, 2013.
4. Welzer H. *Climate Wars: What People Will Be Killed For in the 21st Century*. London: Polity, 2012.
5. Robin MM. *The World According to Monsanto—Pollution, Corruption, and the Control of the World's Food Supply*. New York: New Press, 2010.
6. Carson R. *Primavera Silenciosa*. São Paulo: Gaia Editora, 2010.
7. Carson R. *Silent Spring*. Boston, MA: Houghton Mifflin, 1962.
8. Londres F. *Agrotóxicos no Brasil: um guia para ação em defesa da vida*. Rio de Janeiro: Assessoria e Serviços a Projetos em Agricultura Alternativa, 2011.
9. ABRASCO (Associação Brasileira de Saúde Coletiva) CARNEIRO, Fernando Ferreira (Org.) *Dossiê ABRASCO: um alerta sobre os impactos dos agrotóxicos na saúde/Organização de Fernando Ferreira Carneiro, Lia Giraldo da Silva Augusto, Raquel Maria Rigotto, Karen Friedrich e André Campos Búrigo*. Rio de Janeiro: EPSJV; São Paulo: Expressão Popular, 2015.
10. Gunnell D, Eddleston M. Suicide by intentional ingestion of pesticides: a continuing tragedy in developing countries. *Int J Epidemiol* 2003; 32: 902–909.
11. Bertolote JM, Fleischmann A, Eddleston M, Gunnell D. Deaths from pesticide poisoning: are we lacking a global response? *Br J Psychiatry* 2006; 189: 201–203.
12. Bertolote JM, Fleischmann A, Butchart A, Besbelli N. Suicide, suicide attempts and pesticides: a major hidden public health problem. *Bull World Health Organ* 2006; 84: 257–336.
13. World Health Organization. Suicide data. Available at: http://www.who.int/mental_health/prevention/suicide/suicideprevent/en/ (last accessed 27 February 2018).
14. Beard JD, Umbach DM, Hoppin JA, et al. Pesticide exposure and depression among male private pesticide applicators in the agricultural health study. *Environ Health Perspect* 2014; 122: 984–991.
15. Santos BS. *A gramática do tempo: para uma nova cultura política*. 2nd ed. São Paulo: Cortez, 2008.
16. Nunes JA. Saúde, direito à saúde e justiça sanitária. *Rev Crit Cien Soc* 2009; 87: 143–169.
17. Porto MFS. *Uma ecologia política dos riscos: princípios para integrarmos o local e o global na promoção da saúde e da justiça ambiental*. Rio de Janeiro: Editoria Fiocruz, 2012.
18. Porto MF, Pacheco T, Leroy JP (eds). *Injustiça Ambiental e Saúde no Brasil: o mapa dos conflitos*. Rio de Janeiro: Editora Fiocruz, 2013.
19. Rigotto RM. Os conflitos entre o agronegócio e os direitos das populações: o papel do campo científico. *Agroecologia* 2013; 7: 133–142.
20. Falk JW, Carvalho LA, Silva LR, Pinheiro S. Suicídio e doença mental em Venâncio Aires—RS: consequência do uso de agrotóxicos organofosforados? In: Comiss. Cidadania e Dir. Humanos AL/RS (ed.). *Relatório azul: garantias e violações dos direitos humanos no Rio Grande do Sul—1995*. Porto Alegre RS: CORAG/Assembléia Legislativa do RS, 1996, pp. 244–262.
21. Faria NMX, Facchini LA, Fassa AG, Tomasi E. Estudo transversal sobre saúde mental de agricultores da Serra Gaúcha (Brasil). *Rev Saude Publ* 1999; 33: 391–400.
22. London L, Beseler C, Bouchard MF, et al. Neurobehavioural and neurodevelopmental effects of pesticide exposures. *Neurotoxicology* 2012; 33: 887–896.

23. Idrovo AJ, Sanín LH. Resultados adversos em la procreación em mujeres trabajadoras em la floricultura colombiana: un resumen de la evidencia mediante metanálisis. *Biomedica* 2007; 27: 490–497.

24. Handal AJ, Lozoff B, Breilh J, Harlow SD. Neurobehavioural development in children with potential exposure to pesticides. *Epidemiology* 2007; 18: 312–320.

25. Roberts EM, English PB, Grether JK, Windham GC, Somberg L, Wolff C. Maternal residence near agricultural pesticide applications and autism spectrum disorders among children in the California Central Valley. *Environ Health Perspect* 2007; 115: 1482–1489.

26. Environmental Health Perspectives. Autism and agricultural pesticides—integrating data to track trends. *Environnews/Science Selections* 2007; 115: A504–A505.

27. Landrigan P, Lambertini L, Birnbaum L. A research strategy to discover the environmental causes of autism and neurodevelopmental disabilities. *Environ Health Perspect* 2012; 120: A258–A260.

28. Nevison CD. A comparison of temporal trends in United States autism prevalence to trends in suspected environmental factors. *Environ Health* 2014, 13: 73.

29. Persico AM, Bourgeron T. Searching for ways out of the autism maze: genetic, epigenetic and environmental clues. Trends Neurosci 2006; 29: 349–358.

30. Rossignol DA, Genius SJ, Frye RE. Environmental toxicants and autism spectrum disorders: a systematic review. *Transl Psychiatry* 2014; 4: e360.

31. Shelton JF, Hertz-Picciotto I, Pessah IN. Tipping the balance of autism risk: potencial mechanisms linking pesticides and autism. *Environ Health Perspect* 2012; 120: 944–951.

32. Deth R, Muratore C, Benzecry J, Power-Charnitsky VA, Waly M. How environmental and genetic factors combine to cause autism: a redox/methylation hypothesis. *Neurotoxicology* 2008; 29: 190–201.

33. James SJ, Cutler P, Melnyk S, et al. Metabolic biomarkers of increased oxidative stress and impaired methylation capacity in children with autism. *Am J Clin Nutr* 2004; 80: 1611–1617.

34. Eskenazi B, Marks AR, Bradman A, et al. Organophosphate pesticide exposure and neurodevelopment in young Mexican-American children. *Environ Health Perspect* 2007; 115: 792–798.

35. Sarich C. MIT Scientist Exposes Consequence of Monsanto's Glyphosate & Aluminum Cocktail. Available at: http://naturalsociety.com/dr-stephanie-seneff-mit-scientist-explains-synergistic-effect-aluminum-glyphosate-poisoning-cause-skyrocketing-autism/ (2014, accessed 27 February 2018).

36. Seneff S, Swanson N, Li C. Aluminium and glyphosate can synergistically induce pineal gland pathology: connection to gut dysbiosis and neurological disease. *Agric Sci* 2015; 6: 42–70.

37. Seneff S, Davidson RM, Liu J. Empirical Data confirm autism symptoms related to aluminium and acetaminophen exposure. *Entropy* 2012; 14: 2227–2253.

38. Beecham J, Seneff S. The possible link between autism and glyphosate acting as glycine mimetic—a review of evidence from the literature with analysis. *Mol Genet Med* 2015; 9: 4.

39. Beecham JE, Seneff S. Is there a link between autism and glyphosate-formulated herbicides? *J Autism* 2016; 3: 1.

40. Tygel AF, Folgado C, Castro FP, et al. Campanha Permanente Contra os Agrotóxicos e Pela Vida: construção da resistência brasileira ao avanço do capital no campo. In: Tobar FR, Bazzi AP (eds) *Revista SALTAR LA BARRERA—Crisis socio-ambiental, resistencias populares y construcción de alternativas latinoamericanas al Neoliberalismo*. Chile: Instituto de Ciencias Alejandro Lipschutz/Fundación Rosa Luxemburgo, 2014, pp. 147–178.

41. Ministério da Saúde, Instituto Nacional do Câncer, Coordenação de Programas de Controle do Câncer. *Pro-Onco. O Problema do Câncer no Brasil*, 3rd ed. *Edição revisada e atualizada*. Rio de Janeiro: INCA/Pro-Onco, 1995.

42. Davidson RM, Lauritzen A, Seneff S. Biological water dynamics and entropy: a biophysical origin of cancer and other diseases. *Entropy* 2013; 15: 3822–3876.

43. Guyton KZ, Loomis D, Grosse Y, et al. Carcinogenicity of tetrachlorvinphos, parathion, malathion, diazinon, and glyphosate. *Lancet Oncol* 2015; 16: 490–491.

44. PACS. *Baía de Sepetiba: fronteira do desenvolvimentismo e os limites para a construção de alternativas. PACS—Instituto Políticas Alternativas para o Cone Sul*, 2nd ed. Rio de Janeiro: PACS, 2016.

45. Rigotto RM, Augusto LGS. Saúde e ambiente no Brasil: desenvolvimento, território e iniqüidade social. *Cad Saude Publica* 2007; 23(Suppl. 4): S475–S501.

46. Revista TEMPUS Actas de Saúde Coletiva. *Volume 8—n. 2: Ecologia de Saberes e Saúde do Campo, da Floresta e das Águas. Núcleo de Estudos em Saúde Pública da Universidade de Brasília*. Brasília: NESP, 2014.

47. Araújo JNG, Greggio MR, Pinheiro TMM. Agrotóxicos: a semente plantada no corpo e na mente dos trabalhadores rurais. *Psicol Rev* 2013; 19: 389–406.

48. Conselho Nacional de Segurança Alimentar e Nutricional (CONSEA). Comida de verdade no Campo e na Cidade. Caderno de Orientações—5a. Conferência Nacional de Segurança Alimentar e Nutricional. Documento Final—versão pós-plenária. Brasília: CONSEA, 2015.

49. Mapa de Conflitos envolvendo Injustiça Ambiental e Saúde no Brasil. Available at: www.conflitoambiental.icict.fiocruz.br (accessed 27 February 2018).

50. Porto MF. A tragédia da mineração e a experiência da caravana territorial da bacia do rio Doce: encontro de saberes e práticas para a transformação. *Cienc Cult* 2016; 68: 46–50.

51. Martin S, Griswold W. *Human Health Effects of Heavy Metals. Environmental Science and Technology Briefs for Citizens. Center for Hazardous Substance Research*. Manhattan, KS: Kansas State University, 2009.

52. Angell M. *The Truth About the Drug Companies: How They Deceive Us and What to do About it*. New York: Random House Publishing Group, 2004.

53. Whitaker R, Cosgrove L. *Psychiatry Under The Influence: Institutional Corruption, Social Injury, and Prescriptions for Reform*. New York: Palgrave Macmillan, 2015.

54. Frances A. *Saving Normal: An Insider's Revolt against Out-of-Control Psychiatric Diagnosis, DSM-5, Big Pharma, and the Medicalization of Ordinary Life*. New York: William Morrow Paperbacks, 2014.

55. Amarante P, Freitas F. *Medicalização em Psiquiatria. Coleção Temas em Saúde*. Rio de Janeiro: Editora Fiocruz, 2015.

56. Amarante PDC, Torre EHG. Medicalização e Determinação Social dos Transtornos Mentais: a questão da indústria de medicamentos na produção de saber e políticas. In: Nogueira RP (ed.) *Determinação Social da Saúde e Reforma Sanitária*. Rio de Janeiro: CEBES, 2010, pp. 151–160.

57. Mendes EV. As redes de atenção à saúde. *Cienc Saude Coletiva* 2010; 15: 2297–2305.

58. Polônio MLT, Peres F. Consumo de aditivos alimentares e efeitos à saúde: desafios para a saúde pública brasileira. *Cad Saude Publica* 2009; 25:1653–1666.

59. Declaração de Nyéléni. Foro Mundial pela Soberania Alimentar, Nyéléni, Selingue, Malí, 28 de fevereiro de 2007. [Declaration of the Forum for Food Sovereignty, Nyéléni 2007]. Available at: https://nyeleni.org/spip.php?article290 (accessed 27 February 2018).

60. Wezel A, Bellon S, Doré T, Francis C, Vallod D, David C. Agroecology as a science, a movement and a practice: a review. *Agron Sustain Dev* 2009; 29: 503–515.

Special groups

CHAPTER 24

Family, marriage, and mental health

Fasli Sidheek, Veena A. Satyanarayana, and Geetha Desai

Introduction

A family is far more than a collection of individuals sharing a unique physical and psychological environment. The definition of families are varied in the present culture with difficulty in confining them based on specific differences in structure, form, language, culture, and the like. Yet, all of them continue to share some common properties of having defined set of rules, specific interactional styles, and properties that are unique to them [1].

Family is a unit tied together with a system of unique heritage, shared history, set of values, shared internalized perceptions and assumptions about the world, a sense of we, and a shared sense of purpose. A family provides psychological and social milieu for character formation of its individual members. Thus, the context of relationships becomes immensely important in the developmental course of an individual especially for their sense of well-being.

Ludwig von Bertalanffy proposed the general systems theory as a way of understanding systems, including the family system [2]. Family systems are open systems, governed by certain set of rules that tend to reach steady states, or homeostasis. This is made possible by communication and feedback mechanisms. Circular causality is another important concept in understanding family dynamics [3]. It means that any interaction should be understood in terms of reciprocal sequences and not as linear. Thus, systems thinking reduces the emphasis placed on individual psychopathology and helps understand the family as a whole.

Family life-cycle stages

As we all grow and enter into different stages of life, certain unique challenges are faced by us in each of these stages and successful achievement of tasks results in smooth transition to the next phase. Theorists, like Eric Erikson, have described different psychosocial stages that we pass through. Similarly, most families progress through a series of stages over time, which all are associated with unique developmental tasks. Duvall and Hill [4] first proposed a developmental framework for studying families. It was Carter and McGoldrick's [5] model that received much attention owing to its multidimensional approach including individual, family and sociocultural perspectives. There are specific markers (family stage marker) that cue transition from one stage to another [6]. These markers are events that demand change and a new adaptation, for example, birth of twins, separation, and so on.

Some families fail to move to subsequent stages and as a result get stuck in the previous life-cycle stage or get derailed in their life-cycle stages. Therapy aims to restore and re-establish appropriate developmental tasks by utilizing a family's unused potentials, thus helping them attain mastery and resolution.

Life-cycle stages are not linear wherein a family moves from one stage to the next. At a given time, families can be going through different life stages based on the individual members and generations in the family. As the life-cycle advances in stages, the transition follows a change and adaptation. As they pass through stages all families go through a certain amount of stress before effectively adapting to it and attaining stability. Dysfunctional families tend to deal with this in a less effective fashion and bring about an ample amount of stress in individual members [7].

Contemporary issues in marriage and family therapy

Extramarital involvement

Marriage is based on an unwritten contract of commitment and faithfulness between a couple. When a violation by one of the partners occurs in this contract great distress ensues. Secrecy is the core of an extramarital involvement (EMI) and discovery of it can be equally traumatic for the partner involved and the discoverer. EMI can be of varied nature: primarily emotional, primarily sexual, and a combination of both [8]. People who engage in affairs can have diverse motivations ranging from sexual gratification to novelty to counteracting feelings of dissatisfaction in the marriage to pursuit behaviors. There are no gender differences found in people seeking extramarital relationships. However, studies show there is a gender difference in the consequences of an EMI when revealed, with men being more harsh and less forgiving than women. Betrayal of trust is what intensifies the reaction to the discovery of an EMI. Thus, restoration of trust becomes an important goal in treatment. The involved partner is worked with to address issues of grief and adjustment to the loss of an affair. They are also encouraged to validate and support the uninvolved partner. Once the partners are able to work successfully on this issue and find closure, there is greater intimacy noted between the partners [9].

Violence

Violence here is discussed mostly in terms of partner violence and violence affecting children; other aspects of violence, although important, are not addressed. Intimate partner violence refers to any behaviour within an intimate relationship that causes physical, psychological, or sexual harm to those in the relationship [10]. While discussing violence it is often assumed that the 'victim' is a female and the perpetrator is a male. However, research shows that women can be perpetrators too, although the data are minimal. Also, while exploring the intentions behind violence initiated by both sexes and looking at the consequences, including the extent of injury caused, men are held responsible for the act. As violence is not reported spontaneously, it is advisable to look for warning signs when a couple comes for treatment. A set of screening questions to check the presence of violence is always helpful. One other problem that lies with issue of violence is that most people ignore psychological or emotional violence, as it is not 'visible' as other forms of violence. Many women fail to realize that they are at the receiving end of emotional abuse. Proper screening measures and adequate interventions help women deal with this issue effectively. Children in the family are also affected by either parental violence or violence directed towards them. Studies show that the impact on children who witness violence at home is equivalent to children who are the direct victims of violence [11]. Long-term effects of it on children can include low self-esteem, anxiety, and issues in future relationships. In some children effects do not show up immediately and surface only years later, a condition termed the sleeper effect. Group therapy for children, play therapy, and filial therapy are some of the ways to address these issues.

Divorce

Divorce is one of a few different ways to end an unsatisfactory marriage. It is an unscheduled transition in the life-cycle stages that interrupts the successful attainment of developmental tasks [5]. The effect it has is multifold and pervades all spheres of the involved members' lives. It has implications on many major decisions, transformations, and adjustments [12]. There are varied aspects to divorce, including legal, emotional, and financial implications. How one handles divorce is very important in determining its consequences. Interactional styles of partners, valence of emotional exchanges during conflict, process of decision-making regarding divorce, and who initiates the process all determine the reactions and acceptance of one's divorce. If there was enough preparation time before the decision was made adults and especially children in the family will be less affected. Increased financial independence in women and changing gender roles are thought to be reasons for higher divorce rates [13].

Same-sex marriages

Data from surveys conducted in the USA among therapists concluded that a large proportion of therapists were not adequately prepared to deal with lesbians or gay men in therapy [14–16]. This is an alarming state of affairs as therapists who handle same-sex couples should be aware of the unique challenges faced by such couples.

These couples may enter therapy to resolve same-sex couple-related issues or with common psychiatric problems. Their unique issues can arise from the prejudice and discrimination they face in society, and difficulty in 'coming out' to friends and family members, or society at large. Homophobia or an anti-gay attitude is a reason for this discrimination. 'Internalized homophobia' happens when lesbian and gay people have acquired others' negative feelings towards them. These, in turn, cause further couple problems such as unnecessary arguments resulting from frustration, difficulties, or sexual dysfunction, and depression. The definition of couple-hood itself becomes problematic in lesbian/gay couples as traditional expectations or role definitions are lacking in their relationships. The differences in expectations become apparent when the couple starts living together and this sudden change can cause hurt and anger in partners [17].

Feminist and gay-affirmative therapies address possible issues in lesbian/gay relationships. Mobilizing a social support system and helping members build 'families of choice' aid in reducing stigma towards them and also curbs internalized homophobia.

Theories of family therapy

Behavioural family therapy

Behavioural family therapy (BFT) began in the late 1960s with the application of learning principles to deal with problems in families. Reinforcement principles and social exchange theory were utilized to conceptualize issues between family members. Frequency and a range of positive behaviours were assessed to understand the cost–benefit ratio in the family. According to the theory, equal and mutual exchange of positive behaviours result in positive outcomes among family members. Operant conditioning techniques were also employed to increase positive behaviours among the family members, thus increasing the satisfaction experienced. Communication skills training and problem solving are also integral parts of BFT. In his work with families, Robert P. Liberman used elements from a social learning framework, like role rehearsal and modelling of alternative interpersonal communication patterns. Negative exchanges in the family are believed to reinforce the undesirable behaviour in the system. Operant conditioning has also been used in modifying children's behavioural issues. In couples, problems are viewed as a result of lack of or inadequate interpersonal skills that create intimacy. These include problem-solving skills, positive behaviour changes, effective communication, and so on. Disturbances in these domains can be either because of a skill deficit or as a result of the absence of an adequate environment to express these skills. By 'adequate environment' theorists mean a couple relationship evinced by reciprocal and circular interactions wherein a partner's behavior simultaneously affects and influences each other. Although studies have consistently shown effectiveness, some of the outcome studies have revealed that despite improvements in partner behaviours and communication skills, it did not show an equivalent change in relationship satisfaction. Also, there were discrepancies in the subjective report of what was termed 'positive behaviours' by partners. Thus, it became important to address interpretations and appraisals of self and other behaviours in relationships. Components of cognitive theory were also included in treating families. It required individuals to be aware of and monitor one's thoughts, evaluations, and judgements of each other that might result in negative interactions. In turn, modifying these results in positive behaviours; likewise, improvements in interactions among family members are thought to improve underlying cognitions and emotions.

Object relations family therapy

Object relations family therapy has its roots in object relations theory, group psychology, systems theory, and developmental psychology. Object relations theory assumes object relations to be internal and unconscious representations of an individual's experiences in the past that colours his/her current relationships. Thus, an individual relates not just to the other person, but also to the subjective, internal representation of the other. As the initial object representation of an infant is mother, the infant internalizes its mother as both a good and bad object, based on its caregiving experiences. This process, termed 'splitting', is re-awakened in one's relationship with a potential partner.

Family therapists look at how splitting is manifested in marital relationships. Object relations therapists believe that people bring with them their unique psychological heritage into marriage. Partners often see their split-offs in the other person and react to it. Based on one's internal objects, inner experiences and beliefs, others' behaviours are understood rather than based on their true behaviours. To resolve current family issues, exploration of early object relations is important.

One of the major reasons for marital disharmony is viewed as projective identification. Partners tend to project disowned parts of their self onto the other and blame their partner for possessing those characteristics. James Framo believed that families should be taken through different stages of individual and conjoint sessions to resolve these early issues.

Therapy aims at bringing out the material in the unconscious to the conscious. Insight, transference, countertransference, and projective identification are important elements of object relations family therapy. Along with the real interpersonal relationships of individual family members it also looks into internal object relations of each individual and the shared internal object relations of the entire family.

Systemic approaches

Brief strategic therapy

Strategic therapy is based on the assumption that 'ironic processes', which are a result of a constant effort to solve certain patterns or problems, need to be identified and interrupted. Therapy aims at resolving the problem at hand as quickly and efficiently as possible. Uncovering deep-rooted issues, improving relational concerns, and so on, are not looked at in therapy; instead, 'here-and-now' problems are addressed. According to this theory, there are no normative families, meaning maladaptive strategies adopted by certain families are unique to them and might serve some purpose. Unlike other marital therapies, strategic therapy even has provisions to see partners individually. Even when looking at individual members, an interactional model is adopted. Problems within individual members are considered to be a problem and worked upon rather than problems between individual members.

Problems are looked at not from a causal perspective; rather, attention is paid to what or how the problem is being maintained. The very attempts at controlling or solving problems are thought to maintain it. Given this, the therapist tries to identify and deliberately interrupt these 'ironic processes' thereby breaking the perpetuating cycle of problems, and creating a window to try out newer and effective solutions. Treatment techniques include identifying symptoms, interrupting repetitive patterns of interaction, or prescribing symptoms.

Structural family therapy

Contrary to the psychoanalytic understanding of human problems as originating from intra-psychic difficulties, Salvador Minuchin and colleagues followed an 'outside-in' approach to understanding human behaviour. Structure, subsystems, and boundaries are the essential components of structural family theory. Family structure is an organized pattern in which family members interact and is reinforced by the expectations that establish rules in the family [18]. Based on this theory, the family is defined as a system that comprises of several subsystems. This can include parental and child subsystems based on generational differences, sibling subsystems, and the like. These subsystems, according to Minuchin, are demarcated by 'boundaries'. Boundaries are invisible lines that differentiate individual members in the family (or a system) that governs the rules of functioning in the system. The permeability of these boundaries can vary from being rigid to diffuse. The exchange of resources can be quite permissive to the extent of deprivation in systems with diffused boundaries, whereas transfer does not happen adequately in systems with rigid boundaries. Together, the systems, subsystems, and boundaries collectively form the 'structure' of the family.

Problems arise in families when there is a problem in family structure. Strategies of structural family therapy include joining and accommodating, working with interaction, structural mapping, highlighting and modifying interactions, boundary-making, unbalancing, and challenging unproductive assumptions.

Experiential approaches

Narrative therapy

One of the newer approaches to family therapy include narrative therapy. The core idea behind this approach is that our sense of reality is constructed through stories (or narratives) that we create of ourselves, and the society that we live in. These stories are formed from the way people interpret certain situations and link various sequences through their lens so that it makes a meaningful story to them. The story created thus involves ones' abilities, actions, relationships, achievements, and failures [19]. And therefore, depending on the stories generated, families might find themselves entangled in the web of problems.

According to narrative therapists, families can be helped to liberate themselves from problem-saturated stories by deconstructing the stories that they have formed and also by helping them to gain access to other stories. Families need to create and internalize new stories of their life by rewriting the whole script [1]. Families are believed to be the experts and that they have inherent capacity to construct positive stories about themselves. What usually happens when new events happen in life is that one tends to fit it into the existing frame of stories. This whole exercise of viewing their already-written life story through a new lens gives them an opportunity to see things differently. In their attempts to make sense of their lives, people arrange their experiences over a course of time to attain a meaningful sense of self, thus maintaining continuity and meaning [20].

Narrative therapist's efforts are directed at relieving the family members from ideas of hopelessness and redirecting them to the brighter but hidden plots or subplots of their story. They utilize techniques like mapping the problem domains, externalization of problem, seeking unique outcomes, and spreading the news. They also employ therapeutic ceremonies, creating an opportunity for clients to tell their stories to an audience of outside witnesses like friends, family members, other therapists or community members. Therapists also send letters to clients in supplementing and extending therapeutic sessions [21].

Emotionally focused therapy

Emotionally focused therapy (EFT) is one of the relatively newer forms of therapy that is empirically based. EFT is an integration of an experiential or gestalt within systems approach [22]. In earlier approaches, emotions—if addressed at all—was not given much importance. Emotions were seen as the consequence of a behaviour or cognition, rather than an important event. In EFT, emotion is seen as the core of relationship and also as the cause of distress. Therapists focus on the here and now and reconstruct the experiences of clients [23].

EFT uses emotion in destructing negative cycles of interaction among partners. Clients are helped to identify, express, and modify their emotional responses, thus helping them develop new and appropriate emotional responses. This aids in working on broken bonds and the couple moves together in their new interactional pattern, forming a secure bond. EFT looks at distressed relationships from the framework of attachment insecurity and separation anxiety [23]. When there is a threat to attachment security, people often react in anger as a means to regain proximity towards the attachment figure. To deal with the distress involved in separation, one tends to cling. And if that does not result in expected outcome, it in turn results in despair results in despair. When in distress partners tends to engage in destructive, interactional styles, which only deteriorates their relationship further. The three tasks of EFT are (i) to create a safe and collaborative alliance; (ii) to access and expand the emotional responses that guide the couple's interactions; and (iii) to restructure those interactions in the direction of accessibility and responsiveness [22]. Change is seen as a process that happens over a series of steps during therapist–client interaction, assessment, and cycle de-escalation; changing interactional positions; and consolidation and integration.

Marriage and family therapy process and outcome research

Research in marital therapy began with the aim of assessing the efficacy of marital therapy for a variety of mental disorders and problems. Both efficacy and effectiveness research have concluded without exception that marital therapy is effective [24, 25]. Because of the methodological issues in terms of eclectic orientation in therapies, more attention is paid to change process research to determine clinically representative therapy.

Process Research in marriage and family therapy

Process research lends itself to explanation of interventions, to predicting certain results, and describing how certain specific therapeutic interventions bring about change. This becomes important for clinicians as it has direct applications to therapy. Greenberg and Pinsof [26] define process research as the study of the interaction between patient and therapist systems with the goal of identification of change processes as these systems interact. It examines variables like therapist behaviours, client behaviours, and interactions between therapists and clients during treatment to study the therapy process [27].

Blow et al. [28] conducted a single case-study design to understand how the process of change occurs during marriage and family therapy. Both quantitative and qualitative methods were employed for data collection. The therapist was an advanced doctoral student favouring an emotion-focused approach. Couples attended 15 sessions of therapy over a 13-month period. Findings revealed that the important variables that affected the process of change were the role of client factors and extra-therapeutic events; the therapeutic alliance factors; hope and expectancy factors; therapist factors; and specific techniques used by the therapist. The importance of the therapist was also identified in the process of change.

Davis and Piercy [29, 30] investigated common factors across various therapy models. Semi-structured, open-ended, qualitative interviews were conducted with three different marriage and family therapy (MFT) model developers (EFT, cognitive behavioural therapy, and internal family systems therapy), their former students, and each of their former clients who had terminated therapy successfully. Data analysis using modified grounded theory resulted in two groups of common factors: model-dependent factors and model-independent factors. Model-dependent factors included common conceptualizations (family of origin influences, interactional cycles, etc.) and common interventions (insight facilitation, altering the cycle using affective and cognitive elements, etc.). Model-independent themes included therapist variables; client-related variables; therapeutic alliance; therapeutic process; and expectancy and motivational factors.

A study by Helmeke and Sprenkle [31] looked at clients' perception of key elements in couples' therapy. The sample included three couples and a therapist. Data collection included in-depth interviews, non-participant observation, and document analysis. Sources of data were audio and video recordings, questionnaires, field notes, and a reflective journal belonging to the therapist. The findings revealed that although clients could identify key elements, a lack of congruence between husband and wife, and between therapist and client, was noted. Thus, the key elements identified in therapy were highly individualized experiences.

Outcome research in marriage and family therapy

Betty Carter [32] undertook a single case study with a young man and his family, where the primary diagnosis was schizophrenia. Assessment included a diagnostic interview based on the *Diagnostic and Statistical Manual of Mental Disorders*, 4th Edition (DSM-IV) and administration of the Sixteen Personality Factor Questionnaire before and after the therapy process. Therapy was conducted in the format of structural family therapy. At the end of therapy sessions, significant changes were noted in factors such as warmth, emotional stability, dominance, liveliness, rule consciousness, vigilance, openness to change, self-reliance, self-control, and tension. The changes were consistent even at the 4-month follow-up.

In a review of outcome research on MFT in the treatment of alcoholism, O'Farrell and Clements [33] concluded that family therapy aids in the effective treatment of alcoholic families. The review included mostly randomized controlled trials and some quasi-experimental studies on MFT efficacy research published between 2002 and mid-2010. Studies on family members of the alcoholic individual, when the person dependent on alcohol was unwilling to seek help, showed that MFT was effective in helping the family cope better and aided the patient in entering treatment. When the alcohol-dependent person sought help, MFT and behavioural couples therapy (BCT) were more effective than individual treatment for increasing abstinence and improving relationship function.

Another systematic review examined outcomes of a specific programme of BCT for the treatment of alcohol and drug abuse devised by O'Farrell et al. [34]. Twenty-three studies, published in peer-reviewed journals that examined this specific programme of BCT, were included in the review. Results demonstrated that BCT reduced substance use behaviour, improved dyadic adjustment and child psychosocial outcomes, and reduced intimate partner violence. Family-based treatment was consistently found to be more efficacious than individual treatment for substance abuse.

Conclusions

Families are social systems where membership is less of a choice (except in marriages), and entry is mostly through birth, adoption, or fostering. The members are tied with attachments of emotion, and share similar sets of values and assumptions about the world. Family as a whole passes through a series of stages, termed family life-cycle stages, each characterized by a set of tasks family members must complete to progress to the next stage. Failure to complete tasks may lead to adjustment problems. Problems were thought to occur mainly in interpersonal domains rather than intrapersonal issues. Thus, their solution also had to be interpersonal in approach. Family relationships became the focus of intervention as these are of greater significance than most other relationships in people's social networks. Therapy targeting family relationships should be grounded in theoretical frameworks, which take account of the family as a social organization. Different schools of family therapy took different stances about the importance of the role of family relationships in problem formation, the maintenance of problems, and problem resolution. And, based on these, different schools of family therapy emerged: looking at interrupting problematic patterns of interaction, modifying beliefs and interpretations of interpersonal behaviours, and viewing experiences of families as socially constructed. When dealing with so-called normative groups there arise special groups requiring specific attention. Divorce, separation, same-sex marriages, violence, and EMI are some of these special issues. Although these are not extreme cases, they require advanced and sensitive skills for effective handling of the problems. Clinical research can either be described in terms of process or outcome. Research studies have shown effectiveness of various modalities of MFT across various psychiatric conditions.

References

1. Goldenberg H, Goldenberg I. *Family Therapy: An Overview*. Boston, MA: Cengage Learning, 2012.
2. Barker P, Chang J. *Basic Family Therapy*. Hoboken, NJ: John Wiley & Sons, 2013.
3. Barker P. *Basic Family Therapy*. Hoboken, NJ: John Wiley & Sons, 2007.
4. Duvall EM, Hill R. *Report to the Committee on the Dynamics of Family Interaction*. Washington, DC: National Conference on Family Life, 1948.
5. Carter EA, McGoldrick M (eds). *The Expanded Family Life Cycle: Individual, Family, and Social Perspectives*. Boston, MA: Allyn & Bacon, 1999.
6. Zilbach JJ. The family life cycle: a framework for understanding children in family therapy. In: Cornbrink-Graham L (ed.). *Children in Family Contexts*. New York: Guilford Press, 1989, pp. 46–56.
7. Glantz MD, and Johnson JL (eds). *Resilience and Development: Positive Life Adaptations*. Berlin: Springer Science & Business Media, 1999.
8. Glass SP, Wright TL. Justifications for extramarital relationships: the association between attitudes, behaviors, and gender. *J Sex Res* 1992; 29: 361–387.
9. Keitner GI, Heru AM, Glick ID. *Clinical Manual of Couples and Family Therapy*. Washington, DC: American Psychiatric Association Publishing, 2009.
10. World Health Organization (WHO). *Understanding and Addressing Violence Against Women: Intimate Partner Violence*. Geneva: WHO, 2012.
11. Anderson SA, Cramer-Benjamin DB. The impact of couple violence on parenting and children: an overview and clinical implications. *Am J Fam Ther* 1999; 27: 1–9.
12. Wetchler JL, Hecker LL. *An Introduction to Marriage and Family Therapy*. New York: Routledge, 2014.
13. Bumpass LL. What's happening to the family? Interactions between demographic and institutional change. *Demography* 1990; 27: 483–498.
14. Garnets L, Hancock KA, Cochran SD, Goodchilds J, Peplau LA. Issues in psychotherapy with lesbians and gay men: a survey of psychologists. *Am Psychol* 1991; 46: 964.
15. Green SK, Bobele M. Family therapists' response to aids: an examination of attitudes, knowledge, and contact. *J Marital Fam Ther* 1994; 20: 349–367.
16. Doherty WJ, Simmons DS. Clinical practice patterns of marriage and family therapists: a national survey of therapists and their clients. *J Marital Fam Ther* 1996; 22: 9–25.
17. Alonzo DJ. Working with same-sex couples. In: Harway M (ed.) *Handbook of Couples Therapy*. Hobokon, NJ: Wiley, 2005, pp 370–385.
18. Nichols MP, Schwartz RC, Minuchin S. *Family Therapy: Concepts and Methods*. New York: Gardner Press, 1984.
19. Morgan A. *What is Narrative Therapy*. Adelaide: Dulwich Centre Publications, 2000.
20. Carr A. *Family Therapy: Concepts, Process and Practice*. Hoboken, NJ: John Wiley & Sons;,2012.
21. Nichols MP. *The Essentials of Family Therapy*, 4th ed. Boston, MA: Pearson Education, 2009.
22. Johnson SM. Emotionally focussed couple therapy. In: Gurman AS, Lebow JL, Snyder DK (eds). *Clinical Handbook of Couple Therapy*. New York: Guilford Publications, 2015, pp. 107–137.
23. Johnson SM. Listening to the music: emotion as a natural part of systems theory. *J Syst Ther* 1998; 17: 1–7.
24. Hazelrigg MD, Cooper HM, Borduin CM. Evaluating the effectiveness of family therapies: an integrative review and analysis. *Psychol Bull* 1987; 101: 428–442.
25. Shadish WR, Montgomery LM, Wilson P, Wilson MR, Bright I, Okwumabua T. Effects of family and marital psychotherapies: a meta-analysis. *J Consult Clin Psychol* 1993; 61: 992–1002.
26. Greenberg LS, Pinsof WM. *The Psychotherapeutic Process: A Research Handbook*. New York: Guilford Press, 1986.
27. Lambert MJ, Hill CE. Assessing psychotherapy outcomes and processes. In: Bergin BE, Garfield SL (eds). *Handbook of Psychotherapy and Behaviour Change*. Oxford: John Wiley & Sons, 1994, pp. 72–113.
28. Blow AJ, Morrison NC, Tamaren K, Wright K, Schaafsma M, Nadaud A. Change processes in couple therapy: An intensive case analysis of one couple using a common factors lens. *J Martial Fam Ther* 2009; 35: 350–368.

29. Davis SD, Piercy FP. What clients of couple therapy model developers and their former students say about change, part I: model-dependent common factors across three models. *J Marital Fam Ther* 2007; 33: 318–343.

30. Davis SD, Piercy FP. What clients of couple therapy model developers and their former students say about change, part II: model-independent common factors and an integrative framework. *J Martial Fam Ther* 2007; 33: 344–363.

31. Helmeke KB, Sprenkle DH. Clients'perceptions of pivotal moments in couples therapy: a qualitative study of change in therapy. *J Marital Fam Ther* 2000; 26: 469–483.

32. Carter DJ. Case study: a structural model for schizophrenia and family collaboration. *Clin Case Stud* 2011; 10: 147–158.

33. O'Farrell TJ, Clements K. Review of outcome research on marital and family therapy in treatment for alcoholism. *J Marital Fam Ther* 2012; 38: 122–144.

34. Ruff S, McComb JL, Coker CJ, Sprenkle DH. Behavioral couples therapy for the treatment of substance abuse: a substantive and methodological review of O'Farrell, Fals-Stewart, and colleagues' program of research. *Fam Process* 2010; 49: 439–456.

CHAPTER 25

Prisoners and mental health

Kenneth L. Appelbaum

Introduction

Incarceration presents great challenges and opportunities for public mental health and safety. Many inmates have mental health needs that the conditions of confinement and availability of services can either mitigate or exacerbate. This chapter examines the effect on public mental health and safety of five areas of policy and services for inmates: treatment in prison; treatment after community re-entry; general conditions of confinement; programming to address criminogenic factors and recidivism; and alternatives to incarceration. Although the chapter focuses primarily on prisons, the same considerations apply to varying extents to jails.

This chapter takes a broad perspective on the relationship between prisons and public mental health. Criminal justice policies and practices can profoundly affect society beyond a narrow focus on public mental health, or even public safety. They can reinforce or rend the social fabric. Families and communities can be strengthened or torn apart depending on how we approach crime, punishment, and rehabilitation. Economic considerations include where we choose to allocate scarce resources and whether we encourage or impede the financial stability of offenders, their families, and their communities. How we approach criminal justice also influences the political health of a society. A heavy-handed embrace of law-and-order rhetoric with an excessive focus on retribution can lead to missed opportunities to build more functional and secure communities. There are evidence-based practices that lessen criminal risk, but the political climate needs to support dispassionate research and dialogue about what does and does not work. We know that some programmes successfully rehabilitate offenders, humane conditions of confinement are safer for everyone, and alternatives to incarceration have fiscal and long-term public safety benefits for many offenders. We should now realize that mass incarceration under harsh conditions results in large numbers of embittered former inmates who are ill-prepared to re-enter society successfully.

For these reasons, this chapter focuses on individual, public, and societal mental health. Policies and practices can make societies as a whole sicker or healthier. This is perhaps nowhere more evident than with the effects of a criminal justice system. As described in this chapter, prisons are only one component of this. Dostoevsky said that the degree of civilization in a society can be judged by entering its prisons. Something similar might be said about whether a society relies exclusively on prisons or uses alternatives to incarceration when appropriate.

Mental health treatment in prison

For many inmates, at least in the USA, incarceration offers a rare opportunity to receive comprehensive medical and mental health care [1]. These individuals arrive in jails and prisons having had little to no prior access to clinical services. Not all correctional systems provide prisoners with adequate healthcare services, but systems that have sufficient resources can find themselves addressing long neglected mental health needs. Although treatment in prison, as in the community, has the primary purpose of relief of suffering, it also has potentially substantial public health benefits.

In addition to causing distress, untreated mental disorders significantly impair functioning. Cognitive, affective, perceptual, and behavioural symptoms can interfere with an inmate's ability to participate in and benefit from educational, vocational, and other programming. Absence of treatment results in a lost opportunity to gain skills that prepare inmates to lead more law-abiding and productive lives. Effective treatment that enables inmates with mental illness to engage in constructive activities and programming has benefits for the patient and society.

Mental health treatment services can also support facility operations. Inmates with mental illness have higher rates of misconduct and disciplinary problems [2]. Symptomatic inmates may have difficulty understanding and following rules. This can result in behaviours and incidents that disrupt normal institutional activities and divert the time and attention of staff. Providing needed treatment to these inmates improves environmental stability and efficiency for everyone, whether staff or other inmates.

In extreme instances, disruptive behaviours by inmates put the safety of other persons at risk. This occurs when untreated severe mental illness directly contributes to assaultive behaviours or indirectly causes harm to others when inmates engage in self-injurious behaviours. Even when they are not the direct targets of assaults, third parties can sustain physical injuries or exposure to infectious body fluids while responding to self-injurious inmates. Treatment that helps stabilize inmates who have these dangerous behaviours has the added benefit of lessening the risk of physical and psychological trauma to others in their environment.

When inmates fail to comply with expectations or commands by correctional officers, they are also more likely to incur disciplinary sanctions that include placement in restrictive housing units. It has long been known that inmates with mental illness have higher rates of disciplinary infractions and account for a disproportionate percentage of infractions [3, 4]. Officers might misinterpret as willful disobedience of orders any delayed or absent response by inmates whose poor compliance stems from problems with attention, memory, perception, impulsivity, or other symptoms of psychiatric disorder. Many correctional officers do not have the training to recognize symptoms of mental illness, especially more subtle symptoms, or the skills to work effectively with impaired individuals. Correctional officers have a greater tendency toward hierarchical, instead of collaborative and therapeutic, relationships. Mistaken interpretations of seemingly uncooperative behavior and misattribution of inmate motive may lead custody officials to impose unjustified sanctions. This results in an excessive number of punitive findings against inmates with serious mental illness. While the prevalence of mental disorders in correctional settings already exceeds prevalence in the community, the greatest over-representation occurs in disciplinary segregation and high-security supermax units [2, 5].

Provision of effective mental health services during incarceration mitigates many of the broader public health and safety problems associated with serious mental illness among inmates. In addition to providing direct treatment services, correctional mental health clinicians can offer training, liaison, and consultation that result in greater sensitivity, appropriate referrals, and less overall stress for correctional officers. The resulting public health benefits extend beyond the primary goal of relieving the patient's distress. Treatment better enables inmates to participate in non-clinical programming, lessens disruptions in the institution, enhances safety for everyone, and helps avoid unwarranted disciplinary sanctions.

Mental health treatment after community re-entry

Whatever benefits an inmate gains from mental health treatment during incarceration can be lost without continuity of care after release. For similar reasons to treatment while in custody, access to clinical services in the community can help relieve individual distress and enhance public mental health and safety. Might these services also lessen the likelihood of offender recidivism? The answer is not straightforward.

Problems arise with the definition, measurement, and interpretation of recidivism. The outcomes that define recidivism range from rearrest to reconviction to reincarceration. Not everyone who commits a crime, however, is arrested, not everyone who has been rearrested is found guilty, and not everyone who has been reincarcerated has committed a new crime. Individuals on parole, for example, may be returned to prison based solely on technical violations of their parole conditions. Casting the broadest net, recidivism would include any new contact with the criminal justice system, including arrests that do not result in convictions and returns to prison that do not arise from new criminal activity. A more restrictive definition might be limited only to new crimes that result in new prison sentences.

Regardless of definition, measurement of recidivism presents its own problems. Over what time frame does one measure? The calculated rate will rise as the period of monitoring lengthens. What data sources does one use and how reliable are they? Without comprehensive and well-matched monitoring of individuals across all jurisdictions, many instances of recidivism may go undetected. Monitoring limited to the original jurisdiction, for example, will fail to identify former inmates who are arrested in other states or even other countries.

Finally, the interpretation of recidivism data requires caution. Assessing the efficacy of a rehabilitative intervention involves comparisons of relative outcomes using comparable definitions, time frames, data sources, and populations. As described later in this chapter, much of the early literature on rehabilitation and recidivism lacked reliable methodology, but research quality has improved dramatically in recent decades.

Mitigating the factors associated with recidivism has great relevance to public health and safety. At least 95% of state prisoners in the USA eventually return to the community [6]. Effective planning for a prisoner's re-entry to society has parallels to planning for a patient's discharge from hospital. It begins at the time of admission, comprehensively addresses the individual's needs, and has goals that include a successful transition to lessen the likelihood of the person returning to the institution. The parole system in the USA has often failed in this mission owing largely to inadequate policies and services [7]. For example, conditions of parole often include boilerplate requirements, such as participation in substance use treatment, regardless of individual needs, which can interfere with employment schedules or other important life activities that enhance successful re-entry. Parole supervision sometimes involves little more than monitoring of compliance with technical requirements instead of provision of individualized supportive services. The move toward determinate sentences and away from discretionary parole in recent years has only exacerbated the shortcomings of parole as a tool to aide re-entry. By 2012, more than one in five released inmates left prison unconditionally and without community supervision because they had served their full sentences [8].

Whether mandated as a condition of parole or sought voluntarily, mental health treatment after community re-entry from prison may not be the most robust factor in preventing recidivism. Poverty is an important moderator of many of the social problems, including criminality, associated with mental illness [9]. According to a meta-analysis, offenders with or without mental disorder have the same major predictors of recidivism [10]. The analysis identified that criminal history, antisocial personality, substance abuse, and family dysfunction have significant predictive value, but clinical factors have little relevance to long-term risk of recidivism. Additional studies have found that symptoms of mental illness contribute little to criminal behaviour [11], and others have found that most predictors for recidivism are similar for all released prisoners, although participation in treatment can play a protective role for some offenders with mental illness [12, 13]. In contrast, an increasing number of studies have shown that routine outpatient treatment and access to medications does reduce the likelihood of arrest among patients with serious mental illness [14–19]. Taken as a whole, the literature indicates that social factors play a substantial role in the risk of criminality independent of the presence of mental illness, but effective treatment services for persons with serious mental illness can help them to avoid additional risk of arrest and incarceration.

Conditions of confinement

Independent of the role of mental health treatment services during and after incarceration, the conditions of confinement in a correctional facility exercise a sometimes underappreciated effect on public mental health and safety. Those conditions can foster positive changes in behaviour or they can harm and embitter inmates in a way that increases the likelihood of future criminality. Unfortunately, the latter outcome occurs far too often.

Although prisons can provide interventions that enhance mental health and reduce recidivism, they can also inadvertently make matters much worse. A prime example of misguided policy and practice involves the use of solitary confinement under extreme conditions that deprive inmates of programming, educational activities, diversions, or meaningful human contact for prolonged periods that can last months, years, or even decades. Often touted in systems that use it as an essential tool for safety and positive behaviour change, solitary confinement accomplishes neither of these goals [20].

The belief that such extreme conditions of isolation enhance prison safety has been deemed 'largely speculative' [21]. A blue-ribbon commission in the USA went further by declaring that these conditions are 'counter-productive, often causing violence inside facilities and contributing to recidivism after release' [22]. Improvements in safety after elimination or significant reduction in the use of solitary confinement have been reported by several correctional systems in the USA and the UK [23–28]. Countries that have successfully eliminated the use of prolonged solitary confinement include Germany, the Netherlands, England, and Wales [29, 30].

Intensive security does not require absence of programming, restrictions of diversions and activities, or severe social isolation. The relatively few inmates who pose a substantial risk of serious harm to other inmates or staff can be kept safe without resorting to these deprivations.

Instead of relying on harsh and punitive conditions to punish unwanted behaviours, prisons are more likely to shape inmate behaviour in the desired direction by using rewards and reinforcement. Correctional practices in Germany, for example, restrict use of solitary confinement and emphasize positive reinforcement [29]. Facilities that encourage inmate responsibility and self-governance experience less disorder than facilities with a greater focus on control and punitive sanctions [31].

How a society views the purpose of incarceration can profoundly influence the conditions in its jails and prisons. The purpose of criminal sanctions in general, and of incarceration in particular, fall into four primary categories: retribution, deterrence, incapacitation, and rehabilitation [32]. With the exception of retribution, each of these rationales has prevention of future crime as its purpose. Retribution uniquely looks only backward toward the crime already committed. Having violated the social contract, offenders must pay the set penalty, regardless of whether doing so will discourage further criminal activity. This 'just deserts' approach to criminal sanctions underlies much of criminal justice policy in recent decades, including determinate sentencing. The nature of the crime determines the amount of time that an inmate serves, not whether the inmate has been reformed.

The other rationales for criminal sanctions look primarily to the future. Incapacitation renders the offender unable to commit further crimes, in the community at least, while confined. Deterrence seeks to dissuade further criminal activity by the offender (specific deterrence) through the unpleasant experience of punishment and by other citizens (general deterrence) through the awareness of the punishment of criminals. The final rationale for criminal

consequences, rehabilitation, however, has perhaps the greatest potential for enhancing public safety and mental health.

The popularity of rehabilitation as a criminal justice goal has waxed and waned over the years. For much of the twentieth century rehabilitation served as the predominant concept behind the criminal justice system in the USA [33]. Many correctional practices that persist, such as probation and parole, have their origins in the rehabilitative ideal. Other practices, such as indeterminate sentences that allow linkage of the duration of incarceration to the time it takes to rehabilitate the offender, have gradually been abandoned.

Even the use of the term 'corrections' has its origins in the rehabilitative movement. In 1954 the American Prison Association, the oldest organization of correctional professionals in the USA, changed its name to the American Correctional Association, to reflect the philosophy of prisons as reformative institutions [34]. Perhaps the high watermark in the USA in this movement to view prisons as places to habilitate offenders came in 1967 with publication of a 342-page report by the President's Commission on Law Enforcement and Administration of Justice, commissioned by Lyndon Johnson [35]. The Commission decried the often 'brutal and degrading' (p. 159) conditions in penal institutions and the resulting failure to rehabilitate inmates. They called 'for a revolution in the way America thinks about crime'(p. v) and recommended that '[a]ll institutions should be run to the greatest possible extent with rehabilitation a joint responsibility of staff and inmates' (p. 174). The report described innovative and successful rehabilitation programmes for offenders, and it challenged the criminal justice system in the USA 'to reexamine old ways of doing things, to reform itself, to experiment, to run risks, to dare' (p. 12). In short, the commissioners said that the system 'needs vision' supported by a broad public and private commitment to conduct research as the instrument to drive reforms focused on the goal of rehabilitation. Other than a few nascent initiatives, however, the call to action by the commission went largely unheeded.

At the time of the Commission's report, much of the research literature on the efficacy of correctional treatment to reduce criminal behaviour had significant methodological shortcomings. A 1966 review of 100 studies published between 1940 and 1960 found positive results in about half of them, but most of the reviewed studies had serious design flaws that limited their validity [36]. The authors of the review concluded that the evidence of effectiveness of correctional treatment was 'slight, inconsistent, and of questionable validity' (p. 157). A similar review in 1972 of 100 published studies concluded that not one of the studies meet even 'the most minimal standards of scientific design'[37, p. 380]. Thus, the Commission's belief in 1967 in the established efficacy of rehabilitation programmes may have been based, in large part, on their relatively uncritical acceptance of the positive claims made in a literature rife with inadequate controls and other serious methodological flaws.

A watershed moment occurred in 1974 with the publication of a paper by Robert Martinson [38]. Martinson, a sociology researcher, analysed more than 20 years of data on effectiveness of rehabilitation programmes in reducing recidivism. He concluded that with few exceptions the programmes did not work. Rehabilitation quickly fell into disfavour as politicians, the news media, and the general public all latched onto Martinson's deduction. Within 5 years, however, Martinson published a new analysis finding that some programmes did show success in reducing recidivism [39], but the damage had been done. Doubts about the efficacy of rehabilitative programmes persist to this day, despite a growing body of more recent and better evidence to the contrary.

What is one to make of all these conflicting older analyses and conclusions? The simple answer is that the early literature on rehabilitation programmes included many claims of efficacy, but these claims arose from methodologically unreliable studies. Consequently, few dependable conclusions about efficacy can be drawn from these early studies. The same lack of reliability does not apply to more recent studies.

A survey of over 200 published studies conducted from 1981 to 1987 found many well-controlled research projects that demonstrated success in rehabilitating offenders [40]. A broad and growing array of interventions has been shown in well-designed research in recent decades to reduce significantly recidivism for targeted populations of offenders [41]. A comprehensive review of dozens of published meta-analyses based on hundreds of experimental studies has led to at least two overarching conclusions [42]. Firstly, increasing the severity of punitive sanctions results, at best, in modest reduction in recidivism and, at worst, in increased recidivism. Secondly, rehabilitation treatment is consistently found to lower recidivism. The gap between the effects of sanctions versus treatment is prominent. The reduction in recidivism found even in the least-positive meta-analyses of rehabilitation treatment still exceeds the largest reductions in recidivism found in meta-analyses of increasing sanctions. In other words, the poorest results with treatment exceed the best results with punishment.

Rehabilitative programming to address criminogenic factors

Programmes that enhance public health and safety by helping to reduce criminal recidivism can take place during or following incarceration and fall into several categories, including educational and vocational programming, risk–needs–responsivity model, cognitive–behavioural interventions, therapeutic communities, and re-entry programmes.

Educational and vocational programming

The most commonly used forms of correctional rehabilitation programming involve educational and vocational activities. These programmes, however, poorly mirror the more effective interventions found in the research literature [42]. Educational activities and work assignments for inmates have merit, but they do not take advantage of better-studied interventions with demonstrated efficacy.

Risk–needs–responsivity model

The risk–needs–responsivity model consists of three core principles that effectively target criminogenic factors [43]. The risk principle matches level of service to the offender's probability of reoffending. The need principle targets treatment to criminogenic needs, which consist of dynamic and remediable factors that contribute to criminal behaviour. The responsivity principle focuses on effective ways to teach new behaviours and tailors interventions to the strengths, motivation, personality, and other characteristics of the offender.

Cognitive–behavioral therapy interventions

The basic elements of cognitive–behavioural therapy (CBT) involve identifying and mitigating maladaptive thinking and attitudes and changing problematic behaviours. CBT has potential benefits for psychiatric, behavioural, and substance-related disorders. Reductions in recidivism have been found with high-quality programmes that include anger control and interpersonal problem-solving with higher-risk offenders [44].

Therapeutic communities

Perhaps the most progressive and intensive example of innovative changes in conditions of incarceration involve the use of therapeutic communities. Therapeutic communities are distinct housing units where residents and staff actively participate in running the unit and treatment sessions. These programmes combine confrontation of antisocial attitudes and behaviours with support of efforts toward growth and positive change. Incarceration-based drug treatment therapeutic communities have shown great efficacy in reducing criminal recidivism and drug relapse [45]. Although staff- and resource-intensive, these programmes can lead to other cost savings. A therapeutic community focused on substance abuse treatment generated lower administrative costs by diminishing disciplinary problems, disruptive incidents, and inmate grievances [46]. This approach has achieved significant improvement in violent behaviour with highly assaultive and disruptive inmates [47].

Re-entry programs

Re-entry programmes seek specifically to prepare inmates for successful return to the community. These can take place during incarceration, during the time immediately before and after release, or during an extended period after release. Some of the elements associated with success in reducing recidivism include duration of at least 6 months, location primarily in community settings, and use predominantly of positive reinforcement and cognitive–behavioral techniques [48].

When considering interventions to reduce recidivism some caveats apply [41]. For example, recidivism increases among individuals at low risk of reoffending when they are included in programmes with higher-risk individuals. Boot camps and wilderness programmes do not reduce recidivism, and 'scared straight' or other shock-type programmes can actually increase recidivism.

Alternatives to incarceration

An even more fundamental question involves whether incarceration itself, regardless of the conditions of that confinement, advances or hinders public safety and mental health. The estimated worldwide rate of incarceration is 144 per 100,000 population, but the rate in the USA is almost five times greater at 698 per 100,000 [49]. Only one other nation, the sparsely populated Republic of Seychelles, has a higher known rate of incarceration. Almost one-quarter of the 10.35 million prisoners in the world reside in the USA. With over two million prisoners, the USA has more people in penal settings than any other country, including China. In 2012 the USA spent $83 billion on incarceration, with at least 11 states spending more on corrections than on higher education [50]. The available evidence suggests that incarceration on this scale has done very little to reduce crime [50, 51]. The crime control benefits of soaring rates of incarceration have diminished to the point of being undetectable. In other words, escalating rates of incarceration have not been accompanied by comparable declines in rates of crime. This heavy-handed approach to criminal justice probably has done more to compromise, instead of advance, public health and safety.

Sending offenders to prison or increasing the severity of punishment also have little, if any, deterrent effect. The National Institute of Justice of the United States Department of Justice has concluded that 'The *certainty* of being caught is a vastly more powerful deterrent than the punishment' (original emphasis) [52]. Although the existing research has limitations in its size and quality, several empirical studies and meta-analyses of the literature both within and outside the USA have found that spending time in prison appears to increase the likelihood of future criminal behaviour compared with non-custodial sanctions [53, 54]. Three out of four state prisoners are rearrested within 5 years of their release [55]. The overall social experience of incarceration can include trauma, loss of community connections, and stigmatization that make society less safe by fostering future criminality when inmates return to the community [56]. Inmates placed in higher-security prisons have been found to have increased recidivism compared with similar inmates who serve time in lower-level settings [57]. Thus, the available data indicate that incarceration may exacerbate criminal tendencies, and independent of other variables, the risk goes up in conjunction with the security level in which the inmates reside.

The apparent counterproductive influence of incarceration on recidivism is closely associated with the harsh conditions that prevail in many prisons. As already noted, specific rehabilitative interventions for targeted populations can work, even though stark prison conditions and excessive use of high security do not promote prosocial behavior. Thus, humane conditions of confinement combined with evidence-based rehabilitation programmes either inside or outside of prison are more likely to have a net positive effect.

In contrast to institutional confinement, community corrections typically involve non-custodial interventions as part of either pre-trial, probation, or parole management. Pre-trial diversion occurs in lieu of prosecution, probation provides community supervision after conviction as an alternative to incarceration, and parole involves supervised conditional release from prison. At the end of 2014 the USA had about 1 in 52 adults, or close to 5 million people, under community supervision [58]. These alternatives to incarceration can have fiscal and public safety advantages [59], but the cost–benefit ratio varies among programmes and target populations [60, 61].

Illustrative programmes

Diversion programs

Diversion of individuals who come into contact with the criminal justice system can occur either before or after police booking. Pre-booking programmes rely on the police and seek to avoid arrest typically through transfers to crisis intervention services. Post-booking programmes involve the courts and divert offenders to community services after arrest.

Mental health Crisis Interventions Teams are a prime example of a pre-booking diversion programme. These programmes use specially trained police officers to respond to situations concerning individuals with mental illness. Although more and better research is needed, studies suggest that the training improves officer comfort and efficacy when dealing with persons with serious mental illness and that Crisis Interventions Teams in communities with accessible

treatment services result in lower arrest rates and criminal justice system costs [62].

Drug courts comprise the most widespread model for post-booking diversion programmes. As of the end of 2009, the USA had 2459 drug courts, with extensive documentation of their efficacy in cost-effective crime reduction [63]. Eligible participants may have charges of drug possession or other offenses that relate to or support their substance use. A judge-led multidisciplinary team of legal, clinical, and law-enforcement professionals work with the offender to maintain abstinence and make positive life changes. As a conservative estimate, every dollar spent for addiction treatment programmes, in general, saves up to $7 in criminal justice-related costs alone and over $12 if healthcare savings are included [64].

Similar to drug courts, over 1000 other problem-solving courts in the USA focus on issues such as domestic violence, gambling, homelessness, truancy, and mental illness [63]. Mental health courts were initially developed to serve defendants charged with misdemeanors, but some now include individuals charged with felonies. They have been shown to reduce recidivism and to increase participation in community treatment [65, 66].

Managing offenders in the community instead of prison has potential advantages beyond the positive effects on the offender's rehabilitation and mental health. Incarceration causes collateral damage to the family and friends of inmates, with especially adverse effect on mental and physical health of children. Parental incarceration has been found to have an independent association with attention deficit and attention deficit hyperactivity disorders, and with behavioural, learning, conduct, developmental, speech, and language problems in the children of inmates [67]. Other risk factors associated with parental imprisonment include child anti-social behaviour, offending, mental health problems, drug abuse, school failure, and unemployment [68]. The detrimental effects of paternal incarceration exceed those of other forms of father absence and occur even for children who did not live with their fathers prior to the incarceration [69]. Adverse effects extend at least into young adulthood with significantly associated health problems that include depression, post-traumatic stress disorder, anxiety, high cholesterol, asthma, and migraines [70]. As of 2009, an estimated 2.7 million children under the age of 18 years in the USA had a parent in jail or prison [71]. This represented 1 in every 28 children. Twenty-five years earlier, only 1 in 125 children had an incarcerated parent. The number of children who have lived with a parent who was incarcerated at any time after the child's birth goes up to 1 in 14 [72]. Researchers and policymakers are paying increasing attention to the negative influence of parental incarceration on children [73]. These consequences must be taken into account when calculating the public health and mental health effects of the massive growth in imprisonment.

In addition to health-related consequences, the collateral harm to children of inmates includes potentially lifelong financial disadvantages that push them down the socio-economic ladder [71]. The risk of having an imprisoned parent falls disproportionately among children who are black or have a low-education parent [74]. The damage to children is not limited to instances of parental incarceration. Economic strain and negative school outcomes occur among children who have anyone in their household, even non-immediate family members, incarcerated [75].

When community-based programmes are not an option, prison nurseries can at least mitigate the harm that results from incarceration of mothers with infant children. In addition to facilitating more positive developmental outcomes for their infants, mothers who participate in prison nurseries have been found to have large reductions in recidivism [76].

The enormous financial costs of mass incarceration also cause societal damage. In 2010 alone, the USA spent $80 billion on incarceration [77]. Every dollar spent on prisons means one less dollar available for other public needs. Money that could be used to support infrastructure, education, general health care, social safety nets, and a myriad of other services ends up consumed in the prison industry. Many of these other services help advance overall public mental health and safety. Funding prisons at their expense doubles the harm.

Individuals who appear to fail in a community corrections placement do not necessarily represent a threat to public safety. For example, a 9% rate of reincarceration has been reported among adults on parole, but less than a third of the reincarcerated parolees returned to prison because of a new offense [58]. Most of the parolees who returned to prison did so because of violations of conditions of supervision (e.g. failure to keep appointments or maintain employment) unrelated to new criminal activity. Supervision programmes that focus primarily on surveillance, with revocation of parole often for technical violations, do not generally have the same economic and crime-reduction benefits as treatment-oriented intensive supervision programmes [60].

Although research indicates that specific programmes result in sustained reductions in recidivism among targeted populations of offenders, these interventions have been underused in the USA [78].

Conclusions

Mental health treatment for inmates during incarceration and after community re-entry has benefits for the individual and for society. Correctional institutions function more safely and more efficiently when inmates receive the clinical care that they need and everyone benefits if those services facilitate successful transition from prison. Even in the absence of these broader benefits, however, compassion and justice dictate that everyone, including inmates, has access to basic mental and physical health care. Programmes that specifically target criminogenic risk factors extend beyond these fundamental clinical services. Whether these programmes work has been the focus of controversy and confusion, but the evidence shows that targeted and well-designed interventions can effectively reduce recidivism. Policymakers need to understand and act upon this evidence if they truly care about public health and safety. They also must recognize that the long experiment with mass incarceration has been a fiscal, societal, and public mental health and safety failure. We have reaped little-to-no benefit in crime reduction from the explosive growth in prison populations or from the vast sums of money diverted to the correctional industry. The harsh and excessively punitive conditions in most prisons only add to the problem by making inmates worse, not better. Their families, children, and communities also pay a heavy price in their own fiscal and social stability and their mental health. All this can change, however. We know much about what does work. We have successful models to draw upon. We can make more effective use of our prisons and the criminal justice system in general. They can become fiscally responsible interventions that enhance, instead of compromise,

public mental health and safety. We know how to reshape prison policy to make things better. We need only the will and wisdom to get it done.

References

1. Marks JS, Turner N. The critical link between health care and jails. *Health Aff (Millwood)* 2014; 33: 443–447.
2. Abramsky S, Fellner J, Human Rights Watch (Organization). *Ill-Equipped: U.S. Prisons and Offenders With Mental Illness.* New York: Human Rights Watch, 2003.
3. Adams K. The disciplinary experiences of mentally disordered inmates. *Crim Justice Behav* 1986; 13: 297–316.
4. Lovell D, Jemelka R. When inmates misbehave: the costs of discipline. *Prison J* 1996; 76: 165–179.
5. Lovell D. Patterns of disturbed behavior in a supermax population. *Crim Justice Behav* 2008; 35: 985–1004.
6. Hughes T, Wilson DJ. *Reentry Trends in the United States.* Washington, DC: U.S. Department of Justice, Office of Justice Programs, Bureau of Justice Statistics, 2002.
7. Petersilia J. Prisoner reentry: public safety and reintegration challenges. *Prison J* 2001; 81: 360–375.
8. The Pew Charitable Trusts. *Max Out: The Rise in Prison Inmates Released Without Supervision.* Washington, DC: The Pew Charitable Trusts, 2014.
9. Draine J, Salzer MS, Culhane DP, Hadley TR. Role of social disadvantage in crime, joblessness, and homelessness among persons with serious mental illness. *Psychiatr Serv* 2002; 53: 565–573.
10. Bonta J, Law M, Hanson K. The prediction of criminal and violent recidivism among mentally disordered offenders: a meta-analysis. *Psychol Bull* 1998; 123: 123–142.
11. Junginger J, Claypoole K, Laygo R, Crisanti A. Effects of serious mental illness and substance abuse on criminal offenses. *Psychiatr Serv* 2006; 57: 879–882.
12. Hall DL, Miraglia RP, Lee LW, Chard-Wierschem D, Sawyer D. Predictors of general and violent recidivism among SMI prisoners returning to communities in New York State. *J Am Acad Psychiatry Law* 2012; 40: 221–231.
13. Peterson J, Skeem JL, Hart E, Vidal S, Keith F. Analyzing offense patterns as a function of mental illness to test the criminalization hypothesis. *Psychiatr Serv* 2010; 61: 1217–1222.
14. Constantine R, Petrila J, Andel R, et al. Arrest trajectories of adult offenders with a serious mental illness. *Psychol Public Policy Law* 2010; 16: 319–339.
15. Constantine RJ, Robst J, Andel R, Teague G. The impact of mental health services on arrests of offenders with a serious mental illness. *Law Hum Behav* 2012; 36: 170–176.
16. Gilbert AR, Moser LL, Van Dorn RA, et al. Reductions in arrest under assisted outpatient treatment in New York. *Psychiatr Serv* 2010; 61: 996–999.
17. Robst J, Constantine R, Andel R, Boaz T, Howe A. Factors related to criminal justice expenditure trajectories for adults with serious mental illness. *Crim Behav Ment Health* 2011; 21: 350–362.
18. Van Dorn RA, Andel R, Boaz TL, et al. Risk of arrest in persons with schizophrenia and bipolar disorder in a Florida Medicaid program: the role of atypical antipsychotics, conventional neuroleptics, and routine outpatient behavioral health services. *J Clin Psychiatry* 2011; 72: 502–508.
19. Van Dorn RA, Desmarais SL, Petrila J, Haynes D, Singh JP. Effects of outpatient treatment on risk of arrest of adults with serious mental illness and associated costs. *Psychiatr Serv* 2013; 64: 856–862.
20. Appelbaum KL. American psychiatry should join the call to abolish solitary confinement. *J Am Acad Psychiatry Law* 2015; 43: 406–415.
21. Briggs CS, Sundt JL, Castellano TC. The effect of supermaximum security prisons on aggregate levels of institutional violence. *Criminology* 2003; 41: 1341–1376.

22. Gibbons JJ, Katzenbach ND. *Confronting Confinement: A Report of the Commission on Safety and Abuse in America's Prisons.* New York: Vera Institute of Justice, 2006.

23. Shames A, Wilcox J, Subramanian R. Solitary Confinement: Common Misconceptions and Emerging Safe Alternatives. Available at: http://www.vera.org/pubs/solitary-confinement-misconceptions-safe-alternatives (2015, accessed 28 February 2018).

24. Vera Institute of Justice. Mississippi DOC's Emmitt Sparkman on reducing the use of segregation in prisons. Available at: http://www.vera.org/blog/mississippi-docs-emmitt-sparkman-reducing-use-segregation-prisons (2011, accessed 31 August 2015).

25. McCleland J. The High Costs of High Security at Supermax Prisons. Available at: http://www.npr.org/2012/06/19/155359553/the-high-costs-of-high-security-at-supermax-prisons (2012, accessed 4 July 2015).

26. Commission on Safety and Abuse in America's Prisons. Confronting confinement: testimony of James Burton, former warden Oak Park Heights prison, 2006.

27. Kupers TA, Dronet T, Winter M, et al. Beyond supermax administrative segregation: Mississippi's experience rethinking prison classification and creating alternative mental health programs. *Crim Justice Behav* 2009; 36: 1037–1050.

28. McClatchey C. HMP Grendon: Therapy for dangerous prisoners. Available at: http://www.bbc.com/news/uk-11947481 (2011, accessed 4 July 2015).

29. Subramanian R, Shames A. *Sentencing and Prison Practices in Germany and the Netherlands: Implications for the United States.* New York: Vera Institute of Justice, 2013.

30. Franks T. Forty years in solitary confinement and counting. Available at: http://www.bbc.co.uk/news/magazine-17564805 (2012, accessed 28 February 2018).

31. Reisig MD. Rates of disorder in higher-custody state prisons: a comparative analysis of managerial practices. *Crime Delinq* 1998; 44: 229.

32. Packer HL. *The Limits of the Criminal Sanction.* Stanford, CA: Stanford University Press, 1968.

33. Cullen FT, Gendreau P. Assessing correctional rehabilitation: policy, practice, and prospects. *Crim Justice* 2000; 3: 299–370.

34. American Correctional Association. The history of the American Correctional Association Available at: http://www.aca.org/ACA_Prod_IMIS/ACA_Member/About_Us/Our_History/ACA_Member/AboutUs/AboutUs_Home.aspx?hkey=0c9cb058-e3d5-4bb0-ba7c-be29f9b34380 (2016, accessed 3 June 2016).

35. President's Commission on Law Enforcement and Administration of Justice. *The Challenge of Crime in a Free Society.* Washington, DC: United States Government Printing Office, 1967.

36. Bailey WC. Correctional outcome: an evaluation of 100 reports. *J Crim Law Criminol Police Sci* 1966; 57: 153–160.

37. Logan CH. Evaluation research in crime and delinquency: a reappraisal. *J Crim Law Criminol Police Sci* 1972; 63: 378–387.

38. Martinson R. What works?—Questions and answers about prison reform. *Public Interest* 1974; 35: 22–54.

39. Martinson R. New findings, new views: a note of caution regarding sentencing reform. *Hofstra Law Rev* 1979; 7: 243–258.

40. Gendreau P, Ross R. Revivification of rehabilitation: evidence from the 1980s. *Justice Q* 1987; 4: 349–407.

41. Warren R, Crime and Justice Institute. *Evidence-Based Practice to Reduce Recidivism: Implications for State Judiciaries.* Washington, DC: United States Department of Justice, National Institute of Corrections, 2007.

42. Lipsey MW, Cullen FT. The effectiveness of correctional rehabilitation: a review of systematic reviews. *Annu Rev Law Soc Sci* 2007; 3: 297–320.

43. Bonta J, Andrews DA. *Risk-Need-Responsivity Model for Offender Assessment and Rehabilitation.* Public Safety Canada, 2007 Cat. No.: PS3-1/2007-6.

44. Landenberger NA, Lipsey MW. The positive effects of cognitive–behavioral programs for offenders: a meta-analysis of factors associated with effective treatment. *J Exp Criminol* 2005; 1: 451–476.

45. Mitchell O, Wilson DB, MacKenzie DL. Does incarceration-based drug treatment reduce recidivism? A meta-analytic synthesis of the research. *J Exp Criminol* 2007; 3: 353–375.

46. Zhang SX, Roberts REL, McCollister KE. An economic analysis of the in-prison therapeutic community model on prison management costs. *J Crim Just* 2009; 37: 388–395.

47. Cooke DJ. Containing violent prisoners: an analysis of the Barlinnie Special Unit. *Br J Criminol* 1989; 29: 129–143.

48. Petersilia J. What works in prisoner reentry? Reviewing and questioning the evidence. *Fed Probat* 2004; 68: 4–8.

49. Walmsley R. World Prison Population List, eleventh edition. Available at: http://www.icpr.org.uk/media/41356/world_prison_population_list_11th_edition.pdf (2015, accessed 28 February 2018).

50. Council of Economic Advisors. *Economic Perspectives on Incarceration and the Criminal Justice System.* Washington, DC: Executive Office of the President of the United States, 2016.

51. Roeder O, Eisen L-B, Bowling J. *What Caused the Crime Decline?* New York: Brennan Center for Justice, New York University School of Law, 2015.

52. National Institute of Justice. Five Things about Deterrence. Available at: https://www.ncjrs.gov/pdffiles1/nij/247350.pdf (2016, accessed 20 June 2016).

53. National Research Council. *The Growth of Incarceration in the United States: Exploring Causes and Consequences.* Washington, DC: National Academy of Sciences, 2014.

54. Nagin DS, Cullen FT, Lero Jonson C. Imprisonment and reoffending. *Crime Just* 2009; 38: 115–200.

55. Durose MR, Cooper AD, Snyder HN. *Recidivism of Prisoners Released in 30 States in 2005: Patterns from 2005 to 2010.* Washington, DC: Bureau of Justice Statistics, Office of Justice Programs, U.S. Department of Justice, 2014.

56. Cullen FT, Jonson CL, Nagin DS. Prisons do not reduce recidivism: the high cost of ignoring science. *Prison J* 2011; 91(3 Suppl.): 48S–65S.

57. Gaes GG, Camp SD. Unintended consequences: experimental evidence for the criminogenic effect of prison security level placement on post-release recidivism. *J Exp Criminol* 2009; 5: 139–162.

58. Kaeble D, Maruschak LM, Bonczar TP. *Probation and Parole in the United States, 2014.* Washington, DC: U.S. Department of Justice, Office of Justice Programs, Bureau of Justice Statistics, 2015.

59. Justice Policy Institute. *Pruning Prisons: How Cutting Corrections Can Save Money and Protect Public Safety.* Washington, DC: Justice Policy Institute, 2009.

60. Aos S, Phipps P, Barnoski R, Lieb R. *The Comparative Costs and Benefits of Programs to Reduce Crime.* Olympia, WA: Washington State Institute for Public Policy, 2001.

61. Aos S, Drake E. *Prison, Police, and Programs: Evidence-based Options That Reduce Crime and Save Money.* Olympia, WA: Washington State Institute for Public Policy, 2013.

62. Compton MT, Bahora M, Watson AC, Oliva JR. A comprehensive review of extant research on Crisis Intervention Team (CIT) programs. *J Am Acad Psychiatry Law* 2008; 36: 47–55.

63. Huddleston W, Marlowe DB. *Painting the Current Picture: A National Report on Drug Courts and Other Problem-Solving Court Programs in the United States.* Washington, DC: Office of National Drug Control Policy, Bureau of Justice Assistance, and the National Drug Court Institute, 2011.

64. National Institute on Drug Abuse. *Principles of Drug Addiction Treatment: A Research-based Guide*, 3rd ed. Bethesda, MD: National Institutes of Health, U.S. Department of Health and Human Services, 2012.

65. Goodale G, Callahan L, Steadman HJ. Law & psychiatry: what can we say about mental health courts today? *Psychiatr Serv* 2013; 64: 298–300.

66. Steadman HJ, Redlich A, Callahan L, Robbins PC, Vesselinov R. Effect of mental health courts on arrests and jail days: a multisite study. *Arch Gen Psychiatry* 2011; 68: 167–172.

67. Turney K. Stress proliferation across generations? Examining the relationship between parental incarceration and childhood health. *J Health Soc Behav* 2014; 55: 302–319.

68. Murray J, Farrington DP. The effects of parental imprisonment on children. *Crime Just* 2008; 37: 133–206.

69. Geller A, Cooper CE, Garfinkel I, Schwartz-Soicher O, Mincy RB. Beyond absenteeism: father incarceration and child development. *Demography* 2012; 49: 49–76.

70. Lee RD, Fang X, Luo F. The impact of parental incarceration on the physical and mental health of young adults. *Pediatrics* 2013; 131: e1188–1195.

71. The Pew Charitable Trusts. *Collateral Costs: Incarceration's Effect on Economic Mobility*. Washington, DC: The Pew Charitable Trusts, 2010.

72. Murphey D, Cooper PM. *Parents Behind Bars: What Happens to Their Children?* Available at: https://www.childtrends.org/publications/parents-behind-bars-what-happens-to-their-children/ (2015, accessed 28 February 2018).

73. Uggen C, McElrath S. Parental incarceration: what we know and where we need to go. *J Crim Law Crim* 2014; 104: 597–604.

74. Wildeman C. Parental imprisonment, the prison boom, and the concentration of childhood disadvantage. *Demography* 2009; 46: 265–280.

75. Nichols EB, Loper AB. Incarceration in the household: academic outcomes of adolescents with an incarcerated household member. *J Youth Adolesc* 2012; 41: 1455–1471.

76. Goshin LS, Byrne MW. Converging streams of opportunity for prison nursery programs in the United States. *J Offend Rehabil* 2009; 48: 271–295.

77. Department of Justice. *Smart on Crime: Reforming the Criminal Justice System for the 21st Century*. Washington, DC: United States Department of Justice, 2013.

78. National Institute of Corrections and Crime and Justice Institute. *Implementing Evidence-Based Practice in Community Corrections: The Principles of Effective Intervention*. Washington, DC: National Institute of Corrections and Crime and Justice Institute, 2004.

CHAPTER 26

LGBTI and mental health

Martin Plöderl, Lieselotte Mahler,
Timo O. Nieder, and Götz Mundle

LGBTI—and other colours of the rainbow

The acronym LGBTI stands for lesbian, gay, bisexual, trans(-gender), and inter(-sex), and was established over the years as a description of sexual and gender minorities. We will use LGBTI in this chapter, although it is conceptually problematic because lesbian, gay, and bisexual are certain sexual orientations, whereas trans(-gender) relates to various gender identities and inter(-sex) to diverse sex characteristics. Thus, trans(-gender) and inter(-sex) should be considered independently from one's sexual orientation. Although causes for mental health issues are specific for each of the LGBTI subgroups, there are also important shared causes that justify recognizing LGBTI groups together in this chapter. We first give an overview of the diverse subgroups, which are subsumed under the umbrella term LGBTI.

Sexual minorities

Individuals can be characterized by their sexual orientation on at least three important dimensions: identity, behaviour, and attraction. Based on the identity dimension, individuals are sexual minorities if they identify other than heterosexual, for example as lesbian, gay, bisexual (LGB), bisexual, asexual, pansexual, queer, or if they are questioning their sexual identity. With the behavioural or attraction dimensions, someone belongs to a sexual minority if the person is not exclusively having sex with someone of the other sex, or if the sexual attraction is not exclusively heterosexual.

Whereas the three dimensions of sexual orientation correlate substantially (e.g. [1]), the association is not perfect. In one study, only few (≤ 1%) adolescents identified or behaved exclusively homosexual in contrast to approximately 5% who were same-sex attracted [2]. In another study on adult men who had sex with men, the majority identified as heterosexual [3]. Thus, the different dimensions of sexual orientation cover largely overlapping but also distinct groups.

Trans(-gender)

The term 'trans' or 'transgender' (for the rest of this chapter, simply 'trans') is an umbrella term covering a range of individuals who identify not in congruence with what would be expected based on their primary sex characteristics (either male or female). In line with this, trans individuals differ from cis(-gendered) individuals, who experience their gender in congruence with their primary sex characteristics. There is no universal definition of trans and the term is dynamic. It includes transgender people, i.e. persons whose gender identity differs from the sex assigned them at birth, who are not exclusively masculine or feminine (genderqueer, non-binary, pangender), who refuse to belong to any gender (agender, gender neutral) or who belong to a third gender, and cross-dressers, independent of the underlying motives [4]. Some of these groups are still classified as mental disorders in the International Classification of Diseases (ICD) 10th Revision (ICD-10). Transsexualism (F64.0), for example, refers to the persistent desire to live and be accepted as the opposite sex that is linked to the clinical need for transition-related medical interventions (e.g. hormone treatment, surgeries). Dual Role Transvestitism (F64.1) refers to the wearing of clothes of the opposite sex in order to enjoy the temporary experience of one's membership of the opposite sex without any desire for a permanent sex change. Gender Identity Disorder of Childhood (F64.2) refers to the distress with one's sex and the desire to belong to the other sex in childhood. It has been proposed to change Transsexualism to Gender Incongruence in the upcoming ICD 11th Revision (ICD-11) [5]. Moreover, there is significant debate concerning the need for a specific diagnosis of Gender Incongruence in Childhood [6, 7]. In the *Diagnostic and Statistical Manual of Mental Disorders* (DSM), Transsexualism was first replaced with Gender Identity Disorder in the fourth edition and then with Gender Dysphoria in the more recent fifth edition. In line with the fifth edition, the American Psychiatric Association stated for the first time that the incongruence between sex and gender is not a matter of pathology, but rather a human variation. Even the World Medical Association (WMA) has followed this same direction and recently published a statement on transgender people emphasizing that gender incongruence is not in itself a mental disorder [8].

Inter(-sex)

For some individuals, binary male/female categories of sex are not appropriate because biological variations do not allow such simplifying and misleading categorization. Commonly, sex is determined by sex chromosomes, types of gonads, sex hormones, internal reproductive anatomy, and, usually, at birth by the appearance of external genitalia. Individuals are intersex or 'inter' (used throughout the rest of this chapter for simplicity) if one or more of these characteristics are not typically male or female. In medicine, inter conditions such as congenital adrenal hyperplasia (CAH) or complete androgen insensitivity (CAIS) are often labelled as disorders of sex development (DSD) and are listed in the ICD, a practice that is criticized by nearly all support groups [9], as well as critical sex researchers (i.e. [10]) because of its stigmatizing and pathologizing implications. Instead, 'diverse sex developments' or 'differences of sex development' are preferred terms [11].

Trans, inter, and necessary reconsiderations of sexual orientation

As discussed in the previous section, trans and inter are both conceptually different from sexual orientation. Both the terms *other sex* and *heterosexual* are problematic for trans and inter people. For example, some trans and inter people identify as heterosexual men or women, thus they do not necessarily belong to a sexual minority with respect to their the identity dimension of sexual orientation. It remains open to individual decisions if an inter person self-describes as heterosexual and what it means to the person. Similar yet different, trans people might label themselves as hetero- or homosexual pre-transition and vice versa post-transition. Therefore, at least in a scientific context, terms referring to the sexual object only without referring to the sexual subject should be favoured [12]. According to this, the sexual orientation of a person of any gender or sex who is sexually attracted to women or to femininity can be described as gynephile or gynophilic. The sexual orientation of a person of any gender or sex who is sexually attracted to men or to masculinity can be described as androphile or androphilic.

LGBTI and mental health

Sexual minorities

Mental health problems among LGB individuals were documented 100 years ago by Magnus Hirschfeld [13], who observed high rates of suicide attempts (25%) and suicides (3%) among 10,000 German homosexual men that he knew of [8]. Before its removal from the DSM in 1973 and from the ICD in 1992, homosexuality was classified as a mental disorder. Theories of homosexuality assumed pathological mechanisms as cause for homosexuality or homosexuality as expression of an immature development [14].

In an influential study, Evelyn Hooker [15] found that psychiatrists could not distinguish Rorschach interpretations of gay men from those of heterosexual men, supporting the idea that gay men are not inherently pathological. This finding and other studies reporting no significant differences based on sexual orientation were important for depathologizing homosexuality [16].

However, studies continued to report increased mental health problems among LGB participants [16]. Saghir and Robins [17], for example, reported elevated levels of alcohol and drug abuse. Most of these early studies, however, lacked heterosexual control groups and recruited participants from the gay community, resulting in a possible bias that may over- or underestimate the prevalence of mental health problems among LGB individuals [18–21]. Since the 1990s, the quality of studies has substantially improved by using innovative research methodologies such as birth cohorts [22, 23], prospective designs [24, 25], twin registries [26, 27], matching LGB individuals with their heterosexual siblings [28], and using multiple dimensions of sexual orientation [1, 2, 29–32], or combined dimensions of sexual orientation [33]. In these improved studies, LGB individuals continued to report increased mental health problems and suicidality compared with heterosexuals.

Of special importance are recent studies using large, representative samples including enough LGB participants to achieve adequate statistical power, different dimensions of sexual orientation, and valid methods to assess mental health problems. Several meta-analyses of these studies reported statistically significant disparities between LGB and heterosexual individuals for substance use problems, most assessed mental health disorders, and suicidality [21, 34–37]. However, these meta-analyses often collapsed sexual minorities into one group to increase statistical power, or because some studies did not report results for sexual minority subgroups. This could have distorted the differences between subgroups [38]. For example, bisexual individuals commonly have higher levels of mental health problems than lesbian and gay individuals [21, 36, 37]. Moreover, studies have often used different dimensions of sexual orientation (identification, behaviour, attraction), which affects the differences in sexual orientation [31]. Furthermore, sexual orientation differences have varied with gender and type of mental health problem [34, 37].

A recent systematic review of population-based studies took into account sexual orientation subgroup differences, gender, year of publication, region, and study quality [39]. The majority of studies, including recent ones, reported increased levels of mental health problems for sexual minority individuals compared with heterosexuals, including depression, anxiety, suicide attempts/suicides, and drug-related mental health problems. A different picture emerged for alcohol-related problems, where the majority of studies reported no differences or lower rates among gay and bisexual males. However, in the majority of higher-quality studies that used clinical diagnoses of alcohol dependency, gay and bisexual males again had increased rates. The differences between LGB and heterosexual individuals were largest for attempting suicides and deaths by suicides, where most of the effect sizes were large (odds ratios > 3.5), and they were smallest for alcohol-related mental health problems. The increase of risk varied in magnitude but existed across sexual minority subgroups in all dimensions of sexual orientation (behaviour, attraction, identity), for men and women, age groups, regions, and in more recent studies. In the majority of studies, levels of mental health problems were higher for bisexuals than for lesbian and gay individuals, and comparable or smaller for mostly heterosexuals and questioning individuals. The review also supports the previously reported larger sexual orientation differences for males than females for all disorders except substance-related disorders, where the majority of studies reported larger sexual orientation differences for females. In summary, the sexual orientation discrepancies for different mental health problems remain a robust finding in studies of the past decades.

To avoid unjustified pathologization, it should be pointed out that despite the robust sexual orientation differences in mental health, a clear majority of LGB people do *not* suffer from mental health problems. For example, the most recent meta-analysis of studies on adults reported that 11–20% of LGB adults (depending on sampling method) reported having attempted suicide versus 4% heterosexual attempters [21].

Trans

Fewer studies about the mental health of trans individuals exist than studies on LGB individuals, and, to our knowledge, there are only four population surveys about mental health problems for trans people [40–43]. In a recent systematic review of 38 studies using samples of people diagnosed with gender dysphoria by health professionals, most cross-sectional studies found increased rates of mental disorders or psychopathology versus the general population, documenting the vulnerability of this population [44]. However, only few studies used matched control groups and most of the 11 longitudinal studies reported an improvement of mental health following transition-related medical interventions. Another recent review of 31 papers reported clearly higher prevalence of non-suicidal self-injury, suicide ideation, suicide attempts, and suicides for trans individuals versus the general population or cisgendered controls [45]. The increased suicide risk was also reported in longitudinal studies. The most recent review of 116 studies in 30 countries reported increased rates of mental health problems (including depression, post-traumatic stress disorder, and substance use) among trans adults [46]. As with LGB individuals, to avoid unjust pathologization, it should be pointed out that the majority of trans individuals who seek transition-related care do not suffer from axis I (male to female 38%, female to male 37%) or axis II (15%) disorders [47]. In line with this, the WMA published a statement in 2015, that 'being transgender does not in itself imply any mental impairment' and that 'gender incongruence is not in itself a mental disorder' [8].

Inter

Only a few studies on the mental health of inter people are available and these are mostly based on small samples from a clinical context, from inter organizations, or support groups. Thus, it is impossible to draw firm conclusions for the many different types of inter conditions. An early review of 11 studies published up until 2005 reported increased mental health problems, with the exception of CAH across different types of inter [48]. Another review of 35 studies on individuals with female or ambiguous genitalia from CAIS or partial androgen insensitivity syndrome, 5α-reductase 2 deficiency and 17-β-hydroxysteroid dehydrogenase deficiency found that psychological distress and suicidality are an issue [49]. Increased levels of symptoms related to mental health were also reported in more current studies [48, 50–56] but not in others [57–59]. Of note, levels of suicide ideation were higher for those with gonadectomy than those without (61 vs 23%) [48]. Repeated genital surgeries correlated with dissatisfaction with physical appearance [10]. In one of the few non-Western studies, more internalizing symptoms, including depression, were reported in an Indonesian sample with late identified inter conditions, but no differences were found for several other symptoms [60]. Five of 40 inter Africans aged 3 months–16 years attempted suicide [61], which is a very high rate given that many were not old enough to consider suicide.

CAH

Increased rates of mental health problems were reported in some studies [58, 62–64] but not in others [48, 65, 66]. The most reliable studies are likely to be those which followed Swedish participants since they were newborns diagnosed with different forms of CAH. For those who lived as women, a 1.9-fold increased risk for any of the assessed mental disorder, compared with matched female controls, and a non-significantly lower rate of suicides or suicide attempts were reported [67]. Differences between the subtypes were generally negligible. For males with CAH, increased rates of most mental disorders and fatal and non-fatal suicidal behaviours

were reported, but with variations for different subtypes of CAH [68]. Another study using the Swedish register found similar rates of suicides as causes of death among those with CAH, compared with matched controls [69].

Surgical procedures and mental health

A review of longitudinal studies evaluating the psychological impact of surgical procedures of inter conditions only revealed 13 studies [70]. Most of the studies failed to use reliable measures, considering only the clinicians view of success, assessing only sexual satisfaction as outcome, or taking a heterosexist view of sexuality and appropriate bodies: 'Therefore, when female genitalia are evaluated, it is in the sense of being able to accommodate a regular-sized penis. In those cases, alternative sexual orientations or practices are not accounted for, even when sexual satisfaction is evaluated' (p. 4). Machado et al. [70] further claim that in most circumstances, there is no medical urgency for surgical sex assignment but instead a social urgency, resulting from rigid, binary gender norms. In addition, there are documented negative outcomes from surgical procedures. Thus, a solely biomedical approach to inter conditions raises serious problems. Fortunately, this is clearly acknowledged in a recent consensus statement [9], wherein the goal is to improve quality of life, and the views of intersex organizations are also taken into account. It is acknowledged that 'There is still no consensual attitude regarding indications, timing, procedure and evaluation of outcome of DSD surgery' (p. 19) and the resulting need for shared decision-making. Coercive surgical procedures have been acknowledged as human rights violations by the World Health Organization [71].

To sum up, the majority, but not all, of the studies reported increased mental health problems for inter people compared with the general population.

Methodological problems with LGBTI populations

As with all hidden populations, estimating the prevalence of mental disorders among LGBTI individuals remains inherently limited [19]. For example, LGBTI people may not participate or choose to disclose their status in studies, and the associated bias may lead to over- or underestimation of the prevalence rates, even in 'representative' population-based samples. Studies have also used different dimensions or constructs to assess LGBTI status, making the results hardly comparable across studies [39]. Most population-based studies did not differ between sex assigned at birth and gender identity, and did not assess inter conditions. Additionally, online and in-person data collection methods reach respondents with tremendously different health and life experiences (for trans persons, see [72]). Large and costly samples are needed to reach sufficient numbers of LGBTI individuals, which may be a reason why there are almost no population-based studies outside of Western cultures. Therefore, convenience samples from LGBTI communities remain an important alternative despite the possible biases [73, 74]. Similarly, studies on the mental health of trans and inter people use clinical samples and the results are likely different from those of the general trans and inter population. However, as the treatment paradigm for trans people in the twentieth century was restrictive and excluding, leaving trans people without appropriate care (cf. [75]), non-clinical samples might display the present trans population much closer to reality than clinical samples. The intersection of LGBTI status with other minority categories (e.g. race, religion, disability) may be crucial for understanding individual mental health, and related research is emerging [76–79] but are beyond the scope of this chapter.

Explanatory models of LGBTI and mental health

Current theoretical models about LGBTI health disparities focus on the noxious effects of society's rigid norms of gender and sexuality, with the resulting homonegativity (also referred to as homophobia), binegativity, transnegativity, and internegativity (LGBTI negativity will be used for the rest of the chapter) with their various expressions on different levels of society and within the individual.

The most prominent model to explain LGB health disparities is Ilan Meyer's minority stress model [80]. According to this model (Fig. 26.1), LGB people are, besides experiencing general stressors, also burdened by minority specific stressors. These include distal minority stress, for example actual discrimination and violence, and proximal stressors, such as hiding one's sexual minority status, fear of coming out, or devaluating one's sexual orientation (internalized homonegativity). The negative impact of these stressors can be buffered by social support and coping abilities and are influenced by contextual factors, such as prominence, valence, or integration of the minority status.

The underlying pathogenic mechanisms are further elaborated in the psychological mediation model of Mark Hatzenbuehler [81]: distal minority stress not only impacts mental health directly, but also indirectly by having a negative effect on general mental processes such as coping, emotion regulation, social, and cognitive processes. Minority stress can also affect group specific processes (expectations of rejection, concealment, and internalized homonegativity). General and group-specific processes influence each other.

Ron Stall's syndemics model was originally developed to explain why urban gay men are at risk for a variety of health and psychosocial problems but has been applied to transgender women too [82, 83]. The developmental approach is a strength of the model: early in life, long before coming out, boys are socially penalized for not fulfilling masculine norms due to actual or ascribed gender nonconformity. This is followed by the coming out process, internalization of homonegativity, and acquirement of proto-gay social skills. Gay men may move to 'gay ghettos' as a reaction to a homophobic social context, which comes with chances (connecting, support) and risks (drugs, rejection), and may lead to a snowball effect of developing different health problems.

Social constructionist theorists criticize the minority stress models presented so far for their biomedical viewpoint, i.e. that the emotional distress of LGB individuals is pathologized and that the risk is placed within the individual, neglecting the complex interconnection of social, economical, and cultural factors [84]. Furthermore, the models cannot explain why some LGB people are still at risk for mental health problems despite the widespread removal of legal and policy barriers, increased gay-affirmative attitudes, and the Internet as new resource for young LGB people. Two current social constructionist perspectives highlight that queer youth are constructed as vulnerable, uncertain type of people, confronted with minority stress, who just have to pass through a difficult youth ('it gets better') and then may become a stable, acknowledged person who perhaps lives in a city and marries another person of the same sex [84, 85]. This may actually put more pressure onto youth. Explaining mental problems of LGB youth mainly through bullying experiences downplays the actual problem of being LGB in a heteronormative culture [85]. Shame, other distressing feelings, and suicidality can be logical but not pathological reactions from forming a non-normative identity, with being LGBTI as a special violation of gender and sexuality norms. This violation of norms and their psychosocial consequences unify LGBTI groups, despite their uniqueness.

Trans people face unique challenges, but many risk factors are comparable to LGB people. A review found that victimization (social stigma, trans-negativity, discrimination, and violence, etc.), difficulties accessing health care, interpersonal problems, and lack

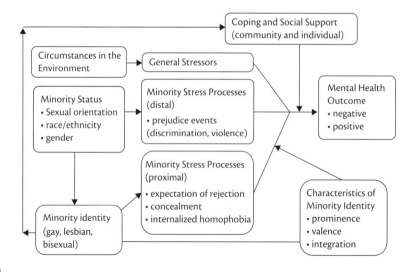

Fig. 26.1 Minority stress model.
Source: Reproduced from Psychological Bulletin, 129(5), Meyer, I. H, Prejudice, social stress, and mental health in lesbian, gay, and bisexual populations: Conceptual issues and research evidence, pp. 674-97, Copyright (2003), with permission from American Psychological Association.

of social support were risk factors, whereas social support and transition-related medical care were protective factors [44]. The minority stress model and the syndemics models have been applied for trans people, but there is less research about proximal gender minority stressors [46, 86]. However, it is also necessary to understand how 'health is shaped by the distribution of power along lines of gender' [46].

For inter individuals, theoretical models about mental health are, to our knowledge, lacking. However, the models described earlier appear to be useful because some stressors and pathogenic processes may be comparable. In a qualitative study, mental health-related challenges are partly similar to those of LGB (challenges related to self-awareness, coming out and identity management, identity formation with respect to gender role and/or sexual orientation, connecting to other women with CAH). Nevertheless, there are also notable differences: distress when receiving the diagnosis, acceptance of the inter condition, difficult physical consequences, infertility, fear of being rejected in relationships, body image, self-perception or perception of others as man or woman, everyday and sexual functioning, medication and medical crisis, and finding adequate medical care [11, 87]. Social support from parents and having had somebody to talk to about intersex in childhood were important protective factors for symptoms affecting mental health, suicidality, and satisfaction with the body [10]. One very specific potential risk factor for intersex individuals is early coercive surgical alterations of the genitals that may be associated with later mental health or other problems [9, 48, 70]. Empirical studies about the relative impact of the inter-specific stressors on mental health are sparse. However, social support and related treatment experiences appear to influence adult well-being [10].

Importantly, not only LGBTI individuals are affected by LGBTI negativity and rigid gender norms, but also those who are perceived as LGBTI, independent of their actual LGBTI status. For example, heterosexual youth who experience homophobic discrimination outnumber LGB victims and they have elevated levels of suicide attempts, similar to actual LGB youth [88]. Furthermore, homophobic bullying is one of the most frequent forms of bullying and is more strongly associated with suicide ideation than other forms of bullying [89]. Gender atypical youth of any sexual orientation had increased levels of depression [90], and of young people who attempted suicide, 75% were LGBT and/or experienced bullying because of gender atypicality [91]. Thus, the negative impact of LGBTI negativity and rigid gender norms goes beyond LGBTI people and is a general public health problem.

LGBTI-specific intervention and prevention

As societal LGBTI negativity and the underlying rigid gender norms play a crucial role in the development of mental health problems of LGBTI individuals, intervention and prevention efforts cannot be restricted to LGBTI individuals but need to be applied to the social context. Prevention programmes for LGBTI youth were realized decades ago [92], but empirical data for their effectiveness are emerging only recently.

Individual approaches

Psychotherapeutic interventions specifically designed for LGBTI individuals are emerging and were found to be effective [93, 94]. Cognitive behavioural interventions for gay and bisexual men can

successfully be inferred from minority stress and syndemics model [95, 96]. Besides LGBTI-tailored interventions, there are facilities specialized for LGBTI individuals, such as the Trevor Project (http://www.thetrevorproject.org/), a telephone helpline and online platform for suicidal LGBTI youth, or the It Gets Better Project (http://www.itgetsbetter.org/) where famous and ordinary people try to deliver hope for LGBTI youth in crisis via online video messages. Of special note are voluntary LGBTI organizations worldwide who are pioneers in providing LGBTI-affirmative support and safe places, in times when being LGBTI was or still is criminalized, punished, or pathologized, even in (mental) health care.

Social approaches

Family

Family support is an important protective factor for LGBTI youth [10, 97, 98], but LGBT individuals report lower levels of family support [41, 97], and a non-accepting family was the number one problem mentioned by LGBT youth [99]. The project 'Lead With Love' provides a free online video for parents whose children come out as LGBT and educates parents how to react positively and how to deal with overwhelming feelings [100]. A modified attachment-based psychotherapy focuses on an improvement of the adolescent-parent relationship to reduce suicidality of LGB youth [101], which seems to work even for some persistently non-accepting parents [102].

School

School can be a risky place for LGBTI youth, as anti-gay bullying is frequent and harmful, as described earlier. However, schools can do much to make it a safer and healthier place for LGBTI youth. In a retrospective study, half of the gay and bisexual suicide attempters associated the problematic situation at school with respect to being gay or bisexual with their suicide attempt, but those who felt accepted at school much less likely attempted suicide [103]. LGBT-supportive high-school environments correlated with less depression and suicidality for sexual minority boys but not significantly so among girls [104]. For LGBT youth, the presence of gay-straight alliances (GSA) were associated with less homophobic victimization and fewer homophobic remarks, reduced fear for safety [105], reduced depression [106], and less drug abuse [107, 108]. Participating in GSAs also seemed to buffer the effect of anti-LGBT victimization on depression and suicide attempts, at least for lower levels of victimization [106]. The existence of anti-bullying policies, including homophobic bullying were associated with less suicidal behaviour of lesbian and gay youth [109], especially in combination with GSAs [110].

Societal approaches at the macro-level

The public-health impact of structural stigma has been highlighted in several studies. Sexual minority individuals living in homophobic regions had an increased risk of suicide, dying earlier by suicide, and an increased overall mortality translating into 12 years shorter life-expectancy compared with less homophobic regions [111]. Of note, heterosexuals living in homophobic regions had a lower life expectancy than heterosexual in the least homophobic regions, indicating that homonegativity is a general public health problem [112]. A recent study reported lower perceived stigma for transgender individuals living in states with non-discrimination laws compared with other states, and lower perceived stigma was associated with reduced mental health problems [113]. As these studies are cross-sectional, a causal effect of structural stigma on mental health cannot be inferred. However, one impressive quasi-experimental study investigated mental health before and after the introduction of the 'gay marriage ban' [114]. Whereas no or small changes occurred among heterosexuals or among LGB individuals in states without the gay marriage ban, the prevalence of mental disorders significantly increased for LGB individuals in states where the gay marriage ban was introduced. Similarly, legalizing same-sex marriages in Massachusetts was associated with a reduced general and mental health care use among gay and bisexual males [115]. The causal mechanisms of how structural discrimination impacts the mental health of LGB individuals is highlighted by Hatzenbuehler [116]. For example, denying marriage can deprive LGB individuals of financial and social support relevant for mental health. However, allowing gay marriage or ending 'don't ask don't tell' may positively alter intra-individual processes described in the minority stress models mentioned earlier.

Removing barriers in (mental) health care

Structural LGBTI negativity also affects (mental) health care, where LGBTI patients seem to face personal and structural barriers [117]. On a personal level, there may be experiences of discrimination, microaggression, harsh language or behaviour, rejection, denial of service, attempts to change sexual orientation, silencing LGBTI issues, or implicit biases [117–124], or there may be expectations of such behaviour, hindering disclosure to health professionals [117]. Furthermore, healthcare providers often lack cultural competency with respect to LGBTI topics [117, 125–128]. Given these barriers, it is not surprising that LGBTI patients report having been dissatisfied with mental health care [129], and frequently remain disclosed or avoided LGBTI issues [119, 130–132]. Improving mental health care by LGBTI-affirming policies and adequate training is thus an important step to reduce health disparities in LGBTI individuals. Positive signals in this direction are the statements of the WMA on natural variations of human sexuality and transgender people [8, 133], the statement of the World Psychiatry Organization on gender identity and same-sex orientation [134], and other statements, guidelines, and recommendations for LGBTI-affirmative health care that have appeared in recent years [9, 117, 135–138]. Of note, these guidelines and this chapter have been written from a 'western' viewpoint. The situation is dramatically different in countries where LGBTI is still criminalized or pathologized. For example, homosexuality is still be punished by death in Iran, Mauritania, Nigeria, Qatar, Saudi Arabia, Afghanistan, Somalia, Sudan, United Arab Emirates, and Yemen, or by imprisonment in many other countries [139]. Providing LGBTI-affirmative mental health care may be challenging in those countries and may place healthcare professionals at risk. Thus, removing barriers and providing appropriate, LGBTI-affirmative health care is closely linked to the societal situation for LGBTI individuals.

Conclusions

Most current studies report that LGBTI individuals are at an increased risk for mental health issues and disorders. This risk can be explained well with the pathogenic effect of LGBTI negativity, leading to minority stressors that are a burden for LGBTI individuals and increase their risk for developing a mental disorder

or suicidality. Next to this, trans people suffering from body dysphoria related to the sex characteristics and inter people suffering from coercive genital surgeries are further reasons for severe mental problems. Eliminating LGBTI negativity on different levels of society, interventions, and prevention efforts tailored for LGBTI individuals, providing access to adequate transition-related (mental) health care (e.g. hormones and surgeries) and protecting inter individuals from unconsented genital surgeries are crucial steps to remove the LGBTI health disparities and support LGBTI (mental) health.

Acknowledgements

We thank Gorji Marzban for critical reading of this paper from the intersex point of view.

References

1. Plöderl M, Kralovec K, Fartacek R. The relation between sexual orientation and suicide attempts in Austria. *Arch Sex Behav* 2010; 39: 1403–1414.
2. Priebe G, Svedin CG. Operationalization of three dimensions of sexual orientation in a national survey of late adolescents. *J Sex Res* 2013; 50: 727–738.
3. Pathela P, Hajat A, Schillinger J, Blank S, Sell R, Mostashari F. Discordance between sexual behavior and self-reported sexual identity: A population-based survey of New York City men. *Ann Intern Med* 2006; 145: 416–425.
4. Richards C, Bouman WP, Seal L, Barker MJ, Nieder TO, T'Sjoen G. Non-binary or genderqueer genders. *Int Rev Psychiatry* 2016; 28: 95–102.
5. Drescher J, Cohen-Kettenis P, Winter S. Minding the body: situating gender identity diagnoses in the ICD-11. *Int Rev Psychiatry* 2012; 24: 568–577.
6. Drescher J, Cohen-Kettenis PT, Reed GM. Gender incongruence of childhood in the ICD-11: controversies, proposal, and rationale. *Lancet Psychiatry* 2016; 3: 297–304.
7. Winter S, De Cuypere G, Green J, Kane R, Knudson G. The proposed ICD-11 gender incongruence of childhood diagnosis: a World Professional Association for transgender health membership survey. *Arch Sex Behav* 2016; 45: 1605–1614.
8. World Medical Association. WMA statement on on transgender people. Adopted by the 66th WMA General Assembly, Moscow, Russia, October 2015. Available at: https://www.wma.net/policies-post/wma-statement-on-transgender-people/ (accessed 28 February 2018).
9. Lee PA, Nordenstrom A, Houk CP, et al. Global disorders of sex development update since 2006: perceptions, approach and care. *Horm Res Paediatr* 2016; 85: 158–180.
10. Schweizer K, Brunner F, Gedrose B, Handford C, Richter-Appelt H. Coping with diverse sex development: treatment experiences and psychosocial support during childhood and adolescence and adult well-being. *J Pediatr Psychol* 2017; 42: 504–519.
11. van Lisdonk J. *Living With Intersex/DSD. An Exploratory Study of the Social Situation of Persons With Intersex/DSD*. The Hague: Sociaal en Cultureel Planbureau, 2014.
12. Nieder TO, Elaut E, Richards C, Dekker A. Sexual orientation of trans adults is not linked to outcome of transition-related health care, but worth asking. *Int Rev Psychiatry* 2016; 28: 103–111.
13. Hirschfeld M. *Die Homosexualität des Mannes und des Weibes. Handbuch der Gesamten Sexualwissenschaften in Einzeldarstellungen*. Berlin: Louis Marcus Verlagsbuchhandlung, 1914.
14. Drescher J. Out of DSM: depathologizing homosexuality. *Behav Sci* 2015; 5: 565–575.
15. Hooker E. The adjustment of the male overt homosexual. *J Project Techn* 1957; 21: 18–31.

16. Gonsiorek JC. The empirical basis for the demis of the illness model of homosexuality. In: Gonsiorek JC, Weinrich JD (eds). *Homosexuality Research Implications for Public Policy*. Newbury Park, CA: SAGE, 1991, pp. 115–136.

17. Saghir M, Robins E. *Male and Female Homosexuality*. Baltimore, MD: Williams and Wilkins, 1973.

18. Savin-Williams RC. Suicide attempts among sexual-minority youths: population and measurement issues. *J Consult Clin Psych* 2001; 69: 983–991.

19. Plöderl M, Wagenmakers EJ, Tremblay P, et al. Suicide risk and sexual orientation: a critical review. *Arch Sex Behav* 2013; 42: 715–727.

20. Kuyper L, Fernee H, Keuzenkamp S. A comparative analysis of a community and general sample of lesbian, gay, and bisexual individuals. *Arch Sex Behav* 2016; 45: 683–693.

21. Hottes TS, Bogaert L, Rhodes AE, Brennan DJ, Gesink D. Lifetime prevalence of suicide attempts among sexual minority adults by study sampling strategies: a systematic review and meta-analysis. *Am J Public Health* 2016; 106: 921.

22. Fergusson DM, Horwood LJ, Beautrais AL. Is sexual orientation related to mental health problems and suicidality in young people? *Arch Gen Psychiatry* 1999; 56: 876–880.

23. Fergusson DM, Horwood LJ, Ridder EM, Beautrais AL. Sexual orientation and mental health in a birth cohort of young adults. *Psychol Med* 2005; 35: 971–981.

24. Wichstrom L, Hegna K. Sexual orientation and suicide attempt: a longitudinal study of the general Norwegian adolescent population. *J Abnorm Psychol* 2003; 112: 144–151.

25. Marshal MP, Dermody SS, Cheong J, Burton CM, Friedman MS, Aranda F, et al. Trajectories of depressive symptoms and suicidality among heterosexual and sexual minority youth. *J Youth Adolesc* 2013; 42: 1243–1256.

26. Herrell R, Goldberg J, True WR, et al. Sexual orientation and suicidality—a co-twin control study in adult men. *Arch Gen Psychiatry* 1999; 56: 867–874.

27. Frisell T, Lichtenstein P, Rahman Q, Langstrom N. Psychiatric morbidity associated with same-sex sexual behaviour: influence of minority stress and familial factors. *Psychol Med* 2010; 40: 315–324.

28. Balsam KF, Beauchaine TP, Mickey RM, Rothblum ED. Mental health of lesbian, gay, bisexual, and heterosexual siblings: effects of gender, sexual orientation, and family. *J Abnorm Psychol* 2005; 114: 471–476.

29. McCabe SE, Hughes TL, Bostwick W, Boyd CJ. Assessment of difference in dimensions of sexual orientation: implications for substance use research in a college-age population. *J Stud Alcohol* 2005; 66: 620–629.

30. Drabble L, Midanik LT, Trocki K. Reports of alcohol consumption and alcohol-related problems among homosexual, bisexual and heterosexual respondents: results from the 2000 National Alcohol Survey. *J Stud Alcohol* 2005; 66: 111–120.

31. Bostwick WB, Boyd CJ, Hughes TL, McCabe SE. Dimensions of sexual orientation and the prevalence of mood and anxiety disorders in the United States. *Am J Public Health* 2010; 100: 468–475.

32. Kann L, Olsen EO, McManus T, et al. Sexual identity, sex of sexual contacts, and health-risk behaviors among students in grades 9-12—youth risk behavior surveillance, selected sites, United States, 2001–2009. *MMWR Surveill Summ* 2011; 60: 1–133.

33. Gattis MN, Sacco P, Cunningham-Williams RM. Substance use and mental health disorders among heterosexual identified men and women who have same-sex partners or same-sex attraction: results from the national epidemiological survey on alcohol and related conditions. *Arch Sex Behav* 2012; 41: 1185–1197.

34. Plöderl M, Sauer J, Fartacek R. Suizidalität und psychische Gesundheit von homo-und bisexuellen Männern und Frauen. Eine Metaanalyse internationaler Zufallsstichproben. *Verhaltensther Psychosoz Prax* 2006; 38: 283–302.

35. King M, Semlyen J, Tai SS, et al. A systematic review of mental disorder, suicide, and deliberate self harm in lesbian, gay and bisexual people. *BMC Psychiatry* 2008; 8: 70.

36. Marshal MP, Dietz LJ, Friedman MS, et al. Suicidality and depression disparities between sexual minority and heterosexual youth: a meta-analytic review. *J Adolesc Health* 2011; 49: 115–123.

37. Marshal MP, Friedman MS, Stall R, et al. Sexual orientation and adolescent substance use: a meta-analysis and methodological review. *Addiction* 2008; 103: 546–556.

38. Savin-Williams RC. Then and now: recruitment, definition, diversity, and positive attributes of same-sex populations. *Dev Psychol* 2008; 44: 135–138.

39. Plöderl M, Tremblay P. Mental health of sexual minorities. A systematic review. *Int Rev Psychiatry* 2015; 27: 367–385.

40. Rath JM, Villanti AC, Rubenstein RA, Vallone DM. Tobacco use by sexual identity among young adults in the United States. *Nicotine Tob Res* 2013; 15: 1822–1831.

41. Clark TC, Lucassen MFG, Bullen P, et al. The health and well-being of transgender high school students: results from the New Zealand Adolescent Health Survey (Youth'12). *J Adolesc Health* 2014; 55: 93–99.

42. Effrig JC, Bieschke KJ, Locke BD. Examining victimization and psychological distress in transgender college students. *J Coll Counsel* 2011; 14: 143–157.

43. Robinson JP, Espelage DL. Inequities in educational and psychological outcomes between LGBTQ and straight students in middle and high school. *Educ Researcher* 2011; 40: 315–330.

44. Dhejne C, Van Vlerken R, Heylens G, Arcelus J. Mental health and gender dysphoria: a review of the literature. *Int Rev Psychiatry* 2016; 28: 44–57.

45. Marshall E, Claes L, Bouman WP, Witcomb GL, Arcelus J. Non-suicidal self-injury and suicidality in trans people: a systematic review of the literature. *Int Rev Psychiatry* 2016; 28: 58–69.

46. Reisner SL, Poteat T, Keatley J, et al. Global health burden and needs of transgender populations: a review. *Lancet* 2016; 388: 412–436.

47. Heylens G, Elaut E, Kreukels BP, et al. Psychiatric characteristics in transsexual individuals: multicentre study in four European countries. *Br J Psychiatry* 2014; 204: 151–156.

48. Schutzmann K, Brinkmann L, Schacht M, Richter-Appelt H. Psychological distress, self-harming behavior, and suicidal tendencies in adults with disorders of sex development. *Arch Sex Behav* 2009; 38: 16–33.

49. Wisniewski AB, Mazur T. 46,XY DSD with female or ambiguous external genitalia at birth due to Androgen Insensitivity Syndrome, 5alpha-Reductase-2 Deficiency, or 17beta-Hydroxysteroid Dehydrogenase Deficiency: a review of quality of life outcomes. *Int J Pediatr Endocrinol* 2009; 2009: 567430.

50. D'Alberton F, Assante MT, Foresti M, et al. Quality of life and psychological adjustment of women living with 46,XY differences of sex development. *J Sex Med* 2015; 12: 1440–1449.

51. Thyen U, Lux A, Jurgensen M, Hiort O, Kohler B. Utilization of health care services and satisfaction with care in adults affected by disorders of sex development (DSD). *J Gen Intern Med* 2014; 29(Suppl. 3): S752–S759.

52. Fliegner M, Krupp K, Brunner F, et al. Sexual life and sexual wellness in individuals with complete androgen insensitivity syndrome (CAIS) and Mayer-Rokitansky-Kuster-Hauser Syndrome (MRKHS). *J Sex Med* 2014; 11: 729–742.

53. Boks MP, de Vette MH, Sommer IE, et al. Psychiatric morbidity and X-chromosomal origin in a Klinefelter sample. *Schizophr Res* 2007; 93: 399–402.

54. Close S, Fennoy I, Smaldone A, Reame N. Phenotype and adverse quality of life in boys with Klinefelter syndrome. *J Pediatr* 2015; 167: 650–657.

55. Turriff A, Levy HP, Biesecker B. Prevalence and psychosocial correlates of depressive symptoms among adolescents and adults with Klinefelter syndrome. *Genet Med* 2011; 13: 966–972.

56. Herlihy AS, McLachlan RI, Gillam L, Cock ML, Collins V, Halliday JL. The psychosocial impact of Klinefelter syndrome and factors influencing quality of life. *Genet Med* 2011; 13: 632–642.

57. Kleinemeier E, Jurgensen M, Lux A, Widenka PM, Thyen U, Disorders of Sex Development Network Working Group. Psychological adjustment and sexual development of adolescents with disorders of sex development. *J Adolesc Health* 2010; 47: 463–471.

58. Johannsen TH, Ripa CP, Mortensen EL, Main KM. Quality of life in 70 women with disorders of sex development. *Eur J Endocrinol* 2006; 155: 877–885.

59. Fagerholm R, Mattila AK, Roine RP, Sintonen H, Taskinen S. Mental health and quality of life after feminizing genitoplasty. *J Pediatr Surg* 2012; 47: 747–751.

60. Ediati A, Faradz SM, Juniarto AZ, van der Ende J, Drop SL, Dessens AB. Emotional and behavioral problems in late-identified Indonesian patients with disorders of sex development. *J Psychosom Res* 2015; 79: 76–84.

61. Osifo OD, Amusan TI. Female children with ambiguous genitalia in awareness-poor subregion. *Afr J Reprod Health* 2009; 13: 129–136.

62. Mueller SC, Ng P, Sinaii N, et al. Psychiatric characterization of children with genetic causes of hyperandrogenism. *Eur J Endocrinol* 2010; 163: 801–810.

63. Liang HY, Chang HL, Chen CY, Chang PY, Lo FS, Lee LW. Psychiatric manifestations in young females with congenital adrenal hyperplasia in Taiwan. *Chang Gung Med J* 2008; 31: 66–73.

64. Krysiak R, Drosdzol-Cop A, Skrzypulec-Plinta V, Okopien B. Sexual function and depressive symptoms in young women with nonclassic congenital adrenal hyperplasia. *J Sex Med* 2016; 13: 34–39.

65. Morgan JF, Murphy H, Lacey JH, Conway G. Long term psychological outcome for women with congenital adrenal hyperplasia: cross sectional survey. *BMJ* 2005; 330: 340–341.

66. Reisch N, Hahner S, Bleicken B, et al. Quality of life is less impaired in adults with congenital adrenal hyperplasia because of 21-hydroxylase deficiency than in patients with primary adrenal insufficiency. *Clin Endocrinol* 2011; 74: 166–173.

67. Engberg H, Butwicka A, Nordenstrom A, et al. Congenital adrenal hyperplasia and risk for psychiatric disorders in girls and women born between 1915 and 2010: a total population study. *Psychoneuroendocrinology* 2015; 60: 195–205.

68. Falhammar H, Butwicka A, Landen M, et al. Increased psychiatric morbidity in men with congenital adrenal hyperplasia due to 21-hydroxylase deficiency. *J Clin Endocrinol Metab* 2014; 99: E554–E560.

69. Falhammar H, Frisen L, Norrby C, et al. Increased mortality in patients with congenital adrenal hyperplasia due to 21-hydroxylase deficiency. *J Clin Endocrinol Metab* 2014; 99: E2715–E2721.

70. Machado PS, Costa AB, Nardi HC, Fontanari AM, Araujo IR, Knauth DR. Follow-up of psychological outcomes of interventions in patients diagnosed with disorders of sexual development: a systematic review. *J Health Psychol* 2016; 21: 2195–2206.

71. OHCHR, UN Women, UNAIDS, UNDP, UNFPA, UNICEF and WHO. Eliminating Forced, Coercive and Otherwise Involuntary Sterilization: An Interagency Statement. Available at: http://www.who.int/reproductivehealth/publications/gender_rights/eliminating-forced-sterilization/en/ (2014, accessed 28 February 2018).

72. Reisner SL, Conron K, Scout N, Mimiaga MJ, Haneuse S, Austin SB. Comparing in-person and online survey respondents in the U.S. National Transgender Discrimination Survey: implications for transgender health research. *LGBT Health* 2014; 1: 98–106.

73. European Union Agency for Fundamental Rights. Being Trans in the EU – Comparative analysis of EU LGBT survey data. Available at: http://fra.europa.eu/en/publication/2014/being-trans-eu-comparative-analysis-eu-lgbt-survey-data (2014, accessed 28 February 2018).

74. Grant JM, Mottet LA, Tanis J, Harrison J, Herman J, Keisling M. *Injustice at Every Turn: A Report of the National Transgender Discrimination Survey*. Washington, DC: National Center for Transgender Equality and National Gay and Lesbian Task Force, 2011.

75. Nieder TO, Richter-Appelt H. Tertium non datur – either/or reactions to transsexualism amongst health care professionals: the situation past and present, and its relevance to the future. *Psychol Sex* 2011; 2: 224–243.

76. McCann E, Lee R, Brown M. The experiences and support needs of people with intellectual disabilities who identify as LGBT: a review of the literature. *Res Dev Disabil* 2016; 57: 39–53.

77. Lytle MC, De Luca SM, Blosnich JR. The influence of intersecting identities on self-harm, suicidal behaviors, and depression among lesbian, gay, and bisexual individuals. *Suicide Life Threat Behav* 2014; 44: 384–391.

78. Rodriguez EM. At the intersection of church and gay: a review of the psychological research on gay and lesbian christians. *J Homosex* 2010; 57: 5–38.

79. Meyer IH. Identity, stress, and resilience in lesbians, gay men, and bisexuals of color. *Couns Psychol* 2010; 38: 442–454.

80. Meyer IH. Prejudice, social stress, and mental health in lesbian, gay, and bisexual populations: Conceptual issues and research evidence. *Psychol Bull* 2003; 129: 674–697.

81. Hatzenbuehler ML. How does sexual minority stigma 'get under the skin'? A psychological mediation framework. *Psychol Bull* 2009; 135: 707–730.

82. Stall R, Friedman M, Catania JA. Interacting epidemics and gay men's health: a theory of syndemic production among urban gay men. In: Wolitski RJ, Stall R, Valdiserri RO (eds). *Unequal Opportunity: Health Disparities Affecting Gay and Bisexual Men in the United States*. New York: Oxford University Press, 2008, pp. 251–274.

83. Operario D, Yang MF, Reisner SL, Iwamoto M, Nemoto T. Stigma and the syndemic of HIV-related health risk behaviors in a diverse sample of transgender women. *J Community Psychol* 2014; 42: 544–557.

84. McDermott E, Roen K. *Queer Youth, Suicide and Self-harm*. Basingstoke: Palgrave Macmillan, 2016.

85. Cover R. *Queer Youth Suicide, Culture and Identity: Unliveable Lives?* London: Routledge, 2016.

86. Hendricks ML, Testa RJ. A conceptual framework for clinical work with transgender and gender nonconforming clients: an adaptation of the minority stress model. *Prof Psychol Res Pract* 2012; 43: 460–467.

87. Malouf MA, Inman AG, Carr AG, Franco J, Brooks LM. Health-related quality of life, mental health and psychotherapeutic considerations for women diagnosed with a disorder of sexual development: congenital adrenal hyperplasia. *Int J Pediatr Endocrinol* 2010; 2010: 253465.

88. Reis E, Saewyc E. *83,000 Youth: Select Findings of Eight Population-based Studies as They Pertain to Anti-gay Harassment and the Safety and Wellbeing of Sexual Minority Students*. Seattle, WA: Safe Schools Coalition of Washington, 1999.

89. Patrick DL, Bell JF, Huang JY, Lazarakis NC, Edwards TC. Bullying and quality of life in youths perceived as gay, lesbian, or bisexual in Washington State, 2010. *Am J Public Health* 2013; 103: 1255–1261.

90. Roberts AL, Rosario M, Slopen N, Calzo JP, Austin SB. Childhood gender nonconformity, bullying victimization, and depressive symptoms across adolescence and early adulthood: an 11-year longitudinal study. *J Am Acad Child Adolesc Psychiatry* 2013; 52: 143–152.

91. Ioerger M, Henry KL, Chen PY, Cigularov KP, Tomazic RG. Beyond same-sex attraction: gender-variant-based victimization is associated with suicidal behavior and substance use for other-sex attracted adolescents. *PLOS ONE* 2015; 10(9).

92. Commonwealth of Australia. *Community Matters. Working With Diversity for Well-being*. Carlton South: Commenwealth of Australia, 2001.

93. Kaysen D, Lostutter TW, Goines MA. Cognitive processing therapy for acute stress disorder resulting from an anti-gay assault. *Cogn Behav Pract* 2005; 12: 278–289.

94. Jaffe A, Shoptaw S, Stein J, Reback CJ, Rotheram-Fuller E. Depression ratings, reported sexual risk behaviors, and methamphetamine use: latent growth curve models of positive change among gay and bisexual men in an outpatient treatment program. *Exp Clin Psychopharmacol* 2007; 15: 301–307.

95. Pachankis JE. A transdiagnostic minority stress treatment approach for gay and bisexual men's syndemic health conditions. *Arch Sex Behav* 2015; 44: 1843–1860.

96. Pachankis JE, Hatzenbuehler ML, Rendina HJ, Safren SA, Parsons JT. LGB-affirmative cognitive-behavioral therapy for young adult gay and bisexual men: a randomized controlled trial of a transdiagnostic minority stress approach. *J Consult Clin Psychol* 2015; 83: 875–889.

97. Plöderl M, Fartacek R. Suicidality and associated risk factors among lesbian, gay, and bisexual compared to heterosexual Austrian adults. *Suicide Life Threat Behav* 2005; 35: 661–670.

98. Ryan C, Russell ST, Huebner D, Diaz R, Sanchez J. Family acceptance in adolescence and the health of LGBT young adults. *J Child Adolesc Psychiatr Nurs* 2010; 23: 205–213.

99. Human Rights Campaign. Growing up LGBT in America. HRC youth survey report. Key findings. Available at: http://hrc-assets.s3-website-us-east-1.amazonaws.com//files/assets/resources/Growing-Up-LGBT-in-America_Report.pdf (2012, accessed 28 February 2018).

100. Huebner DM, Rullo JE, Thoma BC, McGarrity LA, Mackenzie J. Piloting lead with love: a film-based intervention to improve parents' responses to their lesbian, gay, and bisexual children. *J Prim Prev* 2013; 34: 359–369.

101. Diamond GM, Diamond GS, Levy S, Closs C, Ladipo T, Siqueland L. Attachment-based family therapy for suicidal lesbian, gay, and bisexual adolescents: a treatment development study and open trial with preliminary findings. *Psychotherapy* 2012; 49: 62–71.

102. Diamond GM, Shpigel MS. Attachment-based family therapy for lesbian and gay young adults and their persistently nonaccepting parents. *Prof Psychol Res Pract* 2014; 45: 258–268.

103. Plöderl M, Faistauer G, Fartacek R. The contribution of school to the feeling of acceptance and the risk of suicide attempts among Austrian gay and bisexual males. *J Homosex* 2010; 57: 819–841.

104. Denny S, Lucassen MF, Stuart J, et al. The association between supportive high school environments and depressive symptoms and suicidality among sexual minority students. *J Clin Child Adolesc Psychol* 2016; 45: 248–261.

105. Marx RA, Kettrey HH. Gay-straight alliances are associated with lower levels of school-based victimization of LGBTQ plus youth: a systematic review and meta-analysis. *J Youth Adolesc* 2016; 45: 1269–1282.

106. Toomey RB, Ryan C, Diaz RM, Russell ST. High school gay-straight alliances (GSAs) and young adult well-being: an examination of GSA presence, participation, and perceived effectiveness. *Appl Dev Sci* 2011; 15: 175–185.

107. Heck NC, Livingston NA, Flentje A, Oost K, Stewart BT, Cochran BN. Reducing risk for illicit drug use and prescription drug misuse: High school gay-straight alliances and lesbian, gay, bisexual, and transgender youth. *Addict Behav* 2014; 39: 824–828.

108. Konishi C, Saewyc E, Homma Y, Poon C. Population-level evaluation of school-based interventions to prevent problem substance use among gay, lesbian and bisexual adolescents in Canada. *Prev Med* 2013; 57: 929–933.

109. Hatzenbuehler ML, Keyes KM. Inclusive anti-bullying policies and reduced risk of suicide attempts in lesbian and gay youth. *J Adolesc Health* 2013; 53: S21–S26.

110. Saewyc E, Konishi C, Rose H, Homma Y. School-based strategies to reduce suicidal ideation, suicide attempts, and discrimination among sexual minority and heterosexual adolescents in Western Canada. *Int J Child Youth Fam Stud* 2014; 5: 89–112.

111. Hatzenbuehler ML, Bellatorre A, Lee Y, Finch BK, Muennig P, Fiscella K. Structural stigma and all-cause mortality in sexual minority populations. *Soc Sci Med* 2014; 103: 33–41.

112. Hatzenbuehler ML, Bellatorre A, Muennig P. Anti-gay prejudice and all-cause mortality among heterosexuals in the United States. *Am J Public Health* 2014; 104: 332–337.

113. Gleason HA, Livingston NA, Peters MM, Oost KM, Reely E, Cochran BN. Effects of state nondiscrimination laws on transgender and gender nonconforming individuals' perceived community stigma and mental health. *J Gay Lesbian Ment Health* 2016; 20: 350–362.

114. Hatzenbuehler ML, McLaughlin KA, Keyes KM, Hasin DS. The impact of institutional discrimination on psychiatric disorders in lesbian, gay, and bisexual populations: a prospective study. *Am J Public Health* 2010; 100: 452–459.

115. Hatzenbuehler ML, O'Cleirigh C, Grasso C, Mayer K, Safren S, Bradford J. Effect of same-sex marriage laws on health care use and expenditures in sexual minority men: a quasi-natural experiment. *Am J Public Health* 2012; 102: 285–291.

116. Hatzenbuehler ML. Social factors as determinants of mental health disparities in LGB populations: implications for public policy. *Soc Iss Policy Rev* 2010; 4: 31–62.

117. Institute of Medicine. *The Health of Lesbian, Gay, Bisexual, and Transgender People: Building a Foundation for Better Understanding.* Washington, DC: The National Academic Press, 2011.

118. Cant B. Exploring the implications for health professionals of men coming out as gay in healthcare settings. *Health Soc Care Community* 2006; 14: 9–16.

119. Eliason MJ, Schope R. Original Research: Does 'Don't Ask Don't Tell' apply to health care? Lesbian, gay, and bisexual people's disclosure to health care providers. *J Gay Lesbian Med Assoc* 2001; 5: 125–134.

120. Eliason MJ, Dibble SL, Robertson PA. Lesbian, gay, bisexual, and transgender (LGBT) physicians' experiences in the workplace. *J Homosex* 2011; 58: 1355–1371.

121. Bartlett A, Smith G, King M. The response of mental health professionals to clients seeking help to change or redirect same-sex sexual orientation. *BMC Psychiatry* 2009; 9: 11.

122. Lambda Legal. *When Health Care Isn't Caring: Lambda Legal's Survey of Discrimination Against LGBT People and People with HIV.* New York: Lambda Legal, 2010.

123. Willging CE, Salvador M, Kano M. Unequal treatment: mental health care for sexual and gender minority groups in a rural state. *Psychiatr Serv* 2006; 57: 867–870.

124. Dean MA, Victor E, Grimes LG. Inhospitable healthcare spaces: why diversity training on LGBTQIA issues is not enough. *J Bioeth Inq* 2016; 13: 557–570.

125. Hinchliff S, Gott M, Galena E. 'I daresay I might find it embarrassing': general practitioners' perspectives on discussing sexual health issues with lesbian and gay patients. *Health Soc Care Comm* 2005; 13: 345–353.

126. Parameshwaran V, Cockbain BC, Hillyard M, Price JR. Is the lack of specific lesbian, gay, bisexual, transgender and queer/questioning (LGBTQ) healthcare education in medical school a cause for concern? Evidence from a survey of knowledge and practice amongst UK medical students. J Homosex 2017; 64: 357–381.

127. Khan A, Plummer D, Hussain R, Minichiello V. Does physician bias affect the quality of care they deliver? Evidence in the care of sexually transmitted infections. *Sex Transm Infect* 2008; 84: 150–151.

128. East JA, El Rayess F. Pediatricians' approach to the health care of lesbian, gay, and bisexual youth. *J Adolesc Health* 1998; 23: 191–193.

129. Elliott MN, Kanouse DE, Burkhart Q, et al. Sexual minorities in England have poorer health and worse health care experiences: a national survey. *J Gen Intern Med* 2015; 30: 9–16.

130. Bernstein KT, Liu KL, Begier EM, Koblin B, Karpati A, Murrill C. Same-sex attraction disclosure to health care providers among New York City men who have sex with men: implications for HIV testing approaches. *Arch Intern Med* 2008; 168: 1458–1464.

131. Law M, Mathai A, Veinot P, Webster F, Mylopoulos M. Exploring lesbian, gay, bisexual, and queer (LGBQ) people's experiences with disclosure of sexual identity to primary care physicians: a qualitative study. *BMC Fam Pract* 2015; 16.

132. Willging CE, Salvador M, Kano M. Pragmatic help seeking: How sexual and gender minority groups access mental health care in a rural state. *Psychiatr Serv* 2006; 57: 871–874.

133. World Medical Association. WMA statement on natural variations of human sexuality. Available at: https://www.wma.net/policies-post/wma-statement-on-natural-variations-of-human-sexuality/ (2013, accessed 28 February 2018).

134. World Psychiatric Association. WPA Position Statement on Gender Identity and Same-Sex Orientation, Attraction, and Behaviours. Available at: http://www.wpanet.org/detail.php?section_id=7&content_id=1807 (2016, accessed 28 February 2018).

135. Makadon HJ. *The Fenway Guide to Lesbian, Gay, Bisexual, and Transgender Health*. Philadelphia, PA: ACP Press, 2008.

136. American Psychological Association. Guidelines for psychological practice with lesbian, gay, and bisexual clients. *Am Psychol* 2012; 67: 10–42.

137. Coleman E, Bockting W, Botzer M, et al. Standards of care for the health of transsexual, transgender, and gender-nonconforming people, version 7. *Int J Transgenderism* 2012; 13: 165–232.

138. Hollenbach AD, Eckstrand KL, Dreger AD. *Implementing Curricular and Institutional Climate Changes to Improve Health Care for Individuals Who Are LGBT, Gender Nonconforming, or Born With DSD: A Resource for Medical Educators*. Washington, DC: Association of American Medical Colleges, 2014.

139. ILGA. Sexual orientation laws. Available at: http://ilga.org/maps-sexual-orientation-laws (2016, accessed 28 February 2018).

CHAPTER 27

Sexual minority adolescents and mental health

Richard Montoro

Introduction

Two factors distinguish the sexual minority population from other stigmatized minorities: the need to self-declare and, for most, not having parents that belong to the same stigmatized minority. Combined with stigma, these three factors provide the basic elements to understanding the protective factors and risk factors behind the mental health disparities, as well as the clinical interventions and public health measures that can be useful with this population.

The lack of teaching in medical schools on sexual orientation and gender minorities is a vacuum that is quickly filled by the healthcare practitioner's ambient culture—which may not be entirely accurate [1, 2]. Thus, the first part of this chapter will focus on definitions: a basic glossary and current conceptualizations of sexual orientation and gender identity—which will be essential to understanding the rest of the chapter. The process of self-declaration ('coming out') is entwined with the parental relationship and will be discussed together. An overview of stigma theory and the minority stress model will be presented before outlining the literature on the mental health disparities of the sexual minority population. The chapter will then conclude with proposed interventions to help reduce the mental health disparities of this population.

There is an important caveat: although same-sex erotic behaviour has been present in most societies, ancient and contemporary [3], gender identity and sexual orientation are cultural constructs that will vary from one society to the next. For example, several Latin American countries will define the receptive partner in male same-sex sexual activity as homosexual, but not necessarily the insertive partner. Genders outside the Western male–female binary are well entrenched in several cultures, such as the Fa'afafine of Samoa and the Two-Spirit of some indigenous North American groups. Even within Western culture, as shall be discussed later in this chapter, non-binary genders are increasingly recognized.

Nonetheless, although definitions of sexual minorities vary in the global literature, the health disparities of adolescents who indicate some form of non-heterosexual orientation are remarkably similar [4]. Current access to electronic communications is rapidly removing existing barriers between different cultures, particularly among young people and it would appear that young people from different cultures are more similar to each other in their views on sexuality than to their particular cultural background [5].

Therefore, please be advised that much of the conceptual material, research, and suggested interventions described herein are based on a Western cultural context. Generalizability of the interplay between sexual minority youth and their ambient society will vary based on either's proximity to Western culture.

Sexual minority youth: a glossary

Identities are cultural constructs, and as such are always in evolution. Sexual minority youth are no exception. Broadly defined, a sexual minority is anyone whose sexual orientation and/or gender identity are not of the majority. The majority being comprised of individuals who are *cisgendered*, where someone's internal sense of gender matches the gender assigned at birth, *and heterosexual*—where someone is attracted to the 'opposite' sex as conceived in the binary view of gender (man vs woman).

The term *sexual minority* is often used as an alternate to LGBTQ (lesbian, gay, bisexual, trans, and queer), but it also allows for the inclusion of those that decline categorization, as well as those who do not fit neatly into any of the LGBTQ categories. As their issues are not identical, gender and sexual orientation minorities will be discussed separately where appropriate, although, of course, many gender minorities also have a minority sexual orientation. When discussing terms such as homosexual or heterosexual with a transgender individual, it is the chosen gender (and not the assigned gender) that is used for self-identification purposes. For example, a male-to-female transwoman who is attracted to women will self-identify as lesbian personally and socially. Unfortunately, there is a classification scheme of gender identity disorder in the literature that uses the terms homosexual and heterosexual subtypes as they relate to the person's *assigned* gender [6], which can understandably lead to confusion between clinicians and their patients.

As sexual minorities often define themselves in the face of stigma, many prefer a more tailored self-identity label to the mainstream LGBTQ identities that are often assigned. Box 27.1 is a glossary of common terms used by sexual minority youth and has been partly sourced from several excellent glossaries [7–9], but as with any culture-bound glossary, it is to be expected that terms will be used differently in different areas and evolve over time. Thus, as with any identity term, it is always best to trust the person's definition of how they are using the term over any glossary.

Box 27.1 Glossary of common terms used by gender and sexual orientation minorities

Agender: a person who does not have a felt sense of gender.

Androphilic/androsexual: a person of any gender identity who can experience sexual, emotional, and/or romantic attraction for men and/or masculinity (*see* Homosexual, Heterosexual).

Asexual: a person who has little-to-no interest in sexual relationships and behaviour; however, not all asexual people are aromantic (*see* Romantic).

Assigned gender/assigned sex: the gender assigned to a child, generally at or soon after birth.

Bisexual: a person who can experience sexual, emotional, and/or romantic attraction for men and women but not necessarily simultaneously or equally. Sometimes used to describe sexual attraction component only (*see* Romantic).

Cisgender: a person whose gender identity matches the gender assigned at birth.

FtM, F2M: a female-to-male transgender person; a transman.

Gay: a man who can experience sexual, emotional, and/or romantic attraction only for men. Colloquially used as an umbrella term to include all LGBTQ people.

Gender dysphoria: a Diagnostic and Statistical Manual of Mental Disorders, 5th Edition (DSM-5) diagnosis describing the distress caused by a discrepancy between a person's gender identity and their assigned gender. Once the distress has resolved, usually through social and/or medical interventions, the person no longer has the diagnosis (*see* Gender identity disorder).

Gender expression: the way in which a person expresses their gender identity through clothing, behaviour, posture, mannerisms, speech patterns, activities, etc.

Gender fluid: a person whose gender identification and presentation shifts, whether within or outside of societal, gender-based expectations.

Gender identity: a person's internal sense of gender, which may or may not be the same as one's gender assigned at birth.

Gender identity disorder: Previous diagnostic term used in the International Classification of Diseases, 10th Revision (ICD-10) and DSM, 4th Edition (DSM-IV) for persons whose gender identity was different from their assigned gender. The term fell into disfavour as the person would continue to be pathologized even once their transition was complete (*see* Gender dysphoria).

Genderqueer: a catch-all term for a person with a gender identity other than man and woman.

Gender non-conforming: a person who does not conform to society's expectations of gender expression based on the gender binary, expectations of masculinity and femininity, or how they should identify their gender.

Gender role: norms determined by societies regarding how male and female persons should behave; expecting people to have personality characteristics and/or behaviours based on their assigned gender.

Gender variance: behaviours, appearance, or identity of individuals who do not conform to culturally defined norms for their assigned gender.

Gynephilic/gynesexual: a person of any gender identity who can experience sexual, emotional, and/or romantic attraction for women and/or femininity (*see* Homosexual, Heterosexual).

Heterosexual: a person who can experience sexual, emotional, and/or romantic attraction only for people of the 'opposite sex', as conceived in the binary view of gender (man vs woman). Sometimes used to describe sexual attraction component only (*see* Romantic).

Homosexual: a person who can experience sexual, emotional, and/or romantic attraction only for people of the same gender. Sometimes used to describe sexual attraction component only (*see* Romantic).

Intersex: a general term used for a variety of conditions in which a person is born with a reproductive or sexual anatomy that do not fit the typical definitions of female or male. Gender identities in this population are heterogeneous and can be male, female, or non-binary.

Lesbian: a woman who can experience sexual, emotional, and/or romantic attraction only for women.

MtF, M2F: a male-to-female transgender person; a transwoman.

Non-binary: a person whose gender identity is neither male nor female, but rather a combination of both or neither.

Pansexual: a person who can experience sexual, emotional, and/or romantic attraction for people of all gender identities.

Queer: a person will often state they are queer if they feel that they do not fit into dominant norms, owing to their own gender identity/expression, their sexual practices, their relationship style, etc. Sometimes used as an umbrella term to refer to all non-heterosexual or non-cisgender identities.

Romantic (used with prefixes *a, bi, hetero, homo,* or *pan*): a specifier to more accurately represent someone's sexual orientation by separating sexual and romantic components, e.g. *Alex is bisexual and homoromantic; Pat is asexual and heteroromantic.*

Skoliosexual: a person who can experience sexual, emotional, and/or romantic attraction only for people with non-binary gender identities.

Transgender/trans: a person whose gender identity differs from their gender assigned at birth. This term is more encompassing and has replaced the term transsexual. If the term trans is joined with a gender, it is the person's gender identity that is used and not the assigned gender (e.g. transman).

Transvestite: a person who regularly or occasionally wears the clothing socially assigned to a gender not their own but is generally comfortable with their assigned gender and does not wish to change it.

Sexual orientation

Basic constructs

Sexual orientation has traditionally been described as a categorical variable (e.g. homosexual, heterosexual) each with a mutually exclusive membership; each group homogenous and uniformly different from the other groups in how they experience and enact their sexual desire. However, it is more accurate to conceptualize sexual orientation as being composed of multiple dimensions. The three most commonly described are *sexual attraction, sexual behaviour,* and *self-identification*. Treating sexual orientation as a category implies that these dimensions must always go together, but research has shown this to be incorrect [10–12]. And, indeed, one

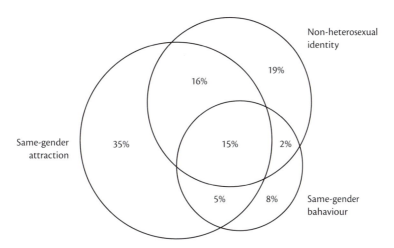

Fig. 27.1 Dimensions of sexual orientation in a sample of sexual minority adolescents.

Source: Adapted from *J Adolesc Health*, 45(6), Igartua K, Thombs BD, Burgos G, Montoro R. Concordance and discrepancy in sexual identity, attraction, and behavior among adolescents, pp. 602–8, Copyright (2009), with permission from Elsevier.

can easily think of cases where only one, or different combinations of two dimensions occur: an individual with same-gender behaviour may not endorse same-gender attraction; a self-identified heterosexual person may have same-gender attractions and so on.

Our Canadian study with adolescents supports this [11]. Sexual orientation dimensions were surveyed in 1951 Montreal high school students aged 14–18 years. Twelve per cent of the sample endorsed at least one of the sexual orientation minority dimensions. A non-heterosexual identity was endorsed by 6.8% of the total sample, evenly split between those with a lesbian, gay, or bisexual (LGB) identity and those that were unsure of their sexual orientation. Same-gender attraction was endorsed by 9.0% of the total sample and 4.0% reported same-gender behaviour. When these dimensions are mapped out graphically, the representation in Fig. 27.1 is drawn. As shown, no single dimension effectively captured the sexual orientation minority population and there was no consistent pattern of overlap between the three measures. The question on attraction identified 71%; identity identified 52%; and behaviour only 31% of the sexual orientation minority subgroup, making it clear that any one question is a poor screen for sexual orientation minority status.

Given the youth of our adolescent sample, it is tempting to assume that adolescents in the throes of identity formation may simply be giving contradictory responses, a reflection of their own uncertainty. However, the National Health and Social Life Survey conducted on adults over the age of 18 years showed a similar pattern of dimension overlap, yielding an overall sexual orientation minority prevalence of 9.3% [10].

The recent American health statistics report from the 2011–2013 National Survey of Family Growth did not publish results that allowed for an overall prevalence of sexual orientation minorities [12], but it reported that sexual attraction and self-identified sexual orientation correlated closely but not completely with sexual behaviour. Published rates for each dimension were as follows: same-gender attraction present in 17.3% of women and 7.0% of men; current homosexual or bisexual identity in 5.2% of women and 2.8% of men; and same-gender sexual behaviour as an adult in 14.2% of women and 5.5% of men. The preponderance of women endorsing a same-gender sexuality dimension is a consistent

pattern over the last decade and may reflect a greater relaxation of female gender roles and reduced social stigma in this regard. This gender pattern was noted in our own study with adolescents [11], as shown in Table 27.1.

It is important to note that older statistics in North America show the inverse gender ratio in surveys of same-gender attraction and same-gender sexual behaviour, as well as overall lower rates [10, 13]. Whether this reflects an actual change in these dimensions, or simply a change in the under-reporting bias common to all socially undesirable survey items, or a little of both, is unclear.

Coming out

The process of sexual orientation identity formation is commonly referred to as 'coming out' and is a unique developmental task for sexual orientation minorities. Despite the moniker, coming out is not a discrete event but starts in childhood or early adolescence with the onset of same-gender romantic or sexual attractions. Because of the presumed heterosexuality of children, as well as the social stigma associated with non-heterosexual sexual orientations, the individual often meets the dawning of these same-gender attractions with confusion and trepidation. Parental support around coming out is generally absent before the child informs the parent(s) about their sexual orientation.

Table 27.1 Gender pattern in dimensions of sexual orientation in a sample of sexual minority adolescents

	Girls (%)	Boys (%)
Same-gender attraction	13.1	5.0
Same-gender behaviour	4.9	2.9
Gay, lesbian, bisexual identity	4.2	2.2
Unsure identity	4.1	2.6

Source: Adapted from *J Adolesc Health*, 45(6), Igartua K, Thombs BD, Burgos G, Montoro R. Concordance and discrepancy in sexual identity, attraction, and behavior among adolescents, pp. 602–8, Copyright (2009), with permission from Elsevier.

For most stigmatized minorities, parents and their children share the same minority status, whether racial or religious. Parents can thus serve as role models and teach stigma-related coping skills to their children. Children with disabilities and adopted children of a visible minority still benefit from the parents' awareness of their challenges and efforts to help them cope with them. The invisibility of LGB sexual orientation in childhood generally means that most LGB individuals were parented with the presumption of a heterosexual identity, leading to missed opportunities for LGB-specific guidance and supervision as these adolescents embark on their first romantic and sexual relationships. To make matters worse, parents as a group will hold, on average, the same attitudes and beliefs towards LGB individuals as their culture does. Thus, many LGB people will have heard anti-LGB sentiments from their parents during their childhood, and may also have been received verbal or physical remonstrations if they happened to also have been gender variant. By the time the first same-gender attractions appear, many of these children will have integrated the same anti-LGB sentiments as their parents.

There have been several models of sexual orientation formation (e.g. [14, 15]) that posit linear pathways of minority sexual orientation development generally moving from *awareness* of same-gender attractions to *confusion* at having these stigmatized feelings to *acceptance* of one's sexual orientation, and, finally, to *integration* of one's sexual orientation into one's public identity and broader social relationships. More recent research seems to indicate that the coming out trajectories are not the same for everyone [16, 17]. Although both genders have, on average, a 10-year period between awareness and acceptance, girls had a higher rate of self-identifying prior to engaging in same-gender sexual activity, whereas the inverse order was more often endorsed in boys. Compared with Caucasian adolescents, African American and Latino teens had similar trajectories but delays in public disclosure and LGBTQ community involvement [18].

Those who come out younger have an increased comfort with their sexual orientation but were at increased risk for rejection and harassment from family and schoolmates [19]. Rejection by parents is not inconsequential. Compared with adults, adolescents have a limited capacity to exert a change in their environment. It is therefore unsurprising to find that approximately one-third of homeless high-school students were either unsure as to their sexual orientation or endorsed a sexual minority status [20].

A recent study of American high-school students showed not only that those LGBTQ students that were out were more victimized, but also had higher self-esteem and lower depression [21]. Although the positive effects of being out did not vary by community, the rates of victimization were higher in rural students than their urban and suburban peers—potentially outweighing the benefits. This brings home the importance of evaluating the community when analysing the risks and rewards of disclosure in LGBTQ youth. In societies where an LGBTQ public identity puts one at serious risk of violence or imprisonment, the compartmentalization of one's sexual orientation from one's public self may be the only viable option until such time, if ever, that the individual can leave the unsafe environment.

Gender identity

Much like sexual orientation, gender identity is often assumed to be categorical (male or female), each with a mutually exclusive membership; each group homogenous and uniformly different in terms of gender role and expression, gender of their sexual partners, and, most notably, their genitals. However, when one understands that gender identity relies *only* on an individual's felt sense of gender and that this internal sense of gender is the only attribute common to all individuals of that gender, then the diversity of representations for any given gender identity is to be expected, as it is for all other identities (e.g. Catholic, Iranian, mother, boss, etc.).

Gender identity in childhood

Self-awareness of one's assigned gender and gender identity evolves gradually in childhood. Most children develop the ability to identify their own assigned gender, as well as that of others, between 18 and 24 months of age. Children can start voicing a strong preference for opposite-gender clothes, toys, activities, and even gender as early as 2 years of age, all the while correctly identifying the gender assigned to their bodies.

It is important to note that gender-variant behaviour—behaviour that does not conform to culturally defined norms expected of their assigned gender—is common in childhood. A large-scale study of Dutch twins at 7 and 10 years of age found that opposite-gender behaviour was more common (2.4–5.2%) than wishing to be the opposite-gender (0.9–1.7%) [22]. Although girls were more likely to have opposite-gender behaviours, the gender ratio neared equality in terms of actually wishing to be the opposite gender.

Gender identity in adolescence

Of the children who do receive a diagnosis of gender dysphoria, only a minority will continue to have gender dysphoria into adolescence. Studies of persistence rates of childhood gender identity disorder (see Box 27.1) into adolescence are in the range of 12–37% [23–25]. So far it has not been possible to identify consistently which children will persist. Studies have pointed to the amount of childhood opposite-gender behaviour [24, 25] and the intensity of self-identification [25] as the opposite gender to be most predictive of adolescent gender dysphoria. Natal girls were more likely to persist than natal boys. Natal boys were more likely to persist if they were older at their initial assessment and had a childhood role transition—factors that were not more associated with persistence in natal girls [25]. It is important to note that some gender dysphoric children will desist in adolescence, only to re-enter transitioning services in adulthood. This represented 10% of the overall persistence rate in one Dutch sample, where 27% of the 150 dysphoric children persisted and an additional 3% returned as adults after desisting in adolescence [26].

In a qualitative follow-up study of children with gender identity disorder into adolescence, the teenagers recalled retrospectively that the period between 10 and 13 years of age was crucial to their later gender identity [27], regardless of whether or not the transgender identification had persisted. Three sets of experiences seemed to have the largest influence: (i) the onset of puberty and secondary sexual characteristics; (ii) the introduction to the high-school environment with its explicit differences in how genders are treated; and (iii) the discovery of sexuality and romantic experiences. The exploration, reflection, and evaluation of themselves through these experiences seemed to be pivotal in the consolidation of their gender identity. Whether pubertal hormones themselves have a direct role on gender identity consolidation, other than driving puberty forward, is unclear, but clinically it does seem that gender identity is more malleable in childhood than later in life [28].

After this initial pubertal period, it is generally thought that the persistence rates from adolescence to adulthood is high [29], although epidemiological studies are lacking. There are, however, three follow-up studies of adolescents in a Dutch gender clinic consulting for gender dysphoria. After a full diagnostic assessment, those who received puberty suppression and/or cross-gender hormones all went on to gender-affirming surgery [30–32].

Some individuals present with gender dysphoria for the first time in adolescence. Many will recollect some cross-gender behaviour in their early years, although they have no formal childhood history of gender dysphoria. There have been efforts to determine if those with adolescent onset represent a different subgroup from those with a childhood onset, but the results have been conflicting [29]. The impetus to understand this distinction is that adult studies have shown that natal males, with late-onset gender dysphoria, and sexual attraction to persons different from one's assigned gender can predict a more challenging course [6, 33]. It is possible that much of these adults' difficulties may be related to the poor social acceptability of being a recognizable transwoman with continued physical markers of male gender from a full male puberty (deep voice, broad chest, large hands and feet), combined with the negative effects of misogyny and anti-gay stigma related to their post-transition sexual orientation.

Given how quickly the gender landscape is changing, recent studies show significant differences with the older literature. A study of two gender identity clinics, one in Toronto and one in Amsterdam [34], looked at referrals of adolescents to their services between two cohort periods: prior to 2006 and between 2006 and 2013. Both centres showed a large increase in adolescent referrals per year, as well as a sex ratio favouring natal females—which is an inversion of the sex ratio from the older data set. In their discussion, they note that the increased visibility of transgendered persons in the media and availability of information on the Internet has probably contributed to lower social stigma and an overall increase in adolescents seeking clinical care for gender dysphoria. They hypothesize that the inversion of the sex ratio may be because despite the lower social stigma for transgender people overall, feminine behaviour in natal boys still carries more disapproval than masculine behaviour in natal girls.

A recent estimate of gender dysphoria in adults is in the range of 0.3% [35], which is considerably larger than traditional estimates based on gender reassignment clinics [36, 37]. New Zealand has been the first to conduct a nationally representative survey of adolescents that included a question on being transgender. It indicated that 1.2% of high-school students identified as transgender and 2.5% were unsure about their gender. Furthermore, just over half of the transgender students reported they had first wondered about being transgendered after the age of 12 years [38]. Whether this reflects an actual change in prevalence is unclear given the lack of prior transgender population data outside of gender reassignment clinics. The larger prevalence in the New Zealand study most probably includes individuals who identify under the broader terms of transgender or gender queer, and who may not present to specialized gender clinics for gender reassignment interventions. How this broader population compares with the traditionally studied gender dysphoria population has yet to be determined.

Stigma

Stigma is often seen as emanating from a characteristic in a group that is outside the norm, thereby making the group undesirable. However, it is the power that lies in the dominant group of a given society that determines which minority characteristics are deserving of stigma and which are inconsequential [39]. The labelled differences are then associated with negative stereotypes and the identified individuals are split off from 'us' into 'them', facilitating status loss and discrimination.

Grounded in stigma theory, the *minority stress model* posits that the excess stress subjected to individuals in a stigmatized minority is responsible for health disparities in that group rather than any characteristic of the minority per se [40]. The components described in the minority stress model are threefold: (i) the presence of external, objective stressful events and conditions related to the minority status (chronic, as well as acute), (ii) the expectation of such events and the vigilance this engenders; and (iii) the internalization of negative societal attitudes. It is important to note that the model does not rest on individual events or experiences—it is socially based. It rests on laws and policies, so the stress is chronic rather than episodic. And the stresses are unique to that group, requiring additional coping above and beyond those needed to deal with the stresses to which everyone is exposed. Although the minority stress model was elucidated around mental health disparities in the LGB population, similar factors are thought to be at play in the health disparities of gender minorities [41, 42].

Mental health disparities in sexual orientation minority youth

There have been several meta-analyses of mental health disparities in sexual orientation minority adolescents. A meta-analysis of studies on substance abuse showed that sexual orientation minority adolescents had an overall odds ratio (OR) of 2.89 [43]. Another meta-analysis on the rate of sex while intoxicated showed than sexual orientation minority youth were almost twice as likely to report sex while under the influence of drugs or alcohol [44]. Data from the Youth Risk Behaviour Survey indicated that purging and diet pill use was elevated in girls and boys with an LGB identity (OR range 1.9–6.8) and the risk of obesity compared with same-gender heterosexuals was twice as high in bisexual boys and girls [45]. A meta-analysis of rates of violence and victimization in adolescence showed that sexual orientation minorities were, on average, 3.8 times more likely to experience sexual abuse, 1.2 times more likely to have parental physical abuse, 1.7 times more likely to suffer assault at school, and 2.4 times more likely to miss school because of fear [46].

All of these factors are, of course, risk factors in themselves of suicide. A recent meta-analysis showed that sexual orientation minority youth reported significantly higher rates of overall suicidality (OR 2.92) compared with heterosexual youth [47]. The disparities increased with each increase in the severity of the suicidality: suicidal ideation (OR 1.96), suicidal intent/plans (OR 2.20), suicide attempts (OR 3.18), and suicide attempts requiring medical attention (OR 4.17). Effects did not vary across gender, recruitment source, and sexual orientation definition used in these studies. It is important to note that the sexual orientation definitions were most often based on one question, and occasionally two, in the included studies—making elucidation of *which* sexual orientation dimension (attraction, behaviour, or identity) is responsible for the mental health disparity impossible.

Given the minority stress model, one would predict that the closer one identifies to the minority, the larger the impact of minority stress [40]. In our study of 1856 Montreal high-school students, we examined each sexual orientation dimension with respect to suicidality outcomes [48]. LGBQ and unsure sexual orientation identities, regardless of same-sex attraction or behaviour, had over twice the odds of suicidal ideation and suicide attempts than the reference group of heterosexually identified youth *without* same-sex attraction or behaviour. Interestingly, heterosexually identified youth *with* same-sex attraction or behaviour were not at increased risk. This suggests that it is the identification with a sexual minority that carries the increased risk and not the same-sex attractions and behaviours themselves. Moreover, when the impact of bullying on the sample was examined, students with a heterosexual identity *with* same-sex attraction or behaviour had similar increases in the odds of their suicide parameters than the reference group of heterosexually identified youth *without* same-sex attraction or behaviour [49]. In contrast, even after controlling for independent risk factors such as depressed mood, fighting, physical and sexual abuse, and age of first sexual contact, the increased odds were much higher in the students with LGBQ or unsure identities, regardless of behaviour or attraction, who were subject to bullying.

Other studies on sexual orientation minority youth have shown a correlation between enacted stigma (bullying, harassment, exclusion, and violence) and increased rates of mental health problems such as depression, post-traumatic stress disorder, and suicidality [50–52]. A similar correlation exists between stigma and health risk behaviours, such as substance use [53, 54] and at-risk sexual behaviours, including teenage pregnancy [54, 55]. Cyberbullying, or bullying via electronic means such as social networks, emails and text messages, is increasing among adolescents [50, 56]. Cyberbullying is more destructive than in-person bullying in important ways: (i) the aggression tends to be more virulent as the perpetrator is hidden behind a keyboard and not bound by in-person interaction; (ii) mass dissemination of the bullying or humiliation is easy and nearly instantaneous; and (iii) it can be without reprieve as the aggression can continue even in the relative safety of the victim's home. These factors may explain why cyberbullying has been found to be associated with more depression and suicidal ideation [57], even when controlling for the presence of co-occurring in-person bullying. Again, as with in-person bullying, sexual minority youth are at increased risk versus their heterosexual peers, particularly in girls [50].

Family rejection after coming out has been relatively less studied as a risk factor, although it has been associated with significantly higher rates of depression, suicide attempts, substance use and unprotected sex [58]. Disclosure of sexual orientation by LGBQ youth to at least one parent was associated with more verbal and physical abuse as well as suicidality than in their closeted peers [59]. Sexual orientation disclosure in general for LGBQ youth was associated with more negative responses, which, in turn, predicted greater unsafe sex and substance use [60]. Family rejection may lead to homelessness as many sexual minority youth are either kicked out of the home or they choose to leave an unsafe home environment. Data from the 2005 and 2007 Massachusetts Youth Risk Behavior Survey found that 25% of lesbian and gay, 15% of bisexual, and 3% of exclusively heterosexual public high school students were homeless; this greater likelihood was driven by their increased risk of living apart from their parents or guardians [20]. Furthermore, it would seem that LGBTQ street youth had higher rates of victimization, substance use, mental health disorders, and sexual partners than their heterosexual peers [61]. Other studies have found increased risk of risky sexual behaviours, involvement in prostitution, survival sex, and teen pregnancy in LGBQ homeless youth [55, 62, 63].

Protective factors in sexual orientation minority youth

Although it is vital to address these disparities, it is important to acknowledge that most sexual orientation minority youth do not experience mental health problems and that resilience in this population is the rule rather than the exception [64]. Nonetheless, a recent review of the literature found that sexual orientation minority youth were less likely to have access to known protective factors than heterosexually identified youth, reporting lower connectedness to family, school, peers, and adults outside the family [4]. Of the usual protective factors, only religiosity has been shown to not protect sexual orientation minority youth from suicidality [65]. Given the anti-LGBTQ stance of several religions, it is possible that sexual minority teens may turn away from their religious affiliation as an adaptive strategy.

Parental acceptance has been shown to safeguard youth with same-sex attractions or gender non-conformity from psychological distress and social anxiety. Interestingly, for gender non-conforming boys it was high levels of paternal acceptance, but not maternal acceptance, that protected against psychological distress and social anxiety. For girls with same-sex attraction, those with median-to-high levels of maternal acceptance, but not paternal acceptance, were protected against social anxiety [66]. In another study of LGBQ youth, parental support was shown to reduce the psychological distress associated with homophobic victimization, although it did not lessen the impact of victimization on internalized homophobia [67].

In a study on resilience factors, LGBQ adolescents and adults showed different patterns of response to support from family and friends, LGBTQ community connectedness, and having a steady partner. In terms of well-being, family support was the strongest predictor of well-being in adolescents, whereas it was friend support that was the strongest predictor of well-being among adults. LGBTQ community connectedness was also associated with well-being in LGBQ adults but not LGBQ adolescents. This may be owing to the fact that most adults can move away from unsupportive families, and garner their support in the community—unlike their adolescent counterparts for whom family support is critical [68].

As for school resources specific to LGBQ youth, it has been shown that adolescents in schools with LGBQ support groups reported lower rates of victimization and suicide attempts. In their logistic regression analysis, the relationship between LGBQ support groups and suicidality became non-significant once victimization, anti-bullying policies and perceived availability of staff (all significantly protective) were included. This suggests that the effect of the LGBQ support groups is largely via their influence on the school environment, as opposed to the support they offer the individuals in the support group [69].

In a study that grouped American school climates on a city or state level, LGB students living in areas with more protective school climates reported fewer past-year suicidal thoughts. Each school was scored on eight items, which included protected environments (e.g. gay–straight alliances), as well as curricula and services that addressed the unique concerns of LGB students. The sexual orientation disparities were nearly eliminated in states and cities with the most protective school climates [70].

In another study, the impact of anti-bullying policies was examined at a county level. The anti-bullying policies, when present, of each school district in the county needed to name sexual orientation as a protected class to be considered 'inclusive'. The counties with the highest proportion of school districts with inclusive anti-bullying policies had a significantly reduced risk for suicide attempts in lesbian and gay youth, even after controlling for exposure to peer victimization and sociodemographic characteristics. Anti-bullying policies that did not mention sexual orientation did not buffer lesbian and gay youths from attempting suicide. Interestingly, heterosexual and bisexual youths were unaffected by the proportion of inclusive anti-bullying policies [71].

One author used a four-item composite index of anti-LGBQ structural stigma in the different counties of Oregon. The composite index was based on objective measures of the density of same-sex couples, the proportion of registered Democrats (a more liberal political party), the proportion of public high schools with gay–straight alliances, and LGB protective school policies on bullying and discrimination. LGB youth living in unsupportive environments had a 20% greater risk of attempting suicide than their peers living in supportive environments [72]. Using a similar four-item composite index, the same author compared various American states and found that high structural anti-LGBQ stigma was related to more pronounced sexual orientation disparities in marijuana and other substance use than low structural anti-LGBQ stigma states [73].

Mental health disparities in gender minorities

In contrast to the literature on LGBQ youth, the research on health disparities among transgender youth is relatively less developed. The recent New Zealand nationally representative survey of high-school students found mental health disparities for transgender students in terms of depressive symptoms (OR 5.7) and suicide attempts (OR 5.0). School bullying was higher in the transgender students (OR 4.5) and the perception that one parent cared about them was lower (OR 0.3) [38]. Smaller youth population studies that asked about transgender identity had numbers too small to analyse separately from LGBQ youth [51]. This leads to the assumption that LGBQ health disparities can be generalized to gender minorities, which is sure to be only partly accurate at best; current thinking is that gender minorities are at an even greater risk of health disparities than LGBQ youth, given that they face more stigma.

Non-population-based research in this field includes a retrospective cohort study to examine the mental health records of 180 transgender teenagers and young adults. These transgender youth had a two- to three-fold increased risk of depression, anxiety disorder, self-harm, and suicidal ideation and attempt compared with cisgender matched controls [74]. Other studies only examine convenience samples and are limited in their ability to describe relative risk. One of the largest was an online survey used to collect data on a non-probability sample of 923 transgender youth. It indicated that 65% of the transgender teenagers aged 14–18 years had considered suicide in the past year and three-quarters had self-harmed. Only a quarter of participants reported their mental health as good or excellent [75]. In a smaller study, of 55 transgender youth interviewed, nearly half reported serious suicidal ideation and one-quarter had attempted suicide. Risk factors in this sample for suicide attempts were suicidal thoughts related to transgender identity, past parental verbal and physical abuse, and lower body esteem [76].

Protective factors in gender minorities

For gender minorities, there are some recent encouraging studies where children and adolescents confirmed in their chosen gender seem to fair reasonably well. Socially transitioned children with gender dysphoria who are supported in their preferred gender identity have been shown to have developmentally normative levels of depression and only minimal elevations in anxiety, in sharp contrast to the increased rates of internalizing psychopathology in children with gender dysphoria living in their natal sex [77].

Another study followed 55 adolescents with gender dysphoria prior to puberty suppression (mean age 13.6 years), at the introduction of cross-sex hormones (mean age 16.7 years), and at least 1 year after gender reassignment surgery (mean age 20.7 years). All psychological measures improved over the time course of the study, and as young adults their well-being was comparable with same-age adults from the general population [32]. Again, these results are in sharp contrast with the mental health disparities outlined earlier for gender minorities. The difference may be owing to the access to specialized health care in the study population. Additionally, and possibly more significantly, the families of the study subjects were involved and supportive of the process—which is not the case for many transgender children and adolescents.

Interventions

Interventions aimed at reducing the mental health disparities of the sexual minority population must address the different levels in which stigma exists. A single intervention is unlikely to have lasting impact as there are multiple mutually reinforcing mechanisms linking attitudes and beliefs of the dominant groups to an array of negative outcomes for stigmatized persons [39]. Thus, interventions need not only be multifaceted and multi-level, but they would ideally produce fundamental changes in attitudes and beliefs of powerful groups, or limit the power of such groups to make their distinctions the dominant ones. An example of how certain interventions can produce changes is laws protecting the civil rights of LGBTQ persons. These laws have multiple effects in multiple instances, which lead to LGBTQ persons being able to live openly within their family of origin, their place of work, and the larger community, which then impacts on the dominant group's ability to *other* LGBTQ persons as they are now visibly part of the fabric of every social sphere.

Interventions can be conceptualized loosely as belonging to three different levels: (i) the structural level (e.g. societal norms, laws, and policies); (ii) the interpersonal level (e.g. bullying, microaggressions); and (iii) the individual level (e.g. negative beliefs and behaviours) [78]. Table 27.2 provides a non-exhaustive collection of possible interventions most relevant to sexual minority youth at each of these levels.

Table 27.2 Interventions aimed at reducing stigma for lesbian, gay, bisexual, trans, and queer (LGBTQ) youth

Structural	
State	Policies and laws to protect individuals from discrimination and harassment based on sexual orientation and/or gender identity
	Policies requiring medical insurance plans to include gender-affirming medical care
	Promotion and support of LGBTQ community groups
School	Anti-bullying policies inclusive of sexual orientation and gender identity
	Creation of gay–straight alliances and/or safe spaces
	Teaching and printed documentation on HIV, sexually transmitted infections, and pregnancy prevention relevant to LGBTQ youth
	Access to a gender-neutral bathroom or usage of bathroom facilities based on gender identity
Healthcare setting	Availability of healthcare providers who are competent in providing care to people with sexual orientation or gender-related issues
	Visible posted policies on confidentiality and non-discrimination, as well as visible markers that the setting is LGBTQ friendly (e.g. LGBTQ-inclusive posters)
	Documentation in the waiting room about relevant LGBTQ healthcare issues
	Gender-neutral bathrooms or a visible policy on gender usage of the bathroom being based on gender identity
	Administrative and medical questionnaires inclusive of sexual orientation and gender diversity (e.g. mother/father)
Interpersonal	
Parents	Public health campaigns sensitizing parents to sexual orientation and gender diversity, and their role in optimizing their LGBTQ child's mental health
	Support groups for parents of LGBTQ children (e.g. PFLAG)
Healthcare providers	Individual marker of LGBTQ awareness (e.g. rainbow flag pin or poster)
	Profession-specific training on LGBTQ-related health issues
	History taking inclusive of sexual orientation and gender diversity
Individual	
Increase coping capacity and decrease Internalized stigma	LGBTQ youth groups in the community, virtual support groups
	Gay–straight alliances in schools
	Psychoeducation and psychotherapy aimed at identifying sources of stigma, recognizing its negative impact, and learning how to handle it more effectively

Note: PFLAG: Parents and Friends of Lesbians and Gays.

Structural interventions

State

Sexual minority youth are embedded in their society. Laws protecting certain minorities and not others signal to citizens which groups have inherent value and which do not. State laws and policies on LGBTQ access to marriage and adoption, hate crime protection, employment non-discrimination, immigration equality, and anti-bullying powerfully shape the health of sexual minority populations [79]. For example, sexual minority youth living in areas with a high rate of LGBTQ hate crimes had higher rates of suicidal ideation and attempts than their peers living in low LGBTQ hate crime areas. Sexual minority youth suicidality did not vary with overall violent and property crimes, suggesting specificity of the LGBTQ hate crimes as a risk factor [80]. Laws also provide the framework within which more specific settings, such as schools, can feel free to intervene to protect their LGBTQ youth.

School

School is often considered the primary target for structural interventions as this is the principal social arena for most adolescents outside the home. Explicit naming of sexual orientation and gender minorities in anti-bullying efforts have promoted the discussion of anti-LGBTQ bias in highs schools and allowed youth with current or possibly developing LGBTQ identities to be able to identify adult allies and feel that their safety is important to the authorities in their schools. Teaching and documentation relevant to LGBTQ youth health concerns can help serve these functions as well. Laws that protect the job safety of LGBTQ teachers will allow them to serve as role models for their students.

Gender minorities often feel unsafe using public bathrooms, in general, and at school, in particular. Different schools have found different solutions, including gender-neutral bathrooms (generally the staff bathroom) for transgender youth, gender-neutral bathrooms for everyone, and explicit policies explaining that access to gendered bathrooms are based on the student's gender identity, or comfort with a gender in the case of students with a non-binary gender. Again explicit handling of this issue allows gender minorities to feel that their needs are important and that adults take them seriously.

Gay–straight alliances in schools are student-led groups, generally with a faculty advisor, intended to provide a safe, supportive environment for sexual minority youth and those who are perceived as such, and their straight allies where they can socialize, receive support, and engage in advocacy efforts. Schools with gay–straight alliances have lower rates of smoking, drinking, truancy, suicide attempts, and sex with casual partners in their sexual minority students [81]. Interestingly, although the effect was most pronounced in sexual minority students, heterosexual students also benefited from having a gay–straight alliance in their school—possibly because they address issues that are relevant to all youth.

Healthcare settings

Health care has the potential to provide respite from victimization and be a resource for sexual minority youth facing mental health challenges. However, health care providers often forget that before a youth enters the office, they have already collected a certain amount of information on how LGBTQ-friendly a setting will be. Rather than risk exposing themselves to a healthcare provider, sexual minority youth will take their cue from how LGBTQ inclusive administrative staff, waiting room documentation, questionnaires, and posted policies are. Training of front-line staff in LGBTQ awareness and revision of all documentation can help the healthcare setting better meet the needs of sexual minority youth [82].

Interpersonal interventions

Parents

Family support is one of the most protective factors for sexual minority youth [66–68]. Public health campaigns targeting parents have been the most common method for reaching this population in the general public, with follow-up resources for parents to contact, be they educational or psychotherapeutic. Additionally, there are community groups for parents of LGBTQ and gender-variant children that offer a safe space for parents to discuss feelings, challenges, and strategies around parenting these children. In areas that do not have access to these community resources, the Internet offers equivalent support groups virtually. Parents and Friends of Lesbians and Gays (PFLAG) is a well-respected organization that has chapters in many English-speaking countries.

Healthcare providers

One of the major barriers to care is the lack of physicians competent in LGBTQ health care. The median reported time in American and Canadian medical school curricula dedicated to LGBTQ-related content was 5 hours [81]. Lack of education means physicians will often be uncertain and ambivalent in their interaction with sexual minority patients, and sexual minority patients often anticipate that the healthcare providers will not be able to meet their needs. This upsets the usual balance of power in the provider–patient relationships and interpersonal stigma is often enacted to reinforce the power and authority of the medical provider during these interactions [82].

Adolescents can be reluctant to discuss sexual orientation or gender identity issues if they are unsure of the reception they will receive. Many teens will withhold this information until they are confident enough that the healthcare provider is LGBTQ-friendly. Outward signs can include a rainbow pin or posted materials in the office stating that it is an LGBTQ-friendly space. The next-most-noted signal is language, particularly in the history taking. Questions such as 'Do you have a boyfriend?' should be replaced by 'Are you in a relationship?' Open-ended questions about identity will elicit terms with which the person feels comfortable—it is always best to use their term in the encounter rather than substituting

another term (e.g. *homosexual*, when the patient described herself as *lesbian*).

Confidentiality is important in any clinical encounter, but LGBTQ youth are even more sensitive to it than their heterosexual peers. Realistic reassurance as to the confidentiality of the information they choose to share can help encourage disclosure. As sexual minority youth can choose to be invisible in terms of these differences, a universal approach with all youth becomes essential, including sexual history and gender identity questions. It is important to remember that many heterosexually identified youth, as well as gay and lesbian youth, will have had sexual experiences or attractions to both genders.

Clinicians can sometimes feel awkward when a young person shares that they are gender questioning or transgender, particularly if they had assumed the young person's gender based on their gender presentation. Handling these kinds of errors directly is best, by simply recognizing the mistake and asking for the young person's preferred pronouns and preferred name. Some gender questioning youth may wish to continue using their assigned names and pronouns for the time being, but asking their preference helps to establish the clinician as LGBTQ aware.

Individual interventions

Most of the interventions studied have been at the individual level. Multiple psychotherapeutic approaches have been adapted to be explicitly LGBTQ-affirmative [83]. They generally aim to increase resilience in the face of anti-LGBTQ stigma and address the internalized stigma through educational and cognitive behavioural strategies.

Community and school support groups can also serve this function. One example is Hatch Youth, a social support group for 13–20-year-old sexual minority youth in Houston, Texas [84]. Hatch Youth provides services four nights a week in a supportive environment where youth can learn about their health, interact with LGBTQ adult mentors, and, perhaps most importantly, interact with other LGBTQ youth. Each Hatch Youth meeting is organized into three 1-hour sections: unstructured social time, education, and a youth-led peer support group. Those who attended Hatch Youth for more than 1 month reported higher social support, which, in turn, led to decreased depressive symptoms, increased self-esteem and coping ability.

Online interventions have also been tested. Queer Sex Ed is aimed at 16–20-year-old sexual minority youth and is comprised of five modules of online multimedia sexual health interventions. Almost all ($n = 15/17$) of the study outcomes were significantly improved on measures of self-acceptance, sexual health knowledge, relationship variables, and safer sex [85]. The major positive feedback was that it included information about relationship skills and sexual functioning, rather than focusing on sexually transmitted infections and scare tactics often used in school-based sex education. The major negative feedback was the length of the intervention (just under 2 hours) and any material that was not highly interactive or video.

Conclusion

Mental health disparities of sexual minority adolescents are well established and the smoking gun seems to lie at the feet of stigma and minority stress. Sadly, the medical profession has historically played a significant role in generating stigma for sexual minority youth on both interpersonal and structural levels by pathologizing their identities. It is likely that the medical profession can now play a role in eliminating this stigma and improving the mental health of their sexual minority youth population by supporting interventions at the personal, interpersonal, and structural levels. Future research is needed on these multi-level interventions, as well as on ways to address and deconstruct anti-LGBTQ stigma in the broader population.

Acknowledgements

The author would like to thank Dr Karine Igartua for her invaluable suggestions and assistance in preparation of this chapter.

References

1. Stoddard J, Leibowitz SF, Ton H, Snowdon S. Improving medical education about gender-variant youth and transgender adolescents. *Child Adolesc Psychiatr Clin N Am* 2011; 20: 779–791.

2. Rubin R. Minimizing health disparities among LGBT patients. *JAMA* 2015; 313: 15–17.

3. Kirkpatrick RC, Plato, Levi-Strauss C. The evolution of human homosexual behavior. *Curr Anthropol* 2000; 41: 385–413.

4. Saewyc EM. Research on adolescent sexual orientation: development, health disparities, stigma and resilience. *J Res Adolesc* 2011; 21: 256–272.

5. Wood PL. Teenage sexuality in different cultures. *J Pediatr Adolesc Gynecol* 2012; 25: 228–232.

6. Lawrence AA. Sexual orientation versus age of onset as bases for typologies (subtypes) for gender identity disorder in adolescents and adults. *Arch Sex Behav* 2010; 39: 514–545.

7. Veltman A, Chaimowitz G. mental health care for people who identify as lesbian, gay, bisexual, transgender, and (or) queer. *Can J Psychiatry* 2014;5 9: 1–7.

8. UCSF Lesbian, Gay, Bisexual and Transgender Resource Center. General definitions. Available at: https://lgbt.ucsf.edu/glossary-terms (accessed 20 March 2017).

9. RAINBOW. Glossary of LGBT Terms. Available at: http://www.rainbowproject.eu/material/en/glossary.htm (accessed 20 March 2017).

10. Laumann EO. *The Social Organization of Sexuality: Sexual Practices in the United States*. Chicago, IL: University of Chicago Press, 1994.

11. Igartua K, Thombs BD, Burgos G, Montoro R. Concordance and discrepancy in sexual identity, attraction, and behavior among adolescents. *J Adolesc Health* 2009; 45: 602–608.

12. Copen CE, Chandra A, Febo-Vazquez I. Sexual behavior, sexual attraction, and sexual orientation among adults aged 18-44 in the United States: data from the 2011-2013 National Survey of Family Growth. *Natl Health Stat Report* 2016; (88): 1–14.

13. Michaels S. The prevalence of homosexuality in the United States. In: Cabaj RP, Stein TS (eds). *Textbook of Homosexuality and Mental Health*. Arlington, VA: American Psychiatric Association, 1996, pp. 43–63.

14. Cass V. Sexual orientation identity formation: a Western phenomenon. In: Cabaj RP, Stein TS (eds). *Textbook of Homosexuality and Mental Health*. Arlington, VA: American Psychiatric Association, 1996, pp. 227–251.

15. Troiden RR. The formation of homosexual identities. In: Garnets LD, Kimmel DC (eds). *Psychological Perspectives on Lesbian and Gay Male Experiences*. New York: Columbia University Press, 1993, pp. 191–217.

16. Rosario M, Meyer-Bahlburg HF, Hunter J, Exner TM, Gwadz M, Keller AM. The psychosexual development of urban lesbian, gay, and bisexual youths. *J Sex Res* 1996; 33: 113–126.

17. Savin-Williams RC, Diamond LM. Sexual identity trajectories among sexual-minority youths: gender comparisons. *Arch Sex Behav* 2000; 29: 607–627.

18. Rosario M, Schrimshaw EW, Hunter J. Ethnic/racial differences in the coming-out process of lesbian, gay, and bisexual youths: a comparison of sexual identity development over time. *Cultur Divers Ethnic Minor Psychol* 2004; 10: 215–228.

19. Floyd FJ, Stein TS. Sexual orientation identity formation among gay, lesbian, and bisexual youths: multiple patterns of milestone experiences. *J Res Adolesc* 2002; 12: 167–191.

20. Corliss HL, Goodenow CS, Nichols L, Austin SB. High burden of homelessness among sexual-minority adolescents: findings from a representative Massachusetts high school sample. *Am J Public Health* 2011; 101: 1683–1689.

21. Kosciw JG, Palmer NA, Kull RM. Reflecting resiliency: openness about sexual orientation and/or gender identity and its relationship to well-being and educational outcomes for LGBT students. *Am J Community Psychol* 2015; 55: 167–178.

22. van Beijsterveldt CE, Hudziak JJ, Boomsma DI. Genetic and environmental influences on cross-gender behavior and relation to behavior problems: a study of Dutch twins at ages 7 and 10 years. *Arch Sex Behav* 2006; 35: 647–658.

23. Drummond KD, Bradley SJ, Peterson-Badali M, Zucker KJ. A follow-up study of girls with gender identity disorder. *Dev Psychol* 2008; 44: 34–45.

24. Wallien MS, Cohen-Kettenis PT. Psychosexual outcome of gender-dysphoric children. *J Am Acad Child Adolesc Psychiatry* 2008; 47: 1413–1423.

25. Steensma TD, McGuire JK, Kreukels BP, Beekman AJ, Cohen-Kettenis PT. Factors associated with desistence and persistence of childhood gender dysphoria: a quantitative follow-up study. *J Am Acad Child Adolesc Psychiatry* 2013; 52: 582–590.

26. Steensma TD, Cohen-Kettenis PT. More than two developmental pathways in children with gender dysphoria? *J Am Acad Child Adolesc Psychiatry* 2015; 54: 147–148.

27. Steensma TD, Biemond R, de Boer F, Cohen-Kettenis PT. Desisting and persisting gender dysphoria after childhood: a qualitative follow-up study. *Clin Child Psychol Psychiatry* 2011; 16: 499–516.

28. Byne W, Bradley SJ, Coleman E, et al. Report of the American Psychiatric Association Task Force on Treatment of Gender Identity Disorder. *Arch Sex Behav* 2012; 41: 759–796.

29. Leibowitz S, de Vries ALC. Gender dysphoria in adolescence. *Int Rev Psychiatry* 2016; 28: 21–35.

30. Cohen-Kettenis PTPD, Van Goozen SHMPD. Sex reassignment of adolescent transsexuals: a follow-up study. *J Am Acad Child Adolesc Psychiatry* 1997; 36: 263–271.

31. Smith YLS, Van Goozen SHM, Kuiper AJ, Cohen-Kettenis PT. Sex reassignment: outcomes and predictors of treatment for adolescent and adult transsexuals. *Psychol Med* 2005; 35: 89–99.

32. de Vries AL, McGuire JK, Steensma TD, Wagenaar EC, Doreleijers TA, Cohen-Kettenis PT. Young adult psychological outcome after puberty suppression and gender reassignment. *Pediatrics* 2014; 134: 696–704.

33. Smith YLS, van Goozen SHM, Kuiper AJ, Cohen-Kettenis PT. Transsexual subtypes: clinical and theoretical significance. *Psychiatry Res* 2005; 137: 151–160.

34. Aitken M, Steensma TD, Blanchard R, et al. Evidence for an altered sex ratio in clinic-referred adolescents with gender dysphoria. *J Sex Med* 2015; 12: 756–763.

35. Gates G. How Many People are Lesbian, Gay, Bisexual and Transgender. Available at: https://williamsinstitute.law.ucla.edu/research/census-lgbt-demographics-studies/how-many-people-are-lesbian-gay-bisexual-and-transgender/ (accessed 20 March 2017).

36. Zucker KJ, Lawrence AA. Epidemiology of gender identity disorder: recommendations for the standards of care of the world professional association for transgender health. *Int J Transgenderism* 2009; 11: 8–18.

37. De Cuypere G, Van Hemelrijck M, Michel A, et al. Prevalence and demography of transsexualism in Belgium. *Eur Psychiatry* 2007; 22: 137–141.

38. Clark TC, Lucassen MF, Bullen P, et al. The health and well-being of transgender high school students: results from the New Zealand adolescent health survey (Youth'12). *J Adolesc Health* 2014; 55: 93–99.

39. Link BG, Phelan JC. Conceptualizing stigma. *Annu Rev Sociol* 2001; 27: 363–385.

40. Meyer IH. Prejudice, social stress, and mental health in lesbian, gay, and bisexual populations: conceptual issues and research evidence. *Psychol Bull* 2003; 129: 674–697.

41. White Hughto JM, Reisner SL, Pachankis JE. Transgender stigma and health: a critical review of stigma determinants, mechanisms, and interventions. *Soc Sci Med* 2015; 147: 222–231.

42. Hendricks ML, Testa RJ. A conceptual framework for clinical work with transgender and gender nonconforming clients: an adaptation of the Minority Stress Model. *Prof Psychol* 2012; 43: 460–467.

43. Marshal MP, Friedman MS, Stall R, et al. Sexual orientation and adolescent substance use: a meta-analysis and methodological review. *Addiction* 2008; 103: 546–556.

44. Herrick AL, Marshal MP, Smith HA, Sucato G, Stall RD. Sex while intoxicated: a meta-analysis comparing heterosexual and sexual minority youth. *J Adolesc Health* 2011; 48: 306–309.

45. Austin SB, Nelson LA, Birkett MA, Calzo JP, Everett B. Eating disorder symptoms and obesity at the intersections of gender, ethnicity, and sexual orientation in US high school students. *Am J Public Health* 2013; 103: e16–e22.

46. Friedman MS, Marshal MP, Guadamuz TE, et al. A meta-analysis of disparities in childhood sexual abuse, parental physical abuse, and peer victimization among sexual minority and sexual nonminority individuals. *Am J Public Health* 2011; 101: 1481–1494.

47. Marshal MP, Dietz LJ, Friedman MS, et al. Suicidality and depression disparities between sexual minority and heterosexual youth: a meta-analytic review. *J Adolesc Health* 2011; 49: 115–123.

48. Zhao Y, Montoro R, Igartua K, Thombs BD. Suicidal ideation and attempt among adolescents reporting 'unsure' sexual identity or heterosexual identity plus same-sex attraction or behavior: forgotten groups? *J Am Acad Child Adolesc Psychiatry* 2010; 49: 104–113.

49. Montoro R, Thombs B, Igartua KJ. [The association of bullying with suicide ideation, plan, and attempt among adolescents with GLB or unsure sexual identity, heterosexual identity with same-sex attraction or behavior, or heterosexual identity without same-sex attraction or behavior]. *Sante Ment Que* 2015; 40: 55–75 (in French).

50. Cenat JM, Blais M, Hebert M, Lavoie F, Guerrier M. Correlates of bullying in Quebec high school students: the vulnerability of sexual-minority youth. *J Affect Disord* 2015; 183: 315–321.

51. Almeida J, Johnson RM, Corliss HL, Molnar BE, Azrael D. Emotional Distress among LGBT youth: the influence of perceived discrimination based on sexual orientation. *J Youth Adolesc* 2009; 38: 1001–1014.

52. D'Augelli AR, Grossman AH, Starks MT. Childhood gender atypicality, victimization, and PTSD among lesbian, gay, and bisexual youth. *J Interpers Violence* 2006; 21: 1462–11482.

53. Birkett M, Espelage DL, Koenig B. LGB and questioning students in schools: the moderating effects of homophobic bullying and school climate on negative outcomes. *J Youth Adolesc* 2009; 38: 989–1000.

54. Bontempo DE, D'Augelli AR. Effects of at-school victimization and sexual orientation on lesbian, gay, or bisexual youths' health risk behavior. *J Adolesc Health* 2002; 30: 364–374.

55. Saewyc EM, Poon CS, Homma Y, Skay CL. Stigma management? The links between enacted stigma and teen pregnancy trends among gay, lesbian, and bisexual students in British Columbia. *Can J Hum Sex* 2008; 17: 123–139.

56. Rice E, Petering R, Rhoades H, et al. Cyberbullying perpetration and victimization among middle-school students. *Am J Public Health* 2015; 105: e66–e72.

57. Perren S, Dooley J, Shaw T, Cross D. Bullying in school and cyberspace: associations with depressive symptoms in Swiss and Australian adolescents. *Child Adolesc Psychiatry Ment Health* 2010; 4: 28.

58. Ryan C, Huebner D, Diaz RM, Sanchez J. Family rejection as a predictor of negative health outcomes in white and Latino lesbian, gay, and bisexual young adults. *Pediatrics* 2009; 123: 346–352.

59. D'Augelli AR, Hershberger SL, Pilkington NW. Lesbian, gay, and bisexual youth and their families: disclosure of sexual orientation and its consequences. *Am J Orthopsychiatry* 1998; 68: 361–371.

60. Rosario M, Schrimshaw EW, Hunter J. A model of sexual risk behaviors among young gay and bisexual men: longitudinal associations of mental health, substance abuse, sexual abuse, and the coming-out process. *AIDS Educ Prev* 2006; 18: 444–460.

61. Cochran BN, Stewart AJ, Ginzler JA, Cauce AM. Challenges faced by homeless sexual minorities: comparison of gay, lesbian, bisexual, and transgender homeless adolescents with their heterosexual counterparts. *Am J Public Health* 2002; 92: 773–777.

62. Coker TR, Austin SB, Schuster MA. The health and health care of lesbian, gay, and bisexual adolescents. *Annu Rev Public Health* 2010; 31: 457–477.

63. Rew L, Whittaker TA, Taylor-Seehafer MA, Smith LR. Sexual health risks and protective resources in gay, lesbian, bisexual, and heterosexual homeless youth. *J Spec Pediatr Nurs* 2005; 10: 11–19.

64. Herrick AL, Egan JE, Coulter RW, Friedman MR, Stall R. Raising sexual minority youths' health levels by incorporating resiliencies into health promotion efforts. *Am J Public Health* 2014; 104: 206–210.

65. Rostosky SS, Danner F, Riggle ED. Is religiosity a protective factor against substance use in young adulthood? Only if you're straight! *J Adolesc Health* 2007; 40: 440–447.

66. van Beusekom G, Bos HM, Overbeek G, Sandfort TG. Same-sex attraction, gender nonconformity, and mental health: the protective role of parental acceptance. *Psychol Sex Orientat Gend Divers* 2015; 2: 307–312.

67. Bergeron FA, Blais M, Hebert M. [The role of parental support in the relationship between homophobic bullying, internalized homophobia and psychological distress among sexual-minority youths (SMY): a moderated mediation approach]. *Sante Ment Que* 2015; 40: 109–127 (in French).

68. Shilo G, Antebi N, Mor Z. Individual and community resilience factors among lesbian, gay, bisexual, queer and questioning youth and adults in Israel. *Am J Community Psychol* 2015; 55: 215–227.

69. Goodenow C, Szalacha L, Westheimer K. School support groups, other school factors, and the safety of sexual minority adolescents. *Psychol Schs* 2006; 43: 573–589.

70. Hatzenbuehler ML, Birkett M, Van Wagenen A, Meyer IH. Protective school climates and reduced risk for suicide ideation in sexual minority youths. *Am J Public Health* 2014; 104: 279–286.

71. Hatzenbuehler ML, Keyes KM. Inclusive anti-bullying policies and reduced risk of suicide attempts in lesbian and gay youth. *J Adolesc Health* 2013; 53(1 Suppl.): S21–S26.

72. Hatzenbuehler ML. The social environment and suicide attempts in lesbian, gay, and bisexual youth. *Pediatrics* 2011; 127: 896–903.

73. Hatzenbuehler ML, Jun HJ, Corliss HL, Bryn Austin S. Structural stigma and sexual orientation disparities in adolescent drug use. *Addict Behav* 2015; 46: 14–18.

74. Reisner SL, Vetters R, Leclerc M, et al. Mental health of transgender youth in care at an adolescent urban community health center: a matched retrospective cohort study. *J Adolesc Health* 2015; 56: 274–279.

75. Veale JF, Watson RJ, Peter T, Saewyc EM. Mental health disparities among Canadian transgender youth. *J Adolesc Health* 2017; 60: 44–49.

76. Grossman AH, D'Augelli AR. Transgender youth and life-threatening behaviors. *Suicide Life Threat Behav* 2007; 37: 527–537.

77. Olson KR, Durwood L, DeMeules M, McLaughlin KA. Mental health of transgender children who are supported in their identities. *Pediatrics* 2016; 137: e20153223.

78. Hatzenbuehler ML, Pachankis JE. Stigma and minority stress as social determinants of health among lesbian, gay, bisexual, and transgender

youth: research evidence and clinical implications. *Pediatr Clin North Am* 2016; 63: 985–997.

79. Mustanski B, Birkett M, Greene GJ, Hatzenbuehler ML, Newcomb ME. Envisioning an America without sexual orientation inequities in adolescent health. *Am J Public Health* 2014; 104: 218–225.

80. Duncan DT, Hatzenbuehler ML. Lesbian, gay, bisexual, and transgender hate crimes and suicidality among a population-based sample of sexual-minority adolescents in Boston. *Am J Public Health* 2014; 104: 272–278.

81. Poteat V, Sinclair KO, DiGiovanni CD, Koenig BW, Russell ST. Gay–straight alliances are associated with student health: a multischool comparison of LGBTQ and heterosexual youth. *J Res Adolesc* 2013; 23: 319–330.

82. Steever JB, Cooper-Serber E. A review of gay, lesbian, bisexual, and transgender youth issues for the pediatrician. *Pediatr Ann* 2013; 42: 34–39.

83. Craig SL, Austin A, Alessi E. Gay affirmative cognitive behavioral therapy for sexual minority youth: a clinical adaptation. *Clin Soc Work J* 2013; 41: 258–266.

84. Wilkerson JM, Schick VR, Romijnders KA, Bauldry J, Butame SA, Montrose C. Social support, depression, self-esteem, and coping among LGBTQ adolescents participating in hatch youth. *Health Promot Pract* 2016; 23: 23.

85. Mustanski B, Greene GJ, Ryan D, Whitton SW. Feasibility, acceptability, and initial efficacy of an online sexual health promotion program for LGBT youth: the Queer Sex Ed intervention. *J Sex Res* 2015; 52: 220–230.

CHAPTER 28

Children and adolescents

Jessica L. Plauché and Bennett L. Leventhal

Introduction

Addressing matters related to child and adolescent mental health, particularly in the public context, is a relatively new concept. Until the late nineteenth century, children were largely considered to be property; they were more important as members of the family and community workforce than they were as developing members of society. Lacking basic human rights and societal protections, children could be victimized, maltreated, and even killed without legal repercussions. Indeed, global rates of child mortality were remarkably high until recent decades, resulting in little motivation for communities or caregivers to invest in nurturing the cognitive and emotional needs of their children during the first 5 years of life—a period that we now understand to be critical for brain development and future health outcomes. Hence, until recent times, there was no clear societal commitment to provide healthcare services for children, let alone address their mental health needs.

In the late nineteenth century, the field of paediatrics emerged as a specialized area of clinical medicine, and increasing knowledge and service within primary healthcare systems led to subsequent efforts to improve nutrition, fight infectious disease, and reduce childhood mortality. Global public health measures in the twentieth century resulted in the dissemination of effective vaccines, and evidence-based medications such as antibiotics and insulin, and proper hygiene; in more developed countries, improved access to maternal–infant care resulted in significantly reduced rates of early childhood mortality. While it is important that these achievements in public health measures continue for the rapidly increasing global population of children, a growing body of research over the last few decades has demonstrated that adequate health care must also include mental health. And, thus, from a public health perspective, in order to prevent illness effectively, reduce morbidity and mortality, and promote well-being in the twenty-first century, we must recognize that child and adolescent mental health is, indeed, a critical public health issue that deserves our fullest attention.

Until recently, various other public systems, in addition to health care, did not recognize that childhood and adolescence represents a special period of development. For example, major shifts in public legislation within the United States' criminal justice, education, and child protective systems supporting the notion that children and teenagers should not be treated as simply 'little adults' began little more than a century ago. Prior to the inauguration of the first juvenile court in Cook County, Illinois, in 1899, children over the age of 7 years were often tried and convicted as adults for criminal activity. The implementation of a separate juvenile justice system, with goals of rehabilitation rather than punishment, was

an important initial step in the public recognition that children and adolescents have a unique set of developmental and mental health needs that differ significantly from those of adults. Following shortly after the juvenile justice movement, compulsory public education became statutory across all states in the USA in 1918, although public laws did not provide the same rights for children with special needs or disabilities. It was not until 1975 that the US government determined that education was a *right* for *all* children by enacting Public Law (PL) 94-142, The Education for All Handicapped Children's Act, which required that all children receive a free and appropriate education, at public expense, in the least restrictive environment.

The history of progress in child protection laws against abuse and neglect is also a recent phenomenon. Prior to the nineteenth century, there seemed to be little concern about children being involved in forced labour and all manner of abuse. A landmark case in the USA took place in the mid-1800s when an abused child by the name of Mary Ellen Wilson was removed from her home and protected under 'The Prevention of Cruelty to Animals Act' because, at the time, although there were protections for animals, no such legal prohibitions against abuse existed with respect to the abuse of children [1]. And it was not until 1962, with the publication of C. Henry Kempe's paper, 'The battered-child syndrome' [2], that there was recognition of child abuse by the medical profession. This ultimately led to meaningful legislation to protect children in the USA.

Beyond the USA, global efforts to provide legal protections for basic human rights for children have only emerged in the last few decades. As an example, the United Nations Convention on the Rights of Children, the first international treaty designed to protect the human rights of children, was not ratified by the required number of nations until 1990. It was ultimately ratified by all members of the United Nations, except the USA, which has signed but not ratified it. For the first time, at an international level, children (defined by the Convention as those under the age of 18 years, with the exception of countries with national laws that specify an earlier age of majority) were recognized as deserving of human rights, while also placing protective responsibility on parents and governments. While it may seem to be a bit astonishing, it took two separate 'optional' protocols, in the year 2000, to protect children from two additional forms of abuse: (i) children could not be parties to war as combatants; and (ii) children could not be bought or sold.

With this brief history in mind, it is clear that concern about the 'public mental health' of children and adolescents is a relatively new concept with many elements evolving in the past century, and most in only the last few decades. Accordingly, there is much room for improvement in the public mental health of children and adolescents in both the developing and developed parts of our world.

Because this is such a broad topic with many possible areas for study and advancement, this chapter cannot be comprehensive. Instead, we have chosen to narrow our discussion to five selected, but important, areas, which represent the breadth but hardly the depth of the areas of study and progress: (i) developmental epidemiology; (ii) concepts of healthy development and mental well-being; (iii) access to care; (iv) adverse childhood experiences/child maltreatment; (v) paediatric psychopharmacology.

Developmental epidemiology

For much of the history of medicine, there has been little understanding or appreciation of the developmental aspects of disease and, in particular, the role of development in psychiatric illness. In fact, prior to the eighteenth century, there was little-to-no acknowledgement of childhood psychiatric illness in the medical or scientific literature. Explanations for childhood behavioural problems were often based on religious theories or the presence of supernatural phenomena. It was commonly believed that children were too young to have reasoning, manageable emotions, or the capacity to have mental illness. English physician–philosopher John Locke (1632–1704) posited that children entered the world as a blank slate or *tabula rasa*; that is, children were without the inherent capacity to develop reasoning or pathology and that one's mind and personality are entirely shaped by sensations and reflections from the environment [3]. Importantly, Locke also emphasized the need for more humane childrearing practices, suggesting that without nurture, children would suffer emotional damage. His ideas were later incorporated as a cornerstone of psychoanalytic theories of the late nineteenth and early twentieth centuries.

Psychoanalytically oriented theorists, such as Sigmund Freud (1856–1939), Anna Freud (1895–1982), Melanie Klein (1882–1960), Erik Erikson (1902–94), and Jean Piaget (1896–1980), to name but a few, were among the first to contextualize psychopathology developmentally by linking it with early childhood experiences. In this evolving work, various frameworks were proposed with the goal of understanding how the development of human drives, behaviours, emotions, and cognitions are associated with mental illness. However, aside from single case reports, at the time there was a limited scientific evidence base for many of these theories—psychoanalytical or otherwise. Indeed, some of these models were quite misleading. For example, in observing infants and their caregivers, Margaret Mahler (1897–1985) suggested that children progress through six developmental stages in order to individuate from caregivers. She initially suggested that there was a 'normal autistic' phase of development from birth to 2 months of age, during which infants are detached and self-absorbed as a means of self-protection from the chaos of the world. It was suggested that it was the mother's job to bring the child out of this isolation and into the bigger world, and that failure to do so was the cause of autism [4]. Mahler later abandoned the 'normal autistic' phase as advances in child development research disproved its existence, but the remnants of this notion remain. Similar suggestions about failures in parenting, especially by mothers, as a primary cause of developmental psychopathology were a part of the early conceptual

framework in the field. For example, the term 'schizophrenogenic mother' was used to suggest that schizophrenia resulted from maternal behaviour [5]. This misinformed attribution of causality to poor parenting practices has had a devastating and lasting impact on public perceptions of child and adolescent psychiatric disorders, as well as on those who have developed public policy.

In addition to gross historical misconceptions about the aetiology of childhood psychiatric disorders, their prevalence and clinical presentation were also not well understood. Prior to the publication of the Diagnostic and Statistical Manual of Mental Disorders, Third Edition (DSM-III), which incorporated a group of disorders 'usually first present in infancy, childhood, or adolescence', including autistic disorder, reactive attachment disorder, and separation anxiety disorder, to name a few, there was little attention paid to a nosology for mental disorders relevant to children [6]; official classifications in DSM, Second Edition (DSM-II), referred only to 'behavioral disorders of childhood and adolescence' [7]. Furthermore, it was often inaccurately assumed that children could not be informants about their own thoughts and behaviours. One such example was the notion that children lacked the capacity to have depression. Only in the 1960s and 1970s did it become apparent that mood disorders and a wide range of psychopathology could be present in childhood and adolescence [8]. Indeed, the last 40 years have seen the application of increasingly sophisticated scientific methods that have been successful in demonstrating that developmental psychopathology is driven by a complex and dynamic interplay between genetic predispositions and the social and physical environment.

Over the last four or five decades there has been a revolution in concepts of developmental psychopathology, with validation of a specific nosology and clinical presentation for childhood and adolescent psychiatric disorders. With advancements in a commonly accepted nosology has come an opportunity to conduct epidemiological studies of the prevalence of psychiatric disorders in paediatric populations. This began with the landmark Isle of Wight study, in which nearly all children living on the island (*n* = 2307) who were born during a 2-year period (from September 1953 to August 1955) were screened for psychiatric and educational problems, using standardized teacher and parent questionnaires (such questionnaires were also a novelty) [9]. The same cohort was again assessed in adolescence (aged 14–15 years) and in adulthood (aged 44–45 years). Of note, the population living on the island, located off the southern coast of England, was and continues to be broadly representative of the UK's population today. The authors of the study found the overall rate of psychiatric disorders in children aged 9–11 years to be 6–8%, and also demonstrated the validity of standard assessment questionnaires in the diagnosis of childhood-onset psychiatric disorders. Many other longitudinal studies, such as the National Institutes of Health National Comorbidity Studies, and the Great Smoky Mountains Study, have demonstrated that psychiatric disorders in children are highly prevalent and often continuous over time; children who have a disorder at an early period are at least three times more likely to suffer from a psychiatric disorder at follow-up and that comorbidity with two or more concomitant diagnoses is common. Not surprisingly, differences in developmental trajectories of disorders have been found to be different between males and females [10, 11].

Recent epidemiological studies have demonstrated that not only is child and adolescent psychopathology common, but it is also highly likely to be an antecedent to psychopathology in adulthood [12]. Many of the most prevalent psychiatric problems—including depressive disorders, anxiety disorders, substance abuse, suicidal ideation, self-injurious behaviours, and suicide attempts—are first present in childhood and adolescence. In landmark work by Ronald Kessler, Kathleen Merikangas, and colleagues, it was demonstrated that 48% of the population has a diagnosable psychiatric disorder at some point in their lifetime. More striking is the finding that 50% of all psychiatric disorders begin before the age of 14 years and 75% begin before the age of 24 years [13, 14]. Reported rates of the global point prevalence of any childhood psychiatric disorder vary between studies, although best estimates demonstrate that 20–40% of all children worldwide have a clinically diagnosable psychiatric disorder, and that even more children demonstrate subclinical problems [15–17]. While these remarkable findings have changed the public, clinical, and scientific views of child and adolescent psychiatric disorders, there have not been adequate improvements in policy or professional training—particularly for primary care practitioners, who are often the sole providers of mental health care for children, despite insufficient training in this area of practice—thus adding to the public health burden associated with childhood-onset psychiatric disorders.

Psychiatric illness is now among the greatest causes of lifetime health-related burden for people aged 10–24 years. The leading causes of disability-adjusted life years for this age group include unipolar depressive disorders (8.2%), road traffic accidents (5.4%), schizophrenia (4.1%), bipolar disorder (3.8%), and violence (3.5%) [18, 19]. Longitudinal studies have found that childhood depression is associated with academic problems, suicidal behaviour, substance abuse, welfare dependence, and unemployment later in life [20, 21]. Furthermore, psychiatric illnesses are associated with other adverse health outcomes by increasing the risk for communicable and non-communicable diseases, and contributing to intentional and accidental injury [22].

Some have argued against these findings, whereas others have raised concerns about epidemics of disorders such as autism spectrum disorder with best-estimated prevalence rates of 2.2–2.6%—a threefold increase from 0.8% in the last 30 years. However, careful studies of autism spectrum disorder and other psychiatric diagnoses (attention deficit hyperactivity disorder (ADHD), anorexia nervosa) indicate that rather than rising incidence, better identification and case finding are likely to be the principal causes of advances in prevalence.

In summary, the very fact that methods now exist for epidemiological studies of developmental psychopathology is a major advance. The developmental epidemiology of psychiatric disorders allows for several critical conclusions:

1. Psychiatric disorders are among the most common causes of morbidity and impairment in all human populations—children, adolescents, and adults.

2. Many, if not most, psychiatric illnesses present in adults are likely to be developmental disorders that begin early in life.

3. Owing to their high prevalence, severity, and chronicity, child and adolescent psychiatric disorders comprise one of the most significant public health burdens in the world and, given the lack of services, represent a global public mental health crisis.

4. Prevention and early intervention for developmental psychopathology has the potential to reduce the lifetime burden of overall (psychiatric *and* medical) morbidity and mortality.

5. More evidence-based strategies and additional resources that are broadly available around the world (not just in urban areas) are needed to reduce this enormous burden of disease through prevention, early intervention, and chronic disease models of care.

Concepts of healthy development and mental well-being

While interest in child and adolescent health, and in particular mental health, is a relatively recent phenomenon, the rapid expansion of knowledge in developmental neuroscience, developmental psychology, and other disciplines has offered a solid base on which to build a structure for understanding typical, healthy development and its perturbations. The rapidly expanding conceptual framework is opening up new opportunities for guidance with respect to supporting healthy development, as well as prevention of disorders.

Childhood and adolescence begins with conception and, by various definitions, ends sometime between 18 and 26 years of age. It is the period in the human life cycle during which the most rapid change and growth occurs in all developmental domains. As children and young people grow up, they acquire increasingly sophisticated motor, cognitive, social, and emotional skills and capacities; they transition from being completely dependent on caretakers for survival to functioning as relatively autonomous individuals. This distinctive progression through typical developmental milestones is mediated by brain development, which involves a complex and dynamic interplay between an individual's genes and environment. During this process, small and large perturbations have the potential to create profound and lasting impacts on the trajectory of one's lifelong health and well-being. As an example, adverse childhood experiences, including child maltreatment, often have long-lasting consequences on both physical and psychological health outcomes in adulthood. When examining health and wellness, it is also important to consider the types of stimulation, experiences, caregiving, and interventions that are necessary and/or sufficient for human development to go 'right'. In other words, what promotes children's health and well-being, and what can be done to ameliorate disruptions in development in order to improve a child's capacity for adaptive functioning?

Mental well-being is not simply the absence of psychopathology [23]. According to the World Health Organization, 'a state of well-being [is one] in which every individual realizes his or her own potential, can cope with the normal stresses of life, can work productively, and is able to contribute to their community'[24]. However, this definition, with its emphasis on realizing one's potential and working productively, appears more applicable to adults. Child development takes place within a complex network of systems, often including a child's family, educational system, peers, community, and broader cultural influences. Therefore, a definition of mental well-being for children and adolescents must include the context of the cultural norms, values, and expectations of the important systems at play in the child's life, and how well they align and interact with each other and with the child's own emerging sense of self/identity (values, coping strategies, strengths, activities, etc.). There are individual, family, and contextual factors that are associated with mental well-being for children and adolescents [25]. One large cohort study in the UK included over 12,000 eleven-year-old children to examine a variety of ecological factors (including individual characteristics such as gender and ethnicity, socio-economic status, perceived socio-economic status, cognitive factors, health factors, family structure, home environment, parent health, social relationships, and wider environmental factors.) Using these data, investigators calculated separate standardized mental illness and well-being scores for all participants. The authors, Patalay and Fitzsimons [26], found that mental illness and well-being scores were weakly correlated among the children in the study, suggesting that these concepts should be considered separately. For example, while some variables were associated with higher levels of mental illness symptoms and a corresponding decrease in overall well-being (e.g. residing in a single-parent household, being bullied by siblings, and having peer problems), other determinants differed in the degree to which they were associated to mental illness and well-being. In general, well-being for children in this age group was more closely associated with positive social relationships and environmental factors (e.g. school connectedness and the perception of living in a safe neighbourhood), whereas greater mental illness symptoms were more closely correlated with communication difficulties, special education needs, chronic illness, frequent altercations with caregivers, and difficulties in peer relationships. Notably, higher family income was correlated with lower levels of mental illness but not with positive well-being. Perhaps even more interesting was that perceived inequality (and particularly when perceived to be wealthier than peers) was one of the strongest determinants associated with lower well-being scores. These findings make a clearer case that the absence of mental illness is not equivalent to having a positive sense of well-being (and vice versa).

Considering recent global trends that generally threaten the health and wellness of young people (e.g. poverty, political unrest, isolation, terrorism, child trafficking, forced migration, consumerism to the point of disregard for the natural environment) [27], it may appear easier and more important to focus efforts on improving underlying structural barriers and social conditions that are known to perpetuate negative health outcomes rather than consider the elements of wellness or positive mental health. However, a growing body of public mental health research argues that both are necessary, important, and not mutually exclusive. For example, despite growing up with various types of adversity, it is still possible for individuals to demonstrate incredible resilience, successfully navigate through challenging experiences, and ultimately achieve a sense of mental well-being.

In order to have the greatest opportunity for healthy development and mental well-being, children should be provided with certain basic needs by their caregivers and the broader community and ecological framework in which they live. As the head is still a part of the body, the necessities of good physical development will help the brain in its developmental journey. This begins well before pregnancy and includes family planning and for prospective mothers to be of proper childbearing age before conceiving. While outcomes for the child and mother certainly depend on a variety of factors, a growing body of literature has found that children of teenage mothers are more likely to experience a variety of negative developmental outcomes, such as violent and non-violent criminal convictions, poor academic performance, and problems related to

substance abuse [28–31]. Family planning not only allows women to prepare for pregnancy, but also to have appropriate inter-pregnancy intervals necessary for the physical and mental health of the baby and the mother. This should be followed by good prenatal care, which includes nutrition and appropriate professional supervision of the pregnancy, and interventions when necessary. Early postnatal care includes adequate nutrition for the mother and child (with encouragement of breastfeeding), clean and sanitary conditions (including clean water), vaccinations, maintenance of homeostasis (temperature, satiation, etc.), and regular follow-up with primary healthcare providers to monitor developmental progress in the child and the family, and provide anticipatory guidance for caregivers. Monitoring for developmental milestones is crucial, along with early interventions, which includes screening for maternal depression and connecting mothers with appropriate treatment for postpartum depression when needed.

The brain does not develop well under conditions of under- or overstimulation (which includes all five senses plus somatic sensations). From the first days of life, children's brains are hardwired for social learning, and require interesting, varied, and appropriate stimuli, which is mediated through secure bonding and attachment with primary caregivers; accordingly, caregiver attunement and responsiveness is associated with higher infant cognitive ability and reduced levels of early behavioural problems [32]. The need for age-appropriate stimulation and experiences continues throughout childhood and adolescence. There are two extremes from this standard that create high risk for poor development outcomes. The first is virtually no stimulation during early, critical periods in development. First observed in rhesus monkeys by Harry and Margaret Harlow [33], and modelled at a cellular level studying the visual cortex in kittens in the Nobel Prize-winning work by David Hubel and Torsten Wiesel [34], stimulation is necessary for the brain to develop properly. The devastating clinical manifestations resulting from a lack of stimulation was observed by Rene Spitz in his descriptions of emotional deprivation (which he referred to as 'anaclitic depression') in hospitalized infants and later observed in the Romanian Adoptees Study, where the absence of physical contact and other necessary stimulation during a critical early period yielded disastrous results [35, 36]. At the other extreme is overstimulation, which can lead to stress that the developing child is ill-equipped to manage. Prolonged, severe, or unpredictable stress in one's environment, associated with perceived lack of physical and psychological safety, interferes with a child's ability to maintain homeostasis and leaves the protective systems such as the autonomic nervous and other systems depleted or unresponsive, and disrupts cellular migration and dendrification [37].

In addition to appropriately dosed and varied stimulation, children also need consistency and predictability in their environments. Schedules and routines for basic activities, such as regular meals, sleep, and social interactions, are crucial. These social interactions begin in the home with primary caretakers and immediate family, and rapidly expand to extended family and members of the community, including peers. Thus, having a place to call home that is relatively safe and reliable in structure, where one does not have to be constantly vigilant about environmental threats, enables children to be curious about their surrounding environment and use their brains in more creative ways to learn about the world around them. This is augmented by access to adequate nutrition, education, and health care, and so on, all of which serves to reinforce this developmental progress.

In recent decades, there have been significant advances in the understanding of brain development, resulting in a greater appreciation of the importance of the prenatal period and the first few years of life. A more detailed account of brain development is beyond the scope of this chapter; what follows is a broad overview. Brain development, characterized by a series of overlapping processes, begins shortly after conception and continues into early adulthood. The major processes include (i) neurogenesis (production of brain cells or neurons); (ii) migration (neurons move to their final destination); (iii) neuronal differentiation (growth of axons and dendrites); (iv) synaptogenesis (forming connections/networks with other cells); (v) pruning and apoptosis (refining and downsizing the number of neurons and connections); and (vi) myelination and/or gliagenesis (important for speeding up connections/communication). Babies are born with approximately 100 billion neurons, much more than the adult brain, and with the exception of neurons in the olfactory bulb, neurogenesis peaks in the third to fourth prenatal months and substantially declines after, roughly, the second trimester. As a result of synaptogenesis, connectivity between neurons increases from approximately 2500 synapses per neuron at birth to roughly 15,000 synapses per neuron by 2–3 years of age. The phrase 'neurons that fire together wire together' underlies the process of synaptic pruning, during which the synapses that are used are strengthened and those that are not used are ultimately eliminated. Additionally, programmed cell death, or apoptosis, results in the planned pruning of approximately 40–60% of redundant neurons (depending on the brain region) after birth. The final step, myelination of the frontal lobes, occurs primarily during adolescence and into early adulthood. Each of these steps is essential to the successful development of well-being in the child. And each reflects a complex set of interactions between genes and other biological events, as well as powerful interactions between the biological processes and the environment: biology alters experience and experience alters biology [38].

The complexity of brain development creates a cradle of opportunity when it comes to wellness, healthy development, and mental well-being. It does not happen by accident and we are far enough along scientifically to appreciate the major risk factors, as well as those that will foster health development and even resilience—the ultimate goal for all developing individuals.

Taken together, healthy development and well-being, as well as good health, are the result of a complex but thoroughly integrated process. It is the primary responsibility of parents and other caregivers but requires the support of a robust set of public, environmental, and social supports and policies—parents cannot complete this process alone. When successful, healthy development creates enormous potential for individuals and communities. However, when development is disrupted, the potential outcomes can be devastating on an individual and societal level. Public commitment to healthy child and adolescent development is the best preventive exercise and a necessity for all communities and nations.

Access to care

Despite the massive public health burden associated with child and adolescent psychiatric disorders, most healthcare systems around the world are not adequately responding to this crisis [39]. A report

by the World Health Organization, *Mental Health Atlas 2011*, indicated that there are significant discrepancies between high-income countries and low-and-middle-income countries with respect to child and adolescent mental health needs and resources for treatment [40]. In a multicentre study of service use in Brazil, it was found that less than 20% of youth with psychiatric disorders accessed any care in the previous 12 months [41]. However, even in high-income countries, there are significant delays in accessing any type of treatment and high rates of unmet need for mental health services. A study examining three nationally representative household surveys in the USA found that nearly 80% of children and adolescents in need of mental health services *did not receive any type of care* [42]. Even when children with mental health disorders are referred for services, many do not receive appropriate treatment. As an example, one study demonstrated that approximately half of children with identified ADHD receiving treatment in mental healthcare settings in the USA did not receive care that followed recommended treatment guidelines [43]. Furthermore, children with psychiatric disorders are often identified and initially 'treated' in the education, social service (child welfare), or juvenile/adult justice systems, which historically have not been collaborative or well-informed by evidence-based mental health practices [44, 45]. Indeed, even in the USA, the largest public psychiatric treatment facilities are the jail and prison systems [46].

There is a major discrepancy between the need for mental health services and the availability of trained service providers for the majority of the global population of young people. There are approximately 2.2 billion children and adolescents under the age of 18 years in the world—roughly a third of the world population—and 90% reside in low-and-middle income countries where there are scarce resources for many services, especially mental health. By comparison, there are only approximately 20,000 child and adolescent psychiatrists in the world, with an estimated 50% of these residing in the USA, where most settle in urban, affluent areas and go into private practice. Even in a developed country such as the USA, there are thousands of counties without access to a single child and adolescent psychiatrist. And many of these counties do not have child psychologists, social workers, and other professional service providers appropriately trained to address the mental health needs of children. This situation is even more abysmal elsewhere in the world. India, the second most populous country in the world, has fewer than 10 child psychiatrists and, as of 2005, in the whole of Sub-Saharan Africa excluding South Africa, there were fewer than 10 psychiatrists who were trained to work with children.

The current situation is nothing short of an international healthcare crisis. And this crisis will get worse because the lack of providers to diagnose and treat developmental psychopathology makes it appear as though 'it does not exist'; and 'if it does not exist' it is not a problem to the healthcare systems, policymakers, and others charged with improving public health.

The United States' Federal Bureau of Health Professions has declared child and adolescent psychiatry as the most underserved field of all medical subspecialties for a good reason, and this only serves to reinforce the reality that public mental health with respect to children and adolescents is a major problem for healthcare systems worldwide [47, 48].

It is apparent that barriers to access for care include (i) a dearth of adequately trained providers; (ii) the maldistribution of child and adolescent psychiatrists with respect to countries, as well as urban versus non-urban settings; (iii) a dearth of appropriate public policy and resources to support the development of public mental health systems for children and adolescents; (iv) fragmented models of care that do not integrate child mental health services into other systems of care for children (including other healthcare systems, education, child welfare and juvenile justice systems); and (v) pervasive stigma and misinformation regarding psychiatric illness, in general, but more specifically, child and adolescent psychiatric illness.

There is no easy solution to the monumental challenges we face with global shortages of professionals and many other reasons (e.g. geographical, organizational, and economic) for limiting access to child and adolescent mental health services. It is probably not realistic to think that, in the near future, there will be enough child psychiatrists and psychologists trained or distributed appropriately to address the world's growing population of children, nor will there be adequately disseminated global public policy changes or increases in resources and collaboration between systems of care.

Given the many barriers, a public health approach is the only logical strategy to promote mental well-being, prevent mental illness, and improve health outcomes and access to care. A fundamental tenet of this approach must include the recognition that for all people, and particularly for children and adolescents, the pursuit of health and mental well-being is closely tied to social justice and human rights [49]. Furthermore, it is important to highlight the indivisibility between physical and mental health and the fact that *there is no health without mental health* [50]. To meaningfully improve public health across the lifespan, policies are needed that address children's basic environmental needs, which include reducing poverty, providing universal education, providing primary health care (including vaccines), and access to clean water and adequate nutrition [51]. Additional recommendations include improving education and training for those on the 'front lines' in the community who are working with children—including primary care providers, teachers, social workers, and parents. Efforts should also be mobilized to change public perceptions of mental illness. It should be seen as a part of 'physical' and neurological illness. Finally, efforts must be undertaken to address pernicious bias and stigma against those with psychiatric illness, including stopping the attribution of 'blame' and discrimination toward individuals who are in need treatment.

Adverse childhood experiences

Child maltreatment is a serious public health concern around the world [52, 53]. Estimates of the past-year prevalence of violence against children taken from 38 reports, representing 96 countries, revealed that globally, over 50% of all children, aged 2–17 years—*one billion children worldwide*—experienced at least one type of violent victimization [54]. An international study, which included 24 developing countries, indicated that, on average, 63% of caregivers reported that a household member had used physical violence with their child during the past month, ranging from 28% in Bosnia and Herzegovina to 84% in Jamaica [55]. While physical discipline seems to be largely less effective than other means of discipline and is potentially dangerous, it is important to note that there are cultural differences in the acceptability of the use of physical discipline in childrearing. This affects both social and legal definitions of what constitutes physical abuse and maltreatment

and, by extension, the data from different countries and cultures. The existing literature uses various names for child maltreatment, including but not limited to childhood trauma, child abuse, adverse childhood experiences (ACEs), and, put more simply, violence. For the purposes of this chapter, we have chosen to use these terms interchangeably as they reflect a spectrum of events that may have a significant adverse impact on child and adolescent development. These include physical, sexual, and emotional forms of abuse, neglect, maltreatment, or exploitation, as well as exposure to violence between adults. The groundbreaking Adverse Childhood Experiences Study by Vincent J. Felitti and colleagues identified 10 categories of adverse events, which, in addition to those already listed, included living with household members with a history of substance abuse, mental illness, or incarceration [56]. The authors of the study found a strong association between the cumulative number of ACE exposures and the risk of later developing some of the leading causes of morbidity and mortality.

Unfortunately, these adverse childhood experiences and the negative consequences they may have on a child's well-being often go unrecognized [57]. As an example, a global meta-analysis, including 10 million children, estimated that, compared with official reports, the actual self-reported prevalence of child sexual abuse is over 30 times higher and over 75 times higher for physical abuse [58, 59].

The failure to recognize ACEs as a major public mental health concern comes at a great cost to society from a moral and ethical perspective: it is an outrageous indignity not to protect children from harm. If that were not enough, from a socio-economic perspective, such damage to children has a huge societal and economic cost. Rigorous economic studies indicate that the lifelong consequences of childhood exposure to violence result in $120 billion annually in lost productivity in the USA and up to 3.5% of the gross domestic product in subregions of East Asia [60]. A burgeoning body of literature on the topic of ACEs and resulting neurobiological underpinnings has helped improve our understanding of the mechanisms connecting ACEs with lifelong adverse outcomes. In turn, this improvement in understanding has led to growing evidence for effective approaches to prevention and intervention.

It is important to recognize that exposure to a traumatic experience can have a variable impact on an individual's functioning and that adverse events often occur in the lives of most individuals [61]. Fortunately, the majority of individuals who experience a discrete traumatic event do not subsequently develop adverse health consequences or psychopathology, such as post-traumatic stress disorder. An individual's stress response to adversity depends largely on the nature of the traumatic experience (in terms of timing, severity, frequency, and proximity in space and time), characteristics of the individual (developmental, genetic, and neurobiological), the environmental context, and the available social supports, or lack thereof. Compared with adults, children are more vulnerable to the effects of adversity by nature of their age, lack of experience, and still-developing cognitive functioning. Children rely on the adults in their lives for protection and security, and in the face of certain adverse experiences, may develop greater feelings of powerlessness and loss of control.

Advances in developmental neuroscience have begun to illuminate the mechanisms that drive the normative process of child brain development, as well as the changes in brain architecture and function that can result from chronic and repeated adverse experiences. There has been increasing interest in the concept of *allostatic load* [62], a term that refers to the process by which chronic or repeated stress results in the dysregulation and potentially irreversible physiologic disruptions, especially affecting the biological stress-regulatory systems. Additionally, an increasing number of longitudinal studies have shown that the graduated experience of enduring multiple (i.e. ≥ 3) forms of adverse experiences (i.e. ACEs) in the early childhood period increases an individual's risk of lifelong difficulties in a dose–response fashion with educational achievement, economic productivity, health status, and mortality. The Fragile Families and Child Wellbeing Study, a prospective cohort study, followed nearly 5000 children born between 1998 and 2000 in urban US settings, with follow-up interviews with parents 1, 3, 5, and 9 years after the child's birth (recorded ACEs reported in the mother's 5-year follow-up interview and teacher-reported school performance in the child's last month of kindergarten) [63]. A secondary analysis of data from this study sample included 1007 children and demonstrated that experiencing three or more ACEs in the first 5 years of life was associated with teacher-reported delays in language, literacy, and mathematic skills, as well as attention problems, social problems, and aggression [64].

Multiple studies have suggested that childhood exposure to one type of ACE increases the risk of exposure to additional ACEs, as well as the risk of repeated exposure over time. This can lead to *toxic stress*, defined as the extreme, frequent, or extended activation of the stress response system that causes distress for the child and may lead to negative psychological and physiological results, as well as a variety of adverse health outcomes [65].

Based on current research, exposure to ACEs allows for modest ability to estimate risk to children with a variety of exposures in the course of development. Other longitudinal studies over the last 50 years have identified an even broader group of primary risk factors for childhood psychopathology and other adverse outcomes, including poverty, malnutrition, loss of caregivers (through death, illness, or domestic disruptions), neglectful or abusive caregiving, directly experiencing or witnessing violence, parental mental illness, homelessness, community disasters, early pregnancy, neonatal complications, refugee status, and exposure to war. Despite trends toward economic improvement in many parts of the world, poverty continues to affect a disproportionate number of children globally, as children represent one-third of the world population but comprise 50% of those living in extreme poverty. One in five American children (or 21.3% of those under 18 years of age) lives in poverty [66]. Studies have shown that this same percentage of children raised with low socio-economic status will endure more than half of the medical and psychiatric morbidities within the population, and will consume the majority of American health and dental care expenses [67]. Growing up in poverty is also correlated with numerous other adverse outcomes that can negatively affect mental health, including lower educational achievement, decreased earning potential, limited access to health care, malnutrition, parental divorce or separation, and higher rates of exposure to violence [68].

The mechanisms by which adverse childhood experiences increase the risk for poor health outcomes are not yet fully understood. Indeed, more research is needed to help identify if there are particularly sensitive periods for the effects of early 'trauma' or stress; this will then allow for the identification of appropriate methods and timing for interventions. To accomplish this there will be a need to better understand the undoubtedly complex interplay between an individual's neurobiology/genetics and the developmental parameters that affect vulnerability to psychopathology.

Felitti proposed the following [69]: two broad mechanisms exist by which adverse childhood experiences transform into biomedical disease:

- disease as the delayed consequence of various coping devices like overeating, smoking, drug use, and promiscuity; for example, ACEs → depression or anxiety → overeating → type 2 diabetes → coronary artery disease;

- disease caused by chronic stress mediated by chronic hypercortisolemia and proinflammatory cytokines; for example, chronic headache or back pain, primary pulmonary fibrosis, osteoporosis, coronary artery disease.

It appears that there is a tremendous public health opportunity associated with interventions that reduce the risk for developmental psychopathology and other adverse outcomes for those children who have been exposed to excessive stress, ACEs, and/or traumatic events. In the current world, public mental health must pay particular attention to those children and adolescents living in poverty, those who are victims of war and/or exposed to chronic, high levels of violence, and those who are refugees. These are the children who are often 'missed' by traditional public mental health systems.

As with most public health strategies, the first efforts should be clearly focused on prevention—providing safe, healthy environments for developing children and adolescents. The second set of strategies should target early assessment and early intervention for children and adolescents exposed to adverse events; this will require the use of evidence-based tools in the hands or properly trained personnel. Whenever possible, this work should include family members, as well as the affected child (particularly in the case of caregiver illness); in addition to therapies, for most children appropriate nutrition, clean water, sanitation, and general health care will be necessary. This should also include re-establishment of stability and routines in the life of the child with school and age and culturally appropriate education and social opportunities.

ACEs are critical events that affect the lives of children and families. As this is a pervasive matter that affects families from all countries, rich and poor, prevention programmes must be universally available, as should evidence-based interventions. This is clearly a case in which the field knows what to do but lack public policy support and the resources to do it.

Paediatric psychopharmacology

The history of child and adolescent psychiatry has largely focused on psychological and psychosocial intervention, even more so than adult psychiatry. Indeed, there was a brief period of time in the 1970s when a medical internship was not felt to be necessary for psychiatrists and it was, hence, not required by the American Board of Psychiatry and Neurology. That situation has changed dramatically with the advent of psychopharmacology, primarily for adult psychiatric disorders, with downward extension into child and adolescent psychiatry. This is ironic as one of the first truly effective psychotropic medications was used in children. In his 1937 paper,

Charles Bradley wrote about the relatively successful use of the stimulant, Benzedrine, in the treatment of behavior problems [70]:

> The most striking change in behavior occurred in the school activities … of these patients. There appeared a definite 'drive' to accomplish as much as possible. Fifteen of the 30 children responded to Benzedrine by becoming distinctly subdued in their emotional responses … this was an improvement from the social viewpoint.

In retrospect, this landmark paper raised questions about what was developmentally appropriate and inappropriate behaviour and to what extent medical interventions were appropriate for behaviour concerns in youth. While Bradley was clear that medications should play a supportive role in the care of children, it marked the beginning of changes in care for children in which some physicians became 'psychopharmacologists' playing little or no role in other aspects of the evaluation and treatment of children and adolescents.

The use of psychotropic medications to treat psychiatric illness in children and adolescents has significantly increased in the past four decades, particularly in the USA [71, 72]. As the result of an explosion in research on 'paediatric psychopharmacology' there are data to support the use of psychotropic medications for a wide variety of child and adolescent psychiatric disorders, including ADHD, depression and anxiety (particularly when moderate to severe or treatment refractory), obsessive–compulsive disorder, Tourette's disorder, bipolar disorder, autism spectrum disorder and childhood-onset schizophrenia [73]. The most commonly prescribed classes of psychotropic medications for children and adolescents include stimulant, antidepressant (primarily the selective serotonin reuptake inhibitors), and antipsychotic medications, as well as various mood stabilizers, including lithium and valproic acid. Many large-scale placebo-controlled studies have shown encouraging evidence for medication treatments for children and adolescents. The number and quality of these studies are too numerous to review, but the reader is directed to a selected group of seminal studies for consideration:

1. CAMS—the Child/Adolescent Anxiety Multimodal Study [74].

2. CoLT—the Collaborative Lithium Trials for bipolar disorder in children [75].

3. MTA—Multimodal Treatment Study of Children with ADHD [76].

4. PATS—Preschool ADHD Treatment Study + (PATS 6 Year Follow-up) [77].

5. POTS I and POTS II—Pediatric OCD Treatment Study [78].

6. Risperidone for Core Symptom Domains of Autism [79].

7. TADS—the Treatment for Adolescents with Depression Study [80].

8. TASA—the Treatment of Adolescent Suicide Attempters Study [81].

9. TEAM—the Treatment of Early-Age Mania [82].

10. TEOSS—treatment of Early Onset Schizophrenia Study [83].

11. TORDIA—treatment of Resistant Depression in Adolescents [84].

There are certainly many other studies to consider. But, based on this growing body of work, there is a strong consensus that psychopharmacology can play a critical role in the care of children and adolescents with psychiatric disorders. However, there is some

controversy, as well. This is for many reasons, including the lack of biological markers for disorders and treatment responses, limited data on long-term outcomes, and significant side effects in some instances. This is further complicated by a variety of clinical features, including syndromal heterogeneity, high rates of comorbidity, and, of course, stigma and bias that limit insurance coverage and availability of medications.

What does remain clear is that, when prescribed and monitored properly by a trained professional, medications can be an important, if not life-saving component of the treatment of psychiatric disorders in children and adolescents. This is even more compelling when the medications are combined with other evidence-based therapeutic interventions; together, a combined approach can often alleviate suffering and expedite recovery from psychiatric illness.

While medications alone as treatment are rarely warranted, the relative ease of dispensing a prescription and the lack of trained personnel to both monitor treatment outcomes, as well as administer other evidence-based treatments, there is a disturbing and growing trend to 'just prescribe'. Public and private payers of psychiatric services often cover medications but significantly limit access to other services. This creates a problem for patients and practitioners and, in particular, often makes it impossible to follow evidence-based practice parameters or guidelines. There are additional challenges facing the evidence-based, ethical use of psychotropic medications in children and adolescents:

1. Many psychotropic medications are prescribed for children and adolescents 'off-label'; this means that they are not approved as safe and effective by the relevant regulatory agency with regard to a given age, indication, dose, safety, administration form, or duration of treatment for a particular disorder or symptom [85]. Furthermore, some off-label prescriptions have alarmingly limited evidence to support their use.

2. Despite an improved understanding and evidence base for the short-term efficacy and safety of some classes of psychotropic medications for young people, few controlled studies have investigated the long-term safety and efficacy outcomes of psychotropic medications or of multi-class psychotropic treatment regimens.

3. There have been increasing trends toward 'polypharmacy' or co-prescribing two or more medications for young populations. This includes the use of multiple medications in the same class for which there is no evidence.

4. The increasing rate of prescribing medications (often stimulant medications) for certain populations of children—e.g. preschool-age children, as well as higher percentages of children in institutional settings or foster care—is particularly worrisome [86].

5. The increased use of atypical antipsychotic medications in paediatric patients appears to be a developing problem as this class of medications has been shown to increase the risk for obesity and metabolic problems [87–89].

In the final analysis, psychotropic medications appear to play an ever-expanding role in the treatment of the entire spectrum of psychiatric disorders in children and adolescents. As the evidence becomes available, medications can and should be fully integrated in the treatment armamentarium for children and adolescents. While some extremists argue that we are 'drugging children', there are effective medications that can be used safely in the care of children and adolescents. To not use them when indicated is as unethical as it is to use the medications inappropriately. For many reasons, the future of paediatric psychopharmacology is promising if the research continues and professionals are trained to provide evidence-based treatments.

Public health concerns regarding the safety and efficacy of medications for paediatric populations has led to important governmental regulations and legislation. As public mental health policies evolve, it is critical that the practice of psychopharmacology be integrated into child and adolescent mental health care research, training, and public policy. This should be intrinsic to the standard of care for children. Such public policies must include the availability of psychotropic medication for which there is a solid evidence base, just as there should be access to other evidenced-based treatments. And, finally, public policies should be developed to make sure that medications and other forms of treatment can be provided jointly so as to improve the outcomes for children and adolescents with psychiatric disorders.

Child and adolescent mental health is a relatively new concern in the public arena. Despite this short history, there has been tremendous progress on this long and arduous journey. Our understanding of the requisites for mental health and wellness in developing children and adolescents has improved enormously, and neuroscience (developmental, behavioural, and cognitive), as well as environmental science and psychology, along with the other social sciences, are advancing rapidly. Concepts of normal development and its perturbations are changing rapidly as is the evidence base for prevention, diagnosis, and treatment of psychiatric disorders. These changes will lead to novel, evidence-based interventions that will greatly improve the lives of children and adolescents around the world.

As the complexity of human biology has grown, especially with respect to the central nervous system, it has become clear that simple mechanistic, molecular, or cellular models will likely yield much more limited progress in understanding basic human biology, as well as human function in health and disease. Traditional approaches to understanding human biology have largely been reductionistic, with a tendency to reduce each function to the lowest operating unit such as a cell, organelle, molecule, gene, fibre, and so on. While this approach has yielded significant progress in the study of human function in health and disease, there are apparent limits, especially when trying to understand the functioning of whole organisms, as well as more complex biological events and behaviour. As a result, new systems models are developing and opening new opportunities for further progress. Systems biology essentially adopts engineering strategies to create biologically based, interdisciplinary approaches to study the complex interactions of the many, diverse elements of biological systems. The major opportunity in systems biology is the possibility of multidimensional examinations of whole systems of biological function and how they relate to behaviour, cognition, and other manifestations of biological activity.

Systems biology requires the broadest view of what is a system. In the case of human development, the system must include the totality of the environment in which we live. This includes all the natural features of the environment, such as air and soil, but it also must encompass the derivative elements such as social structures and culture. It is this complexity that makes public mental health at once both simple and, all-too-often, a failure. The simplicity comes from focusing on just one element in biology or the environment. This leads to plans and policies that are doomed to fail. It is hard to make integrated models that are clear enough to form the basis of sound policy and practice. But, as the knowledge base is broadening, so is the capacity to make systems changes that will improve the lives and futures for children and adolescents with and without mental disorders.

Systems-biology approaches to neural function are particularly exciting, especially for studying the brain and its function, the latter of which coalesces as systems neuroscience. However, to be successful, it requires investigators with disparate training who often lack a common language discourse to establish close and enduring collaborative programmes of research. Disciplines in systems biology of neuroscience include biologists, physicists, mathematicians, statisticians, engineers, computational scientists, and many more. Identifying and developing working collaborations for systems neuroscience are both scientific and educational goals of this project. Specifically, we will identify the necessary scientists to form a team that will develop a common working language and integrate models for investigation. We will train each other to provide the necessary tools for productive investigations. Equally importantly, we will use this opportunity to model and develop educational opportunities—both didactic and in the laboratory—to train the next generation of systems neuroscientists and to help the world public health infrastructure better serve the mental health needs of children and adolescents.

Conclusions

Unfortunately, public policy and, hence, public mental health rarely keeps up with the rapid advancement of both basic and clinical science. But, with planning and preparation, anticipation of these advances can help policymakers implement change more quickly and effectively. With this in mind, there are several key concepts and strategies to emphasize:

1. Well-being and mental health are both important.

   a. Wellness is not the absence of mental illness and demands equal attention in order to facilitate health development.

   b. The prevention and treatment of mental illness in children and adolescence is a pressing public health challenge that must be coupled with improving the well-being of young people.

2. Public education.

   a. Directed at parents, professionals, policymakers, and the media.

   b. Developmental models are essential for understanding children and adolescents and the mental health problems they face.

   c. Repeat the facts:

      i. Child and adolescent mental disorders are among the most prevalent illnesses affecting children.

      ii. Child and adolescent mental disorders, without adequate treatment, lead to a lifetime of disability and suffering.

      iii. Child and adolescent mental disorders, without adequate treatment, add enormous costs to many public systems: health care, education, juvenile and criminal justice, child welfare, etc.

      iv. Child and adolescent mental disorders are responsive to a multitude of evidence-based treatments.

3. Healthcare must be integrated and accessible.

   a. General health care without mental health care is inadequate.

   b. Clinical services must be integrated and coordinated.

   c. New models of health care are necessary for non-urban settings and in low- and middle-income countries.

4. Stigma and discrimination toward mental illness is persistent and damaging.

   a. Public repudiation of stigma against mental illness is essential for improving the acceptability of accessing treatment.

   b. Public policy must not yield to bias and stigma.

5. Children and adolescents constitute a specialized population with respect to public health and mental health.

   a. The rapid pace of early development makes them particularly vulnerable to adverse environmental events.

   b. The rapid pace of early development creates extraordinary opportunities for prevention and early intervention.

6. Training is crucial.

   a. It takes skilled professionals of many sorts to provide health care and mental health care.

   b. Child and adolescent health needs many more clinicians and investigators; systems are necessary to increase the numbers of trained professionals, as well as their distribution in underserved areas.

   c. Training skilled basic and applied researchers is as important as training clinicians.

7. Research is still important.

   a. While there is often a preference for providing services, services cannot improve without research.

   b. There is a pressing need to advance both clinical and basic knowledge in child and adolescent development, developmental psychopathology, and developmentally oriented prevention and treatment services.

Public mental health for children and adolescents is a critical investment in our future. It is the shared responsibility of many: parents, families, community members, clinicians, educators, and policymakers. While each has a special role, it is only together that we can achieve the best for children and adolescents. Working together will make it possible for public mental health for children and adolescents to join and become a full partner and integral part of the general healthcare system of the twenty-first century.

References

1. Mallon GP. The legend of Mary Ellen Wilson and Etta Wheeler: child maltreatment and protection today. *Child Welfare* 2013; 92: 9–11.
2. Kempe CH, Silverman FN, Steele BF, Droegemueller W, Silver HK. The battered-child syndrome. *JAMA* 1962; 181: 17–24.
3. Locke J, Winkler K. *An Essay Concerning Human Understanding: Abridged and Edited, With an Introduction and Notes.* Indianapolis, IN: Hackett Pub, 1996.
4. Mahler MS. Autism and symbiosis, two extreme disturbances of identity. *Int J Psychoanal* 1958; 39: 77–83.
5. Fromm-Reichmann F. Notes on the development of treatment of schizophrenics by psychoanalytic psychotherapy. *Psychiatry* 1948; 11: 263–273.
6. American Psychiatric Association. *Diagnostic and Statistical Manual of Mental Disorders*, 3rd ed. Washington, DC: American Psychiatric Association, 1980.
7. American Psychiatric Association. *Committee on Nomenclature and Statistics. DSM-II, Diagnostic and Statistical Manual of Mental Disorders*, 2nd ed. Washington, DC: American Psychiatric Association, 1968.
8. Cytryn L, McKnew DH, Jr. Proposed classification of childhood depression. *Am J Psychiatry* 1972; 129: 149–155.
9. Rutter M, Tizard J, Yule W, Graham P, Whitmore K. Research report: Isle of Wight Studies, 1964–1974. *Psychol Med* 1976; 6: 313–332.
10. Costello EJ, Mustillo S, Erkanli A, Keeler G, Angold A. Prevalence and development of psychiatric disorders in childhood and adolescence. *Arch Gen Psychiatry* 2003; 60: 837–844.
11. Copeland WE, Wolke D, Shanahan L, Costello EJ. Adult functional outcomes of common childhood psychiatric problems: a prospective, longitudinal study. *JAMA Psychiatry* 2015; 72: 892–899.
12. Ravens-Sieberer U, Wille N, Erhart M, et al. Prevalence of mental health problems among children and adolescents in Germany: results of the BELLA study within the National Health Interview and Examination Survey. *Eur Child Adolesc Psychiatry* 2008; 17(Suppl. 1): 22–33.
13. Kessler RC, Berglund P, Demler O, Jin R, Merikangas KR, Walters EE. Lifetime prevalence and age-of-onset distributions of DSM-IV disorders in the National Comorbidity Survey Replication. *Arch Gen Psychiatry* 2005; 62: 593–602.
14. Kessler RC, Chiu WT, Demler O, Merikangas KR, Walters EE. Prevalence, severity, and comorbidity of 12-month DSM-IV disorders in the National Comorbidity Survey Replication. *Arch Gen Psychiatry* 2005; 62: 617–627.
15. Belfer ML. Child and adolescent mental disorders: the magnitude of the problem across the globe. *J Child Psychol Psychiatry* 2008; 49: 226–236.
16. Kessler RC, Avenevoli S, Costello J, et al. Severity of 12-month DSM-IV disorders in the National Comorbidity Survey Replication Adolescent Supplement. *Arch Gen Psychiatry* 2012; 69: 381–389.
17. Merikangas KR, He JP, Brody D, Fisher PW, Bourdon K, Koretz DS. Prevalence and treatment of mental disorders among US children in the 2001–2004 NHANES. *Pediatrics* 2010; 125: 75–81.
18. Gore FM, Bloem PJ, Patton GC, et al. Global burden of disease in young people aged 10-24 years: a systematic analysis. *Lancet* 2011; 377: 2093–2102.
19. Murray CJ, Vos T, Lozano R, et al. Disability-adjusted life years (DALYs) for 291 diseases and injuries in 21 regions, 1990–2010: a systematic analysis for the Global Burden of Disease Study 2010. *Lancet* 2012; 380: 2197–2223.
20. Fergusson DM, Woodward LJ. Mental health, educational, and social role outcomes of adolescents with depression. *Arch Gen Psychiatry* 2002; 59: 225–231.
21. Fergusson DM, Boden JM, Horwood LJ. Recurrence of major depression in adolescence and early adulthood, and later mental health, educational and economic outcomes. *Br J Psychiatry* 2007; 191: 335–342.
22. O'Connor TG, Davies L, Dunn J, Golding J. Distribution of accidents, injuries, and illnesses by family type. ALSPAC Study Team. Avon Longitudinal Study of Pregnancy and Childhood. *Pediatrics* 2000; 106: E68.
23. Keyes CL. The mental health continuum: from languishing to flourishing in life. *J Health Soc Behav* 2002; 43: 207–222.
24. World Health Organization. *Constitution of the World Health Organization.* Geneva: World Health Organization, 1946.
25. Viner RM, Ozer EM, Denny S, et al. Adolescence and the social determinants of health. *Lancet* 2012; 379: 1641–1652.

26. Patalay P, Fitzsimons E. Correlates of mental illness and wellbeing in children: are they the same? Results from the UK Millennium Cohort Study. *J Am Acad Child Adolesc Psychiatry* 2016; 55: 771–783.

27. Kasser T, Kanner AD. Psychology and consumer culture the struggle for a good life in a materialistic world. Available at: http://www.loc.gov/catdir/toc/fy041/2003004965.html (2004, accessed 2 March 2018).

28. Coley RL, Chase-Lansdale PL. Adolescent pregnancy and parenthood. Recent evidence and future directions. *Am Psychol* 1998; 53: 152–166.

29. Coyne CA, D'Onofrio BM. Some (but not much) progress toward understanding teenage childbearing: a review of research from the past decade. *Adv Child Dev Behav* 2012; 42: 113–152.

30. Jaffee S, Caspi A, Moffitt TE, Belsky J, Silva P. Why are children born to teen mothers at risk for adverse outcomes in young adulthood? Results from a 20-year longitudinal study. *Dev Psychopathol* 2001; 13: 377–397.

31. Jaffee SR, Strait LB, Odgers CL. From correlates to causes: can quasi-experimental studies and statistical innovations bring us closer to identifying the causes of antisocial behavior? *Psychol Bull* 2012; 138: 272–295.

32. Walker SP, Wachs TD, Gardner JM, et al. Child development: risk factors for adverse outcomes in developing countries. *Lancet* 2007; 369: 145–157.

33. Harlow HF, Harlow M. Social deprivation in monkeys. *Sci Am* 1962; 207: 136–146.

34. Hubel DH, Wiesel TN. Receptive fields, binocular interaction and functional architecture in the cat's visual cortex. *J Physiol* 1962; 160: 106–154.

35. Spitz RA. Anaclitic depression; an inquiry into the genesis of psychiatric conditions in early childhood. *Psychoanal Study Child* 1946; 2: 313–342.

36. Rutter M. Developmental catch-up, and deficit, following adoption after severe global early privation. English and Romanian Adoptees (ERA) Study Team. *J Child Psychol Psychiatry* 1998; 39: 465–476.

37. Stevens JS, van Rooij SJ, Jovanovic T. Developmental contributors to trauma response: the importance of sensitive periods, early environment, and sex differences. *Curr Top Behav Neurosci* 2016 Nov 10 (Epub ahead of print).

38. Shonkoff JP, Phillips DA (eds); Committee on Integrating the Science of Early Childhood Development, Board on Children, Youth, and Families. *From Neurons to Neighborhoods: The Science of Early Childhood Development*. Washington, DC: National Academies Press.

39. Belfer ML, Saxena S. WHO Child Atlas project. *Lancet* 2006; 367: 551–552.

40. World Health Organization (WHO). *Department of Mental Health and Substance Abuse. Mental Health Atlas 2011.* Geneva: WHO, 2011.

41. Paula CS, Bordin IA, Mari JJ, Velasque L, Rohde LA, Coutinho ES. The mental health care gap among children and adolescents: data from an epidemiological survey from four Brazilian regions. *PLOS ONE* 2014; 9: e88241.

42. Kataoka SH, Zhang L, Wells KB. Unmet need for mental health care among U.S. children: variation by ethnicity and insurance status. *Am J Psychiatry* 2002; 159: 1548–1555.

43. Hoagwood K, Kelleher KJ, Feil M, Comer DM. Treatment services for children with ADHD: a national perspective. *J Am Acad Child Adolesc Psychiatry* 2000; 39: 198–206.

44. Burns BJ, Costello EJ, Angold A, et al. Children's mental health service use across service sectors. *Health Aff (Millwood)* 1995; 14: 147–159.

45. Hamoda HM, Belfer ML. Challenges in international collaboration in child and adolescent psychiatry. *J Child Adolesc Mental Health* 2010; 22: 83–89.

46. Earley P. *Crazy: A Father's Search Through America's Mental Health Madness.* New York: Berkley, 2006.

47. Kim WJ. Child and adolescent psychiatry workforce: a critical shortage and national challenge. *Acad Psychiatry* 2003; 27: 277–282.

48. Thomas CR, Holzer CE, 3rd. The continuing shortage of child and adolescent psychiatrists. *J Am Acad Child Adolesc Psychiatry* 2006; 45: 1023–1031.

49. Patel V, Prince M. Global mental health: a new global health field comes of age. *JAMA* 2010; 303: 1976–1977.

50. Prince M, Patel V, Saxena S, et al. No health without mental health. *Lancet* 2007; 370: 859–877.

51. Eisenberg L, Belfer M. Prerequisites for global child and adolescent mental health. *J Child Psychol Psychiatry* 2009; 50: 26–35.

52. Gilbert R, Widom CS, Browne K, Fergusson D, Webb E, Janson S. Burden and consequences of child maltreatment in high-income countries. *Lancet* 2009; 373: 68–81.

53. Butchart A, Mikton C, World Health Organization (WHO), United Nations Office on Drugs and Crime, United Nations Development Programme. *Global Status Report on Violence Prevention, 2014.* Geneva: WHO, 2014.

54. Hillis S, Mercy J, Amobi A, Kress H. Global prevalence of past-year violence against children: a systematic review and minimum estimates. *Pediatrics* 2016; 137: e20154079.

55. Lansford JE, Deater-Deckard K. Childrearing discipline and violence in developing countries. *Child Dev* 2012; 83: 62–75.

56. Felitti VJ, Anda RF, Nordenberg D, et al. Relationship of childhood abuse and household dysfunction to many of the leading causes of death in adults. The Adverse Childhood Experiences (ACE) Study. *Am J Prev Med* 1998; 14: 245–258.

57. Mercy JA, Vivolo-Kantor AM. The Center for Disease Control and Prevention's (CDC) Youth Violence Prevention Centers: paving the way to prevention. *J Prim Prev* 2016; 37: 209–214.

58. Stoltenborgh M, van Ijzendoorn MH, Euser EM, Bakermans-Kranenburg MJ. A global perspective on child sexual abuse: meta-analysis of prevalence around the world. *Child Maltreat* 2011; 16: 79–101.

59. Stoltenborgh M, Bakermans-Kranenburg MJ, van Ijzendoorn MH. The neglect of child neglect: a meta-analytic review of the prevalence of neglect. *Soc Psychiatry Psychiatr Epidemiol* 2013; 48: 345–355.

60. Hillis S, Mercy J, Saul J, Gleckel J, Abad N, Kress H. THRIVES: using the best evidence to prevent violence against children. *J Public Health Policy* 2016; 37(Suppl. 1): 51–65.

61. Flaherty EG, Thompson R, Litrownik AJ, et al. Adverse childhood exposures and reported child health at age 12. *Acad Pediatr* 2009; 9: 150–156.

62. McEwen BS. Stress, adaptation, and disease. Allostasis and allostatic load. *Ann N Y Acad Sci* 1998; 840: 33–44.

63. McLanahan S, Bendheim-Thoman Center for Research on Child Wellbeing, Columbia University, Social Indicators Survey Center. *The Fragile Families and Child Wellbeing Study. National Report.* Princeton, NJ, New York: Center for Research on Child Wellbeing Social Indicators Survey Center, Columbia University School of Social Work, 2001.

64. Jimenez ME, Wade R, Jr., Lin Y, Morrow LM, Reichman NE. Adverse experiences in early childhood and kindergarten outcomes. *Pediatrics* 2016; 137: e20151839.

65. Johnson SB, Riley AW, Granger DA, Riis J. The science of early life toxic stress for pediatric practice and advocacy. *Pediatrics* 2013; 131: 319–327.

66. Dreyer B, Chung PJ, Szilagyi P, Wong S. Child poverty in the United States today: introduction and executive summary. *Acad Pediatr* 2016; 16(3 Suppl.): S1–S5.

67. Boyce WT. The lifelong effects of early childhood adversity and toxic stress. *Pediatr Dent* 2014; 36: 102–108.

68. Mash EJ, Wolfe DA. *Abnormal Child Psychology*, 6th ed. Boston, MA: Cengage Learning, 2016.

69. Felitti VJ. Adverse childhood experiences and adult health. *Acad Pediatr* 2009; 9: 131–132.

70. Bradley C. The behavior of children receiving benzedrine *Am J Psychiatry* 1937; 94: 577–581.

71. Zito JM, Safer DJ. Recent child pharmacoepidemiological findings. *J Child Adoles Psychopharmacol* 2005; 15: 5–9.

72. Zito JM, Safer DJ, de Jong-van den Berg LT, et al. A three-country comparison of psychotropic medication prevalence in youth. *Child Adolesc Psychiatry Ment Health* 2008; 2: 26.

73. Rapoport JL. Pediatric psychopharmacology: too much or too little? *World Psychiatry* 2013; 12: 118–123.

74. Piacentini J, Bennett S, Compton SN, et al. 24- and 36-week outcomes for the Child/Adolescent Anxiety Multimodal Study (CAMS). *J Am Acad Child Adolesc Psychiatry* 2014; 53: 297–310.

75. Findling RL, Frazier JA, Kafantaris V, et al. The Collaborative Lithium Trials (CoLT): specific aims, methods, and implementation. *Child Adolesc Psychiatry Ment Health* 2008; 2: 21.

76. Molina BS, Hinshaw SP, Swanson JM, et al. The MTA at 8 years: prospective follow-up of children treated for combined-type ADHD in a multisite study. *J Am Acad Child Adolesc Psychiatry* 2009; 48: 484–500.

77. Riddle MA, Yershova K, Lazzaretto D, et al. The Preschool Attention-Deficit/Hyperactivity Disorder Treatment Study (PATS) 6-year follow-up. *J Am Acad Child Adolesc Psychiatry* 2013; 52: 264–278.e2.

78. Cognitive-behavior therapy, sertraline, and their combination for children and adolescents with obsessive-compulsive disorder: the Pediatric OCD Treatment Study (POTS) randomized controlled trial. *JAMA* 2004; 292: 1969–1976.

79. McDougle CJ, Scahill L, Aman MG, et al. Risperidone for the core symptom domains of autism: results from the study by the autism network of the research units on pediatric psychopharmacology. *Am J Psychiatry* 2005; 162: 1142–1148.

80. March JS, Silva S, Petrycki S, et al. The Treatment for Adolescents With Depression Study (TADS): long-term effectiveness and safety outcomes. *Arch Gen Psychiatry* 2007; 64: 1132–1143.

81. Brent DA, Greenhill LL, Compton S, et al. The Treatment of Adolescent Suicide Attempters study (TASA): predictors of suicidal events in an open treatment trial. *J Am Acad Child Adolesc Psychiatry* 2009; 48: 987–996.

82. Walkup JT, Wagner KD, Miller L, et al. Treatment of early-age mania: outcomes for partial and nonresponders to initial treatment. *J Am Acad Child Adolesc Psychiatry* 2015; 54: 1008–1019.

83. Sikich L, Frazier JA, McClellan J, et al. Double-blind comparison of first- and second-generation antipsychotics in early-onset schizophrenia and schizo-affective disorder: findings from the treatment of early-onset schizophrenia spectrum disorders (TEOSS) study. *Am J Psychiatry* 2008; 165: 1420–1431.

84. Emslie GJ, Mayes T, Porta G, et al. Treatment of Resistant Depression in Adolescents (TORDIA): week 24 outcomes. *Am J Psychiatry* 2010; 167: 782–791.

85. Brauner JV, Johansen LM, Roesbjerg T, Pagsberg AK. Off-label prescription of psychopharmacological drugs in child and adolescent psychiatry. *J Child Psychopharmacol* 2016; 36: 500–507.

86. Zito JM, Safer DJ, dosReis S, Gardner JF, Boles M, Lynch F. Trends in the prescribing of psychotropic medications to preschoolers. *JAMA* 2000; 283: 1025–1030.

87. Cooper WO, Arbogast PG, Ding H, Hickson GB, Fuchs DC, Ray WA. Trends in prescribing of antipsychotic medications for US children. *Ambul Pediatr* 2006; 6: 79–83.

88. Olfson M, Blanco C, Liu L, Moreno C, Laje G. National trends in the outpatient treatment of children and adolescents with antipsychotic drugs. *Arch Gen Psychiatry* 2006; 63: 679–685.

89. Patel NC, Crismon ML, Hoagwood K, et al. Trends in the use of typical and atypical antipsychotics in children and adolescents. *J Am Acad Child Adolesc Psychiatry* 2005; 44: 548–556.

CHAPTER 29

Recognizing mental health problems in the ageing community

Linda Chiu Wa Lam and Wai Chi Chan

Improvement in public health and medical care has greatly increased the chance of surviving previously fatal diseases. According to World Health Statistics 2016, the global life expectancy by birth for children born in 2015 was 71.4 years (73.8 years for females and 69.1 years for males). Although the figure varies significantly across different countries, it was reported that life expectancy increased by 5 years between 2000 and 2015, the fastest increase since the1960s [1]. In 2010, about 8% of the population were aged 65 years or over. It is estimated that the proportion of the older population will rise to 16% by 2050, resulting in a tripling of the size of the old-age community. Most developed countries are still expected to have the highest proportion of an ageing population. But the greatest increase is expected to come from developing regions, with a rise of almost 250% projected [2].

Longevity represents the success of medical care. However, advancing age is associated with a higher likelihood of chronic non-communicable and degenerative diseases affecting one's everyday functioning and quality of life. These conditions also pose a great burden of care on the affected individuals, their families, and the community. Mental health problems are as prevalent as physical diseases in late life. Degenerative processes in the body and the brain, changes in psychosocial situations, and long-term predispositions are important factors that shape the mental health profiles of the older community.

Mental disorders commonly occurring in older adults

Dementia and other neurocognitive disorders

Dementia, the prevalence of which increases exponentially after 65 years of age, is a highly significant public health problem. Dementia, referred to as a neurocognitive disorder in the fifth edition of *the Diagnostic and Statistical Manual of Mental Disorders*, represent the cognitive, mental, and physical disturbances due to different pathological changes [3]. Alzheimer's disease and vascular dementia are the commonest types of dementia, and their incidence increases dramatically after the age of 65 years [4].

The syndromes of dementia are generally represented by progressive global cognitive impairment, neuropsychiatric symptoms, and behavioural disturbances, as well as physical and functional deterioration. The trajectories of decline or disease course are highly variable. Disease mechanisms in different dementia subtypes influence symptom manifestations, but individual variability in physical health and environmental factors also modulate physical and mental symptoms.

Cognitive decline is part of the dementing process. However, it is frequently not the most distressing symptoms, either to the patients or their caregivers. Neuropsychiatric symptoms and the associated behavioural disturbances are reported to be associated with caregiver burden, morbidity, and decision for hospitalization. Mood disturbances like depression, apathy, and anxiety are highly prevalent and may occur in over 60% of the patients suffering from dementia. Psychotic features such as delusions, while less common, are also regularly reported in about one-third of patients. Other disturbances such as disorganized psychomotor activities peak in the moderate phase of dementia, occurring in about 50% of patients with different types of dementia [5–7].

To examine the mental morbidity associated with dementia, it is pertinent that the attention should not be focused on the prevalence of diagnoses only. As many studies have revealed, the cognitive and neuropsychiatric symptomatology, functional impact, morbidity, and mortality associated with dementia constitute the main bulk of public health burden [8–10].

Depression and anxiety disorders in late life

The European MentDis_ICF65+ study assessed 3142 older people aged 65–84 years in different European countries and identified that nearly a quarter of the sample was diagnosed with any current mental disorder (23.3%; 95% confidence interval (CI) 19.9–26.7). The most prevalent category was anxiety disorders (11.4%; 95% CI 9.1–13.6), followed by affective disorders (8.0%; 95% CI 6.3–9.6) and substance-related disorders (4.6%; 95% CI 3.7–5.6) [11]. The EURODEP concerted action examined 14,200 participants (aged 60–104 years) in seven European countries with the Geriatric Mental State examination, which revealed that anxiety symptoms were found in 32% of participants who were not depressed, 67% in those with subthreshold depression, and 87% for those with case-level depression [12]. Apart from being highly prevalent, depressive and anxiety symptoms frequently coexist in the community, even in people who do not reach the diagnostic thresholds.

Depressive disorders

Prospective studies evaluating the trajectories of depressive disorders in late life have suggested that baseline depression is associated with a high risk of recurrence. However, a significant proportion of people with pre-existing depressive symptoms will remit. A prospective study reported 341 subjects with subthreshold depression followed up for 15 years in Amsterdam: 44.9% recovered from subthreshold symptoms, 40.5% remained chronically at the subthreshold level, and 14.7% developed major depressive disorder. Psychosocial stressors and physical health play roles in modulating the onset and remissions of depression in late life [13].

It is also suggested that depression in mid-life is an independent risk factor for neurodegeneration and development of dementia decades later. In a study that examined the data of 30,902 subjects who were followed-up for a maximum of 27 years, there was a 35% increase in risks of dementia among those reporting mental distress in a fully adjusted model (odds ratio 1.35; 95% CI 1.01–1.80). The authors also reported that the interactions with age suggested that risks were associated with early mid-life mental distress compared with late mid-life participants [14].

Depression in late life frequently presents with significant cognitive impairment. Frontal executive dysfunction is often reported in older adults suffering from depression. The comorbidity between depressive symptoms and cognitive impairment makes it difficult to differentiate if elderly depression is a risk factor for dementia, or a symptom of degeneration that happens early in the clinical phase. The analytic cohort of the Health, Aging, and Body Composition study included 2488 black and white older adults. During the 5 years of prospective observation, three depressive symptom trajectories were identified:

> … persistent minimal symptoms, moderate and increasing symptoms, and high and increasing symptoms. Compared with the minimal symptom group, the high and increasing depressive symptom group was associated with significantly increased risk of dementia (fully adjusted hazard ratio 1.94; 95% CI 1.30–2.90), while the moderate and increasing trajectory was not associated with an elevated risk of dementia [15].

Among all putative factors, cerebrovascular diseases are found to be positively associated with depressive disorders in late life. Depression adversely affects the outcomes of myocardial infarctions and is associated with an increased incidence of stroke. From 2004 to 2013, the China Kadoorie Biobank Cohort observed 199,294 men and 288,083 women aged 30–79 years without a history of stroke or heart disease. Past year depression was marginally associated with a 15% increased risk of stroke (adjusted hazard ratio 1.15; 95% CI 0.99–1.33), with a positive dose–response relationship between the number of depression symptoms and increased stroke risk [16].

Anxiety disorders

As mentioned earlier, anxiety disorders are prevalent across the life-span. Old age is no exception to this. People with anxiety disorders have more physical complaints and poorer quality of life. Among different types of anxiety disorders, generalized anxiety disorder is usually the most prevalent, whereas panic disorder and specific phobias are less common.

In contrast to depression, anxiety disorders in late life have received much less research attention. Anxiety symptoms in older adults without dementia are not uncommonly considered as the 'worried well'. Recently, there have been reports suggesting that anxiety disorders are not as benign as generally perceived. They are associated with increased reports of suicidal feelings even after being adjusted for depressive symptoms [17].

More interestingly, it is also observed that anxiety symptoms are associated with specific cognitive impairment consistent with that observed in Alzheimer's disease. Anxious people may have poor attention and worse cognitive performance. However, it is not clear if this suboptimal cognitive performance represents the effects of anxious mood on cognition, or is an index of underlying degeneration. The Rotterdam study prospectively examined 5877 subjects for over 15 years. Baseline anxiety symptoms were associated with impaired cognitive performance. However, the presence of anxiety did not affect cognitive decline over the follow-up period [18]. In the Australian Imaging, Biomarkers, and Lifestyle (AIBL) Study, the presence of amyloid plaques, as revealed by positron emission tomography imaging, in non-demented individuals was associated with cognitive decline over 3 years. The presence of anxiety symptoms at baseline accelerated the trajectories of decline [19]. Anxiety symptoms may be alleviated with different modalities of intervention. If anxiety symptoms alter the trajectories of cognitive decline in older adults, this common but largely ignored condition in late life should be revisited with new knowledge and enthusiasm for its public health implications.

Negative perceptions about life

Sense of uselessness and thoughts of death are not uncommon in late life. At an advanced age, negative perceptions about life are not infrequently reported with rationality in the face of disabilities and chronic degenerative diseases. Thoughts of death are associated with depressive disorders. In psychological autopsy studies of older people who committed suicide, major psychiatric disorders with depression, in particular, were reported in the majority of people. Most of the suicide completers had a pre-suicidal plan, or sought help and expressed their death wishes to others before their actual attempts [20, 21].

Depressive ideas and negative cognition are also very common in persons with dementia. However, the prevalence of self-harm in dementia is less well studied. Conventional exploration of the factors associated with deliberate self-harm in clients with major depressive disorder may not be applicable to people living with dementia. In the context of cognitive impairment, judgement may be more impaired and behaviours may not be easily correlated with the contextual factors. In a systematic review of suicidal risks in patients with Alzheimer's disease, the authors reviewed publications from 1980 to 2015. They identified that suicide occurs in these individuals even many years after the diagnosis of dementia, and patients who have attempted suicide once are at a higher risk of dying from suicide [22].

Negative perceptions about life are not only associated with poor psychological states, but may also be linked to worse physical outcomes. Depression has been associated with higher mortality after myocardial infarction. The Religious Orders Study is a longitudinal cohort study of older persons conducted between 1994 and 2002 on 851 Catholic clergy members in the USA. The investigators examined the association between negative affect and all-cause mortality, and identified that negative affect in older persons, especially internally experienced distress, were associated with increased mortality. On the contrary, measures of externally directed negative affect, such as the tendencies to be angry with others and to express anger overtly, were not associated with an increased mortality risk [23].

There may be shared physiological mechanisms for mood and physical disorders such as coronary heart disease. It has been suggested that platelet dysfunction is implicated in the development of depressive mood, and also confers cerebrovascular risks. The chronic stress associated with mood disorders is associated with altered cortisol response and this has implications on immunity and inflammatory reactions of the body. A multidimensional conceptual framework may help to delineate the association between mood and physical disorders [24].

Insights from long-term prospective cohort studies

Large-scale prospective studies conducted since the last century offer important information on the potential modulating factors that influence mental health in late life.

The Grant Study is one of the longest prospective studies exploring the predictors of healthy ageing. A group of 268 men at Harvard College was recruited for regular psychosocial and cognitive assessment from 1939, with another group of non-delinquent men recruited in Boston area as control. The study recorded childhood environment, dominant personality traits, mental and physical health over time, smoking, alcohol abuse, and depression. Questionnaires were distributed and completed by the participants every 2 years and physical examinations of the participants were carried out every 5 years. Cognitive status was assessed at 80, 85, and 90 years of age. The study observed few predictors with a strong association with either intact cognition ($n = 40$) or dementia ($n = 44$) at 90 years of age. Three factors were found to be significant in determining intact cognition, namely warm childhood relationship with mother, exercise at 60 years of age, and high maternal education [25].

The British 1946 cohort recruited 5362 people born in 1946 (The National Survey of Health and Development). The participants were followed-up for the 70 years after birth. Birth history, early childhood history, intelligence, psychosocial situation, and adult and midlife factors were collected periodically. Some of the participants had been followed-up for over 20 times. Many constitutional and lifestyle factors were found to be associated with cognitive function and mental health in late life. Weight at birth, age of developmental milestones, economic deprivation in early childhood, acute stressors in childhood, and adulthood and socio-economic status in adulthood were assessed for their direct and indirect effects on adolescent (age 13 and 15 years) and adult (age 36, 43, and 53 years) measures of depressive symptoms. Childhood deprivation and stressors had important direct and indirect effects on depression. Stressors in adulthood were strongly associated with adult depression. The cohort also examined the association between lifestyles at 36 and 43 years of age, change in these behaviours over time, and decline in verbal memory and visual search speed between 43 and 60–64 years in 1018 participants. Their findings suggested that healthy dietary choices and physical activity were associated with slower memory and visual search speed decline over 20 years, with evidence that increasing physical activity was important [26–28].

The Rotterdam Study is a prospective, population-based cohort that started in 1990, conducted among inhabitants, aged 55 years

and older, of a district of Rotterdam, The Netherlands. In a study of the association between mild cognitive impairment at baseline and mood disorders, the findings suggested that persons with mild cognitive impairment had more depressive and anxiety disorders and also a higher risk of developing depressive disorder and anxiety disorder. However, the same study did not identify any significant association between anxiety and risk of cognitive decline. These findings suggested that there may be common pathological pathways for cognitive and psychiatric outcomes [18, 29].

The Prospective Population Study of Women in Gothenburg began in 1968 with a representative sample of 1462 women (participation rate 90%) living in Gothenburg of Sweden. The participants were born in 1908, 1914, 1918, 1922, and 1930. Women participated from 1968 to 2000, when they were aged 78–92 years. Original birth records containing birth weight, length, head circumference, and gestational time, as well as social factors were obtained. Lifetime depression was diagnosed via multiple information sources. Over their lifetime, 44.6% of women in this sample experienced depression. Birth weights ≤3500 g and shorter gestational time were independently associated with higher odds of lifetime depression in a logistic regression model adjusted for age. Eight hundred women had baseline assessment for depression, with follow-up assessment conducted in 527 women at 2005. At baseline, lower levels of physical activity were related to higher depression scores. Participants with decreasing physical activity over time evidenced higher depression scores at 32-year follow-up. The results highlighted that there are significant interactions between depression and physical activity in the long term and both neurodevelopmental and environmental contributions to lifetime depression should not be ignored [30, 31].

After decades of systematic exploration and longitudinal observations, it is now widely recognized that cognitive impairment and mental health status in old age are affected by multiple factors that would best be perceived with a life course approach. Many lifestyle factors, such as physical activity, social engagement, and cerebrovascular risks, are implicated in midlife and have an enduring influence on mental health in late life. From an individual perspective, modifications of these factors may attenuate the risks of different mental health and cognitive problems. From a public health perspective, these studies do have implications on promotion for healthy ageing.

Public health strategies

Mental health status in adulthood

It is increasingly recognized that mental and physical health conditions in later life are related to developmental and psychosocial factors that operate early in life. Depression and anxiety in adult life are associated with adverse psychosocial situations, which could be both the cause and the consequences of psychological disturbances. However, as studies revealed, these conditions also impact on late-life cognitive function, mental health, and physical outcomes. As the recognition of common mood disorders is still low in many countries, it is important to boost community awareness and early interventions for these health conditions in all age groups. Recognizing mental health problems in the older community would help to alleviate mental morbidity and optimize life quality. More accessible treatments for adults, especially the self-help stress reduction strategies available to the wider community, may have an impact on one's mental health in later life.

Physical activity

Physical activity, in particular regular exercise habits, has been recognized as an important determining factor of cardiovascular health. The American Heart Association has stipulated clear guidelines as to how physical exercise may help to control blood pressure and other cardiovascular risk factors. However, standard guidelines as to how much and what types of exercise will help with cognition remains uncertain.

The adoption of continuous aerobic exercise could be challenging for older adults with chronic physical conditions, as they may suffer from limitations that hinder the practice of such exercise. As the physiological mechanisms for exercise-related brain health may be different from that for physical well-being, other exercise modalities may also be helpful. Recent studies do suggest that resistance training may have beneficial effects on executive function in older adults [32, 33]. A 1-year randomized controlled trial of mind body (tai chi) exercise intervention in Chinese older adults at risk of cognitive decline showed that practising tai chi 3 days a week helped to attenuate the cognitive decline and development of dementia. It is of interest to note that tai chi practice also reduced the depression symptom scores in this group of non-depressed participants [34].

Physical exercise and its effects on depression, as well as anxiety, have been studied for a number of years. The association between physical exercise and lessen risks of depression has been postulated with a number of physiological mechanisms. People suffering from depression are reported to have lower levels of brain-derived neurotrophic factor (BDNF), which may affect their neuronal protective mechanisms. However, physical exercise is positively associated with BDNF activity, thus drawing a link between physical exercise and depression. More interestingly, polymorphisms of the *BDNF* gene may confer differential response to exercise. Further research may help to explore the advice of exercise strategies as a potential adjuvant intervention for depression and related mood disorders [35–37].

Active social engagement and healthy lifestyles

Active engagement in social activity boosts self-efficacy, allows for cognitive stimulation, and provides as an asset for peer support. While passive social participation may not offer major benefits in cognitive enhancement, it may help to restore positive emotional reactions. In a prospective study of 239 postmenopausal, non-smoking, disease-free women, accumulation of major life stressors across a 1-year period predicted telomere attrition. Interestingly, telomere attritions were moderated by high scores of health behaviours (leisure time activity, diet, and sleep) and appeared to be protected when they were exposed to stress. This study highlighted that a physiological marker of cell ageing—telomere length—could be modulated with health behaviours [38].

Conclusions

Mental health problems are common across the lifespan. The problem will be compounded by the emergence of neurocognitive disorders at old age. As there are complex interactions between mental health problems, cognitive impairments, and physical morbidity, clinicians have to consider the different perspectives that affect the person's mental well-being, as well as functional independence, when formulating the management plans.

To consider preventive approaches, the optimization of cerebrovascular health from midlife will certainly play a role in depression and dementia. Healthy lifestyles with attention to being physical active and mentally positive in adulthood may have enduring influence on mental health in late life. Community education to improve the awareness of symptoms of mental distress, and facilitation of a beneficial lifestyle would, hopefully, re-map the landscape of societal burden for mental disorders in late life.

References

1. World Health Organization. World Health Statistics 2016: Monitoring health for the SDGs. Available at: http://www.who.int/gho/publications/world_health_statistics/2016/en/ (accessed 18 October 2016).
2. World Health Organization. Global health and ageing. Available at: http://www.who.int/ageing/publications/global_health/en/ (accessed 18 October 2016).
3. American Psychiatric Association. *Diagnostic and Statistical Manual of Mental Disorders*, 5th ed. Arlington, VA: American Psychiatric Association, 2013.
4. Qiu C, De Ronchi D, Fratiglioni L. The epidemiology of the dementias: an update. *Curr Opin Psychiatry* 2007; 20: 380–385.
5. Lyketsos CG, Lopez O, Jones B, Fitzpatrick AL, Breitner J, DeKosky S. Prevalence of neuropsychiatric symptoms in dementia and mild cognitive impairment: results from the cardiovascular health study. *JAMA* 2002; 288: 1475–1483.
6. Brodaty H, Connors MH, Xu J, Woodward M, Ames D; PRIME study group. The course of neuropsychiatric symptoms in dementia: a 3-year longitudinal study. *J Am Med Dir Assoc* 2015; 16: 380–387.
7. Lautenschlager NT. Progress in BPSD research: analyzing individual BPSD might hold the key to better support caregivers. *Int Psychogeriatr* 2016; 28: 1759–1760.
8. Schulz R, Belle SH, Czaja SJ, McGinnis KA, Stevens A, Zhang S. Long-term care placement of dementia patients and caregiver health and well-being. *JAMA* 2004; 292: 961–967.
9. Nagata T, Nakajima S, Shinagawa S, et al. Psychosocial or clinico demographic factors related to neuropsychiatric symptoms in patients with Alzheimer's disease needing interventional treatment: analysis of the CATIE-AD study. *Int J Geriatr Psychiatry* 2017; 32: 1264–1271.
10. Feast A, Moniz-Cook E, Stoner C, Charlesworth G, Orrell M. A systematic review of the relationship between behavioral and psychological symptoms (BPSD) and caregiver well-being. *Int Psychogeriatr* 2016; 28: 1751–1774.
11. Andreas S, Schulz H, Volkert J, et al. Prevalence of mental disorders in elderly people: the European MentDis_ICF65+ study. *Br J Psychiatry* 2017; 210: 125–131.
12. Braam AW, Copeland JR, Delespaul PA, et al. Depression, subthreshold depression and comorbid anxiety symptoms in older Europeans: results from the EURODEP concerted action. *J Affect Disord* 2014; 155: 266–272.
13. Jeuring HW, Huisman M, Comijs HC, Stek ML, Beekman ATF. The long-term outcome of subthreshold depression in later life. *Psychol Med* 2016; 46: 2855–2865.
14. Skogen JC, Bergh S, Stewart R, Knudsen AK, Bjerkeset O. Midlife mental distress and risk for dementia up to 27 years later: the Nord-Trøndelag Health Study (HUNT) in linkage with a dementia registry in Norway. *BMC Geriatr* 2015; 15: 23.
15. Kaup AR, Byers AL, Falvey C, et al. Trajectories of depressive symptoms in older adults and risk of dementia. *JAMA Psychiatry* 2016; 73: 525–531.

16. Sun J, Ma H, Yu C, et al. Association of major depressive episodes with stroke risk in a prospective study of 0.5 Million Chinese adults. *Stroke* 2016; 47: 2203–2208.

17. Jonson M, Skoog I, Marlow T, Fässberg MM, Waern M. Anxiety symptoms and suicidal feelings in a population sample of 70-year-olds without dementia. *Int Psychogeriatr* 2010; 24: 1865–1871.

18. de Bruijn RF, Direk N, Mirza SS, et al. Anxiety is not associated with the risk of dementia or cognitive decline: the Rotterdam Study. *Am J Geriatr Psychiatry* 2014; 22: 1382e1390.

19. Pietrzak RH, Lim YY, Neumeister A, et al. Amyloid-β, anxiety, and cognitive decline in preclinical Alzheimer disease: a multicenter, prospective cohort study. *JAMA Psychiatry* 2015; 72: 284–291.

20. Ho RC, Ho EC, Tai BC, Ng WY, Chia BH. Elderly suicide with and without a history of suicidal behavior: implications for suicide prevention and management. *Arch Suicide Res* 2014; 18: 363–375.

21. Van Orden KA, Simning A, Conwell Y, Marlow T, Skoog I, Waern M. Characteristics and comorbid symptoms of older adults reporting death ideation. *Am J Geriatr Psychiatry* 2013; 21: 803–810.

22. Serafini G, Calcagno P, Lester D, Girardi P, Amore M, Pompili M. Suicide risk in Alzheimer's disease: a systematic review. *Curr Alzheimer Res* 2016; 13: 1083–1099.

23. Wilson RS, Bienias JL, Mendes de Leon CF, Evans DA, Bennett DA. Negative affect and mortality in older persons. *Am J Epidemiol* 2003; 158: 827–835.

24. Granville Smith I, Parker G, Rourke P, Cvejic E, Vollmer-Conna U. Acute coronary syndrome and depression: a review of shared pathophysiological pathways. *Aust N Z J Psychiatry* 2015; 49: 994–1005.

25. Vaillant GE, Okereke OI, Mukamal K, Waldinger RJ. Antecedents of intact cognition and dementia at age 90: a prospective study. *Int J Geriatr Psychiatry* 2014; 29: 1278–1285.

26. Davis D, Cooper R, Terrera GM, Hardy R, Richards M, Kuh D. Verbal memory and search speed in early midlife are associated with mortality over 25 years' follow-up, independently of health status and early life factors: a British birth cohort study. *Int J Epidemiol* 2016; 45: 1216–1225.

27. Colman I, Jones PB, Kuh D, et al. Early development, stress and depression across the life course: pathways to depression in a national British birth cohort. *Psychol Med* 2014; 44: 2845–2854.

28. Cadar D, Pikhart H, Mishra G, Stephen A, Kuh D, Richards M. The role of lifestyle behaviors on 20-year cognitive decline. *J Aging Res* 2012; 2012: 304014.

29. Mirza SS, Ikram MA, Bos D, Mihaescu R, Hofman A, Tiemeier H. Mild cognitive impairment and risk of depression and anxiety: a population-based study. *Alzheimers Dement* 2017; 13: 130–139.

30. Gudmundsson P, Andersson S, Gustafson D, et al. Depression in Swedish women: relationship to factors at birth. *Eur J Epidemiol* 2011; 26: 55–60.

31. Gudmundsson P, Lindwall PM, Gustafson DR, et al. Longitudinal associations between physical activity and depression scores in Swedish women followed 32 years. *Acta Psychiatr Scand* 2015; 132: 451–458.

32. Best JR, Chiu BK, Liang Hsu C, Nagamatsu LS, Liu-Ambrose T. Long-term effects of resistance exercise training on cognition and brain volume in older women: results from a randomized controlled trial. *J Int Neuropsychol Soc* 2015; 21: 745–756.

33. Suo C, Singh MF, Gates N, et al. Therapeutically relevant structural and functional mechanisms triggered by physical and cognitive exercise. *Mol Psychiatry* 2016; 21: 1633–1642.

34. Lam LC, Chau RC, Wong BM, et al. A 1-year randomized controlled trial comparing mind body exercise (Tai Chi) with stretching and toning exercise on cognitive function in older Chinese adults at risk of cognitive decline. *J Am Med Dir Assoc* 2012; 13: 568.e15–20.

35. Hallgren M, Helgadóttir B, Herring MP, et al. Exercise and internet-based cognitive-behavioural therapy for depression: multicentre randomised controlled trial with 12-month follow-up. *Br J Psychiatry* 2016; 209: 414–420.

36. Polyakova M, Stuke K, Schuemberg K, Mueller K, Schoenknecht P, Schroeter ML. BDNF as a biomarker for successful treatment of mood disorders: a systematic & quantitative meta-analysis. *J Affect Disord* 2015; 174: 432–440.

37. Dotson VM, Hsu FC, Langaee TY, et al. Genetic moderators of the impact of physical activity on depressive symptoms. *J Frailty Aging* 2016; 5: 6–14.

38. Puterman E, Lin J, Krauss J, Blackburn EH, Epel ES. Determinants of telomere attrition over 1 year in healthy older women: stress and health behaviors matter. *Mol Psychiatry* 2015; 20: 529–535.

CHAPTER 30

Mental health in intellectual disability

Sabyasachi Bhaumik, Dasari Mohan Michael, Reza Kiani, Avinash Hiremath, Shweta Gangavati, and Amala Jesu

Introduction

Public health data on people with intellectual disability (ID) has mainly focused on the physical health aspects and the health inequalities this population experiences. Information on the public health perspective of mental health has been very limited and has largely been dependent on published epidemiological research in people with intellectual disability.

The Public Health England Learning Disability Observatory estimated that in 2015, there were 1,087,100 people with learning disabilities in England [1]. However, it acknowledges the fact that the number of people with learning disabilities recorded in health and welfare systems is much lower.

The Observatory has information on the extent to which people with learning disabilities access a range of services. For example, people with learning disabilities are now more likely to use a wide range of general hospital services and the number of people with learning disabilities in England eligible for and receiving a learning disability annual health check continues to rise (52.2% coverage for 2014–15), but there are substantial geographical variations in that respect.

Similarly, the report from the Observatory reveals that there are substantial geographical variations in the provision of every form of social care service, and expenditure on social care support. For example in 2013–14, the Observatory reported that, overall, 117,025 adults with learning disabilities were using some form of community services, most commonly day services, home care, professional support, and equipment and adaptations. The biggest category of long-term support expenditure has been reported for residential care (£1.7 billion), followed by supported living (£933 million), other long-term community support (£613.2 million), direct payments (£454 million), home care (£349 million), supported accommodation (£274 million), and nursing care (£58 million).

The Observatory report shows that despite the number of completed Deprivation of Liberty Safeguards applications for adults with learning disabilities between 2009–10 to 2013–14 remaining stable; following the 'Cheshire West' Supreme Court judgment in 2014, the number of Deprivation of Liberty Safeguards applications increased substantially. The data also show that over half of surveyed family carers spent more than 100 hours a week providing care for their loved ones; almost a third were not in paid employment as a result of their caring responsibilities.

The presence of health inequalities for people with ID is a common occurrence across the globe. People with ID have complex healthcare needs and the quality of services available to them leaves much to be desired. There have been global concerns raised regarding avoidable mortality and morbidity in people with ID due to the paucity of care while emphasizing the need to recognize the basic principles for any individual in all healthcare settings, which consist of being treated with respect, dignity, and to be included in any health service development work.

This chapter aims to highlight the health inequalities that exist in people with ID, along with measures to improve care and promote good mental and physical health.

Definition of intellectual disability

ID can be defined as a developmental condition, which has resulted in the impairment of global mental abilities that may impact on an individual's adaptive functioning in three areas. Based on the individual's ability to perform daily activities, these areas can be described as follows [2]:

1. The ability to use language, read and write, use mathematical calculations, general knowledge, memory for detail and the ability to reason. These functions are dependent on the ability of an individual to *conceptualize*.

2. The ability to empathize with others, make judgements in social interactions, demonstrate appropriate interpersonal communication, and make and keep relationships/friendships. These functions are dependent on the ability of an individual to *socialize*.

3. The ability to carry out practical tasks such as to manage their own money, find and hold a job successfully, take part in leisure and recreational activities, their personal appearance and personal hygiene, and study or work activities. These functions are dependent on the ability of an individual to *organize*.

The International Classification of Mental and Diseases and Related Problems, 10th Revision (ICD-10) [3] defines ID (mental retardation) as a condition of arrested or incomplete development of the mind that is especially characterized by impairment of skills manifested during the developmental period, which contributes to the overall level of intelligence, i.e. cognitive, language, motor, and social abilities. The ICD-10 also classifies ID into categories based on IQ, with a score less than two standard deviations below the population mean of 100 as the cut-off (i.e. IQ < 70).

The *Diagnostic and Statistical Manual of Mental Disorders, Fifth Edition* (DSM-5) [4] defines ID (intellectual developmental disorder) as a disorder with onset during the developmental period that includes both intellectual and adaptive functioning deficits in conceptual, social, and practical domains.

The forthcoming eleventh revision of the ICD (ICD-11) [5] has chosen the new terminology of 'Developmental Intellectual Disability' to define ID.

While ID does not have a specific age requirement, an individual's symptoms must begin during the developmental period and ID is diagnosed based on the severity of deficits in adaptive functioning. The causation of ID can be broadly categorized based on the developmental phase when the damage to the brain has occurred. Therefore, it is possible that the damage may have occurred during the prenatal period and may be attributable to malnutrition (intra-uterine growth restriction), iatrogenic causes (radiation), and intra-uterine infections (TORCH infections, i.e. Toxoplasmosis, Other (syphilis, varicella-zoster, parvovirus B19), Rubella, Cytomegalovirus, and Herpes infections); during the perinatal period and may be attributable to birth asphyxia resulting in anoxic brain damage or brain haemorrhage due to a traumatic delivery; and during the postnatal period and may be attributable to insults to the brain due to kernicterus, meningo-encephalitis, and so on [6].

Epidemiology

Studies of the prevalence of ID give varying rates, depending on the parameters used, definition, and system of classification. The term ID denotes a heterogeneous group of individuals with a varying range of abilities. The diagnosis of ID is dependent on a systematic assessment of both intellectual and adaptive functioning. It is sometimes problematic to carry out an IQ assessment, and clinicians may need to depend on the assessment of adaptive functioning in order to ascertain the diagnosis and degree of ID. Individuals may not have access to an IQ assessment, especially in low-and-middle-income countries (LAMICs) and scales such as Glasgow Level of Ability and Development scale (GLADS) [7], which measures adaptive functioning, may help to diagnose and also sub-classify. The term ID, although used synonymously with learning disability, should not be confused with the term 'learning difficulty', which includes reading, writing, and numeracy problems such as dyslexia, specific scholastic disorders, and so on. It has been estimated that 2% of the adult population may be suffering from an ID [8]. A meta-analysis by Pallab et al. [9] arrived at an overall prevalence figure of 10.37 per 1000 population, with LAMICs having almost twice the prevalence as that of high-income countries. The administrative prevalence is 0.47% of the adult population, meaning that only a quarter of people use specialist ID services; however, one study reported a global prevalence of 1–3% [10]. Administrative prevalence is calculated based on the number of individuals who access ID services, which is lower than population-based prevalence studies that have screened whole populations for ID.

Based on IQ and level of adaptive functioning, ID can be further sub-categorized into mild (IQ 50–69, mental age equivalent 9–12 years), moderate (IQ 35–49, mental age equivalent 6–9 years), severe (IQ 20–34, mental age equivalent 3–6 years), and profound (IQ < 20, mental age equivalent < 3 years). King et al. [11] reported that of all the people with ID, 85% had mild ID, 10% moderate, 4% severe, and 2% profound ID.

Mental health problems in people with intellectual disability

In comparison with the general population, the lifetime prevalence of all mental health problems is higher in people with ID. The primary factor is underlying brain damage, which has been shown to predispose individuals to mental health problems, more than the general population [12]. People with ID experience the same range of mental disorders as that of the general population. The prevalence of enduring mental health problems, including schizophrenia, is reported to be approximately 2–3 times higher in people with ID than in the general population [13]. There are multiple factors that influence this, including congenital malformations, developmental disorders, and neurological and genetic disorders. Apart from these, there are also other reasons that may contribute to the increased risk and these can be attributed to low self-esteem, deficits in social skills, communication difficulties, frequent changes in care delivery, poor environment, and shortfalls in the availability of quality health services. In addition, a very high proportion of people with ID present with challenging behaviours, which may or may not be associated with any underlying mental or physical health problems. These behaviours may manifest as aggression, self-injurious behaviour, disruptive or destructive behaviour, and occasionally anti-social behaviour. The association of dementia of Alzheimer's type with Down syndrome is also well known, and is more prevalent in this population than in the general population.

Current estimates of the prevalence of mental health problems in people with ID indicate an overall prevalence figure of 40% [6]. Other prevalence figures are as follows: schizophrenic illness (3%), depressive illness (4%), bipolar affective disorder (~1.5%), and dementia (20%).

Population health characteristics and inequalities

Although research shows that people with ID are more likely to have medical and mental health problems than the general population [14, 15], they are particularly at risk of delayed diagnosis [16]. These delays may be related to people with ID having communication difficulties, sensory impairments, and being reliant on family and carers to recognize their symptoms and seek medical help [17]. They may be unable to complain of symptoms, or may display challenging behaviour [18], which clinicians or staff attribute to other causes (diagnostic overshadowing). Lack of awareness of how this client group might present, negative attitudes of professionals towards this client group, and institutional discrimination are some of the other barriers in accessing appropriate treatment modalities in general hospitals where professionals may not have experience in dealing with people with ID (Box 30.1) [19].

The Improving Health and Lives Learning Disabilities Observatory has published several reports on health inequalities

Box 30.1 Barriers to accessing health care by people with intellectual disability

Barriers related to service users

Co-morbid physical disability, autism, and mental ill health.
Severity of intellectual disability and communication difficulties.
Atypical presentation of physical ailments through change in behaviour.
Fear of hospital and investigation.
Some people with intellectual disabilities might not understand the importance of their symptoms.

Barriers related to service provision

Lack of accessible/pictorial information.
Poor access to the clinics and general hospitals.
Environmental barriers.
Not taking into consideration needs of individuals with special needs.

Barriers related to healthcare professionals and carers

Attitudes and assumptions.
Lack of awareness and training.
Institutional discrimination
Perceived difficulties in obtaining informed consent

Source: Data from Marston G, Perry D, Intellectual disabilities. In: Cormac I, Gray D (eds), *Essentials of Physical Health in Psychiatry*, pp. 372–382, Copyright (2013), Royal College of Psychiatrists.

and their causes in people with ID [20]; these reports highlight five determinants of health inequalities faced by children with ID that are potentially amenable to intervention:

• social (e.g. poverty);

• genetic and biological (e.g. various genetic syndromes, e.g. Down syndrome);

• communication difficulties (e.g. deafness);

• personal (e.g. lack of exercise, poor diet, substance misuse);

• limited access to, and the quality of healthcare provision (e.g. lack of appropriate access to hospitals, diagnostic overshadowing, institutional discrimination, lack of reasonable adjustments, low uptake of screening and health-promoting activities, e.g. cancer screening, dental procedures, visual and hearing assessment).

Premature mortality in people with intellectual disability

Over the last few decades studies have consistently revealed that people with ID have a shorter life expectancy and die more prematurely than the general population [21–23]. For example, one study reported high standard mortality ratios (SMRs) in the ID population caused by congenital abnormalities (85.60), diseases of the nervous system and sense organs (16.30), mental disorders (other than dementia; 11.41), and bronchopneumonia (6.47) [24]. Excess

deaths were also reported for diseases of the genitourinary system and digestive system, cerebrovascular disease, other respiratory infections, dementia, other circulatory system diseases, and accidental deaths [24].

Premature death occurs more often in those with severe ID than in those who have mild ID [25–30]. The intrinsic risk factors for premature mortality in this population consist of medical co-morbidities (e.g. epilepsy), which are related to the more severe degree of ID. For example, a study by Forsgren et al. [25] determined that the SMR in those with only ID was significantly increased to 1.6 compared with that of the general population. In those with ID and epilepsy, the SMR was 5.0, and if they had additional cerebral palsy the SMR increased to 5.8. In patients with ID who had epilepsy, pneumonia was the most common cause of death.

A study by Kiani et al. [31] found all-cause specific SMRs were 2.2 and 2.8 for men and women with ID, respectively. SMRs were 3.2 and 5.6 for men and women with epilepsy and ID, respectively. The SMRs for 'sudden unexpected death in epilepsy' (SUDEP) in patients with ID were 37.6 for men and 52.0 for women. The study also found that in the majority of cases of ID there was little detailed documentation on the circumstances surrounding deaths, no communication with patients/carers about risk of SUDEP, and an absence of carers' referral for bereavement counselling.

A recent study on mortality of people with ID is also in line with the previous literature in this area over the past few decades, in that this population has a higher mortality rate than the general population (hazard ratio (HR) 3.6) [32]. The risk remained high when adjusted for comorbidities, smoking, and deprivation (HR 3.1); the HR was higher among adults with ID and Down syndrome or epilepsy. The study also found that over a third of all deaths among adults with ID were classified as being amenable to healthcare intervention versus 22.5% in the general population (HR 5.9). The authors concluded that this mortality disparity suggests the need to improve access to, and quality of, health care among people with ID [32].

The extrinsic risk factors that contribute to the higher rates of premature mortality in this population are related to the environment they are living in, the provision of care, polypharmacy and access to healthcare services, and discrimination [33, 34], some of which is highlighted in the 'Death by Indifference' report by Mencap. Although the report originally (2007) focused on the death of five individuals as a result of institutional/healthcare discriminations [35], the follow-up report (2012) provided more details on the death of more people with ID ('Death by Indifference: 74 and Counting'). The reports highlighted lack of basic care, poor communication, delayed diagnosis and treatment, and the inappropriate use of the Mental Capacity Act 2005 and do not attempt to resuscitate orders. 'Death by Indifference' triggered an independent inquiry/investigation by the Parliamentary and Health Service Ombudsman. This resulted in the government establishing strategies for improvement in access of people with ID to health services: Valuing People Now (2009) and the Six Lives progress report (2010) [36, 37].

The Confidential Inquiry Into Premature Deaths of People with Learning Disabilities (CIPOLD) [23], commissioned by the Department of Health in England, reported a two-times increase in the mortality of those with mild-to-profound ID, with nearly a quarter of people being younger than 50 years of age when they died versus about 9% of the general population. People with ID were also found likely to die, on average, 16 years earlier than the general population. This study also showed that although the risk of dying at an early age was greatest for people with more severe ID, the median age at death of people with mild ID was still substantially younger than that of the general population and twice as many deaths were deemed avoidable in the ID group compared with the general population. Those with more severe ID, congenital and chromosomal abnormalities, and those without the support of family members/friends were more likely to have premature deaths that could have been prevented with good-quality health care.

The CIPOLD study found a range of potentially modifiable factors related to care and service provision, such as problems in advanced care planning, adherence to the Mental Capacity Act 2005, living in inappropriate accommodation, adjustment of care, and carers not feeling listened to, which could have been targeted to reduce premature mortality in people with ID.

Measures to improve health

Assessing health problems in individuals with ID is challenging. The hurdles faced by the clinicians when trying to obtain a comprehensive history and conduct a physical examination on people with ID can only be overcome by having a robust understanding of the principles of communication in people with ID. It cannot be emphasized enough the need to be empathic and to treat the person with due respect and dignity, thereby shifting the focus from their disabilities to their abilities by making information accessible to them and thereby improving their understanding of the illness. Sometimes clinicians need to rely on a presumptive definitive diagnosis and a diagnosis may become evident with the passage of time. While doing this, every effort should be made to gain an understanding of the individual's normal pattern of behaviour and any deviation due to illness. This will help to establish and gauge the optimum treatment response to be achieved.

When an individual with ID is first seen by the specialist team, it is critical that the clinician makes every effort to gather as much information as possible from all relevant sources, such as the affected person's family, school, day centre, and place of work. Following the completion of the assessment, and once a working diagnosis has been established the information should be shared with the individual and their family in a user-friendly format. Other professionals, such as a speech and language therapist, may be asked for support when conveying information, in order to ensure effective facilitation of their communication.

In the longer term, appropriate policies and procedures consistent with Valuing People Now [36] should facilitate people with ID accessing generic health services through coordinated multidisciplinary team working, annual health checks, health action plans, communication passports, and health facilitation.

The 2005 Mental Capacity Act provides a legal framework to enable the clinician to treat those vulnerable patients who lack capacity to consent to appropriate health interventions in hospital settings. The Department of Health has made it explicit that all healthcare providers should make reasonable adjustments to service delivery to meet the complex needs of vulnerable groups of service users in accordance with the Equality Act [38]. Following one of the recommendations of the Independent Inquiry into Access to Healthcare for People with ID ([38], the Learning Disabilities Observatory has been set up, which aims to provide better and more accessible information on the health of people with ID. It will also help hospitals and other providers to better understand the complex needs of people with ID and their carers, which, in turn, should improve outcomes for this vulnerable client group (www.improvinghealthandlives.org.uk/).

The observatory has published recommendations for health and social care providers and commissioners of the services to address the health inequalities experienced by people with ID. Some of these recommendations are reducing the chances that people with ID will be exposed to variables that damage their health (e.g. poverty, poor housing conditions, unemployment, discrimination); increasing the uptake of annual health checks, and cervical and breast screening (in women); helping unpaid and paid carers to better understand the health needs of people with ID; and making 'reasonable adjustments' to health services (e.g. through providing more accessible information and longer appointment times) [39].

Reports such as 'Healthcare for All' [38] and 'Death by Indifference' [35] have given increasing recognition to the substandard levels of health care experienced by people with ID. The follow-up report to 'Death by Indifference, Six Lives' [37] determined that there were serious questions about how well equipped the National Health Service and local authorities are to provide services tailored to the needs of people with ID. The provision of high-quality health care for this client group is therefore a national priority, as highlighted by 'Valuing People Now' [36]. On a similar note, developing local and national databases, publication of research projects on the mortality of people with ID, for example those related to cancer [40], involving service users and their carers in service planning, and mandatory incorporation of ID teaching in undergraduate and postgraduate clinical training curricula can equip future healthcare professionals with the skill set to address the complex needs of people with ID in various settings [41].

CIPOLD subsequently proposed 18 recommendations (Box 30.2) that, if implemented, would reduce the risk of premature death in people with ID [23]. Tyrer et al. [24] also recommended that strategies to reduce health inequalities in people with ID should focus on decreasing mortality from potentially preventable causes, such as respiratory infections and cardiovascular system diseases.

Prevention strategies

Ensuring that high-quality health care for individuals with ID is both available and accessible should be made an international priority. A World Health Organization (WHO) initiative, Mental Health Gap Action Programme (mhGAP) [42] has highlighted differences in the availability of health services between the high-income countries and LAMICs as the latter appear to have a patchy, variable, and lower provision. These differences only re-emphasise the need that reasonable adjustments are made for individuals with ID so that they can be enabled to access mainstream health services. The health status of individuals with ID can only be improved if this is made a priority.

Health promotion

When describing health promotion in people with ID, it is imperative that both physical and mental health issues and the interface between them are discussed. The morbidity and mortality rates, physical health, and health inequalities in people with ID have

Box 30.2 Some of the recommendations of the Confidential Inquiry Into Premature Deaths of People with Learning Disabilities

Identification of people with intellectual disability (ID) on the National Health Service central registration system and healthcare record systems.

Reasonable adjustments to be audited annually and examples of best practice to be shared with other organizations.

A named coordinator to be allocated to people with complex health needs, or two or more long-term conditions.

Standardization of annual health checks and a clear pathway between these and health action plans.

People with ID to have access to the same investigations and treatments as anyone else.

Barriers to individuals' access to health care to be addressed.

Adults with ID to be considered high-risk for deaths from respiratory problems.

Mental Capacity Act advice to be easily available in hospital setting and training and regular updates to be mandatory for staff.

Do not attempt resuscitation guidelines to be more clearly defined and standardized.

Referred to a specialist palliative care team when needed.

Improved collection of mortality data about people with ID.

Systems in place to ensure that local ID mortality data are analysed and published.

Establishment of a national ID mortality review group.

Source: Data from Heslop P, Blair P, Fleming P et al., Confidential Inquiry into premature deaths of people with learning disabilities (CIPOLD): Final report, Copyright (2013), Norah Fry Research Centre.

been previously discussed in this chapter. Here, more details are provided for health promotion strategies.

The planning of health promotion should begin with recognizing the main barriers that individuals with ID experience (Box 30.1). Health promotion includes actions to create living conditions and environments that support and promote mental and physical health, and allow people to adopt and maintain healthy lifestyles. Many people with ID are exposed to abuse, stigmatization, marginalization, humiliation, and discrimination; however, there has been a delay in developing and applying appropriate norms to meet their needs. People with ID are a vulnerable group with complex health needs and co-morbidities, and who experience significant health inequalities when compared with the general population [43].

Although there is a paucity of robust evidence on health promotion in people with ID, research is available, such as that undertaken by Beange et al. [44], which highlights the unmet healthcare needs of people with ID. In 2006, Krahn et al. [33] identified a range of contributing factors, which they attributed to the poor health of people with ID. These factors included complex health conditions that have been poorly managed; frequent changes in direct care that have resulted in inattention to health status and care needs; behaviour problems that have been poorly assessed, understood, and managed; insufficient or inadequate attention being paid to individual health promotion behaviours; and difficulties encountered when implementing clinical preventative services.

The foundations for health promotion, clearly laid out in the Ottawa Charter by the WHO [45] highlighted several issues, some of which are discussed in the following paragraphs.

Promoting healthy behaviours in people with ID should include activities, such as education and support in making healthy choices, which, in turn, improve the quality of life of people with ID. People with ID may have limited opportunities to learn about the importance of healthy lifestyles, including maintaining a normal weight, maintaining a good diet, ensuring regular exercise, and the implications and risks that result from smoking, consumption of alcohol and other illicit substances. Regular medical reviews and appropriate investigations will ensure that people with ID maintain health and lead healthy lives. It is not sufficient to target education and training at people with ID; it is equally important that health care professionals receive appropriate education regarding ID.

Raising the awareness of primary healthcare staff, and staff in educational establishments and non-governmental organizations will go a long way in ensuring that health promotion is kept at the top of the agenda of all initiatives undertaken by these organizations. In addition, people with ID must be given opportunities to participate in healthy lifestyles; and being supported in that process by carers, family members, and champions goes a long way to ensuring the person with ID leads a healthy life, which promotes mental health well-being. Educating carers and providing them with information regarding healthy lifestyles and their positive impact on the life of the person with ID, is crucial in addition to providing user-friendly information to people with ID, for example the importance of physical exercise (regular walking, if possible), engagement in gainful activity (reducing boredom), and making the right choices regarding food. These individuals therefore require support from advocates and a structured programme of regular medical reviews through annual health checks.

Awareness of co-morbid conditions in ID should lead to regular screening in order to prevent or treat these comorbidities in a proactive manner. People with ID may sometimes find it difficult to understand the reasoning behind screening tests and therefore health promotion must include health education prioritizing careful explanation and preparation by the staff or family members. This will ensure that the individual receives support and assistance. In turn, staff and family members, along with the people who have ID, should also be provided with accessible and user-friendly information, which will help with improving their understanding.

Mental health promotion should also include efforts focused at promoting a positive sense of self for the individual supported by family, carers, and professionals alike. Providing opportunities to learn and help to apply new skills, which promote autonomy and participation will promote a sense of dignity and acceptance as valued members of society, which, in turn, contribute to a sense of well-being. The environment can be enhanced to promote this through improving access, inclusion, better understanding, due respect, and appropriate support.

The UK's Department of Health has suggested a two-stage model aimed at promoting health through (i) reducing risk factors such as unemployment, deprivation, poverty, isolation, and so on; and (ii) increasing protective factors, which include improving self-esteem and promoting empowerment, facilitating social participation, improving environments, and so on.

The response from the WHO includes the creation of a comprehensive mental health action plan for 2013–20. The action plan's overall aim is to promote health well-being, prevent mental disorders, provide care, enhance recovery, and promote human rights, and in doing so reduce the mortality, morbidity, and disability for individuals with mental disorders, and focuses on four key objectives:

1. To strengthen effective leadership and governance for mental health.

2. To provide comprehensive, integrated and responsive mental health and social care services in community-based settings.

3. To implement strategies for promotion and prevention in mental health.

4. To strengthen information systems, evidence, and research for mental health.

In order to achieve these objectives, the implementation of the action plan should require and include clear actions for governments, international partners, and the WHO. Ministries of health will need to take a leadership role and collaborate closely with the WHO to work with them and with international and national partners, including civil society, to implement the plan. As there is no action that fits all countries, each government will need to adapt the action plan to its specific national circumstances.

Implementation of the action plan will enable persons with ID to find it easier to access mental health and social care services; have availability of treatment in general healthcare settings; participate in the reorganization of the delivery and evaluation of services so that care and treatment becomes more responsive to their needs; and gain greater access to health services. The WHO's mhGAP action programme facilitates this process. This is further supported by the development of the mhGAP action programme for ID [46], which can be rolled out to all skilled healthcare professionals in general healthcare settings. The mhGAP training programme for ID is aimed at training frontline healthcare workers on all aspects of mental health care for people with ID, thereby raising awareness, early detection, and appropriate signposting for individuals in need. This programme is currently being rolled out in many LAMICs in a phased manner and the feedback so far has been highly positive. Eventually, a sustainable plan for the future will be delivered through the programme of training the trainers.

Our own experience in Sri Lanka and India, where mhGAP training has been provided to two cohorts of frontline care workers [46], demonstrated a marked increase in knowledge and understanding of the mental health problems that people with ID experience. Overall, the training programme was received very positively and there was a palpable enthusiasm in making a difference to the quality of clinical care that healthcare workers can provide in rural areas. However, it remains to be established whether this training has translated into a real difference in actual clinical practice. The next stage of our programme is going to address this particular issue through the assessment of the actual clinical practice of the frontline healthcare workers. At the same time we need to be aware that mhGAP in ID training is not cost neutral and depends on the goodwill and resources made available to the training providers. For this reason the emphasis should be on training the trainers so that it becomes sustainable within the country's healthcare workforce. Many LAMICs have extremely limited resources and are unable to provide sustainable training programmes for their staff members owing to limited resources; however, there is no single solution to such a major issue and hence a powerful government initiative especially for this highly marginalized and discriminated population will be a key factor in making any real difference.

Conclusions

Health promotion (including mental and physical health) and prevention in people with ID is, at present, at a rudimentary stage in many parts of the world, although there has been a greater awareness in the health system about the health needs of people with ID, which is encouraging.

In this chapter we have identified the issues relating to current definitions; however, the fundamental problem that exists in this area is that of a lack of formal diagnostic process for many, especially in low-resource countries. There are initiatives to develop a universal culture-fair rating scale, which can be used by field workers and which may help in identifying the at-risk population for further signposting and management. A current field trial of this work (GLADS) is being undertaken in Europe and the Asian subcontinent in order to look at its specificity, reliability, and sensitivity [7].

The high prevalence of mental and physical health problems in people with ID has many causes; however, case identification can be extremely difficult owing to communication difficulties, atypical presentations, and the interface between mental and physical health co-morbidities; hence, the problem of diagnostic overshadowing is difficult to overcome, unless the person is assessed by a specialist healthcare worker. Use of specialist rating scales in these areas have their significant limitations and need sustainable training programmes for all mental healthcare workers, which may be resource intensive.

Alternatively, a resource-effective option might be to disseminate, via the route of training the trainers, the mhGAP programme ID modules in all LAMICs. This plan should not be left to individual charitable organizations and should be incorporated in physical and mental health planning processes for each country where resources are extremely limited. However, we need to recognize that in many LAMICs, family members play an important role in the care provision for individuals with ID. Threfore, an emphasis on disseminating the knowledge and skills through family and carers will be needed to make progress sustainable. In turn, this endeavour should result in an effective process of health promotion, prevention, and early identification at the grass-roots level.

The current picture of mortality and morbidity in people with ID for both children and adults is worrying and highlights the significant gaps that exist in our health systems worldwide. Although steps have been taken in some Western countries to try and rectify this problem, an approach that really addresses the issue of a shift in the culture of the health professionals in this regard is yet to be seen. There is ample evidence to suggest that despite the publication of reports such as 'Six Lives' [37] and 'Death by Indifference' [35], many people with ID continue to be the recipients of poor-quality care in mainstream settings. The current initiatives to rectify this including establishing acute care pathways and employing liaison nurses in acute care settings are to be lauded but should be supplemented by an information-based health promotion addressed to the general public, including schools, colleges, educational institutions, and care settings. For low-resourced countries, effective use of a disability discrimination act or similar acts should ensure that accessibility to services should not remain a barrier. In addition, other health policy initiatives should include a clear reference to this marginalized population and their needs so that reasonable adjustments in their care can be provided.

There is a tendency among some governments to delegate the development and provision of services for people with ID to the social services departments; however, the provision of services for people with ID has a significant health component and therefore as a first step there needs to be a joint responsibility between both health care and social services to deliver their care. The next step will be to identify specific resource allocation for the care of people with ID in all health and social care policies. It will then be important to create champions at each organization level who will ensure implementation of awareness-raising programmes, which will eventually help to develop a care pathway-based approach with input from clinical staff in the organization.

Non-government organizations also play a significant role in low-resource countries in raising awareness and by promoting mental and physical health, and providing support to people with ID in the absence of a clear government policy. Their roles can be strengthened as partners in these new initiatives right from the start, which, hopefully, will reduce the need for high-level resource allocation in LAMICs in competition with other population health needs.

References

1. Public Health England. Learning Disabilities Observatory. People with learning disabilities in England. 2015: Main report. Available at: https://www.gov.uk/government/uploads/system/uploads/attachment_data/file/613182/PWLDIE_2015_main_report_NB090517.pdf (accessed 20 June 2017).
2. American Association of Intellectual and Developmental Disabilities. Definition of Intellectual Disability. Available at: http://aaidd.org/intellectual-disability/definition#.V5zkcvkrK01/ (accessed 20 July 2016).
3. World Health Organization (WHO). *The ICD-10 Classification of Mental and Behavioural Disorders*. Geneva: WHO, 1992.
4. American Psychiatric Association (APA). *Diagnostic and Statistical Manual of Mental Disorders, Fifth Edition (DSM-5)*. Washington DC: APA, 2013.
5. Cooray S, Bhaumik S, Roy A, Devapriam J, Rai R, Alexander R. Intellectual disability and the ICD-11: towards clinical utility. *Adv Ment Health Care Intellect Disabil* 2015; 9: 3–8.
6. Bhaumik S, Kiani R, Gangavati S, Khan S. Management of intellectual disability. In: Fiorillo A, Volpe U, Bhugra D (eds). *Psychiatry in Practice. Education, Experience and Expertise*. Oxford: Oxford University Press, 2015, pp. 359–376.
7. Cooray S, Cooper S-A, Weber G, et al. The clinical utility of the Glasgow Level of Ability and Development Scale in screening for disorders of intellectual development: a multicentre international study. *J Intellect Disabil Res* 2016; 60: 775.
8. Emerson E, Hatton C. Centre for Disability.People with Learning Disabilities in England. Available at: http://www.lancaster.ac.uk/staff/emersone/FASSWeb/Emerson_08_PWLDinEngland.pdf (accessed 19 October 2016).
9. Pallab K, Maulik MN, Mascarenhas Colin D, Mathers TD, Shekhar S. Prevalence of intellectual disability: a meta-analysis of population-based studies. *Res Dev Disabil* 2011; 32: 419–436.
10. Harris JC. *Intellectual Disability. Understanding its Development, Causes, Classification, Evaluation and Treatment*. New York: Oxford University Press, 2006.
11. King BH, Toth KE, Hodapp RM, Dykins EM. Intellectual disability. In: Sadock BJ, Ruiz P (eds). *Comprehensive Textbook of Psychiatry*, 9th ed. Philadelphia, PA: Lippincott Williams & Wilkins, 2009, pp. 3444–3474.
12. Rutter M, Bishop DVM, Pine DS, et al. *Rutter's Child and Adolescent Psychiatry*. Oxford: Oxford University Press, 2008.
13. Cooper SA, Smiley E, Morrison J, Williamson A, Allan L. Mental ill-health in adults with intellectual disabilities: prevalence and associated factors. *Br J Psychiatry* 2007; 190: 27–35.
14. van Schrojenstein Lantman De Valk HM, Metsemakers JF, Haveman MJ, Crebolder HF. Health problems in people with intellectual disability in general practice: a comparative study. *Fam Pract* 2000; 17: 405–407.
15. van Schrojenstein Lantman-de Valk HMJ, Noonan Walsh P. Managing health problems in people with intellectual disabilities. *BMJ* 2008; 337: a2507.
16. Tuffrey-Wijne I, Bernal J, Hubert J, Butler G, Hollins S. People with learning disabilities who have cancer: an ethnographic study. *Br J Gen Pract* 2009; 59: 503–509.
17. Alborz A, McNally R, Glendinning C. Access to healthcare for people with learning disabilities: mapping the issues and reviewing the evidence. *J Health Serv Policy* 2005; 10:173–182.
18. Lindsey M. Comprehensive health care services for people with learning disabilities. *Adv Psychiatr Treat* 2002; 8: 138–147.
19. Marston G, Perry D. Intellectual disabilities. In: Cormac I, Gray D (eds). *Essentials of Physical Health in Psychiatry*. Glasgow: Bell & Bain, 2013, pp 372–382.
20. Public Health England. The determinants of health inequities experienced by children with learning disabilities. Available at: https://www.ldag.info/media/294672/determinants_of_child_health_inequalities.pdf (accessed 19 October 2016).
21. Eyman RK, Grossman HJ, Chaney RH, Call, TL. The life expectancy of profoundly handicapped people with mental retardation. *N Engl J Med* 1990; 323: 584–589.
22. Cohen A, Asor E, Tirosh E. Predictive factors of early mortality in children with developmental disabilities: a case-comparison analysis. *J Child Neurol* 2008; 23: 536–542.
23. Heslop P, Blair P, Fleming P, Hoghton M, Marriott A, Russ L. Confidential Inquiry into premature deaths of people with learning disabilities (CIPOLD). *Lancet* 2014; 383: 889–895.
24. Tyrer F, McGrother C. Cause-specific mortality and death certificate reporting in adults with moderate to profound intellectual disability. *J Intellect Disabil Res* 2009; 53: 898–904.
25. Forsgren L, Edvinsson SO, Nyström L, Blomquist HK. Influence of epilepsy on mortality in mental retardation: an epidemiologic study. *Epilepsia* 1996; 37: 956–963.
26. Hollins S, Attard MT, von Fraunhofer N, McGuigan S, Sedgwick P. Mortality in people with learning disability: risks, causes, and death certification findings in London. *Dev Med Child Neurol* 1998; 40: 50–56.
27. Patja K, Iivanainen M, Vesala H, Oksanen H, Ruoppila I. Life expectancy of people with intellectual disability: a 35-year follow-up study. *J Intellect Disabil Res* 2000; 44: 591–599.
28. Patja K, Mölsä P, Iivanainen M. Cause-specific mortality of people with intellectual disability in a population-based, 35-year follow-up study. *J Intellect Disabil Res* 2001; 45: 30–40.
29. Lavin KE, McGuire BE, Hogan MJ. Age at death of people with an intellectual disability in Ireland. *J Intellect Disabil* 2006; 10: 155–164.
30. Tyrer F, Smith LK, McGrother CW. Mortality in adults with moderate to profound intellectual disability: a population-based study. *J Intellect Disabil Res* 2007; 51: 520–527.
31. Kiani R, Tyrer F, Jesu A, et al. Mortality from sudden unexpected death in epilepsy (SUDEP) in a cohort of adults with intellectual disability. *J Intellect Disabil Res* 2013; 58: 508–520.
32. Hosking FJ, Crey IM, Shah SM, Harris T, DeWilde S, Beighton C, Cook DG. Mortality among adults with intellectual disability in England: comparisons with the general population. *Am J Public Health* 2016; 106: 1483–1490.

33. Krahn GL, Hammond L, Turner A. A cascade of disparities: health and health care access for people with intellectual disabilities. *Ment Retard Dev Disabil Res Rev* 2006; 12: 70–82.

34. Ouellette-Kuntz H. Understanding health disparities and inequities faced by Individuals with intellectual disabilities. *J Appl Res Intellect Disabil* 2005; 18: 113–121.

35. Mencap. *Death by Indifference*. London: Mencap, 2007.

36. Department of Health. *Valuing People Now: A New Three-year Strategy for People with Learning Disabilities*. London: Department of Health.

37. Local Government Ombudsman and Health Service Ombudsman. *Six Lives: The Provision of Public Services to People with Learning Disabilities*. London: The Stationery Office, 2009.

38. Michael J. *Healthcare for All: Report of the Independent Inquiry into Access to Healthcare for People with Learning Disabilities*. London: Department of Health, 2008.

39. Emerson E, Baines S, Allerton L, Welch V. Health Inequalities & People with Learning Disabilities in the UK: 2012. Available at: http://cdn.basw.co.uk/upload/basw_14846-4.pdf (accessed 20 July 2016).

40. Satge D, Merrick J. *Cancer in Children and Adults with Intellectual Disabilities, Current Research Aspects*. New York: Nova Science, 2011.

41. Kiani R, Vahabzadeh A, Hepplewhite, EA, et al. Overcoming challenges in diagnosing and treating cancers in people with intellectual disability: a case analysis. *Tiz Learn Disabil Rev* 2014; 19: 51–58.

42. World Health Organization. WHO Mental Health Gap Action Programme (mhGAP). Available at: http://www.who.int/mental_health/mhgap/en/ (accessed 20 July 2016).

43. Scheepers M, Kerr M, O'Hara D, et al. Reducing health disparity in people with intellectual disabilities: a report from Health Issues Special Interest Research Group of the International Association for the Scientific Study of Intellectual Disabilities. *J Policy Pract Intellect Disabil* 2005; 2: 249–255.

44. Beange H, Mc Elduff A, Baker W. Medical disorders of adults with mental retardation: a population study. *Am J Ment Retard* 1995; 99: 595–604.

45. World Health Organization. The Ottowa Charter for Health Promotion 1986. Available at: http://www.euro.who.int/__data/assets/pdf_file/0004/129532/Ottawa_Charter.pdf (accessed 19 July 2016).

46. Gumber R, Gangavati S, Bhaumik S, et al. The WHO mhGAP Intervention Guide for people with intellectual disability: the Sri Lankan experience. *Br J Psychiatry* 2015; 12(Suppl. S1): S-19-S-23.

CHAPTER 31

Physical and psychiatric co-morbidity

Niels Okkels, Christina Blanner Kristiansen, and Povl Munk-Jørgensen

Introduction

Co-morbidity: Disease(s) that coexist(s) in a study participant in addition to the index condition that is the subject of study [1].

In the 1934 book *Mortality of People with Mental Disease*, Benjamin Malzberg gives a detailed account of the increased mortality among institutionalized psychiatric patients [2]. He recognized that the increased mortality was, at least in part, owing to a high co-occurrence of physical illness. In fact, he accurately stated that the leading cause of death was disease of the heart—as it is today—almost a century later [3].

Compared with the general population, the average lifespan of psychiatric patients is decreased by 15–20 years [3–6]. Coexisting physical and mental illness is common and increases the complexity of treatment, costs of health care, and risk of polypharmacy [7]. It worsens the prognosis and increases the risk of complications. Co-occurrence of disorders worsens the prognosis of all diseases involved to a significantly greater extent than simply the addition of problems related to the diseases involved [7]. As such, co-morbidity is one of the most important, current challenges to public mental health and modern medicine in general [8–11].

Despite an abundance of documentation, the increased mortality from physical illness in psychiatric patients has not improved. In fact, in recent decades, the mortality gap has worsened, likely reflecting that patients with severe mental illness have not fully benefited from the improvements in health outcomes available to the general population [11, 12]. The gap reflects a great discrepancy between available knowledge and clinical reality [13]. Malzberg's book proves that academic medicine has long been aware that people with mental illness suffer from higher rates of physical illness than the general population. Why has this knowledge not been implemented? Why do psychiatric patients still die prematurely?

In this chapter we explain the concept of co-morbidity, and outline the impact of physical co-morbidity on mortality, health care, and the economy. We then present examples of prevalent physical illnesses in psychiatric patients. Then, we discuss the pathways by which two separate illnesses may come to co-occur in one individual, such as co-occurrence by chance, or when one illness causes the other. The chapter ends with a discussion of the challenges posed by co-morbidity, such as caring for complex patients in a (sub)specialized healthcare system, and the tendency of clinical trials to exclude patients with co-morbidity.

The solutions to these challenges may include education of healthcare professionals, integrated health care with more emphasis on generalists and collaboration, and targeting of risk factors that are common to both physical and mental illnesses.

What is co-morbidity?

Co-morbidity is the co-occurrence of two or more disorders [14]. Although the knowledge of increased mortality and physical co-morbidity in psychiatric patients is old, the concept of co-morbidity is relatively young. It was first described in the scientific literature by Richard Feinstein in 1970 [15], and it was not until 1990 that it was introduced as a search term in the large electronic medical database PubMed [16].

Timing and sequence

Imagine a patient with diabetes (index disease) who later develops severe depression (co-morbid illness), or vice versa, a patient with depression (index disease) who develops diabetes (co-morbid illness). For a patient with co-morbid depression and diabetes it might seem arbitrary to discuss which disease is the index, and which is the co-morbid. However, the sequence of the diseases is important for several reasons. Firstly, the aetiology of the co-morbid illness may relate to the index disease. As we will see in the section 'Pathways to co-morbidity', there are several ways in which diabetes can increase the risk of developing depression, and vice versa [17]. Secondly, the sequence may be important to our treatment strategy. For example, a patient with periodic depression may have been treated with a diabetogenic psychotropic drug for years, and the first step in a treatment plan would be to discontinue the drug and find a suitable replacement.

Thus, the sequence of co-morbidity is important in considerations about aetiology and treatment. Another important point is that the field of co-morbidity primarily considers chronic, incurable diseases, that become more prevalent with old age.

Co-morbidity versus multi-morbidity

Co-morbidity is closely related to multi-morbidity. *Co-morbidity* considers one disease to be an index disease and thus gives weight to the sequence in which the diseases arise [14]. As such, co-morbidity is sensitive to the perspective of the clinician, and carries a risk of losing the perspective of the 'whole patient'. *Multi-morbidity*, however, simply considers a patient with 'many diseases' [18]. As such, multi-morbidity gives equal weight to all diseases. It points the attention to the common challenges of caring for patients with two or more diseases, such as polypharmacy, inadequacy of clinical guidelines considering only one disease, and barriers to integrated care. Also, multi-morbidity may be a more meaningful term to patients, who do not care about 'index' diseases but more about what it means to live with two diseases co-existing and its implications to treatment and life in general. In this sense, multi-morbidity emphasizes a holistic and patient-centred approach.

Coexisting diseases

Psychiatric diagnoses have diagnostic criteria that establish a hierarchy between physical and mental illness [19]. For example, the diagnostic criteria for depression dictate that significant organic (i.e. physical) disease must be ruled out, such as severe hypothyroidism or acute anaemia, causing symptoms that resemble depression. In practice, however, separating disease entities is not easy. Consider a patient with symptoms of both asthma and anxiety. Anxiety is both a well-defined disease and a symptom related to other disorders, such as when experiencing an asthmatic attack. Should the clinician then diagnose asthma *and* anxiety (co-morbidities), or should he or she consider the patient's anxiety as part of the condition of asthma? There is no unified answer to this problem, which illustrates that the concept of co-morbidity depends on how we define and classify disease. As such, there is an increasing challenge of distinguishing a differential diagnosis from a co-morbidity from a symptom that is integrated in the index disease. This is partly owing to an increasing number of available diagnoses [20].

We have now considered *what* co-morbidity is. Now we will discuss *why* co-morbidity is an important issue to discuss.

Impact of co-morbidity

Co-morbidity impacts on the individual, diagnosis and treatment, healthcare systems, and society [7, 9]. Compared with a patient with diabetes only, a patient with co-morbid diabetes *and* depression may experience delayed diagnosis, polypharmacy, increased complications, more morbidity, and worse outcome [17]. Consequences on a societal level include lost work days, expenditures for medication and treatment, readmissions, and prolonged hospital stays. This section will focus on two outcomes that are important from a public mental health perspective: mortality and economic costs.

Increased mortality

Most disorders, both physical and mental, are associated with an increased mortality. Evidently, having two disorders increases mortality, as compared with having one disorder. But, in fact, having two disorders increases mortality more than the combined mortality from the disorders, yielding a 2 + 2 = 5 effect. As an example, an individual suffering from both depression and diabetes does not have an increased mortality corresponding to the sum: the coexistence of the disorders increases mortality even more than the sum of the disorders.

What explains this excess mortality? Having one disease may delay diagnosis of a second (co-morbid) disease. Imagine a patient suffering from diabetes who complains about low energy, weight gain, and difficulties concentrating. These three complaints may easily be attributed to the clinical syndrome of diabetes. But if, in fact, this patient has a co-morbid depression, the diagnosis may be delayed because of misattribution of symptoms to the index disease [21]. The other way around a patient suffering from depression may consult his doctor with complaints that are interpreted as symptoms of depression, when, in fact, the patient has developed a physical illness, such as hypothyroidism. There is a well-documented tendency among clinicians to attribute physical symptoms to a patient's mental illness, thus 'covering up' the co-morbidity and delaying diagnosis [22, 23]. For example, a study using data from the extensive Swedish health service registers followed 8277 patients with schizophrenia over 7 years [5]. They found that male patients died, on average, 15 years earlier and females 12 years earlier than the background population, and that a leading cause was cardiovascular disease. Worryingly, the patients with schizophrenia who died from cardiovascular disease were less likely to have been diagnosed earlier, despite having twice as many contacts to the healthcare system in total.

Another explanation for excess mortality is polypharmacy, defined as the use of four or more medications by a patient [24]. Having co-morbid diseases increases the risk of polypharmacy, which again increases the risk of adverse drug reactions, interactions, and side effects. We will discuss polypharmacy in more depth in the section 'Management of co-morbidity'.

A third explanation may be undesirable interactions between two diseases, or between a drug and a disease. Having paranoid schizophrenia may complicate treatment of co-morbid cardiovascular disease if the patient is sceptical about the cardiologist's diagnosis and refuses to take heart medication (disease–disease interaction). Also, the antipsychotic medication may directly worsen the prognosis of cardiovascular recovery (drug–disease interaction) [25].

Compared with the general population, people with schizophrenia have a 2–3-fold increased risk of dying. The differential mortality gap between people with schizophrenia and the general population has worsened in recent decades, likely reflecting that patients with severe mental illness have not fully benefited from the improvements in health outcomes available to the general population [12]. Another explanation may be the introduction of second-generation antipsychotics. The increased mortality implicates a public mental health failure: that we have not succeeded in closing the mortality gap between people with severe mental illness and the general population. In the following subsection we will discuss another severe consequence of co-morbidity: the economic costs.

Economic costs

Co-morbid physical and mental illnesses challenge our healthcare systems and economies by prolonged recovery, increased length of hospital stays, more complications, increased rates of hospitalization, and more frequent emergency department visits. Having a co-morbid physical illness increases costs by a factor of 1.3–2.3 verus having a mental illness alone, according to a recent review [26]. However, having a co-morbid mental illness increases costs by a factor of 1.5–1.8 versus having a physical illness alone.

A report from 2016 concludes that the cost of co-morbid physical illness is AUD$15 billion in Australia (approximately £9 billion) and NZD$3.1 billion in New Zealand (approximately £1.8 billion) [27]. If the burden of substance abuse is included, the cost is AUD$45.4 billion and NZD$6.2 billion, respectively, corresponding to approximately £28 billion and £3.6 billion. Looking at indirect costs, physical and psychiatric co-morbidity is associated with high rates of absenteeism and poor functioning at work. Again, the combined effect of co-morbidity is higher than each condition individually.

Among patients with co-morbid diabetes and depression, systematic depression treatment increases time free of depression and appears to have substantial economic benefits [28]. The authors of the study recommend screening for depression to be integrated in the routine clinical care of patients with diabetes.

Pathways to co-morbidity

There are several hypotheses of why physical and mental illness frequently co-occur. These include common risk factors such as growing up in a socio-economically deprived environment, excess alcohol consumption, and a sedentary lifestyle. Other factors contributing to a high occurrence of co-morbidity is stigma and difficult access to treatment, low confidence among mental health workers in managing mental illnesses, and lack of funding to mental health institutions [7]. A higher co-occurrence than expected from the prevalence in the background population implies an association between physical and mental illness that can reveal aspects of aetiology, common risk factors, pathophysiological interplay, and perhaps even direct causation [29]. In the following subsections we present a non-exhaustive series of situations to illustrate some of the pathways [30].

How diseases co-occur

Consider the following theoretical situations: one disease co-occurs by chance with another disease [14]. As an example consider cancer and schizophrenia, where the prevalence appears equal to that in the general population, with some occurring more frequently, and others less frequently [31, 32]. By statistical chance there must be an overlap that can be calculated as the prevalence of cancer multiplied by the prevalence of schizophrenia. If the point prevalence of cancer is 10% and the point prevalence of schizophrenia is 1%, the combined prevalence is $0.1 \times 0.01 = 0.001$, that is, approximately 0.1% of the population will have co-morbid cancer and schizophrenia, assuming independence between the two.

In another situation, one disease *induces* the other. As an example consider a patient with anorexia nervosa who develops osteoporosis. Prolonged under-nutrition may result in loss of bone mass and, ultimately, osteoporosis [33]. Note the unidirectional association; osteoporosis cannot (as far as we know) induce anorexia nervosa. Another example of co-morbid disorders with an unidirectional relationship could be cirrhosis caused by chronic alcohol abuse.

A third situation: two disorders have a bidirectional relationship where both disorders affect each other. One disorder affects the other and vice versa. As an example, consider asthma and anxiety [34]. In the acute setting, having an asthma attack may induce symptoms of anxiety; or the other way around, having an attack of anxiety may induce difficulty breathing. Another example of diseases with a bidirectional relationship could be diabetes and depression, which both affect each other in complex ways [17]. Suffering from a chronic disease such as diabetes may come with decreased function that limits participation in daily routines, social activities, and work. The burdens of diabetes management, including insulin injection, regular doctor's appointments, dietary restrictions, and glucose self-monitoring, can lead to negative emotions and loss of interest, poor sleep, and concentration. In sum, diabetes may lead to loss of function in areas that are central to life and have a negative impact on general well-being and mood. Further, it is hypothesized that the chronic state of inflammation can contribute to the development of depression. As such there are both psychological, social, and biological factors that may explain how diabetes can induce depression [35]. How, then, can depression lead to diabetes? Depression is associated with alterations in the hypothalamic–pituitary–adrenal axis, which plays a central role in the complex metabolic pathology of many chronic diseases, including diabetes. Also, psychotropic medications may predispose an individual to develop metabolic illness, including diabetes [36].

In a fourth situation, two disorders seem related, but their association can be explained by a third factor. As an example, consider the association between schizophrenia and lung cancer, which may be explained by the fact that people with schizophrenia smoke more than the general population [37]. Schizophrenia is associated with smoking, which is associated with lung cancer. In other words, smoking 'confounds' the association between schizophrenia and lung cancer. Another example could be severe mental illness and HIV, which can be explained by the association of severe mental illness with intravenous substance abuse, which is associated with HIV [38].

In another situation, a risk factor increases the risk of two co-morbid disorders. As an example, consider sedentary behaviour, which is an independent risk factor for both depression and cardiovascular disease [39, 40].

Finally, consider a situation where two risk factors are mutually associated. As an example consider traumatic experiences and low socio-economic status [41]. The first predispose a person to develop bipolar disorder [42], and the second predispose a person to develop cardiovascular disease [43].

Physical illnesses in psychiatric patients

To improve our treatment and prevention of co-morbid physical illness in patients with mental illness, the first and most important premise is to know what to look for. We will therefore, in this section, present knowledge about the co-morbidity between the most common mental illnesses and the most important physical illnesses.

Epidemiology

The worldwide prevalence of co-morbidity of all disorders is estimated to be 60% and perhaps greater than 80% in people aged > 85 years [44]. Co-morbidity occurs 10–15 years earlier in people who are socio-economically deprived, and social deprivation is particularly associated with psychiatric co-morbidity [45]. The prevalence of both physical and mental illness is 11% in the most deprived versus 5.9% in the least deprived. Also, the presence of a mental illness increases with the number of physical co-morbidities.

Table 31.1 Physical illnesses that are more common in patients with severe mental illness than in the general population

Group	Specific diseases
Cardiovascular diseases	Ischaemic heart disease
	Stroke
	Hypertension
Infectious diseases	HIV
	Hepatitis
	Tuberculosis
Endocrine diseases	Diabetes
	Obesity
	Metabolic syndrome
	Osteoporosis
	Hyperlipidaemia
Dermatological diseases	Psoriasis
	Atopic dermatitis
Autoimmune diseases	
Respiratory disease	Chronic obstructive pulmonary disease
	Pneumonia
Urogenital diseases	Sexual dysfunction
Gynaecological diseases	Obstetric complications

Source: Adapted from World psychiatry, 10(1), Hert M, Correll CU, Bobes J, et al., Physical illness in patients with severe mental disorders. I. Prevalence, impact of medications and disparities in health care, pp. 52–77, Copyright (2011), with permission from John Wiley and Sons.

In the course of a lifetime, approximately 30% of a population will come into contact with the mental health services [46]. Thus, the group of 'psychiatric patients' is very large and heterogeneous, spanning age groups, genders, socio-economic strata, and cultures. This heterogeneity is reflected in physical illnesses: there is not just one or two diseases that can explain the excess mortality. In fact, there is a long list of physical illnesses that are more commonly co-morbid in psychiatric patients, including diabetes [47], ischaemic heart disease [48, 49], stroke [50], hypertension [51], infectious diseases [52], osteoporosis [33], autoimmune diseases [53], respiratory illnesses [48], dermatological disorders [54], and chronic kidney failure [31]. Table 31.1 presents an overview of physical illnesses that are more prevalent in psychiatric patients compared with the background population. The list is diverse and includes illnesses from all organ systems and medical specialties. A second conclusion may be that the diseases fall into two clusters: diseases that are related to substance abuse, and diseases that develop because of a lifestyle with smoking, little exercise, and being overweight.

A very common co-morbidity to mental illness is not listed in Table 31.1, namely substance abuse. Co-morbid mental illness and substance abuse is common and presents a great challenge to mental health care [55]. In fact, this co-morbidity has its own expression, 'dual diagnosis'. Substance abuse is, per definition, a mental illness, however, and therefore not a 'co-morbid physical illness', and we will not elaborate further on this concept in this chapter.

Clearly, a comprehensive review of all physical illnesses co-morbid to mental illnesses is beyond the scope of this chapter. In the following, we present three that are very important from a public mental health point of view; diabetes, metabolic syndrome, and cardiovascular disease.

Diabetes

The prevalence of diabetes is 2–3 times as prevalent in people with schizophrenia, bipolar disorder, and schizoaffective disorder than in the general population. In patients with depression the prevalence of diabetes is 1.2–2.6 times higher than in people without depression [31]. Looking at severe mental illness broadly, including schizophrenia, bipolar disorder, and severe depression, the prevalence of type 2 diabetes mellitus is approximately 1 in 10, and the risk is almost doubled compared with matched controls [47]. For people with severe mental illness, the risk of type 2 diabetes mellitus is consistently elevated across age groups and gender compared with the general population. Multi-episode mental illness (compared with first episode) is a significant predictor of developing type 2 diabetes mellitus, and the prevalence is higher among individuals prescribed antipsychotics. Among patients with diabetes, both minor and major depression is associated with increased mortality compared with patients with diabetes alone [56].

In summary, there seems to be a strong association between severe mental illness and diabetes. It is possible that this relation can be explained, at least partly, by long-term exposure to unhealthy lifestyle risk factors that are common to both patients with diabetes and severe mental illness, such as sedentary behaviour [47, 56].

Metabolic syndrome

The overall prevalence of metabolic syndrome among patients with schizophrenia, bipolar disorder, and depression, is about one in three [57]. The relative risk compared with the general population is about 1.5. As for diabetes, there is no difference in prevalence when comparing patients with schizophrenia, bipolar disorder, or depression. Old age, obesity, and treatment with antipsychotic medications are important moderators of this relationship. In fact, the risk of metabolic syndrome differs across commonly used antipsychotic drugs [25]. However, despite this knowledge, and dissemination of clinical guidelines, patients on antipsychotic medications are under-assessed for metabolic and cardiac risk factors, such as weight and blood pressure [58]. Similarly to diabetes, multi-episode mental illness appears to be an important risk factor in developing metabolic syndrome. There are geographical differences with the highest prevalences found in Australia, New Zealand, and North America. This finding may be affected by the diagnostic criteria that are used for metabolic syndrome; however, it could reflect environmental and perhaps genetic differences. The authors of a large review on metabolic syndrome and severe mental illness conclude that screening for risk factors, including lifestyle and certain antipsychotic medications, should be a key priority in the interdisciplinary treatment of people with severe mental illness [57].

Cardiovascular disease

The mortality from heart disease in people with severe mental illness is increased by approximately a factor three compared with the general population. In contrast, the rate of *diagnosed* heart disease in this population is only slightly increased compared with the general population [59]. This indicates that heart disease is under-diagnosed in this patient group. In the years following a diagnosis of heart disease, patients with severe mental illness have increased mortality but undergo fewer invasive procedures than the general population. This under-treatment contributes to the excess mortality.

A study from the UK demonstrated that patients with severe mental illness have a marked excess mortality from cardiovascular disease across all age groups [48]. Thus, there is a threefold increase of dying from coronary heart disease or stroke among persons younger than 50 years of age, and a twofold increase among those aged 50–70 years. The risk remains increased even when adjusting for prescription of antipsychotic medication; however, a higher presribed dosage predicted higher risk of mortality from cardiovascular disease.

An Australian study followed more than 200,000 people with mental illness for almost two decades [60]. They found that death from ischaemic heart disease was the leading cause of death, and that the mortality rate from ischaemic heart disease has not declined over time. There is little difference in admission rates for ischaemic heart disease between psychiatric patients and the general population; however, much fewer revascularization procedures are performed in psychiatric patients, particularly in people with psychosis. Thus, patients with mental illness and cardiovascular disease are also under-treated when diagnosed.

Management of co-morbidity

A wealthy man I know went from doctor to doctor to try to find a reason for his fatigue. Each doctor looked in depth at the organ in which (s)he was an expert. Each did the latest tests … And the patient, the person, got worse [61].

Co-morbidity poses significant challenges to the patient, daily clinical care, our healthcare systems, and public mental health [7, 9]. Research is designed to answer questions about single disease and often exclude participants that are complex [62]. Medical schools teach students mostly about single diseases and typical case examples from textbooks illustrate patients with single diseases [45]. Clinical guidelines have been developed to improve clinical decision-making and help clinicians follow best evidence-based practice but fail to consider management of patients with more than one disease [63]. In the following, we will go through the inadequacies of guidelines and polypharmacy and then turn to some potential approaches to manage co-morbidity: integrated care, collaborative care, and goal-oriented care.

Inadequacy of guidelines

Clinical guidelines are typically developed by specialist groups for the management of single diseases, such as guidelines developed by endocrinologists for managing diabetes [63]. Guidelines rarely deal with co-morbidity and they are developed based on evidence from clinical trials that usually exclude patients with co-morbid conditions [62]. Applying recent UK clinical guideline recommendations to a hypothetical 78-year-old woman with depression, previous myocardial infarction, type 2 diabetes, osteoarthritis, and chronic obstructive pulmonary disease would yield 11 prescriptions with up to 10 other drugs routinely recommended, engagement in nine lifestyle interventions, and expectations to attend 8–10 routine primary care appointments and 8–30 consultations for depression

[63]. Thus, every recommendation in a guideline in isolation may be sound, but the sum of all recommendations in an individual is not [64]. This problem represents a significant challenge in measuring clinical care on a public mental health scale [65].

Polypharmacy

Following single-disease guidelines in the treatment of patients with co-morbidities may lead to polypharmacy as defined by concomitant use of four or more medications in a patient [24]. Polypharmacy is a common problem and it is estimated that 30% of people in developed countries aged 65 years or older are prescribed five or more drugs [66]. Polypharmacy increases the risk of drug interactions, side effects, and overall mortality. Within the field of psychiatry, a national survey on prescription from office-based psychiatrists in the USA found an increase in visits where two or more psychotropic drugs were prescribed from 43% in 1996 to 60% in 2005–06 [67]. In the same time period, the median number of medications prescribed in each visit increased from one to two. The basic principles of assessing patients with polypharmacy include assessing reasons for all drugs that a patient is currently taking, considering the overall risk of drug-induced harm, and assess each drug with respect to its potential benefit and harms [24]. There have been public health initiatives to reduce polypharmacy in elderly patients, and perhaps it is time to consider similar initiatives aimed at psychotropic medications specifically.

Integrated care

Over the past decades our healthcare system has become increasingly sub-specialized, both on a clinical and structural level. This fragmentation of health care creates a range of challenges for patients with co-morbidity. In a fragmented healthcare system we risk losing sight of the 'whole' patient. Patients are more dissatisfied with health care in more fragmented healthcare systems [61]. From the patients' perspective this has partly to do with an experience of not being considered a person, when encountering a clinician that assumes responsibility for only a technical skill, procedure, or body part. From the clinician's perspective, the lack of responsibility and relation to patients may lead clinicians to report frequent feelings of inadequacy, dissatisfaction, and frustration.

Solving the future challenges of co-morbidity requires involvement of generalist physicians that can incorporate the patient's perspective and personal health status, integrate disease-specific guidelines to the unique personal situation of the patient, and integrate the personal goals and preferences of the patients with the medical priorities, thereby shifting the focus from problem-oriented to goal-oriented [68, 69]. Also, general practitioners can follow patients over time, be attentive to the fact that the goals of patients can change over time, involve other healthcare providers, and participate in shared decision-making. A holistic approach requires that the clinician establishes a relationship with the patient and takes responsibility of the whole patient, and not just a technical detail or single disease [61]. This approach will likely also lead to better health and higher satisfaction in patients, and less frustration in healthcare professionals.

Overcoming the de-integration of health care will likely require large-scale structural changes based on political and public mental health initiatives. Two recent reviews conclude that it is difficult to improve outcomes for people with multiple conditions [70, 71]. There is emerging evidence for the improvement, however, if interventions can be targeted at common risk factors such as depression, or on difficulties that people experience with daily functioning. Authorities in public mental health argue for an integrated understanding between mental illnesses and other health conditions. Mental illness interacts with health conditions in complex ways and should be integrated in the policy framework for health improvement, as underlined by an influential review published in *The Lancet*, 'No health without mental health' [9].

Goal-oriented care

Often, healthcare professionals aim to help their patients fix a *problem*—usually cure a disease or prevent death. There is plenty of evidence that physicians and patients are good at identifying problems: today, more patients than ever before have a diagnosis, undergo procedures, and have medical treatment, such as drug therapy. A problem-oriented approach may work well for acute or curable illnesses, such as acute pneumonia in a young patient. However, for chronic conditions that cannot be cured, it may be more fruitful to focus on the patient's needs and goals for life in general [68]. The goal-oriented model focuses on health in a broad sense and includes the patient's preferences. The model places a greater emphasis on patient's resources and strengths. The patient is invited to define what health means to him, thus encouraging a shared patient-physician collaboration. Naturally, to have the patients share their needs, goals, and expectations will require good communication skills from the physician.

Collaborative care

Collaboration is the involvement of non-medical specialists to improve the care of patients in a primary care setting. It involves a range of interventions from simple and brief encounters, such as telephone calls, to encourage compliance with medication, to more complex and lasting interventions, such as follow-up home visits from a nurse. A study comparing the collaborative care model to usual treatment for patients with co-morbid depression and diabetes found improved satisfaction with care, higher patient-rated improvement, fewer depressive symptoms, and more adequate dosing of antidepressant medication [72]. The intervention consisted of a specialist clinical nurse in collaboration with the primary care physician focusing on problem-solving therapy, and education and support of antidepressant medication treatment. The trial underlined that depression can be treated in the context of major physical illness. Other interventions to help improve the management of patients with co-morbidities are peer support, improved self-management, and problem-solving skills.

Research in co-morbidity

The randomized clinical trial is perhaps the strongest research method for informing evidence-based decision-making. Patients with co-morbidities, however, receive little attention in chronic disease trials, and are often excluded from samples [62, 73]. The reason is that researchers wish to homogenize their study sample in order to better evaluate the effect of their intervention. For example, a study evaluating the effect of an antidepressant would typically exclude patients with chronic severe physical co-morbidity, as the prognosis of significant co-morbidity may alter the post-treatment evaluation, and be impossible to distinguish from the effects of the treatment [15]. In short, the pretreatment characteristics of patients must be sufficiently similar in order to evaluate the effects of a treatment. The results from this 'homogeneous' or 'purified' population, however, cannot be extrapolated to the heterogeneous world of clinical reality, in the words of Richard Feinstein [15]. Apart from excluding patients with common co-morbidities, there is a tendency to give a limited report on co-morbidities of trial participants. Inclusion and exclusion criteria are often difficult to interpret, and studies generally do not discuss what effect the presence of co-morbidity may have on treatment [73].

There exist other considerable challenges to research in co-morbidity, particularly in relation to its definition and methods of measuring [74]. Also, there is a lack of qualitative research into the effects of co-morbidity on processes of care and what constitutes 'best care' for these patients [8].

Conclusions

Co-morbidity represents one of the most important challenges to today's health care (Box 31.1). Physical and psychiatric co-morbidity increase mortality, complexity in diagnostics and treatment, risk of polypharmacy, and economic costs. The first papers documenting increased mortality in psychiatric patients were published in the early years of the twentieth century. Despite the availability of this knowledge for almost a century now, the problem has not improved. In fact, it seems mortality due to increased prevalence of physical illness may be increasing. As such, physical and psychiatric co-morbidity presents both a historical scandal and an acute challenge. Potential solutions are emerging as interventions in collaborative care proves to decrease morbidity and mortality, and even economic expenses.

Specialization and single-disease focus have, indeed, provided great discoveries and progress in fields such as interventional cardiology, cancer treatment, and infectious medicine. However, in an age with increasing lifetimes and the rising prevalence of chronic, incurable diseases, the fragmented approach is sustaining inequity and increased mortality in psychiatric patients. This is, in part, due to single-disease guidelines, a siloed healthcare system, and clinical trials excluding patients with co-morbidities. Thus, we need to challenge the single-disease framework, apply a holistic approach, and engage generalists in collaborative care. Furthermore, researchers must design trials that include a heterogeneous patient

---

Box 31.1 Take-home message

- Physical and psychiatric co-morbidity is common: it increases mortality, increases complexity in diagnostics and treatment, increases the risk of polypharmacy, and increases economic costs.

- Challenges include single-disease guidelines, a siloed healthcare system, and clinical trials excluding patients with co-morbidities.

- Promising initiatives include collaborative care, goal-oriented care, and integrated care.

- We suggest revising medical education, clinical care, approach to research, and public health initiatives to take a broader approach on health and illness.

population to reflect a 'real-world' clinical population, or, at a minimum, describe how their findings relate to patients with co-morbidity. Also, there is a need for qualitative studies into the needs, expectations, and goals of patients with co-morbidity. On a public mental health scale we must support generalists in collaborating with other healthcare workers to provide comprehensive care, especially in socio-economically deprived areas.

As such, we must completely revise medical education, clinical care of patients with co-morbidity, approach to clinical research, and public health initiatives, to take a broader approach on health and illness: an approach that focuses on patients and goals, and less on diseases and problems.

Further reading

For more information on common risk factors and prevention we suggest the chapter in this book, 'Mental and physical health' (Chapter 21). For further reading on physical and psychiatric co-morbidity we suggest the book *Comorbidity of Mental and Physical Disorders*, edited by Norman Sartorius and colleagues. Also, we recommend the interested reader consults *Medical and Psychiatric Comorbidity Over the Course of Life*, edited by William W. Eaton, and *Global Perspectives on Mental–Physical Comorbidity*, a compilation of studies from the World Health Organization Mental Health Surveys. For the clinician, we recommend the *Handbook of Medicine in Psychiatry*, by Peter Manu and Corey Karlin-Zysman.

Acknowledgements

Linda Marie Kai and Clara Reece Medici commented on previous drafts of this chapter.

References

1. Oxford University Press. *A Dictionary of Epidemiology*, 6th ed. New York: Oxford University Press, 2014.
2. Malzberg B. *Mortality Among Patients With Mental Disease*. Utica, NY: State Hospitals Press, 1934.
3. Lawrence D, Kisely S, Pais J. The epidemiology of excess mortality in people with mental illness. *Can J Psychiatry* 2010; 55: 752–760.
4. Joukamaa M, Heliovaara M, Knekt P, Aromaa A, Raitasalo R, Lehtinen V. Mental disorders and cause-specific mortality. *Br J Psychiatry* 2001; 179: 498–502.
5. Crump C, Winkleby MA, Sundquist K, Sundquist J. Comorbidities and mortality in persons with schizophrenia: a Swedish national cohort study. *Am J Psychiatry* 2013; 170: 324–333.
6. Olfson M, Gerhard T, Huang C, Crystal S, Stroup TS. Premature mortality among adults with schizophrenia in the United States. *JAMA Psychiatry* 2015; 72: 1172–1181.
7. Sartorius N, Holt RIG, Maj M (eds). *Comorbidity of Mental and Physical Disorders*. Basel: Karger, 2015.
8. Fortin M, Soubhi H, Hudon C, Bayliss EA, van den Akker M. Multimorbidity's many challenges. *BMJ* 2007; 334: 1016–1017.
9. Prince M, Patel V, Saxena S, et al. No health without mental health. *Lancet* 2007; 370: 859–877.
10. Thornicroft G. Physical health disparities and mental illness: the scandal of premature mortality. *Br J Psychiatry* 2011; 199: 441–442.
11. Sartorius N. Comorbidity of mental and physical disorders: a main challenge to medicine in the 21st century. *Psychiatr Danub* 2013; 25(Suppl. 1): 4–5.
12. Saha S, Chant D, McGrath J. A systematic review of mortality in schizophrenia: is the differential mortality gap worsening over time? *Arch Gen Psychiatry* 2007; 64: 1123–1131.

13. Munk-Jorgensen P, Blanner Kristiansen C, Uwawke R, et al. The gap between available knowledge and its use in clinical psychiatry. *Acta Psychiatr Scand* 2015; 132: 441–450.
14. Valderas JM, Starfield B, Sibbald B, Salisbury C, Roland M. Defining comorbidity: implications for understanding health and health services. *Ann Fam Med* 2009; 7: 357–363.
15. Feinstein AR. The pre-therapeutic classification of co-morbidity in chronic disease. *J Chron Dis* 1970; 23: 455–468.
16. NCBI. MeSH term: Comorbidity. Available at: https://www.ncbi.nlm.nih.gov/mesh/?term=comorbidity (accessed 5 March 2018).
17. Katon W, Maj M, Sartorius N (eds). *Depression and Diabetes*. Chichester: Wiley-Blackwell, 2011.
18. van den Akker M, Buntinx F, Knottnerus JA. Comorbidity or multimorbidity. *Eur J Gen Pract* 1996; 2: 65–70.
19. World Health Organization (WHO). *The ICD-10 Classification of Mental and Behavioural Disorders: Clinical Descriptions and Diagnostic Guidelines*. Geneva: WHO, 1992.
20. Craddock N, Mynors-Wallis L. Psychiatric diagnosis: impersonal, imperfect and important. *Br J Psychiatry* 2014; 204: 93–95.
21. Levenson JL. *Essentials of Psychosomatic Medicine*. Washington, DC: American Psychiatric Association Publishing, 2007.
22. Koranyi EK. Morbidity and rate of undiagnosed physical illnesses in a psychiatric clinic population. *Arch Gen Psychiatry* 1979; 36: 414–419.
23. Jones S, Howard L, Thornicroft G. 'Diagnostic overshadowing': worse physical health care for people with mental illness. *Acta Psychiatr Scand* 2008; 118: 169–171.
24. Scott IA, Hilmer SN, Reeve E, et al. Reducing inappropriate polypharmacy: the process of deprescribing. *JAMA Intern Med* 2015; 175: 827–834.
25. De Hert M, Detraux J, van Winkel R, Yu W, Correll CU. Metabolic and cardiovascular adverse effects associated with antipsychotic drugs. *Nat Rev Endocrinol* 2012; 8: 114–126.
26. McDaid D, Park A-L. *Counting All the Costs: The Economic Impact of Comorbidity*. Berlin: Karger Publishers, 2014.
27. The Royal Australian & New Zealand College of Psychiatrists. The Economic Costs of Serious Mental Illness and Comorbidities in Australia and New Zealand. Available at: https://www.ranzcp.org/Files/Publications/RANZCP-Serious-Mental-Illness.aspx (accessed 5 March 2018).
28. Simon GE, Katon WJ, Lin EH, et al. Cost-effectiveness of systematic depression treatment among people with diabetes mellitus. *Arch Gen Psychiatry* 2007; 64: 65–72.
29. Prados-Torres A, Calderon-Larranaga A, Hancco-Saavedra J, Poblador-Plou B, van den Akker M. Multimorbidity patterns: a systematic review *J Clin Epidemiol* 2014; 67: 254–266.
30. Klein DN, Riso, Lawrence P. Psychiatric disorders: problems of boundaries and comorbidity. In: Costello CG (ed.). *Basic Issues in Psychopathology*. New York: Guilford Press, 1993, pp. 19–66.
31. de Hert M, Correll CU, Bobes J, et al. Physical illness in patients with severe mental disorders. I. Prevalence, impact of medications and disparities in health care. *World Psychiatry* 2011; 10: 52–77.
32. Ji J, Sundquist K, Ning Y, Kendler KS, Sundquist J, Chen X. Incidence of cancer in patients with schizophrenia and their first-degree relatives: a population-based study in Sweden. *Schizophr Bull* 2013; 39: 527–536.
33. Solmi M, Veronese N, Correll CU, et al. Bone mineral density, osteoporosis, and fractures among people with eating disorders: a systematic review and meta-analysis. *Acta Psychiatr Scand* 2016; 133: 341–351.
34. Katon WJ, Richardson L, Lozano P, McCauley E. The relationship of asthma and anxiety disorders. *Psychosom Med* 2004; 66: 349–355.
35. Fisher EB, Chan JC, Kowitt S, Nan H, Sartorius N, Oldenburg B. Conceptual perspectives on the co-occurrence of mental and physical disease: diabetes and depression as a model. In: Sartorius N, Holt RIG, Maj M (eds). *Comorbidity of Mental and Physical Disorders*. Berlin: Karger Publishers, 2014, pp. 1–14.

36. De Hert M, Detraux J, Van Winkel R, Yu W, Correll CU. Metabolic and cardiovascular adverse effects associated with antipsychotic drugs. *Nat Rev Endocrinol* 2012; 8: 114–126.

37. Lasser K, Boyd JW, Woolhandler S, Himmelstein DU, McCormick D, Bor DH. Smoking and mental illness: a population-based prevalence study. *JAMA* 2000; 284: 2606–2610.

38. Rosenberg SD, Goodman LA, Osher FC, et al. Prevalence of HIV, hepatitis B, and hepatitis C in people with severe mental illness. *Am J Public Health* 2001; 91: 31–37.

39. Ford ES, Caspersen CJ. Sedentary behaviour and cardiovascular disease: a review of prospective studies. *Int J Epidemiol* 2012; 41: 1338–1353.

40. Zhai L, Zhang Y, Zhang D. Sedentary behaviour and the risk of depression: a meta-analysis. *Br J Sports Med* 2015; 49: 705–709.

41. Felitti VJ, Anda RF, Nordenberg D, et al. Relationship of childhood abuse and household dysfunction to many of the leading causes of death in adults. The Adverse Childhood Experiences (ACE) Study. *Am J Prev Med* 1998; 14: 245–258.

42. Okkels N, Trabjerg B, Arendt M, Pedersen CB. Traumatic stress disorders and risk of subsequent schizophrenia spectrum disorder or bipolar disorder: a nationwide cohort study. *Schizophr Bull* 2017; 43: 180–186.

43. Winkleby MA, Jatulis DE, Frank E, Fortmann SP. Socioeconomic status and health: how education, income, and occupation contribute to risk factors for cardiovascular disease. *Am J Public Health* 1992; 82: 816–820.

44. Salive ME. Multimorbidity in older adults. *Epidemiol Rev* 2013; 35: 75–83.

45. Barnett K, Mercer SW, Norbury M, Watt G, Wyke S, Guthrie B. Epidemiology of multimorbidity and implications for health care, research, and medical education: a cross-sectional study. *Lancet* 2012; 380: 37–43.

46. Pedersen CB, Mors O, Bertelsen A, et al. A comprehensive nationwide study of the incidence rate and lifetime risk for treated mental disorders. *JAMA Psychiatry* 2014; 71: 573–581.

47. Vancampfort D, Correll CU, Galling B, et al. Diabetes mellitus in people with schizophrenia, bipolar disorder and major depressive disorder: a systematic review and large scale meta-analysis. *World Psychiatry* 2016; 15: 166–174.

48. Osborn DP, Levy G, Nazareth I, Petersen I, Islam A, King MB. Relative risk of cardiovascular and cancer mortality in people with severe mental illness from the United Kingdom's General Practice Rsearch Database. *Arch Gen Psychiatry* 2007; 64: 242–249.

49. Jakobsen AH, Foldager L, Parker G, Munk-Jorgensen P. Quantifying links between acute myocardial infarction and depression, anxiety and schizophrenia using case register databases. *J Affect Disord* 2008; 109: 177–181.

50. Jorgensen TS, Wium-Andersen IK, Wium-Andersen MK, et al. Incidence of depression after stroke, and associated risk factors and mortality outcomes, in a large cohort of Danish patients. *JAMA Psychiatry* 2016; 73: 1032–1040.

51. Johannessen L, Strudsholm U, Foldager L, Munk-Jorgensen P. Increased risk of hypertension in patients with bipolar disorder and patients with anxiety compared to background population and patients with schizophrenia. *J Affect Disord* 2006; 95: 13–17.

52. Andersson NW, Goodwin RD, Okkels N, et al. Depression and the risk of severe infections: prospective analyses on a nationwide representative sample. *Int J Epidemiol* 2016; 45: 131–139.

53. Andersson NW, Gustafsson LN, Okkels N, et al. Depression and the risk of autoimmune disease: a nationally representative, prospective longitudinal study. *Psychol Med* 2015; 45: 3559–3569.

54. Gupta MA, Gupta AK. Psychiatric and psychological co-morbidity in patients with dermatologic disorders: epidemiology and management. *Am J Clin Dermatol* 2003; 4: 833–842.

55. Kessler RC. The epidemiology of dual diagnosis. *Biol Psychiatry* 2004; 56: 730–737.

56. Katon WJ, Rutter C, Simon G, et al. The association of comorbid depression with mortality in patients with type 2 diabetes. *Diabetes Care* 2005; 28: 2668–2672.

57. Vancampfort D, Stubbs B, Mitchell AJ, et al. Risk of metabolic syndrome and its components in people with schizophrenia and related psychotic disorders, bipolar disorder and major depressive disorder: a systematic review and meta-analysis. *World Psychiatry* 2015; 14: 339–347.

58. Okkels N, Thygesen NB, Jensen B, Munk-Jorgensen P. Evaluation of somatic health care practices in psychiatric inpatient wards. *Aust N Z J Psychiatry* 2013; 47: 579–581.

59. Laursen TM, Munk-Olsen T, Agerbo E, Gasse C, Mortensen PB. Somatic hospital contacts, invasive cardiac procedures, and mortality from heart disease in patients with severe mental disorder. *Arch Gen Psychiatry* 2009; 66: 713–720.

60. Lawrence DM, Holman CD, Jablensky AV, Hobbs MS. Death rate from ischaemic heart disease in Western Australian psychiatric patients 1980–1998. *Br J Psychiatry* 2003; 182: 31–36.

61. Stange KC. The problem of fragmentation and the need for integrative solutions. *Ann Fam Med* 2009; 7: 100–103.

62. Fortin M, Smith SM. Improving the external validity of clinical trials: the case of multiple chronic conditions. *J Comorbid* 2013; 3: 30–35.

63. Hughes LD, McMurdo ME, Guthrie B. Guidelines for people not for diseases: the challenges of applying UK clinical guidelines to people with multimorbidity. *Age Ageing* 2013; 42: 62–69.

64. Wallace E, Salisbury C, Guthrie B, Lewis C, Fahey T, Smith SM. Managing patients with multimorbidity in primary care. *BMJ* 2015; 350: h176.

65. Boyd CM, Darer J, Boult C, Fried LP, Boult L, Wu AW. Clinical practice guidelines and quality of care for older patients with multiple comorbid diseases: implications for pay for performance. *JAMA* 2005; 294: 716–724.

66. Qato DM, Alexander GC, Conti RM, Johnson M, Schumm P, Lindau ST. Use of prescription and over-the-counter medications and dietary supplements among older adults in the United States. *JAMA* 2008; 300: 2867–2878.

67. Mojtabai R, Olfson M. National trends in psychotropic medication polypharmacy in office-based psychiatry. *Arch Gen Psychiatry* 2010; 67: 26–36.

68. Mold JW, Blake GH, Becker LA. Goal-oriented medical care. *Fam Med* 1991; 23: 46–51.

69. Boeckxstaens P, De Maeseneer J, De Sutter A. The role of general practitioners and family physicians in the management of multimorbidity. In: Sartorius N, Holt RIG, Maj M (eds). *Comorbidity of Mental and Physical Disorders*. Berlin: Karger Publishers, 2014, pp. 129–136.

70. Smith SM, Soubhi H, Fortin M, Hudon C, O'Dowd T. Managing patients with multimorbidity: systematic review of interventions in primary care and community settings. *BMJ* 2012; 345: e5205.

71. Smith SM, Wallace E, O'Dowd T, Fortin M. Interventions for improving outcomes in patients with multimorbidity in primary care and community settings. *Cochrane Database Syst Rev* 2016; 3: CD006560.

72. Katon WJ, Von Korff M, Lin EH, et al. The pathways study: a randomized trial of collaborative care in patients with diabetesand depression. *Arch Gen Psychiatry* 2004; 61: 1042–1049.

73. Boyd CM, Vollenweider D, Puhan MA. Informing evidence-based decision-making for patients with comorbidity: availability of necessary information in clinical trials for chronic diseases. *PLOS ONE* 2012; 7: e41601.

74. Boeckxstaens P, De Sutter A, Vaes B, Degryse JM. Should we keep on measuring multimorbidity? *J Clin Epidemiol* 2016; 71: 113–114.

CHAPTER 32

Globalization, migration, and mental health
A conceptual model for health research

Vishal Bhavsar, Shuo Zhang, and Dinesh Bhugra

Introduction

Globalization has become an oft-used term to describe a collection of processes all involving social economic and cultural *exchange*. It is a term with wide currency, and one used prominently in debates about economics, development, international relations, and, increasingly, health; however, there remain differences in what is meant by the term among those who use it. Moreover, definitions of globalization have tended to emphasize the material impacts of development, and downplay dynamic processes affecting the movement of people, goods, services, and ideas, including those ideas that pertain to health care. The construct of health is broadly defined by the World Health Organization (WHO) as the absence of illness, and mental health as 'a state of well-being in which every individual realizes his or her own potential, can cope with the normal stresses of life, can work productively and fruitfully, and is able to make a contribution to her or his community'. Although previous literature has conceptualized globalization as influencing health at multiple levels, few have theorized the impact of globalization on mental health, even though mental health has largely been overlooked in terms of resources, policy-making, and provision in global circles of influence for much of the past 30 years. For mental health, the impact of changing economic and social relations introduces particular problems, including:

1. The external and inter-cultural validity of psychiatric diagnosis; in comparison to physical health, the definition of good mental health is even more complex and disputed.

2. The rapidly changing circumstances within which people live, work, and develop and maintain relationships with each other is particularly important for mental health; these factors are inherently tied up with normative processes of forming and maintaining one's identity, and social/family relationships, which are fundamental to mental health.

3. Specificity: factors that influence the occurrence of mental health problems may or may not be the same as for physical disorders, and could require distinct policy responses.

We argue that, although mental health is ordinarily regarded as one particular aspect of general health and well-being, mental health presents distinctive and problematic challenges for understanding the effects of globalization on living and functioning.

Migration

Although people have been migrating for millennia, in recent times these have been more obvious and frequent, particularly from rural areas to urban areas as a result of urbanization, which can be seen as direct response to globalization. Across nations migration can be attributed to educational, economic, and political reasons. Migrants may be pulled in one direction or pushed from another one. The stages of migration can be preparatory phase or pre-migration, actual physical migration, and post-migration or settlement phase, which may go on for several years or even generations. During this phase of acculturation individuals may shrink their own cultural values while expanding on cultural values of the receiving country. A key aspect is to recognize that individual migration experiences can vary tremendously, and researchers and clinicians need to make allowances for these. Models of health and well-being will also vary across cultures. Despite the centrality of mental health to overall well-being, the pervasiveness of globalization [1], and the distinct challenges by mental health in terms of treatment and policy-making, theories of how globalization itself influences mental health are poorly characterized. Empirical research into mental health and care across the globe has been driven mainly by economic considerations, and findings have been understood within, and taken to reinforce, Western disease frameworks. This is most telling in the emergent policy and research field of global mental health [2], which has come under recent fire for conflating Western psychiatric categories with universal human distress [3]. Global mental health as a concept perhaps fits better with managing infectious diseases, as was evident from controlling the spread of severe acute respiratory syndrome or Ebola. For mental health, care must be taken not to dilute cultural relativism. Cultures determine and very strongly influence idioms of distress and also individuals' explanatory models where they seek help from. For example, in many traditional societies, the first port of call may be alternative or complementary therapies, which often do not appear in the global mental health agenda. With increasing levels of migration globally, partly due to increased linking with globalization, the explanatory models and expectations of treatment can move across borders.

Although mental health research has gathered a great deal of evidence about changing patterns of psychiatric morbidity around the world, explicit theoretical models are necessary in science in order to understand what is happening beneath the surface of empirical observations. Causal knowledge is needed to intervene meaningfully in human health; therefore, given the significant possible impacts of globalization on health, it is incumbent on researchers and policymakers to reflect on how we can mitigate/influence the impact of globalization.

Thus, in this chapter, we review theoretical models for globalization and health from the literature, before developing and presenting our own model. Then we present a conceptual model for the effects of globalization on mental health and identify some action points for future research and policy-making. Importantly, our model frames Western biomedical approaches as, broadly, strongly evidenced hypotheses that require testing, validation, and specification in varied and multiple locales. Cross-disciplinary research in mental health and development is lacking and this model provides a framework for doing so.

Methods for the development of this framework

We first review previous literature presenting conceptual models for globalization and health, identifying references to mental health-related outcomes such as suicide and depression. From the epidemiological literature on these specific outcomes we identify prevailing theoretical models for these outcomes, and develop a conceptual framework for testing hypotheses related to the way in which globalization could affect mental health. As a result, we then develop on this previous work by proposing a multi-level model of globalization and mental health, extending previous work in relation to health as a whole.

Descriptions of previous models

Models of globalization and health in the literature tend to develop and commit to a top-down approach. Cornia's formulation [4] of the impact of globalization attributes health gains in Asian tiger economies to domestic deregulation and the removal of international trade and finance barriers, and recommends gradual integration of poor countries into the world economy and the creation of democratic institutions. As well as Cornia, Woodward et al. [5] also emphasize direct material effects of economic globalization on health—globalization's effects are mediated through population-level health influences, influences on separate health sectors, and national economies, politics, and society, through to a 'lower' level involving individual risk of ill health, changes to the household economy, and alteration to the healthcare system. Beaglehole and Yach [6] address the implications of globalization for the governance of health, calling for an appropriate governmental response to growing tobacco and alcohol use in low- and middle-income countries, but points to increasing global advocacy, the development of global norms, protocols and safeguards, the reorientation of health services, an increase in resources, and enhanced transnational cooperation to this end. Labonté and Torgerson's model [7] is slightly more holistic—it conceptualizes globalization's effect on population health as a series of '-scapes', which create forces for change in political, social, cultural, and economic spheres, across a range of regional levels, which, in turn, affect health across the life course of individuals, and result in health outcomes measured at different levels of organization.

In a major recent model of the health impact of globalization, Huynen et al. [8] propose a multi-level framework for the purposes of development of future scenarios and empirically testable hypotheses. Their approach aims to build on previous models that have focused on material and economic aspects of development [5, 7], and address a broader understanding of health, and of globalization itself. Central to the model is the 'complex multicausality of population health', where the production of health reflects the interplay of networks of causal factors ranged across levels of organization and proximity to health outcomes—proximate causes being the more immediate causes of health problems, and more distal causes being the more fundamental influences on health that have a greater number of intermediate connections with other factors. This is joined with a broad definition of globalization, which comprises governance, markets, communication, mobility, cultural interaction, and environmental change. A model is presented that frames population health as having institutional, economic, sociocultural, and environmental influences, mediated proximally through health services, 'social environment lifestyle' and physical environment, water, and food.

Thus, for migrants, too, multi-causality models need to be taken into account. A web of causation needs to be understood in this context. There are multiple factors: genetic, social, psychological, and behavioural, which can all play a role in causing distress and illness. It must be recognized that clinicians are interested and, indeed, trained in dealing with diseases ('dis-ease') where the pathology lies, but patients are much more interested in making sense of social and functioning aspects of their distress, which stops them from forming relationships, working, earning a living, and so on. Therefore, migrants may carry with them their cultural values and expectations that will strongly affect where and when they seek help from. Any strategy in educating and managing such distress will need to take these idioms of distress into account.

A social model of globalization and mental health

Such a model is applicable not only to migrants, but also countries as a whole. Across the models of globalization and mental health reviewed earlier, we note the following:

1. Limited, if any, mention is made of mental health or how this might relate to globalization processes.

2. The role of reciprocal social interaction and exchange in the maintenance of health is not made explicit.

3. Despite a focus on the impact of development on poor countries, the interplay of social, cultural, religious, and other identities in these models is overlooked.

4. Models do not make explicit or examine the connection between evolving flows of people, media, technologies, ideologies, and capital, and the definitions and response to mental health problems.

Review of these theoretical frameworks revealed a number of limitations when applied to mental health problems. These are outlined in the following paragraphs, and summarized in Fig. 32.1.

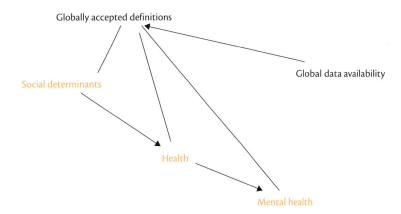

Fig. 32.1 A simple schematic diagram showing the relationship between globalization and mental health based on previous models.

Previous theoretical approaches to globalization have adopted a multi-level approach to health and its relationship to social life [9, 10]. These approaches emphasize pathways that involve risk factors and processes that are ranged across levels of organization beyond the individual, often framed to operate at institutional or neighbourhood levels [8]. For example, there is clear evidence from Western countries that the ethnic composition of one's neighbourhood has an influence on mental health if you are from an ethnic minority; in an analysis of health survey data from England, a 10% decrease in the proportion of people from one's own ethnic group living in one's neighbourhood was accompanied by a small but statistically significant increase in the odds of reporting psychotic-like experiences [11]. But, more generally, what does a multi-level theoretical model for globalization and development mean for mental health outcomes, and how do we test them? Influential social epidemiologists Kawachi and Subramanian [12] point out the role of deprivation at the level of the individual and of the neighbourhood is important in understanding the effects of development on health. Epidemiological evidence suggests that effects of social context might be more significant for mental health outcomes [13, 14], but that the definitions of levels are clearly stated but poorly specified; for example, there is strong evidence that neighbourhoods of residence are important, but how and where neighbourhoods are drawn is unclear [15], and little work on the role of neighbourhoods and mental health is available outside rich country settings. We make global asymmetry in available data on social context and mental health explicit in our model. It is worth noting that most migrants may well end up in urban settings where the quality of accommodation and social support networks may, indeed, be very poor.

In addition to overcrowding and poverty in these settings, there is strong evidence that health status is driven by employment [16, 17], income [18], and educational opportunities [19], and all models of globalization and health appreciated the role for these conditions as fundamental causes of ill health [20]. Furthermore, previous models also display complexity in terms of the temporal delineation of factors. Temporal resolution is a fine thing to plan for in rich countries, but such factors are difficult to determine within the scope of current data collection methods in low- and middle-income countries. In fact, such models reflect a key way in which theoretical models involve implicit statements regarding the availability of data. Therefore, data need to improve in low- and middle-income

countries, in a way that is determined by the communities that produce the data and not by external agencies. Thus, we need to bring the availability and quality of data on mental health into the debate on the widening impact of social and economic change, so we can understand what is going on with mental health around the world in response to social and economic change.

For example, in *Social Determinants of Health* [21], Marmot and Wilkinson lay out a series of ways in which social and economic environments influence health. Social stratification, along the lines of ethnicity, geographical location, sexual identity, and economic and political power is presented as a dynamic process, interrelating with an individual's development. The psychosocial environment at work is considered crucial. Although evidence is strong for the social determinants of health, evaluating and intervening on such determinants (e.g. education, employment, job opportunities, living conditions, access to healthy food) requires good data, which we argue need to be part of theoretical models. Migrants will face social stratification, poor or uncertain employment, and poverty, among other factors.

Building on this, it is evident that prior theoretical models of globalization and health emphasize proximal influences on health such as smoking, alcohol, substance use, unhealthy eating, and underemphasize life experiences of violence, trauma, loss, privation, and destitution, which we consider to crucial to understanding both development and health [22]. Although stress is sometimes located in these models [4], experiences of particular events and processes and stress overlap, but are not identical concepts; for example, the experience of abuse during childhood leads not only to stress, but also to institutionalization, stigma, and further violent adversity in adulthood, which may, in turn, drive important changes in behaviour in relation to health. Empirical research in social and economic influences on mental health require models that are sensitive to the broad ways in which life events, linked to higher-level structural processes in countries, such as war, recession, inter-sectarian conflicts, and political/electoral transitions, are experienced, rather than merely considering traumatic events as being black boxes.

Life events in globalization and mental health

For example, it is clear that the psychological effects of a bereavement are not only understandable in terms of the type of event, but also about the meaning attached to the deceased, and the broader social, economic, and cultural repercussions of the bereavement—similar arguments can be made about drastic changes to one's work, family life, food availability, sex life, and recreational pattern. The same range of arguments can be made about the experiences of migrants related to conflict, and exposure to physical violence, in particular. In addition, they may face cultural bereavement and culture shock, which bring with them additional problems related to acculturation and adjustment. Culture conflict may be noted with the majority or the new culture and across generations within the same culture, thereby adding to the series of life events. Such life experiences, including those of violence at different levels, as presented in our model, may be said to *embody* structural conditions and link them inextricably with the individual's experience of the world and the people in it [23]. For example, violence is and always has been part of the effects of development on people, a perhaps inevitable (albeit decreasingly rare, according to Pinker [24]) by-product of cultural exchange. However, the health effects of development that might be explained by changes in the dynamics of violence, at global, inter-personal, and inter-ethnic levels, remain poorly understood. Cougle et al. [25] present a conceptual flow of violence through to health problems using injury, stress, and distress as main explanations, which, in turn, relate to the development of chronic physical health conditions, increased biological vulnerability/sensitivity to health problems, and lifestyle changes and differences in the use of health care. The interplay of these forces with contextual factors also shapes the prevalence of violence/threatening environments [26]. We propose a broader role for supportive/caring contexts at the interpersonal, family/household/local, and country levels in coping with violence exposure.

On this basis, fundamental issues emerge in the integration of violence into ongoing health/development debates in an empirically testable way. Pre-existing models have seen difficulty in integrating violence/crime into economic/social/cultural processes. What is necessary is a theoretical perspective that is sensitive to the relationship between development processes at different levels and mental health. Implications of this work could be that violence prevention must understand the different pathways by which violence affects health and healthcare/counselling provision should be integrated into conflict management solutions [27]. Furthermore, the intersections of violence with binaries of ethnicity and gender will also come into play, raising important questions—as cultural exchange drives and influences identity formation in our global melting pot, how does identity tension emerge and how is this implicated in mental health problems and the response to violence as a crucial mediator? The mental response to events is intimately concerned not only with how life is experienced, but also how it is communicated to others. Models of understanding how people are likely to respond to joblessness, environmental hazards, or conflict are likely to involve awareness of patterns of communication in these places, including the rapidly expanding and established role of social media.

Although previous models have identified social context as important, few models have made testable theories explicit—for example, family structures: single parent, two grandparents only—may have specific effects on particular outcomes. For migrants who may have lost family members in the conflict or who may have left families behind, these issues become extremely important. There may also be survivor guilt. There is good and clear evidence that marital and relationship status is related to health and that this is bi-directional over time [28, 29]. Moreover, household structure has been linked to the development of mental health problems and resilience [30]. These potential mechanisms for the influence of development on health require urgent testing and theorization. As a result of migration family structures may well have changed dramatically.

A public mental health case study: children in China

We have reviewed models of globalization and health, and identified some respects in which they may be limited in explaining and investigating the mental health of people around the world, highlighting the role of structural conditions, deprivation, adverse experiences, and global asymmetries in the availability of data on health determinants. A conceptualization of globalization and mental health that locates these factors as central could be empirically useful. For example, it could help identify causal factors for changing mental health patterns in locales where economic transitions have occurred rapidly, such as China. There is some observational evidence that the epidemiological patterns in depression and severe mental illness in China could be considerably different from those seen in other countries—Pearson notes higher rates of suicides and schizophrenia incidence in women [31]. Compounding this disparity, large proportions of rural Chinese families are disrupted by economic factors—nearly one-fifth of schoolchildren have a parent working away from home. Multivariate analyses indicated that these children had more unhealthy lifestyles, including irregular eating patterns, inactivity, smoking, and suicidal ideation. In particular, girls with this parental structure were 1.5 times more likely to report feeling unhappy most of the time or always, and more than 2.5 times more likely to report binge drinking [32]. However, the absence of poverty or wealth explanations in this analysis is striking, and may be responsible for many of the associations seen. Indeed, socio-economic associations appear to be stronger if the mother leaves the home, rather than the father; in a study of 592 children left behind in three rural Chinese communities, mother-absent children displayed stronger associations of socio-economic status with depression and anxiety [33]. So, although children left behind may be considered an at-risk group in the context of rapid economic and demographic transition, Biao [34] emphasizes that purely epidemiological approaches have a tendency to pathologize women and children themselves, rather than focus attention on the economic exclusion of rural Chinese communities as a whole. One potential mechanism could involve the economic inactivity of unguarded children and young adults—in one survey of students in Macheng, China, 40% of subjects were left behind, and had nearly twice the annual prevalence of unintentional injury than those who were not. Similarly, a representative survey of a county of Shandong province estimated the prevalence of children left behind to be 54%, with associations with emotional, social, and school functioning [35]. These two results indicate, assuming causality that left-behind status is a prevalent characteristic in Chinese rural communities, that interventions involving this group should form part of a comprehensive public mental health strategy that could have important effects on both economic productivity and educational attainment. One study estimated the total cost of depression in China to be USD$6,264 million (at 2002 prices and exchange rates [36]). These observations suggest that the mental health of rural communities in China is an urgent issue, and one that is only partially understood by applying individual-based models of risk and intervention, or top-down models emphasizing economic and institutional dynamics.

In particular, understanding the process of identity formation in different local contexts is likely to be crucial. For example, Cheng and Berman [37] examine the unique experience of Chinese adolescents in a globalizing China with a different value structure. Measurement and detailed qualitative investigation of these processes in relation to dynamic family arrangements and economic tensions will be crucial for improving explanatory and predictive models, and then policy. Thus, internal migration itself can contribute to distress and increased burden, which may be related to lack of social support.

Constructs and definitions of mental disorder and its causes

Definitions in general, and the definitions one chooses to use, carry with them certain meanings. We note that previous theoretical models of the effects of globalization and development on health have left the definitions of health, and of well-being [38], uncontested, and therefore not admitting the possibility that these definitions themselves might be under the influences of forces of development, globalization, and cultural exchange. In this day and age surely absence of disease cannot be the only definition of health as millions of people around the world live with multiple complex co-morbidities? For example, those with bipolar disorder or diabetes in between episodes can function reasonably well. Although articulated as a resource to mitigate the effects of work intensification, increasing employment insecurity, and an increasingly competitive world, the concept of well-being is similarly packaged [38], and also lacks almost any investigation in low- and middle-income countries, as well as among migrants, whether they are within the same country or move across nations.

Similarly, the diagnosis of intermittent explosive disorder is a category identified in the USA that has been exported to other parts of the rich world, and thereafter to low- and middle-income countries [39], but whose definitions have been left largely disputed and reinforce the idea of a universal mental state [40]. This hypothesis has evidence, but this evidence is incomplete; uncritical acceptance of universal psychopathology risks overlooking processes of defining and measuring abnormality, which urgently need to come under the spotlight. As another example: how is social media impacting the definition and ascription of disordered/dysfunctional eating in low- and middle-income countries [41]?

Further, people disagree about the materiality of mental disorders, i.e. whether they have a basis in neurobiology or not. This debate has often taken place across lines of culture, language, and theoretical background. It is seen, for example, between the lines in the argument over the utility of cognitive–behavioural therapy for psychosis [42, 43]. Insofar as mental disorders inherently involve addressing the experiences of distress, identity, and selfhood in patients, how these notions work in different places is necessary to understanding what is going on underneath the 'global epidemiology' of mental disorders [44]. The incorporation of conceptions of selfhood and mental wellness are necessary to understand the local elaboration and occurrence of mental disorder. Increasing rates of attention deficit hyperactivity disorder diagnoses [45], the construction of intermittent explosive disorder [46], and dangerous and severe personality disorder as psychiatric problems [47], and the changing relevance of dependence diagnoses for understanding

the global use of drugs such as alcohol and opiates, are all examples of how disease constructs are arrived at through a complicated prism of economic and social–cultural–political concerns.

Development affects not only definitions of illness, but also of wellness. Angry disagreement over the utility and ethics of the UK government's welfare-to-work schemes raise clear questions about what it is to be well enough to work, above and beyond what it means to be ill [48, 49]. There are clear and apparently increasing tensions within popular notions of illness, work capability, and well-being. Both within the workforce and outside it, there is good evidence that austerity has negatively affected mental health [50, 51]. Therefore we can hypothesize a causal pathway linking global economic recession, welfare policy change, revisions of collective notions of wellness, increasing morbidity, and, ultimately, increased pressure on structurally underfunded mental health services together with increasing burden on these services. Theoretical approaches to the effect of global social and economic shifts on mental health require sensitivity to issues of definition, and how stakeholders engage with these definitions. These notions are left unexamined by WHO pronouncements on global health, such as the definition cited at the beginning of this chapter. The question of culture-sensitive definitions not only applies to what constitutes mental health in low- and middle-income countries, but also relates to reference point categories like exposure to violence and trauma. The development and establishment of cross-cultural concepts of trauma and trauma-related mental health problems is crucial, as are the ways that they play out through the experience of violence at different levels, as we discussed in previous sections. We suggest that attention should be paid to how these contests play out in different locales (Fig. 32.2).

Drawing together the points discussed, we identify a number of intervening levels between individual mental health and macroeconomic processes. We frame globalization as manifest not only in these processes, but also affecting levels and patterns of migration. However, such factors also influence communication, mobility, and conflict operating across countries and geopolitical units. In addition, we propose that global measurement is a further manifestation of development and the increasing inter-connectedness of people.

The model frames population mental health as being under the dynamic influence of causes ranged across a number of levels, but we attempt to avoid prioritizing higher levels by emphasizing the importance of migration, which we consider to be a factor under the influence of processes operating across levels. Themes across levels are that of the close connection between economic and cultural resources, the importance of geographical movement of individuals (whether that is between countries, regions, or neighbourhoods) and the role of violence and conflict, which can, again, be considered as a product of discrete global, regional/national, or local circumstances. Data are considered central to the development of coherent effective definitions, and to the implementation of effective evaluation and policy programmes.

Implications for 'global mental health' and global programmes

With the promise of improving global health, there now exist a series of international programmes that aim to measure, evaluate, and ultimately influence health around the world [44, 52, 53]. In

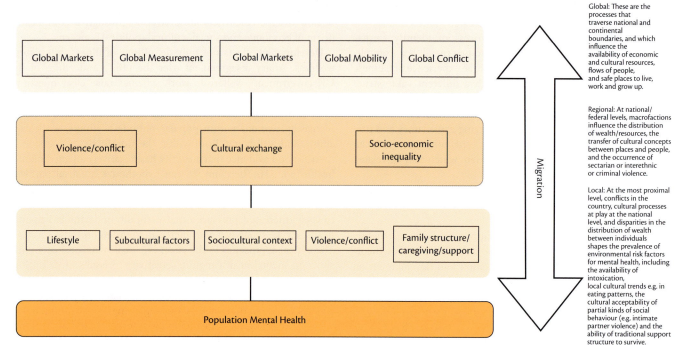

Fig. 32.2 Presentation and description of model.

particular, major attempts to improve the mental health of people living in poor countries have been under way for some time, under the banner of the movement for global mental health [2]. These programmes have recently come under strong criticism for perpetuating styles of enquiry that are inherently colonial, for neglecting the historical construction of poverty and injustice, and undermining and excluding local models of healing and health, limiting clinical benefit [3]. Although we suggest that the work of global mental health to empower lay mental health workers to deliver clinically and cost-effective mental health interventions, and to understand the aetiology of mental health problems in the developing world needs closer attention to the social determinants of health, we also argue that many of these determinants need to be considered through local prisms of data availability and definitions. As movements like the Global Burden of Disease project and global mental health continue to grow at speed, ensuring mechanisms by which they remain investigative and hypothesis driven, and responsive to a changing world, including evolving landscapes of conflict, and economic shift, and not under the control of biased and determined convictions in a particular disease model is important. These are particularly applicable to migrants.

We may therefore tentatively argue for a empirical approach to global mental health that locates Western disease models as hypotheses for evidencing, not merely as reference points for the implementation of broad policy and service changes on people who, in some cases, have not asked for them.

In a previous paper we have argued that globalization and its effects on industry, the development and structure of cities, and media are important influences on idioms of distress in depressive illness around the globe [54]. In the model presented here, we consider models for evaluating not only how depression is expressed, but also how it is diagnosed, and transitions of categories over time. We have commented in previous papers that migration, downward

social mobility, and enduring disadvantage over time are important considerations in understanding of the worlds of people exposed to social economic transitions in low- and middle-income countries. We have extended these observations by trying to suggest routes towards better empirical understanding of these associations [55]. These observations could be useful in defining new predictions for mental health burden in a rapidly changing global milieu. Others have pointed out a startling lack of a health dimension to global scenario studies [8]; there is a particular and urgent need for forecasting and scenario work on mental illness in light of potential sociocultural, economic, and environmental change. Prediction of the future requires solid empirical evidence based in strong theoretical frameworks.

Conclusions

Global health projects to define, measure, and intervene on human disease have done much good, and the world is a better place for having them. However, funding for these programmes is increasingly in dispute, and evaluations of these models themselves lacks theoretic rigour, as applied to mental health. It is our contention that these models, such as those reflected in the Global Burden of Disease project, and so on, require explicit theoretic adaptation in order to have explanatory power in relation to mental health. In terms of policy and implementation, the development and roll-out of policy programmes about mental health require integrated understandings of local scenarios and set-ups in relation to the economics, the flow of people, and culture. Again, global mental health initiatives can sometimes overlook this. An integrated understanding of how mental health, as a product of personal experience shaped through family and childhood and collectively shared understandings, is influenced by the social and economic environment. Although we are among those who are worried about the impact of social media, and so on, on identities and identity formation, clearly there is an evidence/methodological gap in this area and there needs to be work to identify how globalization is influencing concepts of mental health, how globalization is changing conceptualizations of violence, and the real ways in which the experience of violence itself and sociocultural stressors/changes are influencing population mental health. The rise of populist political movements may augur a new period of provincialism and nationalism [56], providing important new challenges for understanding the interplay between local and national processes in shaping our mental health. Recent political upheavals in many countries, including Brexit in the UK, can be attributed to the impact of perceived and real migration and globalization, which has made people in the new or receiving countries more hostile, leading to additional stress on migrants. The search for targets to blame continues and the migrants are often easy to identify. Understanding the impact of individual and global migration and the impact of immigration on the political and economic landscapes of receiving countries is important in order to plan and deliver services.

References

1. Bhavsar V, Bhugra D. Globalization: mental health and social economic factors. *Glob Soc Policy* 2008; 8: 378–396.
2. Patel V, Prince M. Global mental health: a new global health field comes of age. *JAMA* 2010; 303: 1976–1977.
3. Summerfield D. How scientifically valid is the knowledge base of global mental health? *BMJ* 2008; 336: 992–994.
4. Cornia GA. Globalization and health: results and options. *Bull World Health Organ* 2001; 79: 834–841.
5. Woodward D, Drager N, Beaglehole R, Lipson D. Globalization and health: a framework for analysis and action. *Bull World Health Organ* 2001; 79: 875–881.
6. Beaglehole R, Yach D. Globalisation and the prevention and control of non-communicable disease: the neglected chronic diseases of adults. *Lancet* 2003; 362: 903–908.
7. Labonte R, Torgerson R. Interrogating globalization, health and development: Towards a comprehensive framework for research, policy and political action. *Crit Public Health* 2005; 15: 157–179.
8. Huynen MM, Martens P, Hilderink HB. The health impacts of globalization: a conceptual framework. *Global Health* 2005; 1: 14.
9. Pickett KE, Pearl M. Multilevel analyses of neighbourhood socioeconomic context and health outcomes: a critical review. *J Epidemiol Community Health* 2001; 55: 111–122.
10. Diez-Roux AV. Bringing context back into epidemiology: variables and fallacies in multilevel analysis. *Am J Public Health* 1998; 88: 216–222.
11. Das-Munshi J, Becares L, Boydell JE, et al. Ethnic density as a buffer for psychotic experiences: findings from a national survey (EMPIRIC). *Br J Psychiatry* 2012; 201: 282–290.
12. Kawachi I, Subramanian S. Neighbourhood influences on health. *J Epidemiol Community Health* 2007; 61: 3–4.
13. Diez Roux AV. Investigating neighborhood and area effects on health. *Am J Public Health* 2001; 91: 1783–1789.
14. March D, Hatch SL, Morgan C, et al. Psychosis and place. *Epidemiol Rev* 2008; 30: 84–100.
15. Becares L, Cormack D, Harris R. Ethnic density and area deprivation: neighbourhood effects on Maori health and racial discrimination in Aotearoa/New Zealand. *Soc Sci Med* 2013; 88: 76–82.
16. Roelfs DJ, Shor E, Davidson KW, Schwartz JE. Losing life and livelihood: a systematic review and meta-analysis of unemployment and all-cause mortality. *Soc Sci Med* 2011; 72: 840–854.
17. Paul KI, Moser K. Unemployment impairs mental health: meta-analyses. *J Vocat Behav* 2009; 74: 264–282.
18. Kondo N, Sembajwe G, Kawachi I, van Dam RM, Subramanian S, Yamagata Z. Income inequality, mortality, and self rated health: meta-analysis of multilevel studies. *BMJ* 2009; 339: b4471.
19. Calvin CM, Deary IJ, Fenton C, et al. Intelligence in youth and all-cause-mortality: systematic review with meta-analysis. *Int J Epidemiol* 2011; 40: 626–644.
20. Link BG, Phelan J. Social conditions as fundamental causes of disease. *J Health Soc Behav* 1995; Spec No: 80–94.
21. Marmot M, Wilkinson R. *Social Determinants of Health.* Oxford: Oxford University Press, 2005.
22. Appadurai A. *Modernity at Large: Cultural Dimensions of Globalization.* Minneapolis: University of Minnesota Press, 1996.
23. Krieger N. Embodiment: a conceptual glossary for epidemiology. *J Epidemiol Community Health* 2005; 59: 350–355.
24. Pinker S. Decline of violence: taming the devil within us. *Nature* 2011; 478: 309–311.
25. Cougle JR, Resnick H, Kilpatrick DG. Factors associated with chronicity in posttraumatic stress disorder: a prospective analysis of a national sample of women. *Psychol Trauma* 2013; 5: 43–49.
26. Sampson RJ, Raudenbush SW, Earls F. Neighborhoods and violent crime: a multilevel study of collective efficacy. *Science* 1997; 277: 918–924.
27. Tol WA, Patel V, Tomlinson M, et al. Relevance or excellence? Setting research priorities for mental health and psychosocial support in humanitarian settings. *Harv Rev Psychiatry* 2012; 20: 25–36.
28. Amato PR, Keith B. *Parental Divorce and the Well-being of Children: A Meta-analysis.* Washington, DC: American Psychological Association, 1991.
29. Amato PR, Keith B. Parental divorce and adult well-being: a meta-analysis. *J Marriage Fam* 1991; 53: 43–58.
30. Weitoft GR, Hjern A, Haglund B, Rosén M. Mortality, severe morbidity, and injury in children living with single parents in Sweden: a population-based study. *Lancet* 2003; 361: 289–295.
31. Pearson V. The mental health of women in China. *Hong Kong J Psychiatry* 1998; 8: 3–8.
32. Gao Y, Li LP, Kim JH, Congdon N, Lau J, Griffiths S. The impact of parental migration on health status and health behaviours among left behind adolescent school children in China. *BMC Public Health* 2010; 10: 1.
33. Liu Z, Li X, Ge X. Left too early: the effects of age at separation from parents on Chinese rural children's symptoms of anxiety and depression. *Am J Public Health* 2009; 99: 2049–2054.
34. Biao X. How far are the left-behind left behind? A preliminary study in rural China. *Popul Space Place* 2007; 13: 179–191.
35. Jia Z, Shi L, Cao Y, Delancey J, Tian W. Health-related quality of life of 'left-behind children': a cross-sectional survey in rural China. *Qual Life Res* 2010; 19: 775–780.
36. Hu T-w, He Y, Zhang M, Chen N. Economic costs of depression in China. *Soc Psychiatry Psychiatr Epidemiol* 2007; 42: 110–116.
37. Cheng M, Berman SL. Globalization and identity development: a Chinese perspective. *New Dir Child Adolesc Dev* 2012; 2012: 103–121.
38. Foresight. *Mental capital and wellbeing: making the most of ourselves in the 21st century.* Available at: https://www.gov.uk/government/publications/mental-capital-and-wellbeing-making-the-most-of-ourselves-in-the-21st-century (2008, accessed 6 March 2018).
39. Silove D, Brooks R, Steel CRB, et al. Explosive anger as a response to human rights violations in post-conflict Timor-Leste. *Soc Sci Med* 2009; 69: 670–677.
40. Wakefield J. DSM-5, psychiatric epidemiology and the false positives problem. *Epidemiol Psychiatr Sci* 2015; 24: 188–196.
41. McLaren L, DeGroot J, Adair C, Russell-Mayhew S. Socioeconomic position, social inequality, and weight-related issues. In: McVey G, Levine P, Piran N, Ferguson HB (eds). *Preventing Eating-related and Weigh-related Disorders: Collaborative Research, Advocacy, and Policy Change.* Waterloo: Wilfred Press, 2012, pp. 249–267.
42. Jauhar S, McKenna P, Radua J, Fung E, Salvador R, Laws K. Cognitive-behavioural therapy for the symptoms of schizophrenia: systematic review and meta-analysis with examination of potential bias. *Br J Psychiatry* 2014; 204: 20–29.

43. Birchwood M, Shiers D, Smith J. CBT for psychosis: not a 'quasi-neuroleptic'. *Br J Psychiatry* 2014; 204: 488–489.

44. Whiteford HA, Degenhardt L, Rehm J, et al. Global burden of disease attributable to mental and substance use disorders: findings from the Global Burden of Disease Study 2010. *Lancet* 2013; 382: 1575–1586.

45. Mandell DS, Thompson WW, Weintraub ES, DeStefano F, Blank MB. Trends in diagnosis rates for autism and ADHD at hospital discharge in the context of other psychiatric diagnoses. *Psychiatr Serv* 2005; 56: 56–62.

46. Rees S, Silove D, Verdial T, et al. Intermittent explosive disorder amongst women in conflict affected Timor-Leste: associations with human rights trauma, ongoing violence, poverty, and injustice. *PLOS ONE* 2013; 8: e69207.

47. Duggan C. Dangerous and severe personality disorder. *Br J Psychiatry* 2011; 198: 431–433.

48. Curnock E, Leyland AH, Popham F. The impact on health of employment and welfare transitions for those receiving out-of-work disability benefits in the UK. *Soc Sci Med* 2016; 162: 1–10.

49. Butler P. Welfare to work programme failing disabled and ill jobseekers, say charities. Available at: https://www.theguardian.com/politics/2015/sep/17/welfare-to-work-programme-failing-disabled-and-ill-jobseekers-say-charities (2015, accessed 6 March 2018).

50. Hawton K, Bergen H, Geulayov G, et al. Impact of the recent recession on self-harm: Longitudinal ecological and patient-level investigation from the Multicentre Study of Self-harm in England. *J Affect Disord* 2016; 191: 132–138.

51. Barnes M, Gunnell D, Davies R, et al. Understanding vulnerability to self-harm in times of economic hardship and austerity: a qualitative study. *BMJ Open* 2016; 6: e010131.

52. Murray CJ, Lopez AD. Mortality by cause for eight regions of the world: Global Burden of Disease Study. *Lancet* 1997; 349: 1269–1276.

53. Prince M, Patel V, Saxena S, et al. No health without mental health. *Lancet* 2007; 370: 859–877.

54. Bhugra D, Mastrogianni A. Globalisation and mental disorders. *Br J Psychiatry* 2004; 184: 10–20.

55. Gupta S, Bhugra D. Globalization, economic factors and prevalence of psychiatric disorders. *Int J Ment Health* 2009; 38: 53–65.

56. Parker C. The end of globalization? Davos disagrees. Available at: https://www.weforum.org/agenda/2017/01/the-end-of-globalization-davos-disagrees/ (2017, accessed 6 March 2018).

CHAPTER 33

Treatment of mental health problems in refugees and asylum seekers

Giulia Cossu, Antonio Preti, and Mauro Giovanni Carta

Introduction

The refugees who flee to a host country have often experienced a range of traumatic events well before being forced to leave: war trauma, persecution, humiliation, gender-based violence, human rights violations, and significant family losses. 'Communities have been destroyed by disrupting core attachments to families, friends and cultural systems' [1]. Many immigrants have experienced displacement and hardship in transit countries, and dangerous travels. Lack of information about immigration status, potential hostility, and undignified and protracted detention are all potentially traumatic and stressful events. Not surprisingly, asylum seekers and refugees can be exposed to events that could influence their mental health [2].

According to the fifth edition of the *Diagnostic and Statistical Manual of Mental Disorders* (DSM-5) [3], 'Trauma' and 'Stressor-Related Disorder' include disorders that arise from exposure to a traumatic or stressful event. These include reactive attachment disorder, disinhibited social engagement disorder, post-traumatic stress disorder (PTSD), acute stress disorder, and adjustment disorders. Many individuals who have been exposed to a traumatic or stressful event exhibit anxiety, fear-based symptoms, and prominent clinical characteristics, such as anhedonic and dysphoric symptoms, externalizing angry and aggressive symptoms, or dissociative symptoms [3]; most of these symptoms evolve into a structured disorder. Other frequently diagnosed disorders among asylum seekers are depression and anxiety disorders [4].

In order to provide a complete framework that could best illustrate the incidence of mental disorders among refugee populations, two comprehensive systematic reviews and meta-analyses showed that they are about 10 times more likely than the general population to have PTSD, with a higher incidence rate in younger people [5, 6]. Specifically, the consequences of war on mental health in refugees should be evaluated seriously. The studies by Mollica et al. [7, 8] on Bosnian refugees has shown that after 3 years, 45% of people suffering from PTSD still present significant symptoms. Devastating effects have been found more than 10 years after exposure to traumatic events [7, 8]. The high risk of psychiatric disorders has also been documented in the Lebanese population in the study by Karam et al. [9], 20 years after the Lebanese war, and in particular among those who were children at that time.

If it is clear that civilians are paying the highest price for the brutality of war, it should be underlined that even military personnel are not immune to long-term consequences: no less than half of the Israeli soldiers who took part in the war operations in Lebanon suffer lifetime experiences of triple co-morbidity (PTSD + anxiety + depression) and almost 20% suffer from PTSD with very late onset [10].

Interestingly, the effects of trauma on Syrian refugees in Turkey are similar to the findings of the cited studies in Lebanon [11]. In Lebanon, large groups of the population were affected by the war, but not all citizens, as is now the case in Syria. This helps us assume the long-term consequences of the current wars on these populations. Furthermore, some mental conditions that may result from conflict exposure are probably underestimated in diagnostic practices. As a matter of fact, diagnostic assessment practices among refugees tend to focus mainly on PTSD, without considering the overall disorder spectrum that stressful and traumatic events can trigger. For instance, adjustment disorder is scarcely investigated, and very few hints are available about its treatment [12], despite its prevalence of 5–20% in psychiatric consultation services for adults, and up to 40% in psychological consultation services. Diagnostic and therapeutic practices aimed to refugees tend to neglect adjustment disorder. Insomnia is very frequent among refugees [13], but only a few trials have underlined insomnia as a single disorder, when it is generally considered a symptom of depression and PTSD [14]. Although somatic symptoms are frequently associated with psychological distress and early traumatic experiences (e.g. violence, abuse, deprivation) [3], 'Somatic Symptom and Related Disorders' are understated in psychiatric medical practices addressed at refugees [15]. Complicated grief was included in the DSM-5 as a diagnostic category requiring more study and research, and it could actually prove useful when working with refugees. A stronger focus on the dimensional perspective of the whole disorders spectrum linked to stressful and traumatic experiences—and not solely targeted at PTSD—would be recommended in clinical practices treating refugee populations.

The mental health of refugees in camps, in temporary accommodation centres, and in host countries

The refugee population is not homogeneous. Health status differences may depend upon the cultural and political situation in the country of origin, upon cultural and integration policies in the host country, and upon the situation the migrants are in when they require medical attention and political asylum. Quality of life during the integration experience can also affect refugee health.

The living conditions experienced by the refugees in camps may differ substantially from the living conditions of those who have reached the first host country, or who live permanently in a country. These differences can affect the mental health of refugees with different outcomes.

For instance, it is easily understood how the experience of instability and difficulties in a refugee camp may differ from that of a refugee who has obtained political asylum and is integrated in the host country. Among other things, such differences concern living conditions, freedom, and reunion with family members.

Studies on the mental health of refugee populations who lived in camps for some time have shown that the prevalence rates of mental disorders are higher than in other refugee populations. One study on 408 Malian refugees in a camp in Burkina Faso has revealed that around 60% of the interviewed sample met the criteria for 'Trauma and Stress-Related Disorders' [16]. This prevalence further rose to 90% among those experiencing difficulties in getting food and adequate housing. Although not all the refugee camps generate the same troubles concerning livelihood, this condition is more common than one might think in most camps [17, 18]. Similar outcomes have been found in 820 Syrian refugees living in the camp on the border of Turkey with Syria. In total, 688 (83.9%) of these 820 refugees had scores on the Impact of Event Scale-Revised (IES-R) above the predetermined cut-off point (> 33) of probable PTSD [11]. It is likely that both acute and chronic stressors, like these, act as risk factors, increasing the chance that a mental disorder would develop.

A study recently conducted in Sardinia, an Italian island that often greets new arrivals from migration waves, has shown that 22.1% of a sample of 860 refugees living in a camp were positive for at least one screener of depressive, bipolar disorder, or PTSD [19]. These results are very low compared with the aforementioned results. This might be explained by the hypothesis that the people who are able to start a long, dangerous journey in makeshift boats and land illegally in foreign lands, may be the ones who have a better mental health status than those who decide not to leave. In any case, the share of psychopathology incidence in this sample of refugees could be explained by the range of traumatic experiences they may have been exposed during the journey.

Collecting information about the mental health of refugees who have reached a good level of integration and social inclusion in the host countries over the time is difficult. A good integration process is likely to become an important protection factor or to reduce the onset, development, and course of mental disorders and psychopathological burden.

On the contrary, if the asylum process is inefficient, and integration in the host society is poor, asylum seekers and refugees are more exposed to developing mental suffering.

Some studies have shown that even after many years spent in the host country, refugees show some critical mental conditions. The mental health status of 586 Cambodian refugees two decades after their resettlement in the USA has been assessed [20]. All participants had been exposed to trauma before immigration and 70% reported exposure to violence after settlement in the USA. High rates of PTSD (62%, weighted) and major depression (51%, weighted) were found with high co-morbidity between PTSD and major depression (42%, weighted).

Objectives of the study

Assessing the effectiveness of treatments among refugee populations

We aim to provide an investigation of the clinical practices and critically assess the effectiveness of selected interventions aimed at treating symptoms of mental disorders among refugee populations, as they are reported in the scientific literature. We include and analyse only the studies on adult refugees who have received a psychiatric diagnosis, through a systematic review of randomized controlled trial (RCT). The final part discusses potential preventative measures and treatment effectiveness in order to prevent the onset and development of mental disorders among refugees.

Several different kinds of treatment of trauma among refugee populations have been applied, and some approaches have received more specific attention. In order to provide an overview of the results reported in the literature about refugee populations with psychosocial disabilities, we will first illustrate some of the major approaches dealt with in this specific issue. Some approaches have seen the use of group techniques, including community, family member, or individual session therapy, which in some cases were integrated and used in a multidisciplinary way [21].

Community-based interventions

Many community-based interventions are focused on the community as a health tool, providing family and community cohesion, support, and collective identity, which, in turn, serve as key potential protective factors to reduce the overall burden of mental illnesses [22]. Community-based health interventions aim to empower local community groups to take an active part and true participation in diagnosing and solving their own health problems [23, 24].

According to these models, participation in health outcomes can be implemented in a variety of forms. Some studies have shown that the community could request the support of medical services in some steps of the process, such as the planning or implementation of the intervention. Formats of community-based interventions mainly focus on outreach, workshops, train-the-trainer models, employment of refugees, and mentoring programmes oriented to having a strong social impact and social inclusion [25–27].

Trauma-focused cognitive–behavioural therapy

Trauma-focused cognitive–behavioural therapy (CBT) is a components-based psychosocial treatment model that integrates elements of cognitive–behavioural, attachment, humanistic, empowerment, and caregiver therapy models. Psychoeducation is provided to patients and their caregivers about the impact of trauma and common reactions. Relaxation and stress training skills are provided to help identify and cope with a range of emotions and behavioural adjustments. Cognitive coping and processing are enhanced by illustrating the relationships among feelings, behaviours, and thoughts about the trauma, and providing help to modify inaccurate or unhelpful thoughts. Another important component of trauma-focused CBT is trauma narration, when patients describe their personal traumatic experiences [28, 29].

Narrative exposure therapy

Narrative approaches seem ideally suited to cross-cultural applications. Narrative exposure therapy (NET) has been considered a short and pragmatic PTSD treatment. It is designed to be easy to implement, even when provided by trained laypersons with a minimal background in medicine and psychology. It should be applicable across cultures, and fit the social and political background of the setting [30]. Instead of defining a single traumatic event as a therapeutic target, in NET the patient constructs a narrative of his or her whole life, from his or her birth to present day, recording a new biography with the therapist's support. NET is not used for a single traumatic event; patients are encouraged to reconstruct a narration of their lives in order to elaborate traumatic experiences and contextualize them in a more social-justice and emotionally aware framework. In NET, narration is necessary because memories and emotional processing are not always accurate in traumatic report; the assumption is that emotional responses associated with memory could be reconstructed in a better and more sustainable way ([28, 30].

Interpersonal psychotherapy

Interpersonal psychotherapy (IPT) is a time-limited psychotherapy that focuses on interpersonal issues, which are understood to be a factor in the genesis and maintenance of psychological distress. The targets of IPT are symptom resolution, improved interpersonal functioning, and increased social support. IPT aims to discuss and analyse specifically current social functioning with consequent benefits for quality of life and mood symptom experience. IPT focus is not retelling or narrating past traumatic experiences; the target is to change current relationships for the better, in order to control and improve mood symptoms. The patient's interpersonal functioning problems are analysed and structured in four areas: interpersonal disputes, role transitions, grief, and interpersonal deficits. The very first part of the therapy is targeted at obtaining the 'interpersonal inventory assessment', an important starting point of IPT. In order to enable the person to manage the emotional and social skills learned as goals for the future, therapy works through identifying dispute, role transition, or grief and linking them with emotional and interpersonal accomplishments occurring during the final part of IPT treatment. Despite the growing body of evidence concerning the effectiveness of this therapy in a range of mental disorders [31], few studies have addressed its effectiveness among refugee populations subjected to traumatic experiences [32].

Eye movement desensitization and reprocessing

Eye movement desensitization and reprocessing (EMDR) is a non-traditional type of psychotherapy. It is known particularly for treating PTSD after traumatic experiences. The aim of EMDR is to alleviate the distress associated with traumatic memories, facilitating access to and processing of traumatic experiences and

other adverse life events, and bringing them to an adaptive resolution. The therapeutic goal is to relieve distress, reformulate negative beliefs, and reduce physiological arousal. During EMDR therapy, the patient attends to emotionally disturbing material in brief sequential doses while simultaneously focusing on an external stimulus. The therapist directs lateral eye movements, or uses hand-tapping or audio stimulation. EMDR therapy facilitates access to the traumatic memory network, targeting memory and its corresponding negative and positive cognitions, emotions, and location of distress, so that information processing is enhanced, with new associations being forged between the traumatic memory and more adaptive emotions or information [33]. EMDR with traumatized refugees is receiving a lot of attention [34].

This approach is used as the main therapeutic intervention or as part of a phased-in multi-modal approach. Several trials describe the successful use of EMDR with refugees from diverse cultural backgrounds [35–37].

Systematic review

Previous reviews have examined the efficacy of various treatments on refugees [38–40]. This chapter focuses specifically on the evidence of RCTs in order to assess the effectiveness of various approaches to adult refugee populations. For this systematic review, only treatments involving adults were chosen, because young refugee populations deserve further attention. Young refugee populations have shown differences in the course of mental illness related to stressful and traumatic events [5, 6]. We have also decided not to choose RCTs that have established the effectiveness of treatment studies on refugees subjected to torture because these deserve specific evaluation, as has already been demonstrated [38]. It can be assumed that there is a level of institutional or structural violence—although this is often considered more abstract and less direct than torture [41], which can even cause traumatic experiences and determine a psychopathological burden. Therefore, this review includes only the studies where less than 50% of the clinical population was made up of tortured refugees. The time range has been set to the latest 10 years given the increasing number of treatments following massive mental health request, which, in turn, is the result of global forced migration processes, and also because practices tend to evolve and improve fast.

Methods

A number of strategies were used. This chapter presents not only the findings of systematic reviews, but also careful sifting of evidence.

Bibliographic databases and trial registers were searched from the start of database coverage to 26 July 2016: Ovid PsycINFO, MEDLINE, Embase, Entrez-PubMed, Web of Science, and Google Scholar. Other sources were the reference lists of reviews resulting from the searches, reference lists from the final set of the included studies, and tables of contents from the top 10 most frequently cited papers. We used the following keywords: 'refugees, mental health'.

The following inclusion criteria were adopted: (i) clinical population aged 18 years and older; (ii) refugees who had not suffered torture (> 50% of the clinical population examine); (iii) available in English; (iv) only refugees or asylum seekers; (v) only RCTs; (vi) time range from 2006 to 2016.

A study was considered for inclusion if it described an RCT of any pharmacological or psychological intervention designed to reduce symptoms of mental disorders in refugees or asylum seekers, who were given a diagnosis according to DSM or *International Classification of Diseases* (ICD) criteria. Studies could include participants with co-morbidity, but the main outcome of any trial had to be the treatment of mental disorders symptoms, rather than treatment of co-morbidity or ancillary outcomes.

For it to be included, a pharmacological RCT had to compare a drug treatment combined with or versus a psychosocial or psychotherapy approach in one of the treatment group conditions, including placebo or an active comparator. A psychological trial had to compare one psychotherapy approach with another active treatment, or with a non-specific control group, or a waitlist group.

We reviewed the abstracts of all the studies identified by the review search strategy. We reviewed the full texts of all intervention studies and decided which articles should be included, based on the inclusion and exclusion criteria specified herein.

Results

Study characteristics

The search strategy identified 22 potentially relevant RCTs. Eleven were excluded. Six of these examined clinical populations mostly composed of refugees who had undergone torture [27, 37, 42–45]. Another was a further analysis of the same clinical population examined in a study already included in the review [46]. Two trials analysd, respectively, the predictors of treatment outcome and the study protocol [47, 48]. Two more studies did not fulfil the randomization procedures criteria [49, 50].

Features of the included studies
Geographical setting of the included studies
Eleven trials met the criteria for inclusion as shown in Table 33.1. Four trials involved adults who had refugee status in Germany [51–54]. Three studies were conducted in the USA [55–57]. One of the trials was conducted in Norway [58]. One trial involved Sudanese refugees living in Cairo, Egypt [32]. One study was carried out in a refugee camp located on the border between Turkey and Syria [11], and one in Denmark [59].

Outcomes of the included studies
All the clinical population had undergone clinical evaluations at the time of assessment, with the main aim of detecting PTSD symptoms according to ICD-10 or DSM. A reduction in symptoms of PTSD emerged as the main outcome shared by all the included studies; Table 33.1 shows the measures used to assess PTSD severity and the other chosen outcome measures. Eight of 11 studies added a measure concerning PTSD severity to the outcome, and related to depression symptoms [11, 32, 52–55, 57, 58]. One of the studies reported, among the main outcome measures, cortical activation following aversive picture presentation with neuromagnetic oscillatory brain activity (steady-state visual evoked fields) [53]. Post-traumatic growth [60] and well-being were included among the main outcomes in one trial [57].

Post-traumatic growth is the experience of positive change that develops as a result of highly traumatic stressful experiences. It is manifested in a variety of attitudes: a change in priorities, an increased appreciation for life and interpersonal relationships, and a greater sense of personal strength [60]. Outcome measures

concerning severity of violence toward household and emotional reaction of anger were examined, among the main outcome measures, in one study [32]. The measure of physical illness was chosen among the main outcomes in two trials [51, 54]. One of these assessed the number of mental health visits [56]. One study investigated the effect of psychotherapy treatment in immunological alterations [54], whereas another one included the systolic blood pressure response [55].

Types of treatment in the included trials
In six studies the effectiveness of NET was examined in comparison with control conditions [51–54, 57, 58]; one of these has compared NET with IPT [52], and another with trauma counseling [51]. In two studies the effectiveness of culturally adapted CBT was assessed in comparison with waitlist control condition [55, 59], whereas in another trial it was matched with psychopharmacological treatment and medical consultations [59]. Treatment group—consisting of Coffee and Family Education and Support (CAFES) in multiple-family groups—was chosen as the experimental condition and compared with an inactive control group in one study [56]. IPT versus waitlist control group condition was compared in one trial [32]. One study verified the differences in efficacy between EMDR treatment and waitlist condition [11].

Effectiveness of treatments
Overall, the studies included in the review confirm the effectiveness of the implemented treatments, with differences in strength and duration of outcome measures variation. The one exception was a trial that did not detect any statistically significant efficacy between experimental conditions—i.e. flexible CBT and antidepressants—and control group conditions [59].

Effectiveness of narrative exposure therapy
One trial involved Somali and Rwandan refugees; it compared manualized NET with the more flexible trauma counseling, and with a no-treatment monitoring group. Both active treatment groups were statistically and clinically superior to the monitoring group on PTSD symptoms, and on physical health regression at post-test and follow-up. The active treatment groups did not differ one from the other in PTSD symptoms and in physical health regression at post-test and at the 6-month follow-up [51].

The aim of one of the included studies was to evaluate the efficacy of treatment modules for trauma spectrum disorders in a sample of Rwandan genocide orphans, who, at the time, were already older than 18 years of age. There were two active treatment conditions: NET and IPT; at post-test, the finding was of no significant group differences between NET and IPT on any of the examined outcome measures. At the 6-month follow-up, only 25% of NET, and 71% of IPT participants still fulfilled PTSD criteria. The study also found a significant time × treatment interaction at post-test and at the 6-month follow-up, in which NET participants showed a significant higher improvement than IPT participants on the severity of symptoms of PTSD and depression [52].

In a group of 34 refugees from the Middle East, East-Central Europe, the Balkans, and Africa treated with NET, PTSD symptom severity significantly decreased at the 4-month post-test ($P < 0.001$), whereas the participants in the waiting list condition showed no significant improvement ($P = 0.11$). Moreover, an interaction effect for time × treatment was found for the Hamilton Depression Rating Scale ($F(1, 17) = 13.2$, $P < 0.005$). The NET participants

Table 33.1 Measures, interventions, and timing of assessments in the included trials

First author, country [ref.]	Sample	Duration	Treatment group vs control	Primary outcome measures	General findings	Type of analysis	Effect sizes
Neuner, Germany [51]	277 Somali and Rwandan refugee participants	◆ 3-week treatment (six sessions, usually two sessions per week) ◆ 6-month follow-up	NET condition TC condition MG condition	◆ PDS, PTSD Diagnostic Scale [73] ◆ Physical health checklist of cough, diarrhoea, flu, pain, fever, and headache	Groups that received active treatment developed statistically and clinically better health status on the PTSD scales than did a non-treated monitoring group. The comparison of NET and TC showed no significant difference between the approaches. Efficacy has been also established for both active treatments at follow-up	Within-treatment effect sizes (Cohen's d) of the outcome variables by group	PDS, PTSD: ◆ NET, d (pre to post) = 1.4 ◆ NET, d (pre to follow-up) = 1.4 ◆ TC, d (pre to post) = 1.5 ◆ TC, d (pre to follow-up) = 1.5 ◆ MG, d (pre to post) = not assessed ◆ MG, d (pre to follow-up) = 0.8 Physical symptom score: ◆ NET, d (pre to post) = 0.1 ◆ NET, d (pre to follow-up) = 0.9 ◆ TC, d (pre to post) = 0.2 ◆ TC, d (pre to follow-up) = 0.5 ◆ MG, d (pre to post) = not assessed ◆ MG, d (pre to follow-up) = −0.2
Hinton, USA [55]	24 Cambodian refugee participants	◆ 12-week treatment ◆ 3-month follow-up	CBT (culturally adapted CBT condition) WL	◆ CAPS ◆ Emotion Regulation Scale ◆ O-PASS ◆ O-FSS ◆ O-CCSS ◆ Systolic BP Δ score ◆ Diastolic BP Δ score ◆ Heart rate Δ score	The patients randomized to CBT had much greater improvement than patients in the waitlist condition on all psychometric measures and on one physiological measure. After receiving CBT, the delayed treatment group improved on all measures, including the systolic BP response to orthostasis. The CBT treatment's reduction of PTSD severity was significantly mediated by improvement in orthostatic panic and emotion regulation ability	Between-group effect sizes, comparing the IT and DT groups at the second assessment (post-treatment) using Cohen's d, no statistical significance was found at follow-up	Between-group effect size, based on second assessment, Cohen's d CAPS: IT, DT d = 1.98 Emotion regulation scale: IT, DT d = 2.53 O-PASS: IT, DT d = 2.84 O-FSS: IT, DT d = 1.18 O-CCSS: ItIT, DT d = 2.79 Systolic BPΔ score: IT, DT d = 1.31 Diastolic BP Δ score: IT, DT d = 0.30 Heart rate Δ score: IT, DT d = 0.10 At the second assessment no difference was found

(Continued)

Table 33.1 Continued

First author, country [ref.]	Sample	Duration	Treatment group vs control	Primary outcome measures	General findings	Type of analysis	Effect sizes
Schaal, Germany [52]	26 Rwandan genocide orphans (mean age of participants at pre-test 19.42 years)	◆ 4-week treatment (one session per week) ◆ 3-month post-test ◆ 6-month follow-up	IPT condition NET condition	◆ CAPS ◆ HAM-D ◆ Mini-International Neuropsychiatric Interview	At post-test, there were no significant group differences between NET and IPT on any of the examined outcome measures. There was a significant time × treatment interaction in the severity of PTSD and depression symptoms. At follow-up, NET participants showed a significantly higher improvement than IPT participants on severity of PTSD symptoms and depression	Three assessment periods (pre-test, post-test, and follow-up) in outcome measures were calculated using Cochran's Q tests, Friedman tests, and ANOVA. For significant results, changes within the particular treatment conditions from pre-test to post-test and from pre-test to follow-up were analysed using binomial tests, paired t-tests, and Wilcoxon tests. Effect sizes ($\dot{\eta}2$) were computed for both treatment conditions (pre-test/post-test and pre-test/follow-up)	CAPS severity score NET: ◆ $\dot{\eta}2$ (pre–post) 0.39 ◆ $\dot{\eta}2$ (pre–follow-up) 0.71 IPT: ◆ $\dot{\eta}2$ (pre–post) 0.23 ◆ $\dot{\eta}2$ (pre–follow-up) 0.00 MINI depression score: NET: ◆ $\dot{\eta}2$ (pre–post) 0.12 ◆ $\dot{\eta}2$ (pre–follow-up) 0.52 IPT: ◆ $\dot{\eta}2$ (pre–post) 0.28 ◆ $\dot{\eta}2$ (pre–follow-up) 0.41 Hamilton score: NET: ◆ $\dot{\eta}2$ (pre–post) 0.45 ◆ $\dot{\eta}2$ (pre–follow-up) 0.75 IPT: ◆ $\dot{\eta}2$ (pre–post) 0.35 ◆ $\dot{\eta}2$ (pre–follow-up) 0.43 Between-group differences in post-traumatic stress symptomatology and depression symptomatology at follow-up (*$P < 0.05$; **$P < 0.01$) CAPS severity score, $F_{(1,23)} = 7.68$**, $B = -28.28$ MINI depression score, $F_{(1,23)} = 3047$*, $B = -1.83$, $t_{(23)} = -1.86$* Hamilton score $F_{(1,23)} = 5.20$*, $B = -7.57$, $t_{(23)} = -2.28$*

Study	Participants	Design	Groups	Measures	Results	Analysis	Statistical details
Weine, USA [56]	197 refugee participants from Bosnia-Herzegovina and their families	◆ 16 week treatment (nine multiple-family group sessions) ◆ 6-, 12-, and 18-month follow-up	CAFES CG (received no intervention condition)	Number of mental health visits as a function of group intervention Mediators: The PTSD Symptoms Scale [73] A subscale for avoidance in PTSD The Center for Epidemiological Studies Depression Scale	The results indicated that a multiple-family group was effective in increasing access to mental health services and that depression and family comfort with discussing trauma mediated the intervention effect	Longitudinal analysis of mental health visits at the three post-intervention time points (6, 12, and 18 months), with random-effect regression models for mental health visits	Three models were considered: linear, quadratic, and linear with subjects clustered in families. Results of the linear model analysis indicated significance in the following two coefficients: a higher average difference in the group's trend line ($b2 = 3.17; P < 0.0049$); a higher average difference with elevated pre-intervention mental health visits ($b4 = 4.44; P < 0.0056$) The quadratic model had no significantly improved fit over the linear model ($LRv2 = 3684.9 - 3683.9 = 1.0$, which on two degrees of freedom is not significant)
Adenauer, Germany [53]	34 refugee participants from the Middle East, Central East, The Balkans, Africa	◆ 12-week treatment ◆ 4-month follow-up (single assessment to the post-treatment)	NET WL	◆ CAPS ◆ HAM-D ◆ Cortical activation following aversive picture presentation with neuromagnetic oscillatory brain activity (ssVEF)	In patients treated with NET, PTSD symptom severity significantly declined at the 4-month post-test ($P < 0.001$), whereas the WL group showed no significant improvement ($P = 0.11$). Moreover, an interaction effect for time × treatment was found for the HAM-D ($F(1, 17) = 13.2, P < 0.005$). The NET group reported significantly less depressive symptom severity at post-test ($P < 0.001$), whereas depressive symptoms remained unchanged in the WL group. Only in the NET group, parietal and occipital activity towards threatening pictures increased significantly after therapy	Changes in clinical symptoms were evaluated using repeated-measures ANOVA with treatment condition (NET and WL) as between-factor, and time (pre-test and post-test) as within-factor Threat effect (cortical activation following aversive picture presentation) with MAG was assessed by permutation test and calculated with unpaired t-tests within this region of interest in both recording sessions	PTSD symptoms CAPS score NET ($n = 11$) Pre-test, post-test $P = < 0.001$ WL ($n = 8$) Pre-test, post-test $P = NS$ Depressive symptoms HAM-D score NET ($n = 11$) Pre-test, post-test $P = < 0.001$ WL ($n = 8$) Pre-test, post-test $P = NS$ Threat effect (cortical activation following aversive picture presentation) group differences in pre- to post-treatment change revealed a significant effect in the superior parietal cortex (pre-test: $t = 0.31, P = 0.76$, post-test: $t = 2.58, P = 0.02$)

Table 33.1 Continued

First author, country [ref.]	Sample	Duration	Treatment group vs control	Primary outcome measures	General findings	Type of analysis	Effect sizes
Stenmark, Norway [58]	81 refugees and asylum seekers from Afghanistan, Iraq, the Middle East, Africa, and other countries (all participating)	◆ 9 week treatment (nine sessions, one session per week) ◆ 6-month follow-up	NET TAU (CBT psychotherapy) condition	◆ CAPS ◆ HAM-D	Both NET and TAU gave clinically relevant symptom reduction both in PTSD and in depression. NET gave significantly more symptom reduction compared with TAU, as well as significantly more reduction in participants with PTSD diagnoses at post-treatment and at follow-up	Mixed-effect models of longitudinal data were used; within-group effect sizes (Hedges' g and 95% CIs in brackets) of CAPS total scores (PTSD) and HAM-D scores (depression) displayed separately for all refugees (n =35) who had completed their treatments	CAPS total score NET: Refugees (n = 21) ◆ 1 month after treatment 1.37 (0.70–2.04) ◆ 6 months after treatment 1.53 (0.85–2.22) Asylum seekers (n = 12) ◆ 1 month after treatment 0.90(0.06–1.74) ◆ 6 months after treatment) 0.93 (0.09–1.77) TAU: Refugees (n = 14) ◆ 1 month after treatment 0.42 (−0.33 to 1.16) ◆ 6 months after treatment 0.57 (−0.19 to 1.33) Asylum seekers (n = 7) ◆ 1 month after treatment 0.82 (−0.28 to 1.91) ◆ 6 months after treatment 0.31 (−0.75 to 1.36) HAM-D score NET: Refugees (n = 21) ◆ 1 month after treatment 0.89 (0.26–1.52) ◆ 6 months after treatment 1.07 (0.42–1.71) Asylum seekers (n = 12) ◆ 1 month after treatment 0.72 (−0.11 to 1.54) ◆ 6 months after treatment 0.31 (−0.49 to 1.12) TAU Refugees (n=14) ◆ 1 month after treatment 0.60 (−0.16 to 1.36) ◆ 6 months after treatment 0.57 (−0.18 to 1.33) Asylum seekers (n = 7) ◆ 1 month after treatment 1.10 (−0.03 to 2.22) ◆ 6 months after treatment −0.32 (−1.37 to 0.74)

Study	Participants	Conditions	Treatment	Measures	Results	Analysis	Effect sizes
Meffert, Egypt [32]	◆ 22 Sudanese refugee participants	IPT WL	◆ 3/4-week treatment (twice a week) ◆ No follow-up	HTQ (PTSD) BDI–II CTSYVL STAXIS TAXIT	The effect sizes of IPT treatment for PTSD symptoms, depression, state anger, trait anger, and CTSYVL were −2.52, −2.38, −1.21, −1.43, and −0.84, respectively. IPT predicted a significant decrease in symptoms of PTSD, state anger, and depression using a conservative ITT analysis	Change scores were calculated for IPT and waitlist groups. Effect size was determined by dividing mean change scores by the SD of the change scores. Linear regression was used to assess the relative predictive value of baseline measures and group assignment. Because the sample size was small and scores on most of the outcome measures were not normally distributed, we used non-parametric bootstrap resampling to estimate regression standard errors and P-values [74]	Change score effect sizes Cohen's d Effect size for IPT group change score HTQ, IPT d = −2.52 HTQ, WL d = −0.75 BDI–II, IPT d = −2.38 BDI–II, WL d = −0.47 STAXIS, IPT d = −1.21 STAXIS, WL d = −0.41 STAXIT, IPT d = −1.43 STAXIT, WL d = −0.32 CTSYVL, IPT d = −0.84 CTSYVL, WL d = −0.53
Hijazi, USA [57]	◆ 63 Iraqi refugee participants	B-NET WCG	◆ 3-week treatment (one session per week) ◆ 2- and 4-month follow-up	PTGI [60] WHO-5 [75] PTSD assessed by two sections of the HTQ translated into Arabic [76] Arabic translation [77] of the 21-item BDI–II [78] Somatic symptoms were assessed by using the PHQ-15 [79]	Significant condition × time interactions showed that those receiving brief NET had greater post-traumatic growth and well-being through 4 months than controls. B-NET reduced symptoms of post-traumatic stress and depression more but only at 2 months; symptoms of controls also decreased from 2 to 4 months, eliminating condition differences at 4 months	Primary analyses of the effects of B-NET vs control were conducted using a mixed design (between-within) repeated measures ANOVA assessing between-condition differences from baseline to follow-up. The two follow-up assessment points were analysed separately. If there was a significant condition × time interaction, within-condition, paired t-tests were conducted to determine how each condition changed over time. Effect sizes both within and between conditions were calculated. Within Cohen's d	Within- and between-condition comparisons of outcomes from baseline to 2-month and 4-month follow-ups PTG: Brief NET treatment ◆ 2-month d = 0.23 ◆ 4-month d = 0.52** Waitlist controls ◆ 2-month d = −0.26 ◆ 4-month d = −0.36 Well-being: Brief NET treatment ◆ 2-month d = 0.65** ◆ 4-month d = 0.92*** Waitlist controls ◆ 2-month d = −0.02 ◆ 4-month d = 0.24 Trauma symptoms: Brief NET treatment ◆ 2-month d = −0.39** ◆ 4-month d = −0.50**

(Continued)

Table 33.1 Continued

First author, country [ref.]	Sample	Treatment group vs control	Duration	Primary outcome measures	General findings	Type of analysis	Effect sizes
							Waitlist controls ♦ 2-month d = −0.01 ♦ 4-month d = −0.26 Depressive symptoms: Brief NET treatment ♦ 2-month d = −0.62*** ♦ 4-month d = −0.84*** Waitlist controls ♦ 2-month d = 0.17 ♦ 4-month d = −0.53** Somatic symptoms: Brief NET treatment ♦ 2-month d = −0.53** ♦ 4-month d = −0.57*** Waitlist controls ♦ 2-month d = −0.22 ♦ 4-month d = −0.41 Condition × time Interaction PTG: ♦ 2-month ES = 0.48* ♦ 4-month ES = 0.83*** Well-being: ♦ 2-month ES = 0.56* ♦ 4-month ES = 0.54* Trauma symptoms: ♦ 2-month ES = −0.48* ♦ 4-month ES = −0.32 ♦ Depressive symptoms:2-month ES = −0.46* ♦ 4-month ES = −0.27 Somatic symptoms: 2-month ES = −0.32 4-month ES = −0.13

Study	Sample	Intervention / Comparison	Duration & follow-up	Outcome measures	Results	Statistical analysis	Statistics
Morath, Germany [54]	34 refugee participants from Africa, the Balkans, and the Middle East	NET / WL	◆ 12-week treatment (one session per week) ◆ 4- and 12-month follow-up	◆ PTSD symptom severity (CAPS score) ◆ Depressive symptoms (HAM D score) ◆ Somatic complaints (SOMS 7 score) ◆ Classes of T cells: ◆ Naïve ◆ Immune responses to novopathogenic organisms CD45RA(+) CCR7(+) ◆ Memory ◆ Central memory (CM) CD45RA(−) CCR7(+) ◆ Effector memory (EM) CD45RA(−) CCR7(−) ◆ TEMRA CD45RA(+) CCR7(−) ◆ Treg ◆ CD4(+) CD25(+) FoxP3(+)	PTSD symptoms were significantly reduced only in the NET group, 4 months post-therapy (effect size: Hedges' g = 1.61). One year after therapy, PTSD symptoms were improved even further in the NET group compared to baseline (Hedges' g = 1.96). This symptom improvement was mirrored in an increase in the originally reduced proportion of Tregs in the NET group at the 1-year follow-up, when comparing subgroups matched for baseline Treg numbers. However, no changes were found for the initially reduced proportion of CD45RA+ CCR7+ naïve T lymphocytes	Linear mixed models were used to analyse changes in clinical characteristics and lymphocyte differentiations from t.0 to t.1	CAPS, $F_{(1,32)}$ 16.90, $P = 0.0003$ HAM-D $F_{(1,32)}$ 0.89, $P = 0.35$ SOMS $F_{(1,31)}$ 6.19, $P = 0.02$ Classes of T cells % CD3 total a $F_{(1,25)}$ 0.17, $P = 0.68$ % CD3 naïve $F_{(1,26)}$ 0.00, $P = 0.98$ %CD3 memory $F_{(1,26)}$ 0.08, $P = 0.78$ % CD8 total $F_{(1,26)}$ 0.34, $P = 0.56$ % CD8 naïve $F_{(1,25)}$ 0.07, $P = 0.80$ % CD8 memory a $F_{(1,25)}$ 0.60, $P = 0.45$ % CD4 total $F_{(1,25)}$ 0.05, $P = 0.83$ % CD4 naïve $F_{(1,25)}$ 0.29, $P = 0.61$ % CD4 memory $F_{(1,25)}$ 0.05, $P = 0.82$ % T reg $F_{(1,23)}$ 3.06, $P = 0.09$
Acarturk, Turkey [11]	29 Syrian refugee participants living in a camp	EMDR / WL	◆ 7-week treatment ◆ 1-month follow-up	◆ PTSD symptoms IES-R and depression symptoms ◆ BDI	The pilot RCT indicated that EMDR may be effective in reducing PTSD and depression symptoms among refugees. ANCOVA showed that the EMDR group had significantly lower trauma scores at post-treatment as compared with the wait-list group (d = 1.78, 95% CI 0.92–2.64), but the same result was not found at follow-up. The EMDR group had also a lower depression score after treatment as compared with the waitlist group (d = 1.14, 95% CI 0.35–1.92)	Repeated measurement ANOVA was used to compare change over time in target measures	Statistical comparisons across time and groups pB0.05; **pB0.01; ***pB0.001. BDI Time df= 1, 25, F-value = 7.023* Time × group df = 1, 25, F-value = 7.35* IES Time and time × group not reported

(Continued)

Table 33.1 Continued

First author, country [ref.]	Sample	Duration	Treatment group vs control	Primary outcome measures	General findings	Type of analysis	Effect sizes
Buhmann, Denmark [59]	280 refugee participants from Iraq, Iran, Lebanon, former Yugoslavia, Afghanistan, and other countries	◆ 24-week treatment ◆ No clear follow-up time	CT (CBT, psychopharmacological treatment, and consultations) PFT (and psychoeducation) c CBT WL	◆ PTSD severity ◆ measured by the HTQ	In a pragmatic clinical setting, there was no effect of flexible CBT and antidepressants on PTSD	FIML was used in the analyses based on a structural equation modeling in STATA. Effect sizes (Cohen's d) were calculated as the ratio of the post-treatment regression coefficients to the pretreatment SD	Outcomes: pre- and post-treatment scores for each intervention group HTQ Medication vs no medication regression coefficient (95% CI) Pretreatment 0.02 (−0.12 to 0.16) P = 0.83 Post-treatment 0.07 (−0.08 to 0.22) P = 0.39 Therapy vs. no therapy regression coefficient (95% CI) Pre-treatment −0.07 (−0.21 to 0.07) P = 0.31 Post-treatment 0.06 (−0.09 to 0.21) P = 0.46

NET: narrative exposure therapy; TC: trauma counselling; MG: monitoring group; PTSD: post-traumatic stress disorder; WL: waitlist delayed treatment group; CAPS: Clinician-Administered PTSD Scale; O-PASS: Orthostatic-PA Severity Scale; O-FSS: Orthostatic-PA Flashback Severity Scale; O-CCSS: Orthostatic-PA Catastrophic Cognition Severity Scale; BP: blood pressure; IT: immediate treatment; DT: delayed treatment; IPT: interpersonal psychotherapy; HAM-D: Hamilton Rating Scale for Depression; ANOVA: one-way analysis of variance; CAFES: Coffee and Family Education and Support; CG: control group; ssVEF: steady-state visual evoked fields; NS: not significant; TAU: treatment as usual; CI: confidence interval; HTQ: Harvard Trauma Questionnaire; BDI-II: Beck Depression Index II; CTSYVL: Conflict Tactics Scale – Violence Toward Household; STAXIS: State Anger Scale; TAXIT: Trait Anger Scale; ITT: intention-to-treat; SD: standard deviation; B-NET: brief NET; WCG: waitlist control group; PTGI: Posttraumatic Growth Inventory; WHO-5: World Health Organization Well-being Index (Arabic translation); PHQ-15: 15-item Patient Health Questionnaire; Treg: regulatory T cells; EMDR: eye movement desensitization and reprocessing IED-R: Impact of Event Scale Revised; RCT: randomized controlled trial; ANCOVA: analysis of covariance; CT: combination treatment; PFT: psychopharmacological treatment; FIML: full information maximum likelihood.

*P < 0.05; **P < 0.01; ***P < 0.001

reported significantly less depressive symptom severity at post-test ($P < 0.001$), whereas depressive symptoms remained unchanged in the waiting list conditions group. Considering that one of the main outcomes measures assessed in this study was occipital activity towards threatening pictures, the results confirm a significant increase after NET therapy at post-treatment [53].

One study, in particular, was driven by the requirement to validate the efficacy differences between the experimental condition and the control one, dividing the clinical population into two groups: refugees and asylum seekers. For the purposes of this review, we considered only data relating to participating refugees. The study showed clinically relevant symptom reduction in both PTSD and depression in the NET group, compared with treatment as usual (TAU), as well as a significantly higher reduction in participants with PTSD diagnoses. At the 6-month follow-up of the participating refugees, the effect size of the between-group (NET vs TAU) for the Clinician-Administered PTSD Scale (CAPS) scores was 0.77 (confidence interval (CI) 0.07–1.47) and the between-group effect size (NET vs TAU) for the Hamilton Rating Scale for Depression (HAM-D) scores at the 6-month follow-up was 0.52 (CI –0.17 to 1.21) [58].

A recent study involving 63 Iraqi refugees analysed the significant condition by time interactions, and found that those receiving brief NET had greater post-traumatic growth and well-being after 4 months than the control group in the waitlist condition [57].

The brief version of NET reduced the symptoms of post-traumatic stress and depression more, but only at 2 months. Also, the symptoms in the control waitlist condition group decreased from 2 to 4 months, eliminating condition differences at the 4-month follow-up. Conversely in an equally recent study [54], PTSD symptoms were significantly reduced only in the NET group, 4 months after the therapy (effect size: Hedges' g = 1.61) and 1 year after the therapy compared with baseline (Hedges' g = 1.96). This symptom improvement was mirrored in an increase in the reduced proportion of regulatory T cells outcome in the NET group at the 1-year follow up.

Cognitive–behaviour therapy

Culturally adapted CBT was chosen as the treatment group condition in two of the included studies. One revealed greater improvement in the culturally adapted CBT group versus the waitlist condition on the decrease of PTSD symptoms and systolic blood pressure response to orthostasis [55]. In the study perspective, the reduction of PTSD severity achieved by CBT treatment was significantly mediated by improvement in orthostatic panic and emotion regulation ability, chosen as other outcomes. The other study concerning CBT did not detect any statistically significant efficacy between the experimental conditions, which consisted of flexible CBT and antidepressants, and the control group conditions (psychopharmacological treatment with psychoeducation; CBT: cognitive–behavioural psychotherapeutic treatment without psychopharmacological treatment; and waitlist condition) regarding the decrease in PTSD symptoms [59].

Interpersonal psychotherapy

Two studies tested the effectiveness of interpersonal psychotherapy on a refugee group, obtaining different results. A group of 22 Sudanese refugee participants was divided into two subgroups: one received IPT, the other was in the waitlist control condition. The study revealed IPT as an effective treatment for PTSD symptoms, depression, state anger, trait anger, and Conflict Tactics Scale – Violence Toward Household as the main outcomes [32]. The other trial compared two active treatment conditions: NET and IPT, finding no significant group differences between NET and IPT at post-test but an improvement on the severity of symptoms of PTSD and depression at the 6-month follow-up in NET participants [52].

Family-focused treatment

One trial started by considering that multiple-family groups may function by facilitating the ability of persons with mental illness to receive appropriate treatment from mental illness services. The study used the technique of a family-focused education group (CAFES), involving 197 refugees from Bosnia and Herzegovina suffering from depression and PTSD, and their families. The results indicated that a multiple-family group has been effective in increasing access to mental health services, and that depression and family comfort with discussing trauma could mediate the intervention effect [56].

Eye movement desensitization and reprocessing

Only one pilot RCT was found involving a refugee population in EMDR treatment [11]. In this trial, 29 Syrian refugees living in a camp were assigned to treatment or to a waitlist condition. The trial has indicated that EMDR may be effective in reducing PTSD and depression symptoms among refugees. Analysis of covariance showed that the EMDR group had significantly lower trauma scores at post-treatment compared with the waitlist group (d = 1.78, 95% CI 0.92–2.64), but the same result was not found at follow-up. The EMDR group also had a lower depression score after treatment than the waitlist group (d = 1.14, 95% CI 0.35–1.92); no result on the follow-up assessment of the decrease in depressive symptoms has been reported.

Discussion

Cultural sensitivity practices and community support role

A preliminary evaluation of the included studies has shown that some kinds of treatments are receiving more attention than others. NET seems to be the most frequently implemented and evaluated approach. Because of its promising results and its relatively short structure (approximately 10 sessions), it might be considered a sustainable treatment for individuals exposed to strongly traumatic events and that can also be implemented in settings that remain volatile and insecure [61]. A recent meta-analysis concerning RCTs of NET revealed that all interventions show a total average effect size of 0.53 (Cohen's d), whereas the effect size was of 1.02 in a trial that actively involved refugees as counsellors in the care process [30]. This fact could suggest that NET, because of its structure, can be easily conducted by a native-speaking counsellor and that, in this specific variation, it can be actually more effective on clinical populations of refugees. The effectiveness of a common cultural background between counsellors and treated refugees might suggest that a culturally sensitive approach could really be considered a key component in the therapeutic process. Therefore, the activation of a refugee community network support is likely to play a crucial role in the effectiveness of the care process. Nevertheless, only two out of all the studies included in this review chose a refugee community member as counsellor or therapist [32, 51].

Among the studies that have verified the NET intervention, one has carried out a specific 6-week training period for lay counsellors from the same community of refugees, with a focus on developing active listening, empathy, and verbalization and managing emotional processing [51].

Other studies on NET have focused on providing support during the assessment phase and the therapeutic process by native speaker professionals or certified translators, who were not from the same refugees' cultural community [57, 58].

One study was carried out with the aim of verifying the effectiveness of a culturally adapted variant of CBT [55]. Culturally adapted CBT consists of a cognitive–behavioural model of PTSD and panic disorder, muscle relaxation and diaphragmatic breathing, mindfulness training, yoga stretching tasks, various exercises to promote emotional regulation, and interoceptive exposure. However, the therapists in this study were not chosen according to a common cultural origin with the refugees.

Because of its structure, IPT appears to be an approach that is less centred on standard clinical protocols and more focused on the quality of individual relations, which is why it is might be considered more adaptable and sensitive to different cultural backgrounds [32, 52]. In one of the included studies involving Sudanese refugees in Cairo receiving IPT treatment, some Sudanese community members were selected as therapists for the treatment according to their emotional intelligence and interpersonal skills [32].

Family support is often recognized as a key context for refugees and their mental health, as it is a resource for adjustment and coping [62].

One of the studies included in this review showed that multiple-family group intervention can be effective in increasing access to mental health services, whereas depression and family support can mediate the intervention effect [56].

Promoting mental health and preventing mental disorder among refugees

Prevention in mental health is one of the most relevant topics. The necessity of reducing incidence, prevalence, and recurrence of mental disorders, and of preventing mental illness risk conditions and decreasing the impact of illness in the affected persons, their families, and the society has been underlined [63]. The migration process exposes refugees to several potential traumatic experiences that increase the risks of developing mental disorders. Refugees' exposure may span generations, with significant negative impacts on public health and socio-economic development [63]. Nevertheless, few studies have verified the effectiveness that prevention programmes could have on the well-being of refugees [64].

Preventative efforts to reduce the onset of mental disorders among migrants should focus on mental health education, restoring human rights, and offering emotional, social, and economic support to address the barriers against traditional mental health services in Western countries, in order to produce positive mental health outcomes [65]. Bearing in mind the factors that have proved crucial for refugees' quality of life, post-migration interventions should provide an integrated approach to promote and prevent mental health. They should include psychological work with trauma, work orientation, language training, support with regard to bureaucratic and political awareness and service accessibility, social and institutional resources, and facilitating the creation of a supportive refugees' network within the host community. Essentially, preventative programmes should consider an institutional level, a social level facilitating community network, and a personal level oriented to psychological well-being. The need for an integrated approach to prevent mental health problems has been acknowledged in the mental health sector. Preventative programmes that take personal experiences and needs into account, and which address the broader social policy contexts in which refugees are placed have been discussed and considered as an extremely valid opportunity [65, 66]. Preventative activities aimed at facilitating and speeding up the integration process have already proved to be a protective factor against experiences of discrimination and mental disease in the perspective of long-term health benefits and lower psychopathological burden [67]. Some studies have been developed to substantiate the preventative approaches that have activated refugees' community networks. Community-oriented intervention offered in the early stages of refugee resettlement—to prevent or detect the initial stages of mental illness—has been performed among young refugees that have resettled in the USA [68]. Results have shown that community-based mental health services seem more effective than the traditional primary-care model. The authors placed particular emphasis on the community-support preventative approach, by highlighting the importance of specifically designed family-based services for refugees, and explaining that preventative mental health interventions based on community collaboration and family involvement, are an effective way to produce positive health outcomes [69, 70]. Not only does community collaboration help build relationships with people and overcome the feeling of being isolated, alone, and discriminated, but it is also a key to turn prevention into a great facilitator of the access to information and resources by refugee community members.

A Comprehensive Service Model programme involving families schools and communities, which has attempted to overcome numerous obstacles to providing culturally competent services and health support, has been described [71]. The finding was that children who had received such services showed improvement over time.

A review has assessed some school-based programmes for refugee and asylum-seeking children [72], showing that interventions to assist immigrant and refugee children might help children adapt themselves in host countries. School-based programmes for younger refugee populations exploit the potential of family support, peer and educational domains, and empowerment. However, the reviewed studies on preventative school interventions have revealed that very few school-based programmes have been implemented with the minimum methodological quality standards, and therefore preventing an effective programme evaluation.

References

1. Lindert J, Carta MG, Schäfer I, Mollica RF. Refugees mental health: a public mental health challenge. *Eur J Public Health* 2016; 26: 374–375.

2. World Health Organization Regional Office for Europe. Mental Health and Psychosocial Support for Refugees, Asylum Seekers and Migrants on the Move in Europe. A multi-agency guidance note (2015). Available at: http://www.euro.who.int/en/health-topics/health-determinants/migration-and-health/publications/2016/mental-health-and-psychosocial-support-for-refugees,-asylum-seekers-and-migrants-on-the-move-in-europe.-a-multi-agency-guidance-note-2015 (accessed 7 March 2018).

3. American Psychiatric Association (APA). *Diagnostic and Statistical Manual of Mental Disorders*, 5th ed. Arlington, VA: APA.

4. Naja WJ, Aoun MP, El Khoury EL, Abdallah FJ, Haddad RS. Prevalence of depression in Syrian refugees and the influence of religiosity. *Compr Psychiatry* 2016; 68: 78–85.

5. Fazel M, Wheeler J, Danesh J. Prevalence of serious mental disorder in 7000 refugees resettled in western countries: a systematic review. *Lancet* 2005; 365: 1309–1314.

6. Bogic M, Njoku A, Priebe S. Long-term mental health of war-refugees: a systematic literature review. *BMC Int Health Hum Rights*2015; 15: 29.

7. Mollica RF, McInnes K, Sarajlić N, Lavelle J, Sarajlić I, Massagli MP. Disability associated with psychiatric comorbidity and health status in Bosnian refugees living in Croatia. *JAMA* 1999; 282: 433–439.

8. Mollica RF, Caridad KR, Massagli MP Longitudinal study of posttraumatic stress disorder, depression, and changes in traumatic memories over time in Bosnian refugees. *J Nerv Ment Dis* 2007; 195: 572–579.

9. Karam EG, Fayyad J, Nasser Karam A, et al. Effectiveness and specificity of a classroom-based group intervention in children and adolescents exposed to war in Lebanon. *World Psychiatry* 2008; 7: 103–109.

10. Ginzburg, Ein-Dor, Solomon, Comorbidity of posttraumatic stress disorder, anxiety and depression: a 20-year longitudinal study of war veterans. *J Affect Disord* 2010; 123: 249–257.

11. Acarturk C, Konuk E, Cetinkaya M, et al. EMDR for Syrian refugees with posttraumatic stress disorder symptoms: results of a pilot randomized controlled trial. *Eur J Psychotraumatol* 2015; 6: 27414.

12. Carta MG, Preti A. Trauma-related disorders. adjustment disorders and their clinical management. *Sci Am Psychiatry* 2017 (in press).

13. Basishvili T, Eliozishvili M, Maisuradze L, et al. Insomnia in a displaced population is related to war-associated remembered stress. *Stress Health* 2012; 28: 186–192.

14. Lee YJG, Jun JY, Lee YJ, et al. Insomnia in North Korean refugees: association with depression and post-traumatic stress symptoms. *Psychiatry Investig* 2016; 13: 67–73.

15. Hinton DE, Kredlow MA, Bui E, Pollack MH, Hofmann SG. Treatment change of somatic symptoms and cultural syndromes among Cambodian refugees with PTSD. *Depress Anxiety* 2012; 29: 147–154.

16. Carta MG, Wallet Oumar F, Moro MF, et al. Trauma and stressor related disorders in the Tuareg refugees of a camp in Burkina Faso. *Clin Pract Epidemiol Ment Health* 2013; 9: 189–195.

17. de Jong JT, Komproe IH, Van Ommeren M. Common mental disorders in postconflict settings. *Lancet* 2003; 361: 2128–2130.

18. Dobricki M, Komproe IH, de Jong JT, Maercker A. Adjustment disorders after severe life-events in four postconflict settings. *Soc Psychiatry Psychiatr Epidemiol* 2010; 45: 39–46.

19. Carta MG, Moro MF, Preti A, et al. Human rights of asylum seekers with psychosocial disabilities in Europe. *Clin Pract Epidemiol Ment Health* 2016; 12: 64–66.

20. Marshall GN, Schell TL, Elliott MN, Berthold SM, Chun CA. Mental health of Cambodian refugees 2 decades after resettlement in the United States. *JAMA* 2005; 294: 571–579.

21. Slobodin O, de Jong JT. Mental health interventions for traumatized asylum seekers and refugees: What do we know about their efficacy? *Int J Soc Psychiatry* 2015; 61: 17–26.

22. Siriwardhana SA, Bayard Roberts S, Stewart R. A systematic review of resilience and mental health outcomes of conflict-driven adult forced migrants. *Conflict Health* 2014; 8: 13.

23. Morgan LM, Community participation in health: perpetual allure, persistent challenge. *Health Policy Plan* 2001; 16: 221–230.

24. Harpham T, Few R. The Dar Es Salaam Urban Health Project, Tanzania: a multi-dimensional evaluation. *J Public Health Med* 2002; 24: 112–119.

25. Stone L. Cultural influences in community participation in health. *Soc Sci Med* 1992; 35: 409–417.

26. Williams ME, Thompson SC. The use of community-based interventions in reducing morbidity from the psychological impact of conflict-related trauma among refugee populations: a systematic review of the literature. *J Immigr Minor Health* 2011; 13: 780–794.

27. Bolton P, Lee C, Haroz EE, et al. A transdiagnostic community-based mental health treatment for comorbid disorders: development and outcomes of a randomized controlled trial among Burmese refugees in Thailand. *PLOS MED* 2014; 11: e1001757.

28. Buhmann CB. Traumatized refugees: morbidity, treatment and predictors of outcome. *Dan Med J* 2014; 61: B4871.

29. Lambert JE, Alhassoon OM, Trauma-focused therapy for refugees: meta-analytic findings. *J Couns Psychol* 2015; 62: 28–37.

30. Gwozdziewycz N, Mehl-Madrona L. Meta-analysis of the use of narrative exposure therapy for the effects of trauma among refugee populations. *Perm J* 2013; 17: 70–76.

31. Swartz HA, Grote G. Brief interpersonal psychotherapy (IPT-B): overview and review of evidence. *Am J Psychother* 2014; 68: 443–462.

32. Meffert SM, Abdo AO, Alla OAA, et al. A pilot randomized controlled trial of interpersonal psychotherapy for Sudanese refugees in Cairo, Egypt. *Psychol Trauma* 2014; 6: 240–249.

33. Shapiro F, Snyker E, Maxfield L. EMDR: Eye movement desensitization and re processing. In: Kaslow FW (ed.). *Comprehensive Handbook of Psychotherapy*. Hoboken, NJ: John Wiley & Sons, 2002, pp. 241–272.

34. World Health Organization. WHO releases guidance on mental health care after trauma. Available at: http://www.who.int/mediacentre/news/releases/2013/trauma_mental_health_20130806/en/ (accessed 7 March 2018).

35. Bower RD, Pahl L, Bernstein MA. Case presentation of a tattoo-mutilated, Bosnian torture survivor. *Torture* 2004; 14: 16–24.

36. Regel S, Berliner P. Current perspectives on assessment and therapy with survivors of torture: the use of a cognitive behavioural approach. *Eur J Psychother Counsel* 2007; 9: 289–299.

37. Ter Heide FJ, Mooren TM, Kleijn W, de Jongh A, Kleber RJ. EMDR versus stabilisation in traumatised asylum seekers and refugees: results of a pilot study. *Eur J Psychotraumatol* 2011; 2.

38. Patel N, Kellezi B, Williams AC. Psychological, social and welfare interventions for psychological health and well-being of torture survivors. *Cochrane Database Syst Rev* 2014; (11): CD009317.

39. Nickerson A, Bryant RA, Silove D, Steel Z. A critical review of psychological treatments of posttraumatic stress disorder in refugees. *Clin Psychol Rev* 2011; 31: 399–417.

40. Crumlish N, O'Rourke K. A systematic review of treatments for post-traumatic stress disorder among refugees and asylum-seekers. *J Nerv Ment Dis* 2010; 198: 237–251.

41. Galtung J. Violence, peace, and peace research. *J Peace Res* 1969; 6: 167–191.

42. Neuner F, Kurreck S, Ruf M, Odenwald M, Elbert T, Schauer M. Can asylum-seekers with posttraumatic stress disorder be successfully treated? A randomized controlled pilot study. *Cogn Behav Ther* 2010; 39: 81–91.

43. Liedl A, Müller J, Morina N, Karl A, Denke C, Knaevelsrud C. Physical activity within a CBT intervention improves coping with pain in traumatized refugees: results of a randomized controlled design. *Pain Med* 2011; 12: 234–245.

44. Dittmann D, Schauer M, Ruf M, Catani C, Odenwald M, Elbert T, Neuner F. Treatment of traumatized victims of war and torture: a randomized controlled comparison of narrative exposure therapy and stress inoculation training. *Psychother Psychosom* 2011; 80: 345–352.

45. Buhmann C, Andersen I, Mortensen EL, Ryberg J, Nordentoft M, Ekstrøm M. Cognitive behavioral psychotherapeutic treatment at a psychiatric trauma clinic for refugees: description and evaluation. *Torture* 2015; 25: 17–32.

46. Halvorsen JØ, Stenmark H, Neuner F, Nordahl HM. Does dissociation moderate treatment outcomes of narrative exposure therapy for PTSD? A secondary analysis from a randomized controlled clinical trial. *Behav Res Ther* 2014; 57: 21–28.

47. Sonne C, Carlsson J, Elklit A, Mortensen EL, Ekstrøm M. Treatment of traumatized refugees with sertraline versus venlafaxine in combination with psychotherapy—study protocol for a randomized clinical trial. *Trials* 2013; 14: 137.

48. Sonne C, Carlsson J, Bech P, Vindbjerg E, Mortensen EL, Elklit A. Psychosocial predictors of treatment outcome for trauma-affected refugees. Eur J *Psychotraumatol* 2016; 7: 30907.

49. Stade K, Skammeritz S, Hjortkjær C, Carlsson J. 'After all the traumas my body has been through, I feel good that it is still working.' —Basic Body Awareness Therapy for traumatised refugees. *Torture* 2015; 25: 33–50.

50. Rees B, Travis F, Shapiro D, Chant R. Reduction in posttraumatic stress symptoms in Congolese refugees practicing transcendental meditation. *J Trauma Stress* 2013; 26: 295–298.

51. Neuner F, Onyut PL, Ertl V, Odenwald M, Schauer E, Elbert T. Treatment of posttraumatic stress disorder by trained lay counselors in an African refugee settlement: a randomized controlled trial. *J Consult Clin Psychol* 2008; 76: 686–694.

52. Schaal S, Elbert T, Neuner F. Narrative exposure therapy versus interpersonal psychotherapy. A pilot randomized controlled trial with Rwandan genocide orphans. *Psychother Psychosom* 2009; 78: 298–306.

53. Adenauer H, Catani C, Gola H, Keil J, Ruf M, Schauer M, Neuner F. Narrative exposure therapy for PTSD increases top-down processing of aversive stimuli—evidence from a randomized controlled treatment trial. *BMC Neurosci* 2011; 12: 127.

54. Morath J, Gola H, Sommershof A, et al. The effect of trauma-focused therapy on the altered T cell distribution in individuals with PTSD: evidence from a randomized controlled trial. *J Psychiatr Res* 2014; 54: 1–10.

55. Hinton DE, Hofmann SG, Pollack MH, Otto MW. Mechanisms of efficacy of CBT for Cambodian refugees with PTSD: improvement in emotion regulation and orthostatic blood pressure response. *CNS Neurosci Ther* 2009; 15: 255–263.

56. Weine S, Kulauzovic Y, Klebic A, et al. Evaluating a multiple-family group access intervention for refugees with PTSD. *J Marital Fam Ther* 2008; 34: 149–164.

57. Hijazi AM, Lumley MA, Ziadni MS, Haddad L, Rapport LJ, Arnetz BB. Brief narrative exposure therapy for posttraumatic stress in Iraqi refugees: a preliminary randomized clinical trial. *J Trauma Stress* 2014; 27: 314–322.

58. Stenmark H, Catani C, Neuner F, Elbert T, Holen A. Treating PTSD in refugees and asylum seekers within the general health care system. A randomized controlled multicenter study. *Behav Res Ther* 2013; 51: 641–647.

59. Buhmann CB, Nordentoft M, Ekstroem M, Carlsson J, Mortensen EL. The effect of flexible cognitive-behavioural therapy and medical treatment, including antidepressants on post-traumatic stress disorder and depression in traumatised refugees: pragmatic randomised controlled clinical trial. *Br J Psychiatry* 2016; 208: 252–259.

60. Tedeschi RG, Calhoun LG. Posttraumatic growth: conceptual foundations and empirical evidence. *Psychol Inq* 2004; 15: 1–18.

61. Robjant K, Fazel M., The emerging evidence for Narrative Exposure Therapy: a review. *Clin Psychol Rev* 2010; 30: 1030–1039.

62. Voulgaridou M, Papadopoulos R, Tomaras V. Working with refugee families in Greece: systemic considerations. *J Fam Ther* 2006; 28: 200–220.

63. World Health Organization. Prevention of Mental Disorders: Effective Interventions and Policy Options: Summary Report. Available at: http://www.who.int/mental_health/evidence/en/prevention_of_mental_disorders_sr.pdf (accessed 7 March 2018).

64. Kirmayer LJ, Narasiah L, Munoz M, et al.; Canadian Collaboration for Immigrant and Refugee Health (CCIRH). Common mental health problems in immigrants and refugees: general approach in primary care. *CMAJ* 2011; 183: E959–E967.

65. Porter M. Global evidence for a biopsychosocial understanding of refugee adaptation. *Transcult Psychiatry* 2007; 44: 418–439.

66. Watters C. Emerging paradigms in the mental health care of refugees. *Soc Sci Med* 2001; 52: 1709–1718.

67. Beiser M, Longitudinal research to promote effective refugee resettlement. *Transcult Psychiatry* 2006; 43: 56–71.

68. Durà-Vilà G, Klasen H, Makatini Z, Rahimi Z, Hodes M. Mental health problems of young refugees: duration of settlement, risk factors and community-based interventions. *Clin Child Psychol Psychiatry* 2013; 18: 604–623.

69. Weine MD. Developing preventive mental health interventions for refugee families in resettlement. *Fam Process* 2011; 50: 410–430.

70. Weine SM, Kulauzovic Y, Besic S, et al. A family beliefs framework for developing socially and culturally specific preventive interventions for refugee families and youth. *Am J Orthopsychiatry* 2006; 76: 1–9.

71. Birman D, Beehler S, Harris EM, et al. International Family, Adult, and Child Enhancement Services (FACES): a community-based comprehensive services model for refugee children in resettlement. *Am J Orthopsychiatry* 2008; 78: 121–132.

72. Tyrer RA, Fazel M. School and community-based interventions for refugee and asylum seeking children: a systematic review. *PLOS ONE* 2014; 9: e89359.

73. Foa EB, Cashman L, Jaycox L, Perry K. The validation of self-report measure of post-traumatic stress disorder: The Post-traumatic Diagnostic Scale. *Psychol Assess* 1995; 9: 445–451.

74. Efron B, Tibshirani RJ. *An Introduction to the Bootstrap.* New York: Chapman and Hall, 1993.

75. Bech P. *Quality of Life in the Psychiatric Patient.* London: Mosby-Wolfe, 1998.

76. Shoeb M, Weinstein H, Mollica R. The Harvard trauma questionnaire: adapting a cross-cultural instrument for measuring torture, trauma and posttraumatic stress disorder in Iraqi refugees. *Int J Soc Psychiatry* 2007; 53: 447–463.

77. Ghareeb A. *Arabic Translation of the Beck Depression Inventory-II.* Cairo: Anglo Egyptian Bookshop, 2000.

78. Beck AT, Steer RA, Brown GK. *Beck Depression Inventory Manual. 2.* San Antonio, TX: Psychological Corporation, 1996.

79. Kroenke K, Spitzer RL, Williams JB. The PHQ-15: Validity of a new measure for evaluating the severity of somatic symptoms. *Psychosom Med* 2002; 64: 258–266.

CHAPTER 34

Lifestyle

Dexing Zhang and Samuel Y. S. Wong

Introduction

The World Health Organization (WHO) has reported that differences in four lifestyle factors—smoking, physical activity, alcohol intake, and diet—can make a major difference in health status [1]. From a health service utilization perspective, the adoption of a healthy lifestyle can be a cost-effective way to reduce the health service burden from both physical and mental health conditions.

Lifestyle

Lifestyle refers to the way of life of an individual, group, or culture. It denotes the set of habits and customs that is influenced by socialization. A healthy lifestyle not only can 'add years to life' by reducing premature mortality and improving life expectancy, but also 'add life to years'—by improving quality of life. Lifestyle activities usually include diet, level of physical activity, substance use, and social and personal interactions, and this chapter focuses on these four lifestyle factors.

Physical activity

Physical activity is movement of the body produced by skeletal muscles requiring energy expenditure more than resting, for example walking, running, dancing, swimming, yoga, and gardening. Exercise is a subset of physical activity that is planned, structured, and repetitive bodily movement to maintain or improve physical fitness—such as stamina, mobility, and strength, which relate to the ability to perform physical activity. Sports are a type of physical activity that involves structured competitive situations governed by rules. It is well established that physical activity is good for mental and physical health, and it plays a role in both the prevention and treatment of health problems and improves overall quality of life, making one more resilient to illness [2]. On the other hand, physical inactivity led to 3.2 million deaths worldwide in 2004 [1]. A conservative estimate found that the healthcare cost due to physical inactivity in 2013 was $53.8 billion worldwide [3]. Physical inactivity was also attributed to 13.4 million disability-adjusted life years (DALYs) and $13.7 billion in productivity losses worldwide in 2013 [3]. However, the role of physical activity and physical inactivity lacks full acknowledgement in mental problems in either clinical or non-clinical populations.

Benefits of physical activity on mental health

Current evidence suggests beneficial effects of exercises on psychological well-being with small-to-moderate effects, for example reducing anxiety and depression and improving mood, affect, sleep, cognition, personality, self-perceptions, and self-esteem [2, 4], although more studies are warranted to make definitive conclusions on its effects with respect to the type, frequency, and intensity of physical activity, and its effects on different populations and conditions [5]. As a rule of thumb, to keep one healthy, a 30-minute daily routine of moderate-intensity physical activity is recommended [2]. Results from a systematic review by Stonerock et al. [6] suggest that for anxiety, aerobic and non-aerobic exercise may be comparable to treatments such as medication or cognitive–behavioural therapy. It is also better than placebo or waitlist control with a small-to-medium effect size although more randomized controlled trials (RCTs) with better methodologies are needed to make definitive conclusions on its effectiveness [6]. Wang et al. [7] found that Qigong is effective in reducing stress and anxiety in healthy adults compared with lecture attendance and structured movements or waitlist control. Exercise training also improves anxiety among patients with a chronic illness and programmes that are less than 12 weeks in duration and lasting for at least 30 minutes in each session seem to show the largest improvements [8]. Exercise is also recommended for patients with cancer during treatment and recovery, to reduce side effects and improve quality of life [9]. However, its effects on psychological outcomes in people with type 2 diabetes are inconclusive, which might be owing to the limited number of studies in this area [10].

People who are physically active have lower levels of depression, as shown in epidemiological studies [11]. Aerobic and non-aerobic exercises can prevent depression [12], and both aerobic and non-aerobic exercises are suggested to be used together with medication for the treatment of major depression [13]. In general, among different exercise types, frequencies, and intensities, supervised aerobic exercise undertaken three times weekly at moderate intensity for a minimum of 9 weeks is recommended in the treatment of depression, although efforts are needed to look into the long-term effects [12, 14]. For older people with clinical symptoms of depression, structured exercise tailored to individual ability can reduce the severity of depression [15]. A systematic review and meta-analysis was conducted to evaluate the effects of exercise on clinically relevant depressive symptoms among elderly [15]. Seven RCTs of exercise for depression were meta-analysed. The exercise type included in this meta-analysis included a mixture of endurance and strength training, and the exercise intervention lasted for 3–4 months, with each session lasting 30–45 minutes, 3–5 times a week. The authors found lower depression severity among participants randomized to the exercise group versus those in the control group, and concluded that mixed exercise (strength and endurance training) had a small but clinically important effect on depressive symptoms. Exercise can also benefit women during menstruation, pregnancy, and menopause [2]. Aerobic and non-aerobic exercises appear to be effective in preventing and treating antenatal depression [16]. However, owing to the heterogeneity of the studies, the beneficial effects of exercise on postnatal depression are uncertain [17]. This is worth further exploration as women are often reluctant to take antidepressants postpartum or approach psychological therapies.

How physical activity works: possible mechanisms

The mechanisms responsible for the effects of physical activity on psychological well-being are still not quite clear. Physical activity might shape how we think, feel, and behave through the mind–body relationship. Potential clinical, psychological, or biological moderators have been suggested [18], which include an increase in core body temperature and endorphins, less tension in muscles, effects on serotonergic systems and neurotransmitters, improved sleep, feeling better, or having a sense of control, which result in improved self-esteem [2].

Sedentary behaviour

Too much sitting is not good for mental health. To define 'sedentary behaviour', one must be expending very little energy (≤ 1.5 metabolic equivalents), sitting or lying down, and be awake [19]. Tudor-Locke and Bassett Jr [20] suggested that, for healthy adults, < 5000 steps/day may be used as a 'sedentary lifestyle index'; 5000–7499 steps/day is typical of daily activity excluding sports/exercise, and might be considered 'low active'; 7500–9999 likely includes some volitional activities (and/or elevated occupational activity demands) and might be considered 'somewhat active'; and $\geq 10\,000$ steps/day indicates the point that should be used to classify individuals as 'active' [20]. For children who are considered to be more active, or elderly who are less active, the index might need to be adjusted to be higher or lower.[20] Common sedentary behaviours include sitting or lying at the time of TV viewing, video game-playing, computer use (collectively termed 'screen time'), driving, reading, studying, writing, or working at a desk. Nowadays, modern people are likely to be much less active than people of previous generations. While physically active people have lower depression levels, sedentary behaviour increases the risk of depression [21]. The review by Zhai et al. [22] confirmed the association between sedentary behaviour and the risk of depression, for example the pooled relative risks (RRs) of depression for sedentary behaviour were 1.31 (95% confidence interval (CI) 1.16–1.48) in cross-sectional studies and 1.14 (95% CI 1.06–1.21) in longitudinal studies. The pooled RRs of depression were 1.13 (95% CI 1.06–1.21) for long-time TV viewing and 1.22 (95% CI 1.10–1.34) for prolonged computer or Internet use [22]. Another review by Teychenne et al. [23] on sedentary behaviour and risk of anxiety suggests the association may also exist, although a definitive conclusion cannot be made owing to a lack of studies.

Sedentary behaviour affects individuals across the whole life span. Some preliminary findings on early childhood (from birth to 5 years of age) physical activity and sedentary behaviour suggest a dose–response relationship in indicating that physical activity is positively, and sedentary behaviour inversely, associated with psychosocial well-being [24]. In school-aged children and adolescents, greater screen time is associated with more hyperactivity/inattention problems and internalizing problems, as well as lower psychological well-being, perceived quality of life, and lower self-esteem [25]. Among older adults, the relationship between sedentary behaviour and mental health is not confirmed [26], but greater sedentary time is related to an increased risk of all-cause mortality, as well as metabolic syndrome, larger waist circumference, and overweight/obesity, which may be indirectly related to poor mental well-being [26].

In our modern world, sitting in an office for long hours has become common practice for many working people. There is a need to examine the combined effects of physical activity and sedentary behaviours on health and to explore whether physical activity can offset the negative impacts of sedentary behaviours on health. The systematic review by Biswas et al. in 2015 [27] concluded that prolonged sedentary time was independently associated with deleterious health outcomes, including all-cause mortality, cancer cardiovascular disease, and diabetes. Sedentary time was associated with a 30% lower relative risk for all-cause mortality among those with high levels of physical activity (pooled hazard ratio (HR) 1.16, 95% CI 0.84–1.59) aversus those with low levels of physical activity (pooled HR 1.46, 95% CI 1.22–1.75) [27]. The Lancet has published two series on physical activity in 2012 and 2016, respectively. One of the papers looked into more than one million people from 16 studies on physical activity and sedentary behaviour with a follow-up period of 2–18 years. It found that those who sat for more than 8 hours a day but had active physical activity above 35.5 metabolic equivalent of task-hours (MET-h) per week did not have higher risk of mortality than those who sat for less than 4 hours per day and with higher physical activity [28]. One MET equals to the rate of energy produced per unit surface area of an average person seated at rest and 30 MET-h per week is about 50–65 min of moderate intensity activity per day, for example walking at 5.6 km/h or cycling for pleasure at 16 km/h each day [28]. However, with respect to mental health outcomes, there is a lack of data to show whether exercise can compensate for the adverse effects of prolonged sedentary behaviour and more studies are needed in this area.

Risks of physical activity

Sudden cardiac death and musculoskeletal injury are the most common adverse outcomes associated with exercise. However, it appears that benefits may outweigh the potential risks [2]. A few people may also become dependent on exercise, but the prevalence rate is likely to be very low [29], with a 0.3–0.5% prevalence rate found in an adult general population survey conducted in Hungary [30].

How to get people more physically active

Public health initiatives to increase physical activity have great potential in improving health and well-being at a population level. These initiatives need multi-sectoral and multidisciplinary efforts taking into account the individual, familial, environmental, cultural, and social factors among different populations. For example, the motivations of participating in physical activities are different across different age and gender groups. In general, children are more likely to be motivated to participate in physical activity for fun and enjoyment, for learning and improving skills, for spending time with friends, and achieving the feelings of success and winning, whereas older youth may also engage in physical activity for weight control and improving body appearance. Adults are more likely to be motivated for potential health benefits, as well as for relaxation and enjoyment [2]. The individual key barriers are lack of time and for young people, issues of safety, and feelings of incompetence [2]. To implement useful physical activity programmes on a large scale, collective work is needed from people working in health, city planning, transport, education, culture, leisure, and environmental sustainability, based on the best evidence from both evidence-to-practice and practice-to-evidence perspectives [31]. The RE-AIM framework (Reach, Effectiveness, Adoption, Implementation, Maintenance) can be a useful reference framework for designing and promoting potential interventions on physical activity [31].

Diet

Healthy diet is eating diverse and balanced foods that give a person the needed nutrients to maintain health and have energy according to different conditions throughout the lifespan. It contains appropriate portions of oils, fruits, vegetables, grains, protein, and dairy, which protect against malnutrition and also prevent non-communicable diseases. From the guidance of the WHO [32] and the Office of Disease Prevention and Health Promotion of the US Department of Health and Human Services [33], in a healthy diet, added sugars should be limited to less than 10% of total energy intake, and a further reduction to less than 5% of total energy intake is advised for additional health benefits; sodium should be limited to 5 g per day; saturated fats should be limited—less than 10% of daily calories should come from saturated fats; processed food should also be avoided. An example of a healthy diet is the Mediterranean diet, which is high in unrefined cereals, fruits, vegetables, legumes, and olive oil. The diet also consists of moderate consumption of dairy, moderate-to-high consumption of fish, and low meat consumption. Breastfeeding has benefits in healthy growth and is also encouraged.

Dietary patterns, nutrition, and mental health

The relationship between dietary patterns and mental health has received attention only recently, although two systematic reviews of epidemiological studies have shown associations between healthy dietary patterns and reduced prevalence of, or risk for, depression [34, 35]. In another cohort study conducted in Japan, it was shown that healthy dietary patterns were associated with a reduced prevalence of suicide [36]. A more recent systematic review conducted in children and adolescents showed that unhealthy dietary patterns were associated with worse mental health in these two populations [37]. Although these studies suggest a relationship between dietary patterns and increased prevalence of depression, well-designed RCTs that evaluated the efficacy of dietary patterns and mental health outcomes were only conducted in recent years. Results from the PREDIMED study [38] suggested a reduced risk for incidence of depression among individuals randomized to a Mediterranean diet supplemented with nuts, with protective effects being more evident among people with type 2 diabetes mellitus. Another study [39], which employed dietary counselling as an indicated prevention intervention, showed that dietary counselling was similar in effectiveness to that of psychotherapy for the prevention of depression among older adults.

Besides dietary patterns, some researchers have studied the role of nutrients in their effects on mental health [40]. Supportive evidence suggests that a deficiency of omega-3 fatty acids, S-adenosyl-methionine, zinc, B vitamins (folic acid, B12, choline), iron, magnesium, amino acids (N-acetyl cysteine), and vitamin D may be associated with various mental health problems [41]. Epidemiological studies also suggest that the relationship between diet and depression may be independent of body mass index or other socio-economic factors [42]. However, the mechanisms of nutrients and their effects on mental health are not fully understood and gut microbiota and inflammatory pathways have been examined the most as potential mechanisms [42].

Nutrients and depression

Reviews indicate that good diet quality or a high intake of fruit, vegetables, fish, and whole grains may be associated with a reduced depression risk [34, 35, 43]. Omega-3 fatty acids may have benefits in patients with major depressive disorder [44, 45], although the results might have been biased [46]. It has been shown that blood zinc concentration levels [47] and vitamin D levels are both lower [48] among individuals with depression. Zinc supplementation may have benefits as a standalone or adjunct treatment to antidepressants for depression [49]. Lomagno et al. [50] found studies supporting zinc supplementation for pre-menopausal women with major depressive disorder, and mood was also improved after iron supplementation in pre-menopausal women [50]. The meta-analysis conducted by Gowda et al. [48] does not find significant reduction in depression after vitamin D supplementation but most of the studies were conducted among people with mild depression and people with normal levels of serum vitamin D at baseline. Spedding [51] found that among individuals with 25 hydroxyvitamin D deficiency at baseline, vitamin D supplementation (above 800 IU/day) had a statistically significant effect (effect size 0.78) in improving depressive symptoms [48]. There was no change in depression levels after the use of folate and vitamin B12 over the short term, but it may be helpful with prolonged intake over weeks to years to reduce depression relapse or prevent clinical symptoms among people at risk of depression [52].

Cognition/dementia

Diet has also been shown to be associated with cognition [53]. Moderate-to-high adherence to a Mediterranean diet was consistently associated with a reduced risk of cognitive impairment (RR 0.60, 95% CI 0.43–0.83) and the development of Alzheimer's disease [35, 54, 55]. Omega-3 fatty acids may help to prevent cognitive decline in the elderly with a decreased rate in the Mini-Mental State Examination (MMSE) score (weighted mean differences (0.15, 95% CI 0.05–0.25) [56], and improvement in attention and processing speed among people with cognitive impairment but without dementia (WMD 0.30, 95% CI 0.02–0.57) [57]. However, the effect may only be relevant in specific cognitive domains and only among people with cognitive impairment but without dementia and not in healthy people or people with Alzheimer's disease [57]. Evidence suggests that low serum vitamin B12 levels are associated with neurodegenerative disease and cognitive impairment [58], but current evidence does not support an effect of folic acid alone or in combination with B vitamins to stabilize or slow decline in cognition, function, behaviour, and global change in patients with mild cognitive impairment or Alzheimer's disease [59]. However, it has been shown that among people receiving a high-dose vitamin B12 supplement (1 mg daily), dementia in a small subset of people (those with pre-existing vitamin B12 deficiency) is reversible [58].

More studies are needed to study the relationship between vitamin B12 deficiency and neurodegenerative disease. Lower vitamin D concentration is also associated with cognitive impairment, but its preventative or treatment effect is yet unknown [60–62]. Zinc and iron supplementation might enhance cognitive functioning among pre-menopausal women; however, further studies are needed to identify the impact on cognition in different populations [50]. There have been mixed findings for the effects of antioxidant intake (vitamins C, vitamin E, flavonoids, carotenoids) on cognitive function or risk of dementia [63].

Neurodevelopmental disorders

Free fatty acid supplementation produces small but significant reductions in symptoms of attention deficit hyperactivity disorder (ADHD) [64, 65], although current evidence is not sufficient in supporting the safety or efficacy of omega-3 fatty acids for people with autism spectrum disorders (ASD) [66]. Vitamin D status (serum 25 hydroxyvitamin D level) in pregnancy or childhood is found to be related to ASD in cross-sectional studies; however, the mechanism is unclear and more preventative studies are needed to confirm this relationship [67]. The effects of mineral supplementation (zinc, magnesium, and iron) have not been confirmed in the treatment of ADHD in children [68].

Moving from findings into actions

Given the high prevalence of common mental disorders and their associated disease burden, slight improvements in mental health through dietary prevention or intervention can result in significant public health gains at the population level, for example by reducing depression and its burden [42]. Dietary prevention and intervention through public health campaigns can result in benefits in fighting against the global burden of both common mental disorders and non-communicable diseases. It is found that one's dietary habits can be influenced early *in utero* by the dietary intake habits of mothers [69]. Targeted interventions on pregnant women are preferred [42, 70]. Pregnancy provides a unique opportunity to advocate for healthy diets with regard to the benefits on offspring as mothers are usually open to health advice and may be more willing to make dietary changes to improve the mental health of their children. Furthermore, early life and adolescence are also regarded as important periods for dietary intervention. However, barriers exist in implementing dietary interventions, especially in deprived countries, for example affordability and access to healthy foods, especially for those living in highly disadvantaged conditions. Furthermore, there is still a great need for evidence-based information to inform the appropriate dosage and the cost-effectiveness of dietary interventions in order to inform policy that can result in changes at population levels.

Substance use

Alcohol use

Alcohol consumption contributes to 3.3 million deaths every year, representing 5.9% of all deaths worldwide [71]. Besides adverse physiological effects such as cancer, liver diseases, and fetal alcohol spectrum disorders, alcohol consumption leads to various mental and psychosocial problems. The mental health effects include alcohol dependence, depression, anxiety, psychosis, cognitive impairment, and increased risk of suicide. The subsequent psychosocial problems are increased risk of driving while drunk, accidents and injuries, violence, decreased work or academic performance, unemployment, and financial, legal, and relationship problems [71–74].

Although there are recommended drinking limits, such as not to exceed two standard drinks per day for healthy adults [75], the WHO has never recommended 'safe' drinking limits. To minimize alcohol-related problems, it is important that healthcare professionals inform patients and the public that alcohol is addictive and also classified by the International Agency for Research on Cancer of the WHO as a Group 1 carcinogen—the same as tobacco smoking, asbestos, and ionizing radiation [76]. In general, the more alcohol one drinks, the higher the chance one will have of alcohol-related problems and there is no 'safe' limit for alcohol consumption.

Alcohol is a causal factor in depression. In some European countries, up to 10% of male depression can be attributed to the drinking of alcohol. Policies that reduce the use of alcohol are likely to be effective in reducing the prevalence of mental disorders [77]. For current drinkers, stopping or reducing drinking can help reduce the risk of getting cancer and many other non-communicable diseases, as well as injuries. As a result, there is a role of healthcare professionals in informing patients of the health risks associated with alcohol drinking and provide advice for reducing or stopping the drinking of alcohol.

Tobacco use

The global health burden of cigarette smoking is large with smoking-related deaths estimated at about 6 million annually [78]. In 2015, over 1.1 billion people smoked tobacco [79]. Tobacco use is notably one of the leading modifiable risk factors related to leading causes of death, such as cardiac disease, cancer, and stroke. Furthermore, premature deaths due to second-hand smoking totalled more than 600,000 in 2004 and most of them occurred in children (28%) and women (47%) as a result of lower respiratory infections, asthma, lung cancer, and ischaemic heart disease, resulting in a significant loss of DALYs—10.9 million annually [80]. Besides harms to physical health, individuals who smoke cigarettes have a higher risk of mental health problems, such as depression, anxiety, and psychosis, than those who do not smoke.

Tobacco control and smoking cessation

Nicotine is the major constituent out of the more than 4000 chemicals in cigarettes and results in smokers becoming addicted to tobacco. It interacts with high-affinity nicotinic acetylcholine receptors and causes the release of dopamine and other neurotransmitters. First-line pharmacotherapy includes nicotine replacement therapy, varenicline, bupropion, and nortriptyline. Other pharmacotherapy options include cytosine [81]. Anti-nicotine vaccines are in development. The vaccines can induce antibodies to bind nicotine in the blood and prevent nicotine from crossing the blood–brain barrier. However, one of the concerns is that it may result in heavier smoking as one may compensate for reduced nicotine levels by getting more nicotine when less of it can travel to the brain [82]. As a result, more studies are needed to examine the effectiveness of the vaccine. Besides pharmacotherapy, supportive care also plays a role in helping smoking cessation through brief advice, individual or group counselling, and self-help materials [81]. There is also a trend to test the benefits of food supplements in smoking cessation.

Examples of these supplements include S-adenosyl-L-methionine, l-acetylcarnitine, N-acetyl-cysteine, and dehydroepiandrosterone, but it may take some time to get conclusive results [82]. E-cigarettes are now also used to deliver nicotine by inhalation; however, regulations are yet to be developed and more evidence is needed on their safety and effectiveness. E-cigarettes may potentially contribute to non-carcinogenic health risks with chemicals such as nicotine, propylene glycol, cadmium, ethylene glycol, nickel, aluminum, and titanium, although some smokers use e-cigarettes to help them stop smoking [83]. Relapse after smoking cessation is common owing to withdrawal symptoms, stress, and weight gain. Withdrawal symptoms during cigarette abstinence often occur as a result of the lack of nicotine occupying the nicotinic acetylcholine receptors, which results in cravings for nicotine to alleviate negative feelings such as depressed mood, insomnia, irritability, headache, sweating, concentration problems, intestinal disorders (cramps, nausea), and tingling in the hands and feet. These withdrawal symptoms usually peak within 2–3 days and go away by two weeks, with some lasting for several months. Most smokers make several attempts to quit before finally achieving successful abstinence [81].

Barriers to smoking cessation exist in both smokers and healthcare professionals. Smokers are usually hesitant to quit smoking owing to a lack of knowledge about the benefits of quitting, high dependence and enjoyment of smoking, psychological or emotional concerns (e.g. stress, depression), fear of weight gain, peer pressure, and living circumstances such as living with other smokers or smoking among their friends and peers. Healthcare professionals may lack the time and skills to help with smoking cessation, and may not offer advice owing to low perceived motivation among patients. However, effective help to stop smoking only takes a few minutes and a substantial abstinence rate of 12–25% can be achieved over 6–12 months [84–86]. The 5As approach (ask, assess, advise, assist, and arrange follow-up) can be used as a structure to provide smoking cessation counselling by healthcare professionals [81].

Besides addressing barriers from individuals and professionals, interventions at the system level can be used to reduce cigarette smoking. At the population level, the WHO has proposed 'MPOWER'—six tobacco control strategies based on evidence from the WHO Framework Convention on Tobacco Control to tackle the tobacco epidemic [87]: Monitor tobacco use and prevention policies (monitoring), Protect people from tobacco smoke (smoke-free environments), Offer help to quit tobacco use (cessation programmes), Warn people about the dangers of tobacco (warning labels), Enforce bans on tobacco advertising, promotion, and sponsorship (mass media, advertising bans), and Raise taxes on tobacco (taxation). National tobacco control programmes are critical to control tobacco use. It is important to build a national capacity to carry out effective and sustainable anti-tobacco policies and programmes with proper monitoring. Governments should establish systems to monitor the use of tobacco and the impact of policies after the implementation. Increasing tobacco taxation to increase tobacco price is the most effective way to reduce tobacco use and encourage people to quit smoking. Warning labels can increase smokers' awareness of health risks and their likelihood of cessation and reducing smoking levels. Policies of mandatory health warning labels on cigarette packages are effective in reducing tobacco use and these policies can be easily implemented at little cost by many countries by increasing the size of warning signs and including pictures rather than text-only warnings. These policies are usually highly supported by the public. Both adults and young people can be more likely to quit smoking or less likely to start smoking after exposure to anti-tobacco mass media campaigns.

Mental health status after cessation

Studies suggest that after smoking cessation, mental health status often improves. Taylor et al. [88] found that when compared with current smokers, people who quit smoking had lower anxiety, depression, mixed depression, and anxiety and stress. Cessation of smoking also leads to better mental health related quality of life and positive affect. These improvements appear in both general population and among those with physical or psychiatric disorders [88].

Smoking among individuals with psychiatric conditions

A less well researched area with respect to cigarette smoking and mental health is mortality attributed to tobacco use among people with psychiatric conditions. Individuals suffering from mental health disorders such as schizophrenia, ADHD, anxiety, and depression are more likely to smoke cigarettes than the general population. For example, people with schizophrenia are five times more likely to smoke and they tend to smoke more heavily. Adolescents and adults with ADHD also have about twice as high a cigarette smoking rate as those without ADHD. A relationship is found between the number of ADHD symptoms and the risk of cigarette smoking, with evidence suggesting more ADHD symptoms are related to earlier onset of cigarette smoking [89]. Cigarette smoking is an important factor that contributes to the shorter life expectancy of people with mental illness [90]. Using the US Patient Discharge Database inpatient data, Callaghan et al. [91] found tobacco-related conditions comprised approximately 53% (n = 23,620/44,469) of total deaths among people with schizophrenia, 48% (n = 6004/12,564) among people with bipolar disorder, and 50% (n = 35,729/71,058) among people with depression [91].

Individuals with psychiatric disorders and cigarette smoking may also face more difficulties in quitting smoking [82, 92]. These individuals are also often excluded from RCTs that evaluate the effectiveness of interventions for smoking cessation, owing to concerns around the potential exacerbation of psychiatric symptoms or difficulty in motivating these populations to quit smoking and getting them to adhere to cessation. Abstinence from tobacco typically does not worsen psychiatric symptoms. Indeed, evidence suggests it may improve psychiatric symptoms [92]. Healthcare professionals are encouraged to promote smoking cessation and provide support to smokers with psychiatric problems and monitor the psychiatric status of smokers during the quitting process.

Social networks

Effects of social ties: the positive and the negative

The relationship between social relationships such as social ties, social networks, and mental health have long been studied by sociologists, and it has been generally agreed by scholars in the field that social ties and social networks are associated with improved mental health and psychological well-being [93, 94]. To better explain the mechanisms responsible for the observed relationships, two models—main effects and stress-buffering—have been proposed by Cohen and Wills [95]. The main effect model proposes that social relationships exert beneficial effects directly on psychological outcomes. These include the adoption of normative health promoting behaviours through social influence such as physical activity, which, in turn, enhances mental health [96]. Participation in a social network also gives meaning and a sense of belonging and security to members within the same social network, which may enhance self-worth and increase motivation for self-care and modulate the neuroendocrine response to stress [97]. Being a member of a social network also increases the chance of having social support when needed, with increased access to health promoting information and informal care. However,, the stress-buffering model proposes that social support is important during the time of stress as it modulates one's response to life stressful events, including a re-appraisal of stressful events [98], and reduced emotional and physiological reactions to said events [99].

Although research has demonstrated the beneficial effects of social support on mental health, not all social support is related to improved mental health. Research has shown that gender and socio-economic position also determines whether social support is related to improved or worsened mental health. For example, Belle [100] noticed that women tended to maintain more intimate social ties than men, which may increase their stress levels when stressful life events occur among people with whom they are closely connected. It has also been suggested that women with lower socio-economic standing may suffer from participation in social networks as they often face difficulty in responding to the needs of other members in the network, and those who need support the most often do not receive the support they need but need to bear the costs of network involvement [101].

Online social networking and mental health

Online social networking happens via social media. Social media, as defined by the Oxford Dictionary, is websites and applications that enable users to view, create, and share content, or to participate in social networking. Billions of people now actively use social media, including Facebook, Twitter, MySpace, WhatsApp, WeChat, LinkedIn, and Google+, in daily life. People interact with each other via social media one to-one, one-to-many, and many-to-many all over the world. Online social networking is relatively new, and many questions related to its impacts on mental well-being are yet to be answered. As the users of social media are increasing, especially in developing countries, any psychological impact found in social media use may have significant public health implications.

By far, research results have indicated mixed impacts of social media use on mental health. People can selectively present themselves on social networking sites. Presenting oneself on social media and getting the true self acknowledged and validated by others is associated with better psychological health [102]. Social media use can broaden one's social networks, especially for shy and socially anxious people. People can also learn and get information from social media. Online support groups provide opportunities for those who are geographically unable to meet with each other to have real-time communication, for example for those with cancers, chronic illness, or those who are part of minority groups. However, use of social media such as Facebook might lead to lower life satisfaction. As there is a tendency for people to only post positive aspects of life on Facebook, users may have the notion that 'they are happier and having better lives than I am' through negative social comparison [103]. In a systematic review by Best et al. [104], the use of social media can either be beneficial or harmful, and most studies reported either mixed or no effects. The reported benefits among adolescents of online communication were increased self-esteem, perceived social support, increased social capital, safe identity experimentation, and increased opportunity for self-disclosure; the harmful effects were reported as increased exposure to harm, social isolation, depression, and cyberbullying [104]. A systematic review by Baker and Algorta in 2016 [105] found that among 11 studies, five showed a positive correlation between online social networking engagement and depression, whereas two studies showed a negative correlation and four studies showed no correlation. Preliminary findings suggested that frequent use of a professional social networking website might be related to increased depression and anxiety. Jones et al. [106] found that among the 1780 young American adults between the age of 19 and 32 years, those who used LinkedIn at least once per week had significantly greater depression and anxiety after adjustment for age, sex, race, relationship status, living situation, household income, education level, and overall social media use compared with those who used the site less than once a week. Moreover, they also found a dose–response relationship between the frequency of LinkedIn use and depression/anxiety [106]. The mixed results suggest that there are many underlying factors that modify or moderate the effects of online social networking on mental health, for example psychological, social, behavioural, and individual factors [105].

An important understudied issue related to online social networking is cyberbullying. People can be victims of cyberbullying, be bullies themselves, or both [107]. Cyberbullying is defined as 'bullying through e-mail, instant messaging, in a chat room, on a website, on an online gaming site, or through digital messages or images '. Unlike traditional bullying that one can be safe after obtaining protection in a physically safe environment, cyberbullying can be hard to eliminate. Cyberbullying can also reach wider audiences in one's social circle than traditional bullying. The mean rate of cyberbullying victimization was 15.5% and the mean rate of cyberbullying perpetration was 16%, based on 80 studies in a systematic review by Modecki et al. [108]. Additionally, one in five children is involved in cyberbullying [109]. Zych et al. [109] conducted a systematic review on bullying and cyberbullying, and showed that both cyberbullying perpetration and victimization can lead to adverse effects such as depression, anxiety, loneliness, lower life satisfaction, and drug and alcohol use problems. Furthermore, suicidal ideation and lower self-esteem can be also associated with cyberbullying victimization [109].

Other lifestyle factors

Many other lifestyle behaviours also have close relationships with mental well-being. Examples of these factors include sleeping habits, engaging with nature, enjoyment of leisure activities, pet ownership, mindfulness practice, religion and spirituality, and contribution and services to others.

Sleep

Sleep health can be defined as 'a multidimensional pattern of sleep-wakefulness, adapted to individual, social, and environmental demands, that promotes physical and mental well-being. Good sleep health is characterized by subjective satisfaction, appropriate timing, adequate duration, high efficiency, and sustained alertness during waking hours' [110]. Insomnia occurs in 6–18% of the general population [111]. More women have insomnia than men, and insomnia symptoms increase with age, although sleep dissatisfaction varies little with age [111]. However, concern has recently arisen with regard to sleep deprivation in adolescents, especially those in Asia [112–114]. Results from surveys revealed that 53% of adolescents' average school-night total sleep time was insufficient (i.e. < 8 hours) [114]. Chronic insomnia is associated with increased risk of physical and mental health problems such as obesity, diabetes, hypertension and heart disease, increased inflammation, poorer cognitive functions, and increased depression, anxiety, and mental distress, as well as all-cause mortality [115]. Insomnia is often a consequence of poor sleep habits, physical condition(s), or psychiatric condition(s). Primary insomnia is insomnia without clear environmental, physical, or psychiatric causes, and is probably due to differences in brain function. Resolving external factors or underlying health problems can relieve insomnia symptoms. If these factors or problems cannot be resolved, cognitive–behavioural therapy and hypnotics can be used as treatment [116].

Nature and leisure activities

Immersing ourselves in natural settings such as the open countryside, fields, remote wilderness, parks, urban green spaces, allotments, and gardens can be beneficial to physical and mental health [117]. Accumulating evidence suggests that the benefits of being in contact with nature include an improvement in self-esteem, attention, cognitive restoration, immunity, and the promotion of physical activity and social contact [118]. Outdoor physical activity also yields better outcomes than doing indoor physical activities [119]. From a public health perspective, including green space in urban areas may have beneficial effects on both the ecosystem and the population's mental well-being, which can result in savings to economy [117, 120].

Participating in enjoyable leisure activities is an important aspect of a healthy lifestyle. Leisure activities may potentially contribute to the prevention of dementia [121]. Older adults who have participated in social and leisure activities are shown to report better physical and mental well-being [122], which may be mediated, in part, by satisfaction with leisure activities [123]. Experimental studies suggest that leisure activity intervention can enhance subjective well-being [123].

Pet ownership

Companion animals may benefit the emotional, social, and cognitive development of children [124]. Early experiences of dog ownership in childhood has been shown to be related to better companionship, social support, and sense of a life worth living in later life [125]. Although there is not enough convincing evidence to suggest companion pet ownership can alleviate loneliness, animal-assisted therapies have been shown to improve loneliness among the elderly [126]. However, based on 11 cross-sectional studies, Islam and Towell [127] did not find a clear association between pet ownership and well-being, although a few of the studies reported that having a cat or dog was related to increased physical activity, overall fitness, or better psychological well-being. It is hard to know if it is pet possession per se or owner characteristics that is responsible for the association observed between pet ownership and positive mental health outcomes, and it would be difficult

to conduct a RCT to examine any potential causal relationship. However, the loss of a pet may induce grief that is similar to the loss of a close friend and may need corresponding management [128].

Religion and spirituality

Spirituality is a broader concept than that of religion. Spirituality generally refers to an individual sense of connectedness to a valued and greater 'whole', such as the universe, together with a sense of belonging and acceptance. Spirituality can be expressed through art, poetry, and myth, as well as religious practice. Religion refers to socially based beliefs and traditions, often associated with ritual and ceremony [129, 130]. Searching for meaning and purpose in life is emphasized in both religion and spirituality. Researchers proposed bio-psychosocial–spiritual models of health to discover the role of religion and spirituality in human well-being [131]. Positive associations have been found between religious and spiritual beliefs and mental and physical well-being [130–132]. Religion may lead to higher levels of compassion, creativity, equanimity, honesty, hope, joy, patience, and perseverance, which can promote good mental health [130]. It may also provide a coping strategy with which to deal with difficulties and adverse life events [130].

Mindfulness practice

Mindfulness is the awareness that arises by paying attention to the present moment, non-judgementally [133]. Mindfulness practices usually involve mindful breathing, walking meditation, sitting meditation, mindful eating, mindful movements and body scanning, focusing the attention on the experience of emotions, thoughts, body sensations, and sounds, and observing them as they arise and subside [133]. Mindfulness practice originates from Buddhism. However, over the last three decades, it has become popular as a secular practice among the general public as a way of improving physical and mental well-being. There are different programmes of mindfulness-based interventions. The mindfulness-based stress reduction programme [134] and mindfulness-based cognitive therapy [135] are the two programmes that are most widely recognized and researched for use in various physical and mental conditions, and research has supported their use especially with regard to their effects on reducing the recurrence of depression [136]. The mechanisms of mindfulness-based practices for improving both physical and mental well-being are not fully understood. Potential mechanisms include changes in mindfulness, a decrease in rumination and worry, and an increase in compassion and self-acceptance, or the cultivation of meta-awareness. Other proposed mechanisms include changes in attention or emotional reactivity [137].

Contribution and services to others

Knight et al. [138] reviewed 13 studies on the giving in non-familial intergenerational interactions, in which there were reciprocal giving of time, skill, knowledge, or self by each generation to the other. They found psychosocial benefits in increased positive attitude and reduced stereotypic thinking towards others, broader views of self, increased social connectedness, reduced depression, and hope for the future [138]. Altruistic volunteering is associated with reduced symptoms of depression, better self-reported health, fewer functional limitations, and lower mortality [139]. The potential reasons might be that volunteering increases social, physical, and cognitive activity, which leads to improved functioning through biological and psychological mechanisms [139].

Lifestyle factors are important determinants of physical and mental well-being. More studies are needed to examine the mechanisms responsible for the relationships between lifestyle factors and mental health. The implementation of evidence-based interventions and policies that encourage and facilitate individuals in adopting health-promoting lifestyles is an effective way to improve public mental health.

References

1. World Health Organization (WHO). *Global Health Risks: Mortality and Burden of Disease Attributable to Selected Major Risks*. Geneva: WHO, 2009.
2. Biddle SJ, Mutrie N. *Psychology of Physical Activity: Determinants, Well-being and Interventions*. New York: Routledge, 2007.
3. Ding D, Lawson KD, Kolbe-Alexander TL, et al. The economic burden of physical inactivity: a global analysis of major non-communicable diseases. *Lancet* 2016; 388: 1311–1324.
4. Sarris S, Moylan S, Camfield DA, et al. Complementary medicine, exercise, meditation, diet, and lifestyle modification for anxiety disorders: a review of current evidence. *Evid Based Compl Alt* 2012; 2012: 809653.
5. Wegner M, Helmich I, Machado S, Nardi AE, Arias-Carrion O, Budde H. Effects of exercise on anxiety and depression disorders: review of meta-analyses and neurobiological mechanisms. *CNS Neurol Disord Drug Targets* 2014; 13: 1002–1014.
6. Stonerock GL, Hoffman BM, Smith PJ, Blumenthal JA. Exercise as treatment for anxiety: systematic review and analysis. *Ann Behav Med* 2015; 49: 542–556.
7. Wang CW, Chan CHY, Ho RTH, Chan JSM, Ng SM, Chan CLW. Managing stress and anxiety through qigong exercise in healthy adults: a systematic review and meta-analysis of randomized controlled trials. *BMC Complem Altern Med* 2014; 14: 8.
8. Herring MP, O'Connor PJ, Dishman RK. The effect of exercise training on anxiety symptoms among patients a systematic review. *Arch Intern Med* 2010; 170: 321–331.
9. Mustian KM, Sprod LK, Janelsins M, Peppone LJ, Mohile S. Exercise recommendations for cancer-related fatigue, cognitive impairment, sleep problems, depression, pain, anxiety, and physical dysfunction: a review. *Oncol Hematol Rev* 2012; 8: 81–88.
10. van der Heijden MMP, van Dooren FEP, Pop VJM, Pouwer F. Effects of exercise training on quality of life, symptoms of depression, symptoms of anxiety and emotional well-being in type 2 diabetes mellitus: a systematic review. *Diabetologia* 2013; 56: 1210–1225.
11. Teychenne M, Ball K, Salmon J. Physical activity and likelihood of depression in adults: a review. *Prev Med* 2008; 46: 397–411.
12. Stanton R, Reaburn P. Exercise and the treatment of depression: a review of the exercise program variables. *J Sci Med Sport* 2014; 17: 177–182.
13. Danielsson L, Noras AM, Waern M, Carlsson J. Exercise in the treatment of major depression: a systematic review grading the quality of evidence. *Physiother Theory Pract* 2013; 29: 573–585.
14. Perraton LG, Kumar S, Machotka Z. Exercise parameters in the treatment of clinical depression: a systematic review of randomized controlled trials. *J Eval Clin Pract* 2010; 16: 597–604.
15. Bridle C, Spanjers K, Patel S, Atherton NM, Lamb SE. Effect of exercise on depression severity in older people systematic review and meta-analysis of randomised controlled trials. *Br J Psychiatry* 2012; 201: 180–185.
16. Daley AJ, Foster L, Long G, et al. The effectiveness of exercise for the prevention and treatment of antenatal depression: systematic review with meta-analysis. *BJOG* 2015; 122: 57–62.
17. Daley A, Jolly K, MacArthur C. The effectiveness of exercise in the management of post-natal depression: systematic review and meta-analysis. *Fam Pract* 2009; 26: 154–162.
18. Schuch FB, Dunn AL, Kanitz AC, Delevatti RS, Fleck MP. Moderators of response in exercise treatment for depression: a systematic review. *J Affect Disorders* 2016; 195: 40–49.
19. Cart L. Letter to the editor: standardized use of the terms 'sedentary' and 'sedentary behaviours'. *Appl Physiol Nutr Metab* 2012; 37: 540.
20. Tudor-Locke C, Bassett Jr DR. How many steps/day are enough? *Sports Med* 2004; 34: 1–8.
21. Teychenne M, Ball K, Salmon J. Sedentary behavior and depression among adults: a review. *Int J Behav Med* 2010; 17: 246–254.
22. Zhai L, Zhang Y, Zhang D. Sedentary behaviour and the risk of depression: a meta-analysis. *Br J Sports Med* 2015; 49: 705–709.
23. Teychenne M, Costigan SA, Parker K. The association between sedentary behaviour and risk of anxiety: a systematic review. *BMC Public Health* 2015; 15(513).
24. Hinkley T, Teychenne M, Downing KL, Ball K, Salmon J, Hesketh KD. Early childhood physical activity, sedentary behaviors and psychosocial well-being: A systematic review: *Prev Med* 2014; 62: 189–192.
25. Suchert V, Hanewinkel R, Isensee B. Sedentary behavior and indicators of mental health in school-aged children and adolescents: a systematic review. *Prev Med* 2015; 76: 48–57.
26. Rezende LFMd, Rey-Lopez JP, Matsudo VKR, Luiz OdC. Sedentary behavior and health outcomes among older adults: a systematic review. *BMC Public Health* 2014; 14(333).
27. Biswas A, Oh PI, Faulkner GE, et al. Sedentary time and its association with risk for disease incidence, mortality, and hospitalization in adults a systematic review and meta-analysis. *Ann Intern Med* 2015; 162: 123–132.
28. Ekelund U, Steene-Johannessen J, Brown WJ, et al. Does physical activity attenuate, or even eliminate, the detrimental association of sitting time with mortality? A harmonised meta-analysis of data from more than 1 million men and women. *Lancet* 2016; 388: 1302–1310.
29. Landolfi E. Exercise addiction. *Sports Med* 2013; 43: 111–119.
30. Mónok K, Berczik K, Urbán R, et al. Psychometric properties and concurrent validity of two exercise addiction measures: A population wide study. *Psychol Sport Exerc* 2012; 13: 739–746.
31. Reis RS, Salvo D, Ogilvie D, Lambert EV, Goenka S, Brownson RC. Scaling up physical activity interventions worldwide: stepping up to larger and smarter approaches to get people moving. *Lancet* 2016; 388: 1337–1348.
32. World Health Organization. Healthy diet fact sheets. Available at: http://www.who.int/mediacentre/factsheets/fs394/en/ (2015, accessed 1 September).
33. U.S. Department of Health and Human Services and U.S. Department of Agriculture. Dietary Guidelines for Americans 2015–2020. 8th Edition. Available at: http://health.gov/dietaryguidelines/2015/guidelines/ (accessed December 2015).
34. Lai JS, Hiles S, Bisquera A, Hure AJ, McEvoy M, Attia J. A systematic review and meta-analysis of dietary patterns and depression in community-dwelling adults. *Am J Clin Nutr* 2014; 99: 181–197.
35. Psaltopoulou T, Sergentanis TN, Panagiotakos DB, Sergentanis IN, Kosti R, Scarmeas N. Mediterranean diet, stroke, cognitive impairment, and depression: a meta-analysis. *Ann Neurol* 2013; 74: 580–591.
36. Nanri A, Mizoue T, Poudel-Tandukar K, et al. Dietary patterns and suicide in Japanese adults: the Japan Public Health Center-based Prospective Study. *Br J Psychiatry* 2013; 203: 422–427.
37. O'Neil A, Quirk SE, Housden S, et al. Relationship between diet and mental health in children and adolescents: a systematic review. *Am J Public Health* 2014; 104: E31–E42.
38. Sanchez-Villegas A, Martinez-Gonzalez MA, Estruch R, et al. Mediterranean dietary pattern and depression: the PREDIMED randomized trial. *BMC Med* 2013; 11: 208.
39. Stahl ST, Albert SM, Dew MA, Lockovich MH, Reynolds CF, 3rd. Coaching in healthy dietary practices in at-risk older adults: a case of indicated depression prevention. *Am J Psychiatry* 2014; 171: 499–505.
40. Sarris J, Logan AC, Akbaraly TN, et al. Nutritional medicine as mainstream in psychiatry. *Lancet Psychiatry* 2015; 2: 271–274.

41. Sarris J, Logan AC, Akbaraly TN, et al. International Society for Nutritional Psychiatry Research consensus position statement: nutritional medicine in modern psychiatry. *World Psychiatry* 2015; 14: 370–371.

42. Dash SR, O'Neil A, Jacka FN. Diet and common mental disorders: the imperative to translate evidence into action. *Front Public Health* 2016; 4.

43. Lai JS, Hiles S, Hure AJ, McEvoy M, Attia J. Systematic review and meta-analysis of dietary patterns and depression: Observational studies. *Ann Nutr Metab* 2013; 63: 428.

44. Grosso G, Pajak A, Marventano S, et al. Role of omega-3 fatty acids in the treatment of depressive disorders: a comprehensive meta-analysis of randomized clinical trials. *PLOS ONE* 2014; 9.

45. Bloch M, Hannestad J. Omega-3 fatty acids for the treatment of depression: Systematic review and meta-analysis. In: 49th Annual Conference of the American College of Neuropsychopharmacology, ACNP 2010. Miami Beach, FL, USA, 5–9 December 2010.

46. Appleton KM, Sallis HM, Perry R, Ness AR, Churchill R. omega - 3 fatty acids for major depressive disorder in adults: an abridged Cochrane review. *BMJ Open* 2016; 6.

47. Swardfager W, Herrmann N, Mazereeuw G, Goldberger K, Harimoto T, Lanctot KL. Zinc in depression: a meta-analysis. *Biol Psychiatry* 2013; 74: 872–878.

48. Gowda U, Mutowo MP, Smith BJ, Wluka AE, Renzaho AM. Vitamin D supplementation to reduce depression in adults: meta-analysis of randomized controlled trials. *Nutrition* 2015; 31: 421–429.

49. Lai J, Moxey A, Nowak G, Vashum K, Bailey K, McEvoy M. The efficacy of zinc supplementation in depression: systematic review of randomised controlled trials. *J Affect Disorders* 2012; 136: e31–e39.

50. Lomagno KA, Hu F, Riddell LJ, et al. Increasing iron and zinc in pre-menopausal women and its effects on mood and cognition: a systematic review. *Nutrients* 2014; 6: 5117–5141.

51. Spedding S. Vitamin D and depression: a systematic review and meta-analysis comparing studies with and without biological flaws. *Nutrients* 2014; 6: 1501–1518.

52. Almeida OP, Ford AH, Flicker L. Systematic review and meta-analysis of randomized placebo-controlled trials of folate and vitamin B12 for depression. *Int Psychogeriatr* 2015; 27: 727–737).

53. Kuczmarski MF, Allegro D, Stave E. The association of healthful diets and cognitive function: a review. *J Nutr Gerontol Geriatr* 2014; 33: 69–90.

54. Opie RS, Ralston RA, Walker KZ. Adherence to a Mediterranean-style diet can slow the rate of cognitive decline and decrease the risk of dementia: a systematic review. *Nutr Diet* 2013; 70: 206–217.

55. Petersson SD, Philippou E. Mediterranean diet, cognitive function, and dementia: a systematic review of the evidence. *Adv Nutr* 2016; 7: 889–904.

56. Zhang XW, Hou WS, Li M, Tang ZY. Omega-3 fatty acids and risk of cognitive decline in the elderly: a meta-analysis of randomized controlled trials. *Aging Clin Exp Res* 2016; 28: 165–166.

57. Mazereeuw G, Lanctot KL, Chau SA, Swardfager W, Herrmann N. Effects of omega-3 fatty acids on cognitive performance: a meta-analysis. *Neurobiol Aging* 2012; 33: e17–e29.

58. Moore E, Mander A, Ames D, Carne R, Sanders K, Watters D. Cognitive impairment and vitamin B12: a review. *Int Psychogeriatr* 2012; 24: 541–556.

59. Li MM, Yu JT, Wang HF, et al. Efficacy of vitamins B supplementation on mild cognitive impairment and Alzheimer's disease: A systematic review and meta-analysis. *Curr Alzheimer Res* 2014; 11: 844–852.

60. Balion CM, Griffith LE, Strifler L, et al. Vitamin D and cognition: a meta-analysis: In: 2011 Meeting of the Canadian Society of Clinical Chemists, Vancouver, BC, Canada, 4–8 June 2011.

61. Annweiler C, Milea D, Whitson HE, et al. Vitamin D insufficiency and cognitive impairment in Asians: a multi-ethnic population-based study and meta-analysis. *J Intern Med* 2016; 280: 300–311.

62. van der Schaft J, Koek HL, Dijkstra E, Verhaar HJJ, van der Schouw YT, Emmelot-Vonk MH. The association between vitamin D and cognition: a systematic review. *Ageing Res Rev* 2013; 12: 1013–1023.

63. Crichton GE, Bryan J, Murphy KJ. Dietary antioxidants, cognitive function and dementia—a systematic review. *Plant Foods Hum Nutr* 2013; 68: 279–292.

64. Sonuga-Barke EJS, Brandeis D, Cortese S, et al. Nonpharmalogical interventions for ADHD: systematic review and meta analyses of randomized controlled trials of dietary and psychological treatments. *Am J Psychiatry* 2013; 170: 275–289.

65. Bozzatello P, Brignolo E, De Grandi E, Bellino S. Supplementation with omega-3 fatty acids in psychiatric disorders: a review of literature data. *J Clin Med* 2016; 5(8).

66. Bent S, Bertoglio K, Hendren RL. Omega-3 fatty acids for autism spectrum disorder: a systematic review. *J Autism Dev Disord* 2009; 39: 1145–1154.

67. Mazahery H, Camargo CA, Conlon C, Beck KL, Kruger MC, von Hurst PR. Vitamin D and autism spectrum disorder: a literature review. *Nutrients* 2016; 8: 57.

68. Hariri M, Azadbakht L. Magnesium, iron, and zinc supplementation for the treatment of attention deficit hyperactivity disorder: a systematic review on the recent literature. *Int J Prev Med* 2015; 6: 83.

69. Savage JS, Fisher JO, Birch LL. Parental influence on eating behavior: conception to adolescence. *J Law Med Ethics* 2007; 35: 22–34.

70. O'Neil A, Itsiopoulos C, Skouteris H, et al. Preventing mental health problems in offspring by targeting dietary intake of pregnant women. *BMC Med* 2014; 12: 1.

71. World Health Organization (WHO). *Global Status Report on Alcohol and Health*. Geneva: WHO, 2014.

72. National Institute for Health and Care Excellence (NICE). Alcohol-Use Disorders: Diagnosis, Assessment and Management of Harmful Drinking and Alcohol Dependence. National Clinical Practice Guidelines 115. Leicester: NICE, 2011.

73. Scottish Intercollegiate Guidelines Network (SIGN). *Guideline 74: The Management of Harmful Drinking and Alcohol Dependence in Primary Care: A National Clinical Guideline*. Edinburgh: SIGN, 2003.

74. Department of Health and Ageing (DHA). *Guidelines for the Treatment of Alcohol Problems*. Canberra: Australian Government, 2009.

75. National Health and Medical Research Council. *Australian Guidelines to Reduce Health Risks from Drinking Alcohol*. Canberra: Commonwealth of Australia, 2009.

76. International Agency for Research on Cancer (IARC). List Of Classifications, Volumes 1–117. Available at: http://monographs.iarc.fr/ENG/Classification/latest_classif.php (2016, accessed 7 March 2018).

77. Jane-Llopis E, Matytsina I. Mental health and alcohol, drugs and tobacco: A review of the comorbidity between mental disorders and the use of alcohol, tobacco and illicit drugs. *Drug Alcohol Rev* 2006; 25: 515–536.

78. World Health Organization (WHO). *WHO Report on the Global Tobacco Epidemic, 2013: Enforcing Bans on Tobacco Advertising, Promotion and Sponsorship*. Geneva: WHO, 2013.

79. World Health Organization (WHO). Prevalence of tobacco smoking. Available at: http://www.who.int/gho/tobacco/use/en/ (2016, accessed 7 March 2018).

80. Öberg M, Woodward A, Jaakkola M, Peruga A, Prüss-Üstün A. Global estimate of the burden of disease from second-hand smoke. Available at: http://apps.who.int/iris/bitstream/10665/44426/1/9789241564076_eng.pdf (accessed 7 March 2018).

81. Zwar N, Richmond R, Borland R, et al. *Supporting Smoking Cessation: A Guide for Health Professionals*. Melbourne: The Royal Australian College of General Practitioners, 2011.

82. Minichino A, Bersani FS, Calo WK, et al. Smoking behaviour and mental health disorders--mutual influences and implications for therapy. *Int J Environ Res Public Health* 2013; 10: 4790–4811.

83. Zulkifli A, Abidin EZ, Abidin NZ, et al. Electronic cigarettes: a systematic review of available studies on health risk assessment. *Rev Environ Health* 2016; 21: 21.

84. Stead LF, Buitrago D, Preciado N, Sanchez G, Hartmann-Boyce J, Lancaster T. Physician advice for smoking cessation. *Cochrane Database Syst Rev* 2013; 5: CD000165.

85. Richmond RL, Makinson RJ, Kehoe LA, Giugni AA, Webster IW. One-year evaluation of three smoking cessation interventions administered by general practitioners. *Addict Behav* 1993; 18: 187–199.

86. Borland R, Balmford J, Bishop N, et al. In-practice management versus quitline referral for enhancing smoking cessation in general practice: a cluster randomized trial. *Fam Pract* 2008; 25: 382–389.

87. World Health Organization (WHO). 2010 Global Progress Report on the Implementation of the WHO Framework Convention on Tobacco Control. Available at: http://apps.who.int/iris/handle/10665/70823 (accessed 7 March 2018).

88. Taylor G, McNeill A, Girling A, Farley A, Lindson-Hawley N, Aveyard P. Change in mental health after smoking cessation: systematic review and meta-analysis. *BMJ* 2014; 348: G1151.

89. Kollins SH, McClernon FJ, Fuemmeler BF. Association between smoking and attention-deficit/hyperactivity disorder symptoms in a population-based sample of young adults. *Arch Gen Psychiat* 2005; 62: 1142–1147.

90. de Leon J, Diaz FJ. A meta-analysis of worldwide studies demonstrates an association between schizophrenia and tobacco smoking behaviors. *Schizophr Res* 2005; 76: 135–157.

91. Callaghan RC, Veldhuizen S, Jeysingh T, et al. Patterns of tobacco-related mortality among individuals diagnosed with schizophrenia, bipolar disorder, or depression. *J Psychiatr Res* 2014; 48: 102–110.

92. Aubin HJ, Rollema H, Svensson TH, Winterer G. Smoking, quitting, and psychiatric disease: a review. *Neurosci Biobehav Rev* 2012; 36: 271–284..

93. Barnett PA, Gotlib IH. Psychosocial functioning and depression: distinguishing among antecedents, concomitants, and consequences. *Psychol Bull* 1988; 104: 97.

94. Santini ZI, Koyanagi A, Tyrovolas S, Mason C, Haro JM. The association between social relationships and depression: a systematic review. *J Affect Disord* 2015; 175: 53–65.

95. Cohen S, Wills TA. Stress, social support, and the buffering hypothesis. *Psychol Bull* 1985; 98: 310.

96. Berkman LF, Glass T. Social integration, social networks, social support, and health. *Soc Epidemiol* 2000; 1: 137–173.

97. Cohen S, Underwood LG, Gottlieb BH. *Social Support Measurement and Intervention: A Guide for Health and Social Scientists.* Oxford: Oxford University Press, 2000.

98. Thoits PA. Social support as coping assistance. *J Consult Clin Psychol* 1986; 54: 416.

99. Kamarck TW, Manuck SB, Jennings JR. Social support reduces cardiovascular reactivity to psychological challenge: a laboratory model. *Psychosom Med* 1990; 52: 42–58.

100. Belle D. Gender differences in the social moderators of stress. *Gender Stress* 1987; 257: 277.

101. Belle DE. The impact of poverty on social networks and supports. *Marriage Fam Rev* 1983; 5: 89–103.

102. Grieve R, Watkinson J. The Psychological benefits of being authentic on Facebook. *Cyberpsychol Behav Soc Netw* 2016; 19: 420–425.

103. Krasnova H, Wenninger H, Widjaja T, Buxmann P. Envy on Facebook: a hidden threat to users' life satisfaction? *Wirtschaftsinformatik* 2013; 92: 1–16.

104. Best P, Manktelow R, Taylor B. Online communication, social media and adolescent wellbeing: a systematic narrative review. *Child Youth Serv Rev* 2014; 41: 27–36.

105. Baker DA, Perez Algorta G. The relationship between online social networking and depression: a systematic review of quantitative studies. *Cyberpsychol Behav Soc Netw* 2016; 19: 638–648.

106. Jones JR, Colditz JB, Shensa A, et al. Associations between internet-based professional social networking and emotional distress. *Cyberpsychol Behav Soc Netw* 2016; 19: 601–608.

107. Slonje R, Smith PK. Cyberbullying: another main type of bullying? *Scand J Psychol* 2008; 49: 147–154.

108. Modecki KL, Minchin J, Harbaugh AG, Guerra NG, Runions KC. Bullying prevalence across contexts: a meta-analysis measuring cyber and traditional bullying. *J Adolesc Health* 2014; 55: 602–611.

109. Zych I, Ortega-Ruiz R, Del Rey R. Systematic review of theoretical studies on bullying and cyberbullying: facts, knowledge, prevention, and intervention. *Aggress Violent Behav* 2015; 23: 1–21.

110. Buysse DJ. Sleep health: can we define it? Does it matter? *Sleep* 2014; 37: 9–U219.

111. Ohayon MM. Epidemiology of insomnia: what we know and what we still need to learn. *Sleep Med Rev* 2002; 6: 97–111.

112. Tarokh L, Saletin JM, Carskadon MA. Sleep in adolescence: physiology, cognition and mental health. *Neurosci Biobehav Rev* 2016; 70: 182–188.

113. Shochat T, Cohen-Zion M, Tzischinsky O. Functional consequences of inadequate sleep in adolescents: a systematic review. *Sleep Med Rev* 2014; 18: 75–87.

114. Gradisar M, Gardner G, Dohnt H. Recent worldwide sleep patterns and problems during adolescence: a review and meta-analysis of age, region, and sleep. *Sleep Med* 2011; 12: 110–118.

115. Irish LA, Kline CE, Gunn HE, Buysse DJ, Hall MH. The role of sleep hygiene in promoting public health: a review of empirical evidence. *Sleep Med Rev* 2015; 22: 23–36.

116. Schutte-Rodin S, Broch L, Buysse D, Dorsey C, Sateia M. Clinical guideline for the evaluation and management of chronic insomnia in adults. *J Clin Sleep Med* 2008; 4: 487–504.

117. Bowler DE, Buyung-Ali LM, Knight TM, Pullin AS. A systematic review of evidence for the added benefits to health of exposure to natural environments. *BMC Public Health* 2010; 10: 456.

118. Bragg R, Wood C, Barton J, Pretty J. Wellbeing benefits from natural environments rich in wildlife. A literature review for The Wildlife Trusts. Available at: http://www.wildlifetrusts.org/sites/default/files/wellbeing-benefits-fr-nat-env-report-290915-final-lo_0.pdf (accessed 7 March 2018).

119. Mitchell R. Is physical activity in natural environments better for mental health than physical activity in other environments? *Soc Sci Med* 2013; 91: 130–134.

120. Tzoulas K, Korpela K, Venn S, et al. Promoting ecosystem and human health in urban areas using Green Infrastructure: a literature review. *Landscape Urban Plan* 2007; 81: 167–178.

121. Fallahpour M, Borell L, Luborsky M, Nygard L. Leisure-activity participation to prevent later-life cognitive decline: a systematic review. *Scand J Occup Ther* 2016; 23: 162–197.

122. Adams KB, Leibbrandt S, Moon H. A critical review of the literature on social and leisure activity and wellbeing in later life. *Ageing Soc* 2011; 31: 683–712.

123. Kuykendall L, Tay L, Ng V. Leisure engagement and subjective well-being: A meta-analysis. *Psychol Bull* 2015; 141: 364–403.

124. Endenburg N, van Lith HA. The influence of animals on the development of children. *Vet J* 2011; 190: 208–214.

125. Nagasawa M, Ohta M. The influence of dog ownership in childhood on the sociality of elderly Japanese men. *Anim Sci J* 2010; 81: 377–383.

126. Gilbey A, Tani K. Companion animals and loneliness: a systematic review of quantitative studies. *Anthrozoos* 2015; 28: 181–197.

127. Islam A, Towell T. Cat and dog companionship and well-being: A systematic review. *Int J Appl Psychol* 2013; 3: 149–155.

128. Stallones L. Pet loss and mental health. *Anthrozoos* 1994; 7: 43–54.

129. Swinton J. *Spirituality and Mental Health Care: Rediscovering a 'Forgotten' Dimension.* London: Jessica Kingsley Publishers, 2001.

130. Dein S, Cook CCH, Koenig H. Religion, spirituality, and mental health current controversies and future directions. *J Nerv Ment Dis* 2012; 200: 852–855.

131. Bertorelli D. Spirituality, religion and mental health. *Aust N Z J Psychiatry* 2014; 48(Suppl.): 100 (abstract).

132. Salsman JM, Pustejovsky JE, Jim HSL, et al. A meta-analytic approach to examining the correlation between religion/spirituality and mental health in cancer. *Cancer* 2015; 121: 3769–3778.

133. Kabat-Zinn J. Mindfulness-based interventions in context: past, present, and future. *Clin Psychol* 2003; 10: 144–156.

134. Kabat-Zinn J. *Full Catastrophe Living*. New York: Delta, 1990.

135. Morgan D. Mindfulness-based cognitive therapy for depression: a new approach to preventing relapse. *Psychother Res* 2003; 13: 123–125.

136. Keng SL, Smoski MJ, Robins CJ. Effects of mindfulness on psychological health: a review of empirical studies. *Clin Psychol Rev* 2011; 31: 1041–1056.

137. van der Velden AM, Kuyken W, Wattar U, et al. A systematic review of mechanisms of change in mindfulness-based cognitive therapy in the treatment of recurrent major depressive disorder. *Clin Psychol Rev* 2015; 37: 26–39.

138. Knight T, Skouteris H, Townsend M, Hooley M. The act of giving: a systematic review of nonfamilial intergenerational interaction. *J Intergener Relatsh* 2014; 12: 257–278.

139. Anderson ND, Damianakis T, Kröger E, et al. The benefits associated with volunteering among seniors: A critical review and recommendations for future research. *Psychol Bull* 2014; 140:1505.

CHAPTER 35

Prevention approaches to reduce alcohol-related harm

William Gilmore, Katherine Brown, and Ian Gilmore

Introduction

Alcohol is a psychoactive drug of potential dependence, and so its use and abuse are inextricably linked to mental health. It may be the primary problem or part of the co-morbidities that accompany mental illness. Alcohol has been embedded in society for thousands of years, and, because it is legal, socially acceptable, and widely available at low cost, it is easy to overlook the burden it places not just on mental health, but on wider health care, on the criminal justice system, and on the overall economy. There is a wealth of evidence to show the value of both preventative public health measures aimed at the whole population and also more targeted approaches towards high-risk groups [1]. However, these approaches often run into significant cultural and political barriers.

A brief history of alcohol consumption

In various beverage forms alcohol has been produced and consumed for thousands of years. Written reference to beer consumption dates back to the earliest civilization around 3000 BC, the Sumerians of Mesopotamia, but it is likely that alcohol has a much longer history than that [2]. Alcohol has been used by individuals and societies throughout time for many reasons ranging from as a medicine, a source of nourishment, a safer alternative to contaminated water, and an intoxicant to an integral part of religious/cultural ceremonies and social occasions. Today we both celebrate and commiserate with alcohol.

Alcohol's intoxicating effect on the individual has been felt for as long as it has been consumed, and examples of attempted regulation of alcohol production, sale, and consumption due to alcohol-related problems can also be traced far back. The Gin Acts of eighteenth-century Britain were a series of legislative interventions, including taxation and control of sale, introduced by Parliament to reduce the observed negative health and social effects, famously portrayed in William Hogarth's print Gin Lane in 1751 (Fig. 35.1), related to the rapid increased production and consumption of the cheap distilled spirit. The Acts and any of their positive impacts, however, were short-lived [3], and while gin consumption was being targeted by government, beer consumption was actually encouraged [4]. The Victorians had higher levels of consumption than in the UK today, despite a strong temperance movement at that time [5], and these levels only began to fall at the turn of the twentieth century (Fig. 35.2). At the outbreak of the First World War, the Defence of the Realm Act was introduced in Britain and included trading hours restrictions on public houses near the vital munitions factories, bans on drinking on public transport, and increases in tax [6]. These measures coincided with a marked reduction in wartime alcohol consumption in Britain (Fig. 35.2), although the fact that a large proportion of young men were away fighting in the trenches may also have been a factor.

The second half of the twentieth century saw UK per capita alcohol consumption begin to steadily increase and it more than doubled between 1950 and 2005 to close to 10 litres of pure alcohol per capita (Fig. 35.2). The affordability of alcohol in the UK followed a similar upward trend [7]. The 1950s onwards was a period of intense globalization, where alcohol producers followed the lead of tobacco and soft-drink companies and became multinational corporations marketing international brands across both the developed and developing worlds [1]. Alcohol consumption in France and Italy dramatically halved during this same period, but started from very high levels of over 20 litres of pure alcohol per capita [8]. In the last 10 years there has been a slight downward trend in UK per capita consumption (Fig. 35.2), which may, in part, be attributed to the economic recession (also observed during the depression of the early 1930s), a government-imposed alcohol excise duty escalator [9], and increasing cultural diversity meaning more abstainers [10]. Despite recent reductions, latest figures from the Organisation for Economic Cooperation and Development rank the UK among the top-20 countries worldwide in terms of their level of alcohol consumption [11].

Per capita consumption figures, based on sale and excise data, are a good indicator of the level of heavy drinking in a population, but information on patterns of alcohol consumption, usually collected in surveys, is also very important in predicting the types of harms a population is likely to encounter. For example, in the UK, younger people (< 45 years of age) are more likely to binge drink and fall victim to short-term harms such as alcohol poisoning, road traffic accidents, and violence, whereas middle-aged and older people (> 45 years of age) are more likely to drink daily and to suffer from conditions related to the long-term use of alcohol, such as cancer, cardiovascular disease, and liver disease [7]. It has been estimated that 20% of the population, approximately 11 million people, consume close to 60% of all alcohol sold and are drinking at levels that increase the risk of harm to their health [12]. The UK has also shifted from a nation of pub goers to a nation predominantly drinking relatively cheap alcohol from supermarkets and off-licences behind closed doors: latest figures from the British Beer and Pub Association show that more than twice the volume of alcohol is bought from the off-licensed trade (5.2 litres of pure

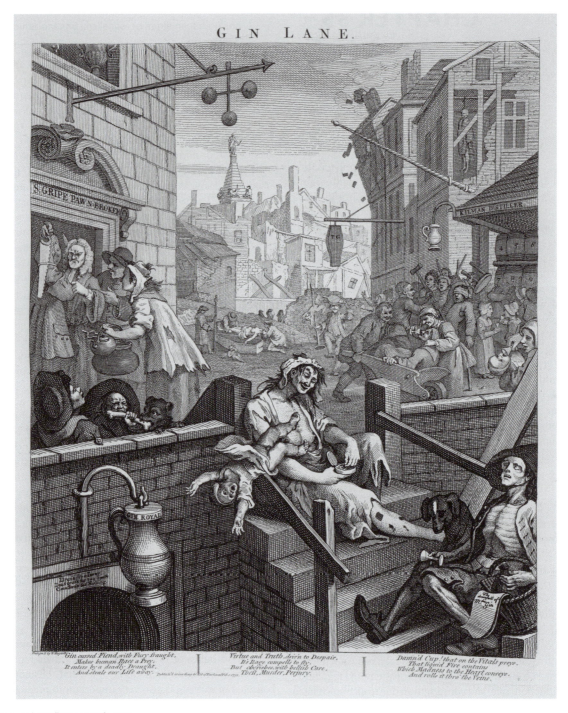

Fig. 35.1 Gin Lane by William Hogarth, 1751.

alcohol per capita) than that bought in pubs, bars, and restaurants (2.5 litres pure alcohol per capita) each year [13].

The burden of alcohol-related harm

The health, social, and economic effects of alcohol use are experienced by drinkers, families, communities, and society at large. Alcohol is associated with more than 60 health conditions, including liver disease, cardiovascular disease, cancers, and a range of mental health problems, and is strongly linked to violence,

accidents, self-harm, suicide, and fetal alcohol spectrum disorder (FASD), affecting both individual drinkers and people who do not drink [14]. Of alcohol's overall population impact, the level of harm inflicted on others has been estimated to be greater than to drinkers themselves [15]. In the UK the government estimates that total costs to society from alcohol use exceed £21 billion each year [16].

Worldwide, alcohol is responsible for 3.3 million deaths each year, which represents 5.9% all deaths, and 5.1% of the global burden of disease and injury is attributable to alcohol, as measured in disability-adjusted life years (DALYs) [14]. In the UK, which is

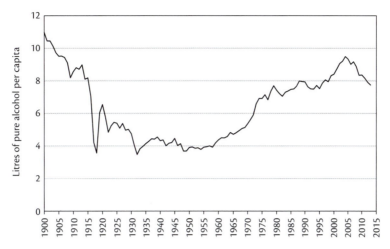

Fig. 35.2 Per capita pure alcohol consumption in the UK, 1900–2013.
Source: Data from British Beer and Pub Association, Copyright (2014).

among the heavier-drinking nations, it is estimated that alcohol is responsible for 10% of the disease burden in terms of DALYs lost [17]. In England there were 1.1 million hospital admissions (20% of which were for mental and behavioural disorders) [7] and 22,000 deaths associated with alcohol in 2014 [18]. Of the 11 million people in England drinking at potentially risky levels, it is estimated that 1.6 million have some degree of alcohol dependency (9% of male and 3% of female drinkers) [19]. Only around 7% of these actually access treatment services [20].

The World Health Organization's (WHO) *International Classification of Diseases*' (ICD) clinical descriptions and diagnostic guidelines describe alcohol dependency as presenting three or more of the following characteristics in the previous year [21]:

1. A strong desire or sense of compulsion to use alcohol.

2. Difficulties in controlling alcohol use, in terms of onset, termination, and levels of consumption.

3. A physiological withdrawal state.

4. Evidence of tolerance.

5. Progressive neglect of alternative pleasures or interests.

6. Persistent drinking despite overtly clear evidence of harmful consequences.

Alcohol use disorders are linked to a number of psychiatric co-morbidities: people suffering from alcohol dependency are at a greater risk of depression, anxiety, drug misuse, nicotine dependence, and self-harm. It is estimated that up to 41% of suicides are attributable to alcohol and 23% of people who engage in deliberate self-harm are alcohol dependent [22].

Chronic alcohol consumption can alter the brain's structure and function, leading to alcohol-related brain damage. One of the side effects commonly associated with alcohol dependency is malnutrition, in particular a deficiency in thiamine (vitamin B1), which can lead to the potentially reversible neurological disorder Wernicke's encephalopathy. Treatment with thiamine can elicit a rapid recovery from Wernicke's encephalopathy; however, if the disorder is left untreated it can develop into Korsakoff syndrome, a severe brain disorder often characterized by anterograde amnesia, with individuals losing the ability to form new memories [23].

Evidence indicates that the harmful effects of alcohol are disproportionately concentrated in low-income and vulnerable groups, indicating that alcohol is a driver of inequalities [24]. Heavy alcohol use is closely linked with a number of social harms and risk factors, including homelessness, social exclusion, domestic abuse, child neglect, and imprisonment, and is often associated with stigma and disadvantage. A 2013 review of patients who died of alcohol-related liver disease in England indicated that this group was more likely to receive suboptimal care in hospital as a result of what appeared to be 'negative and pessimistic attitudes' from healthcare professionals [25].

Prevention measures

The primary and secondary prevention approaches to reduce alcohol-related harm that are presented in the rest of this chapter are among the 10 key areas for national action, as set out in the WHO's evidence-based global alcohol strategy [26]:

1. Leadership, awareness, and commitment.

2. Health services' response.

3. Community action.

4. Drink-driving policies and countermeasures.

5. Availability of alcohol.

6. Marketing of alcoholic beverages.

7. Pricing policies.

8. Reducing the negative consequences of drinking and alcohol intoxication.

9. Reducing the public health impact of illicit alcohol and informally produced alcohol.

10. Monitoring and surveillance.

Primary prevention

In order to have the greatest impact on alcohol-related problems it is necessary to take a population-level approach. Although it is very important to provide treatment services for alcohol-dependent people, this will not address the broader burden of harm caused by

Box 35.1 The Nuffield Council on Bioethics' intervention ladder

Eliminate choice Regulate in such a way as to entirely eliminate choice.

Restrict choice Regulate in such a way as to restrict the options available to people with the aim of protecting them.

Guide choice through disincentives Fiscal and other disincentives can be put in place to influence people not to pursue certain activities.

Guide choice through incentives Regulations can be offered that guide choices by fiscal and other incentives.

Guide choice through changing the default policy Provide a more healthy option as standard.

Enable choice Enable individuals to change their behaviours.

Provide information Inform and educate the public.

Do nothing or simply monitor the current situation.

Source: Reproduced from Nuffield Council on Bioethics, Public health: ethical issues, Chapter 3 Policy process and practice, Copyright (2007) with permission from Nuffield Council on Bioethics.

those that are not dependent. The population-level measures that have the strongest evidence for effectiveness in reducing alcohol-related harm are those that sit within the top half of the Nuffield Council on Bioethics intervention ladder (Box 35.1), and involve government regulation [27]. These primary prevention measures include regulating alcohol affordability, alcohol availability, and alcohol promotion [1, 28–30]. Information and education programmes, although often a popular choice owing to their unobtrusiveness, have largely been shown to be ineffective in isolation but perhaps will have more effect in combination with a suite of regulatory measures and may even have a part to play in generating community support for effective alcohol policies [1, 28–31].

Regulating alcohol affordability

Reducing the affordability of alcohol is by far the most important measure a government is able to take in reducing alcohol consumption and alcohol-related harm at the population level. A 2009 meta-analysis, including 112 international studies, found that a 10% increase in price/tax produced a 4.4% decrease in average alcohol consumption [32]. Price and tax increases are generally politically unpopular and opposed by alcohol industry bodies and heavier drinkers who tend to favour cheaper alcohol products [33, 34]. However, in many countries, alcohol prices are not even keeping up with the cost of living and are thus becoming ever more affordable. In the UK, it has been estimated that alcohol was 61% more affordable in 2012 than it was in 1980 [35]. The government introduced an alcohol excise duty escalator in 2008, keeping the tax rate at 2% above the rate of inflation, but it was abandoned in 2014 [36]. One evidence-based strategy that governments can implement that will strike a balance between raising revenue and reducing alcohol-related harm is minimum unit pricing (a set minimum price under which a 'unit' or 8 g of ethanol cannot be sold).

Minimum unit pricing

Minimum pricing began in Canada, not for public health reasons, but in order for government alcohol monopolies to control revenue across provinces [37]. There are various forms of minimum pricing that are in place across Canada, some based only on beverage volume (per litre) and others on ethanol content by volume. Canadian researchers have conducted numerous evaluations of minimum pricing and shown reductions in alcohol consumption (8%) [38], alcohol-related deaths (32%) [39], and alcohol-related hospitalizations (9%) [40] when minimum prices are increased by 10%. The concept of setting a minimum price per unit of alcohol (MUP) has been borne from this work and has the added advantage of not differentiating between beverage types. It also specifically targets the very cheap alcohol, favoured by heavier drinkers, usually sold for off-premise consumption.

MUP is promoted by the top independent public health bodies in the UK, as the leading intervention in a comprehensive response to tackling alcohol-related problems in the population and resetting the cultural norms surrounding alcohol use [41]. Scotland has taken the lead in recognizing the severity of alcohol's harms and legislated for a MUP in 2012, but, unfortunately it was held up for 5 years by continued legal challenges from the alcohol industry in the Scottish and European courts. Extensive modelling by the University of Sheffield has demonstrated that minimum prices of £0.50 per unit would see reductions in alcohol consumption of 3.5% in Scotland and would have a much larger impact on heavier drinkers than on moderate drinkers. The greatest health outcomes would be experienced by low-income groups, indicating the policy could be an important mechanism for tackling inequalities [42]. Whether England, Wales, and Northern Ireland will follow Scotland's bold step is uncertain at this stage.

Regulating alcohol availability

Alcohol is more readily available now than it has ever been. In England, it is possible to buy a bottle of spirits in the local supermarket together with your bread and milk, or order a pint of beer at a motorway service station on a long journey home, and—since a major relaxation in licensing laws in 2003—purchase alcohol 24 hours a day, 7 days a week. There are a number of ways of restricting the availability of alcohol, but the most effective have been shown to be increasing the legal purchase age, reducing trading hours, and restricting numbers of outlets [1, 28–30].

Purchase age laws

Most countries have laws regarding the minimum age for purchasing alcohol, to protect children and young people. In the UK the minimum age is 18 years, in Portugal it is 16 years (for beer and wine only), and in most states of the US it is 21 years. There is strong evidence from studies investigating both increases and decreases in the legal purchase age of alcohol that shows increases do result in reduced drinking and alcohol-related harm among young people [43]. Of course, in order to optimize the impact, any increase in legal purchase age must be complemented with strict enforcement.

Trading hours

Restrictions on alcohol outlet trading hours can range from a whole day, such as Sunday, through to reducing last orders at bars and clubs by an hour or two in the early hours of the morning. Reviews of the international evidence [44, 45] have concluded that even small reductions in trading hours can have a significant impact on population-level alcohol-related harm, including assault rates.

Outlet density

The evidence base on restricting numbers or the density of outlets in residential communities and night-time economies does not have as long a history as that of trading hours. Despite mixed findings in studies and some criticisms of methodologies used in the literature, three systematic reviews published in recent years have agreed that alcohol outlet densities are positively associated with alcohol-related harm in communities [46–48]. Studies have found positive associations between alcohol outlet densities and a range of harms, including assault and mental health disorders [49, 50]. Owing to licensed outlets having such varied functions and communities being so diverse, how this can be translated into effective regulation is currently unclear. Health evidence, however, is now more routinely considered in licensing decisions, particularly in Scotland where protecting and improving public health has been written into licensing legislation [51].

Regulating alcohol promotion

Product promotion is an integral part of alcohol industry sales strategies. As such, alcohol is heavily promoted worldwide. It has been estimated that in the UK alone over £800 million is spent each year on alcohol advertising [52]. In addition to the more traditional forms of advertising through television, radio, newspapers/magazines, and billboards, alcohol is now promoted through sport and music event sponsorship, the Internet and social media, point-of-sale promotions, and even corporate social responsibility communications [53]. Alcohol products like vodka have also been reinvented (as 'alcopops') and marketed at young people to boost sales [54].

Systematic reviews of the evidence show that exposure to alcohol promotion is associated with the commencement of alcohol consumption among young people and increased levels of consumption among young people who already consume alcohol [55–57].

In most countries, including the UK, alcohol promotion is currently not subject to government regulation. The alcohol industry generally self-regulates by setting voluntary codes of conduct for marketing communications. But there are a number of examples of where this self-regulation fails in protecting young people from exposure to alcohol advertisements [58, 59]. The Loi Évin, introduced in France in 1991, is a rare example of government regulation of alcohol promotion [60]. It is not a blanket ban and it has relaxed over time, but alcohol sponsorship of sporting events and alcohol advertising on television is still prohibited. As host of the Euro 2016 football tournament, however, France's advertising legislation was unable to withstand alcohol industry tactics. Carlsberg, one of the usual tournament sponsors, circumnavigated the ban by replacing its usual pitch-side branding with well-known slogans in the company font [61].

Providing information and education

Education and persuasion strategies are among the most popular measures intended to reduce alcohol harm. It could be argued that the non-restrictive nature of information provision attracts broader support from governments, the public, and alcohol industry groups. It could also be argued that provision of information to consumers about the side effects of products they ingest is a basic right.

Evidence suggests that without the support of other environmental interventions such as controls on affordability, availability, and promotion of alcohol, information and education programmes do not lead to sustained changes in drinking behaviour [62]. In addition, researchers have identified that resources awarded to publicly funded information and awareness campaigns discouraging

underage drinking will always be dwarfed by the positive messages promoted via multimillion-pound advertising campaigns by alcohol companies each year [59].

On balance, it is likely that effective education and information initiatives can play an important role in preventing the harmful use of alcohol as part of a comprehensive strategy. The WHO states that information and education campaigns can support other alcohol policy initiatives, by changing social norms and influencing attitudes [63]. The most commonly used methods of delivering information and education about alcohol include mass media public awareness campaigns, school-based education programmes, and product labelling.

Public awareness campaigns

Public information campaigns designed to prevent harmful use of alcohol can take a variety of forms, but are usually delivered via print, broadcast, and/or digital media, and highlight the negative consequences of excessive consumption. Evidence suggests that campaigns have the most impact in raising awareness of key messages when the audience reach is high and the messages are repeated frequently and supported by public relations or media advocacy initiatives [64]. While campaign evaluations have failed to demonstrate long-term change in drinking behaviours, there is an emerging body of evidence indicating that mass-media campaigns can increase awareness of the negative health consequences associated with drinking, including the link between alcohol and cancer [65]. There is currently no sign, however, that the new UK alcohol guidelines on low-risk drinking [66], released in 2016 and based on the latest evidence, will be supported by effective mass media campaigns. In addition, some studies have shown that advertising campaigns warning about the dangers of drink driving are associated with reductions in alcohol-related traffic accidents when delivered through well-funded mass media and supported by local level prevention efforts such as high-visibility enforcement [67].

School-based education programmes

There is little evidence to show that school-based alcohol education programmes are effective at achieving long-term behaviour change relating to drinking [1]. Studies have shown that some alcohol education initiatives delivered in school settings can increase knowledge about alcohol and shift attitudes about drinking among students [68]. A systematic review of the evidence for success of school-based education programmes found that a small number of generic, universal education programmes that focussed on developing life skills and resilience among students showed more promising results in reductions in drunkenness and binge drinking than alcohol-specific education initiatives [69].

Alcohol product labelling

Studies have shown that health information and warning labels placed on alcohol containers can help to improve consumer awareness and understanding of the health risks associated with drinking, but there is little evidence to link labelling with sustained changes in drinking behaviours [70]. In France, it is mandatory for alcohol containers to display either a text warning or pictogram advising pregnant women not to drink alcohol, with the intention of preventing FASD. While there is no evidence directly linking warning labels with reductions in FASD rates, an evaluation carried out in France 3 years after the introduction of warning labels indicated an associated increase in knowledge and awareness among women about the harmful effects of drinking during pregnancy [71].

Workplace policies

In Europe, the burden of alcohol-related ill health is greatest among adults of working age [63]. It is perhaps not surprising, therefore, that alcohol problems have a significant impact on workplace productivity and that employers can play an important role in preventing alcohol misuse.

Studies have shown that excessive alcohol consumption is associated with increased sickness rates at the population level, with countries reporting higher per capita consumption rates also reporting higher rates of sickness absence [72]. In addition to absenteeism, alcohol use is associated with poor performance in the workplace, sometimes called 'presenteeism'. It is also associated with higher risk of accidents, injury, inappropriate behaviour, poor co-worker behaviour, and low company morale [73]. Conversely, structural factors at the workplace, including high stress and low satisfaction, can increase the risk of alcohol use disorders and alcohol dependence [63].

There is evidence that interventions delivered in workplace settings can help to reduce rates of harmful drinking, and associated negative effects such as poor performance and sickness rates. Programmes that have been associated with reductions in self-reported alcohol consumption or alcohol-related problems include psychosocial skills training, brief interventions and general health check-ups that provide information and advice on a number of risk factors including alcohol such as diet, exercise, stress, depression, and cholesterol [74]. The WHO recommends that efforts are taken in the workplace to reduce alcohol problems, such as policies promoting alcohol-free workplaces, a managerial style that reduces job stress and increases job rewards and optional interventions available on request such as brief advice (see 'Secondary prevention') and alcohol information training [63].

Secondary prevention

As it is likely to take time for the most effective primary prevention measures to gain widespread support and be implemented by governments, there are also secondary prevention measures, involving screening populations at risk, that have been consistently shown to be both effective and cost-effective at changing individual

Table 35.1 The Alcohol Use Disorders Identification Test (AUDIT)

	Scoring system					Score
	0	1	2	3	4	
1. How often do you have a drink containing alcohol?	Never	Monthly or less	2–4 times per month	2–3 times per week	4+ times per week	
2. How many units of alcohol do you drink on a typical day when you are drinking?	1–2	3–4	5–6	7–9	10+	
3. How often have you had 6 or more units on a single occasion in the last year?	Never	Less than monthly	Monthly	Weekly	Daily or almost daily	
4. How often during the last year have you found that you were not able to stop drinking once you had started?	Never	Less than monthly	Monthly	Weekly	Daily or almost daily	
5. How often during the last year have you failed to do what was normally expected from you because of your drinking?	Never	Less than monthly	Monthly	Weekly	Daily or almost daily	
6. How often during the last year have you needed an alcoholic drink in the morning to get yourself going after a heavy drinking session?	Never	Less than monthly	Monthly	Weekly	Daily or almost daily	
7. How often during the last year have you had a feeling of guilt or remorse after drinking?	Never	Less than monthly	Monthly	Weekly	Daily or almost daily	
8. How often during the last year have you been unable to remember what happened the night before because you had been drinking?	Never	Less than monthly	Monthly	Weekly	Daily or almost daily	
9. Have you or somebody else been injured as a result of your drinking?	No		Yes, but not in the last year		Yes, during the last year	
10. Has a relative or friend, doctor or other health worker been concerned about your drinking or suggested that you cut down?	No		Yes, but not in the last year		Yes, during the last year	

AUDIT scoring (all 10 questions):

0–7 Lower risk, 8–15 Increasing risk, 16–19 Higher risk, 20+ Possible dependence.

Note: Provided for educational purposes only.
Source: Reproduced from Babor T, Higgins-Biddle J, Saunders J, et al., The Alcohol Use Disorders Identification Test: Guidelines for use in Primary care, Second edition, Copyright (2001), with permission from World Health Organization.

behaviour and reducing levels of alcohol consumption and related harm [75].

Identification and brief advice

Early identification and brief advice (IBA) typically involves the use of a screening tool to identify hazardous and harmful drinking, followed by short, structured brief advice to encourage drinkers to reduce their consumption. A number of screening tools are used to deliver IBA, and perhaps one of the most common is the Alcohol Use Disorders Identification Test (AUDIT), which consists of 10 multiple choice questions designed to classify drinkers as lower risk, increasing risk, higher risk, or possible alcohol dependence (Table 35.1) [76]. In more time-constrained settings, such as busy hospital emergency departments, shorter screening questionnaires are used. The AUDIT-C, for example, is an abbreviated version of the AUDIT and consists of the first three questions.

For patients who are identified through the AUDIT as possibly alcohol dependent, it is recommended they are referred to specialist alcohol treatment services. For patients identified as increasing or higher risk, it is recommended that feedback and structured advice is given, which can take the form of a sentence or two alongside provision of an information leaflet, or a longer discussion about the individual's drinking and risk levels, depending on what is considered appropriate for the situation and context. However, a recent randomized controlled trial of IBA in primary care showed that brief advice and lifestyle counselling after screening was no more effective in reducing drinking than providing simple feedback and an information leaflet [77].

Studies have shown that delivery of IBA can reduce rates of alcohol consumption among hazardous and harmful drinkers. The strongest evidence is found from IBA delivery in primary care settings; however, there is also evidence to suggest IBA can be effective when delivered in criminal justice settings and emergency departments [78].

Conclusions

The negative effects of alcohol use are wide ranging, and not only do they impact drinkers themselves, but also those around them and society at large. Comprehensive strategies are required to be implemented by governments in order to prevent the huge burden of alcohol-related harm. The most effective interventions that have been shown to reduce population level alcohol-related harm involve regulating alcohol affordability, availability, and promotion. At an individual level early identification and brief advice (IBA) has been shown to be effective in helping drinkers at risk of harm reduce their consumption, particularly in primary care settings.

References

1. Babor T, Caetano R, Casswell S, et al. *Alcohol: No Ordinary Commodity: Research and Public Policy*, 2nd edn. New York: Oxford University Press, 2010.
2. Austin G. *Alcohol in Western Society from Antiquity to 1800: A Chronological History*. Santa Barbara, CA: ABC-Clio Press, 1985.
3. Warner J, Her M, Gmel G, Rehm J. Can legislation prevent debauchery? Mother gin and public health in 18th-century England. *Am J Public Health* 2001; 91: 375–384.
4. Abel E. The gin epidemic: much ado about what? *Alcohol Alcohol* 2001; 36: 401–405.
5. Harrison B. *Drink & the Victorians: the Temperance question in England 1815–1872*. London: Faber & Faber, 1971.
6. McAllister A. The enemy within: the battle over alcohol in World War I. Available at: http://theconversation.com/the-enemy-within-the-battle-over-alcohol-in-world-war-i-30441 (2014, accessed 8 March 2018).
7. Health and Social Care Information Centre. Statistics on Alcohol, England. 2016. Available at: https://digital.nhs.uk/catalogue/PUB20999 (accessed 8 March 2018).
8. World Health Organization. Global information system on alcohol and health, recorded alcohol per capita consumption, 1960–2015 by country. Available at http://apps.who.int/gho/data/node.main.A1022?lang=en (accessed 19 September 2016).
9. Sheron N, Gilmore I. Effect of policy, economics, and the changing alcohol marketplace on alcohol related deaths in England and Wales. *BMJ* 2016; 353: i1860.
10. Bhattacharya A. *Youthful Abandon: Why Are Young People Drinking Less?* London: Institute of Alcohol Studies, 2016.
11. Organisation for Economic Cooperation and Development (OECD). *Health at a Glance 2015: OECD Indicators*. Paris: OECD Publishing, 2015.
12. Bosley S. Problem drinkers account for most of alcohol industry's sales. Available at: https://www.theguardian.com/society/2016/jan/22/problem-drinkers-alcohol-industry-most-sales-figures-reveal (2016, accessed 19 September 2016).
13. British Beer and Pub Association. *Statistical Handbook*. London: BBPA, 2015.
14. World Health Organization (WHO). *Global Status Report on Alcohol and Health*. Geneva: WHO, 2014.
15. Nutt D, King L, Phillips L. Drug harms in the UK: a multicriteria decision analysis. *Lancet* 2010; 376: 1558–1565.
16. Cabinet Office. *Alcohol Misuse: How Much Does it Cost?* London: Cabinet Office, 2003.
17. Department of Health (DoH). *The Evidence on Alcohol Misuse and Harm in England Today. Memorandum to Health Committee Inquiry in the Government's Alcohol Strategy*. London: DoH, 2012.
18. Public Health England. Local Alcohol Profiles for England. Available at http://fingertips.phe.org.uk/local-alcohol-profiles (2016, accessed 19 September 2016).
19. McManus S, Meltzer H, Brugha T, et al. *Adult Psychiatric Morbidity in England, 2007: Results of a Household Survey*. Leeds: NHS Information Centre for Health and Social Care, 2009.
20. Public Health England (PHE). *Adult Alcohol statistics from the National Drug Treatment Monitoring System*. London: PHE, 2014.
21. World Health Organization. The ICD-10 Classification of Mental and Behavioural Disorders: Clinical descriptions and diagnostic guidelines. Available at: http://www.who.int/substance_abuse/terminology/ICD10ClinicalDiagnosis.pdf (2016, accessed 19 September 2016).
22. National Institute for Health and Care Excellence. *Alcohol-Use Disorders: Diagnosis, Assessment and Management of Harmful Drinking and Alcohol Dependence. NICE Clinical Guidelines, No. 115*. Leicester: British Psychological Society, 2011.
23. Zahr NM, Kaufman KL, Harper CG. Clinical and pathological features of alcohol-related brain damage. *Nat Rev Neurol* 2011; 7: 284–294.
24. Smith K, Foster J. Alcohol, Health Inequalities and the Harm Paradox: Why some groups facer greater problems despite consuming less alcohol. Available at http://www.ias.org.uk/uploads/pdf/IAS%20reports/IAS%20report%20Alcohol%20and%20health%20inequalities%20FULL.pdf (2016, accessed 19 September 2016).
25. National Confidential Enquiry into Patient Outcome and Health. Measuring the Units, a review of patients who dies with alcohol-related liver disease. Available at http://www.ncepod.org.uk/2013report1/downloads/MeasuringTheUnits_FullReport.pdf (2013, accessed 19 September 2016).
26. World Health Organization (WHO). Global Strategy to Reduce the Harmful Use of Alcohol. Geneva: WHO, 2010.
27. Nuffield Council on Bioethics. *Public Health: Ethical Issues*. London: Nuffield Council on Bioethics, 2007.

28. Stockwell, T. Alcohol supply, demand, and harm reductions: what is the strongest cocktail? *Int J Drug Policy* 2006; 17: 269–277.

29. Anderson P, Chisholm D, Fuhr D. Effectiveness and cost-effectiveness of policies and programmes to reduce the harm caused by alcohol. *Lancet* 2009; 373: 2234–2246.

30. Gilmore W, Chikritzhs T, Stockwell T, Jernigan D, Naimi T, Gilmore I. Alcohol: taking a population perspective. *Nat Rev Gastroenterol Hepatol* 2016; 13: 426–434.

31. Giesbrecht N. Reducing alcohol-related damage in populations: rethinking the roles of education and persuasion interventions. *Addiction* 2007; 102: 1345–1349.

32. Wagenaar A, Salois M, Komro K. Effects of beverage alcohol price and tax levels on drinking: a meta-analysis of 1003 estimates from 112 studies. *Addiction* 2009; 104: 179–190.

33. Bond L, Daube M, Chikritzhs T. Selling addictions: Similarities in approaches between Big Tobacco and Big Booze. *Australas Med J* 2010; 3: 325–332.

34. Sheron N, Chilcott F, Matthews L, Challoner B, and Thomas M. Impact of minimum price per unit of alcohol on patients with liver disease in UK. *Clin Med* 2014; 14: 396–403.

35. Health and Social Care Information Centre. Statistics on Alcohol, England. Available at: https://digital.nhs.uk/catalogue/PUB10932 (2013, accessed 19 September 2016).

36. Institute of Alcohol Studies. *The Impact of Abolishing the Alcohol Duty Escalator: Can Society Afford for Cheap Drink to Get Cheaper?* London: Institute of Alcohol Studies, 2014.

37. Stockwell T. Minimum unit pricing for alcohol. *BMJ* 2014; 349: g5617.

38. Stockwell T, Zhao J, Giesbrecht N, Macdonald S, Thomas G, Wettlaufer A. The raising of minimum alcohol prices in Saskatchewan, Canada: impacts on consumption and implications for public health. *Am J Public Health* 2012; 102: e103–e110.

39. Zhao J, Stockwell T, Martin G, et al. The relationship between minimum alcohol prices, outlet densities and alcohol-attributable deaths in British Columbia, 2002–2009. *Addiction* 2013; 108: 1059–1069.

40. Stockwell T, Zhao J, Martin G, et al. Minimum alcohol prices and outlet densities in British Columbia, Canada: estimated impacts on alcohol-attributable hospital admissions. *Am J Public Health* 2013; 103: 2014–2020.

41. Gilmore I, Anderson W, Bauld L, et al. *Health First: An Evidence-based Alcohol Strategy for the UK*. Stirling: University of Stirling, 2013.

42. Angus C, Holmes J, Pryce R, Meier P, Brennan A. *Model-based Appraisal of the Comparative Impact of Minimum Unit Pricing and Taxation Policies in Scotland: An Adaptation of the Sheffield Alcohol Policy Model Version 3*. Sheffield: University of Sheffield, 2016.

43. Wagenaar AC, Toomey TL. Effects of minimum drinking age laws: review and analyses of the literature from 1960 to 2000. *J Stud Alcohol Suppl* 2002; (14): 206–225.

44. Stockwell T, Chikritzhs T. Do relaxed trading hours for bars and clubs mean more relaxed drinking? A review of international research on the impacts of changes to permitted hours of drinking. *Crime Prev Commun Saf* 2009; 11: 153–170.

45. Hahn R, Kuzara JL, Elder R, et al. Effectiveness of policies restricting hours of alcohol sales in preventing excessive alcohol consumption and related harms. *Am J Prev Med* 2010; 39: 590–604.

46. Campbell C, Hahn Ra, Elder R, et al. The effectiveness of limiting alcohol outlet density as a means of reducing excessive alcohol consumption and alcohol-related harms. *Am J Prev Med* 2009; 37: 556–569.

47. Popova S, Giesbrecht N, Bekmuradov D, Patra J. Hours and days of sale and density of alcohol outlets: impacts on alcohol consumption and damage: a systematic review. *Alcohol Alcohol* 2009; 44: 500–516.

48. Gmel G, Holmes J, Studer J. Are alcohol outlet densities strongly associated with alcohol-related outcomes? A critical review of recent evidence. *Drug Alcohol Rev* 2015; 35: 40–54.

49. Livingston M. A longitudinal analysis of alcohol outlet density and domestic violence. *Addiction* 2011; 106: 919–925.

50. Pereira G, Wood L, Foster S, Haggar F. Access to alcohol outlets, alcohol consumption and mental health. *PLOS ONE* 2013; 8: e53461.

51. Alcohol Research UK. *Using Licensing to Protect Public Health: From Evidence to Practice*. London: Alcohol Research UK, 2014.

52. Hastings G, Brooks O, Stead M, Angus K, Anker T, Farrell T. Failure of self regulation of UK alcohol advertising. *BMJ* 2010; 340.

53. Yoon S, Lam TH. The illusion of righteousness: corporate social responsibility practices of the alcohol industry. *BMC Public Health* 2013; 13: 630.

54. Mosher J. Joe Camel in a bottle: Diageo, the Smirnoff brand, and the transformation of the youth alcohol market. *Am J Public Health* 2012; 102: 56–63.

55. Anderson P, de Bruijn A, Angus K, Gordon R, Hastings G. Impact of alcohol advertising and media exposure on adolescent alcohol use: a systematic review of longitudinal studies. *Alcohol Alcohol* 2009; 44: 229–243.

56. Smith L, Foxcroft D. The effect of alcohol advertising, marketing and portrayal on drinking behaviour in young people: systematic review of prospective cohort studies. *BMC Public Health* 2009; 9: 1–11.

57. Brown K. Association between alcohol sports sponsorship and consumption: a systematic review. *Alcohol Alcohol* 2016; 51: 747–755.

58. Ross C, Ostroff J, Siegel MB, DeJong W, Naimi TS, Jernigan DH. Youth alcohol brand consumption and exposure to brand advertising in magazines. *J Stud Alcohol Drugs* 2014; 75: 615–622.

59. Hastings G, Brooks O, Stead M, et al. Failure of self-regulation of UK alcohol advertising. *BMJ* 2010; 340: b5650.

60. Rigaud A, Craplet M. The 'Loi Evin': a French exception. Available at http://www.ias.org.uk/What-we-do/Publication-archive/The-Globe/Issue-2-2004-amp-1-2004/The-Loi-Evin-a-French-exception.aspx (2004, accessed 19 September 2016).

61. Surugue L. Euro 2016: Football fans see alcohol adverts once every minute during TV matches. Available at: https://www.ibtimes.co.uk/euro-2016-football-fans-see-alcohol-adverts-once-every-minute-during-tv-matches-1567636 (accessed 8 March 2018).

62. World Health Organization. Evidence for the effectiveness and cost-effectiveness of interventions to reduce alcohol-related harm. Available at: http://www.euro.who.int/__data/assets/pdf_file/0020/43319/E92823.pdf (2009, accessed 19 September 2016).

63. World Health Organization. European action plan to reduce the harmful use of alcohol 2012–2020. Available at http://www.euro.who.int/en/health-topics/disease-prevention/alcohol-use/publications/2012/european-action-plan-to-reduce-the-harmful-use-of-alcohol-20122021 (2012, accessed 8 March 2018).

64. Wakefield, M, Loken, B, Hornik, R. Use of mass media campaigns to change health behaviour. *Lancet* 2010; 376: 1261–1271.

65. Buykx P, Gilligan C, Ward B, et al. Public support for alcohol policies associated with knowledge of cancer risk. *Int J Drug Policy* 2015; 26: 371–379.

66. Department of Health (DoH). *UK Chief Medical Officers' Alcohol Guidelines Review: Summary of the Proposed New Guidelines*. London: DoH, 2015.

67. Edler R, Shults R, Sleet D, et al. Effectiveness of mass media campaigns for reducing drink and driving and alcohol-invovled crashes: a systematic review. *Am J Prev Med* 2004; 27: 57–65.

68. Jones L, James M, Jefferson T, et al. A review of the effectiveness and cost effectiveness of interventions delivered in primary and secondary schools to prevent and/or reduce alcohol use by young people under 18 years old. Available at: https://www.nice.org.uk/guidance/ph7/evidence/effectiveness-and-cost-effectivenessreview-369704701 (2007, accessed 19 September 2016).

69. Foxcroft DR, Tsertsvadze A. Universal school-based prevention programs for alcohol misuse in young people. *Cochrane Database Syst Rev* 2011; (5): CD009113.

70. Wilkinson C, Room R. Warnings on alcohol containers and advertisements: international experience and evidence on effects. *Drug Alcohol Rev* 2009; 28: 426–435.

71. Guillemont J, Léon C. [Committee on National Alcohol Policy and Action (2009). Labelling on alcoholic drinks packaging: The French experience]. Available at: http://inpes.santepubliquefrance.fr/CFESBases/catalogue/pdf/1117.pdf (2009, accessed 8 March 2018; in French).

72. Anderson, P, Baumberg, B. Alcohol in Europe: A public health perspective. Available at: http://ec.europa.eu/health/ph_determinants/life_style/alcohol/documents/alcohol_europe.pdf (2008, accessed 19 September 2016).

73. Pidd K, Berry J, Roche A, et al. Estimating the cost of alcohol-related absenteeism in the Australian workforce: the importance of consumption patters. *Med J Aust* 2006; 185: 637–641.

74. Webb G, Shakeshaft A, Sanson-Fisher R, Harvard A. A systematic review of work-place interventions for alcohol-related problems. *Addiction* 2009; 104: 365–377.

75. Kaner EF, Beyer F, Dickinson HO, et al. Brief interventions for excessive drinkers in primary health care settings. *Cochrane Database Syst Rev* 2007; (2): CD004148.

76. Babor T, Higgins-Biddle J, Saunders J, Moneiro M. AUDIT. The Alcohol Use Disorders Identification Test: Guidelines for Use in Primary care. Available at: http://apps.who.int/iris/bitstream/10665/67205/1/WHO_MSD_MSB_01.6a.pdf (2001, accessed 19 September 2016).

77. Kaner EF, Bland M, Cassidy P, et al. Effectiveness of screening and brief alcohol intervention in primary care (SIPS trial): pragmatic cluster randomised controlled trial. *BMJ* 2013; 346: e8501

78. National Institute for Health and Care Excellence. Alcohol use disorders: prevention. Available at: https://www.nice.org.uk/guidance/ph24?unlid=1595622652016227234415 (2010, accessed 19 September 2016).

CHAPTER 36

Prevention of drug addiction

Olive Mukamana and Patricia Conrod

Introduction

Drug addiction or dependence is a result of problematic use of psychoactive substances, including illicit drugs, such as cannabis, amphetamine-type stimulants, cocaine, opioids and psychoactive medication [1, 2]. The World Health Organization (WHO) defines the dependence syndrome as a:

> cluster of behavioural, cognitive, and physiological phenomena that develop after repeated substance use and that typically include a strong desire to take the drug, difficulties in controlling its use, persisting in its use despite harmful consequences, a higher priority given to drug use than to other activities and obligations, increased tolerance, and sometimes a physical withdrawal state[1] [3].

Based on the same indicators of drug dependence, drug addiction can be categorized as mild, moderate, or severe, as defined by the American Psychiatric Association [2, 4, 5]. In neuroscience, drug addiction is viewed as a 'chronically relapsing disorder' that develops in three stages: (i) experimentation or initiation of use; (ii) transition to consistent heavy use; and (iii) transition to a dependent state of uncontrolled use or relapses [4, 6]. When an individual transitions from the initiation stage to heavy and consistent use, drug-induced neurotoxic effects cause the development of sensitization and tolerance, and they can transition to the addiction stage, during which the effects of drugs on the brain manifest themselves by uncontrolled use, physiological dependence, and related harm [4, 6].

Burden of drug use and drug addiction

According to the United Nations Office on Drugs and Crime (UNODC) 2012 world drug report, an estimated 3.4–6.6% of the world's population (153–300 million people) aged 15–64 years used illicit drugs in 2010 and almost 12% of all illicit drug users suffered from drug dependence and other drug use disorders [7]. According to the same report, and the WHO, cannabis is the most widely used drug worldwide followed by amphetamines, opioids, and cocaine [2, 7]. The literature shows that drug use is not distributed evenly across regions and countries. Its prevalence is shown to be higher in developed countries than in developing countries, although comparable statistics are less available for the latter [1, 2]. The United

Nations and the WHO field surveys conducted in 17 countries of the Americas, Europe, Middle East, Africa, Asia, and Oceania show that the USA has the highest levels of drug use; African and Middle Eastern countries report much lower levels, and the lowest levels are reported in Japan and China [8]. As reported by various authors, the availability of quality data on the prevalence and burden of drug use and drug addiction is limited by challenges of collecting accurate information on an often stigmatized and illegal behaviour like drug use [2, 8, 9]. Nevertheless, available findings show that drug use and addiction are significant public health problems worldwide because of the effects they have on drug users themselves and the society as a whole [2, 7–10].

Problematic drug use is associated with various adverse health effects that contribute considerably to the global burden of disease. Between 99,000 and 253,000 deaths in 2010 were attributable to illicit drug use among those aged 15–64 years worldwide [7]. Drug-related deaths and morbidities include those due to overdose, drug-related crimes, accidents, and injuries, as well as medical conditions caused or worsened by drug use [7, 8, 10]. For example, injection drugs play an important role in the transmission of infectious diseases such as HIV, hepatitis C and hepatitis B; amphetamines can cause fatal arrhythmias or hyperthermia; and cocaine can induce stroke [2, 7]. Chronic or heavy use of cannabis is associated with an increased risk of psychotic symptoms or schizophrenia, particularly in individuals hereditarily predisposed to this disorder [11–13]. Heavy use of cannabis also increases the risk of developing cardiovascular diseases, bronchitis, lung, and digestive tract cancers [1, 10, 14]. In addition, cannabis use increases the risk of using other illicit drugs such as heroin and cocaine [1, 10].

The burden of drug use is more considerable among young people, as shown by various studies reporting greater levels of drug use among adolescents and young adults than in older adults [8, 10]. The UNODC shows that drug use prevalence rates increase during adolescence and peak among people in the 18–25 years age group [7]. Similar trends are reported in other studies showing that in most countries the initiation of drug use is concentrated in mid- and late-teenage years [1, 10]. Drug effects are also more persistent and severe among young users than adult users [1, 10, 14]. For example, 1 in 10 cannabis users in the general population transition to a dependent state, whereas one in three adolescent users develop dependence [1]. The consequences of regular or heavy drug use among young people include psychological and physiological impairment, school drop out, or poor academic performance associated with significant productivity losses and societal costs

---

[1] Reproduced from Health Systems Topics: Substance Abuse, with permission from the World Health Organization. Available from: http://www.who.int/topics/substance_abuse/en/.

[10, 14]. The cost for the treatment of illicit drug use was estimated at $US200–250 billion 2010, equivalent to 0.3–0.4% of the global gross domestic product (GDP) [7]. Productivity losses due to illicit drug use in the USA were estimated at $US120 billion (0.9% of GDP) in 2007 [7]. In Canada, productivity losses were estimated at CAN$8244 million, equivalent to 0.4% of the GDP in 2002 [7, 15], and a similar study in Australia estimated productivity losses at AUS$2.1 billion (0.3% of GDP) in the 2004–05 financial year [7].

Risk factors for drug addiction

Individuals have different levels of vulnerability to transition from experimenting with or occasionally using drugs to using consistently or to reach a dependent state [4, 6]. This vulnerability is related to various factors that are critical in establishing prevention strategies. Two types of risk factors for substance abuse and addiction have been identified: (i) individual factors, including genetic, biological, or psychological factors; and (ii) environmental risk factors, such as policies, the social context, and economic conditions affecting drug access and drug use acceptability [16]. It is important to note that these categories of risk factors are not mutually exclusive as several factors can manifest themselves across various risk dimensions. For example, besides their impact on drug availability and other contextual aspects, laws and norms affect attitudes and behaviours toward drug use [16], and thus exert psychological influences at the individual and interpersonal level.

At the environmental level, the context in which one lives involves parental, peer, or cultural influences mainly affecting drug-related social norms and behaviours, whereas policies such as those regulating drug markets and advertisements affect both drug availability and drug-related social norms [4, 10, 17]. Moreover, poor socio-economic conditions such as unemployment, homelessness, social isolation, and poor academic achievement have been shown to expose individuals to various risky behaviours, including drug use and related harm [10, 16].

At a more individual level, various genetic, biological, or psychological factors explain why the vulnerability of individuals exposed to the same general or environmental factors can vary. Adoption and twin studies have shown that there are several genetic factors involved in various forms of substance misuse [4, 16, 18, 19]. Studies have also demonstrated the role of genetically mediated personality risk factors in predisposing individuals to drug misuse and psychopathological disorders that are often co-morbid with substance use disorders [4, 14, 20, 21]. Castellanos and Conrod [21] proposed a model explaining the vulnerability to substance misuse and psychopathology associated with four personality traits: (i) impulsivity and (ii) sensation-seeking that belong to the disinhibited personality domain; and (iii) hopelessness and (iv) anxiety sensitivity that belong to the inhibited domain (21). Impulsivity is associated with substance misuse and addictive behaviour through poor response inhibition and a weakened capacity to control drug-taking behaviour [4, 14, 21]. Impulsive traits are also associated with externalizing disorders such as antisocial behaviour [4, 14, 21]. Sensation seeking is associated with a sensitivity to drug-induced reward and the reinforcing effect of drugs [14, 21]. These two disinhibited traits are also associated with other risk factors for drug use and misuse such as deviant peer influences [14, 21]. However, hopelessness is associated with substance misuse and mood disorders through a motivational process of coping

with negative affect experienced by individuals high in this trait [14, 21]. Anxiety sensitivity is associated with a high sensitivity to the arousal-dampening effects of drugs, increased withdrawal symptoms, and anxiety disorders [14, 21]. Conrod and Nikolaou [4] proposed a fifth personality profile associated with substance misuse: the psychosis risk. This personality trait is vulnerable to substances of abuse, particularly cannabis, and their exacerbating effect on psychotic-like experiences or psychotic disorders [4]. Psychopathology has also been shown to contribute to individuals' vulnerability to substance misuse and addictive behaviours, and to exacerbate such behaviours in individuals with the abovementioned personality traits [4, 14, 21].

From a developmental point of view, the psychosocial, genetic, and environmental factors that are present from early childhood further increase a child's risk for early drug use initiation, which is also a known risk factor for problematic drug consumption later in adult life [4, 22]. Early onset of drug use potentially contributes to drug use disorders and related harm by disrupting normal brain maturational changes [4, 10], and it has been shown to be an important risk factor for severe or long-term substance misuse, mental health disorders and other psychosocial consequences of drug misuse [1, 22–25]. The transition from childhood to adulthood also represents a common risk factor as biological, cognitive, and social changes occurring during this period predispose adolescents to engage in risky behaviours such as drug use [4]. Research shows that in addition to predisposing adolescents to risky behaviours, these changes make the brain more vulnerable to the pharmacological effects of drugs [4]. Adolescence is also a period during which symptoms of mental health disorders appear, increasing adolescents' vulnerability to problematic drug use [10].

Vulnerabilities at the individual and environmental level interact with themselves and with drug neurotoxic effects when individuals go on to experience heavy and frequent use, further increasing the risk to transition into a dependent state [4, 10, 26].

In the following sections we review prevention strategies targeting the main risk factors for drug addiction and we provide examples of effective interventions. Prevention interventions are categorized as universal when they are provided to the general population, and as selective if they are targeting high-risk populations and indicated as those targeting individuals already experiencing problematic drug use.

Prevention strategies

Universal interventions targeted at the general public

Universal approaches to prevent drug addiction and other drug-related problems mainly include supply-and-demand control policies aimed at limiting drug accessibility and targeting social influences which affect drug acceptability. They also include educational and psychosocial interventions aimed at improving knowledge about the adverse effects of drugs, drug-related attitudes, social skills, and behaviours.

Supply-and-demand control interventions
Law enforcement and pricing policies

Drug supply-and-demand control policies aim to regulate drug markets, to affect suppliers' ability to produce and sell drugs, and to limit consumers' ability to access drugs while protecting non-users from drug exposure [10, 17]. They mainly involve law enforcement and other restrictive measures aimed at regulating drug markets, reducing drug supply and consumption. The literature shows that the illegality of drugs aims to discourage their usage by means of sanctions for those violating drug laws (e.g. arrests and imprisonments) and by limiting their availability on illegal markets, which results in an increase of their retail prices [17]. However, the effect of harsh penalties such as arrests and imprisonments is poorly researched and the evidence showing that such sanctions affect retail prices is weak [16, 17]. Other studies have shown that brief penalties such as overnight incarcerations and coerced abstinence can significantly reduce drug use in offenders under criminal justice supervision [17, 27, 28]. The introduction of laws regulating precursor substances involved in the production of illegal drugs have also been used as a strategy to discourage supply and demand, although findings on their effect on drug usage are mixed [17, 29–31]. Overall, there is little evidence to support the effectiveness of drug-control policies on a reduction in drug use, but the available evidence suggests that when law enforcement raises drug prices and keep them high, the initiation of their use by non-users and consumption among regular users can be reduced [17, 32].

With respect to the non-medical use of prescription psychoactive drugs, prescription regimens are the main control strategies established in developed countries [17]. As reported by Strang et al. [17], those with demonstrated beneficial effects include pricing policies, prescription restrictions, the withdrawal of prescription availability, and the control of opioid substitution therapy administration.

A number of caveats for certain policies have to be noted. The effectiveness of most supply control policies have not been adequately assessed in terms of their effect on the reduction of drug use and drug use initiation, especially in young people, despite the considerable burden of disease associated with drug use by young people [10, 17]. Findings from studies of pricing policies suggest that prices do not affect youth substance use the same way they affect adults' consumption, showing that youth-focused research is still needed to understand how these policies contribute to youth drug use and related harm [10, 33]. Furthermore, studies have shown that some interventions can unintentionally lead to negative outcomes. For example, arrests, imprisonments, school exclusion, and other severe penalties for those violating drug laws lead to marginalization and social isolation, which expose them to additional health and social problems [10, 17]. Policies forcing users to adherence to evidence-based programmes that help them reduce or stop using drugs have been suggested as safer and more-cost effective alternatives to harsh and harmful sanctions, especially among young people [10, 17]. Another example is that of policies aimed to restrict supply and accessibility by raising drug prices, which can lead to an increase in the use of cheaper and unregulated alternatives believed to be as dangerous as, or even more, harmful than the regulated options [10]. With respect to cannabis use in young people, especially in areas where decriminalization processes are underway, it has been suggested that permitting young people to have access to regulated low-potency products can allow to reduce or suppress the use of unregulated and unsafe high-potency alternatives available on the illegal market [10].

Regulating advertisement

Many countries adopted advertisement restrictions for substances such as alcohol and tobacco products, especially in regard to advertising to young people, and similar restrictions should be considered for other substances where decriminalization processes are underway. The rapidly evolving digital marketing strategies also carry various challenges that need to be addressed by advertisement regulations. One challenging characteristic of digital marketing strategies is that they go beyond traditional marketing channels and allow marketers to interact with their targeted audience mainly via social media platforms [10, 34]. Such strategies have the capacity to influence reward-processing behaviours and self-control abilities through the use of social influence, games, and competitions that are particularly relevant to young people [10, 35, 36]. Moreover, studies have shown that Internet-based marketing can reduce the effectiveness of regulating other advertising channels and further increase drug exposure and demand [34, 37]. As the support for cannabis legalization increases, policies should pay particular attention to these strategies, and, most importantly, to the risks they pose to young people.

Educational and psychosocial interventions

Educational and psychosocial interventions are widely provided in universal approaches that generally aim to reduce drug demand by improving knowledge about the adverse effects of drugs and by developing social skills to resist influences to use drugs. Most educational and psychosocial interventions are delivered in school settings where they target the risk factors associated with young people and parental skills [17].

School-based interventions

School-based programmes are recognized for their ability to reach a large number of young people at low cost [10, 38]. Most programmes proven to be effective in preventing drug use focus on the development of general life skills and competencies to resist influences to use drugs [10, 17]. Successful programmes also include the correction of misconceptions about the prevalence and the acceptability of drug use, especially in young people, and they involve interactive techniques such as face-to-face activities, peer interactions, and adult facilitators [10, 17]. For example, a prevention programme that focused on promoting self-esteem, appropriate relationships, and resistance to social influences to use drugs led to a substantial reduction of drug use among high-school students in 56 US public schools [39]. The EU-Dap study conducted in seven European countries also showed that a curriculum-based programme named 'Unplugged', which used a comprehensive social influence approach in addition to life skills components, was associated with a reduction of cannabis use initiation among 12–14-year-old pupils 18 months post-intervention [40, 41]. The 'Good Behaviour Game' is another example of a universal preventive programme that have been shown to have long-term effects [17, 42]. This classroom-based programme used a behaviour management approach in European and US elementary and primary schools, and it has been shown to reduce drug misuse and dependence among males at the age of 19–21 years [42].

Programmes that use didactic educational techniques are mainly effective in improving knowledge about the adverse effects of drugs, but they have smaller effects on behaviour change compared with programmes using interactive techniques [10, 17, 38]. The DARE (Drug Abuse Resistance Education) project is an example of a widely implemented drug education programme in the USA that uses didactic tactics shown to have smaller effect sizes than interactive teaching techniques [43]. Most mass-media campaigns also use didactic educational tactics considered to be the limiting factor of their effectiveness in drug-use prevention [17].

Parental programmes

Parental programmes involve training and support to promote appropriate parental involvement in children activities, communication skills, and abilities to manage child behavioural problems [10, 44]. Most parenting programmes are components of more complex interventions that target other aspects influencing youth behaviours [44]. A systematic review of parenting programmes for preventing substance misuse in young people aged 18 years or younger concluded that the most effective programmes in reducing substance misuse seemed to be those focusing on promoting active parental involvement, the development of social skills and personal responsibility in young people, and those that addressed substance use-related problems [44]. The 'Preparing for the Drug Free Years' and the 'Iowa Strengthening Families Programmes' are examples of parent training programmes coupled with skill building in children with the aim of addressing various risk factors (e.g. poor quality of the relationship between parents and children, poor discipline skills) and protective factors (e.g. peer resistance skills, empathy, and parent–child bonding) [45]. The programmes were rigorously tested and shown to delay substance use initiation and to reduce use among high-school students with small-to-moderate effect sizes [45]. However, the available evidence on parenting programmes shows a lack of interventions addressing the challenges of digital advertisement and social media platforms with regard to their impact on youth drug use [10].

Besides restrictive supply/demand control policies and programmes targeting youth and parenting skills, policies that focus on the physical and the socio-economic environments have been suggested as strategies that can help prevent problematic drug use. These include programmes that allow for better supervision of the environments where young people are most likely to gather (e.g. parks, school playgrounds, etc.) and especially those that allow for better organization of after-school activities, which have been shown to be highly effective in preventing adolescent drug use and antisocial behaviours [10, 46]. Similarly, the link between poor socio-economic conditions (e.g. unemployment, poverty, poor academic achievement, social isolation) and problematic drug use has been demonstrated by various studies [10, 16], suggesting that interventions improving these conditions can help prevent drug-use problems. Research has shown that economic recessions are linked to risky behaviours such as using and selling drugs, particularly among young people [47]. Evans-Lacko et al. [48] also showed that job losses and reduced income greatly affect those with mental health needs, which, in turn, reinforces their vulnerability to severe psychopathology and drug-use disorders. Interventions that help improve socio-economic conditions can therefore contribute to the prevention of drug addiction and related harm, although empirical research on the direct effect of such interventions on drug use is limited. For example, studies have shown that family support interventions promoting early childhood education and easy access to health and social services in low-income families have promising outcomes on antisocial behaviours, school performance, and employment in adolescence [16], suggesting that interventions promoting social and economic well-being can have a significant impact on various vulnerability and protective factors implicated in drug addiction.

Interventions targeting high-risk populations

Some interventions target specific population groups because of the risks they are particularly exposed to compared with the general population, and there is evidence that such selective strategies can be highly effective in preventing or reducing drug use. This is especially true for interventions targeting the previously discussed genetically mediated pathways implicated in drug misuse: the negative affect or the psychopathology pathway, the disinhibited behaviours or impulsive pathway, and the reward-sensitivity pathway. Few prevention programmes target these factors, despite their widely documented role in individuals' predisposition to drug misuse and related harm [4, 20, 21]. We highlight two examples of selective programmes delivered to high-risk groups with personality or behavioural risk factors with demonstrated efficacy. Firstly, the 'Preventure' programme, which mostly targets young people who score high on four personality profiles at risk for addiction and mental health problems: impulsivity, sensation seeking, anxiety sensitivity, and hopelessness [49, 50]. This brief coping skills intervention involves psychoeducational, motivational, and cognitive–behavioural components mainly aimed at building youth resilience in situations where they are prone to engage in risky behaviours such as drug use [50]. It has been rigorously tested in school settings in the UK, Canada, Australia, and the Netherlands, and has been proven effective in delaying the onset of cannabis and cocaine use, as well as reducing the frequency of the drug use with moderate-to-large effect sizes 2 years post-intervention [49, 50]. The programme has also been shown to have herd effects on low-risk students who did not receive it, suggesting that by delaying substance use among the most vulnerable, the programme can exert protective effects at the population level [51].

Another selective programme that has reported strong and long-term effects on youth drug use involved social and problem-solving skills training that was given to kindergarten children with behavioural problems, as well as a child-rearing skills training given to parents [52]. Eight years post-intervention (when those who were selected for the intervention were in their teenage years) the programme was shown to be effective in reducing drug experimentation [52]. This effect was associated with the intervention's influence on pre-adolescent impulsivity, a known risk factor for addiction later in adulthood [21, 52].

Besides their effects on problematic drug use, these programmes were shown to have other beneficial effects, including the prevention and the reduction of youth internalizing and externalizing problems such as depression, anxiety, and antisocial behaviours, which are also risk factors for drug misuse and often co-morbid with drug-use disorders [52, 53].

Beyond primary prevention, which mainly consists of interventions targeted at the general population and high-risk groups as shown by the examples outlined earlier, indicated interventions are targeted at those already experiencing problematic drug use as secondary prevention strategies.

Brief interventions targeting drug users

Studies have shown that regular and heavy drug users have an increased risk of transitioning into a dependent state [4], and interventions targeting such users are necessary to prevent addiction and other consequences of sustained drug use. Most interventions targeting drug users involve screening and brief interventions delivered in primary care and other community settings [17]. They generally use brief motivational interviewing and other brief interventions aimed at increasing the motivation to change drug use behaviours and at providing guidance throughout the change process [10, 17]. Studies have shown that brief cognitive behavioural interventions with the provision of self-help reading material and consultations provided by general practitioners can reduce the frequency of amphetamines and benzodiazepines among regular users [54–56]. Another example consists of a brief motivational intervention delivered by peer educators to cocaine and heroin users who were not receiving any other drug abuse treatment, which was shown to reduce their consumption without the significant involvement of the treatment system [57].

With adolescents and young adults, brief interventions are mainly delivered in school settings and some have been shown to reduce drug use and encourage abstinence in targeted individuals. For example, a 1-hour session of motivational interviewing delivered to college students was proven effective in reducing cannabis use and this reduction was shown to be greater among heavier users and high-risk youth with a low socio-economic status [58]. The Preventure programme, which consists of two sessions of coping skills training, was also proven effective in reducing the use of illicit drugs in high-school students [49]. Outside school settings juvenile drug courts integrating evidence-based contingency management interventions, and family engagement were shown to reduce youth drug use [17, 59].

However, other studies have shown that brief motivational interviewing had no effect among young cocaine and ecstasy users [60], and that in certain cases where positive effects were detected, these deteriorated over time [61]. A more recent study has also shown that screening and brief interventions did not reduce illicit drug use and prescription drug misuse in primary care patients [62]. Findings on the large-scale implementation of these interventions are also mixed [17, 63], suggesting that more efforts should be dedicated to investigating the factors that determine their success in various settings.

Selective prevention strategies are often believed to produce stigma, but this assumption has not been subjected to adequate empirical assessment [10, 64]. Factors that may cause stigma or place programme recipients at particular risk should be thoroughly investigated to identify methods of avoiding such risks and optimizing programmes' beneficial effects.

Comprehensive prevention strategy

Considering the multiple risk factors for drug addiction and the substantial burden of disease associated with youth drug misuse in particular, a comprehensive and youth-focused approach seems to be a promising strategy to address the various risks early enough to avoid the costly consequences of this problem [16, 65].

Effective universal, selective, and indicated prevention programmes can be integrated in a well-resourced and coordinated comprehensive strategy in order to address known risk factors in the general population, among high-risk groups, and among those already experiencing drug-use problems. The integration of these different approaches (universal and selective) is necessary because most universal programmes do not focus on the individual risk factors for drug misuse such as personality and psychopathology, which might explain their small effect on drug-related behaviours,

suggesting that selective interventions focusing on these factors are essential for a successful prevention strategy. Particular attention should therefore be focused on pursuing the evaluation of selective programmes proven to be highly effective in preventing and reducing drug misuse in certain high-risk groups or those proven effective in preventing psychosocial precursors of drug misuse such as mental health and behavioural problems. Most of these programmes have been tested in school settings of developed countries and they should be assessed in other settings to identify the best way they can benefit various high-risk groups in different socio-economic contexts.

Developmental approach

In a comprehensive approach to prevention, the integration of effective universal and selective approaches should account for the developmental course of addiction with a particular attention to the transition period from childhood to young adulthood marked with increased vulnerability. As previously discussed, early drug-use initiation and frequent drug use in this period are widely demonstrated risk factors for addiction and related harm and drug effects have been shown to be more persistent and severe in young users than adults [1, 7, 10]. Howeve, the literature shows that each substance-related problem avoided early in life, or delayed, translates into significant benefits across the lifespan both at the individual and the societal level [17, 66]. Such evidence shows that timing of prevention programme delivery is critical and supports the importance of youth-focused interventions implemented early before substance use problems begin.

Based on Conrod and Nikolaou's [4] description of the developmental process of addiction (Fig. 36.1), universal, selective, and indicated prevention programmes can target the most important factors in each phase of this developmental process. Childhood factors such as the genetic or psychological predisposition to drug use can be addressed by selective interventions proven effective when delivered during childhood or pre-adolescence. The child and parent intervention that significantly reduced drug experimentation during adolescence through its influence on childhood behavioural problems is an example of how a developmentally informed programme can successfully mitigate early vulnerability factors [52]. Universal school and family-based interventions shown to improve child competences and parenting skills can also address important factors such as parent–child relationships and other interpersonal influences related to drug use.

The developmental process of addiction also shows adolescence as a common risk factor for behaviours such as drug experimentation because of the various biological, social, and neural maturation changes that take place in this period [4]. Consequently, adolescence should be the focus of prevention strategies, including universal psychosocial interventions proven to have protective effects on adolescent drug use by promoting general life skills, competences to resist drug use influences, and parenting skills. The 'Good Behaviour Programme' [42], 'Unplugged' [40], the 'Preparing for the Drug Free Years', and the 'Strengthening Families Programmes' [45] are examples of effective universal interventions that are adapted to this developmental period and the risks it represents. For adolescents who are at higher risk of drug misuse owing to various biological, genetic, or psychological factors, there is a need for youth-friendly interventions specifically targeting these risk factors (e.g. early interventions targeting risk factors

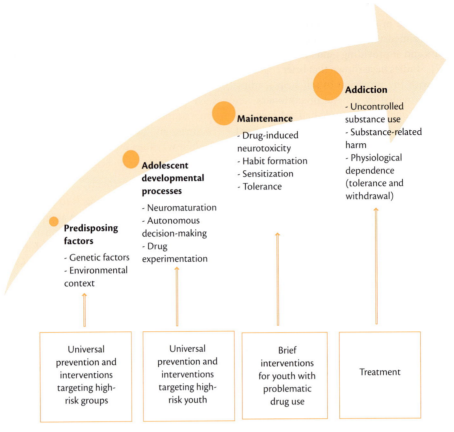

Fig. 36.1 Overview of the developmental process of addiction.

Source: Adapted from *J Child Psychol Psychiatry*, 57(3), Conrod PJ, Nikolaou K, Annual Research Review: On the developmental neuropsychology of substance use disorders, pp. 371-94, Copyright (2016), with permission from John Wiley and Sons.

for drug use and mental health problems), such as the Preventure programme, which not only reduces drug misuse and psychopathology among high-risk younge people, but also has a significant potential to protect low-risk individuals [49–51]. For individuals who progress to drug misuse and reach the maintenance phase during which various pre-existing vulnerabilities interact with drug effects [4], effective and youth-friendly interventions aimed to reduce or stop drug consumption (e.g. [58, 59]) are necessary to prevent the transition into addiction.

Furthermore, considering the demonstrated association between mental health problems, poor socio-economic conditions, and problematic drug use [4, 10, 14, 16], a truly comprehensive strategy should concentrate on the whole person and improve access to integrated health and social services, especially for young people most at risk. The available evidence for the effectiveness of various psychosocial interventions suggests that their integration with other youth health services and initiatives promoting social and economic well-being would result in greater protective effects by addressing a wider range of factors earlier in the trajectory of drug use. Initiatives such as 'Jigsaw', in Ireland [67]; 'Headspace', in Australia [68, 69]; or the 'British Columbia Integrated Youth Services Initiative' (BC-IYSI), in Canada [70] are examples of integrated youth services that have the potential to prevent problematic drug use by targeting various risk and protective factors in young people. Both the Jigsaw and the BC-IYSI are based on the Australian Headspace model of integrated community-based youth

services primarily aimed at improving access to early mental health intervention programmes for adolescents and young adults with integrated services targeting substance use problems, and other health and social issues [67, 69, 70]. Although the efficacy of these initiatives have not yet been rigorously tested, especially regarding youth substance misuse, they have shown promising results with respect to service access, youth psychological distress, and psychosocial functioning [67, 68].

Considering that a large number of young people can be easily and inexpensively reached in schools, we recommend a novel approach that could link such integrated services to evidence-based school interventions and thus proactively engaging the necessary resources for the delivery of early intervention programmes before severe and costly problems begin. As illustrated in Fig. 36.2, school-based universal prevention and a regular well-being assessment can facilitate the identification of youth needs, especially for those most at risk for substance misuse and related problems who can benefit from early. School-based regular needs assessment would also facilitate the delivery of integrated services to those experiencing problems.

In a comprehensive approach to prevention linking integrated services to youth-relevant environments, such services would be more proactive in identifying and preventing potential serious problems, and this would result in reduced bottlenecks as there would be fewer complicated cases that need intensive services. Furthermore, besides reaching a large number of young people at

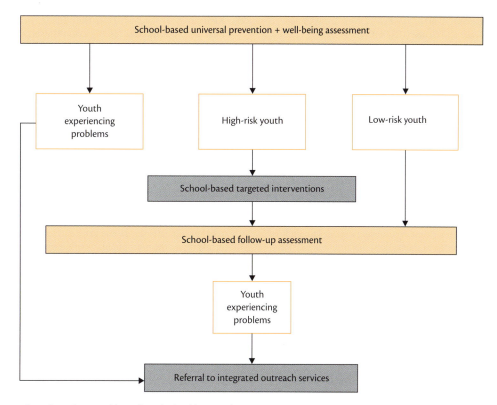

Fig. 36.2 Linking integrated youth services to evidence-based school interventions.

low cost and facilitating a timely delivery of services adapted to their needs, such an approach can normalize mental health interventions and reduce stigma for those receiving them. More generally, this approach can positively impact on young people's school performance and thus promote their well-being across their lifespan.

Conclusions

Investing in research and interventions that allow for the development of youth-focused policies is a promising and cost-effective approach to prevent early drug use and its consequences.

In a comprehensive and developmental approach to prevention, future research should assess how universal and selective interventions can effectively be integrated to reduce early vulnerabilities and enhance protective factors, both in the general population and among high-risk populations.

However, most universal policy measures that target environmental factors, such as drug availability and acceptability, have not been adequately researched, particularly in regard to their effect on youth drug use. Youth-focused assessment is needed to understand what works for this particularly vulnerable population and to develop universal policy measures that effectively prevent early drug misuse. Thorough examination of the costs and benefits of such measures is also needed to avoid or minimize the negative consequences they can inadvertently lead to. However, selective interventions targeting high-risk groups have received less attention in the literature relative to the larger efforts dedicated to universal interventions. Nevertheless, given the evidence showing that selective approaches are highly effective in preventing and reducing drug use in young people [50, 52], more investment should be dedicated to their broader implementation and evaluation in

different cultural and socio-economic contexts. Furthermore, the evidence on the significant potential for selective interventions to exert protective effects at the population level [51] suggests that further investigation is needed to determine whether they could be a more cost-effective solution than the widely implemented universal programmes with little evidence of effectiveness on drug-use behaviours.

The collaboration between researchers, service providers, and decision-makers is thus necessary to establish evidence-based, developmentally informed, and comprehensive strategies to prevent addiction and its costly consequences for individuals and the society as a whole. It is obvious that a successful comprehensive approach to prevention also requires sufficient and long-term investment.

References

1. World Health Organization. *The Health and Social Effects of Nonmedical Cannabis Use*. Geneva: WHO, 2016.
2. Degenhardt L, Hall W. Extent of illicit drug use and dependence, and their contribution to the global burden of disease. *Lancet* 2012; 379: 55–70.
3. World Health Organization. Substance abuse. Available at: http://www.who.int/topics/substance_abuse/en/ (2016, accessed 9 March 2018).
4. J Conrod P, Nikolaou K. Annual research review: on the developmental neuropsychology of substance use disorders. *J Child Psychol Psychiatry* 2016; 57: 371–394.
5. American Psychiatric Association. *Diagnostic and Statistical Manual of Mental Disorders (DSM-5*)*. Arlington, VA: American Psychiatric Publishing, 2013.
6. Le Moal M, Koob GF. Drug addiction: pathways to the disease and pathophysiological perspectives. *Eur Neuropsychopharmacol* 2007; 17: 377–393.

7. World Health Organization. *World Drug Report*. New York: United Nations Offices on Drugs and Crime (UNODC), 2012.

8. Degenhardt L, Chiu W-T, Sampson N, et al. Toward a global view of alcohol, tobacco, cannabis, and cocaine use: findings from the WHO World Mental Health Surveys. *PLOS Med* 2008; 5: e141.

9. Kessler RC, Aguilar-Gaxiola S, Alonso J, et al. The global burden of mental disorders: an update from the WHO World Mental Health (WMH) surveys. *Epidemiol Psichiatr Soc* 2009; 18: 23–33.

10. Anderson P, Braddick F, Conrod P, et al. *The New Governance of Addictive Substances and Behaviours*. Oxford: Oxford University Press, 2016.

11. Arseneault L, Cannon M, Witton J, Murray RM. Causal association between cannabis and psychosis: examination of the evidence. *Br J Psychiatry* 2004; 184: 110–117.

12. Caspi A, Moffitt TE, Cannon M, et al. Moderation of the effect of adolescent-onset cannabis use on adult psychosis by a functional polymorphism in the catechol-O-methyltransferase gene: longitudinal evidence of a gene X environment interaction. *Biol Psychiatry* 2005; 57: 1117–1127.

13. Mackie C, O'Leary-Barrett M, Al-Khudhairy N, et al. Adolescent bullying, cannabis use and emerging psychotic experiences: a longitudinal general population study. *Psychol Med* 2013; 43: 1033–1044.

14. Castellanos-Ryan N, O'Leary-Barrett M, Conrod PJ. Substance-use in childhood and adolescence: a brief overview of developmental processes and their clinical implications. *J Can Acad Child Adolesc Psychiatry* 2013; 22: 41–46.

15. Rehm J, Gnam W, Popova S, et al. The costs of alcohol, illegal drugs, and tobacco in Canada, 2002. *J Stud Alcohol Drugs* 2007; 68: 886–895.

16. Hawkins JD, Catalano RF, Miller JY. Risk and protective factors for alcohol and other drug problems in adolescence and early adulthood: implications for substance abuse prevention. *Psychol Bull* 1992; 112: 64.

17. Strang J, Babor T, Caulkins J, Fischer B, Foxcroft D, Humphreys K. Drug policy and the public good: evidence for effective interventions. *Lancet* 2012; 379: 71–83.

18. Kendler KS, Ohlsson H, Maes HH, Sundquist K, Lichtenstein P, Sundquist J. A population-based Swedish Twin and Sibling Study of cannabis, stimulant and sedative abuse in men. *Drug Alcohol Depend* 2015; 149: 49–54.

19. Lynskey MT, Heath A, Nelson E, et al. Genetic and environmental contributions to cannabis dependence in a national young adult twin sample. *Psychol Med* 2002; 32: 195–207.

20. Sher KJ, Bartholow BD, Wood MD. Personality and substance use disorders: a prospective study. *J Consult Clin Psychol* 2000; 68: 818.

21. Castellanos-Ryan N, Conrod P. Personality and substance misuse: evidence for a four-factor model of vulnerability. In: Verster J, Brady K, Galanter M, Conrod P (eds). *Drug Abuse and Addiction in Medical Illness*. Berlin: Springer, 2012, pp. 47–62.

22. Grant BF, Dawson DA. Age of onset of drug use and its association with DSM-IV drug abuse and dependence: results from the National Longitudinal Alcohol Epidemiologic Survey. *J Subst Abuse* 1998; 10: 163–173.

23. Anthony JC, Petronis KR. Early-onset drug use and risk of later drug problems. *Drug Alcohol Depend* 1995; 40: 9–15.

24. Behrendt S, Wittchen H-U, Höfler M, Lieb R, Beesdo K. Transitions from first substance use to substance use disorders in adolescence: is early onset associated with a rapid escalation? *Drug Alcohol Depend* 2009; 99: 68–78.

25. Teesson M, Degenhardt L, Hall W, Lynskey M, Toumbourou JW, Patton G. Substance use and mental health in longitudinal perspective. In: Stockwell T, Gruenewald P, Toumbourou J, Loxley W (eds). *Preventing Harmful Substance Use: The Evidence Base for Policy and Practice*. New York: Wiley, 2005, p. 43.

26. Byrd AL, Manuck SB. MAOA, childhood maltreatment, and antisocial behavior: meta-analysis of a gene-environment interaction. *Biol Psychiatry* 2014; 75: 9–17.

27. Kleiman M. *When Brute Force Fails: How to Have Less Crime and Less Punishment*. Princeton, NJ: Princeton University Press, 2009.

28. Voas RB, DuPont RL, Talpins SK, Shea CL. Towards a national model for managing impaired driving offenders. *Addiction* 2011; 106: 1221–1227.

29. Cunningham JK, Liu LM. Impacts of federal precursor chemical regulations on methamphetamine arrests. *Addiction* 2005; 100: 479–488.

30. Maher L, Dixon D. Cost of crackdowns: policing cabramatta's herion market. *Current Issues Crim Just* 2001; 13: 5.

31. Day C, Day C, Degenhardt L, Hall W. Changes in the initiation of heroin use after a reduction in heroin supply. *Drug Alcohol Rev* 2006; 25: 307–313.

32. Dave D. The effects of cocaine and heroin price on drug-related emergency department visits. *J Health Econ* 2006; 25: 311–333.

33. Albers AB, DeJong W, Naimi TS, Siegel M, Jernigan DH. The relationship between alcohol price and brand choice among underage drinkers: are the most popular alcoholic brands consumed by youth the cheapest? *Subst Use Misuse* 2014; 49: 1833–1843.

34. Montgomery KC, Chester J, Grier SA, Dorfman L. The new threat of digital marketing. *Pediatr Clin North Am* 2012; 59: 659–675.

35. Casey BJ, Jones RM, Somerville LH. Braking and accelerating of the adolescent brain. *J Res Adolesc* 2011; 21: 21–33.

36. Sowell ER, Thompson PM, Toga AW. Mapping changes in the human cortex throughout the span of life. *Neuroscientist* 2004; 10: 372–392.

37. Goldfarb A, Tucker C. Advertising bans and the substitutability of online and offline advertising. *J Market Res* 2011; 48: 207–227.

38. Mukamana O, Johri M. What is known about school-based interventions for health promotion and their impact in developing countries? A scoping review of the literature. *Health Educ Res* 2016; 31: 587–602.

39. Botvin GJ, Baker E, Dusenbury L, Botvin EM, Diaz T. Long-term follow-up results of a randomized drug abuse prevention trial in a white middle-class population. *JAMA* 1995; 273: 1106–1112.

40. Faggiano F, Richardson C, Bohrn K, Galanti MR; EU-Dap Study Group. A cluster randomized controlled trial of school-based prevention of tobacco, alcohol and drug use: the EU-Dap design and study population. *Prev Med* 2007; 44: 170–173.

41. Faggiano F, Vigna-Tagliani F, Burkhart G, et al. The effectiveness of a school-based substance abuse prevention program: 18-month follow-up of the EU-Dap cluster randomized controlled trial. *Drug Alcohol Depend* 2010; 108: 56–64.

42. Kellam SG, Brown CH, Poduska JM, et al. Effects of a universal classroom behavior management program in first and second grades on young adult behavioral, psychiatric, and social outcomes. *Drug Alcohol Depend* 2008; 95: S5–S28.

43. Ennett ST, Tobler NS, Ringwalt CL, Flewelling RL. How effective is drug abuse resistance education? A meta-analysis of Project DARE outcome evaluations. *Am J Public Health* 1994; 84: 1394–1401.

44. Petrie J, Bunn F, Byrne G. Parenting programmes for preventing tobacco, alcohol or drugs misuse in children < 18: a systematic review. *Health Educ Res* 2007; 22: 177–191.

45. Spoth RL, Redmond C, Shin C. Randomized trial of brief family interventions for general populations: adolescent substance use outcomes 4 years following baseline. *J Consult Clin Psychol* 2001; 69: 627.

46. Gottfredson DC. *Schools and Delinquency*. Cambridge: Cambridge University Press, 2001.

47. Arkes J. Recessions and the participation of youth in the selling and use of illicit drugs. *Int J Drug Policy* 2011; 22: 335–340.

48. Evans-Lacko S, Knapp M, McCrone P, Thornicroft G, Mojtabai R. The mental health consequences of the recession: economic hardship and employment of people with mental health problems in 27 European countries. *PLOS ONE* 2013; 8: e69792.

49. Conrod PJ, Castellanos-Ryan N, Strang J. Brief, personality-targeted coping skills interventions and survival as a non–drug user over a 2-year period during adolescence. *Arch Gen Psychiatry* 2010; 67: 85–93.

50. Mahu IT, Doucet C, O'Leary-Barrett M, Conrod PJ. Can cannabis use be prevented by targeting personality risk in schools? Twenty-four-month outcome of the adventure trial on cannabis use: a cluster-randomized controlled trial. *Addiction* 2015; 110: 1625–1633.

51. Conrod PJ, O'Leary-Barrett M, Newton N, et al. Effectiveness of a selective, personality-targeted prevention program for adolescent alcohol use and misuse: a cluster randomized controlled trial. *JAMA Psychiatry* 2013; 70: 334–342.

52. Castellanos-Ryan N, Séguin JR, Vitaro F, Parent S, Tremblay RE. Impact of a 2-year multimodal intervention for disruptive 6-year-olds on substance use in adolescence: randomised controlled trial. *Br J Psychiatry* 2013; 203: 188–195.

53. O'Leary-Barrett M, Topper L, Al-Khudhairy N, et al. Two-year impact of personality-targeted, teacher-delivered interventions on youth internalizing and externalizing problems: a cluster-randomized trial. *J Am Acad Child Adolesc Psychiatry* 2013; 52: 911–920.

54. Baker A, Lee NK, Claire M, et al. Brief cognitive behavioural interventions for regular amphetamine users: a step in the right direction. *Addiction* 2005; 100: 367–378.

55. Cormack MA, Sweeney KG, Hughes-Jones H, Foot GA. Evaluation of an easy, cost-effective strategy for cutting benzodiazepine use in general practice. *Br J Gen Pract* 1994; 44: 5–8.

56. Bashir K, King M, Ashworth M. Controlled evaluation of brief intervention by general practitioners to reduce chronic use of benzodiazepines. *Br J Gen Pract* 1994; 44: 408–412.

57. Bernstein J, Bernstein E, Tassiopoulos K, Heeren T, Levenson S, Hingson R. Brief motivational intervention at a clinic visit reduces cocaine and heroin use. *Drug Alcohol Depend* 2005; 77: 49–59.

58. McCambridge J, Strang J. The efficacy of single-session motivational interviewing in reducing drug consumption and perceptions of drug-related risk and harm among young people: results from a multi-site cluster randomized trial. *Addiction* 2004; 99: 39–52.

59. Henggeler SW, McCart MR, Cunningham PB, Chapman JE. Enhancing the effectiveness of juvenile drug courts by integrating evidence-based practices. *J Consult Clin Psychol* 2012; 80: 264–275.

60. Marsden J, Stillwell G, Barlow H, et al. An evaluation of a brief motivational intervention among young ecstasy and cocaine users: no effect on substance and alcohol use outcomes. *Addiction* 2006; 101: 1014–1026.

61. McCambridge J, Strang J. Deterioration over time in effect of motivational interviewing in reducing drug consumption and related risk among young people. *Addiction* 2005; 100: 470–478.

62. Saitz R, Palfai TP, Cheng DM, et al. Screening and brief intervention for drug use in primary care: the ASPIRE randomized clinical trial. *JAMA* 2014; 312: 502–513.

63. Gray E, McCambridge J, Strang J. The effectiveness of motivational interviewing delivered by youth workers in reducing drinking, cigarette and cannabis smoking among young people: quasi-experimental pilot study. *Alcohol Alcohol* 2005; 40: 535–539.

64. Rapee RM, Wignall A, Sheffield J, et al. Adolescents' reactions to universal and indicated prevention programs for depression: perceived stigma and consumer satisfaction. *Prev Sci* 2006; 7: 167–177.

65. Spooner C, Mattick R, Noffs W. The nature and treatment of adolescent substance abuse. NDARC monograph. Available at: https://ndarc.med.unsw.edu.au/sites/default/files/ndarc/resources/Mono.40.pdf (1999, accessed 9 March 2018).

66. Hurley SF, Scollo MM, Younie SJ, English DR, Swanson MG. The potential for tobacco control to reduce PBS costs for smoking-related cardiovascular disease. *Med J Aust* 2004; 181: 252–255.

67. O'Keeffe L, O'Reilly A, O'Brien G, Buckley R, Illback R. Description and outcome evaluation of Jigsaw: an emergent Irish mental health early intervention programme for young people. *Irish J Psychol Med* 2015; 32: 71–77.

68. Rickwood DJ, Mazzer KR, Telford NR, Parker AG, Tanti CJ, McGorry PD. Changes in psychological distress and psychosocial functioning in young people visiting headspace centres for mental health problems. *Med J Aust* 2015; 202: 537–542.

69. Muir K, McDermott S, Gendera S, et al. *Independent Evaluation of Headspace: the National Youth Mental Health Foundation: Interim Evaluation Report.* NSW, Australia: Social Policy Research Centre, 2009.

70. British Columbia Integrated Youth Services Initiative. British Columbia Integrated Youth Services Initiative 2015. Available at: http://bciysi.ca/ (accessed 9 March 2018).

CHAPTER 37

Implications of the global mental health and the HIV syndemic on HIV prevention and care

Joseph T. F. LAU, Jinghua Li, Rui She, and Yoo Na Kim

Introduction

The first case of AIDS was identified in San Francisco in 1980 [1]. In 2015, it was estimated that, globally, there were 34.0–39.8 million people living with HIV (PLWH), and, cumulatively, 29.6–40.8 millions of reported deaths, including the 1.1 million deaths reported in that single year [2]. Importantly, the HIV epidemic's nature and course have changed over time. With advances in anti-retroviral treatment (ART), AIDS-related mortality and the rate of progression from HIV to AIDS have declined considerably [3]. HIV/AIDS has now become a chronic disease [4]. Such changes are consequential as some researchers identified the improvements in treatment and decline in mortality as the impetus of the global resurgence of HIV prevalence among men who have sex with men (MSM) [5]. In many cities (e.g. Bangkok in Thailand, and Chongqing and Chengdu in China [6]), HIV prevalence among MSM has exceeded 20% and has continued to increase sharply in recent years [6]. Only in a few areas, such as San Francisco and Zimbabwe, has an early decline in HIV prevalence among MSM been observed [7]. All in all, HIV remains a very serious global health problem.

HIV is often described as a 'social disease' [8], as its transmission is mostly attributed to risk behaviours, which occur in psycho-social and cultural contexts. The complex underlying social nature of HIV distinguishes it from most other infectious or chronic diseases. As vulnerable key populations for HIV prevention (e.g. MSM, drug users, and sex workers) are severely marginalized, they tend to have poor mental health even if they are HIV negative. We will also see in this chapter that psychological problems not only affect well-being and quality of life of the key populations and PLWH [9], they play extremely important roles in HIV transmission, prevention, treatment, and care. We contend that mental health promotion and rehabilitation play important roles in HIV prevention and care.

A syndemic of HIV and mental health problems

A syndemic is defined as 'cases of any two or more health problems that interact synergistically and contribute, as a result of this interaction, to excess burden of disease in a population, particularly under conditions of health and social disparity' [10]. An HIV syndemic is hence defined as the co-occurrence of HIV and other illness/health conditions (e.g. mental disorders, substance use, violence) that interact synergistically and compromise the effectiveness of HIV prevention, treatment, and care [11]. Co-morbidity of HIV and mental health problems is prevalent and is an important nature of the HIV epidemic. In the literature, among PLWH, the prevalence of depression ranges from 12.8% to 78% [12]. For instance, it is 31.8% in low-income countries, 47.4% in middle-income countries, and 37.1% in high-income countries [12]. Prevalence of anxiety among PLWH was found to be 33.9% in low- and middle-income countries and 21.5% in high-income countries [13]. The prevalence of suicidal ideation among PLWH has been found to range from 43% to 59% [14, 15]. Both depression and suicidal ideation are strong predictors of completed suicides [16]. The prevalence of mental health problems is especially high in subgroups of PLWH, such as those who were also MSM [17] and drug users [18]. According to the American Psychological Association, post-traumatic stress disorder (PTSD) is defined as 'an anxiety problem that develops in some people after extremely traumatic events, such as combat, crime, and an accident or natural disaster' [19]. HIV transmission is certainly a traumatic experience. The prevalence of PTSD among PLWH is also high, ranging from 5% to 74% (e.g. 48–57% in the USA [20] and 5–19% in South Africa [20]), according to literature. Hence, problems caused by HIV infection and mental health problems are non-separable.

Another part of the HIV syndemic is the prevalent substance use among PLWH. The prevalence of substance use among PLWH ranges from 5.7% to 82.4% in Europe [21]. Substance use, in the first place, is already prevalent among vulnerable groups such as MSM and female sex workers (FSW) who are HIV negative [22, 23], and it is a risk factor for HIV transmission among these groups [22]. Many of these high-risk substance users continue using substances after contracting HIV, resulting in a high prevalence of substance use among PLWH. Furthermore, substances have been used as a negative coping mechanism to deal with the severe stress faced by PLWH [24], and substance use is associated with non-adherence to ART, which increases HIV viral load and transmissibility [25].

Attention should be paid to the surge in substance use among MSM. For instance, recent studies from mainland China reported a prevalence of 47.3% for nitrates use [26], and the practice was associated with unprotected anal intercourse (UAI). Furthermore, chemsex, or prearranged occasions where drug use and sex (often unprotected) take place, has recently become common among MSM. In the UK and the USA, the prevalence of chemsex among MSM is 20% [27] and 67% [28], respectively. Participation in chemsex is not limited to HIV-negative MSM. A survey of PLWH attending 30 HIV clinics in England and Wales found that nearly a third of HIV-positive MSM reported engaging in chemsex in the past year [29]; the study also reported significantly higher odds of engaging in UAI in the past year among HIV-positive MSM who practised chemsex [29]. Our study, conducted in Hong Kong, showed that 15.7% of HIV-positive MSM ($n = 261$) self-reported having engaged in chemsex since their HIV diagnoses; the figure was probably underestimated. The prevalence of UAI during chemsex among MSM was as high as 68.3% (unpublished data). In that study, the main reasons for participating in chemsex included sensation seeking and stress reduction. The high risk of HIV transmission associated with chemsex activities is an example of how the HIV syndemic conditions interact with each other to impact on HIV prevention.

Factors associated with mental health problems among people living with HIV

The socio-ecological model

Following the multidimensional socio-ecological model [30], we need to look at structural factors (e.g. policy, health services, and culture), interpersonal factors (e.g. social support), as well as individual-level factors (e.g. cognitions and lifestyle) in order to understand factors associated with mental health problems among PLWH. The model reminds us that mental health promotion needs to consider all these interrelated levels. Advocacy and services are both required.

Pre-existing conditions of mental health problems in vulnerable groups

Stressful conditions and prevalent mental health problems among vulnerable groups prior to a diagnosis of HIV may be attributed to the high prevalence of mental health problems among PLWH. For instance, the World Health Organization (WHO) reported that 'MSM had disproportionately high prevalence of psychological problems' [31]. This is a structural problem as these populations are marginalized, stigmatized [32], involved in illegal or socially undesirable behaviours, harassed by police [33], unemployed, and often threatened with violence [34]. These stressors are factors associated with mental health problems among MSM [35], people who inject drugs [36], FSW [37], and transgender women [38]. These vulnerable groups also tend to have lower social and family support [39]. These adversities are certainly intensified by an HIV diagnosis. In some studies, the prevalence of depression and suicidal ideation was as high as 48% among newly diagnosed HIV-positive MSM in mainland China (i.e. those diagnosed for less than 12 months) [40]. Qualitative studies also found that newly diagnosed HIV-positive MSM in mainland China face severe adjustment problems [41]. The high prevalence of mental health problems found among key populations for HIV prevention and PLWH has sequential relationships. Effective improvement of mental health among PLWH must start with structural changes in the social environments and improvements of mental health conditions of the key populations for HIV prevention.

Availability of treatment as one of the structural factors

The availability of ART is another structural factor of mental health problems among PLWH. Although accessibility of ART has improved substantially over the last few decades, about 63% of PLWH, especially those in less developed countries, could not access ART in 2013 [42]. Taking mainland China as an example, many of the PLWH, who are MSM, people who inject drugs, and FSW, are internal migrants. The national policy, however, requires PLWH to receive ART only in their home towns [41], creating a hurdle for treatment. Both quantitative and qualitative studies on newly diagnosed HIV-positive MSM in mainland China showed that non-availability of ART was associated with mental health problems [43, 44].

Socio-environmental factors

Understandably, PLWH may face double, or even triple, sources of stigma, a phenomenon known as 'layered stigma', as they may also be MSM, people who inject drugs, and sex workers [45]. Perceived stigma and enacted stigma not only originate from the general public, but also from sources that are supposed to be caring. These include healthcare professionals and service providers [46], co-workers [47], and family members [48]. Interventions have been successful in increasing empathy and reducing stigma toward PLWH among service providers [49]. Perceived stigma is often internalized and become self-stigma among PLWH [50]. Perceived stigma, enacted stigma [51], and self-stigma [50] have consistently been shown to be strongly associated with various mental health problems, such as depression, anxiety, and suicidal ideation among marginalized populations. Worry about disclosure of one's HIV status is also associated with mental health problems among PLWH [52]. Mental health promotion for PLWH cannot be effective without creation of a supportive environment for PLWH. Structural and complex interventions, fully backed by policies, are required to modify these factors.

Individual-level factors

There is a wide range of individual-level factors associated with mental health problems among PLWH, including sociodemographic factors (e.g. income, unemployment [53]), health and HIV-related factors (e.g. disease progress, treatment [54], and physical health conditions [55]), psychological factors (e.g. HIV-related stigma [50], coping [56], and optimism [57]), and emotional factors (e.g. guilt [58] and shame [59]). However, some of these variables are difficult to modify.

An interesting perspective is to apply the common sense model (also known as the illness perception model and parallel processing model) to understand mental health problems among PLWH. The model is a parallel-processing model in which external and internal stimuli are reasoned to trigger simultaneously cognitive representation and emotional representation. Both emotional and cognitive representation are reasoned to initiate their respective coping procedures, which are further reasoned to influence appraisals of outcomes [60]. The model has been used to explain health outcomes, including psychological outcomes [61] in multiple disease groups (e.g. cancer, diabetes, and cardiovascular disease). Our findings suggest that emotional illness representation and some constructs of cognitive illness representation (e.g. treatment control, illness coherence, consequences, identity, and timeline) were strongly and positively associated with depression and suicidal ideation, and negatively associated with post-traumatic growth among newly diagnosed HIV-positive MSM in China [40]. Previous studies have shown that illness representations could be improved via interventions [62]. Hence, the model points in a new direction for improving mental health among PLWH. Such interventions have not been in place, but with the penetration of social media and development of e-health, self-help online tutorials are potential means for implementing such interventions.

Impact of mental health problems on HIV prevention

Impact on risk behaviours

It is well documented that key populations with mental health problems are more likely than others to engage in HIV-related risk behaviours. Among MSM, depression is associated with UAI with both regular and non-regular male sex partners [63], number of male sex partners, sex work [64], and substance use [65]. Depression is also associated with unprotected sex with sex-work clients [66], as well as their regular and non-regular male sex partners among FSWs [67]. Among people who inject drugs, anxiety is associated with syringe sharing [68]. Mental health problems are also associated with sexual risk behaviours such as patients with sexually transmitted diseases having unprotected sex [69]. On the contrary, risky behaviours have also been reported as risk factors of poor mental health among MSM [64], as risky behaviours might act as potential stressors.

Impact on behavioural interventions for HIV prevention

In general, those who have mental health problems are less interested in and less able to exercise self-care. They are less likely to use preventative measures to maintain or improve health [70]. According to the WHO, HIV testing is one of the four key global strategies for HIV prevention and is the first of the 90–90–90 targets [71]. This first 90–90–90 target set by UNAIDS aims for 90% of all PLWH to know their HIV status by 2020. According to the literature that describes HIV treatment and prevention cascades, a system to monitor the number of PLWH who are receiving medical care and the treatment they need, only around half of PLWH knew about their HIV status [72]. Among MSM—a key population group with high HIV incidence—the HIV testing rate (in the past 12 months) varied from around 30% in Spain [73] to 64% in the USA [74], and is certainly below the 90% target. The literature has shown that mental health problems such as depression, anxiety disorder, and panic disorder are negatively associated with HIV testing [75].

Methadone maintenance treatment (MMT) has been clearly shown to be an effective harm-reduction method that can reduce HIV transmission among people who inject drugs [76]. Mental health problems such as depression have also been shown to be negatively associated with utilization of MMT services [77], retention in MMT programmes, and compliance with methadone intake [78]. Other studies have further shown that mental health problems among key populations such as FSW [79] and transgender people [80] are, again, negatively associated with the utilization of HIV prevention services. Thus, mental health problems are obstacles for HIV prevention.

Impact on biomedical prevention

Despite tremendous efforts made in the last three decades, the progress of vaccine development is still in the early stages. Only one human trial has found a preliminary effect of a vaccine [81]. Until recently, behavioural interventions such as condom promotion, methadone treatment, and needle exchange have been used as the primary means of HIV prevention. In the past few years, however, important evidence for biomedical prevention methods, such as treatment as prevention (TasP) [82], pre-exposure prophylaxis (PrEP) [83], and circumcision of heterosexual males has emerged [84]. TasP refers to a biomedical HIV prevention intervention that uses ART among PLWH to decrease the risk of HIV transmission. ART reduces the HIV viral load in body fluids to a very low level (undetectable), reducing the risk of onward HIV transmission [82]. PrEP is a form of HIV prevention intervention that uses anti-HIV medication to protect HIV-negative people, who are at risk of exposure to HIV, from acquiring HIV [83]. With good adherence, TasP and PrEP could reduce the chance of HIV transmission by 96% and 44%, respectively [82, 83].

Some optimism sparked and the 90–90–90 target [71] that follows the HIV prevention cascade [85] was proposed. Statistical modelling demonstrated that with achievement of the 90–90–90 target by 2020, the HIV epidemic would be under control by 2030 [86]. As behavioural issues are involved when implementing these biomedical preventative measures, combined biomedical and behavioural approaches have been advocated. A meta-analysis found that depression is consistently negatively associated with initiation of ART and with poor adherence to ART among PLWH and can interfere with self-care [87]. Some researchers also contended that mental health problems may affect initiation of PrEP and its adherence in populations such as MSM and substance users [88].

Positive psychology interventions

Recent developments in psychology have extended its emphasis from abnormal psychology to positive psychology. Such a shift in emphasis applies to research targeting PLWH. A number of studies conducted in the USA documented clear trends of post-traumatic growth among PLWH [89], defined as a positive change in one's previous level of functioning as a result of the struggle with the traumatic event [90]. Factors associated with post-traumatic growth included social support [91], resilience [92], enacted stigma, hopefulness, and emotional regulation [91]. It is promising to design mental health promotion interventions based on positive psychology approaches. Examples of effective positive psychology interventions (PPI) targeting PLWH include those promoting resilience [93]. Simple PPI have shown to be effective in reducing depression. Among them, the 'three good things' exercises for improving gratitude, which require participants to record three things in daily life that they are grateful for, for 1–8 weeks, have shown to be effective in improving mental health in various populations (e.g. patients with neuromuscular disease, PLWH, and undergraduates) [94, 95]. We conducted a randomized controlled study on 205 HIV-positive MSM in China and confirmed the effectiveness of the three good things exercises in reducing depression [96]. Other PPI included gratitude visit [94, 95], acts of kindness [94], identifying and using signature strengths [94, 95], best possible selves [97], and savoring [98]. Two meta-analysis showed that PPI have significant effects in reducing depression and enhancing well-being [99, 100]. As compared with traditional psychological and psychiatric services, PPI programmes are easy to practice, require very low expenditure for development and maintenance, and can be practised by participants themselves with minimal instructions. These interventions do not need professional input and can be used in resource-limited countries. It is highly sustainable and scalable in the future. Hence, PPI are a promising approach to promote mental health among PLWH.

Gaps: lack of mental health interventions, services, and personnel

Psychiatric services and treatments are hard to access, even in developed countries [101]. In low-income countries, the ratio of psychiatric doctors to population size is very small: 0.06 per 100,000 population versus 10.5 per 100,000 population in high income-countries [101]. In China, only 9% of depressed patients have access to psychiatric treatment [102], and there are only 1.29 trained psychiatrists, 1.99 psychiatric nurses, and 10.6 'mental health beds' per 100,000 persons nationwide [101]. There is a huge gap between demand and supply of mental health services for PLWH, not to mention tailored services. The same is true for mental health support or promotion services [103]. One obstacle is that PLWH are often managed by clinical staff who are not well trained in dealing with mental health problems or promoting mental health among PLWH [104]. Mental health-related services may not be seen as their primary task, which some of them might narrowly perceive as control of the spread of HIV.

It is also known that, in general, marginalized groups tend to use health services less [105]. Mental health service utilization among PLWH is no exception. Besides availability, worry about stigma [103] and disclosure of their HIV status may increase the reluctance of PLWH to utilize mental health services. Hence, provision of friendly and reliable mental health support services is essential.

Non-governmental organizations (NGOs) can potentially bridge the gap. However, NGOs in many less-developed countries tend to be small and poorly resourced. We surveyed 933 NGO workers who had been providing HIV prevention and care services to HIV-positive MSM in mainland China, and only 62.5% were trained in counselling and 51.8% self-perceived inadequacy in providing mental health support services. Furthermore, 25.0% of these workers (the majority were MSM) had probable depression [106]. About 29.3% reported mild-to-severe anxiety. Around 41.8% had at least one mental health problem [106]. Associative stigma or courtesy stigma, defined as stigma that persons experience not because of their own characteristics, but because they are associated with persons who belong to a stigmatized category in society [107], may affect the mental health of NGO workers who serve PLWH, which may indirectly worsen, instead of improve, the mental health of PLWH served by these NGOs.

According to our literature review, there is a dearth of effective interventions promoting mental health among PLWH. Besides the few PPI mentioned, examples of other effective mental health interventions may include cognitive–behavioural therapy, individual interpersonal therapy, and stress reduction and management [108]. These interventions aim at reducing psychological abnormality (e.g. depression, anxiety, and stress). Some effective resilience-promoting interventions and mindfulness-based stress reduction have also been documented [109, 110]. Mindfulness and resilience are more PPI, but like the other traditional interventions mentioned, they require intensive input from well-trained mental health professionals (e.g. clinical psychologists, counsellors, trainers, and psychiatrists). They are costly and relatively harder to scale up. Mental health-related services at primary, secondary, and tertiary levels are all warranted.

Discussion

The literature clearly identifies a global syndemic of HIV and various psychological problems among PLWH, which reminds us of the multidimensional problems faced by PLWH. The syndemic compromises the effectiveness of HIV prevention and care and increases risk of HIV transmission. Among HIV-negative lesbian, gay, bisexual, and transgender (LGBT) populations such as MSM, mental health problems and drug use problems are prevalent. These prevalent problems partially explain our inability to control spread of HIV among these populations, as to control the spread both effective prevention and treatment of mental health problems and HIV-related interventions are required. The impact of mental health problems may even be larger in resource-limited populations, where psychiatric/psychological care is often hard to access and mental health promotion is not well in place.

The syndemic has deep sociocultural and political roots. For instance, a policy of immediate ART is inconsistent with the limited eligibility by place of residence in mainland China. Cultural sensitivity regarding sexuality and sexual orientations, and laws prohibiting same-sex marriages are potential stressors [111]. We need to acknowledge the complex situations faced by key populations for HIV prevention (e.g. MSM, people who inject drug, and sex workers), and possible adverse consequences on their mental health status. Structural interventions involving interdepartmental efforts are warranted.

Among various sociocultural factors, stigma provides a strong link between HIV and mental health problems. Strong stigma originating from various sources toward key populations for HIV prevention and PLWH represents an important stressor that causes severe mental health problems. Removal of stigma is crucial and needs to be integrated into existing services, but stigma does not seem to have been given its deserved priority. Stigma reduction requires adoption of socio-ecological models for HIV prevention and care [112], and implementation of structural changes. Expectedly or unexpectedly, service providers are seen by many PLWH as one of the sources of stigma. Training to enhance empathy is warranted. Perceived stigma is often internalized as self-stigma. Previous studies have shown that self-stigma can be reduced effectively by using cognitive therapy [113]. There is a dearth of such programmes in the context of HIV.

Policymakers need to be made aware of the close relationships between mental health problems among PLWH/key populations and effectiveness of HIV campaigns. Front-line workers are more concerned about direct public health measures, such as HIV testing, condom use, surveillance, and treatment, and may overlook the importance of mental health promotion and support. The WHO's guideline on prevention and care states that 'People from key populations commonly have multiple co-morbidities and poor social situations. Routine screening and management of mental health disorders (depression and psychosocial stress) should be provided for people from key populations living with HIV in order to optimize health outcomes and improve their adherence to ART' [72]. However, while the WHO has separate guidelines on prevention and treatment issues such as testing (consolidated guidelines on HIV testing services [114], PrEP, and treatment (guideline on when to start ART and on PrEP for HIV [115], it does not have specific guidelines about mental health support toward PLWH. It is an area that requires international guidelines and joint efforts, in addition to policy advocacy.

Capacity gaps may exist. In many places, the training of front-line workers on mental health issues among PLWH and basic counselling skills may not be routine practice. NGOs are important potential sources of mental health support. NGOs in resource-limited countries, however, tend to be small and lack capacity. We have seen that NGOs in mainland China have not been well equipped to provide mental health services to PLWH. Capacity building is greatly needed. An international agenda is needed but apparently non-existent. Comprehensive and successful integrated services that include mental health support have been documented in the USA, Australia, and some other developed countries. However, the model may not be directly transferrable to resource-limited countries, where psychiatrists and clinical psychologists are scarce. New models need to be devised and tested in country-specific settings.

Attention needs to be given to emotional responses among newly diagnosed PLWH, as research showed high levels of distress, PTSD, and suicidal ideation [40], and their coping capacity have long-lasting personal and public health consequences. Basic training should be given to front-line health workers serving PLWH on the detection of severe risk of psychiatric problems, proper disclosure of HIV diagnosis, and psychological first aid. Standard operating procedures should be set up. It is important to understand the representation of emotional illness in newly diagnosed PLWH, who may feel guilty, shameful, angry, or have other negative emotions. Our study showed that emotional representations were related to depression among newly diagnosed PLWH in mainland China. As illness representation is modifiable through interventions [116], illness representation points at a new direction for research and intervention. There is a dearth of such studies.

Primary preventions targeting those at lower risk of contracting HIV, secondary prevention targeting those at high risk, and tertiary prevention targeting those already showing symptoms are all required. Basic primary prevention of mental health problems can be provided to all PLWH; some screening may be installed to detect high-risk individuals requiring secondary prevention. Linkage and referrals between levels of prevention present challenges.

Efforts should be made in developing and implementing new, innovative, and inexpensive means of mental health promotion for PLWH. Health workers should not only look for abnormalities, but also strengths and hopes. Research and interventions should pay attention to the areas of positive psychology, such as building up resilience and post-traumatic growth [90]. Protective effects of such positive developments and related interventions have been documented [99, 100]. We have summarized some preliminary work using simple PPI [96]. Positive psychology exercise has also shown to be effective in reducing depression [99, 100]. These are promising approaches that have good chances of fitting into existing systems.

Mental health services should also be integrated into existing and future HIV preventative services. Clear examples include those of biomedical prevention, such as immediate ART, recommended by the WHO. Many countries, including those that may not have a good capacity to provide mental health support to PLWH, have recently implemented the policy of providing immediate ART to all PLWH [117], whereas they may have little experience handling ART for those with high CD4 cell counts. Mental health problems affect the initiation of ART and adherence to ART among PLWH [87]. Numerous PLWH may be suffering from depression and suicidal ideation; they might not be mindful of taking up ART or adhering to it. Poor ART adherence may lead to drug resistance [118]. PrEP is a hot topic in HIV prevention, and it is also recommended by the WHO for key populations at substantial risk of HIV infection [72]. Implementation of PrEP involves issues of adherence and risk compensation, which may be related to mental health problems. Integration of mental health support and methadone treatment for HIV prevention among people who inject drugs has been shown to be effective [119]. Integration also means collaborations with stakeholders, including mental health professionals and social workers, who have not yet been working in the mainstream of HIV prevention and care.

Besides improving the mental health of PLWH, we need to extend our mental health support to HIV workers, caregivers, and family members of PLWH. Associative stigma is a documented phenomenon [120]. It may be stronger in countries with strong traditional cultures, and possibly also stronger in rural settings, where social norms and control are strong. Our studies on 202 NGOs serving HIV-positive MSM in mainland China showed that 25.0% of their core workers have signs of depression. Yet, these workers are the main forces in providing mental health support to PLWH. The literature has shown that family members and caregivers of PLHW are at risk of developing mental health problems [120]. These people form important social environments of the PLWH. Vicious cycles of poor mental health might be developed.

Last, but not least, we need to raise a caution. We have to be mindful to avoid labelling PLWH as mentally ill. Instead, besides detecting mental health problems, we should focus equally on developing individual strengths, appreciation, and positive personal growth, optimism, and hope. These positive psychology attributes are often yet to be discovered. PLWH are individuals who experience both happiness and distress. PLWH should be supported to overcome difficulties and share their joy.

References

1. McKay RA. 'Patient Zero': the absence of a patient's view of the early North American AIDS epidemic. *Bull Hist Med* 2014; 88: 161–194.
2. UNAIDS. Global HIV statistics. Available at: http://www.unaids.org/sites/default/files/media_asset/UNAIDS_FactSheet_en.pdf (2016, accessed 12 March 2018).
3. Palella FJ, Jr, Baker RK, Moorman AC, et al. Mortality in the highly active antiretroviral therapy era: changing causes of death and disease

in the HIV outpatient study. *J Acquir Immune Defic Syndromes* 2006; 43: 27–34.

4. Deeks SG, Lewin SR, Havlir DV. The end of AIDS: HIV infection as a chronic disease. *Lancet* 2013; 382: 1525–1533.

5. Wolitski RJ, Valdiserri RO, Denning PH, Levine WC. Are we headed for a resurgence of the HIV epidemic among men who have sex with men? *Am J Public Health* 2001; 91: 883–888.

6. Lau JTF, Chow EPF, Li JH, Zhang L. Reflections on public health challenges for the HIV epidemic among men who have sex with men in China. In: Griffiths SM, Tang J, Yeoh EK (eds). *Routledge Handbook of Public Health in Asia: Perspectives on Global Health.* London: Routledge, 2014, pp. 212–229.

7. Halperin DT, Mugurungi O, Hallett TB, et al. A surprising prevention success: why did the HIV epidemic decline in Zimbabwe? *PLOS Med* 2011; 8: e1000414.

8. Velimirovic B. AIDS as a social phenomenon. *Soc Sci Med* 1987; 25: 541–552.

9. Yi S, Tuot S, Chhoun P, Pal K, Choub SC, Mburu G. Mental health among men who have sex with men in Cambodia: Implications for integration of mental health services within HIV programmes. *Int J Equity Health* 2016; 15: 53.

10. Singer M, Clair S. Syndemics and public health: reconceptualizing disease in bio-social context. *Med Anthropol Q* 2003; 17: 423–441.

11. Biello KB, Oldenburg CE, Safren SA, et al. Multiple syndemic psychosocial factors are associated with reduced engagement in HIV care among a multinational, online sample of HIV-infected MSM in Latin America. *AIDS Care* 2016; 28(Suppl. 1): 84–91.

12. Uthman OA, Magidson JF, Safren SA, Nachega JB. Depression and adherence to antiretroviral therapy in low-, middle- and high-income countries: a systematic review and meta-analysis. *Curr HIV/AIDS Rep* 2014; 11: 291–307.

13. Lowther K, Selman L, Harding R, Higginson IJ. Experience of persistent psychological symptoms and perceived stigma among people with HIV on antiretroviral therapy (ART): a systematic review. *Int J Nurs Stud* 2014; 51: 1171–1189.

14. Shelton AJ, Atkinson J, Risser JM, McCurdy SA, Useche B, Padgett PM. The prevalence of suicidal behaviours in a group of HIV-positive men. *AIDS Care* 2006; 18: 574–576.

15. Amiya RM, Poudel KC, Poudel-Tandukar K, Pandey BD, Jimba M. Perceived family support, depression, and suicidal ideation among people living with HIV/AIDS: a cross-sectional study in the Kathmandu Valley, Nepal. *PLOS ONE* 2014; 9: e90959.

16. Lau JT, Yu XN, Mak WW, Cheng YM, Lv YH, Zhang JX. Suicidal ideation among HIV+ former blood and/or plasma donors in rural China. *AIDS Care* 2010; 22: 946–954.

17. Li J, Mo PK, Wu AM, Lau JT. Roles of self-stigma, social support, and positive and negative affects as determinants of depressive symptoms among HIV infected men who have sex with men in China. *AIDS Behav* 2017; 21: 261–273.

18. Walton G, Co SJ, Milloy MJ, Qi J, Kerr T, Wood E. High prevalence of childhood emotional, physical and sexual trauma among a Canadian cohort of HIV-seropositive illicit drug users. *AIDS Care* 2011; 23: 714–721.

19. American Psychological Association. Post-traumatic Stress Disorder. Available at: http://www.apa.org/topics/ptsd/ (2016, accessed 22 September 2016).

20. Sherr L, Nagra N, Kulubya G, Catalan J, Clucas C, Harding R. HIV infection associated post-traumatic stress disorder and post-traumatic growth—a systematic review. *Psychol Health Med* 2011; 16: 612–629.

21. Garin N, Velasco C, De Pourcq JT, et al. Recreational drug use among individuals living with HIV in Europe: review of the prevalence, comparison with the general population and HIV guidelines recommendations. *Front Microbiol* 2015; 6: 690.

22. Wim VB, Christiana N, Marie L. Syndemic and other risk factors for unprotected anal intercourse among an online sample of Belgian HIV negative men who have sex with men. *AIDS Behav* 2014; 18: 50–58.

23. Zhang C, Li X, Hong Y, Su S, Zhou Y. Relationship between female sex workers and gatekeeper: the impact on female sex worker's mental health in China. *Psychol Health Med* 2014; 19: 656–666.

24. Skalski LM, Sikkema KJ, Heckman TG, Meade CS. Coping styles and illicit drug use in older adults with HIV/AIDS. *Psychol Addict Behav* 2013; 27: 1050.

25. Wood E, Montaner JS, Yip B, et al. Adherence and plasma HIV RNA responses to highly active antiretroviral therapy among HIV-1 infected injection drug users. *CMAJ* 2003; 169: 656–661.

26. Li D, Yang X, Zhang Z, et al. Nitrite inhalants use and HIV infection among men who have sex with men in China. *Biomed Res Int* 2014; 2014: 365261.

27. McCall H, Adams N, Mason D, Willis J. What is chemsex and why does it matter? *BMJ* 2015; 351: h5790.

28. Nakamura N, Semple SJ, Strathdee SA, Patterson TL. Methamphetamine initiation among HIV-positive gay and bisexual men. *AIDS Care* 2009; 21: 1176–1184.

29. Pufall EL, Kall M, Shahmanesh M, et al. "Chemsex" and high-risk sexual behaviours in HIV-positive men who have sex with men. Available at: http://www.croiconference.org/sessions/%C2%93chemsex%C2%94-and-high-risk-sexual-behaviours-hiv-positive-men-who-have-sex-men (accessed 12 March 2018).

30. Qiao S, Li X, Zhou Y, Shen Z, Tang Z, Stanton B. Factors influencing the decision-making of parental HIV disclosure: a socio-ecological approach. *AIDS* 2015; 29(Suppl. 1): S25–S34.

31. World Health Organization. Prevention and treatment of HIV and other sexually transmitted infections among men who have sex with men and transgender people: recommendations for a public health approach. Available at: http://www.who.int/hiv/pub/guidelines/msm_guidelines2011/en/ (2011, accessed 12 March 2018).

32. Mahajan AP, Sayles JN, Patel VA, et al. Stigma in the HIV/AIDS epidemic: a review of the literature and recommendations for the way forward. *AIDS* 2008; 22(Suppl. 2): S67–S79.

33. Zhang L, Chow EP, Zhuang X, et al. Methadone maintenance treatment participant retention and behavioural effectiveness in China: a systematic review and meta-analysis. *PLOS ONE* 2013; 8: e68906.

34. LeGrand S, Reif S, Sullivan K, Murray K, Barlow ML, Whetten K. A review of recent literature on trauma among individuals living with HIV. *Curr HIV/AIDS Rep* 2015; 12: 397–405.

35. Klein H. Depression and HIV risk taking among men who have sex with other men and who use the internet to find partners for unprotected sex. *J Gay Lesbian Ment Health* 2014; 18: 164–189.

36. Galea S, Vlahov D. Social determinants and the health of drug users: socioeconomic status, homelessness, and incarceration. *Public Health Rep* 2002; 117(Suppl. 1): S135.

37. Rössler W, Koch U, Lauber C, et al. The mental health of female sex workers. *Acta Psychiatr Scand* 2010; 122: 143–152.

38. Poteat T, Wirtz AL, Radix A, et al. HIV risk and preventive interventions in transgender women sex workers. *Lancet* 2015; 385: 274–286.

39. Williams T, Connolly J, Pepler D, Craig W. Peer victimization, social support, and psychosocial adjustment of sexual minority adolescents. *J Youth Adolesc* 2005; 34: 471–482.

40. Wu X. Mental *Health, Risk Behaviours and Illness Perception among Newly Diagnosed HIV Positive Men Who Have Sex with Men in China.* Hong Kong: The Chinese University of Hong Kong, 2012.

41. Li H, Lau J, Holroyd E. Unmet health service needs of newly diagnosed HIV-positive men who have sex with men in China: results from an ethnography. *J AIDS Clin Res STDs* 2015; 2: 100004.

42. UNAIDS. Global report: UNAIDS report on the global AIDS epidemic 2013. Available at: http://www.unaids.org/sites/default/files/media_asset/UNAIDS_Global_Report_2013_en_1.pdf (2013, accessed 12 March 2018).

43. Wei C, Yan H, Yang C, et al. Accessing HIV testing and treatment among men who have sex with men in China: a qualitative study. *AIDS Care* 2014; 26: 372–378.

44. Liu Y, Ruan Y, Vermund SH, et al. Predictors of antiretroviral therapy initiation: a cross-sectional study among Chinese HIV-infected men who have sex with men. *BMC Infect Dis* 2015; 15: 570.

45. Altman D, Aggleton P, Williams M, et al. Men who have sex with men: stigma and discrimination. *Lancet* 2012; 380: 439–445.

46. Nostlinger C, Rojas Castro D, Platteau T, Dias S, Le Gall J. HIV-Related discrimination in European health care settings. *AIDS Patient Care STDS.* 2014; 28: 155–161.

47. Dray-Spira R, Gueguen A, Lert F. Disease severity, self-reported experience of workplace discrimination and employment loss during the course of chronic HIV disease: differences according to gender and education. *Occup Environ Med* 2008; 65: 112–119.

48. Paxton S, Gonzales G, Uppakaew K, et al. AIDS-related discrimination in Asia. *AIDS Care* 2005; 17: 413–424.

49. Mak WW, Cheng SS, Law RW, Cheng WW, Chan F. Reducing HIV-related stigma among health-care professionals: a game-based experiential approach. *AIDS Care* 2015; 27: 855–859.

50. Mak WW, Cheung RY, Law RW, Woo J, Li PC, Chung RW. Examining attribution model of self-stigma on social support and psychological well-being among people with HIV+/AIDS. *Soc Sci Med* 2007; 64: 1549–1559.

51. Chi P, Li X, Zhao J, Zhao G. Vicious circle of perceived stigma, enacted stigma and depressive symptoms among children affected by HIV/AIDS in China. *AIDS Behav* 2014; 18: 1054–1062.

52. Brown MJ, Serovich JM, Kimberly JA, Hu J. Psychological reactance and HIV-related stigma among women living with HIV. *AIDS Care* 2016; 28: 745–749.

53. Rueda S, Raboud J, Mustard C, Bayoumi A, Lavis JN, Rourke SB. Employment status is associated with both physical and mental health quality of life in people living with HIV. *AIDS Care* 2011; 23: 435–443.

54. Liu C, Johnson L, Ostrow D, Silvestre A, Visscher B, Jacobson LP. Predictors for lower quality of life in the HAART era among HIV-infected men. *J Acquir Immune Defic Syndr* 2006; 42: 470–477.

55. Olley B, Seedat S, Nei D, Stein D. Predictors of major depression in recently diagnosed patients with HIV/AIDS in South Africa. *AIDS Patient Care STDS.* 2004; 18: 481–487.

56. Gibson K, Rueda S, Rourke SB, et al. Mastery and coping moderate the negative effect of acute and chronic stressors on mental health-related quality of life in HIV. *AIDS Patient Care STDS* 2011; 25: 371–381.

57. Liu L, Pang R, Sun W, et al. Functional social support, psychological capital, and depressive and anxiety symptoms among people living with HIV/AIDS employed full-time. *BMC Psychiatry* 2013; 13: 324.

58. Berg MB, Mimiaga MJ, Safren SA. Mental health concerns of HIV-infected gay and bisexual men seeking mental health services: an observational study. *AIDS Patient Care STDS* 2004; 18: 635–643.

59. Bennett DS, Traub K, Mace L, Juarascio A, O'Hayer CV. Shame among people living with HIV: a literature review. *AIDS Care* 2016; 28: 87–91.

60. Leventhal H, Benyamini Y, Brownlee S, et al. Illness representations: theoretical foundations. In: Weinman J, Petrie K (eds). *Perceptions of Health and Illness: Current Research and Applications.* New York: Harwood Acadamic Publishers, 1998, pp. 19–46.

61. Keogh KM, Smith SM, White P, et al. Psychological family intervention for poorly controlled type 2 diabetes. *Am J Manag Care* 2011; 17: 105–113.

62. Jones CJ, Smith HE, Llewellyn CD. A systematic review of the effectiveness of interventions using the Common Sense Self-Regulatory Model to improve adherence behaviours. *J Health Psychol* 2015 [Epub ahead of print].

63. O'Cleirigh C, Newcomb ME, Mayer KH, Skeer M, Traeger L, Safren SA. Moderate levels of depression predict sexual transmission risk in HIV-infected MSM: a longitudinal analysis of data from six sites involved in a 'prevention for positives' study. *AIDS Behav* 2013; 17: 1764–1769.

64. Safren SA, Thomas BE, Mimiaga MJ, et al. Depressive symptoms and human immunodeficiency virus risk behavior among men who have sex with men in Chennai, India. *Psychol Health Med* 2009; 14: 705–715.

65. Tomori C, McFall AM, Srikrishnan AK, et al. Diverse rates of depression among men who have sex with men (MSM) across India: insights from a multi-site mixed method study. *AIDS Behav* 2016; 20: 304–316.

66. Patel SK, Saggurti N, Pachauri S, Prabhakar P. Correlates of mental depression among female sex workers in Southern India. *Asia Pac J Public Health* 2015; 27: 809–819.

67. Ulibarri MD, Roesch S, Rangel MG, Staines H, Amaro H, Strathdee SA. 'Amar te Duele' ('love hurts'): sexual relationship power, intimate partner violence, depression symptoms and HIV risk among female sex workers who use drugs and their non-commercial, steady partners in Mexico. *AIDS Behav* 2015; 19: 9–18.

68. Lundgren LM, Amodeo M, Chassler D. Mental health status, drug treatment use, and needle sharing among injection drug users. *AIDS Educ Prev* 2005; 17: 525–539.

69. Reisner SL, White JM, Mayer KH, Mimiaga MJ. Sexual risk behaviors and psychosocial health concerns of female-to-male transgender men screening for STDs at an urban community health center. *AIDS Care* 2014; 26: 857–864.

70. Knaster ES, Fretts AM, Phillips LE. The association of depression with diabetes management among urban American Indians/Alaska Natives in the United States, 2011. *Ethn Dis* 2015; 25: 83–89.

71. UNAIDS. 90-90-90: An ambitious treatment target to help end the AIDS epidemic. Available at: http://www.unaids.org/sites/default/files/media_asset/90-90-90_en_0.pdf (2014, accessed 12 March 2018).

72. World Health Organization. Consolidated guidelines on HIV prevention, diagnosis, treatment and care for key populations. Available at: http://apps.who.int/iris/bitstream/10665/246200/1/9789241511124-eng.pdf?ua=1 (2016, accessed 12 March 2018).

73. Sullivan PS, Hamouda O, Delpech V, et al. Reemergence of the HIV epidemic among men who have sex with men in North America, Western Europe, and Australia, 1996–2005. *Ann Epidemiol* 2009; 19: 423–431.

74. Centers for Disease Control and Prevention (CDC). HIV prevalence, unrecognized infection, and HIV testing among men who have sex with men--five U.S. cities, June 2004-April 2005. *MMWR.* 2005; 54: 597–601.

75. Mayston R, Lazarus A, Patel V, et al. Pathways to HIV testing and care in Goa, India: exploring psychosocial barriers and facilitators using mixed methods. *BMC Public Health* 2016; 16: 765.

76. Li J, Gilmour S, Zhang H, Koyanagi A, Shibuya K. The epidemiological impact and cost-effectiveness of HIV testing, antiretroviral treatment and harm reduction programs. *AIDS* 2012; 26: 2069–2078.

77. Tran BX, Nguyen LH, Phan HT, Nguyen LK, Latkin CA. Preference of methadone maintenance patients for the integrative and decentralized service delivery models in Vietnam. *Harm Reduct J* 2015; 12: 29.

78. Gu J, Xu H, Lau JT, et al. Situation-specific factors predicting nonadherence to methadone maintenance treatment: a cross-sectional study using the case-crossover design in Guangzhou, China. *AIDS Care* 2014; 26(Suppl. 1): S107–S112.

79. Lau JT, Tsui HY, Ho SP, Wong E, Yang X. Prevalence of psychological problems and relationships with condom use and HIV prevention behaviors among Chinese female sex workers in Hong Kong. *AIDS Care* 2010; 22: 659–668.

80. Nemoto T, Operario D, Keatley J, Han L, Soma T. HIV risk behaviors among male-to-female transgender persons of color in San Francisco. *Am J Public Health* 2004; 94: 1193–1199.

81. Pitisuttithum P, Gilbert P, Gurwith M, et al. Randomized, double-blind, placebo-controlled efficacy trial of a bivalent recombinant glycoprotein 120 HIV-1 vaccine among injection drug users in Bangkok, Thailand. *J Infect Dis* 2006; 194: 1661–1671.

82. Cohen MS, Smith MK, Muessig KE, Hallett TB, Powers KA, Kashuba AD. Antiretroviral treatment of HIV-1 prevents transmission of HIV-1: where do we go from here? *Lancet* 2013; 382: 1515–1524.

83. Grant RM, Lama JR, Anderson PL, et al. Preexposure chemoprophylaxis for HIV prevention in men who have sex with men. *N Engl J Med* 2010; 363: 2587–2599.

84. WHO/UNAIDS Technical Consultation. New data on Male circumcision and HIV prevention: Policy and programme implications. Available at: http://www.who.int/hiv/pub/malecircumcision/research_implications/en/ (2007, accessed 12 March 2018).

85. The GMT Initiative. Emerging HIV Prevention Technologies for Gay Men, Other Men who have se with Men, and Transgender Individuals (GMT). Available at: http://www.amfar.org/uploadedFiles/_amfar.org/Around_the_World/MSM(1)/GMT%20HIV%20Treat%20Cascade%20120213.pdf (2013, accessed 12 March 2018).

86. UNAIDS. The gap report. Available at: http://www.unaids.org/sites/default/files/media_asset/UNAIDS_Gap_report_en.pdf (2014, accessed 12 March 2018).

87. Gonzalez JS, Batchelder AW, Psaros C, Safren SA. Depression and HIV/AIDS treatment nonadherence: a review and meta-analysis. *J Acquir Immune Defic Syndr* 2011; 58: 181–187.

88. Blashill AJ, Ehlinger PP, Mayer KH, Safren SA. Optimizing adherence to preexposure and postexposure prophylaxis: the need for an integrated biobehavioral approach. *Clin Infect Dis* 2015; 60(Suppl. 3): S187–S190.

89. Milam J. Posttraumatic growth and HIV disease progression. *J Consult Clin Psychol* 2006; 74: 817–827.

90. Sawyer A, Ayers S, Field AP. Posttraumatic growth and adjustment among individuals with cancer or HIV/AIDS: a meta-analysis. *Clin Psychol Rev* 2010; 30: 436–447.

91. Wei W, Li X, Tu X, Zhao J, Zhao G. Perceived social support, hopefulness, and emotional regulations as mediators of the relationship between enacted stigma and post-traumatic growth among children affected by parental HIV/AIDS in rural China. *AIDS Care* 2016; 28(Suppl. 1): 99–105.

92. Duan W, Guo P, Gan P. Relationships among trait resilience, virtues, post-traumatic stress disorder, and post-traumatic growth. *PLOS ONE* 2015; 10: e0125707.

93. Springer C, Misurell J, Kranzler A, Liotta L, Gillham J. Resilience interventions for youth. In: Parks AC, Schueller SM (eds). *The Wiley Blackwell Handbook of Positive Psychological Interventions.* Hoboken, NJ: John Wiley & Sons, 2014, Chapter 17.

94. Gander F, Proyer RT, Ruch W, Wyss T. Strength-based positive interventions: further evidence for their potential in enhancing well-being and alleviating depression. *J Happiness Stud* 2013; 14: 1241–1259.

95. Seligman MEP, Steen TA, Park N, Peterson C. Positive psychology progress: empirical validation of interventions. *Am Psychol* 2005; 60: 410–421.

96. Mo P, Lau T, Li J. A Randomized controlled study to evaluate the efficacy of a positive psychology and social networking intervention in reducing depressive symptoms among HIV-infected men who have sex with men in China. In: International Behavioral Health Conference BeHealth 2016 – Multiplicity in Action for Better Health, 16 January 2016, Hong Kong.

97. Sheldon KM, Lyubomirsky S. How to increase and sustain positive emotion: the effects of expressing gratitude and visualizing best possible selves. *J Positive Psychol* 2006; 1: 73–82.

98. Hurley DB, Kwon P. Results of a study to increase savoring the moment: differential impact on positive and negative outcomes. *J Happiness Stud* 2012; 13: 579–588.

99. Bolier L, Haverman M, Westerhof GJ, Riper H, Smit F, Bohlmeijer E. Positive psychology interventions: a meta-analysis of randomized controlled studies. *BMC Public Health* 2013; 13: 119.

100. Sin NL, Lyubomirsky S. Enhancing well-being and alleviating depressive symptoms with positive psychology interventions: a practice-friendly meta-analysis. *J Clin Psychol* 2009; 65: 467–487.

101. Jacob KS, Sharan P, Mirza I, et al. Mental health systems in countries: where are we now? Lancet 2007; 370: 1061–1077.

102. Jin H, Hampton Atkinson J, Yu X, et al. Depression and suicidality in HIV/AIDS in China. *J Affect Disord* 2006; 94: 269–275.

103. Chen YY, Li AT, Fung KP, Wong JP. Improving access to mental health services for racialized immigrants, refugees, and non-status people living with HIV/AIDS. *J Health Care Poor Underserved* 2015; 26: 505–518.

104. Xiang D, Wu D. Comparison of social support and life quality of HIV/AIDS patients- a survey based on commercial blood donors, MSM and FSW. *Soc Sci Front* 2010; 4: 194–200.

105. Currie LB, Patterson ML, Moniruzzaman A, McCandless LC, Somers JM. Examining the relationship between health-related need and the receipt of care by participants experiencing homelessness and mental illness. *BMC Health Serv Res* 2014; 14: 404.

106. Li J, Lau JTF, Wang Z, Cao W, Wang X, Cheng PKM. Needs assessments of staff and volunteers of non-governmental organizations working on HIV prevention among men who have sex with men in China. In: 20th International AIDS Conference. 20–25 July 2014, Melbourne, Australia.

107. Goffman E. *Stigma: Notes on the Management of Spoiled Identity.* Englewood Cliffs, NJ: Prentice Hall, 1963.

108. Brown JL, Vanable PA. Cognitive-behavioral stress management interventions for persons living with HIV: a review and critique of the literature. *Ann Behav Med* 2008; 35: 26–40.

109. Eloff I, Finestone M, Makin JD, et al. A randomized clinical trial of an intervention to promote resilience in young children of HIV-positive mothers in South Africa. *AIDS* 2014; 28(Suppl. 3):S347–S357.

110. Riley KE, Kalichman S. Mindfulness-based stress reduction for people living with HIV/AIDS: preliminary review of intervention trial methodologies and findings. *Health Psychol Rev* 2015; 9: 224–243.

111. Meyer IH. Prejudice, social stress, and mental health in lesbian, gay, and bisexual populations: conceptual issues and research evidence. *Psychol Bull* 2003; 129: 674–697.

112. Grossman CI, Stangl AL. Editorial: Global action to reduce HIV stigma and discrimination. *J Int AIDS Soc* 2013; 16(3 Suppl. 2): 18881.

113. Fung KM, Tsang HW, Cheung WM. Randomized controlled trial of the self-stigma reduction program among individuals with schizophrenia. *Psychiatry Res* 2011; 189: 208–214.

114. World Health Organization. Consolidated guidelines on HIV testing services. Available at: http://apps.who.int/iris/bitstream/10665/179870/1/9789241508926_eng.pdf?ua=1&ua=1 (2015, accessed 12 March 2018).

115. World Health Organization. Guideline on when to start antiretroviral therapy and on pre-exposure prophylaxis for HIV. Available at: http://apps.who.int/iris/bitstream/10665/186275/1/9789241509565_eng.pdf?ua=1 (2015, accessed 12 March 2018).

116. Davies MJ, Heller S, Skinner TC, et al. Effectiveness of the diabetes education and self management for ongoing and newly diagnosed (DESMOND) programme for people with newly diagnosed type 2 diabetes: cluster randomised controlled trial. *BMJ* 2008; 336: 491–495.

117. People's Republic of China National Health and Family Planning Commission. Notice on adjusting the standard of free ART of HIV/AID. Available at: http://www.nhfpc.gov.cn/yzygj/s3594/201606/a4cde43ef1ed466c87821e8f9eb1766e.shtml (2016, accessed 12 March 2018) (in Chinese).

118. Meresse M, March L, Kouanfack C, et al. Patterns of adherence to antiretroviral therapy and HIV drug resistance over time in the Stratall ANRS 12110/ESTHER trial in Cameroon. *HIV Med* 2014; 15: 478–487.

119. Gu J, Lau JT, Xu H, et al. A randomized controlled trial to evaluate the relative efficacy of the addition of a psycho-social intervention to standard-of-care services in reducing attrition and improving attendance among first-time users of methadone maintenance treatment in China. *AIDS Behav* 2013; 17: 2002–2010.

120. Mo PK, Lau JT, Yu X, Gu J. A model of associative stigma on depression and anxiety among children of HIV-infected parents in China. *AIDS Behav* 2015; 19: 50–59.

CHAPTER 38

Suicide and the prevention of suicidal behaviours

Lakshmi Vijayakumar and Morton Silverman

Introduction

Suicide is the tragic and untimely loss of human life that is all the more devastating and perplexing because it is a conscious, volitional act. Suicides have occurred since the beginning of recorded history.

There are compelling reasons why suicide and suicidal behaviour should be considered as a public and global health problem. The primary reason is the enormity of the problem. Globally, over 800,000 people died by suicide in 2012. For each adult who died of suicide there were many more who have attempted suicide [1]. Taking into consideration family members, friends, and work colleagues bereaved by suicide [2], there are many millions of people every year who are affected by suicide and suicide attempts [3].

Globally, lifetime prevalence rates are approximately 9.2% for suicidal ideation and 2.7% for suicide attempt [4]. Suicide ideation and attempts are strongly predictive of suicide deaths; can result in negative consequences such as injury, hospitalization, and loss of liberty; and exert a financial burden of billions of dollars on society [4–6]. Taken together, suicide and suicidal behaviour comprise a major leading cause of global disease burden (i.e. years lost to disability, ill health, and early death). By any measure, there is an urgency to better understand and prevent suicide and suicidal behaviour [7].

Another significant concern is that suicide is a major cause of mortality among young people. The leading cause of death worldwide in 2013 for males aged 10–24 years was road injuries (18.3%), followed by self-harm (7.8%), whereas HIV/AIDS was the leading cause for females (7.5%) followed closely by self-harm (7.4%). For females aged 15–19 years, from 1990 to 2013, self-harm was the leading cause of death, whereas for 20–24-year-old males self-harm was the second leading cause of death. From 1990 to 2013, self-harm was either the first or second leading cause of death for both males and females aged 15–24 years. Loss of young lives is not only a loss to the family, but also to the community and to the economy.

Another compelling reason why suicide and suicidal behaviours are a global health problem is that 75.5% of suicides in the world occur in lower- and lower-to-middle-income countries (LAMICs). It is these countries, bearing the larger part of the global suicide burden, that are relatively less equipped to prevent suicide. They are especially hampered by inadequate infrastructure and scarce economic and human resources. There are only 0.29 mental health professionals per 100,000 population in low-income countries and 2.98 per 100,000 population in low-to-middle-income countries [8]. Hence, only a public health approach would enable a meaningful reduction in suicidal behaviour globally.

There is an increased awareness of the need to address suicide and promote suicide prevention globally. All together, 168 countries have signed the World Health Organization (WHO) Mental Health Action Plan 2013–2020, which commits them to reduce suicide rate in their countries by 10% by the year 2020 [9]. Hence, the first ever WHO report on suicide prevention, *Preventing Suicide: A Global Imperative*, published in September 2014, is a timely call to take action using effective evidence-based interventions. Furthermore, suicide rates are as an indicator for the United Nations' (UN) Sustainable Development Goals (SDG).

Suicidal behaviours (i.e. thoughts and actions) are multidetermined, multifactorial, and multidimensional. Therefore, no one approach, theory or intervention will work in all contexts. Social, psychological, cultural, and other factors can interact to lead a person to engage in suicidal behaviour, but often the stigma attached to mental disorders and suicidal behaviours makes it an impediment to seeking help. Despite the evidence that many deaths are preventable, suicide is too often a low priority for governments and policymakers. Hence, the reduction of suicides and suicidal behaviours should not only be a health objective, but also a social and humanitarian objective. A broad canvas of coordinated and collaborative actions is needed.

Nomenclature and classification

Part of the difficulty in conceptualizing, implementing, and measuring suicide preventative interventions is that there is no internationally agreed-upon set of terms, definitions, or classifications for the range of thoughts, communications, and behaviours that are related to self-injurious behaviours, with or without the intent to die. There is no agreed-upon nomenclature and classification system that currently exists within nations, let alone between and among nations. Nor is there an agreed taxonomy that encompasses the full spectrum of what is clinically defined as suicide-related behaviours. The suicide literature remains replete with confusing (and sometimes derogatory or pejorative) terms, definitions, descriptors, and classifications that make it difficult, if not impossible, to compare and contrast different research studies, clinical reports, or epidemiological surveys [10, 11].

There is an abundance of terms to describe the range of suicidal behaviours and suicide-related behaviours, such as non suicidal self-injury, deliberate self-harm behaviours, and so on. There is no agreement on the terminology, let alone the definitions for the key components of the suicidal process: suicidal ideation (vs death thoughts), intent, motivation, planning, threats, gestures, and behaviours (e.g. preparatory, aborted, interrupted, self-inflicted, non-lethal, lethal, near-lethal, etc.). There remains much confusion about what constitutes suicidal behaviour and what is classified or labelled as other forms of self-injury, accidents, and so on [12–15]. There remains debate about whether the presence/absence of intent should be a qualifying characteristic for labelling self-injurious behaviours as suicidal. There is also debate as to whether the degree of lethality involved in the self-injurious act should serve as the major determinant in categorizing the behaviour as suicidal, non-suicidal, deliberate self-harm, and so on [16].

A uniform nomenclature and classification for suicidal ideation and behaviour has been the subject of considerable international attention and debate [17–20]. Measures of suicide and non-fatal suicidal behaviour (encompassing with this term all self-injurious behaviours inclusive of self-harm and suicide attempt) continue to be hindered by the lack of (i) a standard nomenclature and classification system [19, 21–23]; (ii) clear operational definitions [24–26]; and (iii) standardized lethality measures [16]. It has been pointed out that not only must we use the same terminology and definitions, but also that these terms must be easily understood, applied, and consistent, and should relate to each other in a way that has utility, meaning, and relevance to the real world of at-risk individuals [10, 11].

It is recognized that categorizing self-directed violence behaviour into suicidal and non-suicidal categories can be difficult. This is owing to several considerations: firstly, that the behaviour is multi-dimensional rather that unitary and does not always occur in a dichotomous way (present/absent), meaning that suicidal individuals may perform non-suicidal acts and non-suicidal individuals may perform suicidal acts; and, secondly, that if information is collected only from an individual's self-report, the way the individual perceives his/her intent can change within moments, not to mention the possibility of the intent being disguised or exaggerated [27]. Nevertheless, owing to the essential nature of this information to clinical and public health decision-making, it is critical to try to obtain it.

The WHO defines violence as [28]:

> The intentional use of physical force or power, threatened or actual, against oneself, another person, or against a group or community, that either results in or has a high likelihood of resulting in injury, death, psychological harm, maldevelopment or deprivation (WHO [28] p. 5).

Hence, suicide and suicide attempts are classified as a form of violence. However, self-directed violence encompasses a range of behaviours, including acts of fatal and non-fatal suicidal behaviour and non-suicidal intentional self-harm (i.e. behaviours where the intention is not to kill oneself, as in self-mutilation) [29]. It is important to acknowledge the implications and complexities of including self-harm in the definition of 'suicide attempt'. This means that non-fatal self-harm without suicidal intent is included under this term, which is problematic owing to the possible variations in related behaviours and subsequent interventions. In addition, the inclusion of suicidal ideation in the definition of suicidal behaviour is a complex issue about which there is meaningful ongoing academic dialogue.

In order to conduct its worldwide surveillance studies, the WHO has adopted the following terms and definitions [6]:

Suicide is the act of deliberately killing oneself.

Suicide attempt is used to mean any non-fatal suicidal behaviour and refers to intentional self-inflicted poisoning, injury, or self-harm, which may or may not have a fatal intent or outcome.

Suicidal behaviour refers to a range of behaviours that include thinking about suicide (or ideation), planning for suicide, attempting suicide, and suicide itself.

Epidemiology of suicidal behaviours

Globally, over 800 000 people died by suicide in 2012, according to the WHO Global Health Estimates [6, 30, 31]. This corresponds to a global age-standardized suicide rate of 11.4 per 100,000 population; 15.0 and 8.0 per 100,000 for males and females, respectively. However, as suicidal behaviour is a sensitive issue, and given the stigma often accorded to it—and the illegality of suicidal behaviour in some countries—it is likely that under-reporting and misclassification are greater problems for accurately counting the numbers of suicides than for most other causes of death.

There are many areas of the world where we have little or no information on suicide mortality. For the most part, these areas are among the poorest, and they face numerous social, political, and economic challenges as well [22]. The under-reporting of suicide attempts and deaths by suicide is a major problem worldwide [32, 33], and is particularly problematic in developing countries. Stigma surrounding all forms of suicidal behaviours is believed to be an important matter that can result in under-reporting of suicide, in particular age, gender, and racial/ethnic groups.

The lack of systematic and standardized data collecting and reporting of suicidal behaviours among many countries hinders the development of suicide prevention strategies based on accurate information about the size and extent of the problem. It also prevents a reliable comparison of countries concerning the same problem.

Globally, suicides account for 50% of all violent deaths in men and 71% in women. With regard to age, suicide rates are highest in persons aged 70 years or over for both men and women in almost all regions of the world. In some countries, suicide rates are highest among the young, and, globally, suicide is the second leading cause of death in 15–29 year olds [6]; for young girls, aged 15–19 years, it is the first leading cause of death globally [34]. In more affluent countries, three times as many men die by suicide as do women, but in LAMICs the male : female ratio is much lower (1.5 : 1).

Most studies of suicidal thoughts and behaviours have been conducted within individual Western, high-income countries [35]. Recent studies in several LAMICs, such as China and India, suggest the occurrence of suicidal behaviours may differ markedly from high-income countries [36, 37]. Nock et al. [4] analyzed WHO World Mental Health Surveys conducted in 17 countries, and found that although there is substantial variability in the prevalence of suicidal behaviours cross-nationally, there are important cross-national consistencies in the prevalence and risk factors for suicidal behaviours. The cross-national lifetime prevalence of suicidal ideation, plans, and attempts is 9.2%, 3.1% ,and 2.7%, respectively. Most notably, across all countries examined, 60% of the transitions from suicidal ideation to first suicide attempt occurred within the first year of ideation onset. Moreover, consistent cross-national risk factors included female sex, younger age, fewer years of education, unmarried status, and the presence of a mental disorder, with psychiatric co-morbidity significantly increasing risk. The strongest diagnostic risk factors were mood disorders in high-income countries, but in LAMICs it was impulse control disorders. Nock et al. [4] concluded that there is cross-national variability in the prevalence of suicidal behaviours but strong consistency in the characteristics and risk factors for these behaviours.

Despite a drop in the estimated global age-standardized suicide rate between 2000 and 2012, which may be explained, in part, by an improvement in global health, regionally there have been increases in LAMICs in the African region, and among men in LAMICs in the Eastern Mediterranean Region, emphasizing the need to concentrate and prioritize suicide prevention efforts in LAMICs [6]. However, in some countries, suicide rates are highest among the young [38]. Young adults and elderly women in LAMICs have much higher suicide rates than their counterparts in high-income countries, whereas middle-aged men in high-income countries have much higher suicide rates than middle-aged men in LAMICs.

Not only is death by suicide a global public health problem, but there are also many more individuals who experience suicidal ideation and engage in suicide attempts, which can lead to hospitalizations, permanent disabilities, loss of income, and increased risk of engaging in future suicidal behaviours. In an analysis of WHO Mental Health Surveys, Nock et al. [39] found that a wide range of mental disorders increased the odds of experiencing suicide ideation. However, after controlling for psychiatric co-morbidity, only disorders characterized by anxiety and poor impulse control predicted which people with suicide ideation progress to suicide attempts.

The development of trustworthy surveillance and registration systems have been a central need in several past and present studies on suicide led by the WHO, such as the WHO/EURO Multicentre Study on Suicidal Behavior [40] and the WHO Suicide Prevention Multisite Intervention Study on Suicidal Behaviors (WHO/SUPRE-MISS) [41].

Risk factors

Suicide is contextual, culturally determined, and responsive to economic, political, and social changes, in addition to other factors and/or stresses. Many risk factors have been shown statistically to be correlated with the onset of suicidal ideation, maintenance of suicidal ideation, suicidal intent, suicidal planning, suicide attempts, repeat suicide attempts, and death by suicide. However, these risk factors are not universal, not necessarily related to all suicidal thoughts and behaviours, and differ by age, sex, ethnicity/race, psychiatric disorder, degree of substance abuse, geography, presence of a chronic physical illness, religious belief, sense of connectedness to others, sense of self-worth and self-esteem, and a sense of a future or degree of hope. Undoubtedly, precipitating factors, social contexts, and meanings of suicide differ substantially between countries within any region.

No single factor is sufficient to explain why a person died by suicide: suicidal behaviour is a complex phenomenon that is influenced by several interacting factors, including personal, social, psychological, cultural, biological, and environmental factors. Increasing evidence shows that the specific context is imperative to understanding the risk of suicide. No one risk factor, or set of distinct risk factors, has been shown to cause suicide or suicidal behaviours at the individual or population level.

Many suicides occur impulsively in moments of crisis and, in these circumstances, ready access to the means of suicide, such as pesticides or firearms, can determine whether a person lives or dies. Other risk factors for suicide include a breakdown in the ability to deal with acute or chronic life stresses, such as financial problems. In addition, gender-based violence and child abuse are strongly associated with suicidal behaviour. Suicide rates also vary within countries, with higher rates among those who are minorities or experience discrimination.

Risk factors associated with the *health system and society at large* include difficulties in accessing health care and in receiving the care needed, easy availability of the means for suicide, inappropriate media reporting that sensationalizes suicide and increases the risk of 'copycat' suicides, and stigma against people who seek help for suicidal behaviours, or for mental health and substance abuse problems.

Risk factors linked to the *community and relationships* include war and disaster, stresses of acculturation and dislocation (e.g. among indigenous peoples or displaced persons), discrimination, a sense of isolation and lack of social support, trauma or abuse, violence and conflictual relationships.

Risk factors at the *individual level* include previous suicide attempts, mental disorders, harmful use of alcohol and other substances, job or financial loss, hopelessness, chronic pain and illness, a family history of suicide, and genetic and biological factors.

A number of past studies conducted in non-Western populations have highlighted the importance of life events, and economic and social stress as influences on suicide. For example, studies on South Asian women reveal the proximal influences of gender roles, cultural expectations, family conflict, and domestic violence in female suicide [42], whereas alcohol use, financial issues, and interpersonal conflict are recognized as particularly important risk factors for male suicide in India [43].

An illustration of the many risk factors and how they may interact to heighten the risk for suicidal behaviours, is shown in Fig. 38.1 [44].

Methods for self-injury

There are notable differences in suicide methods between countries, being affected by cultural acceptability, availability, and lethality of means. Pesticide ingestion, hanging, and firearms are among the most common methods of suicide globally; many other methods are used based primarily on their ready accessibility, with the choice of method often varying locally.

Kolves and De Leo [45] analysed and described suicide methods in children and adolescents aged 10–19 years in different countries/territories worldwide. In total, 101 countries or territories have data at least for 5 years between 2000 and 2009. The most frequent suicide method was hanging, followed by poisoning by pesticides for females and firearms for males. Hanging and poisoning by pesticides defined the clusters of countries/territories by

Suicide is an outcome that requires several things to go wrong all at once.
.. There is no one cause of suicide and no single type of suicidal person.

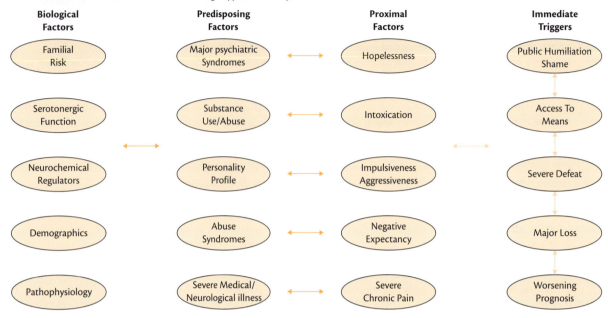

Fig. 38.1 Interaction of multiple risk factors for suicide.
Source: Data from Knesper DJ, American Association of Suicidology & Suicide Prevention Resource Center, Continuity of care for suicide prevention and research: Suicide attempts and suicide deaths subsequent to discharge from the emergency department or psychiatry inpatient unit, Copyright (2010), Education Development Center.

their suicide patterns in young people for both sexes. Overall, the patterns of suicide methods in children and adolescents reflect lethality, availability, and acceptability of suicide means similarly to country-specific patterns of all ages.

Protective factors

In contrast to risk factors, protective factors are believed to guard people against the risk of suicide. Some protective factors counter specific risk factors, whereas others protect individuals against a number of different suicide risk factors. While many interventions are geared towards the reduction of risk factors in suicide prevention, it is equally important to consider and strengthen factors that have been shown to increase resilience and connectedness and that protect against suicidal behaviour. Resilience has a buffering effect on suicide risk; for persons who are highly resilient the association between the risk of suicide and suicidal behaviour is diminished.

Protective factors include strong personal relationships, religious or spiritual beliefs, and lifestyle practice of positive coping strategies and well-being. Well-being is shaped, in part, by personality traits that determine vulnerability for and resilience against stress and trauma. Emotional stability, an optimistic outlook, and a developed self-identity assist in coping with life's difficulties. Good self-esteem, self-efficacy, and effective problem solving-skills, which include the ability to seek help when needed, can mitigate the impact of stressors and childhood adversities. Healthy lifestyle choices that promote mental and physical well-being include regular exercise and sport, adequate sleep and diet, consideration of the impact on health of alcohol and drugs, healthy relationships and social contact, and effective management of stress.

Suicide attempts

A statistically significant risk factor for repeat suicidal behaviours is a history of suicide attempt(s) or non-suicidal self-injury. The research suggests that approximately 10% of people with a history of suicide attempts will eventually die by suicide, and 15% will engage in repetitive suicide attempts within 1 year [46]. It has been estimated that the risk of suicide after deliberate self-harm is about 25 times higher than in the general population [47].

Suicide attempters are an important focus of research, both in their own right and because they are considered a proxy for people who die by suicide [48]. Studies have consistently shown increased rates of stressful or threatening life events, such as interpersonal problems, financial difficulties, mental disorders, physical illness, and disability, in the recent history of individuals who attempt suicide or die by suicide [40, 49, 50]. Interpersonal conflict—with partners, family or friends—has been found to be the most prevalent reason for suicidal behaviour, reported in about 50% of cases [4, 51–54]. Mental health problems are usually the second most common reason [5, 51–54], but can be the most common reason [55].

As part of the Monitoring Suicide in Europe (MONSUE) project [56], data on 4683 suicide attempters from nine European countries were collected. The project found that interpersonal conflict was common for all patients except those widowed, living alone, or retired. Mental health problems were prevalent among over 45 year olds, patients unable to work, and patients with a history of at least three suicide attempts. Financial difficulties were cited more often by patients who were 45–64 years old, divorced or separated, living with children only, and unemployed. Recent bereavement, serious illness, and their own physical illnesses were associated with suicide attempts for those over 65 years of age. Two reasons for suicide attempts—interpersonal conflict and mental health problems—were associated with increased risk of repetition independent of other factors. The authors concluded that suicide attempters have a multitude of problems of varying prevalence depending on age, sex, and other factors. They present a range of clinical profiles that require a multidisciplinary response.

Incorporating the prevention of suicide within a global public health approach

It is not easy to apply the medical model concepts of 'disease' and 'illnesses' to self-harm and self-injury, as they are multifactorial, multidetermined, and multidimensional behaviours that defy simple or universal explanations, making the development, implementation, monitoring, and evaluation of preventative interventions, alone or in combination, difficult at best.

Public health preventative interventions are population-focused, so that those at risk are identified and receive interventions at the community level. Identifying those groups or individuals who are truly at high risk before the expression of suicide ideation or behaviours remains a major challenge for the field of suicide prevention. To date, the majority of approaches have focused on the clinical treatment of those who already have been identified with suicide ideation or who have attempted suicide.

There is an absence of strong epidemiological evidence regarding which risk factors to target for the greatest impact at a population level and evidence regarding the effectiveness of particular approaches. This has led to a recommendation for a multifaceted approach that draws on a range of universal, selective, and indicated strategies, and addresses a broad range of risk factors. Risk factors for suicide attempts and suicide ideation are not completely understood although some factors (being young, female, unmarried, of low socio-economic status, etc.) have been consistently identified as heightening the risk, whereas the evidence is weaker regarding others (being unemployed, having an anxiety disorder, etc.) [57]. Deriving estimates of population-attributable risk is important as it would provide direction as to the nature of preventative programmes that are likely to be successful at both the individual level and the population level.

Inasmuch as suicidal behaviours are often associated with the presence of mental disorders and substance abuse (acute or chronic), some have argued that the best approach to preventing suicide-related thoughts and behaviours is to address, treat, and/or prevent the aetiologies and expression of mental disorders. Effectively treating affective disorders (i.e. major depressive disorder and bipolar disorder) may well be the best prevention intervention for suicide thoughts and behaviours.

Mental health services could have an important part to play in reducing the risk of suicide in those already identified at increased risk for suicide [57–59]. Service-related risk factors for suicide identified in studies include poor continuity of care [60], scarcity of well-developed mental health services in the community [61], short length of inpatient stay [62], reduction of care at final appointment before death [63], and missed appointments with services [57]. However, most studies of the relation between service interventions and suicide rate are limited by small sample sizes, short follow-up periods after intervention, cross-sectional rather than prospective designs, and infrequent collection of data on service-related variables. Nevertheless, the successful prevention of mental illnesses and/or the successful treatment of mental illnesses would contribute to preventing suicidal ideation, suicide attempts, and deaths by suicide.

We know that suicidal individuals share many similar risk profiles with other high-risk groups:

◆ alcohol and substance abuse and dependence;

◆ perpetrators and victims of domestic violence;

◆ victims of early life physical, emotional, and sexual abuse.

Such similarities suggest that the prevention of suicidal behaviours may well rest not only in targeting suicidal behaviours per se, but also in the prevention of childhood adversities, prevention of domestic and intimate partner violence, and prevention of alcohol and substance abuse and dependence. Because of the close relationship between the manifestations of psychiatric disorders and the onset and expression of suicidal behaviours, some have argued that the prevention of the onset and expression of psychiatric disorders, or, at least, the appropriate and timely treatment and management of psychiatric disorders, would have a very positive effect on reducing the incidence and prevalence of suicidal behaviours.

Caine [64] has suggested that addressing adequate housing and consistent care for those with severe mental disorders, integrating the civil and criminal justice systems with community-based mental health services, workplace programmes to promote mental health, providing support to the unemployed, providing outreach programmes to isolated elders and to homeless young people, and providing clinical services to the mentally ill (including alcohol and substance abuse services) will all have direct effects on lowering the suicide rate. Yet addressing one or even a few of these 'proxy measures' will not necessarily reduce the morbidity and mortality associated with suicidal behaviours. Caine argues for recognition of 'common risk' at the community level, including suicide and suicide attempts, alcohol and drug abuse, domestic violence, interpersonal violence (homicides), unemployment, accidental deaths, and workplace losses in productivity.

Such a successful programme was undertaken by the US Air Force Suicide Prevention Program, which adopted a multilayered approach involving 11 initiatives clusters into four areas: increase awareness and knowledge, increase early help-seeking; change social norms; and change selected policies. As a result of this 'community-based' prevention programme there was a 33% reduction in suicide, a 51% reduction in homicide, a 54% reduction in severe family violence, a 30% reduction in moderate family violence, and an 18% reduction in accidental death [65].

Suicide prevention: limitations and challenges to implementation and evaluation

There are several limitations in accessing data on suicide, understanding the complex interaction of risk and protective factors and in identifying appropriate interventions, which are tabulated in Box 38.1.

Suicide is a rare phenomenon with a low base rate. The number of persons required for an effectiveness study is huge.

The limitations in the measurement of suicide prevention interventions are explained in Box 38.2.

Box 38.1 Limitations and challenges to implementation and evaluation

Access to the population: Most suicides are attempted within 1 year of the onset of suicide ideation (60%), and most with serious intent attempt suicide only once; however, over 50% die as a result of their first attempt [35].

Psychology of suicide: As current knowledge about the interactions between cognitions, emotions, and behaviours is limited, it is difficult to devise suicide prevention strategies that address all of them simultaneously.

Identifying appropriate strategies: There is a lack of robust evidence regarding interventions for the greatest impact at a population level. For example, which risk factors to target.

Risk factors for suicide attempts: Knowledge about risk factors for suicide attempts and suicidal ideation is weak for many factors. Existing knowledge is about individual risk rather than at a population level.

Implementing global public health approaches to prevent suicide attempts and deaths by suicide

Public mental health strategies are, by definition, population-based. Hence, most suicide prevention strategies are community-based or nationally based. Currently, there are approximately 28 countries with national suicide prevention strategies. Common to all are the following strategies:

- enhance surveillance and research;
- identify and target vulnerable groups;
- improve the assessment and management of suicidal behaviour;
- promote environmental and individual protective factors;
- increase awareness through public education;
- improve societal attitudes and beliefs, and eliminate stigma towards people with mental disorders or who exhibit suicidal behaviours;
- reduce access to means of suicide;

Box 38.2 Limitations to effective measurement of suicide prevention interventions

As suicide is a low base-rate phenomenon it very difficult to recruit sufficient numbers into the intervention and control groups of a preventative intervention trial to demonstrate effectiveness of an intervention over a short period of time.

This problem also exists—albeit to a lesser extent—in studies where the outcome of interest is suicide attempt rates.

Randomized controlled trials have not identified the most effective intervention strategies to address suicide attempters.

Complex methodologies that advocate a mixed-methods approach that looks to triangulate data from various sources has been recommended as a possible strategy.

- encourage the media to adopt better policies and practices toward reporting suicide;
- support individuals bereaved by suicide.

In addition, all countries should review their legal provisions in relation to suicide to ensure they do not act as a barrier to seeking help.

In a recent comprehensive review of the international literature on effective suicide prevention programs, Zalsman et al. [66] found increasing evidence for restricting access to lethal means in the prevention of suicide, especially with regard to control of analgesics and hotspots for suicide by jumping. School-based awareness programmes have been shown to reduce suicide attempts and suicidal ideation. The anti-suicidal effects of clozapine and lithium have been substantiated but might be less specific than previously thought. Effective pharmacological and psychological treatments of depression are important in prevention. Insufficient evidence exists to assess the possible benefits for suicide prevention of screening in primary care, in general public education, and media guidelines. Other approaches that need further investigation include gatekeeper training, education of physicians, and Internet and helpline support. The paucity of randomized controlled trials is a major limitation in the evaluation of preventative interventions. They concluded that no single strategy clearly stands above the others.

Effective evidence-based interventions in WHO's *Preventing Suicide: A Global Imperative* [6], include highlighting restricting access to means, responsible media reporting, introducing mental health and alcohol policies, early identification and treatment, training of health workers, and follow-up care and community support following a suicide attempt.

Evidence-based interventions
Restricting access to means

Direct access or proximity to means (including pesticides, firearms, heights, railway tracks, poisons, licit and illicit drugs, sources of carbon monoxide such as car exhausts or charcoal, and other hypoxic and poisonous gases) is a major risk factor for suicide. The availability of and preference for specific means of suicide also depend on geographical and cultural contexts [32, 67].

Restricting access to the means of suicide is effective in preventing suicide—particularly impulsive suicide—as it gives those contemplating suicide more time to reconsider and allows time for intervention and change of mind. While mental disorders are diagnosed in around 90% of suicide cases in high-income countries, psychological autopsy studies in China and India revealed only 40–60% had a psychiatric diagnosis, placing an added importance to means restrictions as a universal intervention [36, 68]. Implementation of strategies to restrict means can occur both at the national level, through laws and regulations, and at the local level, for instance by securing risk environments.

Pesticides account for an estimated one-third of the world's suicides [69]. Reducing access to pesticides could significantly impact on reducing impulsive suicide in relevant LAMICs. Suicide by intentional pesticide ingestion primarily occurs in rural and agricultural areas of LAMICs in Africa, Central America, South East Asia, and the Western Pacific. Measures proposed to prevent suicide by pesticides include ratifying, implementing, and enforcing relevant international conventions on hazardous chemicals and wastes; legislating to remove locally problematic pesticides from agricultural practice; enforcing regulations on the sale of pesticides;

reducing access to pesticides through safer storage and disposal by individuals or communities; and reducing the toxicity of pesticides [70, 71].

In addition, the medical management of those who attempt suicide by self-ingestion of pesticides should be optimized, particularly through reduced barriers to immediate care [44, 72, 73]. Suicide by firearms is a highly lethal method, accounting for the majority of suicides in some countries, such as the USA [74, 75]. Available data show a close correlation between the proportions of households owning firearms and the proportion of firearm suicides [76]. Legislation restricting firearm ownership has been associated with a reduction in firearm suicide rates in many countries, including Australia, Canada, New Zealand, Norway, and the UK.

Historically, intentional carbon monoxide poisoning has been one of the most common methods of suicide in some countries. Legislative and pragmatic changes to domestic gas at national and regional levels have substantially reduced suicide by this method. Collectively, evidence indicates that reducing the lethality of carbon monoxide has a direct effect on decreasing overall suicide rates. Charcoal-burning poisoning is a recent method of suicide by toxic gas that has rapidly become a common method in some Asian countries. Removing charcoal packs from open shelves into a controlled area in major store outlets in Hong Kong has significantly reduced charcoal-related suicide deaths [77].

In most European countries, self-poisoning with medication is the second or third most common method of suicide and suicide attempts [78]. Restricting access to and availability of medications that are commonly used in suicide has been shown to be an effective preventative measure [79]. Healthcare providers can play a critical role by restricting the amount of medication dispensed, informing patients and their families about the risks of overdose or prescribed medications, and stressing the importance of adhering to prescribed dosages and disposal of unused tablets.

Responsible media reporting

Inappropriate media reporting practices can sensationalize and glamorize suicide and increase the risk of 'copycat' suicides (imitation of suicides) among vulnerable people. Responsible reporting of suicide in the media has been shown to decrease suicide rates.

Important aspects of responsible reporting include avoiding detailed descriptions of suicidal acts, avoiding sensationalism and glamorization, using responsible language, minimizing the prominence and duration of suicide reports, avoiding oversimplifications, educating the public about suicide and available treatments, and providing information on where to seek help. Media collaboration and participation in the development, dissemination and training of responsible reporting practices are also essential for successfully improving the reporting of suicide and reducing suicide imitation [80]. These improvements were demonstrated in Australia and Austria following active media involvement in the dissemination of media guidelines [81]. Common sense suggests that responsible media reporting about suicide would be effective in all jurisdictions, but further evidence is needed internationally to confirm the value of this type of intervention for reducing suicides in LAMICs.

Introducing mental health and alcohol policies

Whilst mental health should constitute a priority for all governments, suicide prevention efforts should be broadened beyond improving the recognition and treatment of mental disorders. For example, the role of alcohol and substance use disorders in the aetiology of suicidal behaviour has traditionally received much less attention than that of other types of mental disorders such as depression, but it has become increasingly evident that alcohol and drugs are important preventable risk factors for suicide in countries and demographic subgroups within countries where alcohol and drug use are common.

The WHO Mental Health Action Plan 2013–2020 [9] and the WHO Global Strategy to reduce the harmful use of alcohol [82] provide frameworks and guidance on getting started. At the population level, policies to reduce harmful use of alcohol should be developed as a component of a comprehensive suicide prevention strategy, particularly within populations with a high prevalence of alcohol use [83]. In populations with lower levels of drinking, strategies such as awareness-raising can be implemented through general media campaigns, school health promotion activities, or information targeted at vulnerable individuals through health professionals [84, 85]. The alcohol culture of specific regions should be considered carefully before strategies are selected in order to ensure that the strategies are effective in the context. A functioning legal system is also a prerequisite for enforcing these strategies effectively.

Early identification and treatment

Frequently, several risk factors act cumulatively to increase a person's vulnerability to suicide. Early detection and intervention are key activities to ensuring that people receive the care they need. In this regard, all health services should incorporate suicide prevention as a core component.

Asking about suicide gives the opportunity to refer to appropriate care or treatment if required [86]. Protocols for clinical decision-making and management are provided and tools for implementation (including a module for programme planners, situation analysis and adaptation guide, monitoring and evaluation tool, and training materials) are available for implementation primarily in LAMICs. This recommended package of suicide interventions for low-resourced settings was the result of an exhaustive iterative effort by international experts, and its implementation will reveal whether reduced suicides in LAMICs can be demonstrated.

Training of health workers

Education and training of health workers is needed to ensure that psychosocial support is provided to those in need and is a key way forward in suicide prevention. A large number of those who die by suicide have had contact with primary healthcare providers within the month prior to the suicide, and there is a growing number of LAMICs where suicide awareness and skills training has been implemented in primary care services [87]. Educating healthcare workers to recognize depression and other mental and substance use disorders, and to assess imminent risk of suicide are important for determining level of care and referral for treatment, and by that, preventing suicidal behaviour [88, 89]. This can be implemented through the WHO Mental Health Gap Action Programme (mhGAP) Intervention Guide in non-specialized health settings [90]. Training should take place continuously or repeatedly over years, and should involve the majority of health workers in a region or country. It is important to consider local risk factors and to tailor the training programme to these in order for the programme to be successful within countries and cultures.

Follow-up care and community support following a suicide attempt

Recently discharged patients often lack social support and can feel isolated once they leave care. Follow-up and community support have been effective in reducing suicide deaths and attempts among patients who have been recently discharged from the healthcare system [91]. Repeated follow-ups are a recommended low-cost intervention that is easy to implement; existing treatment staff, including trained non-specialized health workers, can implement the intervention and require few resources [90].

This is particularly useful in LAMICs and also recognized in high-income countries. The intervention can involve the use of postcards, telephone calls, or brief in-person visits (informal or formal) to make contact and encourage continued contact [92]. Involving available community support—such as family, friends, colleagues, crisis centres, or local mental health centres—in after-care is important as these can regularly monitor people and en-courage treatment adherence [90]. Communities play a critical role in suicide prevention. In all countries, particularly those with limited resources, the importance of the role of communities in suicide prevention cannot be overstated, particularly in terms of support programmes for vulnerable groups.

The development of integrated suicide prevention strategies that function at the individual, family, community, and societal level are the key to locally relevant and culturally appropriate suicide pre-vention programmes targeting the most vulnerable populations.

In LAMICs, suicide prevention is more a social and public health objective than a traditional exercise in the mental health sector [37, 93, 94]. This approach harnesses community action through building community capacity, while pragmatically recognizing the finite health resources within the primary and secondary health sectors in LAMICs [95, 96].

Having a history of previous suicide attempts is recognized as a strong predictor of subsequent death by suicide. The WHO/SUPRE-MISS [92]– which included a number of LAMICs –and other studies for high-income countries have shown that follow-up services for persons who have attempted suicide can reduce subse-quent suicidal behaviour.

Improving the registration of suicide attempts and developing a support network to follow-up these individuals is, perhaps, the single most practical step low-resourced LAMICs can take to re-duce suicides.

To conclude, the interventions discussed above are all eligible for implementation in LMICs. For universal school-based intervention programmes, evidence is accumulating for their effectiveness in high-income countries, suggesting that they are ready to be tested in LAMICs [97, 98]. Other approaches, such as helplines or gate-keeper training (other than primary healthcare workers), are often used as best-practice approaches, but lack the conclusive evidence of effectiveness on the outcome measures of reduction in suicide or suicide attempts. Approaches like cognitive–behavioural therapy or dialectical behaviour therapy may, at present, be too costly and not feasible owing to the lack of trained personnel.

Community-level strategies that may have potential in preventing suicide in LAMICs include utilizing the services of non-governmental organizations, awareness-raising in schools, commu-nity education around self-immolation, and training of gatekeepers [6, 71, 98–101]; however, there is need for more extensive studies to improve the evidence base for these suggestions in LAMICs before they can be recommended for specific contexts.

An economic investment in suicide prevention programmes

In addition to evidence on the effectiveness of suicide prevention interventions, health planners and decision-makers require in-formation on the expected costs of implementation in different settings, cultures, and contexts, and also on cost-effectiveness, in order to ensure that such strategies represent good value for money in countries with limited resources and can help determine where resources will be best allocated.

For instance, an economic study of self-poisoning in Sri Lanka was able to estimate that resource needs for treatment in the country would amount to US$866,000 in 2004 (each treated case costing an average of US$32) [102].

Globally, there is a lack of robust economic studies to inform planners and policymakers of the budgetary requirements and return on investment associated with efforts to prevent suicide. For national responses to be effective, a comprehensive multi-sectoral suicide prevention strategy, including good-quality data, is essential [96]. A national strategy indicates a government's clear commitment to dealing with the issue of suicide.

Typically, national strategies comprise a range of prevention strategies, such as means restriction, media guidelines and training for health workers. Resources should be allocated for achieving both short-to-medium and long-term objectives; there should be effective planning and the strategy should be regularly evaluated with evaluation findings feeding into future planning.

It is essential that governments assume their role of leadership, as they can bring together a multitude of stakeholders who may not otherwise collaborate. Governments are also in a unique position to develop and strengthen surveillance, resulting in better quality and availability of both suicide and suicide attempt data, and to provide and disseminate data that are necessary to inform action [6].

Future directions

The Millennium Development Goals that expired in 2015 were replaced by Sustainable Development Goals (SDGs) by the UN General Assembly in September 2015 [103]. There are 15 uni-versal goals with 169 targets that are expected to shape the policy decisions of all the countries over the next 15 years. The Inter Agency Expert Group on SDG has announced 230 indicators to measure achievement of the 169 targets. Of particular importance to suicide prevention is target 3.4, which states 'By 2030, reduce by one third premature mortality for NCD's through prevention and treatment and promote mental health and wellbeing. The indicator 3.4.2 is to be suicide mortality rate'.

Hence, every country is challenged to not only improve their data collection, but also to reduce their suicide rates. This presents a unique opportunity to align suicide prevention to SDGs and propel suicide prevention to a broader global canvas.

Of the 19 goals, six goals are related to suicide prevention.

Goal 1: End poverty in all its form everywhere. The target is to build resilience of the poor and those in vulnerable situations and reduce their exposure to climate-related events and other socio-economic, social, and environmental shocks. Providing economic security, reducing unemployment, and enhancing resilience in the community have been targeted in suicide prevention.

Goal 2: End hunger, achieve food security, improve nutrition, and promote sustainable agriculture. Sustainable agriculture can be achieved by banning toxic pesticides, promoting non-pesticide management of pests, limiting access to pesticides by safer storage, all of which have been recommended to reduce suicide rates.

Goal 3: Ensure healthy life and promote well-being for all ages. There are many targets for this particular goal, such as reducing maternal mortality, tuberculosis, HIV, malaria, diabetes, cardiovascular disease, etc. Of particular importance to suicide prevention is Target 3.5, which is to strengthen the prevention and treatment of substance abuse, including narcotic drug abuse and harmful use of alcohol. The WHO has consistently advocated for policies to reduce the harmful use of alcohol as a strategy to reduce suicides.

Goal 5: Achieve gender equality and empower all women and girls. Reduction of domestic violence, child sexual abuse, education, and empowerment has been recommended to reduce suicides particularly in young females.

Goal 11: Make cities and human settlements inclusive, safe, and sustainable. Safe housing, promoting mental health of refugees and internally displaced persona, have been recommended to reduce suicidal behaviour in their communities.

Goal 16: Promote peaceful and inclusive societies for sustainable development, provide access to justice for all and build effective accountable and inclusive institutions at all levels. This aims at reducing discrimination (race, religion) and promoting tolerance and inclusiveness. Decriminalization of suicide could be an important platform for obtaining justice for the distressed individuals who attempt suicide.

Goal 17: Goal 17 is a Venn diagram that incorporates all of the goals (see Fig. 38.2). This representation as it applies to suicide prevention is in synchrony with SDG goals.

Conclusions

Suicide and suicidal behaviours are a global public health problem and solutions can be found only through global attention and communication. Suicide prevention is everybody's business.

Inasmuch as suicide and suicidal behaviours are multidetermined, multifactorial, and occur in all countries and throughout all sectors of the population, a public mental health approach to suicide prevention is the best approach. A multi-level, multifactorial systematic approach is needed to reduce suicide risk comprehensively. This approach requires that components ranging from public health interventions to individual-level interventions are implemented simultaneously in a localized region [104].

Because of the large variation between and among countries in risk factors and rates of suicide, a global approach to improve health overall is needed, while at the same time being sensitive to and taking into account the distinctive features of each culture and country.

Even though many countries have developed a comprehensive national strategy or action plan, there remain real barriers to implementation, monitoring, follow-up, and evaluation.

Not all suicides can be prevented, but a majority can. There are a number of measures that can be taken at community and national levels to reduce the risk, including:

- reducing access to the means of suicide (e.g. pesticides, medication, guns);
- treating people with mental disorders (particularly those with depression, alcoholism, and schizophrenia);
- following-up people who made suicide attempts;
- responsible media reporting;
- training primary healthcare workers.

Evidence for restricting access to lethal means in prevention of suicide has strengthened since 2005, especially with regard to control of analgesics (overall decrease of 43% since 2005) and hotspots for suicide by jumping (reduction of 86% since 2005). If the ultimate goal of means restriction is to reduce the incidence of suicide, the most promising targets are therefore not hotspots, important as these may be, but methods that are commonly used, highly lethal, and readily accessible in or near the home (such as toxic pesticides in developing counties and firearms in the USA).

To be effective in reducing the overall incidence of suicide, however, substitute methods must also be less lethal. Thus, the detoxification of the domestic gas supply in the UK, bans on highly toxic pesticides in Sri Lanka, and decreases in household firearm ownership in the USA were followed by marked reductions in method-specific suicides and overall suicide rates in these countries [105]. These reductions occurred because there was limited substitution by other methods, or, if substitution did occur, less lethal methods were used. Moreover, these reductions were measurable and significant at the population level, because the restricted method accounted for a large proportion of deaths from suicide.

School-based awareness programmes have been shown to reduce suicide attempts and suicidal ideation. The anti-suicidal effects of clozapine and lithium have been substantiated, but might be less specific than previously thought. Effective pharmacological and psychological treatments of depression are important in prevention. Insufficient evidence exists to assess the possible benefits for suicide prevention of screening in primary care, in general public education, and media guidelines. Other approaches that need further investigation include gatekeeper training, education of physicians, and Internet and helpline support. The paucity of randomized controlled trials remains a major limitation in the evaluation of preventative interventions.

There are indications that suicide prevention programmes that contain multiple evidence-informed interventions that are implemented simultaneously may result in reduced levels of suicide and attempted suicide (e.g. European Alliance Against Depression, implementation of mental health service recommendations in the UK). In several culturally different countries where multi-level suicide prevention programmes have been implemented, significant reductions have been observed in suicide and attempted suicide [106–108].

At a more personal level, it is important to know that only a small number of suicides happen without warning. Most people who kill

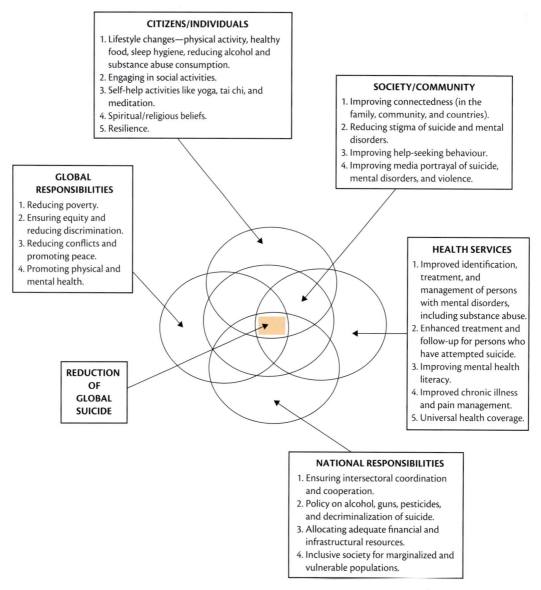

CITIZENS/INDIVIDUALS
1. Lifestyle changes—physical activity, healthy food, sleep hygiene, reducing alcohol and substance abuse consumption.
2. Engaging in social activities.
3. Self-help activities like yoga, tai chi, and meditation.
4. Spiritual/religious beliefs.
5. Resilience.

SOCIETY/COMMUNITY
1. Improving connectedness (in the family, community, and countries).
2. Reducing stigma of suicide and mental disorders.
3. Improving help-seeking behaviour.
4. Improving media portrayal of suicide, mental disorders, and violence.

GLOBAL RESPONSIBILITIES
1. Reducing poverty.
2. Ensuring equity and reducing discrimination.
3. Reducing conflicts and promoting peace.
4. Promoting physical and mental health.

HEALTH SERVICES
1. Improved identification, treatment, and management of persons with mental disorders, including substance abuse.
2. Enhanced treatment and follow-up for persons who have attempted suicide.
3. Improving mental health literacy.
4. Improved chronic illness and pain management.
5. Universal health coverage.

REDUCTION OF GLOBAL SUICIDE

NATIONAL RESPONSIBILITIES
1. Ensuring intersectoral coordination and cooperation.
2. Policy on alcohol, guns, pesticides, and decriminalization of suicide.
3. Allocating adequate financial and infrastructural resources.
4. Inclusive society for marginalized and vulnerable populations.

Fig. 38.2 Suicide prevention in the context of Sustainable Development Goals.

themselves give definite warnings of their intentions. Therefore, all threats of self-harm should be taken seriously. In addition, a majority of people who attempt suicide are ambivalent and not entirely intent on dying.

Key elements in developing a national suicide prevention strategy are to make prevention a multi-sectoral priority that involves not only the health sector, but also education, employment, social welfare, the judiciary, and others. The strategy should be tailored to each country's cultural and social context, establishing best practices and evidence-based interventions in a comprehensive approach.

Resources should be allocated for achieving both short-to-medium and long-term objectives, there should be effective planning, and the strategy should be regularly evaluated, with evaluation findings feeding into future planning. Typical national strategies comprise a range of prevention strategies such as surveillance, means restriction, media guidelines, stigma reduction, and the raising of public awareness, as well as training for health

workers, educators, the police, and other gatekeepers. They also usually include crisis intervention services and postvention.

Indicators that measure a national strategy's progress can include:

◆ a percentage reduction in the suicide rate;

◆ the number of suicide prevention interventions successfully implemented;

◆ a decrease in the number of hospitalized suicide attempts.

While moving forward, two points should be considered. Firstly, suicide prevention activities should be carried out at the same time as data collection. Secondly, even if it is felt that a country is not yet ready to have a national prevention strategy, the process of consulting stakeholders about a national response often generates interest and creates an environment for change. Through the process of creating the national response, stakeholders become committed, public dialogue on stigma is encouraged, vulnerable groups are identified, research priorities are fixed, and public and media awareness are increased.

Key messages

Suicide is a global health problem and reduction of suicide should be a priority in both developing and developed countries.

This requires multi-sectoral interventions at the national, institutional individual, and community level, targeting all sections of the population.

Evidence-based public health interventions to reduce suicides, such as restricting access to lethal means of suicide and policies such as those passed to restrict and control the use of alcohol, need to be implemented in all countries.

Core skills, like identifying and providing interventions to suicidal persons, can be nested within the majority of existing health and welfare programs.

It is essential to improve the collection of data on suicidal behaviour in all countries, to plan, monitor, and evaluate suicide prevention strategies.

References

1. De Leo D, Cerin E, Spathonis K, Burgis S. Lifetime risk of suicide ideation and attempts in an Australian Community: Prevalence, suicidal process, and help-seeking behaviour. *J Affect Disord* 2005; 86: 215–225.
2. Pitman A, Osborn D, King M, Erlangsen A. Effects of suicide bereavement on mental health and suicide risk. *Lancet Psychiatry* 2014; 1: 86–94.
3. Berman AL. Research note: estimating the population of survivors of suicide: seeking an evidence base. *Suicide Life Threat Behav* 2011; 41: 110–116.
4. Nock MK, Borges G, Bromet E, et al. Cross-national prevalence and risk factors for suicidal ideation, plans and attempts. *Br J Psychiatry* 2008; 192: 98–105.
5. Nock MK, Borges G, Bromet EJ, Cha CB, Kessler RC, Lee S. Suicide and suicidal behavior. *Epidemiol Rev* 2008; 30: 133–254.
6. World Health Organization.Preventing suicide: A global imperative. Available at: http://apps.who.int/iris/bitstream/10665/131056/1/9789241564779_eng.pdf?ua=1 (2014, accessed 13 March 2018).
7. Klonsky ED, May AM, Saffer BY. Suicide, suicide attempts, and suicidal ideation. *Annu Rev Clin Psychol* 2016; 12: 14.1–14.24.
8. World Health Organization. WHO Mental Health Atlas. Available at: whqlibdoc.who.int/publications/2011/9799241564359_eng.pdf (2011, accessed 13 March 2018).
9. World Health Organization. Mental Health Action Plan, 2013–2020. Available at: http://apps.who.int/iris/bitstream/10665/89966/1/9789241506021_eng.pdf (2013, accessed 17 October 2014).
10. Silverman MM. The language of suicidology. *Suicide Life Threat Behav* 2006; 36: 519–532.
11. Silverman MM, De Leo D. Why there is a need for an international nomenclature and classification system for suicide. *Crisis* 2016; 37: 83–87.
12. Angelotta C. Defining and refining self-harm. A historical perspective on non-suicidal self-injury. *J Nerv Ment Disord* 2015; 203: 75–80.
13. Beautrais AL. Suicides and serious suicide attempts: two populations or one?. *Psychol Med* 2001; 31: 837–845.
14. De Leo D. Can we rely on suicide mortality data? *Crisis* 2015; 36: 1–3.
15. Linehan MM. Suicidal people: one population or two? *Ann N Y Acad Sci* 1986; 487: 16–33.
16. Berman AL, Shepherd G, Silverman MM. TheLSARS-II: Lethality of suicide attempt rating scale—updated. *Suicide Life Threat Behav* 2003; 33: 261–276.
17. De Leo D, Burgis S, Bertolote JM., Kerkhof, AJFM, Bille-Brahe U. Definitions of suicidal behavior: lessons learned from the WHO/Euro Multicentre Study. *Crisis* 2006; 27: 4–15.
18. O'Carroll PW, Berman AL, Maris RW, Moscicki EK, Tanney BL, Silverman MM. Beyond the tower of babel: a nomenclature for suicidology. *Suicide Life Threat Behav* 1996; 26: 237–252.
19. Silverman MM, Berman AL, Sanddal ND, O'Carroll PW, Joiner TE. Rebuilding the tower of babel: a revised nomenclature for the study of suicide and suicidal behaviors. Part I: background, rationale, and methodology. *Suicide Life Threat Behav* 2007; 37: 248–263.
20. Silverman MM, Berman AL, Sanddal ND, O'Carroll PW, Joiner TE. Rebuilding the tower of babel: a revised nomenclature for the study of suicide and suicidal behaviors. Part II: suicide-related ideations, communications and behaviors. *Suicide Life Threat Behav* 2007; 37: 264–277.
21. De Leo D, Burgis S, Bertolote J, Kerkhof AJFM, Bille-Brahe U. Definitions of suicidal behavior. In: De Leo D, Bille-Brahe U, Kerkhof ADM, Schmidtke A (eds). *Suicidal Behavior: Theories and Research Findings*. Göttingen: Hogrefe & Huber, 2004, pp. 17–39.
22. De Leo D, Milner A. The WHO/START study: promoting suicide prevention for a diverse range of cultural contexts. *Suicide Life Threat Behav* 2010; 40: 99–106.
23. Rudd MD, Joiner TE, Jr. The assessment, management and treatment of suicidality: towards clinically informed and balanced standards of care. *Clin Psychol* 1998; 5: 135–150.
24. Arensman E, Kerkhof AJFM. Classification of attempted suicide: a review of empirical studies, 1963–1993. *Suicide Life Threat Behav* 1996; 26: 46–64.
25. Silverman MM. Challenges to classifying suicidal ideations, communications, and behaviors. In: O'Connor R, Platt S, Gordon J (eds). *International Handbook of Suicide Prevention—Research, Policy & Practice*. Chichester: Wiley Blackwell, 2011, pp. 9–25.
26. Silverman MM. Challenges to defining and classifying suicide and suicidal behaviours. In: O'Connor R, Pirkis J (eds). *International Handbook of Suicide Prevention*, 2nd ed. Chichester: Wiley Blackwell, 2016, pp. 11–35.
27. Silverman MM, Berman AL. Suicide risk assessment and risk formulation Part I: A focus on suicide ideation in assessing suicide risk. *Suicide Life Threat Behav* 2014; 40: 420–431.
28. World Health Organization. World report on violence and health. Available at: whqlibdoc.who.int/publications/2002/9241545615_eng.pdf (2002, accessed 13 March 2018).
29. Hjelmeland H, Knizek BL. Conceptual confusion about intentions and motives of nonfatal suicidal behaviour: a discussion of terms employed in the literature of suicidology. *Arch Suicide Res* 1999; 5: 275–281.
30. World Health Organization. WHO Global Health Estimates. Available at:. http://www.who.int/healthinfo/global_burden_disease/estimates/en/index1.html (2014, accessed 17 October 2014).
31. World Health Organization. WHO methods and data sources for global causes of death 2000–2012. Available at: http://www.who.int/healthinfo/global_burden_disease/GlobalCOD_method_2000_2012.pdf?ua=1 (2014, accessed 17 October 2014).
32. Ajdacic-Gross V, Weiss MG, Ring M, Hepp U, Bopp M, Gutzwiller F, Rössler W. Methods of suicide: international suicide patterns derived from the WHO mortality database. *Bull World Health Organ* 2008; 86: 726–732.
33. De Leo D. Australia revises its mortality data on suicide. *Crisis* 2010; 31: 169–173.
34. World Health Organization. Health for the World's Adolescents. Available at: apps.who.int/iris/bitstream/10665/112750/1/WHO_FWC_MCA_14.05_eng.pdf (2014, accessed 13 March 2018).
35. Kessler RC, Berglund P, Borges G, Nock MK, Wang PS. 'Trends in suicide ideation, plans, gestures, and attempts in the United States, 1990–1992 to 2001–2003. *JAMA* 2005; 293: 2487–2495.
36. Phillips MR, Yang R, Zhang Y, Wang L, Ji H, Zhou M. Risk factors for suicide in China: a national case-control psychological autopsy study. *Lancet* 2002; 108: 392–393.

37. Vijayakumar L. Suicide prevention: the urgent need in developing countries. *World Psychiatry* 2004; 3: 158–159.

38. Rezaeian M. Suicide/homicide ratios in countries of the Eastern Mediterranean Region. *East Mediterr Health J* 2008; 14: 1459–1465.

39. Nock MK, Hwang I, Sampson N, et al. Cross-national analysis of the associations among mental disorders and suicidal behavior: findings from the WHO World Mental Health Surveys. *PLOS Med* 2009; 6: 1–17.

40. Schmidtke A, Bille-Brahe U, De Leo D, et al. Attempted suicide in Europe: rates, trends and sociodemographic characteristics of suicide attempters during the period1989-1992. Results of the WHO/EURO Multicentre Study on Parasuicide. *Acta Psychiatr Scand* 1996; 93: 327–338.

41. Bertolote JM, Fleischmann A, De Leo D, et al. Suicide attempts, plans, and ideation in culturally diverse sites: The WHO SUPRE-MISS community survey. *Psychol Med* 2005; 35: 1457–1465.

42. Bhugra D, Desai M. Attempted suicide in South Asian women. *Adv Psychiatr Treat* 2002; 8: 418–423.

43. Gururaj G., Isaac MK, Subbakrishna DK, Ranjani R. Risk factors for completed suicides: a case–control study from Bangalore, India. *Inj Control Saf Promot* 2004; 11: 183–191.

44. Knesper DJ, American Association of Suicidology and Suicide Prevention Resource Center. *Continuity of Care for Suicide Prevention and Research: Suicide Attempts and Suicide Deaths Subsequent to Discharge from the Emergency Department or Psychiatry Inpatient Unit*. Newton, MA: Education Development Center, 2010.

45. Kolves K, De Leo D. Suicide methods in children and adolescents. *Eur Child Adolesc Psychiatry* 2017; 26: 155–164.

46. Owens D, Horrocks J, House A. Fatal and non-fatal repetition of self-harm. *Br J Psychiatry* 2002; 181: 193–199.

47. Neeleman J. A continuum of premature death. Meta-analysis of competing mortality in the psychosocially vulnerable. *Int J Epidemiol* 2001; 30: 154–162.

48. Saiz P, Bobes J. Suicide prevention in Spain: an uncovered clinical need. *Rev Psiquiatr Salud Ment* 2014; 7: 1–4 (in Spanish).

49. Beautrais AL, Joyce PR, Mulder RT. Precipitating factors and life events in serious suicide attempts among youths aged 13 through 24 year. *J Am Acad Child Adoles Psychiatry* 1997; 36: 1543–1551.

50. Cibis A, Mergl R, Bramesfeld A, et al. Preference of lethal methods is not the only cause for higher suicide rates in males. *J Affect Disord* 2011; 136: 9–16.

51. Heikkinen M, Aro H, Lonnquist J. Recent life events and their role in suicide as seen by the spouses. *Acta Psychiatr Scand* 1992; 86: 489–494.

52. Heikkinen M, Aro H, Lonnquist J. Recent life events, social support and suicide. *Acta Psychiatr Scand* 1994; 377: 65–72.

53. Foster T, Gillespie K, Mcclelland R, Patterson C. Risk factors for suicide independent of DSMIII-R Axis I disorder. *Br J Psychiatry* 1999; 175: 175–179.

54. Paykel E. Life events: effects and genesis. *Psychol Med* 2003; 33: 1145–1148.

55. Cheng A, Chen T, Chen CC, Jenkins R. Psychosocial and psychiatric risk factors for suicide: case-control psychological autopsy study. *Br J Psychiatry* 2000; 177: 360–365.

56. Burón P, Jimenez-Trevino L, Saiz PA, et al. Reasons for attempted suicide in europe: prevalence, associated factors, and risk of repetition. *Arch Suicide Res* 2016; 20: 45–58.

57. Hunt IM, Kapur N, Webb R, et al. Suicide in recently discharged psychiatric patients: a case-control study. *Psychol Med* 2009; 39: 443–449.

58. Gunnell D, Frankel S. Education and debate: prevention of suicide: aspirations and evidence. *BMJ* 1994; 308: 1227–1233.

59. Kapur N, Hunt IM, Webb R, et al. Suicide in psychiatric in-patients in England, 1997 to 2003. *Psychol Med* 2006; 36: 1485–1492.

60. King EA, Baldwin DS, Sinclair JM, Baker NG, Campbell MJ, Thompson C. The Wessex recent in-patient suicide study, 1. Case–control study of 234 recently discharged psychiatric patient suicides. *Br J Psychiatry* 2001; 178: 531–536.

61. Pirkola S, Sund R, Salias E, Wahlbeck K. Community mental-health services and suicide rate in Finland: a nationwide small-area analysis. *Lancet* 2009; 373: 147–153.

62. Bassett D, Tsourtos G. In-patient suicide in a general hospital psychiatric unit: a consequence of inadequate resources? *Gen Hosp Psychiatry* 1993; 15: 301–306.

63. Appleby L, Shaw J, Amos T, et al. Suicide within 12 months of contact with mental health services: national clinical survey. *BMJ,* 1999; 318: 1235–1239.

64. Caine ED. Forging an agenda for suicide prevention in the United States. *Am J Public Health* 2013; 103: 822–829.

65. Knox KL, Litts DA, Talcott GW, Feig JC, Caine ED. Risk of suicide and related adverse outcomes after exposure to a suicide prevention programme in the United States Air Force: cohort study. *BMJ* 2003; 327: 1376–1380.

66. Zalsman G, Hawton K, Wasserman D, et al. Suicide prevention strategies revisited: 10-year systematic review. *Lancet Psychiatry* 2016; 3: 646–659.

67. Mann JJ, Apter A, Bertolote J, et al. Suicide prevention strategies: a systematic review. *JAMA* 2005; 294: 2064–2074.

68. Vijayakumar L, Rajkumar S. Are risk factors forsuicide universal? A case–control study in India. *Acta Psychiatr Scand* 1999; 99: 407–411.

69. Gunnell D, Eddleston M, Phillips MR, Konradsen F. The global distribution of fatal pesticide self-poisoning: systematic review. *BMC Public Health* 2007; 7: 357.

70. Gunnell D, Fernando R, Hewagama M, Priyangika WDD, Konradsen F, Eddleston M. The impact of pesticide regulations on suicide in Sri Lanka. *Int J Epidemiol* 2007; 36: 1235–1242.

71. Vijayakumar L, Jeyaseelan L, Kumar S, Mohanraj R, Devika S, Manikandan S. A central storage facility to reduce pesticide suicides—a feasibility study from India. *BMC Public Health,* 2013; 13: 850.

72. World Health Organization. Clinical Management of Acute Pesticide Intoxication: Prevention of Suicidal Behaviours. Available at: http://whqlibdoc.who.int/publications/2008/9789241597456_eng.pdf (2008, accessed 17 October 2014).

73. National Institute for Health and Care Excellence (NICE). Self-harm in over 8s: long-term management. Available at: http://www.nice.org.uk/guidance/CG133/chapter/introduction (2014, accessed 17 October 2014).

74. Brent DA, Bridge J. Firearms availability and suicide: evidence, interventions, and future directions. *Am Behav Sci* 2003; 46: 1192–1210.

75. Miller M, Warren M, Hemenway D, Azrael D. Firearms and suicide in US cities. *Inj Prev* 2013; 21: 116–119.

76. Anglemyer A, Horvath T, Rutherford G. The accessibility of firearms and risk for suicide and homicide victimization among household members: a systematic review and meta-analysis. *Ann Intern Med* 2014; 160: 101–110.

77. Yip PSF, Law CK, Fu KW, Law YW, Wong PW, Xu Y. Restricting the means of suicide by charcoal burning. *Br J Psychiatry* 2010; 196: 241–242.

78. Hegerl U, Wittenburg L. Focus on mental health carere forms in Europe: the European alliance against depression: a multilevel approach to the prevention of suicidal behaviour. *Psychiatr Serv* 2009; 60: 596–599.

79. Hawton KL, Bergen H, Simkin S, et al. Long term effect of reduced pack sizes of paracetamol on poisoning deaths and liver transplant activity in England and Wales: interrupted time series analyses. *BMJ* 2013; 346: f403.

80. Pirkis J. Suicide and the media. *Psychiatry* 2009; 8: 269–271.

81. Bohanna I, Wang X. Media guidelines for the responsible reporting of suicide. A review of effectiveness. *Crisis* 2012; 33: 190–198.

82. World Health Organization. Global Strategy to Reduce the Harmful use of Alcohol. Available at: http://www.who.int/substance_abuse/activities/gsrhua/en/ (2010, accessed 17 October 2014).

83. World Health Organization. Self-harm and suicide. Available at: http://www.who.int/entity/mental_health/mhgap/evidence/suicide/en/index.html (2015, accessed 19 October 2016).

84. Chisholm D, Rehm J, Van Ommeren M, Monteiro M. Reducing the global burden of hazardous alcohol use: a comparative cost-effectiveness analysis. *J Stud Alcohol* 2004; 65: 782–793.

85. Prince M, Patel V, Saxena S, Maj M, Maselko J, Phillips MR, Rahman A. No health without mental health. *Lancet* 2007; 370: 859–877.

86. Dazzi T, Gribble R, Wessely S, Fear NT. Does asking about suicide and related behaviours induce suicidal ideation? What is the evidence? *Psychol Med* 2014; 44: 3361–3363.

87. World Health Organization. Preventing suicide: A resource for non-fatal suicidal behavior case registration. Available at: apps.who.int/iris/bitstream/10665/112852/1/9789241506717_eng.pdf (2014, accessed 13 March 2018).

88. Wasserman D, Rihmer Z, Rujescu D, et al. The European Psychiatric Association (EPA) guidance on suicide treatment and prevention. *Eur Psychiatry* 2012; 27: 129–141.

89. Kapur N, Steeg S, Webb R, et al. Does clinical management improve outcomes following self-harm? Results from the multicentre study of self-harm in England. *PLOS ONE* 2013; 8: e70434.

90. World Health Organization. mhGAP Intervention Guide for Mental, Neurological and Substance use Disorders in Non-specialized Health Settings: version 1.0. Available at: http://www.who.int/mental_health/publications/mhGAP_intervention_guide/en/ (2011, accessed 17 October 2014).

91. Luxton DD, June JD, Comtois KA. Can post discharge follow-up contacts prevent suicide and suicidal behaviour? A review of the evidence. *Crisis* 2013; 34: 32–41.

92. Fleischmann A, Bertolote JM, Wasserman D, et al. Effectiveness of brief intervention and contact for suicide attempters: a randomized controlled trial in five countries', randomized controlled trial in five countries. *Bull World Health Organ* 2008; 86: 703–709.

93. Pearson M, Zwi A, Buckley N, Manuweera G, et al. Policymaking 'under the radar': a case study of pesticide regulation to prevent intentional poisoning in Sri Lanka. *Health Policy Plan* 2015; 30: 56–67.

94. Malakouti S, Nojomi M, Poshtmashadi M, et al. Integrating a suicide prevention program into the primary health care network: a field trial in Iran. *Med J Islam Repub Iran* 2015; 29: 208.

95. Vijayakumar L, John S, Pirkis J, Whiteford H. Suicide in developing countries (2) risk factors. *Crisis* 2005; 26: 112–119.

96. Vijayakumar L, Pirkis J, Whiteford H. Suicide in developing countries(3) prevention efforts. *Crisis* 2005; 26: 120–124.

97. Aseltine RHJ, James A, Schilling EA, Glanovsky J. Evaluating the SOS suicide prevention program: a replication and extension. *BMC Public Health* 2007; 7: 161. :

98. Wasserman D, Hoven C, Wasserman C, et al. School-based suicide prevention programmes: the SEYLE cluster randomised, controlled trial. *Lancet* 2015; 385: 1536–1544.

99. Vijayakumar L, Nagaraj K, John S. Suicide and Suicide Prevention in Developing Countries. Disease Control Priorities Project Working Paper No 27; 2004.

100. Vijayakumar L, Armsom S. Volunteer perspectives on suicide prevention. In: Hawton K (ed.). *Prevention and Treatment of Suicidal Behaviour: From Science to Practice*. New York: Oxford University Press, 2005, pp. 335– 350.

101. Ahmadi A, Ytterstad B. Prevention of self-immolation by community-based intervention. *Burns* 2007; 33: 1032–1040.

102. Wickramasinghe K, Steele P, Dawson A, et al. Cost to government health-care services of treating acute self-poisonings in a rural district in Sri Lanka. *Bull World Health Organ* 2009; 87: 180–185.

103. United nations. The Sustainable Development Agenda. Available at: http://www.un.org/sustainabledevelopment/development-agenda/ (accessed 13 March 2018).

104. Hegerl U, Rummel-Kluge C, Värnik A, Arensman E, Koburger N. Alliances against depression—a community based approach to target depression and to prevent suicidal behaviour. *Neurosci Biobehav Rev* 2013; 37: 2404–2409.

105. Sarchiapone M, Mandelli L, Losue M, Andrisano C, Roy A. Controlling access to suicide means. *Int J Environ Res Public Health* 2011; 8: 4550–4562.

106. While D, Bickley H, Roscoe A, et al. Implementation of mental health service recommendations in England and Wales and suicide rates, 1997–2006: a cross-sectional and before-and-after observational study. *Lancet* 2012; 379: 1005–1012.

107. Harris FM, Maxwell M, O'Connor RC, et al. Developing social capital in implementing a complex intervention: a process evaluation of the early implementation of a suicide prevention intervention in four European countries. *BMC Public Health* 2013; 13: 158.

108. Székely A, Konkolÿ Thege B, Mergl R, et al. 'How to decrease suicide rates in both genders? an effectiveness study of a community-based intervention (EAAD). *PLOS ONE* 2013; 8: e75081.

CHAPTER 39

Suicidal behaviour among adolescents

Risk and protective factors and universal evidence-based suicide preventive programmes

Danuta Wasserman, Miriam Iosue, and Vladimir Carli

Introduction

Teenage suicide is an important public health issue that affects many adolescents, and also their families, peers, and communities. At least 100,000 adolescents commit suicide worldwide every year, making it the second leading cause of death in 15–29 year olds [1]. To date, it is not possible to predict with certainty if and when an individual is going to commit suicide. Moreover, the known risk factors are non-specific and none of them may be used alone to predict suicide with sufficient accuracy. Nevertheless, suicide can be prevented. Suicide is usually not a sudden act; rather, in most cases, it is the final outcome of a process that is influenced by the interaction of genetic, psychological, environmental, and situational factors [2].

The World Health Organization's (WHO) comprehensive mental health action plan 2013–2020 [3] recognizes suicide prevention as an important priority, setting as a global target a 10% reduction of suicide rate by the year 2020. The action plan identifies young people as one of the most susceptible age groups to suicidal ideation and self-harm, and thus an important target for suicide prevention.

Epidemiology of suicidal behaviours among adolescents

Each year more than 800,000 people die worldwide by suicide. The annual global age-standardized suicide rate is 11.4 per 100,000 population (15.0 for males and 8.0 for females) [1]. However, the real number of suicides may be higher than the statistics show, as suicide is a very sensitive issue surrounded by stigma and for this reason the cause of death can be hidden and death certificates misclassified.

Suicide is uncommon in childhood and early adolescence. According to the WHO report [1], suicide rates are lowest in persons under 15 years of age and highest in those aged 70 years or older. Nevertheless, suicide rates escalate steeply from childhood to middle and late adolescence, with about 100,000 adolescents committing suicide every year. Using the data from the WHO

Mortality Database, Wasserman et al. [4] estimated that the mean suicide rate among adolescents in the 15–19 year age group was 7.4/100,000, with higher suicide rates among males (10.5/100,000) than females (4.1/100,000). Suicide accounts for 8.5% of all deaths among young people aged 15–29 years worldwide [1] and for 17.6% of all deaths among people aged 15–29 years in high-income countries [5].

Most of the research on adolescent suicidal behaviour is performed in developed countries, especially the USA, European countries, and Australia. During 2013 in the USA, suicide was the second leading cause of death for the age group 10–24 years, accounting for 16.8% of all deaths [6]. Suicide is much more common in adolescent and young adult males than females, with a male : female suicide ratio of 5.5 : 1 in 15–24 year olds [7]. According to the Eurostat database [8], in 2013 the crude death rate from suicide among European adolescents aged 15–19 years was 4.51/100,000, with the highest suicide rates in Lithuania (21.38/100,000). Conversely, countries in the Mediterranean region, such as Greece, Italy, Spain, and Portugal, showed lower youth suicide rates. Suicide also represents a serious problem among Australian adolescents, with an age-specific suicide rate for males aged 15–19 years of 12.1/100,000 and of 5.3/100,000 for females [9].

Relatively few countries have reliable data on suicide attempts. Non-fatal suicidal behaviour is more prevalent among younger people than older people and this is owing to the fact that suicide attempts in older age are more serious in both psychological and medical terms [10]. Suicide attempts are more common in girls than boys (1.6 : 1) [7]. According to Beautrais [11], sex differences between completed suicides and suicide attempts can be partly explained by sex differences in methods used to commit suicide. Males seem to choose highly lethal methods (hanging, vehicle exhaust gas, firearms, jumping), whereas females chose less lethal means, particularly self-poisoning. The results of a systematic review indicate that about 9.7% of adolescents report a lifetime suicide attempt [12].

Hultén et al. [13] found that 24% of the individuals who had previously attempted suicide made another attempt within 1 year after the index attempt. The US Youth Risk Behavior Surveillance (YRBS) reported that 8.6% of students had attempted suicide during the 12 months before the survey and 2.8% of students had made a suicide attempt that required medical care [14]. In the Saving and Empowering Young Lives in Europe (SEYLE) study [15], 4.2% of the sample, comprising more than 12,000 pupils, reported lifetime suicide attempts. The frequency of suicide attempts increased with age. Higher rates were found in the European School Survey Project on Alcohol and Other Drugs (ESPAD), with a median rate of 10.5% [16]. In both the YRBS and in SEYLE the prevalence of suicide attempts was higher among females than males (11.6% vs 5.5% and 5.1% vs 3.0%, respectively). Similar gender differences were reported for low- and middle-income countries [17], with an overall prevalence of suicide ideation of 16.2% for females and 12.2% for males, even though some regions showed less or no gender disparity.

The lifetime prevalence of suicidal ideation among adolescents is estimated to be 29.9% [12], which is notably different from 9.2% in the general population [18]. In the YRBS [14], 17.7% of students had seriously considered attempting suicide (23.4% of females vs. 12.2% of males) and 14.6% had made a plan to attempt suicide (19.4% of females vs. 9.8% of males), during the 12 months before the survey. In the SEYLE project [15], suicidal ideation was present in approximately one-third of the sample (32.3%), with a significantly higher prevalence in older pupils and among girls.

Risk factors for adolescent suicidal behaviour

Suicide is a complex, multi-causal phenomenon determined by the interaction of several bio-psychosocial factors. The diathesis–stress model was proposed to explain the complex interactions generating a person's vulnerability to suicidal behaviour. The constitutional predisposition to suicide, determined by genetic make-up, is influenced by acquired environmental factors, such as stress and negative life events [19, 20]. On the other side, protective factors mitigate the effects of risk factors.

Genetic and biological factors

Genetic factors seem to play a role in 30–50% of suicidal behaviours [21, 22]. Strong evidence of a genetic susceptibility to suicidal behaviour comes from twin and adoption studies [22–24]. Similarly to other psychopathological traits, suicidal behaviour inheritance seems to result from the contribution of multiple genes with small effect sizes [25].

The inheritance of suicidal behaviour has proven to be at least partially independent of the inheritance of psychiatric disorders [26]. However, given its strong association with depression, the serotonin system has been the main focus of genetic and biological studies on suicide. Serotonin is associated with increased impulsiveness, impaired control of aggressive behaviours, and suicide attempts. Two meta-analyses [27, 28] confirmed the association between a polymorphism of the TPH1 gene (encoding for the tryptophan hydroxylase, the initial and rate-limiting enzyme in the biosynthesis of serotonin) and suicidal behaviour. A meta-analysis [29] supported the association between the short allele of 5-HTTLPR (the promoter region of the serotonin transporter gene) polymorphism, especially with violent suicidal behaviour in the psychiatric population. Similarly, Wasserman et al. [30] reported a higher occurrence of the short allele among suicide attempters with a high medical damage.

Brain-derived neurotrophic factor (BDNF) is a neutrophin involved in neuronal growth and plasticity of serotonergic and dopaminergic neurons. Tyrosine kinase B (TrkB) is the BDNF receptor. A significant reduction in the mRNA levels of BDNF and TrkB was found in both the prefrontal cortex and hippocampus of adult [31] and teenage suicide subjects [32]. Sarchiapone et al. [33] found a significant association between a single nucleotide polymorphism in the BDNF gene and suicidal behaviour.

Gene–environment interactions may better explain the role of hereditability in suicidality. Caspi et al. [34] showed that the occurrence of stressful life events predicted the onset of newly diagnosed depression or suicidal ideation and attempts among subjects with one or two copies of the short allele of the serotonin transporter promoter polymorphism than individuals homozygous for the long allele. Childhood trauma may interact with low expressing 5-HTTLPR genotypes and increase the risk of suicidal behaviour among patients with substance dependence [35]. Corticotropin-releasing hormone (CRH) is a hypothalamic factor involved in stress response that stimulates the pituitary gland, binding two receptors, CRHR1 and CRHR2. Wasserman et al. [36] described an association between a polymorphism of the CRHR1 gene and suicide attempt in males exposed to low levels of stress. Roy et al. [37] investigated FKBP5, a hypothalamus–pituitary–adrenal axis-regulating gene, suggesting that childhood trauma and variants of FKBP5 may interact to increase suicidality.

Family history of suicidality and mental health problems

Suicidal behaviour aggregates within families and individuals with a family history of suicidal behaviour are at an increased risk of both attempting and committing suicide than individuals without such a family history [26]. Brent et al. [38] reported a sixfold increased risk of suicide attempts in offspring of attempters compared with non-attempters. Among young people aged 10–21 years [39], a parental history of suicide increased the risk of suicide, especially if the mother committed suicide (father suicide odds ratio (OR) 2.30; mother suicide OR 4.75). Similar results were reported by Mittendorfer-Rutz et al. [40], who found twofold increased odds of attempting suicide within 2 years after a maternal suicide attempt in young people aged 15–31 years.

Mittendorfer-Rutz et al. [41] showed that the risk of suicide attempt in adolescents and young adults tends to be associated with familial psychopathology, particularly substance abuse, and affective, neurotic, and personality disorders. The authors found a 2.9 times increased risk of suicide attempt in individuals with a parent or sibling admitted to a hospital due to these disorders. In a study conducted by Gureje et al. [42], parental death by suicide was a strong predictor of persistence of suicide attempts among offspring.

Previous suicide attempts and non-suicidal self-injuries

A previous suicide attempt is one of the strongest predictors of future suicide risk [43]. Hawton et al. [44] found that a previous attempted suicide was associated with the risk of death due to suicide among young people aged 15–24 years (OR 2.3; 95% confidence interval (CI) 1.2–4.4). Hultén et al. [13], analysing 1,720 suicide attempts made by 1,264 individuals aged 15–19 years, found that previous attempted suicide (OR 3.3; 95% CI 2.4–4.4) and use of more lethal methods (OR 1.5; 95% CI 1.1–2.1) were both significantly associated with repetition of attempted suicide. According to Beck [45], previous suicidal experience sensitizes suicide-related thoughts and behaviours, reduces inhibitions, and increases the chance of thoughts to be transferred into behaviours.

Non-suicidal self-injury (NSSI) usually refers to direct and deliberate destruction of one's own body tissue in the absence of intent to die [46]. Several studies described an association between NSSIs and suicidal behaviour among adolescent psychiatric patients [47, 48]. In particular, Nock et al. [46] found that 70% of inpatient adolescents engaging in NSSIs reported a lifetime suicide attempt and 55% reported multiple attempts. A longer history of NSSIs, the use of a greater number of methods, and the absence of physical pain during NSSIs were the variables most strongly associated with suicide attempts.

In the SEYLE sample of European high school adolescents, Brunner et al. [49] studied the prevalence of direct self-injurious behaviour (D-SIB), which is defined as intentional self-inflicted damage to the surface of an individual's body, which includes self-cutting, self-burning, self-biting, self-hitting, and skin damage by other methods, regardless of the suicidal intent. The lifetime prevalence of D-SIB was 27.6%, with 19.7% of the adolescents reporting occasional D-SIB and 7.8% reporting repetitive D-SIB. Strong associations were observed between D-SIB and both psychopathology and risk behaviours, as well as family-related neglect and peer-related rejection/victimization. Suicidality, as well as anxiety and depressive symptoms, had very high ORs for occasional and repetitive D-SIB. Noteworthy, D-SIB cessation reduces risk for suicidal thoughts and behaviour in adolescents [50].

Mental health problems

Youth suicide often occurs in the context of an often treatable mental illness that has frequently gone unrecognized or untreated. Psychological autopsy studies show that approximately 90% of adolescent suicides occur in individuals with a pre-existing psychiatric disorder and in about half of these cases the psychiatric disorder had been present for 2 or more years [51, 52]. Nock et al. [53] reported that 89.3% of adolescents with a lifetime history of suicide ideation and 96.1% with a lifetime history of suicide attempt met lifetime criteria for at least one mental disorder. Major depressive disorder or dysthymia, followed by specific phobia, oppositional-defiant disorder, intermittent explosive disorder, substance abuse, and conduct disorder were the most common disorders found among suicidal adolescents. Psychotic symptoms in non-psychotic young people are important risk markers for a wide range of non-psychotic psychopathological disorders [54]. In the SEYLE Irish cohort, 7% of adolescents who reported positively on the question 'Have you ever heard voices or sounds that no one else can hear?' had a nearly 70-fold increased odds of acute suicide attempts [54]. In a representative sample of 3070 adolescents from 11 European countries in the SEYLE cohort, 12.5% of students were found to require mental healthcare [55]. Adolescents who had been bullied, had severe depressive symptoms, and those with a recent suicide

attempt were more prone to seek help than their peers with other problems [56]. The relationship between mental health problems and suicidal behaviour was also confirmed in two systematic reviews [12, 57]. Receiving care for mental health problems was associated with both suicide and serious suicide attempts. In a case–control study in Denmark [58], a history of psychiatric hospitalization represented a strong risk factor for completed suicide in adolescents and young adults, even after controlling for personal socio-economic status (adjusted OR (AOR) 13.5 for males and 38.9 for females). The risk for suicide was highest immediately after admission or discharge and increased progressively with numbers of psychiatric admissions.

Mood disorders

Mood disorders significantly increase the risk of suicidal behaviours among adolescents [12, 52, 57]. A systematic review on suicidal ideation and suicide attempts in children and adolescents with bipolar disorder, estimated a prevalence of 50.4% for current suicidal ideation and 25.5% for current suicide attempt [59]. Depressive disorders represent the most prevalent condition among adolescent suicide victims, occurring in 49–64% of cases [57]. Nock et al. [53] reported a prevalence of major depressive disorder of 56.8% among suicidal ideators, 69.7% among those who planned to commit suicide, and 75.7% among suicide attempters. Balázs et al. [60] found significant effects of being sub-threshold depressed and depressed on adolescent suicidal ideation. In a case–control study on suicide victims aged 11–18 years, Renaud et al. [61] indicated that the most significant psychiatric disorders associated with child and adolescent suicide were depressive disorders (AOR 39.652, 95% CI 4.501–349.345), followed by substance/alcohol abuse disorders (AOR 7.325, 95% CI 1.127–47.620) and disruptive disorders (AOR 6.464, 95% CI 1.422–29.38).

Substance misuse

While mood disorders are more present in female suicide victims, substance abuse is more present in male victims [57]. Substance use/misuse/abuse represent an important risk factor for attempted and completed suicide among adolescents, especially among older subjects with co-morbid mood disorders or disruptive disorders [12, 52, 53, 61, 62]. Considering that young suicide attempters are more likely to have substance abuse/dependence disorders than suicidal ideators, Gould et al. [63] suggested that substance use may facilitate the transition from ideation to behaviours. Indeed, substance abuse, in the long run, impairs cognitive processes, increases impulsivity and aggression, and lowers the threshold for triggers of suicidal behaviour [2].

Often associated with substance abuse, disruptive disorders carry a 3–6-fold greater risk for youth suicide [52], and a 4–7-fold greater risk for suicide attempts [53].

Anxiety disorders

Anxiety disorders also seem to be associated with suicidal ideation and attempts among adolescents and young adults [64]; however, after controlling for mood disorder and other conditions this association can be significantly attenuated [12, 52]. In the SEYLE European sample, Balázs et al. [60] found an almost two times greater risk for suicidal ideation among sub-threshold anxious and anxious adolescents than non-anxious peers, also when controlling for age, sex, and depressive symptoms.

Psychotic symptoms

Although previous studies showed that psychotic symptoms seemed not to play a major role in adolescent suicidal behaviour [52, 57], Kelleher et al. [65] demonstrated an association between psychotic symptoms and a 10-fold increased odds of suicidal ideation and suicide attempt in early (11–13 years old) and middle (13–15 years old) adolescents. Psychotic symptoms contributed to an increase in the risk of more severe suicidal plans and suicide acts among adolescents with depressive disorders and among those with suicidal ideation.

Eating disorders

A systematic review [66] concluded that there is a strong association between eating disorders and suicidal behaviour during adolescence and young adulthood, although the high rates of comorbid psychopathology, especially mood disorders and substance abuse, may influence this association. Swanson [67] indicated that all subtypes of eating disorders were associated with significantly elevated levels of suicide ideation. More than half of adolescents with bulimia nervosa reported suicide ideation and more than a third reported suicide attempts. Among adolescent students, extreme and less extreme weight control behaviours, as well as body dissatisfaction, were associated with suicidal ideation and attempts [68].

Personal characteristics and personality traits

According to Beck et al. [69], hopelessness is a core characteristic of depression explaining the link between depression and suicide. In adult patients, hopelessness scores differentiate suicidal ideators who eventually died by suicide from those who did not. Among adolescents, some studies [70, 71] found a positive association between hopelessness and suicidality; nevertheless, when controlled for depression, hopelessness was unrelated to suicidal behaviours [72] for boys and only modestly related for girls [73]. In Hong Kong Chinese and white American adolescents, hopelessness was associated with suicidal ideation, even when depressive symptoms were controlled for [74].

Impulsivity can be defined as a predisposition toward rapid, unplanned reactions to internal or external stimuli without regard for the negative consequences of these reactions [75]. Impulsive and aggressive traits have been repeatedly associated with suicidal behaviours among adults [76, 77]. According to Simon et al. [78], inadequate control of aggressive impulses might be an indicator of risk for impulsive suicide attempts. A significant correlation between impulsivity and suicidal behaviour was also described among adolescents [61, 79]. In the study by Renaud et al. [61], impulsive and aggressive behaviours were significantly higher among young suicide victims than among controls, however, this association was not significant when psychiatric disorders, such as depression, alcohol/substance abuse, and disruptive disorders were controlled for.

Sleep difficulties and related problems, such as tiredness and nightmares, also represent a risk factor for suicidal ideation and behaviours [12]. In the SEYLE study [80], reduced sleep was found to be associated with emotional problems, anxiety, suicidal ideation, and conduct problems. Elsewhere, sleep problems were found to predict suicidal ideation among adolescents, even when controlling for depressive symptoms [81].

Homosexual and bisexual orientation was reported to be associated with an increased risk for suicidal ideation and attempts among adolescents and young adults [82, 83]. This association seems to be largely mediated by the presence of risk factors [84] and the lack of protective factors like family connectedness, teacher or other adult caring, and school safety [85]. Five per cent of students in the Irish SEYLE study had concerns regarding their sexual orientation and those students had higher levels of physical assault, sexual assault, attempted suicide, and frequent alcohol use than their peers [83]. In a meta-analysis, Marshal et al. [86] estimated that after controlling for important explanatory variables, sexual minority youth were almost twice as likely to report a history of suicidality as heterosexual youth.

Trauma and stressful life events

Childhood trauma is significantly related to the early onset of suicidal behaviour and repeated suicide attempts. There is strong evidence that childhood sexual and/or physical abuse is a risk factor for suicidal behaviour in clinical [87–89] and community [90, 91] samples of adolescents. Although each form of childhood maltreatment is independently associated with adolescent suicidal ideation and suicide attempts, there is some evidence that sexual and emotional abuse may be relatively more important in explaining suicidal behaviour than physical abuse or neglect [92]. Exposure to violence and sexual assaults are significant risk factors for suicidal behaviour [93] and repeated suicide attempts [94]. Martin et al. [95] described a threefold increased risk of suicidal thoughts and plans in girls who reported current high distress about sexual abuse versus non-abused girls. Moreover, boys who reported current high distress about sexual abuse had a 10-fold increased risk for suicidal plans and threats, and a 15-fold increased risk for suicide attempts, versus non-abused boys.

Negative life events such as loss, change in life situation, and different narcissistic injuries may act as precipitating factors for suicidal behaviour [20, 96]. Stressful life events have been demonstrated to be a significant risk factor for both suicide and serious suicide attempts among adolescents [11]. The presence of life stressors differentiates adolescents with suicidal ideation who engaged in suicidal behaviour from those who do not [97].

Interpersonal problems seem to be particularly important among adolescents. Hawton et al. [98] found that the most frequent stressors underlying suicidal behaviour among adolescents are relationship difficulties with parents, problems with friends, and social isolation. Social isolation from peers significantly increases the risk for suicidal ideation in girls [99]. Reading books and watching films was found in the SEYLE study to be an important protective factor for serious suicidal ideation in adolescents with the lowest levels of social belonging [100]. The perception of a low social support, especially from parents and peers, is associated with adolescent suicidal ideation and attempts both in the community [101] and in the clinical samples [102].

Both victims of bullying and bullies seem to be at increased risk for suicidal ideation [103]. Klomek et al. [104] reported an association of both direct and indirect peer victimization with depression and suicidality. Moreover, the risk increases with the number of peer victimization types the teenager is exposed to. However, the association between victimization and adolescent suicidality may be strongly mediated by other psychological risk factors, such as depression and hopelessness [105]. In the SEYLE study [106], it has been shown that among all different types of bullying, the non-physical victimization is the one most linked to suicidal behaviours. Furthermore, the role of anxiety in addition to depression in the association between bullying and suicide attempts was demonstrated. Above all, it has underscored the significant protective role of parental support in decreasing the risk of suicide attempts associated with peer-maltreatment.

Contagion of suicidal behaviour among adolescents is an important phenomenon to consider. Having a friend who attempted suicide in the past year increases the likelihood of both suicidal ideation and attempts [99]. Between 1% and 5% of adolescent suicides occur in clusters [107]. According to Gould et al. [108], the relative risk of suicide following exposure to another individual's suicide was 2–4 times higher among 15–19 year olds than among other age groups.

In a study of adolescent immigrants, a significantly poorer self-perceived health was found compared with natives. Non-European adolescent migrants, regardless of migrant generation, had higher externalized symptom levels than native adolescents [109].

Risk behaviours

The YRBS [14] identifies six categories of risk behaviours: (i) behaviours that contribute to unintentional injuries and violence; (ii) sexual behaviours that contribute to unintended pregnancy and sexually transmitted diseases, including HIV infection; (iii) alcohol and other drug use; (iv) tobacco use; (v) unhealthy dietary behaviours; and (vi) inadequate physical activity. These behaviours are significantly correlated and often appear in clusters [110], they are usually established during childhood and adolescence and extend into adulthood. Teens engaging in risk behaviours are at increased risk for depression, suicidal ideation, and suicide attempts [111]. According to Epstein and Spirito [112], early onset of alcohol drinking, having had sex before 13 years of age, injection drug use, smoking, fighting, and being forced to have sex are all critical behaviours associated with suicidality. Ruutel et al. [113] explored the importance of role models for alcohol consumption patterns and found that the more adolescents see their family member or role model drunk, the more they drink themselves. An increased risk for suicidal behaviour has been reported among adolescents engaging in bullying [114], delinquent behaviour [115], smoking [116], sexually risky behaviour [117], physical inactivity [118], and poor nutrition [119]. In the SEYLE study, Gambadauro et al. (published, 2017) found that early sexual debut was associated with anxiety, depression, severe suicidal ideation, and suicide attempts. In the SEYLE material, Banzer et al. [120] found that 30.9% of adolescents reported daily smoking and 58% of those reported the onset of smoking under the age of 14 years. Smoking was significantly associated with emotional symptoms, anxiety, previous suicide attempts, conduct problems, hyperactivity, excessive alcohol, and illegal drug use [120].

Using Latent Class Analysis, Carli et al. [15] identified three distinct groups of adolescents regarding risk behaviours: a low-risk group (57.8%), including pupils with low or very low frequency of risk behaviours; a high-risk group (13.2%), including pupils with the highest frequency of all risk behaviours; and an invisible-risk group (29%), comprised of pupils characterized by high media use, sedentary lifestyle, reduced hours of sleep, and a high prevalence of

mental health problems like depression, sub-threshold depression, anxiety, and suicidal ideation. These mental health problems were often overlooked as they were not detected by parents or teachers who were focused mainly on high media use.

Pathological internet use, defined as excessive or poorly controlled preoccupations, urges, or behaviours regarding Internet use, lead to impairment or distress in 5.2% of males and 3.8% of females in the SEYLE cohort [121]. Pathological internet use was significantly higher in adolescents not living with a biological parent or relative, adolescents with a parent or guardian who was unemployed, and in adolescents with parents who did not pay attention to adolescents or did not know what adolescents did in their free time [121]. Kaess et al. [55] found that pathological internet use was significantly associated with depression, suicidal ideation, suicide attempt, conduct problems, hyperactivity, and/or inattention. In the German SEYLE sample, it was demonstrated that pathological internet use and problematic alcohol use share similar psychopathological characteristics, such as conduct problems and depressive symptoms [122].

Access to lethal means

Differences in suicide rates between communities are, at least in part, owing to differences in accessibility to lethal methods of injury [123]. In a case–control study, Brent et al. [124] compared adolescents who died by suicide, inpatient attempters, and psychiatric inpatients who had never attempted suicide. Guns were twice as likely to be found in the homes of suicide victims as in the homes of suicide attempters or psychiatric controls. In a later psychological autopsy study, Brent et al. [125] confirmed that the availability of a gun was a significant risk factor for adolescent suicide. Among gun-owning families, Grossman et al. [126] found an increased risk for suicide in young people living in homes where firearms were less likely to be stored locked, stored separately from ammunition, or to have ammunition that was locked. Barber and Miller [127] reported a 2–5-fold higher risk of suicide in gun-owning homes for all household members. Restricting access to the means of suicide, like minimizing the size of packages and over-the-counter sales of analgesics, locking and withdrawing toxic pesticides, erecting barriers to physically limit access to hot spots like bridges and high buildings, and limiting firearm availability are evidence-based suicide preventive methods [128].

Responsible media reporting prevents copycat suicides and crisis helplines alleviate anxiety and desperation; however, the evidence base for those measures is limited [128].

Protective factors

A protective factor buffers individuals from suicidal thoughts and behaviour, thus reducing the likelihood of suicide. Borowsky et al. [129] estimated that, among adolescents, the presence of protective factors on the individual, family, and community level such as family connectedness and emotional well-being may reduce the risk of a suicide attempt. Resilience has been defined as the capacity for successful adaptation to change, a measure of stress coping ability or emotional stamina, the character of hardiness and invulnerability, the ability to thrive in the face of adversity, or recover from negative events [130]. Roy et al. [131] found that substance abuse patients and prisoners who never attempted suicide had higher resilience scores than those with similar levels of childhood trauma, who had attempted suicide. Similarly, a moderating effect of resilience on suicidal risk was found among adolescent victims of violent life events [132].

Self-esteem has been identified as a key protective factor against suicidality, especially among adolescents and young adults [99, 133, 134]. Cognitive styles related to decision-making and problem-solving may also influence the suicidal process both in adults [135] and adolescents [136].

The literature indicates that social support is associated with decreased likelihood of a lifetime suicide attempt, even after controlling for a variety of other risk factors [137]. Supportive social relations with peers, parents, and school staff has been demonstrated to have a mitigating effect on risk for suicide attempts in boys who had a history of attempting suicide [138]. Perceived family connectedness was also found to be protective against suicide attempts [129]. The SEYLE study showed that pupils with parental support and pro-social behaviours were at a significantly lower risk for engaging in self-injury after being victimized by bullies compared with students without parental support [106]. Religious belief showed a protective effect on suicidality [139], both among adolescents [140] and young adults [141], although this effect may vary in different cultures [12, 142].

In the SEYLE study, several individual protective factors against emotional and suicidal problems like the role of sleep [80], reading books [100], and physical activity [143] were identified. Physical activity has been proven to improve children's mental health [144]. Adolescent suicide attempters were reported to have a negative attitude towards sport activities, lower frequency of involvement in sports, and lower involvement in sports as a coping style for distress [145].

Greater attendance in physical education class was inversely related to suicidal ideation [146, 147]. In the SEYLE study [143], results show that the frequency of physical activity was positively correlated with well-being and negatively correlated with both anxiety and depressive symptoms, up to a threshold of moderate frequency of activity. More frequent activity above moderate level was associated with higher levels of depressive symptoms among girls. Moreover, for girls there were significant differences on the depression, anxiety, and well-being scores between those involved in individual sport/fitness activities and those involved in team sports, with team sport associated with higher well-being and lower anxiety and depressive symptoms. Comparisons between boys involved in individual sport/fitness activities and boys involved in team sports showed no significant differences on the mental health measures [143].

Universal school-based suicide preventive strategies

The WHO report, *Promoting Mental Health: Concepts, Emerging Evidence, Practice* [148], affirmed that 'there is ample empirical evidence that providing universal programmes to groups of students can influence positive mental health outcomes. Several types of interventions at the school level have been identified as achieving improved competence and self-worth, as well as decreasing emotional and behavioural problems' in students.

Ciffone [149] provided evidence that the Sought Elgin High School Suicide Prevention Program changed unwanted attitudes about suicide and improved help-seeking behaviours.

Aseltine et al. [150] examined the effectiveness of the Signs of Suicide (SOS), a school-based prevention programme focusing on two of the most prominent risk factors for suicidal behaviour: underlying mental illness, particularly depression, and problematic use of alcohol. The young people who received the programme were, during 3 months of follow-up, approximately 40% less likely to report a suicide attempt than young people in the control group. The young people exposed to the programme also showed a greater knowledge of depression and suicide and more adaptive attitudes towards these problems. Those results were further confirmed in another study [151].

Wilcox et al. [152] evaluated the effects of the Good Behavior Game (GBG), a programme directed at socializing children for the student role and reducing aggressive and disruptive behaviour. The programme was associated with a significant reduction of risk for suicide ideation and suicide attempts by 19–21 years of age compared with young people in standard control classrooms. Wyman et al. [153] implemented the Sources of Strength, a prevention programme that utilizes peer leaders to increase eight protective factors and encourage adolescents to engage 'trusted adults' to help distressed and suicidal peers. The programme improved the peer leaders' adaptive norms regarding suicide, their connectedness to adults, and their school engagement. The intervention was also able to increase students' perception of adult support for suicidal young people and the acceptability of seeking help.

King et al. [154] assessed the outcomes of the Surviving the Teens Suicide Prevention and Depression Awareness Program, reporting a reduction of suicidal ideation, suicide plans, and attempts, as well as a reduction of depressive symptoms. The programme was able to increase students' self-efficacy and behavioural changes toward help-seeking behaviours.

SEYLE [155, 156] was a randomized controlled trial aimed at evaluating the efficacy of three school-based suicide prevention and mental health promotion interventions compared with a minimal intervention, which served as a control. The active interventions comprised a mental health awareness programme (Youth Aware of Mental Health (YAM) [157]), gatekeeper training (Question Persuade and Refer (QPR) [158]), and professional screening for at-risk adolescents (ProfScreen [55]). At the 12-month follow-up [159], the mental health awareness programme (YAM) was associated with a 50% reduction of incident suicide attempts (OR 0.45, 95% CI 0.24–0.85; $P = 0.014$) and severe suicidal ideation with suicidal plans (OR 0.50, 0.27–0.92; $P = 0.025$) compared with the control group.

Moreover, systematic reviews [160–162] reported the positive outcomes of several school-based suicide prevention programmes in improving knowledge and change of attitudes toward suicide.

Conclusions

The discussed findings have indicated a wide range of risk factors, including youth psychiatric disorders and self-harm, a family history of suicide and mental health problems, stressful life events, impulsivity, aggressiveness, and access to lethal means, as well as suicide preventive possibilities.

A useful model for classifying suicide prevention strategies is the Universal, Selective, and Indicated Prevention [163]. Universal programmes that raise awareness and promote skills training, like SOS, GBG, and YAM, have proven to be effective school-based prevention strategies in significantly reducing suicide attempts. Evidence also supports the usefulness of lethal means restrictions and responsible media reporting in decreasing suicidal behaviours.

Among selective interventions, gatekeeper training and crisis helplines are widely used, but their effectiveness in reducing suicidality has not been proven. Screening programmes, used in the indicated preventive strategies, are implemented worldwide; but the successful outcomes rely on the availability of health and mental health resources.

The prevention of suicidal behaviour among adolescents is possible through the use of evidence-based programs.

References

1. World Health Organization (WHO). *Preventing Suicide: A Global Imperative*. Geneva: WHO, 2014.
2. Wasserman D, Rihmer Z, Rujescu D, et al. The European Psychiatric Association (EPA) guidance on suicide treatment and prevention. *Eur Psychiatry* 2012; 27: 129–141.
3. World Health Organization (WHO). *Mental Health Action Plan 2013–2020*. Geneva: WHO, 2013.
4. Wasserman D, Cheng Q, Jiang G-X. Global suicide rates among young people aged 15–19. *World Psychiatry* 2005; 4: 114–120.
5. World Health Organization (WHO). *Suicide a Leading Cause of Death Among Young Adults in High-income Countries*. Geneva: WHO, 2014.
6. Heron M. Deaths: Leading causes for 2012. *National Vital Statistics Reports* 2015; 64: 1–93.
7. Shaffer D, Pfeffer C. Practice parameter for the assessment and treatment of children and adolescents with suicidal behavior. *J Am Acad Child Adolesc Psychiatry* 2001; 40: 24S–51S.
8. Eurostat. Suicide death rate, by age group. Available at: http://ec.europa.eu/eurostat/web/products-datasets/product?code=tsdph240 (accessed 13 March 2018).
9. Australian Bureau of Statistics. Intentional self-harm by age. Available at: http://www.abs.gov.au/ausstats/abs@.nsf/Lookup/by%20Subject/3303.0~2014~Main%20Features~Intentional%20self-harm%20by%20Age~10051 (accessed 13 March 2018).
10. World Health Organization. World report on violence and health. Available at: http://www.who.int/violence_injury_prevention/violence/world_report/en/ (accessed 13 March 2018).
11. Beautrais A. Suicide and serious suicide attempts in youth: a multiple-group comparison study. *Am J Psychiatry* 2003; 160: 1093–1099.
12. Evans E, Hawton K, Rodham K, Psychol C, Deeks J. The prevalence of suicidal phenomena in adolescents: a systematic review of population-based studies. *Suicide Life Threat Behav* 2005; 35: 239–250.
13. Hultén A, Jiang GX, Wasserman D, et al. Repetition of attempted suicide among teenagers in Europe: frequency, timing and risk factors. *Eur Child Adolesc Psychiatry* 2001; 10: 161–169.
14. Kann L. Youth risk behavior surveillance—United States, 2015. *MMWR Surveillance Summaries* 2016; 65: 1–174.
15. Carli V, Hoven C, Wasserman C, et al. A newly identified group of adolescents at 'invisible' risk for psychopathology and suicidal behavior: findings from the SEYLE study. *World Psychiatry* 2014; 13: 78–86.
16. Kokkevi A, Rotsika V, Arapaki A, Richardson C. Adolescents' self-reported suicide attempts, self-harm thoughts and their correlates across 17 European countries: Self-reported suicide attempts by European adolescents. *J Child Psychol Psychiatry* 2012; 53: 381–389.
17. McKinnon B, Gariépy G, Sentenac M, Elgar F. Adolescent suicidal behaviours in 32 low- and middle-income countries. *Bull World Health Organ* 2016; 94: 340–350F.
18. Nock M, Hwang I, Sampson N, et al. Cross-national analysis of the associations among mental disorders and suicidal behavior: findings from the WHO World Mental Health Surveys. *PLOS Med* 2009; 6: e1000123.
19. Mann J, Oquendo M, Underwood M, Arango V. The neurobiology of suicide risk: a review for the clinician. *J Clin Psychiatry* 1999; 60(Suppl. 2): 7–11.
20. Wasserman D. *Suicide: An Unnecessary Death*, 2nd ed. Oxford: Oxford University Press, 2016.
21. McGuffin P, Marušič A, Farmer A. What can psychiatric genetics offer suicidology? *Crisis* 2001; 22: 61–65.
22. Roy A, Segal N, Sarchiapone M. Attempted suicide among living co-twins of twin suicide victims. *Am J Psychiatry* 1995; 152: 1075–1076.
23. Wender P, Kety S, Rosenthal D, Schulsinger F, Ortmann J, Lunde I. Psychiatric disorders in the biological and adoptive families of adopted individuals with affective disorders. *Arch Gen Psychiatry* 1986; 43: 923–929.
24. Glowinski A, Bucholz K, Nelson E, et al. Suicide attempts in an adolescent female twin sample. *J Am Acad Child Adolesc Psychiatry* 2001; 40: 1300–1307.
25. Sokolowski M, Wasserman J, Wasserman D. Polygenic associations of neurodevelopmental genes in suicide attempt. *Mol Psychiatry* 2016; 21: 1381–1390.
26. Brent D, Mann J. Family genetic studies, suicide, and suicidal behavior. *Am J Med Genet C Semin Med Genet* 2005; 133C: 13–24.
27. Rujescu D, Giegling I, Sato T, Hartmann A, Möller H-J. Genetic variations in tryptophan hydroxylase in suicidal behavior. *Biol Psychiatry* 2003; 54: 465–473.
28. Li D, He L. Further clarification of the contribution of the tryptophan hydroxylase (*TPH*) gene to suicidal behavior using systematic allelic and genotypic meta-analyses. *Hum Genet* 2006; 119: 233–240.
29. Lin P-Y, Tsai G. Association between serotonin transporter gene promoter polymorphism and suicide: results of a meta-analysis. *Biol Psychiatry* 2004; 55: 1023–1030.
30. Wasserman D, Geijer T, Sokolowski M, et al. Association of the serotonin transporter promotor polymorphism with suicide attempters with a high medical damage. *Eur Neuropsychopharmacol* 2007; 17: 230–233.
31. Dwivedi Y, Rizavi H, Conley R, Roberts R, Tamminga C, Pandey G. Altered gene expression of brain-derived neurotrophic factor and receptor tyrosine kinase B in postmortem brain of suicide subjects. *Arch Gen Psychiatry* 2003; 60: 804–815.
32. Pandey G, Ren X, Rizavi H, Conley R, Roberts R, Dwivedi Y. Brain-derived neurotrophic factor and tyrosine kinase B receptor signalling in post-mortem brain of teenage suicide victims. *Int J Neuropsychopharmacol* 2008; 11: 1047–1061.
33. Sarchiapone M, Carli V, Roy A, et al. Association of polymorphism (Val66Met) of brain-derived neurotrophic factor with suicide attempts in depressed patients. *Neuropsychobiology* 2008; 57: 139–145.
34. Caspi A, Sugden K, Moffitt T, et al. Influence of life stress on depression: moderation by a polymorphism in the 5-HTT gene. *Science* 2003; 301: 386–389.
35. Roy A, Hu X-Z, Janal M, Goldman D. Interaction between childhood trauma and serotonin transporter gene variation in suicide. *Neuropsychopharmacology* 2007; 32: 2046–2052.
36. Wasserman D, Sokolowski M, Rozanov V, Wasserman J. The *CRHR1* gene: a marker for suicidality in depressed males exposed to low stress. *Genes Brain Behav* 2008; 7: 14–19.
37. Roy A, Gorodetsky E, Yuan Q, Goldman D, Enoch M-A. Interaction of *FKBP5*, a stress-related gene, with childhood trauma increases the risk for attempting suicide. *Neuropsychopharmacology* 2010; 35: 1674–1683.
38. Brent D, Oquendo M, Birmaher B, et al. Familial pathways to early-onset suicide attempt: risk for suicidal behavior in offspring of mood-disordered suicide attempters. *Arch Gen Psychiatry* 2002; 59: 801–807.
39. Agerbo E, Nordentoft M, Mortensen P. Familial, psychiatric, and socioeconomic risk factors for suicide in young people: nested case-control study. *BMJ* 2002; 325: 74.

40. Mittendorfer-Rutz E, Rasmussen F, Lange T. A life-course study on effects of parental markers of morbidity and mortality on offspring's suicide attempt. *PLOS ONE* 2012; 7: e51585.

41. Mittendorfer-Rutz E, Rasmussen F, Wasserman D. Familial clustering of suicidal behaviour and psychopathology in young suicide attempters. A register-based nested case control study. *Soc Psychiatry Psychiatr Epidemiol* 2008; 43: 28–36.

42. Gureje O, Oladeji B, Hwang I, et al. Parental psychopathology and the risk of suicidal behavior in their offspring: results from the World Mental Health surveys. *Mol Psychiatry* 2011; 16: 1221–1233.

43. Bostwick M, Pabbati C, Geske J, McKean A. Suicide attempt as a risk factor for completed suicide: even more lethal than we knew. *Am J Psychiatry* 2016; 173: 1094–1100.

44. Hawton K, Fagg J, Platt S, Hawkins M. Factors associated with suicide after parasuicide in young people. *BMJ* 1993; 306: 1641–1644.

45. Beck A. *Beyond Belief: A Theory of Modes, Personality, and Psychopathology. Frontiers of Cognitive Therapy*. New York: Guilford Press, 1996.

46. Nock M, Joiner Jr. T, Gordon K, Lloyd-Richardson E, Prinstein M. Non-suicidal self-injury among adolescents: diagnostic correlates and relation to suicide attempts. *Psychiatry Res* 2006; 144: 65–72.

47. Esposito-Smythers C, Goldstein T, Birmaher B, et al. Clinical and psychosocial correlates of non-suicidal self-injury within a sample of children and adolescents with bipolar disorder. *J Affect Disord* 2010; 125: 89–97.

48. Asarnow J, Porta G, Spirito A, et al. Suicide attempts and nonsuicidal self-injury in the treatment of resistant depression in adolescents: findings from the TORDIA study. *J Am Acad Child Adolesc Psychiatry* 2011; 50: 772–781.

49. Brunner R, Kaess M, Parzer P, et al. Life-time prevalence and psychosocial correlates of adolescent direct self-injurious behavior: a comparative study of findings in 11 European countries. *J Child Psychol Psychiatry* 2014; 55: 337–348.

50. Koenig J, Brunner R, Fischer-Waldschmidt G, et al. Prospective risk for suicidal behaviour in adolescents with onset, maintenance or cessation of self-injurious behaviour. *Eur Child Adolesc Psychiatry* 2017; 26: 345–354.

51. Shaffer D, Gould M, Fisher P, et al. Psychiatric diagnosis in child and adolescent suicide. *Arch Gen Psychiatry* 1996; 53: 339–348.

52. Bridge J, Goldstein T, Brent D. Adolescent suicide and suicidal behavior. *J Child Psychol Psychiatry* 2006; 47: 372–394.

53. Nock M, Green J, Hwang I, et al. Prevalence, correlates, and treatment of lifetime suicidal behavior among adolescents: results from the National Comorbidity Survey Replication Adolescent Supplement. *JAMA Psychiatry* 2013; 70: 300–310.

54. Kelleher I, Corcoran P, Keeley H, et al. Psychotic symptoms and population risk for suicide attempt: a prospective cohort study. *JAMA Psychiatry* 2013; 70: 940–948.

55. Kaess M, Brunner R, Parzer P, et al. Risk-behaviour screening for identifying adolescents with mental health problems in Europe. *Eur Child Adolesc Psychiatry* 2014; 23: 611–620.

56. Cotter P, Kaess M, Corcoran P, et al. Help-seeking behaviour following school-based screening for current suicidality among European adolescents. *Soc Psychiatry Psychiatr Epidemiol* 2015; 50: 973–982.

57. Gould M, Greenberg T, Velting D, Shaffer D. Youth suicide risk and preventive interventions: a review of the past 10 years. *J Am Acad Child Adolesc Psychiatry* 2003; 42: 386–405.

58. Stenager K, Qin P. Individual and parental psychiatric history and risk for suicide among adolescents and young adults in Denmark. *Soc Psychiatry Psychiatr Epidemiol* 2008; 43: 920–969.

59. Hauser M, Galling B, Correll C. Suicidal ideation and suicide attempts in children and adolescents with bipolar disorder: a systematic review of prevalence and incidence rates, risk factors, and targeted interventions. *Bipolar Disord* 2013; 15: 507–523.

60. Balázs J, Miklósi M, Keresztény A, et al. Adolescent subthreshold-depression and anxiety: psychopathology, functional impairment and increased suicide risk. *J Child Psychol Psychiatry* 2013; 54: 670–677.

61. Renaud J, Berlim M, McGirr A, Tousignant M, Turecki G. Current psychiatric morbidity, aggression/impulsivity, and personality dimensions in child and adolescent suicide: a case–control study. *J Affect Disord* 2008; 105: 221–228.

62. Galaif E, Sussman S, Newcomb M, Locke T. Suicidality, depression, and alcohol use among adolescents: a review of empirical findings. *Int J Adolesc Med Health* 2007; 19: 27–35.

63. Gould M, King R, Greenwald S, et al. Psychopathology associated with suicidal ideation and attempts among children and adolescents. *J Am Acad Child Adolesc Psychiatry* 1998; 37: 915–923.

64. Boden J, Fergusson D, Horwood L. Anxiety disorders and suicidal behaviours in adolescence and young adulthood: findings from a longitudinal study. *Psychol Med* 2007; 37: 431–440.

65. Kelleher I, Lynch F, Harley M, et al. Psychotic symptoms in adolescence index risk for suicidal behavior: findings from two population-based case–control clinical interview studies. *Arch Gen Psychiatry* 2012; 69: 1277–1283.

66. Dancyger I, Fornari V. A review of eating disorders and suicide risk in adolescence. *Sci World J* 2005; 5: 803–811.

67. Swanson S. Prevalence and correlates of eating disorders in adolescents: results from the national comorbidity survey replication adolescent supplement. *Arch Gen Psychiatry* 2011; 68: 714–723.

68. Crow S, Eisenberg M, Story M, Neumark-Sztainer D. Suicidal behavior in adolescents: relationship to weight status, weight control behaviors, and body dissatisfaction. *Int J Eat Disord* 2008; 41: 82–87.

69. Beck A, Brown G, Berchick R, Stewart B, Steer R. Relationship between hopelessness and ultimate suicide: a replication with psychiatric outpatients. *Am J Psychiatry* 1990; 147: 190–195.

70. Howard-Pitney B, LaFromboise T, Basil M, September B, Johnson M. Psychological and social indicators of suicide ideation and suicide attempts in Zuni adolescents. *J Consult Clin Psychol* 1992; 60: 473–476.

71. Morano C, Cisler R, Lemerond J. Risk factors for adolescent suicidal behavior: loss, insufficient familial support, and hopelessness. *Adolescence* 1993; 28: 851–865.

72. Lewinsohn P, Rohde P, Seeley J. Psychosocial characteristics of adolescents with a history of suicide attempt. *J Am Acad Child Adolesc Psychiatry* 1993; 32: 60–68.

73. Cole D. Psychopathology of adolescent suicide: hopelessness, coping beliefs, and depression. *J Abnorm Psychol* 1989; 98: 248–255.

74. Stewart S, Kennard B, Lee PW, Mayes T, Hughes C, Emslie G. Hopelessness and suicidal ideation among adolescents in two cultures. *J Child Psychol Psychiatry* 2005; 46: 364–372.

75. Moeller F, Barratt E, Dougherty D, Schmitz J, Swann A. Psychiatric aspects of impulsivity. *Am J Psychiatry* 2001; 158: 1783–1793.

76. Turecki G. Dissecting the suicide phenotype: the role of impulsive-aggressive behaviours. *J Psychiatry Neurosci* 2005; 30: 398–408.

77. Sarchiapone M, Carli V, Giannantonio M, Roy A. Risk factors for attempting suicide in prisoners. *Suicide Life Threat Behav* 2009; 39: 343–350.

78. Simon T, Swann A, Powell K, Potter L, Kresnow M-J, O'Carroll P. Characteristics of impulsive suicide attempts and attempters. *Suicide Life Threat Behav* 2001; 32(Suppl. 1): 49–59.

79. Horesh N, Gothelf D, Ofek H, Weizman T, Apter A. Impulsivity as a correlate of suicidal behavior in adolescent psychiatric inpatients. *Crisis* 1999; 20: 8–14.

80. Sarchiapone M, Mandelli L, Carli V, et al. Hours of sleep in adolescents and its association with anxiety, emotional concerns, and suicidal ideation. *Sleep Med* 2014; 15: 248–254.

81. Lee YJ, Cho S-J, Cho IH, Kim SJ. Insufficient sleep and suicidality in adolescents. *Sleep* 2012; 35: 455–460.

82. Silenzio V, Pena J, Duberstein P, Cerel J, Knox K. Sexual orientation and risk factors for suicidal ideation and suicide attempts among adolescents and young adults. *Am J Public Health* 2007; 97: 2017–2019.

83. Cotter P, Corcoran P, McCarthy J, et al. Victimisation and psychosocial difficulties associated with sexual orientation concerns: a school-based study of adolescents. *Irish Med J* 2014; 107: 310–313.

84. Russell S, Joyner K. Adolescent sexual orientation and suicide risk: evidence from a national study. *Am J Public Health* 2001; 91: 1276–1281.

85. Eisenberg M, Resnick M. Suicidality among gay, lesbian and bisexual youth: the role of protective factors. *J Adolesc Health* 2006; 39: 662–668.

86. Marshal M, Dietz L, Friedman M, et al. Suicidality and depression disparities between sexual minority and heterosexual youth: a meta-analytic review. *J Adolesc Health* 2011; 49: 115–123.

87. Grilo C, Sanislow C, Fehon D, Martino S, McGlashan T. Psychological and behavioral functioning in adolescent psychiatric inpatients who report histories of childhood abuse. *Am J Psychiatry* 1999; 156: 538–543.

88. Ben-Efraim Y, Wasserman D, Wasserman J, Sokolowski M. Gene–environment interactions between CRHR1 variants and physical assault in suicide attempts. *Genes Brain Behav* 2011; 10: 663–672.

89. Sokolowski M, Ben-Efraim Y, Wasserman J, Wasserman D. Glutamatergic *GRIN2B* and polyaminergic *ODC1* genes in suicide attempts: associations and gene–environment interactions with childhood/adolescent physical assault. *Mol Psychiatry* 2013; 18: 985–992.

90. Molnar B, Berkman L, Buka S. Psychopathology, childhood sexual abuse and other childhood adversities: relative links to subsequent suicidal behaviour in the US. *Psychol Med* 2001; 31: 965–977.

91. Salzinger S, Rosario M, Feldman R, Ng-Mak D. Adolescent suicidal behavior: associations with preadolescent physical abuse and selected risk and protective factors. *J Am Acad Child Adolesc Psychiatry* 2007; 46: 859–866.

92. Miller A, Esposito-Smythers C, Weismoore J, Renshaw K. The relation between child maltreatment and adolescent suicidal behavior: a systematic review and critical examination of the literature. *Clin Child Fam Psychol* 2013; 16: 146–172.

93. Waldrop A, Hanson R, Resnick H, Kilpatrick D, Naugle A, Saunders B. Risk factors for suicidal behavior among a national sample of adolescents: implications for prevention. *J Trauma Stress* 2007; 20: 869–879.

94. Rosenberg H, Jankowski M, Sengupta A, Wolfe R, Wolford II G, Rosenberg S. Single and multiple suicide attempts and associated health risk factors in new hampshire adolescents. *Suicide Life Threat Behav* 2005; 35: 547–557.

95. Martin G, Bergen H, Richardson A, Roeger L, Allison S. Sexual abuse and suicidality: gender differences in a large community sample of adolescents. *Child Abuse Neglect* 2004; 28: 491–503.

96. Liu R, Miller I. Life events and suicidal ideation and behavior: a systematic review. *Clin Psychol Rev* 2014; 34: 181–192.

97. O'Connor R, Rasmussen S, Hawton K. Distinguishing adolescents who think about self-harm from those who engage in self-harm. *Br J Psychiatry* 2012; 200: 330–335.

98. Hawton K, Fagg J, Simkin S. Deliberate self-poisoning and self-injury in children and adolescents under 16 years of age in Oxford, 1976–1993. *Br J Psychiatry* 1996; 169: 202–208.

99. Bearman P, Moody J. Suicide and friendships among american adolescents. *Am J Public Health* 2004; 94: 89–95.

100. Kasahara-Kiritani M, Hadlaczky G, Westerlund M, et al. Reading books and watching films as a protective factor against suicidal ideation. *Int J Environ Res Public Health* 2015; 12: 15937–15942.

101. Miller A, Esposito-Smythers C, Leichtweis R. Role of social support in adolescent suicidal ideation and suicide attempts. *J Adolesc Health* 2015; 56: 286–292.

102. Prinstein M, Boergers J, Spirito A, Little T, Grapentine W. Peer functioning, family dysfunction, and psychological symptoms in a risk factor model for adolescent inpatients' suicidal ideation severity. *J Clin Child Psychol* 2000; 29: 392–405.

103. Klomek A, Marrocco F, Kleinman M, Schonfeld I, Gould M. Bullying, depression, and suicidality in adolescents. *J Am Acad Child Adolesc Psychiatry* 2007; 46: 40–49.

104. Klomek A, Marrocco F, Kleinman M, Schonfeld I, Gould M. Peer victimization, depression, and suicidiality in adolescents. *Suicide Life Threat Behav* 2008; 38: 166–180.

105. King C, Merchant C. Social and interpersonal factors relating to adolescent suicidality: a review of the literature. *Arch Suicide Res* 2008; 12: 18–196.

106. Barzilay S, Klomek A, Apter A, et al. Bullying victimization and suicide ideation and behaviour among adolescents in Europe: a 10-Country study. *J Adolesc Health* 2017; 61: 179–186.

107. Gould M, Jamieson P, Romer D. Media contagion and suicide among the young. *Am Behav Sci* 2003; 46: 1269–1284.

108. Gould M, Wallenstein S, Kleinman M, O'Carroll P, Mercy J. Suicide clusters: an examination of age-specific effects. *Am J Public Health* 1990; 80: 211–212.

109. McMahon E, Corcoran P, Keeley H, et al. Mental health difficulties and suicidal behaviours among young migrants: multicentre study of European adolescents. *BJPsych Open* 2017; 3: 291–299.

110. Mazur J, Woynarowska B. [Risk behaviors syndrome and subjective health and life satisfaction in youth aged 15 years]. *Med Wieku Rozwoj* 2004; 8: 567–583 (in English).

111. Hallfors D, Waller M, Ford C, Halpern C, Brodish P, Iritani B. Adolescent depression and suicide risk: association with sex and drug behavior. *Am J Prev Med* 2004; 27: 224–231.

112. Epstein J, Spirito A. Gender-specific risk factors for suicidality among high school students. *Arch Suicide Res* 2010; 14: 193–205.

113. Ruutel E, Sisask M, Varnik A, et al. Alcohol consumption patterns among adolescents are related to family structure and exposure to drunkenness within the family: results from the SEYLE project. *Int J Environ Res Public Health* 2014; 11: 12700–12715.

114. Klomek A, Sourander A, Niemelä S, et al. Childhood bullying behaviors as a risk for suicide attempts and completed suicides: a population-based birth cohort study. *J Am Acad Child Adolesc Psychiatry* 2009; 48: 254–261.

115. Brent D, Bridge J. Delinquent accounts: does delinquency account for suicidal behavior? *J Adolesc Health* 2007; 40: 204–205.

116. Bronisch T, Höfler M, Lieb R. Smoking predicts suicidality: findings from a prospective community study. *J Affect Disord* 2008; 108: 135–145.

117. Houck C, Hadley W, Lescano C, Pugatch D, Brown L; Project Shield Study Group. Suicide attempt and sexual risk behavior: relationship among adolescents. *Arch Suicide Res* 2008; 12: 39–49.

118. Brown D, Galuska D, Zhang J, et al. Psychobiology and behavioral strategies. Physical activity, sport participation, and suicidal behavior: U.S. high school students. *Med Sci Sports Exerc* 2007; 39: 2248–2257.

119. Swahn M, Reynolds M, Tice M, Miranda-Pierangeli M, Jones C, Jones I. Perceived overweight, BMI, and risk for suicide attempts: findings from the 2007 Youth Risk Behavior Survey. *J Adolesc Health* 2009; 45: 292–295.

120. Banzer R, Haring C, Buchheim A, et al. Risk factors and comorbidities for occasional and daily smoking in European adolescents: results of the SEYLE Project. *Eur Psychiatry* 2015; 30: 515.

121. Durkee T, Kaess M, Carli V, et al. Prevalence of pathological internet use among adolescents in Europe: demographic and social factors. *Addiction* 2012; 107: 2210–2222.

122. Wartberg L, Brunner R, Kriston L, et al. Psychopathological factors associated with problematic alcohol and problematic Internet use in a sample of adolescents in Germany. *Psychiatry Res* 2016; 240: 272–277.

123. Marzuk P, Leon A, Tardiff K, Morgan E, Stajic M, Mann J. The effect of access to lethal methods of injury on suicide rates. *Arch Gen Psychiatry* 1992; 49: 451–458.

124. Brent D, Perper J, Allman C, Moritz G, Wartella M, Zelenak J. The presence and accessibility of firearms in the homes of adolescent suicides: a case–control study. *JAMA* 1991; 266: 2989–2995.

125. Brent D, Baugher M, Bridge J, Chen T, Chiappetta L. Age- and sex-related risk factors for adolescent suicide. *J Am Acad Child Adolesc Psychiatry* 1999; 38: 1497–1505.

126. Grossman D, Mueller B, Riedy C, et al. Gun storage practices and risk of youth suicide and unintentional firearm injuries. *JAMA* 2005; 293: 707–714.

127. Barber C, Miller M. Reducing a suicidal person's access to lethal means of suicide. *Am J Prev Med* 2014; 47(3 Suppl. 2): S264–272.

128. Zalsman G, Hawton K, Wasserman D, et al. Suicide prevention strategies revisited: 10-year systematic review. *Lancet Psychiatry* 2016; 3: 646–659.

129. Borowsky I, Ireland M, Resnick M. Adolescent suicide attempts: risks and protectors. *Pediatrics* 2001; 107: 485–493.

130. Hoge E, Austin E, Pollack M. Resilience: research evidence and conceptual considerations for posttraumatic stress disorder. *Depress Anxiety* 2007; 24: 139–152.

131. Roy A, Carli V, Sarchiapone M. Resilience mitigates the suicide risk associated with childhood trauma. *J Affect Disord* 2011; 133: 561–594.

132. Nrugham L, Holen A, Sund AM. Associations between attempted suicide, violent life events, depressive symptoms, and resilience in adolescents and young adults. *J Nerv Ment Dis* 2010; 198: 131–136.

133. McGee R, Williams S, Nada-Raja S. Low self-esteem and hopelessness in childhood and suicidal ideation in early adulthood. *J Abnorm Child Psychol* 2001; 29: 281–291.

134. Sharaf A, Thompson E, Walsh E. Protective effects of self-esteem and family support on suicide risk behaviors among at-risk adolescents. *J Child Adolesc Psychiatr Nurs* 2009; 22: 160–168.

135. Jollant F, Bellivier F, Leboyer M, et al. Impaired decision making in suicide attempters. *Am J Psychiatry* 2005; 162: 304–310.

136. Oldershaw A, Grima E, Jollant F, et al. Decision making and problem solving in adolescents who deliberately self-harm. *Psychol Med* 2009; 39: 95–104.

137. Kleiman E, Liu R. Social support as a protective factor in suicide: findings from two nationally representative samples. *J Affect Disord* 2013; 150: 540–545.

138. Kidd S, Henrich C, Brookmeyer K, Davidson L, King R, Shahar G. The social context of adolescent suicide attempts: interactive effects of parent, peer, and school social relations. *Suicide Life Threat Behav* 2006; 36: 386–395.

139. Wu A, Wang J-Y, Jia C-X. Religion and completed suicide: a meta-analysis. *PLOS ONE* 2015; 10: e0131715.

140. Miller L, Gur M. Religiosity, depression, and physical maturation in adolescent girls. *J Am Acad Child Adolesc Psychiatry* 2002; 41: 206–214.

141. Hilton S, Fellingham G, Lyon J. Suicide rates and religious commitment in young adult males in Utah. *Am J Epidemiol* 2002; 155: 413–19.

142. Sisask M, Värnik A, Kloves K, et al. Is religiosity a protective factor against attempted suicide: a cross-cultural case–control study. *Arch Suicide Res* 2010; 14: 44–55.

143. McMahon E, Corcoran P, O'Regan G, et al. Physical activity in European adolescents and associations with anxiety, depression and well-being. *Eur Child Adolesc Psychiatry* 2017; 26: 111–122.

144. Ahn S, Fedewa A. A meta-analysis of the relationship between children's physical activity and mental health. *J Pediatr Psychol* 2011; 36: 385–397.

145. Tomori M, Zalar B, Plesnicar B, Ziherl S, Stergar E. Smoking in relation to psychosocial risk factors in adolescents. *Eur Child Adolesc Psychiatry* 2001; 10: 143–150.

146. Brosnahan J, Steffen L, Lytle L, Patterson J, Boostrom A. The relation between physical activity and mental health among hispanic and non-hispanic white adolescents. *Arch Pediatr Adolesc Med* 2004; 158: 818–823.

147. Taliaferro L, Rienzo B, Miller M, Pigg R, Dodd V. High school youth and suicide risk: exploring protection afforded through physical activity and sport participation. *J School Health* 2008; 78: 545–553.

148. World Health Organization (WHO). *Promoting Mental Health: Concepts, Emerging Evidence, Practice: Summary Report/A Report From the WHO*. Geneva: WHO, 2005.

149. Ciffone J. Suicide prevention: an analysis and replication of a curriculum-based high school program. *Soc Work* 2007; 52: 41–49.

150. Aseltine R, James A, Schilling E, Glanovsky J. Evaluating the SOS suicide prevention program: a replication and extension. *BMC Public Health* 2007; 7: 161.

151. Schilling E, Aseltine R, James A. The SOS suicide prevention program: further evidence of efficacy and effectiveness. *Prev Sci* 2016; 17: 157–166.

152. Wilcox H, Kellam S, Brown C, et al. The impact of two universal randomized first- and second-grade classroom interventions on young adult suicide ideation and attempts. *Drug Alcohol Depend* 2008; 95(Suppl. 1): S60–S73.

153. Wyman P, Brown C, LoMurray M, et al. An outcome evaluation of the Sources of Strength suicide prevention program delivered by adolescent peer leaders in high schools. *Am J Public Health* 2010; 100: 1653–1661.

154. King K, Strunk C, Sorter M. Preliminary effectiveness of Surviving the Teens® suicide prevention and depression awareness program on adolescents' suicidality and self-efficacy in performing help-seeking behaviors. *J School Health* 2011; 81: 581–590.

155. Wasserman D, Carli V, Wasserman C, et al. Saving and empowering young lives in Europe (SEYLE): a randomized controlled trial. *BMC Public Health* 2010; 10: 192.

156. Carli V, Wasserman C, Wasserman D, et al. The Saving and Empowering Young Lives in Europe (SEYLE) randomized controlled trial (RCT): methodological issues and participant characteristics. *BMC Public Health* 2013; 13: 479.

157. Wasserman C, Postuvan V, Herta D, Iosue M, Varnik P, Carli V. Interactions between youth and mental health professionals: the Youth Aware of Mental Health (YAM) program experience. *PLOS ONE* 2018; 13: 1–33.

158. QPR Institute for Suicide Prevention. Practical and proven suicide prevention training. Available at: www.qprinstitute.com (accessed 14 March 2018).

159. Wasserman D, Hoven C, Wasserman C, et al. School-based suicide prevention programmes: the SEYLE cluster-randomised, controlled trial. *Lancet* 2015; 385: 1536–1544.

160. Katz C, Bolton S-L, Katz L, et al. A systematic review of school-based suicide prevention programs. *Depress Anxiety* 2013; 30: 1030–1045.

161. Robinson J, Cox G, Malone A, et al. A systematic review of school-based interventions aimed at preventing, treating, and responding to suicide- related behavior in young people. *Crisis* 2013; 34: 164–182.

162. Cusimano M, Sameem M. The effectiveness of middle and high school-based suicide prevention programmes for adolescents: a systematic review. *Inj Prev* 2011; 17: 43–49.

163. Haggerty R, Mrazek P. Can we prevent mental illness? *Bull N Y Acad Med* 1994; 71: 300–306.

SECTION IV

Interventions: types and places

CHAPTER 40

Parenting skills and promotion of mental health over the lifespan

Stephen Scott

Introduction

Our parents give us everything: our genes and then through up-bringing our values, our nutrition, the first language we speak, and the neighbourhood in which we are brought up. In the centre of this is the moment-to-moment quality of the relationship between parents and children, which can have profound effects on how children grow up to become adults. At one extreme, neglectful and abusive parenting leads to very poor mental health outcomes. At the other, thoughtful, sensitive parenting with firm limits can make it likely that the children are resilient, well-adjusted, and successful.

There are many different theories of what constitutes good parenting, which then leads to different underpinnings for interventions. This chapter concentrates on theories that are empirically well supported and that have led to intervention programmes shown to be effective through randomized controlled trials (RCTs).

Two influential theories of parenting

Social learning theory

Social learning theory developed from general learning theory and behaviourism [1]. The premise is that children's real-life moment-to-moment experiences (rather than the meaning the child may give them) directly shape their behaviour. Because it was a reaction to introspective 'armchair' theories of how humans behave, the theoretical underpinning and related interventions have strongly focused on externally observable behaviour rather than children's inner mental states [2]. Operant behavioural principles of reinforcement and (non-coercive) consequences are applied immediately after the child has acted/responded; there is less emphasis on classical, stimulus-controlled conditioning [3]. Moment-to-moment interactions are central: if a child receives an immediate reward for what they do, such as getting parental attention or approval, then they are more likely to repeat the action, whereas if they are ignored or an unwelcome sanction is applied, then they are less likely to repeat it next time.

Gerald Patterson [2] showed how children's antisocial behaviours were learned from and rewarded by similar negative acts by parents. A negative parenting style has a causal role in the genesis of conduct problems, even after allowing for child factors. The association has been repeatedly found in (i) large-scale epidemiological investigations, such as those in New Zealand and the UK (e.g. Isle of Wight); (ii) intensive clinical investigations such as Patterson's work; and (iii) numerous naturalistic studies of diverse samples

using a mixture of methods (e.g. [4, 5]). The parenting relating styles identified as causing child problem behaviour are high criticism and hostility; harsh punishment; inconsistent discipline; low warmth, involvement, and encouragement; and poor supervision. This involves monitoring where the child is and, as they become older, their activities outside the home. Close supervision and monitoring has greater importance in neighbourhoods where there are many risks such as drugs and violence [6]. Monitoring is more than just a matter of parents being good 'policemen', as knowing the whereabouts of a child depends, in part, on the child trusting the parent enough to tell them where they are going and what they are up to [7]. Therefore, empowering parents to set up effective discipline depends on them also developing a warm, positive relationship so that the child will confide in them, and this is one of the parenting skills included in most modern interventions. These positive elements, such as good communication and listening to a child, promote positive attitudes and feelings towards the parent, so engendering the setting for a more positive relationship context for parental disciplinary interventions. Sensitive responding, warmth, and interest improve child behaviour [8] and attachment [9].

More recently, social learning models have evolved to include inner cognitive or 'mindful' processes such as attributions and expectations that underlie parents' behaviour [10]. Negative attributions about a child predict poorer child outcomes over and above observed parental behaviour [11], and addressing them in interventions leads to better child outcomes [12]. Beliefs can vary considerably across cultures, with more traditional societies showing more authoritarian views, particularly among fathers. Parenting programmes based on 'Western' values need to address different cultural beliefs regarding how best to bring up a child, but if they do this, they can be equally effective in improving parenting in ethnic minority groups [13, 14].

Attachment theory

Attachment theory [15] focuses on the how far the parent protects the child from harm and provides a sense of emotional security, especially when the child is frightened, hurt, upset, or sick. If the parent is there when the child needs, this then leads to what John Bowlby [15] called a 'secure base'. Secure in the knowledge that the parent will look at them when well, this frees the child up to get on with exploring the outside world and learning. The theory suggested that the quality of parental care, particularly sensitivity and responsiveness to the child's emotional needs ('sensitive responding'), promotes a relationship characterized by warm, expressive to-and-fro interchanges ('mutuality'), leading to secure attachment. Mary Ainsworth, in a classical set of studies, separated 12–18-month-old children from their parents and observed what happened on re-union. Those children who sought and received comfort from their parents soon calmed down and were free to get on with exploring the room, whereas there were two so-called 'insecure' reaction patterns. The first was avoidant, where the infant appeared un-concerned by the parent leaving the room but equally did not seek comfort on their return. The second insecure pattern was ambiva-lent, where the child is so cross with the parent on their return that they are preoccupied with the relationship and never appear com-fortable enough to go and play in the room. Abundant evidence has confirmed that sensitive responding is a key parenting dimension in promoting attachment security, but less than initially theorized [16]; longitudinal studies confirm that attachment security does not shape subsequent development deterministically but interacts with child and family factors to influence outcome [17]. In contrast, a particularly detrimental parenting style is frightening and abu-sive parenting, which is associated with 'disorganized' attachment patterns. Here, when the parent returns, the infant reacts in a ra-ther disturbing way, sometimes crawling under a table, sometimes crying, often switching from one response to another. Meta-analyses confirm a strong association of disorganized attachment with maltreatment at the hands of the parent [18]. Disorganization is associated with many forms of child psychopathology, especially conduct problems [19], although it is important to note that it occurs in 15% or more of populations.

Over time, attachment relationships are postulated to be-come internalized and then carried forward in the form of an 'internal working model' to influence expectations for other im-portant relationships. In the last decade, progress has been made in measuring internal working models, in childhood using doll-play story-stems [20], and in adolescence using semi-structured interviews [21]. These measures have shown that insecure patterns of attachment continue to be associated with higher levels of psy-chopathology in middle childhood [20, 22] and adolescence [9], and with less sensitive responding by the parent in both periods [9, 23]. However, some aspects of parenting are not emphasized in attachment accounts of parenting, such as cognitive stimulation or consistent discipline, yet studies of parenting styles associated with child [23] and adolescent [9] attachment security found that con-sistent discipline independently predicted secure attachment, be-yond sensitive responding. Intervention programmes that intend to increase attachment security should also target limit-setting, as well as sensitive responding [24].

Impact of parenting on the child's body

As well as parenting style having an influence over children's thinking, emotions, and behaviour, a wide array of biological processes are also affected. Physiologically, harsh, and abusive parenting often leads to altered stress hormone levels, with chron-ically elevated cortisol and much greater secretion in response to threat or stress, with slower rates of return to normal. Inflammatory responses are also elevated in those who are abused and depressed, and harsh parenting is associated with structural brain changes [25, 26]. Finally, a series of elegant studies in rats led by Michael Meaney, and in chimpanzees by Suomi [27], have shown that harsh and neglectful parenting leads to epigenetic changes (notably

acetylation and methylation) in sections of genes that control pro-tein synthesis [28].

The implications of these biological findings for parenting interventions are not yet clear. The physiological changes may be partly reversible by intervention, thus children taken away from abusive parenting into foster care show improved cortisol secretion patterns [29]. Whether improving the parenting environment leads to measurable epigenetic or brain changes is uncertain at present. Even if biological changes are alterable, they may contribute to be-havioural traits that reduce susceptibility to improved parenting, a subject we now address.

Child traits that can influence susceptibility to parenting effects

The relative contribution to child outcomes of nurture, here typified by parental style, and nature, through genetic inheritance, has long been debated. Until the early 1960s it was assumed that upbringing made all the difference. However, since then behav-ioural geneticists have shown that some child disorders and traits have high heritability, for example attention deficit hyperactivity disorder (ADHD), autism, and callous-unemotional traits, leading some to assume that children with these characteristics will there-fore be less susceptible to parenting and parenting intervention. However, as we shall see, this is not necessarily always the case.

Inherited characteristics and genetic influences

The effects of parenting can differ according to the characteristics of children. In a large follow-up study, Michael Bohman [30] divided early-adopted infants into those whose birth parents had been criminal or alcoholic, representing higher congenital (genetic plus early environmental) risk, versus those who were not. Adopting parents were categorized according to the same criteria (criminal or alcoholic versus not), as a measure of more and less desirable child-rearing conditions. Being known to the police by 17 years of age was 3% versus 12% for children with low versus high congenital risk favourably reared, showing a substantial inherited component to antisocial behaviour under good child-rearing conditions. For those raised in unfavourable conditions, the rates were 7% and 40%, respectively. This study, replicated since, shows that some children have a much greater liability to poorer outcomes under stressful rearing conditions, a so-called diathesis–stress model. In other words, there was a strong interaction whereby children who inherited a more difficult temperament (irritability, lower IQ, poor concentration, etc.) then fared much worse if they were brought up in a less-optimal environment. This then shows that higher con-genital risk do not necessarily condemn a child to poor outcomes; indeed, improving parenting may have larger effects with more vul-nerable children. Better parenting can also help mitigate congenital risk through attachment security. Bergman et al. [31] showed that mothers who had higher amniotic fluid cortisol levels had infants with poorer cognitive development at 17 months, but this effect disappeared if the infant was securely attached due to sensitive ma-ternal responding.

Some parents say, with pride, 'I bring up all my children in the same way, equally', rightly prizing fairness. But so long as one is fair, the evidence suggests that perhaps the statement should be 'I'm proud to bring up each of my children differently'. Longitudinal ob-servational studies suggest that children with different traits may need different parenting styles. Grazyna Kochanska [32] reported that, for temperamentally fearful children, gentle parental control was associated with optimal behavioural and emotional adjustment, whereas temperamentally more aggressive ('fearless') children required firmer control to achieve the same positive results, a finding that has been replicated for children with difficult/irritable temperaments, who do better given firmer control [33].

More recently, the possibility has been explored that rather than just confer liability to poorer outcomes under stressful rearing, some child traits may also confer liability to better outcomes under benign conditions, the so-called *differential susceptibility* hypothesis [34], whereby some children are relatively impermeable to their surroundings, whereas others are more sensitive. Experimentally, Scott and O'Connor [35] found in a RCT that antisocial children who were more emotionally dysregulated (tantrums, anger outbursts) showed a greater response to improved parenting than those who were disobedient in a more controlled way. However, while differential susceptibility is an exciting theory, more replication of findings is necessary to determine the scope and size of its impact.

These results have implications for parenting programmes. Firstly, intervention effects are likely to vary according to child traits, for example children with autistic traits may change less, whereas those with irritable temperaments may change more. Secondly, parenting programmes should not follow a 'one-size-fits-all' rigid approach, but rather the content should be varied according to child characteristics. It was previously believed that an exception to the pattern of child characteristics moderating the effect of parenting quality was attachment security, as this represents the imprint and experience of the child at the hands of their parents. Certainly, twin studies of infants find similar rates in monozygotic and dizygotic twins, suggesting all the variation is owing to environmental influences [36]. However, recent studies in adolescence show that heritable traits account for 40% of the variance in attachment security [37]. It makes sense that some children will be more likely through their natures to continue to trust their parents, whereas others may be more likely to reject them.

Individual genes

In a seminal paper, Caspi et al. [38] found that a variant of a gene coding for the enzyme regulating the level of the central nervous system neurotransmitter monoamine oxidase conferred worse antisocial outcomes in the presence of harsh parenting. The effect has been confirmed in meta-analyses, although it is small. Furthermore, studies are now emerging that identify genotypes that confer differential susceptibility to interventions. However, the field is beset by failure to replicate findings and, if found, authors should demonstrate the specific mechanism of action through which such genes exert their influence.

Interventions

Aims and scope of increasing parenting skills

There are many interventions to improve parenting skills, but those with a strong evidence base go through a systematized curriculum with parents, and are usually referred to as parenting programmes. These typically aim to improve child symptoms, as well as improving the quality of the relationship, but this is not inevitable. Thus, where neglectful or abusive parenting has been uncovered, the goal may be to improve positive parental engagement with the child and reduce harsh emotional and physical practices, whether or not the child

is displaying behavioural or emotional problems. And where there are child problems, parenting programmes may help whether or not suboptimal parenting has contributed to causing the problem. Thus, programmes can help parents to better manage children with problems that are mainly genetically influenced (and so not 'the parent's fault'), such as autism, or children with, say, obsessive–compulsive disorder, even though the quality of parenting is perfectly acceptable at the outset.

Furthermore, where there are child symptoms and parenting is less than optimal, this does not necessarily mean that the parenting caused the child's problems. Parent–child relationships are bi-directional, and more difficult child behaviour can elicit harsher parenting. Several lines of evidence show this, from the classic experiment where parents with relatively well-behaved children were asked to look after children with behavioural problems and became harsher and more critical [39], to experiments showing that where disruptive child behaviour such as ADHD is reduced by medication, parenting quality improves [40]. Two areas of child functioning where parenting has been strongly implicated as causing difficulties are antisocial behaviour (conduct problems) and insecure attachment; these will now be addressed.

Difference between programmes to increase parenting skills and other work with parents

A parenting programme is a particular type of intervention designed to improve the overall quality of parenting that a child receives. Parenting programmes aim to help the way mothers and fathers relate to their child primarily by changing their moment-to-moment interchanges throughout the day, although they also address wider issues such as parental beliefs and feelings. Change is achieved through the training of specific skills such as collaborative play, selective attention, and praise to promote sociable behaviour, and then usually moving onto clear rules backed by consistently applied consequences to reduce misbehaviour. There is a structured sequence of sessions that builds up each of the skills. This approach to intervention is distinct from counselling, where the emphasis is usually on understanding the parent's views and giving them non-directive general support but not increasing their skill level; it is more intensive than psycho-education, where a parent is informed about the nature of the child's problem and given advice on how to manage it but not trained in specific techniques. In family therapy, the therapist typically engages the whole family system, often with a primary emphasis on a deeper understanding of interpersonal processes and meanings; it is the change in understanding, rather than skills, that is postulated to lead to changes in relationships. In contrast, parenting programmes aim to change parenting behaviour directly in the here and now.

The most successful programmes are derived from social learning theory. Characteristics of some of the more widely used programmes are given in Table 40.1, the basic content of a typical programme in Box 40.1, and advantages and disadvantages of group-based versus individual format in Table 40.2.

Programmes to increase parenting skills for children with antisocial behaviour

Effectiveness

Programmes based on social learning theory have continued to develop over the last half-century and there is a larger evidence

Table 40.1 Some evidence-based programmes for increasing parenting skills

Name	Target population	Levels and delivery modes	Evidence	Comments, website, dissemination
Incredible Years	A suite of parent group programmes from babyhood to age 12, including four specific problems such as autism	Universal: 6 weeks Indicated prevention: 14 weeks Treatment: 18–24 weeks	50 RCTs, 10 by developer, 40 independent replications confirm effects	Developer: Carolyn Webster-Stratton. One of the most intensive programmes in clinical process and supervision www.incredibleyears.com
Triple P	A range of programmes at all levels and ages, including ones for special groups such as children with developmental delays	Universal: Online; broadcast media Selective: short one-off sessions up to 4 weeks Indicated: 6–8 weeks More intensive: including specific issues such as parental depression or into parental discord	Over 70 RCTs by developer; some independent replications, a few of which failed to show effects	Developer: Matt Sanders, Comprehensive range of levels; www.triplep.net
Parent–Child Interaction Therapy	Child disruptive behaviour and parenting difficulties, including maltreatment	Parent/child dyad is live coached by therapist over 12–20 sessions.	Several RCTs by developer and independent evaluators show good effects	Developed by Sheila Eyberg, www.pcit.org
Parent Management Training Oregon	Behavioural problems 4–12 years; parents with mental health problems or separating	Individual programme: 19–30 sessions, group 14 sessions	RCTs by programme developer and independents show effects	Developer: Marion Forgatch www.generationpmto.org
Strengthening Families (10–14)	Universal preventive programme for age 10–14 years	Seven 2-hour sessions. which include whole family and separate parent and child groups	Two RCTs by programme developer show some effects	Developer: K. Kumpfer. well developed across many countries https://www.strengtheningfamiliesprogram.org
Nurse Family Partnership	Preventive for young, disadvantaged first-time mothers	Trained nurses home visit mother during pregnancy and first 24 months of child's life	Three RCTs in USA have shown varied and long-lasting effects, but one in UK failed to show any impact	Developer: David Olds www.nursefamilypartnership.org

RCT: randomized controlled trial.

base for this intervention than any other in child mental health. The meta-analysis by the National Institute for Health and Care Excellence (NICE) [41] of 54 RCTs of parenting programmes for indicated prevention or treatment of conduct problems/disorders in 4150 children aged 3–10 years against any control (43 studies vs waiting list or no treatment controls, 11 vs management as usual) found a moderate effect size of 0.54 standard deviations (SD) on parent-rated outcomes, 0.40 SD by independent observation, and 0.69 SD by independent researcher evaluation. Follow-up 1 year later showed persistent effects but a halving of their magnitude. Interestingly, there was no generalization to the school setting—overall, for all programmes, teacher ratings showed no change. No adverse effects or harms were recorded. However, it may be that modest changes in teacher-rated behaviour occur with some more intensive programmes—for example, a recent meta-analysis [42] of 50 trials of Incredible Years found a small but significant effect on classroom behaviour (0.13 SD). Similar findings for parent-reported outcomes were reported in other meta-analyses, for example by the Cochrane Collaboration [43]. The latter also analysed impacts on parental mental health, and found it improved by 0.36 SD. Positive parenting and harsh practices improved, assessed by both parent report and independent observation.

It is not clear how sustainable the effects are in the long term: many trials have used waiting list control groups that are offered the intervention 6 months later. As a result, very few long-term randomized comparisons can be made (e.g. [44, 45]). A small number of trials based on selective prevention samples have retained their randomized control group and have shown good long-term outcomes [46]. A 7– 10-year follow-up by Scott et al. [47] found that, for the more severely affected cases, there were enduring effects, including prevention of emerging antisocial personality disorder traits, but a community sample with milder conduct problems showed no longer-term gains, having reverted to the mean. Perhaps the most famous preventive intervention for conduct problems was carried out by the Conduct Problems Prevention Research Group. However, despite a very intensive intervention with both parenting and also teacher classroom management skills over several years, in early adulthood the sample as a whole (the most antisocial 10% of children in school classes when they were young) showed no effects. Post hoc subgroup analysis did indicate that the more severely antisocial group enjoyed lasting benefits [48], a finding that would appear to be in keeping with that of Scott et al. [47]. In summary, there is convincing evidence that parenting programmes substantially improve parenting practices, parental mental health, and child antisocial behaviour, and, importantly, that behaviour change is seen both by parent report and independent observations. The evidence for longer-term effects requires more studies.

Box 40.1 Session content in a social learning programme

Part 1: Inculcating a child-centred approach

Play is usually covered in depth during the first 2–3 sessions. Instead of giving directions, teaching, and asking questions during play, parents are directed to give a running commentary on their child's actions and let the child choose the activity. Parents are asked to practice these techniques for 10 minutes every day.

Part 2: Increasing acceptable child behaviour

Praise and rewards. The parent is asked to praise their child for lots of simple, desirable everyday behaviours such as playing quietly on their own, eating nicely, getting dressed the first time they are asked, and so on. Later sessions go through the use of reward charts.

Part 3: Giving explicit instructions

Clear commands. Parents are taught to reduce the number of directions but to make them much more authoritative. The manner should be forceful (not sitting down, timidly requesting from the other end of the room; instead, standing over the child, fixing him or her in the eye, and in a clear firm voice giving the command). Directions should specify what the parent *does* want the child to do, not as what the child should *stop* doing ('please speak quietly' rather than 'stop shouting').

Part 4: Strategies to cut down inappropriate child behaviour

Consequences for unacceptable behaviour should be applied within seconds of the undesirable act. They must always be followed through. Simple logical consequences are encouraged: if water is splashed out of the bath, the bath will end; if a child refuses to eat dinner, there will be no pudding, etc.

Ignoring This sounds easy but is a hard skill to teach parents. Whining, arguing, swearing, and tantrums are not dangerous and can usually safely be ignored. The technique is very effective.

Time out from positive reinforcement remains the final 'big one' as a sanction for unacceptable behaviour. The child is put in some boring place for a previously agreed reason (hitting, breaking things, etc.—not minor infringements) for a short time (say, 5 minutes). However, the child must be quiet for the last minute. It is a much more gentle and effective alternative than smacking or demeaning the child.

Comparison with less systematized counselling approach programmes

There have been rather few head-to-head comparisons of social learning theory parenting programmes with non-behavioural, humanistic approaches. For children with severe conduct problems, the classic paper by Bank et al. [49] found that behavioural parent management training was effective, whereas usual family therapy was ineffective on objective measures, despite favourable reports from parents. Most other studies have found that the humanistic approach usually had no effect, whereas the more behavioural programmes changed child outcomes. A trial of a parenting programme based on primarily on emotional communication (the Parenting Puzzle) for mild-to-moderate antisocial behaviour found no effects [50]. Thus, for child behaviour problems, programmes with a practical slant and strong focus on parental behaviour change are more effective.

Programmes to increase parenting skills with infants

Most programmes for infants are based on attachment theory and in the last 30 years or so, several interventions have been developed and validated. The more effective interventions for infants typically last 8–20 sessions and videotape parent–infant interactions and then replay them to the parent. The great strength of this approach is that (i) it allows parents to get an accurate picture of what is actually happening (rather than just talking about their perception of their relationship with their infant, as in traditional parent–infant psychotherapies); (ii) it enables them to see for themselves that when they change their behaviour, this impacts on their infant; (iii) it allows simultaneous exploration of the mother's mental state, so that mental blocks to more sensitive responding can be explored and often overcome. The Leiden group has tested video feedback programmes in RCTs [51].

A good example of a video feedback intervention is the Attachment and Bio-behavioural Catch-up programme [52]. It targets three issues known to affect children's attachment and self-regulation. Firstly, parents are helped to behave in nurturing ways when children are distressed. Secondly, similarly to social learning approaches, parents are helped to follow children's lead, to enable children to better regulate their emotions. Thirdly, parents are helped to reduce frightening behaviour as it is associated with disorganized attachment. These issues are targeted through 10 sessions implemented in families' homes with parents and children present.

Some interventions for infants do not use video feedback. They include more lengthy and intensive psychodynamic ones, for example Slade et al. [53]. David Olds [54], in contrast, developed a home visiting programme delivered by nurses (Nurse Family Partnership), based not on attachment theory, but on systematic evaluation of, and evidence-based interventions for, risk factors from pregnancy to 2 years of age. Thus, parents are encouraged to reduce smoking and alcohol in pregnancy through understanding the effects on their babies; once the baby is born, parent–child interaction is coached, including how to stimulate the baby appropriately, and wider issues such as partner violence and general education for the mother are addressed.

Effectiveness

The meta-analysis by Bakermans-Kranenburg et al. [55] found 81 studies, with over 7000 parent–infant pairs its findings were confirmed in an even-larger meta-analysis by Mountain et al. [56]. Overall, the interventions improved parental sensitivity by 0.33 SD and attachment security by 0.20 SD. The most effective interventions were relatively short (< 26 sessions) and started later (after the infant was 6 months). Both of these finding go against cherished notions that early intervention must be better, and that more effort should lead to more change (mean effect size for long interventions was –0.03). An RCT of the 'ABC' (Attachment and Biobehavioral Catch-up) intervention showed that as well as enhancing child attachment security, it improved diurnal cortisol production, executive functioning, and emotional regulation [52].

For programmes for infants that do not rely on attachment theory, those that focus on specified risk factors seem to fare better. Thus, the Nurse–Family Partnership approach has been evaluated in three RCTs involving over 1000 mother–infant pairs. This has shown benefits for the child in terms of improved cognitive and emotional

Table 40.2 Some advantages and disadvantages of delivering parenting skills interventions individually or in groups

Individual	Group
Case selection	
Can take on special cases unsuitable for groups: shy parents; failed group parenting programmes; high-risk/abusive parents	Can take on a variety of cases, can be hard to stop some parents falling behind
Intensity of work	
Therapist can go into greater depth of skills that need to be taught	Less detailed owing to time constraints and exposure to other parents
Can observe parent interacting with child and pick up styles they are unaware of	Restricted to parents' accounts of what goes on with the child
Can adapt the programme for particular child needs, e.g. attachment problems, autistic tendencies, learning disabilities, ADHD, etc.	
Flexibility	
Flexible order of delivery of programme, e.g. time out can be given early	Fixed order, e.g. limit-setting and time out have to wait until end
Flexible timing to attend to suit parent	Groups held at a fixed time when parent may be busy
Can easily be delivered in the home context	Parents have to come to clinic or community venue
No need to set up a crèche for child	May need to set up a crèche
Support from other parents	
No support from other parents	Other parents can provide validation for their efforts; normalize having a child with problems; enable parents to learn from and support each other
Therapist competence required	
Can work as a solo therapist	Requires a second group leader plus group-management skills
Duration and cost-effectiveness	
Typical programme takes around eight sessions, more complex 10–12	Triple P level 4 has four group sessions plus four telephone sessions; IY minimum 14 sessions, 18–22 recommended for clinical cases
Cost will vary, typically £2000/€2200/$2500	Costs typically lower per case: £1200/€1350/$1800

ADHD: attention deficit hyperactivity disorder; IY: Incredible Years.

development and fewer accidents and injuries, and for the mothers in terms of less harmful health behaviours (e.g. smoking) and higher take up of further education, less use of public handouts, and a longer interval until subsequent pregnancy [54]. However, a word of caution is in order, as a thoroughly carried out UK replication study found no effects [57]. This may be because treatment as usual is less good in poor parts of the USA. Nonetheless, specific skills programmes outperform interventions that draw upon a more general notion that if the parents are supported, then they, in turn, will relate better to their infants. For example, in a trial of a home visiting programme with 97 hours of face-to-face contact with mothers, none of the many mother or child variables measured changed [58]; a similar lack of effectiveness was found for the Oxfordshire Home Visiting project [59].

Parenting skills programmes for other conditions and contexts
Other childhood disorders
Depression, anxiety, and other emotional problems
Evidence supporting a link between quality of parent–child relationships and depression, anxiety and other emotional

problems (e.g. somatic complaints, social withdrawal) is clear, although smaller than that found for disruptive outcomes [60, 61]. Low warmth and conflict are both linked with depression and anxiety; however, the influence of control strategies is generally much weaker. Additionally, emotional symptoms in children are linked with overprotectiveness (e.g. [60]). The elements of parenting programmes aimed primarily at conduct problems are likely to be helpful for children showing emotional symptoms, but, generally, an individual-based intervention should probably be added, although Cartwright-Hatton et al. [62] tested the effects of a group-based parenting programme for diagnosed clinically anxious children (aged 3–9 years) and found strong effects on reducing anxiety disorders. The majority of sessions focused on components of traditional social learning theory-based parent management skills (e.g. child-centred play, rewards, limit-setting), with about one-third of the sessions focusing on components specifically aimed at dealing with anxious children (e.g. anxiety education; fear hierarchies). Importantly, parenting skills programmes can also help *parental* depression [63, 64].

ADHD
A number of parenting programmes designed for conduct problems have also shown improvements in ADHD symptoms [65–69]. Additionally, parenting interventions have been developed and

specifically for children with ADHD, for example The New Forest programme in the UK, which showed good effects on ADHD symptoms in preschoolers in a clinic-based trial but not in routine services [70]. Recent systematic reviews conclude that behavioural parenting interventions are effective for younger children with ADHD, more so than methylphenidate [65], and are probably effective for older children [71]. European and UK guidelines both recommend parenting programmes as the first-line treatment for ADHD [41]. However, Sonuga-Barke et al. [72] found that while effects were good on parent report, they were negligible using direct observation.

Callous unemotional traits

Despite the common belief that children with conduct problems who also show callous unemotional traits are insensitive to parenting, and to parenting interventions, Waller et al. [73] found little evidence to support this belief, either from longitudinal studies or from randomized trials. Nevertheless, specific programmes are being developed for them [74].

Autism spectrum disorders

Reflecting the point made ahead that conditions that are principally genetic can nonetheless be modified by improving the environment, recent research has shown that in autism, intense work improving parent–child interaction can improve core features of autism in the long term [75], as well as the common disruptive behaviour that is associated with it [76].

Specific parental issues and contexts

Involving fathers in parenting skills interventions

Most literature refers to 'parenting skills' as if it makes no difference whether fathers or mothers are involved. While in the great majority of cultures it is more often mothers who spend the most time looking after younger children, fathers do have a particular role, which often increases as children become older [77]. When it comes to parenting interventions, it should not necessarily be assumed that evidence about effectiveness applies equally to mothers and fathers. In practice, however, it is mainly mothers who attend parenting programmes and participate in research evaluations. The under-representation of fathers in these interventions is perhaps surprising, given that in many countries their role now reflects greater equality of gender roles and increased sharing of parenting [78]. Furthermore, there is considerable research suggesting that the amount and quality of father involvement in parenting is beneficial to children's mental health and development, over and above the level of the mother's involvement [77, 79]. A systematic review by Lundahl et al. [80] suggested that where intervention trials involve fathers, they produce stronger effects on child behaviour. Some interventions have been designed to engage couples and fathers, with improved outcomes when couples attend [81]. However, as it would be very difficult to randomize to one versus two parents attending (but see [82]), it is unclear if father attendance per se causes these changes or whether outcomes are better in families with two parents (as found by [83]), and in families where the couple relationship is healthier [81], so fathers are more likely to attend. Irrespective of trial data, it is highly desirable that interventions should involve both parents. Studies of fathers' views [84] suggest a number of barriers (and potential solutions), including time of day of the intervention, and that many interventions are run by women, who may find it easier to communicate with mothers than fathers. This effect can be pronounced in group-based interventions where fathers may feel out of place if they are in a minority.

Parents who abuse their children

There is some promising evidence that social learning theory-based programmes, with some adaptation and extension, can be effective for parents who maltreat their children [85]. For drug-misusing parents, the programme 'Parents under Pressure' has shown promising results [86]. For children in the foster care system, some trials suggest that parenting interventions aimed at foster carers can be effective in reducing problem behaviour in this often very troubled group of young people [87], although other trials have been more disappointing [88, 89], perhaps where the interventions have been less intensive.

Transportability of parenting skills programmes to different cultures and countries

Parenting programmes appear to transport well across cultures, despite different parenting norms and values. A systematic review of programmes developed in the USA and Australia found comparable effect sizes in recipient countries, including Europe and Asia [90]. Surprisingly perhaps, in many cases, 'imported' programmes were more effective in culturally very different settings (e.g. Hong Kong). These findings are consistent with studies of effects in ethnic minority groups within one country. For example, Reid et al. [13], in a large study of low-income families in the USA, found no ethnic differences in outcomes, engagement, or satisfaction across four ethnic groups, and Scott et al. [14] found a similar lack of ethnic differences in outcomes in London.

Given the high levels of international concern about youth crime and violence in developing countries [91], and the loss of children's developmental potential due to poverty and conflict, it is important to know if parenting programmes work in low-and middle-income countries (LAMICs). A recent systematic review [92] found promising evidence from randomized trials that parenting programmes can be effective in LAMICs for improving harsh parenting, and potentially for reducing conduct problems. Broader parenting interventions that also target early cognitive stimulation can be effective for improving parenting skills and children's developmental potential [93, 94]. The World Health Organization (WHO) [91] has begun an important initiative to develop, adapt, and test, via RCTs, programmes in LAMICs, where home-based parenting interventions have already shown good results for infants [92, 95]. There are many other examples of promising practice in developing countries, but very few have been tested in rigorous trials [92], as recommended by the WHO, and sustainability will be challenging.

'Family-peer links': What makes parenting programmes work?

Predictors and moderators of outcome

In a controlled trial, if a characteristic of the participants (e.g. child age or symptom severity) predicts outcome in both the intervention and control groups, then it is a predictor. If, however, there is an interaction with treatment so that one subgroup (say younger children) does better than another (older children) in the intervention group only, then the characteristic is operating as a moderator. Until recently, analyses have mainly been at the level of predictors only, with one or two exceptions. It is crucial that treatment and policy decisions are based on evidence from moderator, rather than predictor, analyses. Without these comparisons between intervention and control group, it is not possible to tell if a group that appears to benefit to a greater extent from treatment (e.g. girls or younger children), would not have done equally well untreated.

Child age and gender

Clinicians often gain the impression that boys and older children, especially adolescents, do worse, and Bank et al. [49] found a smaller effect size with adolescents than with younger children at the same institution. But meta-analyses of interventions for anti-social behaviour are mixed. For example, the Cochrane reviews of parenting interventions for antisocial behaviour found an effect size of 0.56 SD in teenagers [96], 0.53 SD in middle childhood [43], and 0.25 SD in early childhood [97], thus showing *smaller* effects in younger children. Within the middle childhood age range, Furlong et al. [43] found no effect of age on outcome. Teenagers may seem less tractable for a number of reasons. Firstly, many studies on adolescents include the most severe cases [98, 99]. Often, when severity is controlled for, there is no age effect—across a wide age range (2–16 years), Ruma et al. [100] found the adolescent group did slightly less well, but the difference disappeared after taking into account initial severity. Within prepubertal children, there also do not seem to be age effects when using direct observation [101, 102]. In contrast, the meta-analysis by Serketich and Dumas [103] found that across (not within) 36 studies ranging from 3 to 10 years in length effectiveness was *greater* in older children. In summary, it appears that age is not a clear determinant of outcome. Likewise, boys are as likely to improve as girls (e.g. see [102, 104]). There is, therefore, room for some optimism when treating adolescents.

Child psychopathology

The meta-analysis by Reyno and McGrath [105] found that more severe initial antisocial behaviour predicted (not moderated) *less* change, but this was a bivariate association with no controlling for other factors. In contrast, taking other factors into account, Stephen Scott [104] found the opposite, namely that higher initial levels of antisocial behaviour predicted more change. Most recent reviews and meta-analyses tend to concur. Although Furlong et al.'s [43] Cochrane review found no difference by conduct problem severity (coded at the trial level), Shelleby and Shaw's [106] narrative review, and meta-analyses by Lundahl et al. [107] and Leijten et al. [98], found larger effect sizes with higher initial severity. Future studies need to address this issue using multivariate statistics and larger pooled samples. Child ADHD predicts a less good response in some studies [104, 108] but not others [102, 109]. In the Multimodal Treatment Study of Children with ADHD (MTA) study, direct observations in the psychological treatment-only arm showed that parents had changed their behaviour, whereas child ADHD symptoms had not [110]. This suggests that it is the characteristics of the children with ADHD that make them less sensitive to change, rather than parents not implementing more effective parenting practices. In contrast, when studied, co-morbid anxiety appears to predict better treatment response [102]. A broad review by Ollendick et al. [109] concluded that for conduct problem interventions, co-morbidity did not affect outcomes.

Family factors

Demographic predictors of outcome such as single parenthood, lower maternal education, poverty, and larger family size have traditionally been found in meta-analyses to have a small but negative effect on outcomes [105, 107]. However, a recent systematic review [98] that controlled for confounders, especially initial child problem severity, found no diminished effects of parenting interventions in low socio-economic status families, consistent with moderator analyses in recent trials of more flexible interventions [83, 111].

Similarly, reviews have traditionally found that parental psychopathology, especially maternal depression, predicts worse outcomes, as do life events and harsher initial parenting practices [105]. However, Gardner et al. [112] found *larger* child improvement with depressed parents. For mothers with the most negative beliefs about their children, Moira Doolan [11] found no change in child behaviour at all. Overall, these conflicting subgroup findings from small trials suggest that the field would benefit from pooling individual patient-level data from multiple randomized trials [113].

Mediators of change

In recent years, researchers have begun to investigate what mediates outcome, as recommended by Michael Rutter [114]. To mediate treatment outcome, the treatment has to (i) change outcome; (ii) change the mediator; (iii) the mediator has to correlate with outcome; and (iv) the effect of treatment on outcome has to reduce or disappear after controlling for the mediator [115]. It would seem likely that for parenting programmes to change child behaviour, some aspect of parenting would first have to change. This is worth testing as it might not be the case—for example, the parenting programme could make a couple realize that they should say stop arguing in front of their child but still use the same disciplinary strategies.

Beauchaine et al. [102] and Tein et al. [116] found that changes in critical and ineffective parenting mediated child change in antisocial behaviour, whereas several studies have found that positive parenting mediated change [44, 111, 112]. Gardner et al. [45] tested competing mediators, finding that it was change in positive parenting skill, rather than confidence in parenting, that predicted change in child problem behaviour. In adolescents, Eddy and Chamberlain [117] found for parenting, quality of supervision and discipline, and a positive adult–youth relationship all mediated change, as did time spent with deviant peers and the degree of their influence. Taken together, these four factors accounted for a substantial 32% of variance in subsequent antisocial behaviour. Similarly, Huey et al. [118] in a trial of multi-systemic therapy for delinquency showed that a positive relationship and firm discipline mediated outcome, and good supervision mediated deviant peer association which, in turn, mediated subsequent antisocial behaviour. These studies indicate which variables need to change for a good outcome and have led to changes in programmes; for example, there is now a much stronger emphasis on preventing deviant peer association—the OSLC Treatment Fostercare programme penalizes young people for every minute they cannot verifiably account for their whereabouts.

Implementation and dissemination

Implementation

Most of the trials cited in the previous sections were carried using (i) specially recruited cases rather than clinical referrals; (ii) specially trained research therapists rather than regular clinicians; and (iii) university rather than clinical settings. Indeed, John Weisz's studies show that fewer than 5% of psychosocial child mental health trials meet all three 'real-life' criteria [119]. There is therefore considerable concern whether the good effects seen in trials will be replicated in everyday life; where cases have a high degree of co-morbid conditions, most therapists do not use evidence-based approaches and do not get skill-specific supervision. Trials that compared evidence-based approaches in real-life with usual services nonetheless obtained a clear advantage, by 0.3 SDs [119]. The challenge is therefore to disseminate best practice more widely and ensure that it is well implemented [120].

Therapist effects

Therapist performance can be divided into three elements, as follows. (i) The *alliance*, which includes how well client and therapist get on together and agree shared goals. A meta-analysis of youth studies of the alliance found it contributed, on average, an effect size of 0.21 SD to outcome [121]. (ii) *Fidelity* or adherence to specific components of a model that concerns the extent to which the therapist follows the actions prescribed in the manual. In a large, real-life study of the implementation of a family programme for antisocial young people, Sexton and Turner [122] found that therapists who were highly adherent to the model got good results, with a larger effect size on more severe cases, whereas low-adherent therapists actually got poorer results than the control group, implying that they might have done harm. (iii) The *skill* or competence with which the therapist carries out the tasks, that is, how well the therapist performs the actions. Skill can include aspects of the alliance and fidelity. Both Forgatch et al. [123] and Eames et al. [124] found that therapist skill significantly predicted change in independently observed parenting. In summary, there is good evidence that therapist variables make a crucial difference to parenting programmes for antisocial behaviour.

Dissemination

Although formal surveys are lacking in most countries, from the paucity of professionals trained in evidence-based programmes we can conclude that the vast majority of children with conduct problems or insecure attachment are not offered proven approaches. There are examples of initiatives to address this. Norway has set up a national training centre to roll out and support a portfolio of parenting programmes. In England, the National Academy for Parenting Practitioners was set up in 2007 and by 2010 had trained 4000 practitioners in a small number of carefully chosen evidence-based programmes, estimated to have benefited 150,000 children [125]. This was accompanied by a sizeable research programmeme and a detailed evaluation of over 100 parenting programmes, with the results posted on a searchable site for parents and commissioners (http://www.eif.org.uk/publication/commissioning-parenting-and-family-support-for-troubled-families/). For clinically referred cases, the Children and Young People's Increasing Access to Psychological Therapies (CYP-IAPT) initiative is training up to five staff from each local health authority in England in either parent training for conduct problems or cognitive–behavioral therapy for depression and anxiety. The training is intense, 3 days a week over a year, with close supervision of skills. A further element likely to lead to effectiveness is insistence on session-by-session outcome monitoring (https://www.england.nhs.uk/mental-health/cyp/iapt). More is now known about how to achieve successful dissemination, including training managers, as well as clinicians, educating both that regular supervision is necessary, and making the case for the cost-effectiveness of parenting programmes.

Prevention

In an ideal public health preventive strategy, all parents would learn effective parenting skills, which would help to improve parent–child relationships and child well-being, and reduce the population rate of harsh and abusive parents. There would be a tiered set of interventions available in primary and then in increasingly specialist levels of care, to help those with continuing difficulties. This vision has been well articulated by Matthew Sanders [126], and appropriate programmes developed by his group for each level. It is clear that we have good evidence for the effectiveness of parenting interventions for selective and indicated prevention and for treatment of conduct problems. However, it is less clear whether universal prevention parenting programmes work: there have been many successful trials and also many unsuccessful ones [50, 127]. Further studies need to understand under which conditions, and using which delivery mechanisms, universal parenting programmes can be helpful; if they are not, then the conclusion might be that targeted programmes are more useful.

Conclusions

Parenting programmes have developed considerably in recent years. Findings from scores of randomized trials present a positive view of their effectiveness, with widespread implementation in many countries. Recent moderator analyses suggest that for many groups seen as hard to treat, for reasons of social disadvantage or psychopathology, parenting interventions can improve child behaviour. For families with very complex needs, such as those in the child protection system, the evidence is promising. Future developments need to include evaluation of the long-term effects of programmes, and the mechanisms that mediate changes in parenting behaviour. As parenting programmes tend to have small effects on children's behaviour in school, further evidence on school-based programmes is needed. Finally, future studies need to investigate which families can improve with minimal intervention such as computer-based self-instruction.

References

1. Bandura A. *Social Learning Theory*. New York: General Learning Corporation, 1977.
2. Patterson G. *Coercive Family Process*. Eugene, OR: Castalia, 1982.
3. Scott S, Yule W. Behavioural therapies. In: Rutter M, Bishop D, Pine D, Scott S, Stevenson J, Taylor E, Thapar A (eds). *Rutter's Child and Adolescent Psychiatry*, 5th ed. Oxford: Blackwell, 2008, pp. 1009–1025.
4. Denham S, Workman E, Cole PM, Weissbrod C, Kendziora KT, Zahn-Waxler C. Prediction of externalizing behaviour problems from early to middle childhood: Role of parental socialization and emotion expression. *Dev Psychopathol* 2000; 12: 23–45.

5. Gardner F, Sonuga-Barke EJ, Sayal K. Parents anticipating misbehaviour: an observational study of strategies parents use to prevent conflict. *J Child Psychol Psychiatry* 1999; 40: 1185–1196.

6. Pettit G, Bates JE, Dodge KA, Meece DW. The impact of peer contact on adolescent externalizing problems is moderated by parental monitoring, perceived neighborhood safety, and prior adjustment. *Child Dev* 1999; 70: 768–778.

7. Racz SJ, McMahon RJ. The relationship between parental knowledge and monitoring and child conduct problems: 10 year update. *Clin Child Fam Psychol Rev* 2011; 14: 377–398.

8. Gardner F. Positive interaction between mothers and conduct-problem children: Is there training for harmony as well as fighting? *J Abnorm Child Psychol* 1987; 15: 283–293.

9. Scott S, Briskman J, Woolgar M, Humayun S, O'Connor TG. Attachment in adolescence: overlap with parenting and unique prediction of behavioural adjustment. *J Child Psychol Psychiatry* 2011; 52: 1052–1062

10. Snarr J, Slep AM, Grande VP. Validation of a new self-report measure of parental attributions. *Psychol Assess* 2009; 21: 390–401

11. Doolan M. *Mothers' Emotional Valence Representations of Children with Antisocial Behaviour and Their Role in Treatment Outcome.* PhD Thesis, King's College London, 2006.

12. Sanders MR, Pidgeon AM, Gravestock F, Connors MD, Brown S, Young RW. Does parental attributional retraining and anger management enhance the effects of the Triple P-Positive Parenting Programme? *Behav Ther* 2004; 35: 513–535.

13. Reid M, Webster-Stratton C, Beauchaine TP. Parent training in HeadStart: A comparison of response among African-American, Asian-American, Caucasian, and Hispanic mothers. *Prev Sci* 2001; 2: 209–227.

14. Scott S, O'Connor TG, Futh A, Matias C, Price J, Doolan M. Impact of a parenting programme in a high-risk, multi-ethnic community: The PALS trial. *J Child Psychol Psychiatry* 2010; 51: 1331–1341.

15. Bowlby J. *Attachment and Loss: Attachment.* New York: Basic, 1969/1982.

16. De Wolff, M., van IJzendoorn, M. Sensitivity and attachment: a meta-analysis. *Child Dev* 1997; 68: 571–591.

17. Sroufe A, Coffino B, Carlson EA. Conceptualising the role of early experience: lessons from the Minnesota longitudinal study. *Dev Rev* 2010; 30: 36–51.

18. Cyr C, Euser EM, Bakermans-Kranenburg MJ, Van Ijzendoorn MH. Attachment security and disorganization in maltreating and high-risk families: a series of meta-analyses. *Dev Psychopathol* 22: 87–108.

19. Fearon P, Bakermans-Kranenburg MJ, van Ijzendoorn MH, Lapsley AM, Roisman GI. Insecure attachment and disorganization in children's externalizing behaviour: a meta-analysis. *Child Dev* 2010; 81: 435–456.

20. Green J, Stanley C, Peters S. Disorganized attachment representation and atypical parenting in young school age children with externalizing disorder. *Attach Hum Dev* 2007; 9: 207–222.

21. Shmueli-Goetz Y, Target M, Fonagy P, Datta A. The Child Attachment Interview. *Dev Psychol* 2008; 44: 939–956.

22. Futh A, O'Connor TG, Matias C, Green J, Scott S. Attachment narratives and behavioural and emotional symptoms in an ethnically diverse, at-risk sample. *J Am Acad Child Adolesc Psychiatry* 2008; 47: 709–718.

23. Matias C, O'Connor TG, Futh A, Scott S. Observational attachment theory-based parenting measures predict children's attachment narratives. *Attach Hum Dev* 2013; 16: 77–92.

24. O'Connor T, Matias C, Futh A, Tantam G, Scott S. Social learning theory-based parenting intervention promotes attachment-based caregiving: results from a randomized trial. *J Clin Child Adolesc Psychol* 2013; 42: 358–420.

25. Rutter M, Azis Clausen C. Biology of environmental effects. In: Thapar A, Pine D, Leckman J, Scott S, Snowling M, Taylor E (eds). *Rutter's Child and Adolescent Psychiatry*, 6th ed. Oxford: Wiley Blackwell, 2015, pp. 287–302.

26. Danese A, McCrory E. Child maltreatment. In: Thapar A, Pine D, Leckman J, Scott S, Snowling M, Taylor E (eds). *Rutter's Child and Adolescent Psychiatry*, 6th ed. Oxford: Wiley Blackwell, 2015, pp. 365–375.

27. Provençal N, Suderman MJ, Guillemin C, et al. The signature of maternal rearing in the methylome in rhesus macaque prefrontal cortex and T cells. *J Neurosci* 2012; 32: 15626–15642

28. Meaney M. Epigenetics and the biology of gene × environment interactions. In: Tolan P, Leventhal B. *Gene-Environment Interactions in Developmental Psychopathology.* New York: Springer, 2017, pp. 59–94.

29. Fisher P, Gunnar MR, Dozier M, Bruce J, Pears KC. Effects of therapeutic interventions for foster children on behaviour, attachment, and stress regulatory systems. *Ann N Y Acad Sci* 2006; 1094: 215–225.

30. Bohman M. Predisposition to criminality: Swedish adoption studies in retrospect. In: Bock G, Goode J (eds). *Genetics of Criminal and Antisocial Behaviour.* Chichester: Wiley, 1996, pp. 99–114.

31. Bergman K, Sarkar P, Glover V, O'Connor TG. Maternal prenatal cortisol and infant cognitive development: moderation by infant-mother attachment. *Biol Psychiatry* 2010; 67: 1026–1032.

32. Kochanska G. Multiple pathways to conscience for children with different temperaments: from toddlerhood to age 5. *Dev Psychol* 1997; 33: 228–240.

33. Bates JE, Pettit GS, Dodge KA, Ridge B. Interaction of temperamental resistance-to-control and restrictive parenting in the development of externalizing behaviour. *Dev Psychol* 1998; 34: 982–995.

34. Ellis BJ, Boyce WT, Belsky J, Bakermans-Kranenburg MJ, van Ijzendoorn MH. Differential susceptibility to the environment: An evolutionary-neurodevelopmental theory. *Dev Psychopathol* 2011; 23: 7–28.

35. Scott S, O'Connor T. An experimental test of differential susceptibility to parenting among emotionally dysregulated children. *J Child Psychol Psychiatry* 2012; 53: 1184–1193.

36. O'Connor T, Croft C. A twin study of attachment in pre-school children. *Child Dev* 2011; 72: 1501–1511.

37. Fearon P, Shmueli-Goetz Y, Viding E, Fonagy P, Plomin R. Genetic and environmental influences on adolescent attachment. *J Child Psychol Psychiatry* 2014; 55: 1033–1047.

38. Caspi A, McClay J, Moffi TT, Poulton R. Evidence that the cycle of violence in maltreated children depends on genotype. *Science* 2002; 297: 851–854.

39. Anderson KE, Lytton H, Romney DM. Mothers' interactions with normal and conduct disordered boys: who affects whom? *Dev Psychol* 1986; 22: 604–609.

40. Schachar R, Taylor E, Wieselberg M, Thorley G, Rutter M. Changes in family functioning and relationships in children who respond to methylphenidate. *J Am Acad Child Adolesc Psychiatry* 1987; 26: 728–732.

41. National Institute for Health and Care Excellence. *Recognition, Intervention and Management of Antisocial Behaviour and Conduct Disorders in Children & Young People.* London: NICE, 2013.

42. Menting A, Orobio de Castro B, Matthys W. Effectiveness of Incredible Years parent training: meta-analysis. *Clin Psychol Rev* 2013; 33: 901–913.

43. Furlong M, McGilloway S, Bywater T, Hutchings J, Smith SM, Donnelly M. Behavioural/cognitive-behavioural group-based parenting interventions for children age 3-12 with early onset conduct problems. *Cochrane Database Syst Rev* 2012; 2: CD008225.

44. Bywater T, Hutchings J, Daley D, Whitaker C. Long-term effectiveness of the Incredible Years Parenting Programme. *Br J Psychiatry* 2009; 195: 1–7

45. Gardner F, Burton J, Klimes I. RCT of a parenting intervention in the voluntary sector for reducing child conduct problems. *J Child Psychol Psychiatry* 2006; 47: 1123–1132.

46. Forgatch M, Patterson GR, Degarmo DS, Beldavs ZG. Testing the Oregon delinquency model: 9-year follow up of the Oregon Divorce Study. *Dev Psychopathol* 2009; 21: 637–660.

47. Scott S, Briskman J, O'Connor T. Early prevention of antisocial personality: long-term follow-up of two randomized controlled trials comparing indicated and selective approaches *Am J Psychiatry* 2014; 171: 649–657.

48. Conduct Problems Prevention Research Group. The effects of the Fast Track preventive intervention on the development of conduct disorder across childhood. *Child Dev* 2011; 82: 331–345.

49. Bank L, Marlowe JH, Reid JB, Patterson GR, Weinrott MR. Comparative evaluation of parent-training interventions for families of chronic delinquents. *J Abnorm Child Psychol* 1991; 19: 15–33.

50. Simkiss D, Snooks HA, Stallard N, et al. Effectiveness and cost-effectiveness of a universal parenting skills programmeme in deprived communities: multicentre randomised controlled trial. *BMJ Open* 2013; 3: e002851.

51. Velderman M, Bakermans-Kranenburg MJ, Juffer F, Van Ijzendoorn MH, Mangelsdorf SC, Zevalkink J. Preventing preschool externalizing behaviour problems through video-feedback intervention in infancy. *Infant Mental Health Journal* 2006; 27: 466–493.

52. Dozier M, Roben CKP, Caron E, Hoye J, Bernard K. Attachment and biobehavioral catch-up: an evidence-based intervention for vulnerable infants and their families. *Psychother Res* 2016; 28: 18–29.

53. Slade A,Sadler LS, Mayes LC. et al. Minding the baby: enhancing parental reflective functioning in a nursing/mental health home visiting program. In: Berlin L, Ziv Y, Amaya-Jackson L, Greenberg M. l (eds). *Enhancing Early Attachment: Theory, Research, Intervention and Policy*. New York: Guilford, 2005, pp. 152–177.

54. Olds D. The nurse–family partnership: an evidence-based preventive intervention. *Infant Mental Health Journal* 2006; 27: 3–25.

55. Bakermans-Kranenburg MJ, van Ijzendoorn MH, Juffer F . Less is more: meta-analyses of sensitivity and attachment interventions in early childhood. *Psychol Bull* 2003; 129: 195–215.

56. Mountain G, Cahill J, Thorpe H. Sensitivity and attachment interventions in early childhood: a systematic review and meta-analysis. *Infant Behav Dev* 2017; 46: 14–32.

57. Robling M, Bekkers MJ, Bell K, et al. Effectiveness of a nurse-led intensive home-visitation programme for first-time teenage mothers (Building Blocks): a pragmatic randomised controlled trial. *Lancet* 2016; 387: 146–155.

58. Barnes J, MacPherson K, Senior R. The impact on parenting and the home environment of early support to mothers with new babies. *J Child Serv* 2006; 1: 4–20.

59. Barlow J,Davis H, McIntosh E, Jarrett P, Mockford C, Stewart-Brown S. Role of home visiting in improving parenting and health in families at risk of abuse and neglect: Results of a multicentre randomised trial and economic evaluation. *Arch Dis Child* 2007; 92: 229–233.

60. Dadds M, Barrett PM, Rapee RM, Ryan S. Family process, child anxiety and aggression: observational analysis. *J Abnorm Child Psychol* 1996; 24: 715–734.

61. Wood J, McLeod BD, Sigman M, Hwang W-C, Chu BC. Parenting and childhood anxiety. *J Child Psychol Psychiatry* 2003; 44: 134–151.

62. Cartwright-Hatton S, McNally D, Field AP, et al. A new parenting-based group intervention for young anxious children: RCT results. *J Am Acad Child Adolesc Psychiatry* 2011; 50: 242–251.

63. Barlow J, Smailagic N, Huband N, Roloff V, Bennett C. Group-based parenting programmes for improving parental psychosocial health. *Cochrane Systematic Reviews* 2012; 6: CD002020.

64. Hutchings J, Gardner F, Bywater T, et al. Parenting intervention in Sure Start services for children at risk of developing conduct disorder: pragmatic randomised trial. *BMJ* 2007; 334: 678–685.

65. Charach A, Carson P, Fox S, Ali MU, Beckett J, Lim CG. Interventions for preschool children at high risk for ADHD: Comparative effectiveness review. *Pediatrics* 2013; 131: e1584–e1604.

66. Jones K, Daley D, Hutchings J, Eames C. Efficacy of the Incredible Years basic parent training programmeme as an early intervention for children with conduct disorder and ADHD: long-term follow-up. *Child Care Health Dev* 2008; 34: 380–390.

67. Scott S, Spender Q, Doolan M, Jacobs B, Aspland H. Multicentre controlled trial of parenting groups for childhood antisocial behaviour in clinical practice. *BMJ* 2001; 323: 194–201.

68. Scott S, Sylva K, Doolan M, et al. Randomized controlled trial of parenting groups for child antisocial behaviour targeting multiple risk factors: the SPOKES project. *J Child Psychol Psychiatry* 2010; 51: 48–57.

69. Webster-Stratton C, Reid MJ, Beauchaine T. Combining parent and child training for young children with ADHD. *J Clin Child Adoles Psychol* 2011; 40: 191–203.

70. Sonuga-Barke EJ, et al. Parent-based therapies for preschool attention-deficit/hyperactivity disorder: a randomized, controlled trial with a community sample. *J Am Acad Child Adolesc Psychiatry* 2001; 40: 402–408.

71. Zwi M, Jones H, Thorgaard C, York A, Dennis JA. Parent training interventions for ADHD in children aged 5 to 18 years. *Cochrane Database Syst Rev* 2011; 12: CD003018.

72. Sonuga-Barke EJ, Brandeis D, Cortese S, et al. Non-pharmacological interventions for ADHD: systematic review and meta-analyses of randomized controlled trials of dietary and psychological treatments. *Am J Psychiatry,* 2013; 170: 275–289.

73. Waller R, Gardner F, Hyde LW. What are the associations between parenting, callous-unemotional traits, and antisocial behavior in Youth? A systematic review of evidence. *Clin Psychol Rev* 2013; 33: 593–608.

74. Dadds M, Allen JL, McGregor K, Woolgar M, Viding E, Scott S. Callous-unemotional traits in children and mechanisms of impaired eye contact: a treatment target? *J Child Psychol Psychiatry* 2013; 55: 771–780.

75. Pickles A, Le Couteur A, Leadbitter K, et al. Parent-mediated social communication therapy for young children with autism (PACT): long-term follow-up of a randomised controlled trial. *Lancet* 2016; 388: 2501–2509.

76. Scahill L, Bearss K, Lecavalier L, et al. Effect of parent training on adaptive behavior in children with autism spectrum disorder and disruptive behavior: results of a randomized trial. *J Am Acad Child Adolesc Psychiatry* 2016; 55: 602–609.

77. Lamb M. *The Role of the Father in Child Development*. New York: John Wiley, 2004.

78. Maughan B, Gardner F. Families and parenting. In: Smith D (ed.). *A New Response to Youth Crime*. New York: Willan, 2010, pp. 247–286.

79. Ramchandani P, Domoney J, Sethna V, Psychogiou L, Vlachos H, Murray L. Do early father–infant interactions predict onset of externalising behaviours in young children? Findings from a longitudinal cohort study. *J Child Psychol Psychiatry* 2013; 54: 56–64.

80. Lundahl B, Tollefson D, Risser H, Lovejoy MC. A meta-analysis of father involvement in parent training. *Res Soc Work Pract* 2008; 18: 97–108.

81. Cowan P, Cowan CP, Pruett MK, Pruett K, Wong JJ. Promoting fathers' engagement with children: preventive interventions for low income families. *J Marriage Fam* 2009; 71: 663–679.

82. Besnard T, Verlaan P, Vitaro F, Capuano F, Poulin F. Moms and dads count in a prevention programme for kindergarten children with behavioural problems. *Can J School Psychol* 2013; 28: 219–238.

83. Gardner F, Connell A, Trentacosta CJ, Shaw DS, Dishion TJ, Wilson MN. Moderators of outcome in a brief family-centred intervention for preventing early problem behaviour. *J Consult Clin Psychol* 2009; 77: 543–553.

84. Stahlschmidt M, Threlfall J, Seay KD, Lewis EM, Kohl PL . Recruiting fathers to parenting programmes: advice from dads and fatherhood programme providers. *Child Youth Serv Rev* 2013; 35: 1734–1741.

85. MacMillan H, Wathen C, Fergusson D Leventhal J, Taussig H. Interventions to prevent child maltreatment and associated impairment. *Lancet* 2009; 373: 250–66.

86. Dawe S, Harnett P. Reducing potential for child abuse among methadone-maintained parents: results from a randomized trial. *J Subst Abuse Treat* 2007; 32: 381–390.

87. Briskman J, Scott S. *Randomised Controlled Trial of Fostering Changes Parenting Groups for Fostered Children.* London: Department for Education, 2013.

88. Macdonald G, Turner W. An experiment in helping foster-carers manage challenging behaviour. *Br J Soc Work* 2005; 35: 1265–1282.

89. Turner W, Macdonald GM, Dennis JA. Behavioural and cognitive behavioural training interventions for assisting foster carers in the management of difficult behaviour. *Cochrane Database Syst Rev* 2007; 1: CD003760.

90. Gardner F, Montgomery P, Knerr W. Transporting evidence-based parenting programs for child problem behavior (age 3–10) between countries: systematic review and meta-analysis. *J Clin Child Adolesc Psychol* 2015; 53: 1–14.

91. World Health Organization (WHO). *Preventing Violence: Evaluating Outcomes of Parenting Interventions.* Geneva: WHO, 2013.

92. Knerr W, Gardner F, Cluver L. Improving positive parenting skills and reducing harsh and abusive parenting in low- and middle-income countries: a systematic review. *Prev Sci* 2013; 14: 352–363.

93. Rahman A, Iqbal Z, Roberts C, Husain N. Cluster randomized trial of a parent-based intervention to support early development of children in a low-income country. *Child Care Health Dev* 2009; 35: 56–62.

94. Engle P, Black MM, Behrman JR, et al. Child development in developing countries: strategies to avoid the loss of developmental potential in over 200 million children in the developing world. *Lancet* 2007; 369: 229–242.

95. Cooper P, Tomlinson M, Swartz L, et al. Improving quality of mother-infant relationship and infant attachment in South Africa: randomised trial. *BMJ* 2009; 338: b974.

96. Woolfenden S, Williams K, Peat J. Family and parenting interventions in children and adolescents with conduct disorder and delinquency aged 10-17. *Cochrane Database Syst Rev* 2001; 2: CD003015.

97. Barlow J, Smailagic N, Ferriter M, Bennett C, Jones H. Group-based parent-training programmes for improving emotional and behavioural adjustment in children from birth to three. *Cochrane Database Syst Rev* 17; 3: CD003680.

98. Leijten P, Raaijmakers MA, de Castro BO, Matthys W. Does socioeconomic status matter? A meta-analysis on parent training effectiveness for disruptive child behaviour. *J Clin Child Adolesc Psychol* 2013; 42: 384–392.

99. Lipsey M. Those confounded moderators in meta-analysis: Good, bad, and ugly. *Ann Am Acad Polit Soc Sci* 2003; 587: 69–81.

100. Ruma P, Burke RV, Thompson RW. Group parent training: is it effective for children of all ages? *Behav Ther* 1996; 27: 159–169.

101. Dishion T, Patterson G. Age effects in parent training outcome. *Behav Ther* 1992; 23: 719–729.

102. Beauchaine T, Webster-Stratton C, Reid MJ. Mediators, moderators and predictors of 1-year outcomes among children treated for early-onset problems. *J Consult Clin Psychol* 2005; 75: 371–388.

103. Serketich WJ, Dumas JE. The effectiveness of behavioral parent training to modify antisocial behavior in children: a meta-analysis. *J Behav Ther* 1996; 27: 171–186.

104. Scott S. Do parenting programmes for severe child antisocial behaviour work over the longer term, and for whom? 1 year follow up of a multi-centre controlled trial. *Behav Cogn Psychother* 2005; 33: 403–421.

105. Reyno SM, McGrath PJ. Predictors of parent training efficacy for child externalizing behaviour problems—a meta-analytic review. *J Child Psychol Psychiatry* 2006; 47: 99–111.

106. Shelleby E, Shaw D. Outcomes of parenting interventions for child conduct problems: a review of differential effectiveness. *Clin Child Fam Psychol Rev* 45: 628–645.

107. Lundahl B, Risser HJ, Lovejoy MC. A meta-analysis of parent training: moderators and follow-up effects. *Clin Psychol Rev* 2006; 26: 86–104.

108. MTA Cooperative Group. A 14-month RCT of treatment strategies for ADHD: Multimodal Treatment Study of Children with ADHD. *Arch Gen Psychiatry* 1999; 56: 1073–1086.

109. Ollendick TH, Jarrett MA, Grills-Taquechel AE, Hovey LD, Wolff JC. Comorbidity as a predictor and moderator of treatment outcome in youth with anxiety, affective, ADHD, and ODD/CD. *Clin Psychol Rev* 2008; 28: 1447–1471.

110. Wells K, Chi TC, Hinshaw SP, et al. Treatment related changes in objectively measured parent behaviours in the multimodal treatment study of ADHD children. *J Consult Clin Psychol* 2006; 74: 649–657.

111. Dishion T, Shaw D, Connell A, Gardner F, Weaver C, Wilson M. The family check-up: preventing problem behaviour by increasing parents' positive behaviour support. *Child Dev* 2008; 79: 1395–1414.

112. Gardner F, Hutchings J, Bywater T, Whitaker C. Who benefits and how does it work? Moderators and mediators of outcome in an effectiveness trial of a parenting intervention. *J Clin Child Adolesc Psychol* 2010; 39: 568–580.

113. Brown CH, Sloboda Z, Faggiano F, et al. Methods for synthesizing findings on moderation effects across multiple randomized trials. *Prev Sci* 2013; 13: 144–156.

114. Rutter M. Environmentally mediated risks for psychopathology: research strategies and findings. *J Am Acad Child Adolesc Psychiatry* 2005; 44: 3–18.

115. Kraemer H, Wilson GT, Fairburn CG, Agras WS. Mediators and moderators of treatment effects. *Arch Gen Psychiatry* 2002; 59: 877–883.

116. Tein J-Y, Sandler IN, MacKinnon DP, Wolchik SA. Mediation in the context of a moderated prevention effect for children of divorce. *J Consult Clin Psychol* 2004; 72: 617–624.

117. Eddy M, Chamberlain, P. Family management and deviant peer association as mediators of the impact of treatment on youth antisocial behaviour. *J Consult Clin Psychol* 2000; 68: 857–863.

118. Huey SJ, Jr, Henggeler SW, Brondino MJ, Pickrel SG. Mechanisms of change in MST: Reducing delinquent behaviour through therapist adherence and improved family and peer functioning. *J Consult Clin Psychol* 2000; 68: 451–467.

119. Weisz JR, Ng MY, Lau N. Psychological interventions: overview and critical issues for the field. In: Thapar A, Pine D, Leckman J, Scott S, Snowling M, Taylor E (eds). *Rutter's Child and Adolescent Psychiatry*, 6th ed. Oxford: Wiley Blackwell, 2015, pp. 463–482.

120. Fixsen D, Blase KA, Van Dyke MK. Mobilizing communities for implementing evidence based youth violence prevention. *Am J Commun Psychol* 2011; 48: 133–137.

121. Shirk SR, Karver M. Prediction of treatment outcome from relationship variables in child and adolescent therapy: a meta-analytic review. *J Consult Clin Psychol* 2003; 71: 452–464.

122. Sexton T, Turner C. The effectiveness of functional family therapy for youth with behavioural problems. *J Fam Psychol* 2011; 24: 339–348.

123. Forgatch M, Patterson GR, DeGarmo DS, et al. Evaluating fidelity: Predictive validity for a measure of competent adherence to the Oregon model of parent training. *Behav Ther* 2005; 36: 3–13.

124. Eames C, Daley D, Hutchings J, et al. Treatment fidelity as a predictor of behaviour change in parents attending group-based parent-training. *Child Care Health Dev* 2009; 35: 603–612.

125. Scott S. National dissemination of effective parenting programmes to improve child outcomes. *Br J Psychiatry* 2010; 196: 1–3.

126. Sanders M. Triple P-Positive Parenting Programme. *Clin Child Fam Psychol Rev* 1999; 2: 71–90.

127. Malti T, Ribeaud D, Eisner MP. Effectiveness of two universal preventive interventions in reducing children's externalizing behaviour: cluster randomized trial. *J Clin Child Adolesc Psychol* 2011; 40: 677–692

CHAPTER 41

Pregnancy
The earliest opportunity for prevention and early intervention for mental disorders

Philip Boyce, Megan Galbally, and Alain Gregoire

Introduction

The provision of good antenatal care and improved obstetric practice has had a major impact on improving the health outcomes for women and their infants, with lowered maternal and infant mortality. While there have been significant gains in physical health, we still have a long way to go in improving the mental health outcomes of women and their infants. We must pay more attention to the mental health of women during pregnancy, promptly identifying new mental health problems, preventing relapse of pre-existing conditions, and ensuring an optimal environment for fetal and baby development.

Women are in frequent contact with health professionals during pregnancy, providing an ideal opportunity for public health interventions that will benefit the women and, of critical importance, her child. Universal interventions, to reduce the risk of the fetus developing a psychotic disorder in later life can be applied. Reducing morbidity in the mother through targeted interventions has the potential to benefit the woman, as well as optimizing fetal development and reducing the risk of her infant developing later mental health problems. Risk factors for maternal mental illness can be identified and potentially mitigated. For women with a pre-existing disorder, particularly bipolar disorder, interventions can be applied during pregnancy to prevent relapse.

Good antenatal care is essential to good obstetric outcomes, which have been identified as risk factors for the subsequent development of schizophrenia in the offspring [1]. Whether this is causal, or the results of neurodevelopmental problems in the infant, remains unknown. Women with severe mental illness are a group at high risk of poor obstetric outcomes and therefore require particular attention in their antenatal care. This will benefit their mental health and the physical and mental health of their infants, but they often delay antenatal care or feel stigmatized in antenatal clinics. Educating such women about the benefits of antenatal care, and educating professionals on how to best provide care for this high-risk group are essential components of good maternity care.

There are a number of social risk factors during pregnancy that increase the risk of postnatal depression. These include social disadvantage, poor social support, domestic violence, and having experienced childhood adversity or abuse. While some of these risk factors could be modified by targeted interventions, the best way to provide some form of universal intervention would be through changes in social policy, in particular trying to overcome inequality [2], and reduce social disadvantage. Low- and middle-income countries have significantly higher rates of postnatal depression [3], which could be modified, in part, through access to good antenatal care and appropriate support, but can only be fundamentally changed through reducing disadvantage.

Mental illness and psychological distress during pregnancy, in addition to causing significant distress and disability to women, can contribute to adverse pregnancy outcomes [4], have an impact on the developing fetus [5], and the woman's attachment to the fetus, all of which can lead to mental health problems later in life.

Maintaining maternal well-being as a primary prevention strategy

Ensuring women have a healthy diet, coupled with provision of adequate levels of micronutrients (folate, vitamin D, iron, and possibly choline), protecting them against developing viral infections and ceasing smoking are simple universal interventions that may help to reduce the risk of their offspring developing a psychotic disorder.

Schizophrenia [6] and, to an extent, bipolar disorder [7], are, in part, neurodevelopmental in origin. It is therefore worthwhile examining whether there are any potentially reversible extrinsic, pregnancy-related factors (i.e. non-genetic) that could increase the risk for subsequent development of schizophrenia and bipolar disorder. Epidemiological studies have identified three areas that might prove potentially modifiable: (i) deficiencies in micronutrients that are essential for neurodevelopment; (ii) maternal viral infections; and (iii) exposure of the developing fetus to 'toxins', in particular nicotine and alcohol.

There are three lines of evidence that suggest micronutrient deficiency could increase the risk for subsequent psychosis. Firstly, the findings from studies on famine; secondly, findings from the observations regarding season of birth leading to low vitamin D levels; and, finally, the effect of micronutrient supplementation.

The Dutch famine in 1944–45 provided a tragic, but natural, experiment to examine the consequences of famine and fetal development [8, 9]. During the famine, the result of an embargo on transport imposed by the Nazi-occupying force, daily rations yielded fewer than 1000 kcal and malnutrition was the most common cause of death. The birth cohort, conceived during the famine (exposed to the famine in the first trimester of pregnancy), was found to have high rates of congenital abnormalities, such as spina bifida, hydrocephalus, and cerebral palsy. These observations lead to folate supplements being used to prevent neural tube defects. The other critical finding was that there was a significantly increased risk of schizophrenia among this cohort. These findings have been replicated in another 'natural experiment' following the Chinese famine on 1959–1961, again with a twofold increased risk of developing schizophrenia among the offspring of women exposed to the famine while pregnant [10, 11].

Some affective disorders may also have neurodevelopmental origins [7] and higher rates of 'severe affective disorders that required hospitalization' were found among the Dutch famine cohort; however, here the increased risk was to those exposed to famine in the second, and, more significantly, the third trimester of pregnancy [12, 13].

The mechanism whereby famine increases the risk for the development of schizophrenia and affective disorders is, most likely, the result of micronutrient deficiency [14], in particular vitamin D, folic acid, and iron.

Maternal vitamin D deficiency as a possible mechanism for increased risk for developing schizophrenia comes from the intriguing, and consistent, observation that individuals born in winter or spring have an increased risk of developing schizophrenia [15, 16]. This effect increases with distance from the equator [17], suggesting that this seasonal effect is the consequence of the reduced vitamin D levels resulting from reduced sunlight exposure in the latter stages of pregnancy, although a number of explanations have been posited for this observation, including ambient temperature, humidity, and maternal infections [18]. Support for low vitamin D levels comes from a case–control cohort study in which levels of neonatal 25-hydroxyvitamin D (25(OH)D) levels were measured [16]. There was a twofold increased risk of schizophrenia among those neonates with the lowest levels of vitamin D (although the neonates with the highest levels of 25(OH)D also had an increased risk).

Choline is essential for neurodevelopment and deficits have been considered a risk factor for schizophrenia [19]. Ross et al. [19] conducted a randomized placebo-controlled trial of choline (as phosphatidylcholine) supplementation of 100 women in the second trimester of pregnancy and the infants were assessed 5 weeks postpartum. The infants whose mothers had received choline supplementation were more likely to have normal cerebral inhibition, as measured by the auditory P50 cerebral-evoked response, a marker of developmental risk for schizophrenia, and at the 40-month follow-up they had fewer attention and social withdrawal problems [20].

While famine is an uncommon occurrence, malnutrition is not uncommon worldwide, especially among low- to middle-income countries [21], conflict zones, and among refugees. The immediate critical issues among women in such situations are survival and reduction of infant mortality, but attempting to ensure pregnant women are able to get access to adequate nutrition with sufficient micronutrients may go some way to reducing morbidity in their already disadvantaged offspring, and these may be the populations in whom the most gains of this type can be made, as well as those least likely to get good care, if they develop problems.

The general quality of maternal diet is also important for healthy fetal development and subsequent child well-being, including mental health. Jacka et al. [22] found that an unhealthy maternal diet was weakly, but significantly, associated with more externalizing and internalizing problems in their offspring (early markers of subsequent mental health problems) at 18 months old and 3 and 5 years old, independent of all confounding factors examined. Women should be encouraged to have a healthy diet and avoid, to some degree, highly processed foods, 'junk' food, excessive salt, and refined sugars.

Higher rates of schizophrenia have been reported in the offspring of women who were affected by flu in the second trimester of their pregnancy during the 1957 Asian flu epidemic [23, 24]. While this has been a contentious finding because of difficulties of replication, serological evidence found a sevenfold increased risk for schizophrenia for infants exposed to influenza in the first trimester of pregnancy [25] and for affective disorders when exposed in the third trimester [26]. Other infections have been found to increase the risk of schizophrenia, including *Toxoplasma gondii* and possibly herpes simplex type 2 virus [27].

The harmful effects of maternal smoking on obstetric outcomes, and fetal development, as well as effects on the childhood behavioural problems, are well recognized [28, 29]. There is also an increased risk for schizophrenia [30] and bipolar disorder [31] in the offspring of women who smoke during pregnancy, highlighting the pressing need to encourage women to stop smoking while pregnant. The harmful effects of alcohol consumption are also widely recognized [32], and while not being a risk factor for psychotic disorders, led to 'fetal alcohol syndrome', emphasizing the importance modifying alcohol consumption during pregnancy.

Impact of depressive symptoms on the developing fetus

The link between maternal depression in pregnancy and the subsequent child outcomes allows the development of models for prevention and early intervention that benefit both mother and child. The vulnerability of the rapidly developing central nervous system *in utero* supports a focus on depression during pregnancy to identify modifiable risk factors and work towards better mental health into the next generation [33, 34]. While further work is required to understand the exact physiological mechanisms through which maternal depression impacts on fetal development, the emerging paradigm of fetal programming (influences in pregnancy can have lifelong implications for the health and well-being of offspring) has been an increasing focus of research regarding maternal depression and its effects on neonatal, child, adolescent, and adult offspring mental health and emotional well-being [33, 35].

Two meta-analyses have found depression in pregnancy to be associated with an increase in premature delivery [36, 37]. Premature delivery, defined as birth before 37 weeks' gestation, has been consistently associated with an increased risk for poorer developmental outcomes for the infant, making this an important finding if considering effects beyond delivery [38]. The first meta-analysis also found lower birthweight with stronger findings in low-income countries [37]. The second found that antenatal depression was associated with lower breastfeeding initiation [36]. Both of these findings are significant for the long-term health, and well-being, of the offspring. Lower initiation of breastfeeding is significant in reducing an important modifiable risk factor associated with the potential to improve a range of health outcomes for mother and child [39]. The later finding for birthweight is significant in light of broader research into associating low birthweight with long-term poorer health outcomes, starting with the work of Barker et al. and cardiovascular risk [40], but now with findings across a range of other health outcomes, including diabetes, hypertension, and renal function [41–43].

Antenatal depression has been associated with a range of emotional and behavioural symptoms, and mental health and neurodevelopmental outcomes, ranging from adverse effects on internalizing and externalizing symptoms in children, adolescent depression, disorganized attachment, and cognitive development [44–47]. However, some studies have found non-significant associations for many of these outcomes and it should be noted for most associations the effect sizes are small.

In maternal perinatal depression symptoms are frequently continuous or relapsing across pregnancy and the child's early years. Studies that attempted to differentiate effects of antenatal and postnatal depression on child outcomes have produced conflicting results with some finding a stronger effect from pregnancy depression [48] and others showing a stronger effect from depression postnatally [49]. That both periods are important is not surprising given the ongoing rapid neurological development that occurs during the fetus and the infant's first year of life. The mechanisms that may govern fetal programming, such as epigenetic processes, continue, with significant capacity for epigenetic changes identified across infancy [50]. Thus, it is clear that effectively treating maternal mental health problems as early as possible is likely to reduce detrimental outcomes for offspring, including the development of mental disorders. Intervention studies are now needed to identify the potential for modifying these risk factors in a range of populations.

Detection of mental health problems in pregnancy: an opportunity for screening?

Depression and anxiety are common in pregnancy, with rates varying between 4.9% and 17.4% [51]. They also predict subsequent depression and pose a risk for the developing fetus, as discussed earlier [5]. This makes detection and effective treatment of depression and anxiety important public health issues, but rates of both detection and appropriate treatment are poor. Screening for these conditions during pregnancy, using pen-and-paper questionnaires, such as the Edinburth Postnatal Depression Scale (EPDS) or the Patient Health Questionnaire (PHQ), would seem to be an obvious solution.

Screening for depression during pregnancy has been advocated by groups such as the Marcé Society [52], a perinatal research organization, and more recently by the United States Preventative Taskforce [53], as a means to improve the detection, treatment, and risk of subsequent depression. Traditionally, only postpartum screening was considered because of a historical (but unfounded) bias towards postnatal depression in research and clinical practice. However, with the recognition of the high rates of depression and anxiety in pregnancy and its impact on the fetus, screening during pregnancy has been advocated, making use of the opportunity of routine contact with health professionals. For screening programmes to be successful, it is essential that services are put in place to complete an assessment for a woman who may screen positive and then to provide appropriate treatment for her. Screening programmes are acceptable for women [54] and undoubtedly increase the detection of depression [55]; however, evidence for their effects on outcomes are not established [56], and there are risks associated with such programmes [57]. The positive predictive value of screening instruments, such as the EPDS [58], are modest, risking high rates of false-positives being identified, thus stretching limited resources.

While screening programmes may not prove to be the answer, asking women about their mental health, especially about whether they have been treated for a mental disorder in the past should be an essential component of assessment in antenatal clinics to ensure appropriate biopsychosocial management is put in place to reduce morbidity, prevent relapse, and plan for the postpartum period.

Routine screening for modifiable psychosocial risk factors for postnatal depression has also been advocated as a strategy to reduce postnatal depression [52]. However, while these risks can be identified, the predictive value of these risks for developing subsequent postnatal depression still needs to be quantified and effective preventative interventions need further evaluation before such screening is adopted.

Prevention of bipolar relapse

Women with bipolar disorder have a high risk of relapse in the first few weeks following childbirth. Overall, the risk of relapse is 36% [59], making it one of the strongest risk factors (for a defined group of patients) that we are aware of in psychiatry, and the only one for which accurate timing can be predicted months in advance.

Bipolar relapse following childbirth has serious implications for the woman, her baby, and her family. Relapse will often lead to the woman needing to be hospitalized for treatment (for both her safety and for the safety of the infant). This, in turn, can cause a significant disruption to the mother–infant bond unless the woman can be admitted to a specialized mother and baby unit, where specialist care can lead to good outcomes for mother, baby, and their relationship [60]. While the best approach to minimize the risk of relapse should, ideally, involve preconception counselling, preventative measures can be planned during pregnancy.

Prophylactic mood stabilizers are effective in reducing this risk [61], with a recent meta-analysis demonstrating that, overall, the rate of relapse for women taking a mood stabilizer was 23% versus 66% for those not taking a mood stabilizer [59]. It should be noted that sodium valproate did not prevent relapse in one controlled study [62] and should not be taken during pregnancy or in women of child-bearing potential because of the high rates of teratogenicity [63] and the risk of the infant having significant cognitive impairment [64].

While mood stabilizers can reduce the risk of relapse, they are not universally used because of risks to the developing fetus. A detailed risk–benefit analysis (benefit to the woman from not relapsing vs the risk of harms to the infant from exposure to medication *in utero*) needs to be done to determine whether the woman should take a mood stabilizer or not during her pregnancy. There are risks associated with using mood stabilizers during pregnancy [65], first observed with lithium, although that risk had been overestimated [66]. Lithium has to be carefully monitored during pregnancy, and breastfeeding is usually advised against [67]. Second-generation antipsychotics can be used: although there is no evidence for their efficacy in preventing a postpartum relapse, they do have good evidence of efficacy in bipolar disorder generally and have not been associated with adverse fetal outcomes.

Women who have been stable for at least a year, have good social support, and are able to self-manage their bipolar disorder could consider slowly withdrawing from their medication and have a medication-free pregnancy, and if they remain well over the first few weeks postpartum, they could continue to be medication free. Alternatively, they can be started back on mood-stabilizing medication immediately following delivery, to try to prevent relapse [61], especially for women who had a previous postpartum psychosis.

Advocating for better care

The value of preserving maternal mental health as a major contribution to reducing morbidity and mortality during pregnancy and postnatally is now well established. Depression, for example, is the most important cause of life years lost through disability or premature death in women in the reproductive years, in both low- and middle-income countries and in high-income countries [68]. Suicide is a major cause of death in women around the time of childbirth [69]. In addition, as described earlier, the negative effects of poor maternal mental health on the developing child, particularly during pregnancy and in the first year, are significant and long lasting. The scale of these problems and the seriousness of their effects across generations have led to the development of international and national policies and guidance (e.g. [51, 70]). However, even among wealthy nations, there has been little evidence of change in the provision of either services or adequate care for women at this critical time. This reflects the universal discrimination against mental health, from global institutions to individual professionals and the public. This is an irony, given the value we place on our individual mental functioning and the collective importance of this to the productivity and well-being of populations. Across the world, social and health policy and practice in relation to women and parents fare little better.

Recent evidence from the UK has demonstrated the effectiveness of a coordinated campaign to highlight this knowledge and demand specific actions on perinatal mental health: Granville et al. [71] found there were six areas in which the 'Everyone's Business' campaign made a significant impact:

◆ perinatal mental health was made a national political priority;

◆ major funding was received from the English and Welsh governments;

◆ it influenced funding for perinatal mental health by non-statutory national funders;

◆ local health commissioning decisions were induced;

◆ improvements in perinatal mental health services were fostered;

◆ focus on perinatal mental health in Wales, Scotland, and Northern Ireland was increased.

The report highlights the factors that influenced change. A key background factor was the effectiveness of the Maternal Mental Health Alliance (MMHA) [72], which ran the campaign, uniting over 80 national patient and professional organizations with jointly agreed visions, objectives, and strategies. The MMHA combined the efforts of organizations to create a powerful force that was able to attract funding and inspire change. An important influence was the funding body, which supported preparatory work to develop a clear vision and direction.

The report points to a number of highly effective tools used by the campaign:

◆ personal stories to secure emotional commitment of decision-makers [73];

◆ clear, simple, colour-coded maps of patchy or non-existent service provision;

◆ clear graphic illustrations of the evidence base, supporting safety, parity, and equity arguments;

◆ economic evidence, presented in a powerful report commissioned by the campaign, from the London School of Economics and Centre for Mental Health [74], with widely publicized summary infographics;

◆ a comprehensive website of resources and opportunities to harness collective action through networking and communications;

◆ holding politicians and key decision-makers to account through annual roundtables hosted by government ministers;

◆ active and coordinated contributions of many MMHA member organizations and women with lived experience.

Conclusions

It is clear that coordinated, collaborative awareness-raising in the area of maternal mental health, and campaigning for increased provision of services, can lead to success at every level. Across the world, every year, over 130 million women have a baby. Inspired by the successes described herein, a global movement is now forming that could substantially improve outcomes for them and their families.

References

1. Cannon M, Jones PB, Murray RM. Obstetric complications and schizophrenia: historical and meta-analytic review. *Am J Psychiatry* 2002; 159: 1080–1092.

2. Stiglitz JE. *The Price of Inequality*. London: Penguin, 2013.

3. Fisher J, Cabral de Mello M, Patel V, et al. Prevalence and determinants of common perinatal mental disorders in women in low- and lower-middle-income countries: a systematic review. *Bull World Health Organ* 2012; 90: 139G–149G.

4. Boden R, Lundgren M, Brandt L, Reutfors J, Andersen M, Kieler H. Risks of adverse pregnancy and birth outcomes in women treated or not treated with mood stabilisers for bipolar disorder: population based cohort study. *BMJ* 2012; 345: e7085.

5. Stein A, Pearson RM, Goodman SH, et al. Effects of perinatal mental disorders on the fetus and child. *Lancet* 2014; 384: 1800–1819.

6. Rapoport JL, Giedd JN, Gogtay N. Neurodevelopmental model of schizophrenia: update 2012. *Mol Psychiatry* 2012; 17: 1228–1238.

7. van Os J, Jones P, Lewis G, Wadsworth M, Murray R. Developmental precursors of affective illness in a general population birth cohort. *Arch Gen Psychiatry* 1997; 54: 625–631.

8. Susser E, Hoek HW, Brown A. Neurodevelopmental disorders after prenatal famine: the story of the Dutch Famine Study. *Am J Epidemiol* 1998; 147: 213–216.

9. Susser ES, Lin SP. Schizophrenia after prenatal exposure to the Dutch Hunger Winter of 1944–1945. *Arch Gen Psychiatry* 1992; 49: 983–988.

10. Xu MQ, Sun WS, Liu BX, et al. Prenatal malnutrition and adult schizophrenia: further evidence from the 1959–1961 Chinese famine. *Schizophr Bull* 2009; 35: 568–576.

11. St Clair D, Xu M, Wang P, et al. Rates of adult schizophrenia following prenatal exposure to the Chinese famine of 1959–1961. *JAMA* 2005; 294: 557–562.

12. Brown AS, Susser ES, Lin SP, Neugebauer R, Gorman JM. Increased risk of affective disorders in males after second trimester prenatal exposure to the Dutch hunger winter of 1944–45. *Br J Psychiatry* 1995; 166: 601–606.

13. Brown AS, van Os J, Driessens C, Hoek HW, Susser ES. Further evidence of relation between prenatal famine and major affective disorder. *Am J Psychiatry* 2000; 157: 190–195.

14. McGrath J, Brown A, St Clair D. Prevention and schizophrenia—the role of dietary factors. *Schizophr Bull* 2011; 37: 272–283.

15. Torrey EF, Miller J, Rawlings R, Yolken RH. Seasonality of births in schizophrenia and bipolar disorder: a review of the literature. *Schizophr Res* 1997; 28: 1–38.

16. McGrath JJ, Eyles DW, Pedersen CB, et al. Neonatal vitamin D status and risk of schizophrenia: a population-based case-control study. *Arch Gen Psychiatry* 2010; 67: 889–894.

17. Kinney DK, Teixeira P, Hsu D, et al. Relation of schizophrenia prevalence to latitude, climate, fish consumption, infant mortality, and skin color: a role for prenatal vitamin d deficiency and infections? *Schizophr Bull* 2009; 35: 582–595.

18. Tochigi M, Okazaki Y, Kato N, Sasaki T. What causes seasonality of birth in schizophrenia? *Neurosci Res* 2004; 48: 1–11.

19. Ross RG, Hunter SK, McCarthy L, et al. Perinatal choline effects on neonatal pathophysiology related to later schizophrenia risk. *Am J Psychiatry* 2013; 170: 290–298.

20. Ross RG, Hunter SK, Hoffman MC, et al. Perinatal phosphatidylcholine supplementation and early childhood behavior problems: evidence for CHRNA7 moderation. *Am J Psychiatry* 2016; 173: 509–516.

21. Black RE, Victora CG, Walker SP, et al. Maternal and child undernutrition and overweight in low-income and middle-income countries. *Lancet* 2013; 382: 427–451.

22. Jacka FN, Ystrom E, Brantsaeter AL, et al. Maternal and early postnatal nutrition and mental health of offspring by age 5 years: a prospective cohort study. *J Am Acad Child Adolesc Psychiatry* 2013; 52: 1038–1047.

23. Mednick SA, Machon RA, Huttunen MO, Bonett D. Adult schizophrenia following prenatal exposure to an influenza epidemic. *Arch Gen Psychiatry* 1988; 45: 189–192.

24. O'Callaghan E, Sham P, Takei N, Glover G, Murray RM. Schizophrenia after prenatal exposure to 1957 A2 influenza epidemic. *Lancet* 1991; 337: 1248–1250.

25. Brown AS, Begg MD, Gravenstein S, et al. Serologic evidence of prenatal influenza in the etiology of schizophrenia. *Arch Gen Psychiatry* 2004; 61: 774–780.

26. Canetta SE, Bao Y, Co MD, et al. Serological documentation of maternal influenza exposure and bipolar disorder in adult offspring. *Am J Psychiatry* 2014; 171: 557–563.

27. Brown AS, Derkits EJ. Prenatal infection and schizophrenia: a review of epidemiologic and translational studies. *Am J Psychiatry* 2010; 167: 261–280.

28. Mendelsohn C, Gould GS, Oncken C. Management of smoking in pregnant women. *Aust Fam Physician* 2014; 43: 46–51.

29. Gaysina D, Fergusson DM, Leve LD, et al. Maternal smoking during pregnancy and offspring conduct problems: evidence from 3 independent genetically sensitive research designs. *JAMA Psychiatry* 2013; 70: 956–963.

30. Niemela S, Sourander A, Surcel HM, et al. Prenatal nicotine exposure and risk of schizophrenia among offspring in a national birth cohort. *Am J Psychiatry* 2016; 173: 799–806.

31. Talati A, Bao Y, Kaufman J, Shen L, Schaefer CA, Brown AS. Maternal smoking during pregnancy and bipolar disorder in offspring. *Am J Psychiatry* 2013; 170: 1178–1185.

32. Dorrie N, Focker M, Freunscht I, Hebebrand J. Fetal alcohol spectrum disorders. *Eur Child Adolesc Psychiatry* 2014; 23: 863–875.

33. Lewis AJ, Galbally M, Gannon T, Symeonides C. Early life programming as a target for prevention of child and adolescent mental disorders. *BMC Med* 2014; 12: 33.

34. Lewis AJ, Austin E, Knapp R, Vaiano T, Galbally M. Perinatal maternal mental health, fetal programming and child development. *Healthcare* 2015; 3: 1212–1227.

35. Glover V. Annual research review: prenatal stress and the origins of psychopathology: an evolutionary perspective. *J Child Psychol Psychiatry* 2011; 52: 356–367.

36. Grigoriadis S, VonderPorten EH, Mamisashvili L, et al. The impact of maternal depression during pregnancy on perinatal outcomes: a systematic review and meta-analysis. *J Clin Psychiatry* 2013; 74: e321–e341.

37. Grote NK, Bridge JA, Gavin AR, Melville JL, Iyengar S, Katon WJ. A meta-analysis of depression during pregnancy and the risk of preterm birth, low birth weight, and intrauterine growth restriction. *Arch Gen Psychiatry* 2010; 67: 1012.

38. Bhutta AT, Cleves MA, Casey PH, Cradock MM, Anand KJ. Cognitive and behavioral outcomes of school-aged children who were born preterm: a meta-analysis. *JAMA* 2002; 288: 728–737.

39. Eidelman AI. Breastfeeding and the use of human milk: an analysis of the American Academy of Pediatrics 2012 Breastfeeding Policy Statement. *Breastfeed Med* 2012; 7: 323–324.

40. Barker DJ, Osmond C, Simmonds SJ, Wield GA. The relation of small head circumference and thinness at birth to death from cardiovascular disease in adult life. *BMJ* 1993; 306: 422–426.

41. Newsome CA, Shiell AW, Fall CH, Phillips DI, Shier R, Law CM. Is birth weight related to later glucose and insulin metabolism?—A systematic review. *Diabet Med* 2003; 20: 339–348.

42. Huxley RR, Shiell AW, Law CM. The role of size at birth and postnatal catch-up growth in determining systolic blood pressure: a systematic review of the literature. *J Hypertens* 2000; 18: 815–831.

43. Hoy WE, Rees M, Kile E, Mathews JD, Wang Z. A new dimension to the Barker hypothesis: low birthweight and susceptibility to renal disease. *Kidney Int* 1999; 56: 1072–1077.

44. Velders FP, Dieleman G, Henrichs J, et al. Prenatal and postnatal psychological symptoms of parents and family functioning: the impact on child emotional and behavioural problems. *Eur Child Adolesc Psychiatry* 2011; 20: 341–350.

45. Pawlby S, Hay DF, Sharp D, Waters CS, O'Keane V. Antenatal depression predicts depression in adolescent offspring: prospective longitudinal community-based study. *J Affect Disord* 2009; 113: 236–243.

46. Hayes LJ, Goodman SH, Carlson E. Maternal antenatal depression and infant disorganized attachment at 12 months. *Attach Hum Dev* 2013; 15: 133–153.

47. Barker ED, Jaffee SR, Uher R, Maughan B. The contribution of prenatal and postnatal maternal anxiety and depression to child maladjustment. *Depress Anxiety* 2011; 28: 696–702.

48. Deave T, Heron J, Evans J, Emond A. The impact of maternal depression in pregnancy on early child development. *BJOG* 2008; 115: 1043–1051.

49. Hay DF, Pawlby S, Waters CS, Sharp D. Antepartum and postpartum exposure to maternal depression: different effects on different adolescent outcomes. *J Child Psychol Psychiatry* 2008; 49: 1079–1088.

50. Martino D, Loke YJ, Gordon L, et al. Longitudinal, genome-scale analysis of DNA methylation in twins from birth to 18 months of age reveals rapid epigenetic change in early life and pair-specific effects of discordance. *Genome Biol* 2013; 14: R42.

51. National Institute of Health and Care Excellence. *Antenatal and Postnatal Mental Health: The NICE Guideline on Clinical Management*

and Service Guidance. Leicester: The British Psychological Society and The Royal College of Psychiatrists, 2007.

52. Austin MP; Marcé Society Position Statement Advisory Committee. Marcé International Society position statement on psychosocial assessment and depression screening in perinatal women. *Best Pract Res Clin Obstet Gynaecol* 2014; 28: 179–187.

53. Siu AL; US Preventive Services Task Force (USPSTF), Bibbins-Domingo K, Grossman DC, Baumann LC, et al. Screening for depression in adults: US Preventive Services Task Force Recommendation Statement. *JAMA* 2016; 315: 380–387.

54. Buist A, Ellwood D, Brooks J, et al. National program for depression associated with childbirth: the Australian experience. *Best Pract Res Clin Obstet Gynaecol* 2007; 21: 193–206.

55. Avalos LA, Raine-Bennett T, Chen H, Adams AS, Flanagan T. Improved perinatal depression screening, treatment, and outcomes with a universal obstetric program. *Obstet Gynecol* 2016; 127: 917–925.

56. Thombs BD, Arthurs E, Coronado-Montoya S, et al. Depression screening and patient outcomes in pregnancy or postpartum: a systematic review. *J Psychosom Res* 2014; 76: 433–446.

57. Lancet. Screening for perinatal depression: a missed opportunity. *Lancet* 2016; 387: 505.

58. National Institute for Health and Care Excellence. *Antenatal and Postnatal Mental Health: Clinical Management and Service Guidance: Updated Edition.*. Leicester: National Institute for Health and Clinical Excellence: Guidance. Leicester, 2014.

59. Wesseloo R, Kamperman AM, Munk-Olsen T, Pop VJ, Kushner SA, Bergink V. Risk of postpartum relapse in bipolar disorder and postpartum psychosis: a systematic review and meta-analysis. *Am J Psychiatry* 2016; 173: 117–127.

60. Kenny M, Conroy S, Pariante CM, Seneviratne G, Pawlby S. Mother–infant interaction in mother and baby unit patients: before and after treatment. *J Psychiatr Res* 2013; 47: 1192–1198.

61. Bergink V, Bouvy PF, Vervoort JS, Koorengevel KM, Steegers EA, Kushner SA. Prevention of postpartum psychosis and mania in women at high risk. *Am J Psychiatry* 2012; 169: 609–615.

62. Wisner KL, Hanusa BH, Peindl KS, Perel JM. Prevention of postpartum episodes in women with bipolar disorder. *Biol Psychiatry* 2004; 56: 592–596.

63. Hernandez-Diaz S, Smith CR, Shen A, et al. Comparative safety of antiepileptic drugs during pregnancy. *Neurology* 2012; 78: 1692–1699.

64. Meador KJM, Baker GAP, Browning NP, et al. Effects of fetal antiepileptic drug exposure: outcomes at age 4.5 years. *Neurology* 2012; 78: 1207–1214.

65. Snellen M, Malhi G. Bipolar disorder, psychopharmacology, and pregnancy. In: Galbally M, Snellen M, Lewis A (eds). *Psychopharmacology and Pregnancy—Treatment Efficacy, Risks, and Guidelines Treatment Efficacy, Risks, and Guidelines*. Berlin Heidelberg: Springer-Verlag, 2014, pp. 103–118.

66. Diav-Citrin O, Shechtman S, Tahover E, et al. Pregnancy outcome following in utero exposure to lithium: a prospective, comparative, observational study. *Am J Psychiatry* 2014; 171: 785–794.

67. Galbally M, Snellen M, Walker S, Permezel M. Management of antipsychotic and mood stabilizer medication in pregnancy: recommendations for antenatal care. *Aust N Z J Psychiatry* 2010; 44: 99–108.

68. World Health Organization.) Global Burden of Disease, Part 4. Available at: http://www.who.int/healthinfo/global_burden_disease/GBD_report_2004update_part4.pdf (accessed 14 March 2018).

69. MBRRACE. Saving Lives. The Confidential Enquiry into Maternal Deaths. Available at: https://www.npeu.ox.ac.uk/downloads/files/mbrrace-uk/reports/MBRRACE-UK Maternal Report 2015.pdf (accessed 14 March 2018).

70. World Health Organization. Maternal mental health and child health and development in low and middle income countries: report of the meeting held in Geneva, Switzerland, 30 January–1 February, 2008. Available at: http://www.who.int/mental_health/prevention/suicide/mmh_jan08_meeting_report.pdf (14 March 2018).

71. Granville G, Sugarman W, Tedder V. Maternal Mental Health Alliance Everyones Business Campaign: Independent Evaluation Report. Available at: http://everyonesbusiness.org.uk/wp-content/uploads/2016/07/Everyones-Business-Campaign-Independent-Evaluation-Report-Summer-2016.pdf (accessed 14 March 2018).

72. Maternal Mental Health Alliance. Awareness Education Action to improve the lives of mothers and their infants. Available at: http://maternalmentalhealthalliance.org/ (accessed 14 March 2018).

73. Maternal Mental Health Alliance. Everyone's Business: Real Life Stories. Available at: http://everyonesbusiness.org.uk/?page_id=144 (accessed 14 March 2018).

74. Bauer A, Parsonage M, Knapp M, Iemmi V, Adelaja B. Costs of perinatal mental health problems. Available at: https://www.centreformentalhealth.org.uk/costs-of-perinatal-mh-problems (accessed 14 March 2018).

CHAPTER 42

Promoting mental health and well-being
What can schools do?

Katherine Weare

Introduction

Schools are generally expanding their role from the traditional focus on academic learning to include a greater concern with their students' well-being. They are increasingly keen to see their students as whole people, with hearts and bodies, as well as minds and intellects. Many schools routinely use language and concepts such as 'connectedness', 'relationships', 'resilience', 'social and emotional (skills/learning/competences/intelligence), 'values' 'character', 'values', and even 'happiness' [1]. This is part of an overall trend toward emphasizing the positive in approaches to human development: we are seeing an increase in work under headings such as 'thriving', 'flourishing', 'positive psychology', and 'positive mental health [2]. The argument is that we have focused for too long on what is 'wrong' with people, including the young, focusing only on pathologies, problems, and difficulties, and need to explore more deeply on what is 'right'—the positive qualities and strengths that can help meet these challenges [3]. Schools generally welcome this shift, and find it reasonably easy to incorporate, particularly as the links between well-being and learning/attainment become clearer [4].

However, those who are trained to work in educational contexts can become nervous about their capacity to respond to mental health problems, seeing these as extreme states, outside their comfort zone and competence to deal with, and needing the intervention of specialized professionals: they can fear doing harm [5]. Schools need reassurance, support, and advice to develop the confidence to tackle this whole area. We are currently seeing a growth of such advice to schools on mental health, much of it sound and common sense, and based on various types of evidence, some practice based and some from research with various levels of robustness [6].

Schools are increasingly being encouraged to believe in their power to help all students and staff flourish, and to help those in difficulties. This is not just through specialist interventions, but also through the usual everyday work of listening to students and making connections and relationships with them. There is no 'quick fix' or magic bullet: promoting well-being and tackling mental health problems requires a long-term, systemic approach that goes to the heart of the values and processes in the school. School staff are being guided to realize the need to engage in joined-up thinking,

to understand that mental health and well-being are a continuum (they are not separate domains), to understand the links between mental health and learning (to see it as a whole-school issue), and be clear what they can reasonably hope to do themselves, and when and how they need to seek support from parents, families, the community, and the more specialist services to pull together to make mental health and well-being 'everyone's business'. We explore all this in more detail, and the evidence to support it, in this chapter.

The growth of mental health problems in young people

We cannot afford for schools to ignore their vital role in tackling mental health issues, not least because there are not enough specialist resources to tackle such issues adequately. Globally, mental health problems are on the increase in young and old: they constitute a considerable proportion of the world's disease burden, such that they have been called a 'hidden epidemic' [7]. Mental health problems in the adult population typically start before the age of 24 years, and half of lifetime mental illness starts by the age of 14 years [8]. Conduct disorders, which often emerge as 'bad behaviour' and thus not always seen as a mental health issue, will be familiar to schools, but young people also suffer from increasing levels of depression, suicidality, self-harm, anxiety, bipolar affective disorders, substance abuse, schizophrenia, and post-traumatic stress disorder. All of us, including the 'successful', tend to suffer from a ubiquitous sense of stress, fragmentation, and overwhelm, made increasingly acute in our digital age. It is generally estimated that, in developed countries at least (i.e. where we have data), at least 1 out of every 5 young people in the general population will suffer from at least one mental problem in any given year that interferes with their development and learning, with 1 in 10 children and young people having a clinically diagnosed mental health disorder and/or emotional and behaviour problems (often the same children) [7]. Many problems are multiple and many remain undetected, and thus will go untreated unless agencies such as schools take an active role in attempting to identify and respond to students' difficulties. The situation is likely to be similar in more traditional societies, although data are lacking.

Mental health problems and are often deeply stigmatized and neglected, and most nations lack the resources to tackle mental health problems adequately, even in richer developed countries. These problems, and the resultant compromised levels of well-being, underlie many of the personal, educational, and social problems young people experience, such as educational underachievement, crime and violence, and substance abuse [8]. Although multiple agencies are involved, schools, as a primary agent of socialization, have an essential role to play in helping young people to flourish, fulfil their potential and contribute to their communities, working in partnership with families and parents. They need support to recognize and feel able to meet their responsibility and agency as a key part of the overall response.

The growing evidence base for 'what works'

Fortunately, in supporting schools, we now know a good deal about 'what works' and have some solid and practical evidence to build on. Over the last 30 or so years we have seen a major growth in research on the role of the school in promoting mental health and well-being, and tackling mental health problems. This growing evidence base includes evaluations of specific interventions and programmes and we are seeing the emergence of some fairly strong research, including from randomized control trials of specific interventions, with over 50 comprehensive reviews and meta-analyses [9]. Perhaps more helpfully, we are also becoming clearer about the wider educational and social processes that can support well-being and mental health, and the principles that underlie effective work in this area.

This research shows that certain principles and approaches, and some programmes and interventions—when well founded, designed, and implemented—show evidence of clear and positive impacts on a range of outcomes. These outcomes include student well-being [9], social and emotional skills and attitudes [10], the prevention of mental health problems [11], reductions in risky behaviour [12], academic learning and attainment [13], and teacher/staff well-being [14].

This chapter will explore what we can reasonably assume, with our current state of knowledge, are the actions and principles that promote mental health and well-being in schools. As far as space allows, it will include some examples of good practice.

In keeping with the core message that we need a whole-school approach, we will begin by exploring what the school as a whole needs to get right for promoting positive well-being for all its students and staff, which is also the essential basis for tackling mental health problems. We will then look at more specific actions that need to be taken to address mental health problems, within this supportive context.

Take a whole-school approach and implement it carefully

Well-being and mental health involve everyone who works and learns in the school, and in the surrounding community, working together in a joined up, coherent way. There is increasing interest across education in what is variously often called a 'school-wide approach', a 'comprehensive approach', or 'whole-school' approach [15], terms that attempt to encapsulate an approach that recognizes the importance of symbiosis, of working systematically right across the organization, of creating a supportive central culture and ethos, ensuring all parts work together in a coordinated, cohesive,

and coherent way. It is a concept that has been applied with some success to many issues that have been found to work best when integrated at a whole-school level, such as health, well-being, safety, equity, and violence prevention. Such approaches have been shown to be more effective than those that focus on only one or two parts of school life, inclusive of promoting well-being [12]. For example, the evaluation of the nationwide Targeted Mental Health in Schools (TaMHS) project in England and Wales, which developed a very wide range of strategies for tackling mental health issues across many different school-based locations, found making mental health 'everyone's business' was a key strategy and multi-professional teamwork, which aimed at producing engagement and consistency of everyone involved across the school and community, was the core focus of several well-evaluated TaMHS projects [16].

However, the whole-school approach to the promotion of well-being is by no means automatically effective—unless carefully implemented it can become chaotic, diluted, and fragmented [17]. This has demonstrably happened with some whole-school approaches, such as SEAL (social and emotional aspects of learning) in the UK, which, when implemented as intended, was associated with positive outcomes [18], but when carried out in a diffuse way, not so [19]. As a result of evaluations of whole-school programmes, such as SEAL, and also Mind Matters [20], Health Promoting Schools [21], and Communities that Care [22], and of reviews that draw all this together [10, 23], we now know a great deal more than we did about making whole-school approaches effective in the real world.

A whole-school approach needs to be tightly managed, start with a clear vision of the goals, conduct an audit of existing practice and a needs assessment of the students and staff to obtain clarity about current areas of strength and weaknesses, and work with a realistic recognition of the resources of time and money available. Plans for change need to be modest, developed incrementally, and proceed strategically over a sensible time frame with realistic expectations. The whole effort needs strong and committed leadership, energetic and focused staff training, with time and effort spent building up a sense of engagement and ownership in all parts of the school community, and careful and honest evaluation and monitoring.

Develop a 'connected' school and classroom climate and ethos

It has become clear that perhaps the most important aspect of the whole school is also the hardest to pin down and measure—its climate and ethos [1, 24]. In recent years the notions of school well-being [1] and, in particular, school 'connectedness' [25] have come to the fore to summarize the kind of ethos that appears to be the most effective. 'Connectedness' refers to a feeling among members of the school community of being part of and bonded to the school's culture and environment. Connected schools and classrooms are environments in which everyone feels included, involved, listened to, and understood. They are based on a sense of warmth, supportiveness, and responsiveness to students' individual needs; they encourage appropriate expressions of emotion, respectful communication, and problem-solving; and have low levels of conflict and disruptive behaviour as a result [11, 26].

Children come to school from a specific culture and background, and schools need to build a sense of connectedness with all their families and communities. Experiencing connection can help all young people experience a vital sense of cohesion and coherence across their lives and feel a well-rooted sense of belonging, a pride in who they are and where they come, which is highly protective for mental health. Schools can also strengthen family life through helping parents and carers develop their own parenting skills and attitudes, provided this is offered to the whole community of parents, with sensitivity and no judgement [27].

Creating connected school environments is, naturally, a whole-school matter. For example, three school communities in Southeast Queensland, Australia, built school connectedness by fostering interaction among members of the entire school community at both class- and whole-school level, using activities such as strategies to prevent bullying, peer support programmes, extra-curricular activities, support structures for school staff, a fair behaviour management system, collaborative curriculum planning, and partnerships between staff, students, and parents and the community [28].

Supportive school climates are not laissez faire: they are psychologically and physically safe, with clear and high expectations and a sense of strong and positive discipline and boundaries, expressed particularly in the school's policies and practice, to make sure everyone is secure and comfortable [1]. Everyone understands what is acceptable and unacceptable behaviour and are aware of its consequences, experiencing a consistent and proportionate response [29]. Mental health and well-being are particularly affected by the school's policies and practice around diversity—with prejudice and bullying around ability, disability, gender, race, sexual orientation, and perceived social status being actively challenged [30]. Anti-bullying and homophobia policies and practice generally need to be strengthened in many places; for example, a recent inspection report in England and Wales found that the casual use of homophobic and disablist language was alarmingly commonplace. Ignorance about mental health is generally widespread right across society, and schools are being encouraged to be at the forefront of tackling ignorant and pejoratives attitudes, prejudice, and stigma [31].

Tackling risk and building resilience

Mental health is not just an individual matter: many children and young people are routinely exposed to a wide range of risk social factors which undermine their well-being and mental health.

Severe risks emanate from poverty, social marginalization, family fragmentation, and physical or mental illness in the family [32]. Some students will have experienced trauma through abuse, violence, accidents, and injuries. To give an idea of scale, an oft-quoted scenario is that, in an average classroom, 10 young people will have witnessed their parents separate, eight will have experienced severe physical violence, sexual abuse, or neglect, one will have experienced the death of a parent, and seven will have been bullied [33].

Globally, we increasingly need to consider the problems of migration, asylum-seeking, war, conflict, and natural disasters that are impacting on all countries in our interconnected world. Girls and women may be particularly vulnerable, especially in more traditional societies, and, across the globe, young people who identify as different to the mainstream, being lesbian, gay, bisexual, or trans, are very likely to have their mental health compromised through rejection, stigma, and discrimination [34]. These problems are generally worse in low-income countries, where threats are higher, resources to respond are far lower, and prejudiced and stigmatizing attitudes often more entrenched, making the ability to respond even weaker than in more affluent nations, where the problem is bad enough [35].

Low school achievement is a major risk factor, and continues the cycle of deprivation, leading to future poverty, drug use, teenage pregnancy, behaviour problems, and crime [36]. It is clearly the responsibility of the school, and of wider society, to tackle the admittedly very tough challenge of underachievement from children from disadvantaged backgrounds. So recognizing risk of all kinds is not an opportunity for fatalism, or for taking responsibility away from students, it is an opportunity for positive action. As the agency at the front line of the response, there is much schools can do to recognize and tackle disadvantage, and the prejudice and stigma tend to accompany it, and take steps to improve the climate for the acceptance of difference and diversity. Effective schools work with all their students, not only those they find easy to reach. They recognize that their school staff probably come from very different backgrounds themselves and may therefore find the difficulties under which their students labour hard to perceive, identify, and understand. They attempt to reduce their judgements, work with and listen to members of the community, students, and their families, to provide a positive, tailored, and non-discriminatory response.

Schools can help positively to build a protective sense of 'resilience', which means the ability to face, overcome, and be strengthened by difficulties and challenges. Resilience is fostered by the school experience and the intervention of an effective school or teacher can be a turning point for children, especially those with few other supports [37]. Being satisfied with school, having a sense of what is sometimes called school well-being [1], especially having that vital the 'sense of connectedness', which as we have already explored, are major protective factors. They can help students develop their social and emotional skills and has a direct impact on their ability to face difficulties [12].

The Welsh Inspectorate identified the factors that are helping some of their schools tackle risk and promote resilience and succeed in disadvantaged areas, despite facing challenging circumstances. They found that schools that successfully tackled disadvantage had effective leadership and consistently good teaching; attached great importance to extra-curricular and out-of-school-hours provision; had a vibrant curriculum, including vocational courses and the teaching of social and emotional skills; provided extra educational support such as homework clubs, at lunch times, or after school; had high expectations of standards and behaviour, a zero tolerance of excuses for poor provision or underachievement, and a focus in social inclusion without compromising standards; and worked closely with parents and the wider community to reinforce expectations.

Encouraging student participation

We have talked already of the importance of a sense of connectedness as basic for well-being and to protect mental health. Helping students to feel they have a stake in school life through genuine and authentic student participation is core to building this protective sense.

Student connection and engagement can be built into basic pedagogy and curriculum, as students take responsibility for and improve their own learning and development through reflection and inquiry. Through their social and emotional learning they can enhance their sense of self-efficacy, their relationships with others, and develop their social skills. Young people who are struggling or at the margins are both the most important to involve and the least likely to be consulted: schools need to take positive affirmative action in this regard. Peer education is a helpful method to draw on the positive strength of the peer group, helping young people become active players, rather than passive recipients, in the educational process. Students can be effective peer educators in teaching social and emotional skills, particularly social skills, buddying, and conflict resolution [38].

Promoting the mental health and well-being of school personnel

The adage of 'apply your own oxygen mask before trying to help anyone else' applies forcibly to the promotion of well-being in schools. The workforce in the school—teachers and allied professions and support staff—are not going to be motivated to promote the well-being of their students if they feel uncared for and burnt out themselves. A focus on staff well-being has to be central to part of any effort to improve school mental health, and is urgently needed in many places. Schools are notoriously pressurized environments, and research has regularly exposed high levels of stress, anxiety, and depression among the workforce in many countries [39]. As a result, it can be hard to attract people to the teaching and allied professions: many who train never practice; levels of illness, attrition, and early retirement are high; and staff retention is often low. All of this has a knock-on impact on students, including their educational achievements [40].

Well-documented causes of stress among school personnel include a sense of lack of control of the workspace and of workload, a constant sense of pressure, a sense of having no downtime, trying to do too little without sufficient resource, and being overwhelmed by the difficulties of working with hard-to-reach students [39]. Staff suffer from unrealistic expectations from either the outside, or often from their own noble wish to help and fix things. The rise of email and smartphones has attacked an already precarious work–life balance by ensuring that staff can never properly switch off: some school managers think it acceptable for staff to be contacted well after school hours or during vacations.

Schools urgently need to recognize their responsibilities to address the causes of staff stress. They need to create a cultural climate in which mental health problems are not stigmatized and seen as a weakness, but where staff, as well as students, are able to admit when they are not coping, and feel comfortable seeking support and help for their mental health, both within the school—with buddying, mentoring, and line management—and from outside supports. Staff development can help staff build their stress-reduction skills, such as self-efficacy and resilience. Mindfulness, the skill of learning to be in the present, exploring experience with kindness and curiosity rather than negative judgement, is starting to prove to be particularly effective for both staff and student stress [41].

The attitudes, practices, and examples provided by senior managers are pivotal [42]. They can carry out regular reviews of stress levels; they can lead by example and ensure that they are not modelling overwork and a sense of driven-ness themselves; they can encourage staff to have reasonable expectations of themselves, reduce perfectionism, and achieve a sound work–life balance where all can switch off and have a personal life. They can set sensible and sustainable workloads, especially of new and younger staff, or those undergoing difficulties in their personal lives. They can ensure that

their schools take time to celebrate and reward achievement and effort, not just press on to the next target.

Positive approaches to difficult behaviour

How a school tackles 'difficult' behaviour is a critical indicator for the well-being and mental health of students and staff. The national evaluation of the large scale TaMHS project in the UK, mentioned earlier, found that the most strongly endorsed category for tackling mental health difficulties in both primary and secondary schools was work on behaviour management in relation to behavioural difficulties [43].

Out-of=date and non-evidence-based responses do more harm than good. Such responses see student behaviour as entirely negative, emerging in isolation from malevolent intent, a personal challenge to the teacher's authority, and entirely under the student's control. They invariably make the problem worse by failing to find reasons behind the behaviour or to build the vital sense of connection between students and school, which, we are suggesting, is so protective of students' motivation to engage and ultimately to their well-being [44].

Positive behaviour management approaches are more likely to be effective in creating wider well-being and helping students with mental health difficulties: we will summarize here what they involve and how they may be applied [45]. It is not about being soft and laissez faire: appropriate responses provide logical and proportionate consequences for poor behaviour to keep everyone in the context safe, psychologically and physically. But they also see the whole child behind the behaviour, recognize their positive characteristics, and look more deeply to understand and address the underlying meanings and feelings the behaviour represents. They address the potential causes of difficult behaviour, such as an unmet mental health need: it has been estimated that 1 in 10 young people have diagnosable emotional or behaviour difficulty [46]. The behaviour may also be caused by family problems, temporary or long-term, peer difficulties such as harassment and bullying, and learning or medical difficulties. Difficult incidents are seen as opportunities to teach better alternatives [47]: this crucially involves adults modelling more appropriate attitudes and skills in times of difficulty: adults do not take challenges personally, they focus on the student, and stay professional, calm, open-minded and reflective, manage their own emotions and impulses, and seek help with their own associated emotional stress from other adults and not take it out on their students [48]. Mindfulness for school staff is again proving particularly effective in this helping staff attune to students and keep their own cool [41].

Teaching social and emotional skills explicitly

Providing a positive, connected, warm, caring, and boundaried school atmosphere ethos and environment is, we are suggesting, vital. An essential part of this overall context is the development of the skills of those who cultivate such environments through their work and learning.

There are many taxonomies of the skills that promote well-being (sometimes called social and emotional learning (SEL)). They typically comprise self-awareness, emotional regulation, motivation, social skills, and empathy [49]. More recently we can add mindfulness and compassion: mindfulness in schools has a promising evidence base for students and staff, and in the UK has been recommended by an all-party parliamentary group for the training of all teachers [50].

Such skills can act as protective factors, helping prevent the development of mental health problems and risky behaviour in young people, and in school staff, develop their resilience to risk and disadvantage, and assist young people in negotiating the transitions challenges of growing up [12]. SEL skills provide confidence, competence, and the ability to engage. They connected fundamentally with learning, school attainment, and completion, as well as long-term lifetime outcomes of improved adult engagement, health and well-being, career success and earning potential, and lower risk of encounter with the criminal justice system [13, 14].

We know a good deal about how these skills are best transmitted. They are not caught by osmosis: they involve the school taking a conscious, planned, and explicit approach to teaching them energetically, through the overt curriculum, as well as through out-of-class opportunities right across the school and the community. Effective teachers are well trained and keen, not reluctant conscripts, well educated and practiced in social and emotional skills themselves, grasping the relevance of these skills for themselves and their students, and able and willing to embody and model them.

Effective teachers are also well educated in how to transmit these skills in the classroom, and in everyday opportunities across the school. They do not practice 'death by worksheet' or video: they are keen on the subject and positive about its relevance, able to teach these skills with high levels of pedagogic skills, using active and engaging methods, ensuring learning reaches hearts, as well as minds, and impacts on attitudes, values, and feelings [51]. They use low-key and positive approaches, aware that fear, behaviour change, and information are not effective motivators to achieve changes at any kind of deep or long-term level [52].

Manualized programmes and published materials that aim to teach such skills abound. The best of them, with a sound evidence base, in the right context, well taught, and implemented, can make a significant difference to levels of well-being in a school and to mental health problems [9]. Both the 'Friends' programme and the Paths programme (promoting alternative-thinking strategies) have evaluated well across a range of contexts and age groups in both targeted and universal conditions: in the UK they have done best when supported by a whole-school framework, such as SEAL [53, 54].

There is an apparent wealth of programmes to choose from, although the whole field suffers from a degree of over claim, sometimes as a result of commercial interest, that schools need to watch carefully. In light of this concern there have been efforts to review programmes, for example in terms of their type, quality, and the robustness of their evidence base [55]. Many agencies have produced databases and lists of of sources of help and support, and programmes available to support schools at national or local level [6].

Schools can feel overwhelmed by the choice and unsure of what to do and feel under sales pressure from specific programmes. They need to take their time to select any programme they wish to use. They need to ensure that the programme has a solid evidence base, rather than trusting the word of the developers, and claims on websites. They need to put the needs of the school and of the students, not the programme, at the heart of the process, and

to be realistic about the limits that any one, short programme can achieve. The programme needs to fit their context, and be able to be sustained and taught with existing resources.

In any case, and to reiterate a key message, we need to beware of quick-fix, magic-bullet thinking that relying totally on any particular programme can represent. SEL skills are best not seen as a one-off intervention, or as a 'Cinderella subject' in a silo, but are best integrated into the mainstream and supported by the rest of the school experience. Social and emotional skills only start to have a real impact on learning and on wider behaviour when they are reinforced in all interactions across the school [56] and in the longer term. Schools need to ensure the skills they teach are seen as relevant by the students, their families and their communities and their cultures, to the real-life challenges they face. For example, an evaluation of the secondary SEAL programme showed that in more effective schools, social and emotional learning outcomes were extended into activities across the entire educational context with staff, as well as pupils, woven into key learning outcomes through all school activities, and integrated into the fabric of the school in terms of basic school policies and links with other initiatives. Most schools, especially secondary schools, have some way to go in realizing such a vision.

Teaching social and emotional skills to those with mental health issues

Young people with mental health difficulties will need to be taught the same core emotional and social skills as their mainstream fellows but in more explicit, intensive, and extensive ways. Such targeted and skills-based work has been shown to impact clearly on a range of problems, including depression and anxiety, conduct disorders, violence prevention, and conflict resolution, especially when taught in small groups. There are many evidence-based programmes to choose from: PATHS [54] and Friends for Life [53] were tried by the English and Welsh TaMHS programmes and were found to be helpful, in both cases combined with the whole-school framework of SEAL as that was a TaMHS programme basic requirement. Nurture groups have proven to be particularly effective in developing emotional and social well-being in more vulnerable pupils through fostering a sense of safety and belonging, and were promoted in several TaMHS projects [16].

Groups that focus on a particular skill, such as conflict resolution and anger management, can impact on the familiar mental health problems of young people, provided they are good quality, fit the context, and implemented with conviction [11]. Effective approaches often have the same basic mixture of cognitive–behavioural therapy (helping students to re-shape their thinking, learn skills, and alter behaviours), better classroom management, and support for parents: it appears not to matter a great deal which one is chosen, provided it is of good quality, fits the context, and is implemented with conviction.

A long-term approach

We have commented on the natural wish of hard-pressed teachers for a quick fix, for mental health issues in particular. Sadly, there is no such solution and it is clear that one-offs and single, brief interventions, although they may make a short-term splash, do not have any lasting impact. Effective approaches are systemic and long term. Interventions of 6–10 weeks in length have been shown to be effective for promoting specific skills, such as emotional control and milder versions of problems such as conflict and anxiety. More intense interventions, with more sessions per week, generally work better than more diluted ones [57]. However, in the case of more severe problems such as the prevention of mental health difficulties, violence, bullying, anger, and—in the case of broader and deeper areas such as well-being—interventions need time to show benefits, on average at least 9 months to a year [9].

The optimum long-term approach would appear to be a clear intensive intervention followed up by regular revisiting of core learning and top-up sessions in a way that is appropriate for the stage and situation of the learner [51], and integration of the core skills, values, and attitudes across the curriculum and the whole-school experience. Schools often do not provide interventions that are intense or lengthy enough to make a long-term difference, and we need more long-term evaluations of impact—many are only funded for short-term assessment.

A universal approach tackles stigma

We have made it clear that universal approaches are a vital backdrop for work on mental health difficulties, and part of an effective response. The empirical evidence supports starting from a positive focus that emphasizes strengths and capacities—this has been shown to be more effective in the school context than approaches that focus only on problems and difficulties. Targeted approaches work best when they have a solid base of support in universal approaches (for all) provided they are integrated in a coherent way. A backdrop of universal entitlement can avoid the stigma that can attach to more targeted work on mental health problems and particularly to the involvement of specialist services. When schools have a solid, school-wide approach in place, a culture develops in which it is seen as normal and appropriate to talk about mental health difficulties and seek help, and where skills, attitudes, routines, and practices help everyone flourish, including those with more acute levels of need [14].

Identify and start early with mental health interventions

Once a solid backdrop of universal work is in place we need additional interventions and approaches for higher-risk students. In fact, such interventions are likely to have their most dramatic impacts on children with difficulties.

Sadly, schools often delay taking action when students exhibit signs of mental health problems, sometimes from an understandable wish not to 'label', believing that children 'grow out' of it. Unfortunately, the opposite is usually the case [58]. Early intervention using simple, low-key measures can help prevent minor problems from escalating and becoming of clinical significance, and, followed by effective and prompt help, can ensure that problems can be resolved with the least fuss and disruption: the most effective interventions are those that target preschool and early primary years [24].

Anxiety about mental health is creating a concern to identify those with problems, and schools often look to screening tests for support. They can, indeed, be useful if the school is worried about a particular child or young person, as part of the overall picture.

There are many to choose from and the Strengths and Difficulties Questionnaire (SDQ) [59], which has versions for pupils, staff, and parents, to obtain a range of views, is a free-to-use, simple, and well trialled starting point. Some schools, in their anxiety to tackle mental health problems, can hurry to screen the whole school population. Used wisely, screening might be informative as one part of the whole-school picture. However, it has its dangers: mass screening can create complacency, an over-reliance on technology rather than the vital connection and relationships, and problems with the reliability of the test in creating either false-positives or negatives that confuse the picture. Screening and inventories need to be tempered with common sense, listening, and observation by those who work and learn in a school, and their families, to be sensitive to when problems are interfering with children's well-being, learning, behaviour, and social relationships—if they are, the child needs help whatever his or her 'score' suggests.

Teachers can be effective in spotting the early signs of mental health problems, identifying the changes in behaviour, patterns of attainment, or attendance that may suggest a problem. There are concerns that teachers may generally need more help to do this, and find special training and the follow-up use of so-called 'mental health first aid' toolkits useful in this respect, again as a low-key part of a wider whole-school response [5]. Other students often have an acute and first-hand understanding about the difficulties of peers [60], including being alert to problems with the use of social media, which appears to be an increasing source of serious stress and difficulty for young people [61]. Approaches aimed directly at young people that destigmatize mental health problems, spread knowledge about the signs and symptoms of mental health problems, encourage young people to communicate their difficulties, and 'look out' for one another are growing and are welcome [62].

Parents can be a valuable source of information in the early identification of students with difficulties: it is often parental concerns that are the first sign of a problem that needs addressing. Parents should experience the school as welcoming of their concerns and worries, and that they actively participate in decisions taken about their children, with full information and support. We need to recognize that the involvement of school can be a sensitive matter: parents and carers can easily feel patronized, stigmatized, and blamed for their children's difficulties: the school needs to look for strengths in families and try to build on them. This can encourage parents who have had a poor experience of school life, to feel accepted and welcome, and active partners in their children's progress, treatment, and recovery.

Getting specialist help

Once students are identified as having difficulties there needs to be a clear and graduated pathway, with transparent processes for making decisions, to provide support both within the school, and, if necessary, from outside services.

If in-school support is found not to be adequate, students, and their parents and families, need to be encouraged to seek and receive appropriate specialist help. Schools should work closely with other professionals to have a range of support services in place in and linked to schools, and ensure easy and transparent pathways to such services and supportive agencies. These may include school counselling, school-based clinics, psychology, and child and adolescent psychiatry. It is important to make sure that any commissioned counselling or mental health services are fully integrated into the policies, procedures, and referral processes of the school. The young person and their family need to feel at the centre of the process, experiencing care that is responsive to their needs and culture, not passed around, experience long delays without support, or be discharged without the problem being properly addressed.

Conclusions

There is a great deal that schools can do to promote mental health and well-being. Schools can feel confident that a focus on well-being and mental health helps cultivate a healthy and happy school environment for students and staff, which promotes flourishing on all levels, including the promotion of effective learning, as well as preventing and helping manage mental health problems. Mental health and well-being are at the heart of the effective school.

Case study
A whole-school approach to promoting well-being and preventing and tackling mental health issues in a primary school in the UK

King's Hedges Educational Federation

This school was the winner of the Mental Health Coalition's 'Resilience and Results' competition 2013, UK. The following account draws on the judges' comments.

Kings Hedges works hard with its resources to demonstrate exceptional provision for students across all aspects of supporting well-being, with a careful and innovative use of external services and resources, considered measurement and evaluation of achievements, and strong evidence of placing pupils' voices at the heart of decision-making strategies.

The school believes that early intervention is the key. Questionnaires on entry to early years are undertaken as part of a 2-year FAB Project (family happiness and well-being) and this screening process identifies early signs of mental health problems. Home visits are valuable in gaining the parents' perspective on the needs of the child and gives the staff an insight to the child's home and family life.

As a result of a successful Lottery bid, the school has set up 'So to Speak', a group of 20-plus preschool pupils who are demonstrating delayed or limited-speech development. The project aims to minimize the impact of disadvantage by improving factors around expressive language, separation anxiety, and language deficit. The school closely monitors the development of these children and is already seeing that many are exceeding the progress of their peers.

As pupils progress through the school, a rigorous PSHE (personal, social and health education) map gives particular attention to well-being units, including 'keeping safe', 'anti-bullying', and 'sex and relationships education'. Each unit is linked to weekly philosophy sessions which equip pupils with the vocabulary and skills to express their needs and feelings. Pupils are encouraged to talk about their well-being. Issues are discussed by groups of pupils at the school council and pupils

actively support healthy friendships and vulnerable pupils during playtime through the provision of 'buddy stops' and Lunchtime Club.

All staff are given annual safeguarding training and are expected to look out for signs of distress and follow the school's rigorous systems to bring effective and timely support. The school has set up systems such as Talk Time, a school-funded drop-in where children can talk to a trained adult and get advice and help about their worries. If a child has deeper rooted problems or emotional issues then the school can refer them to 'Blue Smile', a counselling/mentoring support service partly funded by the school and charity donations. The Blue Smile team uses play and art therapy techniques to help the child explore difficult emotions, with information about their needs and progress being fed back to the parent or carer. Although initially some parents were nervous about accepting this support, many parents now approach the school when they have concerns about their child as they have heard about the great benefits of the service.

Where staff or parents and carers identify that they need support with family relationships, parenting or behaviour management, the school can refer to 'Red Hen', a charity-funded project that has benefited recently from a successful Lottery bid. It was a project initially set up at King's Hedges and has been extended to provide support to pupils in five local schools.

Useful websites

There are many national and international agencies that offer help, advice, and resources to schools on promoting well-being and addressing mental health issues. Here is a small selection.

- MindEd: https://www.minded.org.uk/ (UK).
- Young Minds: http://www.youngminds.org.uk/ (UK).
- PSHE (Personal, Social and Health Education) Association: https://www.pshe-association.org.uk/ (UK).
- CASEL (Collaborative for Academic, Social and Emotional Learning): http://www.casel.org/ (USA).
- ENSEC (European Network for Social and Emotional Competence): http://enseceurope.org/
- Mental Health Australia: https://mhaustralia.org/tags/young-people
- Mental Health Europe: http://www.mhe-sme.org/
- Mental Health Foundation: https://www.mentalhealth.org.uk/
- SAMSHA (Substance Abuse and Mental Health Services Administration): http://www.samhsa.gov/ (US)
- Schools for Health in Europe: http://www.schools-for-health.eu/she-network
- World Health Organization/Mental Health: http://www.who.int/mental_health/en/
- World Health Organization/Global Schools Health Initiative http://www.who.int/school_youth_health/gshi/en/

References

1. Huebner ES, Kimberly J, Hills KJ, et al. Schooling and children's subjective well-being. In: Ben-Arieh A, Casas F, Frønes I, Korbin JE (eds). *Handbook of Child Well-Being. Theories, Methods and Policies in Global Perspective.* Berlin: Springer, 2014, pp. 797–819.

2. Bok DC. *The Politics of Happiness: What Government Can Learn From the New Research on Well-being.* Princeton, NJ: Princeton University Press, 2010.

3. Suldo SM, Shaffer EJ. Looking beyond psychopathology: the dual-factor model of mental health in youth. *School Psychol Rev* 2008; 37: 52–68.

4. Public Health England. *The Link Between Health and Wellbeing and Attainment. A Briefing for Head Teachers, Schools Governors and Teachers.* London: Public Health England, 2014.

5. Mental Health for England. Mental Health Starts with You. Available at:https://mhfaengland.org/ (accessed 14 March 2017).

6. Children and Young People Mental Health Coalition. Reslience and results: how to improve the mental and emotional wellbeing of children and young people in your school. Available at: http://www.cypmhc.org.uk/media/common/uploads/Final_pdf.pdf (accessed 14 March 2017).

7. Horton R. Launching a new movement for mental health. *Lancet* 2007; 369: 806.

8. Hagell A, Coleman J, Brooks F. *Key Data on Adolescence.* London: Public Health England, 2013.

9. Weare K, Nind M. Mental health promotion and problem prevention in schools: what does the evidence say? *Health Promot Int* 2011; 26 (Suppl 1): 26–69.

10. Durlak JA, Weissberg RP, Dymnicki AB, Taylor RD, Schellinger K. The impact of enhancing students' social and emotional learning: a meta-analysis of school-based universal interventions. *Child Dev* 2011; 82: 474–501.

11. Shucksmith J, Summerbell C, Jones S, Whittaker V. *Mental Wellbeing of Children in Primary Education (targeted/indicated activities).* London: National Institute of Health and Care Excellence, 2007.

12. Catalano, R., Berglund, M.L., Ryan, G.A.M., Lonczak, H.S. and Hawkins, J.D. (2002). Positive youth development in the United States: Research findings on evaluations of positive youth development programs. *Prevention and Treatment*, 5, Article 15.

13. Zins JE, Weissberg RP,Wang M, Walberg HJ. *Building Academic Success on Social and Emotional learning: What Does the Research Say?* New York: Teachers College Press, 2004.

14. Greenberg M, Jennings T. The prosocial classroom: teacher social and emotional competence in relation to student and classroom outcomes. *Rev Educ Res* 2009; 79: 491–525.

15. Weare K. *Promoting Mental, Emotional and Social Health: A Whole School Approach.* London: Routledge, 2000.

16. National Child and Maternal Health Intelligence Network. Findings from the national evaluation of targeted mental health in schools 2008 to 2011. Available at: https://www.gov.uk/government/publications/findings-from-the-national-evaluation-of-targeted-mental-health-in-schools-2008-to-2011 (accessed 15 March 2018).

17. Lendrum A, Humphrey N, Wigelsworth M. Social and emotional aspects of learning (SEAL) for secondary schools: implementation difficulties and their implications for school-based mental health promotion. *Child Adolesc Ment Health* 2013; 18: 158–164.

18. Banerjee R, Weare K, Farr W. Working with 'Social and Emotional Aspects of Learning' (SEAL): associations with school ethos, pupil social experiences, attendance, and attainment. *Br Educ Res J* 2014; 40: 718–742.

19. Department for Education. Social and emotional aspects of learning (SEAL) programme in secondary schools: national evaluation. Available at: https://www.gov.uk/government/publications/social-and-emotional-aspects-of-learning-seal-programme-in-secondary-schools-national-evaluation (accessed 14 March 2017).

20. Rowling L, Mason J. A case study of multimethod evaluation of complex school mental health promotion and prevention: the MindMatters Evaluation Suite. *Aust J Guidance Counsel* 2005; 15: 125–136.

21. Denman S, Moon A, Parsons C, Stears D. *The Health Promoting School: Policy, Research and Practice.* London: Routledge Falmer Press, 2001.

22. Crow I, France A, Hacking S, Hart M. The evaluation of three 'Communities that Care' demonstration projects. Joseph Rowntree Foundation. Available at: https://www.jrf.org.uk/report/evaluation-three-communities-care-demonstration-projects (accessed 14 March 2017).

23. Samdal O, and Rowling L. *The Implementation of Health Promoting Schools: Exploring the Theories of What, Why and How.* London: Routledge, 2014.

24. Greenberg MT, Domitrovich C, Bumbarger B. *Preventing Mental Disorders In School Aged Children. A Review of the Effectiveness of Prevention Programmes.* University Park, PA: Prevention Research Center for the Promotion of Human Development, College of Health and Human Development Pennsylvania State University, 2001.

25. Millings A, Buck R, Montgomery A, Spears M, Stallard P. School connectedness, peer attachment, and self-esteem as predictors of adolescent depression. *J Adolesc* 2012; 35: 1061–1067.

26. McLaughlin C. The Connected School: A Design for Well-being. Available at: http://cdn.basw.co.uk/upload/basw_111244-8.pdf (accessed 14 March 2017).

27. Adi Y, Killoran A, Janmohamed K, Stewart-Brown S. *Systematic Review of the Effectiveness of Interventions to Promotion Mental Wellbeing in Primary Schools.* London: National Institute for Health and Care Excellence, 2007.

28. Rowe F, Stewart D. Promoting connectedness through whole-school approaches: a qualitative study. *Health Education* 2009; 109: 396–413.

29. Department for Education. Behaviour and discipline in schools: advice for headteachers. Available at: https://www.gov.uk/government/publications/behaviour-and-discipline-in-schools (accessed 14 March 2018).

30. National Healthy Schools Programme. Guidance for schools on developing emotional health and wellbeing. Available at: http://www.healthyschoolslondon.org.uk/sites/default/files/EHWB.pdf (accessed 14 March 2017).

31. Young Minds. Stigma, A Review of the Evidence. Available at: https://childhub.org/en/child-protection-online-library/stigma-review-evidence (accessed 14 March 2017).

32. Murali V, Oyebode F. Poverty, social inequality and mental health *Adv Psychiatr Treat* 2004; 10: 216–224.

33. Children and Young People's Mental Health Coalition. Reslience and Results. How to improve the emotional and mental wellbeing of children and young people in your school. Available at: http://www.cypmhc.org.uk/media/common/uploads/Final_pdf.pdf (accessed 14 March 2017).

34. Almeida J, Johnson RM, Corliss HL. Emotional distress among LGBT youth: The influence of perceived discrimination based on sexual orientation. *J Youth Adolesc* 2009; 38: 1001–1014.

35. Patel V, Flisher AJ, Hetrick S, McGorry P. Mental health of young people: a global public-health challenge. *Lancet* 2007; 369: 1302–1313.

36. Rutter M, Hagel A, Giller H. *Anti-Social Behaviour and Young People.* Cambridge: Cambridge University Press, 1998.

37. Gross J (ed). *Getting in Early.* London: Smith Institute and the Centre for Social Justice, 2008.

38. Rones M, Hoagwood K. School-based mental health services: a research review. *Clin Child Fam Psychol Rev* 2000; 3: 223–241.

39. National Union of Teachers. Tackling Stress. Available at: https://www.teachers.org.uk/tackling-stress (accessed 15 March 2018).

40. Bajorek Z, Gulliford J, Taskila T. Healthy teachers, higher marks? Establishing a link between teacher health & wellbeing and student outcomes. Available at: https://www.educationsupportpartnership.

org.uk/sites/default/files/resources/healthy_teachers_higher_marks_
report_0.pdf (accessed 14 March 2017).

41. Weare K. The evidence for mindfulness: impacts on the wellbeing and performance of school staff. Available at: http://mindfulnessinschools. org/research/research-mindfulness-adults-education/ (accessed 14 March 2017).

42. Whitaker T, Whitaker B, Lumpa D. *Motivating and Inspiring Teachers: The Educational Leader's Guide for Building Staff Morale*, 2nd ed. Larchmont, NY: Eye On Education, 2009.

43. Department for Education. Me and My School: Findings from the National Evaluation of Targeted Mental Health in Schools 2008– 2011. Available at: https://www.gov.uk/government/uploads/system/ uploads/attachment_data/file/184060/DFE-RR177.pdf (accessed 14 March 2017).

44. Green J, Howes F, Waters E, Maher E, Oberklaid F. Promoting the social and emotional health of primary school aged children: reviewing the evidence base for school based interventions. *Int J Ment Health Promot* 2005; 7: 30–36.

45. Rogers B. *Classroom Behavior: A Practical Guide to Effective Teaching, Behavior Management and Colleague Support*, 4th ed. Thousand Oaks, CA: Sage, 2015.

46. Green H, McGinnity A, Meltzer H, Ford T, Goodman R. The mental health of young people in Great Britain, 2004. Available at: http://www. esds.ac.uk/doc/5269/mrdoc/pdf/5269technicalreport.pdf (accessed 14 March 2017).

47. Luiselli L, Putnam R, Handler M, Feinberg A. Whole-school positive behaviour support: effects on student discipline problems and academic performance. *Educ Psychol* 2005; 25: 183–198.

48. Boyatzis R. *Resonant Leadership*. Boston, MA: Harvard Business School, 2005.

49. CASEL. CASEL Program Guides: Effective Social and Emotional Learning Programs. Available at: http://www.casel.org/guide/ (accessed 14 March 2017).

50. All Party Parliamentary Group on Wellbeing Economics. Wellbeing in Four Policy Areas. Available at: http://b.3cdn.net/nefoundation/ ccdf9782b6d8700f7c_lcm6i2ed7.pdf (accessed 15 March 2018).

51. Browne G, Gafni A, Roberts J, Byrne C, Majumdar G. Effective/ efficient mental health programs for school-age children: a synthesis of reviews. *Soc Sci Med* 2004; 58: 1367–1384.

52. Merry SN, McDowell HH, Hetrick SE, Bir JJ, Muller N. Psychological and/or educational interventions for the prevention of depression in children and adolescents. *Cochrane Database Syst Rev* 2004; 2: CD003380.

53. Stallard P, Simpson N, Anderson S, Carter T, Osborn C, Bush S. An evaluation of the FRIENDS programme: a cognitive behaviour therapy intervention to promote emotional resilience. *Arch Dis Child* 2005; 90: 1016–1019.

54. Blueprint. Promoting Alternative Thinking Strategies: model programme. Available at: http://www.blueprintsprograms.com/ factsheet/promoting-alternative-thinking-strategies-paths (accessed 15 March 2018).

55. CASEL. CASEL Program Guides. Available at: http://www.casel.org/ guide/ (accessed 14 March 2017).

56. Diekstra R. Effectiveness of school-based social and emotional education programmes worldwide. In: *Social and Emotional Education: An International Analysis*. Santander: Fundacion Marcelino Botin, 2008, pp. 255–284.

56. Garrard W, Lipsey M. Conflict resolution education and anti-social behavior in US schools. A meta-analysis. *Conflict Resolut Q* 2007; 25: 9–37.

57. Department for Education. Mental health and behaviour in schools. Available at: https://www.gov.uk/government/publications/mental-health-and-behaviour-in-schools--2 (accessed 14 March 2017).

58. Youth in Mind. What is the SDQ? Available at: http://www.sdqinfo.org/ a0.html (accessed 15 March 2018).

59. Hennessy E, Heary C. Exploring children's views through focus groups. In: Greene S, Hogan D (eds). *Researching Children's Experience*. London: SAGE, 2005, pp. 236–252.

60. Whiteman H. Social media: how does it affect our mental health and well-being? Available at: http://www.medicalnewstoday.com/articles/ 275361.php (accessed 14 March 2017).

61. Student minds. The student mental health charity. Available at: http://www.studentminds.org.uk/about.html (accessed 14 March 2017).

CHAPTER 43

Early intervention in psychiatry

David J. Castle, Ana Lusicic, and Melissa Petrakis

Introduction

The notion of early intervention has gained substantial traction in recent years in the discipline of psychiatry. It is important to stress that early intervention does not necessarily equate with 'prevention' and also that psychiatry is bedevilled by the inexactitude of diagnosing 'at-risk' or even 'prodromal' states. Furthermore, while there is intuitive appeal in the notion that intervening early in the course of psychiatric disorders—not least in the hope that the longer-term course can be improved—*proving* that such interventions have such beneficial outcomes is fraught with methodological problems and the outcomes of many such studies are equivocal at best. There is also a perennial issue relating to 'how early' intervention should be. This is perhaps most starkly seen in disorders that have a putative neurodevelopmental aetiology, such as autism and schizophrenia, where, arguably, interventions should be from conception, aiming to 'protect' the vulnerable brain *in utero* and early extra-uterine life; yet this would not be feasible except perhaps in a genetic high-risk group. Finally, there are potential downsides to early intervention in terms of labelling, stigma, and exposure to interventions that might carry damaging side effects.

Having said all this, early intervention remains a worthy goal and is reaping some dividends in certain disease areas. This chapter provides a brief overview of selected disorders, encompassing examples of disorders that have an onset in childhood (autism); teenage years/early adulthood (bipolar disorder); and in later life (dementia). We then focus on schizophrenia, as schizophrenia is a disorder with ubiquity across the globe in terms of prevalence, which carries substantial disability and for which there are limited fully effective therapeutic interventions. It is also a disorder in which huge international investment has been made in early intervention, yet with relatively modest returns [1].

Autism spectrum disorders

The so-called autism spectrum disorders (ASD) are characterized by deficits in language and socialization, as well as a range of stereotyped behaviours. They can be enormously impairing for the individual and place a great burden on family members. Signs can be detected in some cases within the first year of life [2], although definitive diagnoses are often delayed and require specialist review and collection of collateral information, notably from parents.

There is emerging evidence that early intervention can be helpful for children with ASD, as well as their families. There is no single specific intervention that is a panacea and a multi-modal multidisciplinary approach is seen as the most effective. Tonge et al. [3] have

recently reviewed this literature and provide a synopsis of validated treatment strategies. They suggest that there are three critical components to such interventions, namely core components, child-focused interventions, and comprehensive interventions. Tonge et al. [3] go on to outline the elements of interventions that fit within these rubrics, and to weigh the evidence for the efficacy and effectiveness thereof. The elements include family involvement, neutral learning environments, coordinated care models, and child-focused interventions.

In terms of *family involvement*, it is acknowledged that parenting a child with ASD is one of the most stressful parenting experiences, partly owing to the lack of affective responsivity and 'warmth' that feeds mutuality in parent–child bonding; and the rigidity and difficulty with any changes to routine that constrict the spontaneity of family excursions and socializing, and which can result in difficult-to-manage behaviours. The impact on unaffected siblings can also be profound. Programs that have included psychoeducation for the family, along with specific strategies to deal with ASD-related behaviours and also promote effective communication, have been shown to be beneficial in reducing children's aberrant behaviours and enhancing parents' confidence [4].

Neutral learning environments are advocated for children with ASD to help integrate learning strategies into the child's everyday routines and to aid socialization [5]. However, unequivocal evidence for the efficacy of such programmes has been elusive [3].

Coordinated and well-articulated care models with excellent communication between team members and with the child and family are seen as crucial in meeting everyone's needs and avoiding mixed messages and confusion [6]. There are a number of specific models—the reader is referred to Tonge et al. [3] for details. It makes clinical and logistic sense that the earlier these elements can be adopted, the better for the individual and the family; however, we are not aware of any definitive data to support differential outcomes according to timing of intervention.

In terms of *child-focused interventions*, Tonge et al. [3] considered the following to have some empirical support, albeit there are a number of conflicting findings in the literature and long-term outcome studies are sparse:

- social skills training, peer training, and social story-based interventions;
- communication skills, termed 'augmentative and alternative communication systems';
- play and behaviour skills;

◆ positive behaviour support, with a focus of environmental manipulations to reduce exposure to environmental triggers and to teach new skills and reward positive behaviours.

Considering the role of *pharmacological interventions*, atypical antipsychotic agents have been employed in people with ASD, largely targeting problematic behaviours [7]. The metabolic side effects of these drugs has been a cause of great concern, expressly for young people and thus some clinicians are hesitant to use them and they would not generally be seen to have a role in early intervention per se (i.e. apart from managing symptoms). Risperidone and aripiprazole have, of the atypical antipsychotics, a relatively benign metabolic signal and have been approved for use in ASD. But even they are not free of weight gain, and monitoring of weight and other parameters is required.

Conclusions

Overall, early intervention in people with ASD and working effectively with a multidisciplinary team and encompassing a number of different parameters of care appears to reap dividends for many if not all cases. The use of medication needs to be weighed against side effect burden and should be used to target specific behaviours or symptoms, with careful and ongoing monitoring. As with many early-intervention trials, those in ASD have been inconsistent in terms of longer-term outcomes and this remains an area of scientific need.

Another fraught question is how to intervene early enough in the trajectory of ASD, to impact most effectively on the developing brain, in an 'at-risk' stage in infancy; as Webb et al. [8] put it, 'before core autism symptoms have emerged [with a view to] alter the developmental trajectory of children at risk for the disorder and impact long-range outcomes'. This is the holy grail of early intervention, and is bedevilled by diagnostic issues; problems with the predictive validity of early signs of disorder; and the difficulties in deploying comprehensive high-fidelity treatments and subjecting them to controlled trial scrutiny and evaluating them over protracted periods.

Bipolar disorder

Bipolar disorder is usually a recurrent illness with a vulnerability to high (hypomanic or manic) and low (depressed) moods. Although technically defined by the manic pole, many sufferers also experience severe and often prolonged depressive episodes. Bipolar disorder usually has an onset in early adulthood and may go undiagnosed for years or even decades. A number of treatments, including an array of medications ('mood stabilizers', e.g. lithium, sodium valproate, lamotrigine; and 'atypical antipsychotics', e.g. quetiapine and olanzapine), as well as different psychological approaches (cognitive–behavioural therapy (CBT), family interventions, psychoeducation) can ameliorate the longer-term course, but all too often patients continue to suffer relapses even if adherent to their treatment regimes [9, 10]. Relapses are damaging to the individual and loved ones, and there is increasing evidence that with each relapse subtle brain damage occurs, with impairment in cognitive functioning [11].

It has been shown that specialist clinical services that ensure optimal care of people with bipolar disorder early in their illness course can be effective in reducing relapse rates—at least as indexed by hospital admissions [12]. However, less clear is whether it is feasible to intervene effectively with individuals at 'high risk' for bipolar disorder before they actually manifest the illness itself. There have been various attempts to delineate individuals at high risk for bipolar disorder. For example, Hafeman et al. [13] used a sample of 359 people whose parents had bipolar disorder, to try to determine early warning signs of bipolar disorder. Only 14.7% actually developed a bipolar spectrum disorder over 8 years of follow-up: the strongest predictors were baseline anxiety/depression, affective lability and proximal affective instability; and manic-like symptoms. The authors suggest that this constellation was associated with a 49% 'conversion rate' to bipolar disorder, but this needs to be seen in the context of a genetically high-risk sampling frame, and how generalizable it is to general population samples is unclear. Also, it is difficult to establish how dimensional constructs such as these can be firmed up enough to differentiate clearly what is 'pathological' from what is normal perturbation of mood as part of child and adolescent development.

It is also not clear what interventions might be effective and safe in putative high-risk cases. Certainly, there is major concern surrounding the use of antipsychotic medications in young children purported to have bipolar disorder: metabolic problems are especially worrying [14, 15]. An arguably more benign strategy has been to provide a family intervention that has been adapted from one used in people with established bipolar disorder. Miklowitz et al. [16] used this approach in a randomized trial of family-focused therapy delivered over a 4-month period, in 40 young people (age range 9–17 years) who were manifesting mood problems and who had a family history of bipolar disorder. Family-focused therapy was—compared with a simple education control intervention—associated with a more rapid resolution of their current mood state and was associated with a more favourable illness course over the ensuing 8 months.

Conclusions

Many authorities in the field point to the impairments associated with youth-onset bipolar, the often long lag before definitive treatment, and the potentially reduced treatment response associated with progressive disorder, as justifying treatment of putative high-risk individuals, essentially using treatments with established utility in people with the full disorder [17]. This is a potentially dangerous approach, given problems with side effects of treatments and the lack of specificity of high-risk criteria, as detailed earlier. There is also a lack of empirical evidence to support any 'preventative' action for any of these interventions. But early provision of psycho-education, monitoring, and family-based interventions do seem to have utility and can, at the very least, serve to engage individuals in a therapeutic manner such that they can access evidence-based medications and other treatments should they progress to a full-blown mood disorder.

The dementias

The dementias are a major problem in ageing societies and place enormous burden on individuals, family members, the healthcare system, and society more broadly. Early diagnosis and intervention has been a goal of clinicians and scientists for decades. One of the barriers is to determine accurately what might be the harbingers of dementia, as opposed to what might be considered normal ageing.

People with dementia often lack awareness of their cognitive decline and it might be only family members who notice the signs and symptoms, which initially might be subtle. Screening measures for dementia, such as the Mini-Mental State Examination [18], have an established place in clinical settings but may miss early disease states and their use in general population settings has been questioned [19].

For individuals who are 'screen positive' or in whom there is clinical evidence of a dementing process, a full diagnostic work-up is required. This should encompass a thorough cognitive assessment with established psychometric tools, as well as evaluation of psychiatric and physical co-morbidities that might be causal or contributory to the cognitive decline: examples of the former include depression, and of the latter, endocrine disorders and malignancies. Delirium is an important differential diagnosis and can also exacerbate cognitive dysfunction in people with dementia. Brian imaging, using computed tomographic scanning or magnetic resonance imaging, is recommended for diagnostic purposes, as well as to establish the subtype of dementia (e.g. Alzheimer's disease vs Lewy body dementia vs cerebrovascular dementia), as prognosis and treatment may differ according to aetiology (e.g. addressing cardiovascular risk issues in cerebrovascular dementia). Subtyping may also be aided by functional neuroimaging, including single photon emission computed tomography [20], as well as positron emission tomography. There has also been recent interest in amyloid imaging and cerebrospinal fluid assays for beta-amyloid and tau, but their place in accurate prediction of who will go on to develop dementia—and which subtype—remains to be determined [19, 21].

If a diagnosis of early dementia is made, there are a number of *medications* that seem to have the ability at least to slow the rate of cognitive decline; in some studies there is evidence of modest improvement in certain aspects of cognition with these agents. Most research has been done in Alzheimer's disease, where acetylcholinesterase inhibitors (donezapil, galantamine, rivastigmine) and the N-methyl-D-aspartic acid receptor antagonists (memantine) have regulatory approval. The acetylcholinesterase inhibitors are used in mild-to-moderate disease, whereas memantine is supposed to be restricted to later illness stages [22].

Certain *non-pharmacological interventions* also have supportive evidence in potentially reducing progression of 'at-risk' individuals to dementia. Perhaps the most compelling, as well as being relatively cheap and easily adopted, is exercise. For example, Lautenschlager et al. [23] randomized 170 people over 50 years of age who reported memory issues but did not meet diagnostic criteria for dementia, to 24 weeks of physical activity and found improved cognitive functioning according to the Alzheimer's Disease Cognitive Assessment Scale–Cognitive Subscale (ADAS-Cog) [24]; controls who did not engage in the exercise regime showed a decline in ADAS-Cog scores. Subsequent research has lent further support to the importance of exercise in at least delaying dementia in at-risk individuals.

Conclusions

The benefits of early intervention in dementia are thus more exciting than one might think. Of course the translation of these findings into general clinical practice remains a challenge, and many of the medications are expensive. The exact stage at which early intervention should begin is difficult to ascertain, as is how long to

continue. Again, more long-term research studies are required, and consideration should be given to whether combinations of different interventions will reap greater dividends than individual interventions, for example a combination of medication plus exercise.

Schizophrenia and related psychoses

Schizophrenia is a disorder that can have a profound effect upon the life of sufferers and their families [25]. It occurs at a rate of around 1% across the globe and often has a protracted course with decline in functioning and a restriction of the ability to engage fully in society. The more severely affected individuals often have an onset in youth or early adulthood, impairing their psychosocial and vocational achievements. There are also common psychiatric co-morbidities such as depression, as well as high rates of illicit substance use. Life expectancy is also dramatically reduced, driven largely by cardiovascular disease and also by suicide.

Given all this, it is again hardly surprising that there has been substantial global investment in early intervention in schizophrenia. Here we review such interventions and weigh the evidence regarding efficacy. Firstly, we address the issue of early detection and duration of untreated psychosis (DUP), and ask whether it is possible to ascertain accurately individuals who are at high risk for schizophrenia.

Early detection and duration of untreated psychosis

Early detection of psychotic disorders, DUP, and its association with prognosis have been among the most intriguing and complex topics in psychosis research over the past three decades. In the early 1990s, Wyatt [26] proposed a 'neurotoxic effect' of psychosis on the brain and reported that patients with long DUP respond less well to treatment. This notion was coupled with ideas that early detection, and medical and social interventions in early, 'critical' stages of illness might modify outcomes of psychotic disorders, notably schizophrenia [27, 28]. Subsequently, DUP has been seen as the most promising potentially modifiable factor that can influence outcome, and, as such, to represent a viable target of public health early detection and intervention services established on a worldwide scale.

Over the years, research findings showing small prognostic relevance of DUP and short-term effects of early detection initiatives increasingly illuminated the need for careful and critical interpretation of evidence [29]. Meta-analyses and critical reviews reported very modest correlations between prolonged, untreated, non-affective psychosis and lower levels of both symptomatic and functional recovery. This is independent of variables known to be associated with poor prognosis and chronic stage of illness (e.g. pre-morbid functioning and mode of onset [30]). Differences between study designs and duration of follow-up limit the reliability of conclusions. Marshall et al. [31] performed a meta-analysis looking at correlations between DUP and an array of symptomatic and functional outcomes in studies with strictly schizophrenia-like disorders, using standardized assessment of DUP and having over 80% follow-up rates. At baseline, the only statistically significant correlations with long DUP were depression/anxiety (correlation coefficient 0.107, 95% confidence interval (CI) 0.025–0.188) and quality of life (correlation coefficient 0.188, CI 0.081–0.290). At the 6- and 12-month follow-up, only weak-to-moderate effects sizes were found for correlations between DUP and all symptoms, depression/anxiety, disorganized, negative and positive symptoms, and overall functioning. Marshall et al. [31] calculated that DUP could explain only 13% of the variance for all symptoms at 6 months. By the 24-month time point, limited data were available, but weak correlations between longer DUP and worse outcome for overall functioning, positive symptoms, and quality of life were maintained, albeit not for social functioning and negative symptoms. Individuals with longer DUP were more likely not to achieve remission at follow-up. Adjustment for pre-morbid potential confounding factors did not alter the results. Limitations noted were lack of blinding to DUP status across studies and insufficient data to permit assessment of publication bias.

Long-term prospective studies are small in number, often presenting contradictory findings, likely as a result of methodological differences between studies. Harris et al. [32] looked at quality of life as an outcome at 8 years in a schizophrenia spectrum sample; 23.9% of outcome variance was explained jointly by predictors such as gender, age of onset of illness, pre-morbid adjustment, education, and duration of prodrome, whereas only 3.3% of outcome variance was explained by DUP. At 12 years, longer DUP predicted poorer remission status, more severe positive and negative symptoms, and greater impairment in general functioning, social functioning, and quality of life, whereas the effect on functioning was largely mediated by concurrent negative symptoms [33]. DUP has been found to be very modestly associated with negative symptoms at longer-term follow-up (5–8 years) [34]. A study examining DUP and long-term symptomatic remission over 13 years showed that the odds of long-term remission was significantly reduced for patients with long DUP compared with people with short DUP, with specific impact on negative symptom remission [35]. Penttilä et al. [36] described a modest correlation between DUP and long-term symptomatic, functional, and global outcomes.

Limited evidence of the correlation of DUP and poor outcome on a range of clinical and functional variables has been a point of debate, partially owing to significant study variations on assessment and definition of DUP; inclusion of broad diagnostic categories encompassing affective psychosis; and lack of reporting on publication bias. DUP has been defined as the period between onset of psychotic symptoms and initiation of pharmacological treatment, but few studies have employed systematized methods of its assessment [31, 37]. Although it is a complex construct, influenced by mode of onset and type of psychotic disorder, in research it has been mostly described as a one-dimensional variable of time, with only modest attempts to examine it comprehensively [38]. Also, cut-off points that define short from long duration of DUP vary significantly between studies, with most reporting associations with outcomes with DUP extending over 3 months [32, 34, 35, 39].

There is an ongoing question as to whether DUP represents a marker or determinant of poor prognosis. The UK-based AESOP (Aetiology and Ethnicity in Schizophrenia and Other Psychoses) study found DUP to be correlated with insidious onset, non-affective psychosis, and reduced social network, all commonly identified as predictors of poor outcome, reflecting the possibility that long, insidious DUP represents an intrinsic feature of a more chronic underlying illness.

Despite the weak correlation between DUP and outcome variable, and the very modest contribution of DUP to determination

of longitudinal trajectory, DUP has been a target of early detection campaigns and intervention strategies with considerable financial investment, despite low clinical benefits. Studies looking at early detection strategies identified a range of different approaches from direct contact via general practitioners (GPs) such as in LEOCAT [40, 41] and REDIRECT [42]; specialized service development (Early Psychosis Prevention and Intervention Centre (EPPIC)); or a multi-targeted approach using multimedia, direct contact, and service development such as in TIPS [43], PEPP [44] and EPIP [45]. Interpretation of results and generalizability of findings are compromised by lack of reliable measurements between intervention and non-intervention areas, issues with assessment of DUP, and study design variation.

Lloyd-Evans et al. [46] concluded that GP education campaigns and specialized early-intervention services do not appear to impact DUP significantly, whereas evidence for parallel different initiatives is mixed. At-risk state criteria have been developed to assist in identifying potential cases in the community, but the low transition rate to psychotic disorder indicate need for ongoing research and critical view of findings, especially in light of non-specific symptoms associated with the prodromal period [47].

Conclusions

The contribution of DUP to outcome in schizophrenia is weak. Early intervention services alone do not have much impact on DUP and there is no convincing evidence that early detection and intervention affect the underlying disease process.

Models of care

There are several models of care introduced in early intervention in psychosis. *Specialist/standalone models* include intensive case management with the aim of having a low case load of up to 10–15 patients per case manager complemented by assertive outreach [48]. The focus is on ensuring the delivery of a range of early-intervention-focused pharmacological and psychosocial interventions. Across established services in Australia, UK, the USA, and Canada, care is delivered for a specific period of time (usually 2–3 years) and mostly target young people and early adult-onset patients (mostly between 15 and 35 years of age). Specialist services include in-patient service, crisis and assertive intervention functions, and continuing care functionality. The pros and cons of such standalone models have been debated, focusing on having limited treatment periods and problems of transfer of patient care to general mental health services; diversion of funding away from general mental health services and deskilling of professionals working in such centres in longer-term care provision; and likewise deskilling clinicians in other services in terms of dealing with early-stage illness [1].

'Hub-and-spoke' models of early-intervention services were developed in part in response to a need to implement specialist skills in rural and remote areas [49]. The 'hub' represents a centre that can provide fundamental support via clinical supervision, as well as training and education for rural specialist staff of different clinical backgrounds ('spokes') who are working in community mental health centres. The central functionality includes management and leadership support and leading relevant public health initiatives. Some advantages of this model include consistency of care, enhancing specialist skills in clinical staff, and lower costs

associated with keeping the model alive. Conversely, limitations of the model include the potential lack of specialist skills and a more limited early-intervention focus [48].

The *specialist outreach model* has been introduced in Canada, for example, to help translate best practice developed in urban centres to rural areas. In an evaluation of this approach, there was no statistically significant difference between specialist outreach clients and hub-and-spoke patients, although the hub-and-spoke model showed a trend towards better community outcomes and fewer hospital admissions [50].

An *integrated* or 'specialist-within-generalist' model seeks to have case managers with skills and training in delivering early intervention embedded into community mental health teams. This has a number of advantages over 'standalone' models and is effective at delivering a high-fidelity service meeting established criteria for the field of early intervention for psychosis [51, 52]. A potential limitation of the model is maintaining the early-intervention ethos and philosophy of care as clinicians might have little contact with others in similar roles and other services demands might divert them [48].

Conclusions

There are a number of different models that aim to achieve comprehensive care for people early in the evolution of their psychotic disorder. No one model has convincingly been shown to be better or worse that another, but standalone models suffer from a number of problems associated with silo effects.

Family-based interventions

The role played by friends and family members in the recovery of individuals with early psychosis is extremely important [53–55]. In addition to helping to create a 'safe, sound and supportive environment to help their loved one with his or her recovery' [56], family members and friends engage in other practical and social tasks such as playing a significant role in first accessing mental health services for their family member [57]. This role extends into encouraging the individual to remain engaged in treatment [56] and in encouraging adherence to their medication regimen, monitoring for signs of depression and suicidality, and identifying and responding to early warning signs of psychotic relapse [57].

An early-intervention approach to service delivery is highly compatible with family work, and early psychosis clinical guidelines stipulate that services should be family inclusive in delivery of psychosocial interventions [58].

The evidence base for family intervention in severe mental illness generally is well recognized. However, it has not yet been established how mental health services can best support and utilize family and friends to meet their full potential as a core component in recovery from early psychosis [59].

The most common family interventions in early psychosis has been the provision of groups, focused on psychoeducation, fostering coping strategies, the improvement of relationships and developing peer support [54, 56, 60]. Groups may be multi-family groups, made up of carers from multiple families and including the person experiencing the psychotic illness, or groups with participants made up of only carers.

Studies of multi-family groups, based on the work of McFarlane and colleagues in Canada since the 1990s [55], have described positive impacts on people having experienced early psychosis, as well as their friends or family members [60, 61]. However, some of the positive outcomes, such as improved knowledge of psychosis, seem not to be specific to the multi-family model as they were also found in studies looking at different group interventions [62].

Despite the appeal of the multi-family approach, a number of early psychosis services have consciously moved away from this model because of an identified need for families and friends to have their own space for support, education, and reflection without the presence of their unwell friend or relative. As with the studies of multi-family groups, positive outcomes have been reported for groups encompassing family and friends without the presence of the person who has experienced psychosis [56, 62–64]. Many participants reported that the informal peer support was greatly valued and they experienced a reduction in perceived stigma, improved knowledge of psychosis, and better coping strategies [56, 62–64]. An advantage of group participation is the benefit of peer support [60, 61, 64]. Lowenstein et al. [64] opined: 'The most important aspects of the groups to carers were learning they were not the only ones experiencing challenges and learning that others have the same thoughts and feelings' (p. 632).

Riley et al. [56] conducted thematic analysis of a focus group for carers who participated in an 8-week group programme. Themes identified were, firstly, friends and family members' feelings about being identified as a 'carer'; and, secondly, identifying some of the barriers to group participation, for example location of the group or anxiety about leaving their unwell relative.

Benefits of peer support for friends and family that occurs naturally in a group setting has been emphasized. The beneficial aspects of peer support in conjunction with a 'sense of collective experience' (p. 99) are also evident in the study of Petrakis et al. [62]. This study explored not only the experiences of carers who participated in the group, but also of those who chose not to participate, as well as the group facilitators and other relevant mental health professionals. Interview data from both carers and their unwell family member emphasized the value of peer support, and that group participation increased understanding of mental illness and treatment. Conclusions drawn were that group participation is associated with a variety of benefits, including increased knowledge about mental illness and enhanced skills for the caring role.

McCann et al. [65] gathered qualitative data from 20 carers to learn about their interactions with mental health clinicians. Responses were largely positive, but carers sometimes felt locked out of treatment decisions. This was attributed to clinicians' concerns about consumer confidentiality. In another study, Naik and Bowden [66] found that carers generally felt that services met their own guidelines but that challenges concerning ease of access to services remained. Sin et al. [57] assessed service developments made in response to an earlier phenomenological study of early psychosis carer needs. These comprised a psychoeducation group, individual family interventions, and the implementation of a care pathway formalizing family-inclusive practice, and referral pathways were implemented. It was noted that these developments improved family inclusiveness in the service.

Despite reported benefits of participating in different types of group interventions, the literature notes very low carer uptake of such groups [57, 60, 62]. Petrakis et al. [62] collected information from carers who chose not to participate in an offered group, and reported barriers including other commitments (e.g. work) and a belief that mental illness matters are private. Cabral and Chaves [61] found that all of the participants in their intervention were women who did not work outside the home; therefore, others, potentially, would not or could not access the group. Finally, Riley et al. [56] noted that many of the participants in their study did not relate to the term 'carer' but preferred to describe their relationship differently, for example as a 'parent' (p. 60). This could represent a further potential barrier to group recruitment.

In assessing outcomes associated with family interventions in early psychosis, two reviews have been published [54, 59]. Bird et al. [54] identified only three pertinent randomized control trials (RCTs), whereas Askey et al. [59] included seven studies, of which five were RCTs. Across the two reviews, there were two studies of group based family interventions; the remainder of the studies were delivered on an individual family basis. Bird et al. [54] concluded that there was consistent evidence supporting the use of family intervention in early psychosis, whereas Askey et al. [59] were more reticent, suggesting that family functioning and stage of illness are factors that must be considered in determining whether to deliver family intervention to prevent a negative impact from the interventions.

Conclusions

Family intervention in the context of early psychosis is promoted in many practice guidelines [58]. However, to date, most of the studies have been small, qualitative studies from early psychosis services, without control groups. Research has predominantly evaluated group-based family support and education as an adjunct to routine service delivery. Studies have argued for greater levels of family intervention in routine service provision [57, 64].

Interventions addressing employment

For people who experience severe mental illness, employment offers benefits, including a reduction in psychotic symptoms, improvement in psychological health and overall well-being, and financial security [67, 68]. Indeed, people who experience mental illness frequently state that securing employment is a key task in their journey to recovery [69, 70]. A focus on work and education as meaningful for self-esteem and as a stepping stone to work is therefore very important in early intervention.

Individual Placement and Support (IPS) is an evidence-based model of supported employment that has been validated in randomized controlled trials (RCTs) and shown itself to be the most successful approach to date for supporting people with a severe mental illness to gain employment [68]. The model comprises the following eight principles [71]:

1. A goal of competitive paid employment.

2. Eligibility is based on client choice.

3. Integrated mental health and employment services.

4. Client preferences are honoured over provider judgements.

5. Rapid job searching.

6. Systematic job development.

7. Time-unlimited and individualized ongoing support.

8. Personalized benefits counselling.

Unemployment has been found to be 10 times higher in young people experiencing first-episode psychosis (FEP) compared with their peers without illness [72]. As age of onset of psychosis often coincides with the transition to further education or employment,

individuals may experience ongoing and prevailing disadvantages in relation to vocational pursuits, particularly if psychosis advances to a more severe and persistent illness [70]. In a modest but promising Australian youth study, Killackey et al. [72] conducted an RCT of a FEP cohort, comparing 6 months of IPS with treatment as usual. Under IPS 65% of individuals ($n = 20$) commenced competitive employment versus only 9.5% of the participants receiving treatment as usual ($n = 21$).

Conclusions

Traditionally, adult models of supported employment have been based on a stepwise approach, whereby patients participate in pre-vocational training and assessment for 'work-readiness' before being placed in work considered appropriate. This approach has been criticized and found to be less effective than individualized placement and support. In working in early intervention it is especially important to harness hope and motivation, working towards personalized job searching and skill development as soon as an individual expresses interest.

Addressing substance-related co-morbidities

In adults experiencing severe and persistent mental illness, smoking and alcohol use are highly prevalent and have been associated with early mortality. In the USA, Hartz et al. [73] undertook a comprehensive analysis of substance use behaviours, drawing on a clinically assessed, diversely ethnic sample of 9142 people with a diagnosis of schizophrenia, bipolar disorder with psychotic features, or schizoaffective disorder, versus 10,195 population controls. They found that for both sexes and all races/ethnicities (with a sample including African Americans, Asians, European Americans, and Hispanic individuals) there were greatly elevated risks for smoking and alcohol use, marijuana use, and drug use in the patient population. Smoking measures were particularly strongly associated with psychotic disorders, with estimated odds ratios (ORs) of 4.61 for smoking more than 100 cigarettes ($P < 1.0 \times 10^{-325}$) and 5.11 for daily smoking for more than 1 month ($P < 1.0 \times 10^{-325}$). Estimated ORs were also highly clinically and statistically significant for alcohol use ($3.96, P = 1.2 \times 10^{-188}$), marijuana use ($3.47, P = 2.6 \times 10^{-254}$), and for recreational drug use ($4.62, P < 1.0 \times 10^{-325}$). Relevant to the early intervention field, it was noted by the authors to be of specific concern that recent public health efforts, while successfully decreasing smoking among people younger than 30 years of age, appear not to have been effective in affecting behaviours in individuals with severe psychotic mental illnesses.

A meta-analysis of studies that examined the prevalence and course of tobacco use specifically in FEP found a high prevalence of tobacco use (58.9%). Patients with FEP had typically smoked for some years prior to the onset of their psychosis; had high use at the time of treatment presentation; and were much more likely to smoke than aged-matched controls [74]. Tobacco cessation programmes and interventions targeted at reducing cardiovascular disease appear not to be producing the hope for reductions in behaviours as the prevalence of tobacco use at intervals between 6 and 120 months following treatment were found to have remained unchanged (OR 0.996; 95% CI 0.907–1.094).

A retrospective medical record study from EPPIC in Melbourne, Australia, reported that a lifetime prevalence of co-morbid substance use disorders of 74% was reduced (during the treatment period) to 36% in patients who completed a full 18 months of treatment within the EPPIC programme [75]. It should be noted, however, that of the 643 patients, 15 experiencing major depressive episodes with psychotic symptoms were omitted from the analyses, as were 273 individuals who did not complete 18 months of treatment at EPPIC. The authors noted that persistent substance use is associated with treatment non-adherence, dropping out of treatment and having low remission rates.

The principles for clinical management of FEP include that all patients with FEP should be screened and monitored for co-morbid substance use; and that early, intensive, specialized pharmacological, and psychosocial interventions should be integrated in a comprehensive longitudinal model of care [76]. In Canada, Addington and Addington [77] noted a high prevalence of substance use disorder (51% overall: 33% with cannabis and 35% with alcohol) in a FEP sample. They reported that with active treatment, numbers with an alcohol substance use disorder declined considerably within 1 year, whereas for cannabis this was possible by 2 years. There remains, however, a substantial problem in engagement of this patient group and a lack of controlled trial data to define which treatments are most effective.

Conclusions

There is an established co-morbid pathology of substance use in people experiencing severe psychotic mental illnesses, across social and cultural groups, and the prevalence has been underestimated. It seems that public health campaigns to reduce substance use have not had a notable impact for those early in the course of a severe psychotic illness. Intervention studies in early intervention have not consistently established efficacious approaches to reduce use of tobacco, alcohol, cannabis, and illicit substances in people experiencing early psychosis. Integration of treatment between specialist mental health and substance use services and systems remains a challenge for people experiencing early psychosis with comorbid substance use conditions.

Psychological interventions

Psychological treatment in psychosis has emerged as an important treatment adjunct to pharmacotherapy aimed at alleviating symptoms of psychosis, co-morbid depressive and anxiety symptoms, and to help improve overall outcomes. In early psychosis, psychological work and research has been conducted in prodromal states, FEP, post-psychotic recovery, co-morbidities (i.e. anxiety, depression, substance use disorders), including family work.

Review studies have identified different targets and gaps for psychological treatments in early-intervention programmes [78–80]. *Indicated prevention* in people who are in prodromal phases of psychotic illness as per predefined criteria has largely focused on the prevention of transition to psychosis [81, 82]. Pharmacotherapy in this patient group has been a controversial issue, especially in the context of previously failed trials, safety, and ethical considerations. In this context, psychological approaches have definite appeal, given their relative lack of side effects.

CBT has established a reasonable evidence base in treatment of depression and anxiety symptoms, commonly encountered in at-risk populations, whereas other research shows promise in treatment of delusions and hallucinations. However, there are few trials of psychological interventions in the early phases of psychosis, and those that have been performed have yielded mixed results in terms of benefits on symptoms and functional

outcomes [83]. Therapeutic goals of CBT are related to managing distress associated with symptoms, an understanding of the psychotic experience, and managing concomitant affective and anxiety symptoms [84]. Studies of CBT in early phases of schizophrenia are scarce, with a few landmark studies in the field showing trends towards improvement of positive symptoms in CBT compared with supportive therapy initially, with comparable advantage to treatment as usual at 18 months on symptom, relapse rate, and hospitalization rate improvement [78, 85]. However, large RCTs such as that of Yung et al. [82] and Morrison et al. [79] have failed to show statistically or clinically robust evidence of efficacy in putatively 'high-risk' individuals.

Cognitive remediation seeks to address cognitive deficits directly and thus has appeal as an intervention, expressly in light of the lack of pharmacological tools effectively tackling cognitive deficits in psychotic disorders. Effect sizes for cognitive remediation treatment in early phases of schizophrenia are smaller than those in trials of people with chronic schizophrenia, but there are meaningful improvements in cognition, symptoms and functioning [86].

Pharmacological interventions

The pharmacological treatment of FEP aims, apart from management of psychotic symptoms, to treat patients in an arguably more 'responsive' stage of illness and thus target underlying neurobiological processes, ultimately improving clinical and functional outcomes. To date, there are few convincing data to support the latter, but this does not detract from judicious use of pharmacotherapy, at the lowest effective dose and with a clear view to minimization of side effects, as a crucial plank in the treatment of patients with early psychosis. It is also important that this is done in the context of a thorough bio-psychosocial formulation, as well as a comprehensive care plan responsive to the developmental stage of the individual.

Clinical practice guidelines recommend pharmacological intervention using a minimal effective dose of conventional or atypical antipsychotics in schizophrenia spectrum disorders for at least 12 months [87–90]. Compared with chronic patients, patients with FEP are considered to have higher response rates; require lower antipsychotic doses; and have a higher sensitivity to adverse effects [91]. Available studies report cumulative response measured at different time points within 8–16 weeks of treatment with a single typical or atypical antipsychotic medication for FEP [92, 93]. Data on treatment with either olanzapine or haloperidol indicates that early responders differ from non-responders by separation in mean Positive and Negative Syndrome Scale (PANSS) score as early as after 1 week of treatment, and late non-responders can be identified with high specificity by the second week of treatment (i.e. 73.9% of late non-responders at week 12 could be been identified at week 2 of treatment). However, after 2 weeks of treatment fewer than half of patients met criteria for minimal response (defined as more than 26.2% improvement in PANSS total score), whereas at week 10, 61% of patients were non-responders according to PANSS total score threshold of > 50% [94]. Kinon et al. [95] describe early response to antipsychotic treatment (i.e. at 2 weeks) as a reliable marker predicting later clinical outcomes at 12 weeks, favouring early switching to another antipsychotic (in that study, from risperidone to olanzapine) although impact on reduction of PANSS score was minimal.

In terms of which antipsychotic to choose in the first episode, Zhang et al. [96] performed a meta-analysis of available randomized trials of FEP and showed similar efficacy in terms of overall symptom reduction and response rates at the 3-month follow-up between first-generation antipsychotics (FGAs; haloperidol, chlorpromazine, molindone, sulpiride, zuclopenthixol) and second-generation antipsychotics (SGA; olanzapine, risperidone, quetiapine, ziprasidone, amisulpride, clozapine) [96]. However, pooled effect sizes showed that SGAs outperformed FGAs on negative symptoms and cognitive composite score, but this effect was lost when adjusted for sponsorship bias: industry-sponsored studies favoured SGAs, whereas non-industry-sponsored studies favoured FGAs.

Given the lack of clear separation between agents in terms of efficacy, clinicians tend to stress tolerability in their decision-making. In the aforementioned meta-analysis, SGAs were, overall, better tolerated than FGAs and showed lower treatment discontinuation rates [96]. However, there is wide diversity of side effect profiles among the SGAs, and clinicians should be wary of using medications 'first line' that carry, for example, a high risk of the metabolic syndrome [90]. The early use of clozapine has also been suggested for some patients who seem to have a treatment unresponsive type of illness, but, again, the metabolic and other side effects associated with that drug need to be entered into the equation [90]. Overall, the adoption of a 'shared decision-making' approach with full consultation with the individual and their family (where appropriate) should underpin antipsychotic prescribing in the first—and indeed subsequent—episodes of psychosis.

It is well known that maintaining adherence is a major challenge in the management of psychiatric illness. Multifactorial determinants of adherence encompass patient, medication, illness, and environmental factors. Good levels of social support and early medication acceptance have been shown to predict non-adherence in the first 6 months of treatment [97]. Ongoing substance abuse, depression, and failure to respond to treatment, along with higher cognitive baseline, ethnicity, and reaching remission status, were significantly related to lower medication adherence [98].

One strategy to enhance adherence in psychotic disorders is the use of long-lasting (injectable) antipsychotics (LAIs). Studies of LAI use in patients with FEP are scarce. A summary of the available evidence suggests effectiveness and safety in the early stages of treatment, with most data available on risperidone LAI compared with olanzapine long-acting injectable and paliperidone palmitate [99]. There is, however, a lack of comparability data between long-acting and oral treatment, as well as head-to-head comparisons between long-acting antipsychotics, in patients with FEP.

Delay in the decision to use antipsychotic medication versus solely psychosocial interventions in FEP has been analysed in light of well-recognized diagnostic heterogeneity in FEP. Some authors consider that this heterogeneity reflects the inclusion of broader patient samples with transdiagnostic psychotic symptoms captured by early detection initiatives [100, 101]. This raises the proposition that delay in antipsychotic treatment or using solely intensive psychosocial intervention via specialized early intervention services is possibly sufficient in a subgroup of patients with psychotic symptoms [100]. Studies in patients considered at ultra-high risk of psychosis exploring use of antipsychotics versus CBT via early-intervention services have not provided sufficiently reliable data for definite conclusions on effectiveness and safety of antipsychotic use in this group of individuals [102].

Conclusions

The appeal of early intervention for psychotic disorders with a hope that one is ameliorating the longitudinal course of the illness cannot be understated. Regrettably, despite substantial research and service investment over the last decade, few robust findings have emerged to support the benefit of such programmes beyond some benefits that accrue during the time that they are actually being delivered; arguably, this could merely be a reflection of good psychiatric care being good for patients, independent of their illness stage. Interventions aimed at 'ultra-high-risk' groups have also largely failed to impact on illness course. Of course, this does not suggest that early intervention is a bad thing. It merely suggests that schizophrenia and related disorders are illnesses in which some people have a particularly pernicious course and require ongoing concerted care. It also suggests that perhaps we should be looking at a much earlier window for intervention. It is well known that *in utero* exposures to adverse environmental factors ranging from maternal smoking to stress to certain infections and nutritional deficiencies, along with certain early-life risk factors (e.g. cannabis use), can increase risk for schizophrenia. Focused targeting of genetically high-risk pregnancies might be a 'best bet' for actual prevention of (at least some cases) of schizophrenia.

Acknowledgements

We are most grateful to Nicola Lautenschlager for useful comments on a previous draft of the 'Dementia' section of this chapter, and to Mary Veljanovska for formatting.

References

1. Castle DJ, Singh SP. Early intervention in psychosis: still the 'best buy'? *Br J Psychiatry* 2015; 207: 288–292.
2. Lord C, Luyster R, Guthrie W, Pickles A. Patterns of developmental trajectories in toddlers with autism spectrum disorder. *J Consult Clin Psychol* 2012; 80: 477.
3. Tonge BJ, Bull K, Brereton A, Wilson R. A review of evidence-based early intervention for behavioural problems in children with autism spectrum disorder: the core components of effective programs, child-focused interventions and comprehensive treatment models. *Curr Opin Psychiatry* 2014 ; 27: 158–165.
4. Roux G, Sofronoff K, Sanders M. A randomized controlled trial of group Stepping Stones Triple P: a mixed-disability trial. *Fam Process* 2013; 52: 411–424.
5. Childress DC. Special instruction and natural environments: Best practices in early intervention. *Infant Young Child* 2004; 17: 162–170.
6. Odom SL, Boyd BA, Hall LJ, Hume K. Evaluation of comprehensive treatment models for individuals with autism spectrum disorders. *J Autism Dev Disord* 2010; 40: 425–436.
7. Cohen D, Raffin M, Canitano R, et al. Risperidone or aripiprazole in children and adolescents with autism and/or intellectual disability: a Bayesian meta-analysis of efficacy and secondary effects. *Res Autism Spectr Disord* 2013; 7: 167–175.
8. Webb SJ, Jones EJ, Kelly J, Dawson G. The motivation for very early intervention for infants at high risk for autism spectrum disorders. *Int J Speech Lang Pathol* 2014; 16: 36–42.
9. Lauder SD, Berk M, Castle DJ, Dodd S, Berk L. The role of psychotherapy in bipolar disorder. *Med J Aust* 2010; 193(4 Suppl.): S31–S35.

10. Malhi GS, Bassett D, Boyce P, et al. Royal Australian and New Zealand College of Psychiatrists clinical practice guidelines for mood disorders. *Aust N Z J Psychiatry* 2015; 49: 1087–1206.

11. Torres IJ, Boudreau VG, Yatham LN. Neuropsychological functioning in euthymic bipolar disorder: a meta-analysis. *Acta Psychiatr Scand* 2007; 116(s434): 17–26.

12. Kessing LV, Hansen HV, Hvenegaard A, et al. Treatment in a specialised out-patient mood disorder clinic v. standard out-patient treatment in the early course of bipolar disorder: randomised clinical trial. *Br J Psychiatry* 2013; 202: 212–219.

13. Hafeman DM, Merranko J, Axelson D, et al. Toward the definition of a bipolar prodrome: dimensional predictors of bipolar spectrum disorders in at-risk youths. *Am J Psychiatry* 2016; 173: 695–704.

14. Frances A, Batstra L. Why so many epidemics of childhood mental disorder?. *J Dev Behav Pediatr* 2013; 34: 291–292.

15. Kowatch RA, Fristad M, Birmaher B, Wagner KD, Findling RL, Hellander M. Treatment guidelines for children and adolescents with bipolar disorder. *J Am Acad Child Adolesc Psychiatry* 2005; 44: 213–235.

16. Miklowitz DJ, Schneck CD, Singh MK, et al. Early intervention for symptomatic youth at risk for bipolar disorder: a randomized trial of family-focused therapy. *J Am Acad Child Adoles Psychiatry* 2013; 52: 121–131.

17. Post RM, Chang K, Frye MA. Commentary: Paradigm shift: preliminary clinical categorization of ultrahigh risk for childhood bipolar disorder to facilitate studies on prevention. *J Clin Psychiatry* 2013; 74: 167–169.

18. Folstein MF, Folstein SE, McHugh PR. 'Mini-mental state': a practical method for grading the cognitive state of patients for the clinician. *J Psychiatr Res* 1975; 12: 189–198.

19. Robinson L, Tang E, Taylor JP. Dementia: timely diagnosis and early intervention. *BMJ* 2015; 350: h3029.

20. Walker Z, Moreno E, Thomas A, et al. Clinical usefulness of dopamine transporter SPECT imaging with 123I-FP-CIT in patients with possible dementia with Lewy bodies: randomised study. *Br J Psychiatry* 2015; 206: 145–152.

21. McKhann GM, Knopman DS, Chertkow H, et al. The diagnosis of dementia due to Alzheimer's disease: Recommendations from the National Institute on Aging-Alzheimer's Association workgroups on diagnostic guidelines for Alzheimer's disease. *Alzheimers Dement* 2011; 7: 263–269.

22. National Institute for Health and Care Excellence (NICE). Donepezil, galantamine, rivastigmine and memantine for the treatment of Alzheimer's disease. Available at: https://www.nice.org.uk/guidance/TA217.

23. Lautenschlager NT, Cox KL, Flicker L, et al. Effect of physical activity on cognitive function in older adults at risk for Alzheimer disease: a randomized trial. *JAMA* 2008; 300: 1027–1037.

24. Rosen WG, Mohs RC, Davis KL. A new rating scale for Alzheimer's disease. Am J Psychiatry 1984; 141: 1356–1364.

25. Castle DJ, Buckley P. *Schizophrenia*, 2nd ed. Oxford: Oxford University Press, 2015.

26. Wyatt RJ. Neuroleptics and the natural course of schizophrenia. *Schizophr Bull* 1991; 17: 325–329.

27. Birchwood M, McGorry P, Jackson H. Early intervention in schizophrenia. *Br J Psychiatry* 1997; 170: 2–11.

28. McGlashan TH. Schizophrenia in translation: is active psychosis neurotoxic?. *Schizophr Bull* 2006; 32: 609–613.

29. Bosanac PE, Patton GC, Castle DJ. Early intervention in psychotic disorders: faith before facts? *Psychol Med* 2010; 40: 353–358.

30. Perkins DO, Gu H, Boteva K, Lieberman JA. Relationship between duration of untreated psychosis and outcome in first-episode schizophrenia: a critical review and meta-analysis. *Am J Psychiatry* 2005; 162: 1785–1804.

31. Marshall M, Lewis S, Lockwood A, Drake R, Jones P, Croudace T. Association between duration of untreated psychosis and outcome in cohorts of first-episode patients: a systematic review. *Arch Gen Psychiatry* 2005; 62: 975–983.

32. Harris MG, Henry LP, Harrigan SM, et al. The relationship between duration of untreated psychosis and outcome: an eight-year prospective study. *Schizophr Res* 2005; 79: 85–93.

33. Hill M, Crumlish N, Clarke M, et al. Prospective relationship of duration of untreated psychosis to psychopathology and functional outcome over 12 years. *Schizophr Res* 2012; 141: 215–221.

34. Boonstra N, Klaassen R, Sytema S, et al. Duration of untreated psychosis and negative symptoms—a systematic review and meta-analysis of individual patient data. *Schizophr Res* 2012; 142: 12–19.

35. Tang JY, Chang WC, Hui CL, et al. Prospective relationship between duration of untreated psychosis and 13-year clinical outcome: a first-episode psychosis study. *Schizophr Res* 2014; 153: 1–8.

36. Penttilä M, Jääskeläinen E, Hirvonen N, Isohanni M, Miettunen J. Duration of untreated psychosis as predictor of long-term outcome in schizophrenia: systematic review and meta-analysis. *Br J Psychiatry* 2014; 205: 88–94.

37. Register-Brown K, Hong LE. Reliability and validity of methods for measuring the duration of untreated psychosis: a quantitative review and meta-analysis. *Schizophr Res* 2014; 160: 20–26.

38. Compton MT, Carter T, Bergner E, et al. Defining, operationalizing and measuring the duration of untreated psychosis: advances, limitations and future directions. *Early Intervent Psychiatry* 2007; 1: 236–250.

39. Schimmelmann BG, Huber CG, Lambert M, Cotton S, McGorry PD, Conus P. Impact of duration of untreated psychosis on pre-treatment, baseline, and outcome characteristics in an epidemiological first-episode psychosis cohort. *J Psychiatr Res* 2008; 42: 982–990.

40. Craig TK, Garety P, Power P, et al. The Lambeth Early Onset (LEO) Team: randomised controlled trial of the effectiveness of specialised care for early psychosis. *BMJ* 2004; 329: 1067.

41. Power P, Iacoponi E, Reynolds N, et al. The Lambeth Early Onset Crisis Assessment Team Study: general practitioner education and access to an early detection team in first-episode psychosis. *Br J Psychiatry* 2007; 191: s133–s139.

42. Lester H, Birchwood M, Freemantle N, Michail M, Tait L. REDIRECT: cluster randomised controlled trial of GP training in first-episode psychosis. *Br J Gen Pract* 2009; 59: e183–e190.

43. Friis S, Vaglum P, Haahr U, et al. Effect of an early detection programme on duration of untreated psychosis. *Br J Psychiatry* 2005; 187: s29–s32.

44. Malla A, Norman R, Scholten D, Manchanda R, McLean T. A community intervention for early identification of First Episode Psychosis. *Soc Psychiatry Psychiatr Epidemiol* 2005; 40: 337–344.

45. Chong SA, Lee C, Bird L, Verma S. A risk reduction approach for schizophrenia: the early psychosis intervention programme. *Ann Acad Med Singapore* 2004; 33: 630–635.

46. Lloyd-Evans B, Crosby M, Stockton S, et al. Initiatives to shorten duration of untreated psychosis: systematic review. *Br J Psychiatry* 2011; 198: 256–263.

47. Castle DJ. Is it appropriate to treat people at high-risk of psychosis before first onset?-no. *Med J Aust* 2012; 196: 557.

48. Behan C, Masterson S, Clarke M. Systematic review of the evidence for service models delivering early intervention in psychosis outside the stand-alone centre. *Early Interv Psychiatry* 2017; 11: 3–13.

49. Welch M, Welch T. Early psychosis in rural areas. *Aust N Z J Psychiatry* 2007; 41: 485–494.

50. Cheng C, Dewa CS, Langill G, Fata M, Loong D. Rural and remote early psychosis intervention services: the Gordian knot of early intervention. *Early Interv Psychiatry* 2014; 8: 396–405.

51. O'Keamey R, Garland G, Welch M, Kanowski L, Fitzgerald S. Factors predicting program fidelity and delivery of an early intervention program for first episode psychosis in rural Australia. *Aust E J Adv Ment Health* 2004; 3: 75–83.

52. Petrakis M, Penno S, Oxley J, Bloom H, Castle D. Early psychosis treatment in an integrated model within an adult mental health service. *Eur Psychiatry* 2012; 27: 483–488

53. Addington J, Collins A, McCleery A, Addington D. The role of family work in early psychosis. *Schizophr Res* 2005; 79: 77–83.

54. Bird V, Premkumar P, Kendall T, Whittington C, Mitchell J, Kuipers E. Early intervention services, cognitive–behavioural therapy and family intervention in early psychosis: systematic review. *Br J Psychiatry* 2010; 197: 350–356.

55. R McFarlane W, Lynch S, Melton R. Family psychoeducation in clinical high risk and first-episode psychosis. *Adoles Psychiatry* 2012; 2: 182–194.

56. Riley G, Gregory N, Bellinger J, Davies N, Mabbott G, Sabourin R. Carer's education groups for relatives with a first episode of psychosis: an evaluation of an eight-week education group. *Early Interv Psychiatry* 2011; 5: 57–63.

57. Sin J, Moone N, Newell J. Developing services for the carers of young adults with early-onset psychosis–implementing evidence-based practice on psycho-educational family intervention. *J Psychiatr Ment Health Nurs* 2007; 14: 282–290.

58. International Early Psychosis Association Writing Group. International clinical practice guidelines for early psychosis. *Br J Psychiatry* 2005; 187: s120–s124.

59. Askey R, Gamble C, Gray R. Family work in first-onset psychosis: a literature review. *J Psychiatr Ment Health Nurs* 2007; 14: 356–365.

60. Nilsen L, Frich JC, Friis S, Røssberg JI. Patients' and family members' experiences of a psychoeducational family intervention after a first episode psychosis: a qualitative study. *Issues Ment Health Nurs* 2014; 35: 58–68.

61. Cabral RR, Chaves AC. Multi-family group intervention in a programme for patients with first-episode psychosis: a Brazilian experience. *Int J Soc Psychiatry* 2010; 56: 527–532.

62. Petrakis M, Bloom H, Oxley J. Family perceptions of benefits and barriers to first episode psychosis carer group participation. *Soc Work Ment Health* 2014; 12: 99–116.

63. So HW, Chen EYH, Chan RCK, et al. Efficacy of a brief intervention for carers of people with first-episode psychosis: a waiting list controlled study. *Hong Kong J Psychiatry* 2006; 16: 92–100.

64. Lowenstein JA, Butler DW, Ashcroft K. The efficacy of a cognitively orientated carers group in an early intervention in psychosis service–a pilot study. *J Psychiatr Ment Health Nurs* 2010; 17: 628–635.

65. McCann TV, Lubman DI, Clark E. Primary caregivers' satisfaction with clinicians' response to them as informal carers of young people with first-episode psychosis: a qualitative study. *J Clin Nurs* 2012; 21: 224–231.

66. Naik VN, Bowden S. Early intervention in psychosis: client and carer perspectives. *Nurs Times* 2008; 104: 32–33.

67. Tsang H, Lam P, Ng B, Leung O. Predictors of employment outcome for people with psychiatric disabilities: a review of literature since the mid'80s. *J Rehabil* 2000; 66: 19.

68. Bond GR, Drake RE. Making the case for IPS supported employment. *Adm Policy Ment Health* 2014; 41: 69–73.

69. Bond GR. Supported employment: evidence for an evidence-based practice. *Psychiatr Rehabil J* 2004; 27: 345.

70. Waghorn G, Lloyd C. The employment of people with mental illness. *Aust E J Adv Ment Health* 2005; 4: 129–171.

71. Drake RE, Bond GR, Becker DR. *Individual Placement and Support: An Evidence-Based Approach to Supported Employment.* Oxford: Oxford University Press, 2012.

72. Killackey E, Jackson HJ, McGorry PD. Vocational intervention in first-episode psychosis: individual placement and support v. treatment as usual. *Br J Psychiatry* 2008; 193: 114–120.

73. Hartz SM, Pato CN, Medeiros H, et al. Comorbidity of severe psychotic disorders with measures of substance use. *JAMA Psychiatry* 2014; 71: 248–254.

74. Myles N, Newall HD, Curtis J, Nielssen O, Shiers D, Large M. Tobacco use before, at, and after first-episode psychosis: a systematic meta-analysis. *J Clin Psychiatry* 2012; 73: 468–475.

75. Lambert M, Conus P, Lubman DI, et al. The impact of substance use disorders on clinical outcome in 643 patients with first-episode psychosis. *Acta Psychiatr Scand* 2005; 112: 141–148.

76. Lubman DI, Sundram S. Substance misuse in patients with schizophrenia: a primary care guide. *Med J Aust* 2003; 178: S71.

77. Addington J, Addington D. Patterns, predictors and impact of substance use in early psychosis: a longitudinal study. *Acta Psychiatr Scand* 2007; 115: 304–309.

78. Tarrier N, Lewis S, Haddock G, et al. Cognitive-behavioural therapy in first-episode and early schizophrenia. *Br J Psychiatry* 2004; 184: 231–239.

79. Morrison AP, French P, Stewart SL, et al. Early detection and intervention evaluation for people at risk of psychosis: multisite randomised controlled trial. *BMJ* 2012; 344: e2233.

80. Addington J, Marshall C, French P. Cognitive behavioral therapy in prodromal psychosis. *Curr Pharm Design* 2012; 18: 558–565.

81. Miller TJ, McGlashan TH, Woods SW, et al. Symptom assessment in schizophrenic prodromal states. *Psychiatr Q* 1999; 70: 273–287.

82. Yung AR, Nelson B, Stanford C, et al. Validation of 'prodromal' criteria to detect individuals at ultra high risk of psychosis: 2 year follow-up. *Schizophr Res* 2008; 105: 10–17.

83. Ochoa S, López-Carrilero R. Early psychological interventions for psychosis. *World J Psychiatry* 2015; 5: 362.

84. Mander H, Kingdon D. The evolution of cognitive–behavioral therapy for psychosis. *Psychol Res Behav Manag* 2015; 8: 63.

85. Lewis S, Tarrier N, Haddock G, et al. Randomised controlled trial of cognitive—behavioural therapy in early schizophrenia: acute-phase outcomes. *Br J Psychiatry* 2002; 181: s91–s97.

86. Revell ER, Neill JC, Harte M, Khan Z, Drake RJ. A systematic review and meta-analysis of cognitive remediation in early schizophrenia. *Schizophr Res* 2015; 168: 213–222.

87. Bassett A, Addington D, Cook P, et al. Canadian clinical practice guidelines for the treatment of schizophrenia. *Can J Psychiatry* 1998; 43: 25S–40S.

88. National Collaborating Centre for Mental Health (UK). Schizophrenia: core interventions in the treatment and management of schizophrenia in primary and secondary care (update) [Internet]. Available at: https://www.ncbi.nlm.nih.gov/pubmed/20704054 (accessed 16 March 2018).

89. Bola JR, Kao DT, Soydan H. Antipsychotic medication for early-episode schizophrenia. *Schizophr Bull* 2011; 38: 23–25.

90. Royal Australian and New Zealand College of Psychiatrists Clinicl Practice Guidelines Team for the Treatment of Schizophrenia and Related Disorders. Royal Australian and New Zealand College of Psychiatrists clinical practice guidelines for the treatment of schizophrenia and related disorders. *Aust N Z J Psychiatry* 2005; 39: 1–30.

91. Robinson DG, Woerner MG, Delman HM, Kane JM. Pharmacological treatments for first-episode schizophrenia. *Schizophr Bull* 2005; 31: 705–722.

92. Emsley R, Rabinowitz J, Medori R. Time course for antipsychotic treatment response in first-episode schizophrenia. *Am J Psychiatry* 2006; 163: 743–745.

93. Gallego JA, Robinson DG, Sevy SM, et al. Time to treatment response in first-episode schizophrenia: should acute treatment trials last several months? *J Clin Psychiatry* 2011; 72: 1691–1696.

94. Stauffer VL, Case M, Kinon BJ, et al. Early response to antipsychotic therapy as a clinical marker of subsequent response in the treatment of patients with first-episode psychosis. *Psychiatry Res* 2011; 187: 42–48.

95. Kinon BJ, Chen L, Ascher-Svanum H, et al. Early response to antipsychotic drug therapy as a clinical marker of subsequent response in the treatment of schizophrenia. *Neuropsychopharmacology* 2010; 35: 581.

96. Zhang JP, Gallego JA, Robinson DG, Malhotra AK, Kane JM, Correll CU. Efficacy and safety of individual second-generation vs. first-generation antipsychotics in first-episode psychosis: a systematic review and meta-analysis. *Int J Neuropsychopharmacol* 2013; 16: 1205–1218.

97. Rabinovitch M, Béchard-Evans L, Schmitz N, Joober R, Malla A. Early predictors of nonadherence to antipsychotic therapy in first-episode psychosis. *Can J Psychiatry* 2009; 54: 28–35.

98. Perkins DO, Gu H, Weiden PJ, McEvoy JP, Hamer RM, Lieberman JA. Predictors of treatment discontinuation and medication nonadherence in patients recovering from a first episode of schizophrenia, schizophreniform disorder, or schizoaffective disorder: a randomized, double-blind, flexible-dose, multicenter study. *J Clin Psychiatry* 2008; 69: 106–113.

99. Emsley R, Chiliza B, Asmal L, Mashile M, Fusar-Poli P. Long-acting injectable antipsychotics in early psychosis: a literature review. *Early Interv Psychiatry* 2013; 7: 247–254.

100. Francey SM, Nelson B, Thompson A, et al. Who needs antipsychotic medication in the earliest stages of psychosis? A reconsideration of benefits, risks, neurobiology and ethics in the era of early intervention. *Schizophr Res* 2010; 119: 1–10.

101. Van Mastrigt S, Addington J, Addington D. Substance misuse at presentation to an early psychosis program. *Soc Psychiatry Psychiatr Epidemiol* 2004; 39: 69–72.

102. De Koning MB, Bloemen OJ, Van Amelsvoort TA, et al. Early intervention in patients at ultra high risk of psychosis: benefits and risks. *Acta Psychiatr Scand* 2009; 119: 426–442.

CHAPTER 44

Anti-stigma interventions
Theory and evidence

Petra C. Gronholm, Claire Henderson,
Tanya Deb, and Graham Thornicroft

Introduction: mental health-related stigma

Mental health-related stigma and discrimination are a world-wide concern. Indeed, it has been noted that there appears to be no known country, society, or culture where people with mental illness would be considered to have the same value and be as acceptable as people without mental illness [1]. People with mental illness often experience reduced well-being and life chances, and it is increasingly recognized that this constitutes a significant public health concern [2, 3]. For example, in UK mental health policy for 2011–15, one of the six key objectives of the Government's mental health strategy specified the need to ensure fewer people experience stigma and discrimination due to their mental illness [4]. Also, at an international level, the vision for the World Health Organizations' Mental Health Action Plan 2013–2020 specifies that people affected by mental illness should be able to participate fully in society and at work, free from stigmatization and discrimination [5].

Definitions and models of stigma and discrimination

The term 'stigma' originates from the Greek word *stigmata*, signifying a visible mark or brand of shame and discredit, physically inflicted onto people like slaves or criminals to publicly indicate their inferior or immoral social status [6].

Current conceptualizations of stigma frequently build on the work by the Canadian sociologist Ervin Goffman, who adopted this concept of a stigmatizing mark in his notion of a 'spoiled identity' [7]. Goffman stated that stigma was the situation of a person disqualified from social acceptance as a result of possessing a deeply discredited attribute that set them apart from others, reducing the stigmatized individual from a whole and usual person to a tainted and discounted one. In the case of mental illness, this discrediting attribute was thought of as a blemish on the individual character, evident through, for example, a label of mental illness or association with mental health services, which indicates that the person has a mental illness.

Key conceptualizations

Since Goffman's seminal definition, the notion of stigma has been the focus of much conceptual and theoretical elaboration and refinement.

Some theorists have taken a social–cognitive perspective on stigma, proposing a model where stigma is defined in terms of: stereotypes (negative beliefs regarding a given group); prejudice (the agreement with negative stereotypes, and/or negative reactions towards a person thought of in these terms); and discrimination (derogatory behaviours due to the prejudice) [8]. Such a perspective of stigma has been considered reflective of problems within three domains, namely knowledge, attitudes, and behaviour [1, 9]. Problems of knowledge reflect a lack of accurate information about mental illness, which can lead to misconceptions about what mental illnesses are and how persons with mental illness should be helped. Lack of knowledge can also perpetuate unhelpful common beliefs, about, for example, what people with mental illness are like or capable of doing. These beliefs reflect agreement with negative stereotypes, such as the belief that persons with mental illness pose a threat to others. Problems of negative attitudes can involve negative thoughts (e.g. beliefs based on stereotypes) and emotions (e.g. anxiety, anger, resentment, hostility, distaste, or disgust) towards persons with mental illness. These negative reactions can, at times, be understood as a result of the anticipated threat a person with mental illness is believed to pose. Problems of behaviour reflect the actual discriminatory actions towards, and the actual experiences of, people with mental illness; for example, social rejection or withdrawal, and loss of opportunities and limited access to social roles.

Another influential conceptualization of stigma builds on a sociological perspective. This frames stigma as a wider societal force, involving both the individual and their broader environment. Namely, stigma is considered to represent the co-occurrence of processes relating to labelling, stereotyping, separation, emotional reactions, status loss, and discrimination, in the presence of a power balance in favour of the stigmatizer over the stigmatized [10, 11]. Thus, this process starts with distinguishing and labelling human differences. Dominant cultural beliefs determine certain labelled differences as undesirable and negative characteristics, or stereotypes, are applied to those who are labelled. The labelled and stereotyped persons are placed in distinct categories, to separate those labelled from the unlabelled; distinguishing 'them' from 'us'. A range of emotional reactions is involved in these processes. The stigmatizers can feel, for example, anger, anxiety, irritation, fear, or pity towards labelled persons. These reactions can shape the stigmatizer's subsequent behaviour towards the stigmatized person, and also signal to a stigmatized person how they are perceived by others. Those who have been stigmatized, however, can experience, for example, embarrassment, shame, fear, alienation, or anger in response to the labelling. Finally, the stereotyping and separation of labelled persons provides a rationale for them to be devalued, rejected, and excluded by others, leading to unequal outcomes through status loss and discrimination. These processes are dependent on social, political, and economic power; this definition of stigma requires the stigmatizer to be in a position of greater power relative to the stigmatized person or group, and through this power difference able to create serious disadvantage and discriminatory consequences for those who are stigmatized.

Different variants of stigma

As evidenced by these conceptualizations, stigma is a broad and multifaceted construct [12, 13]. Consequently, research and intervention with a stigma focus have involved a number of different definitions, targets, and outcomes, all described as reflective of stigma. An overview of these various means of describing, clarifying, and classifying the stigma concept is provided by, for example, Pescosolido and Martin [12]. They outlined two broad perspectives—experiential and action-orientated—through which stigma can be categorized.

The experiential perspective distinguishes between whether stigma is (i) perceived (a belief 'most people' are considered to hold); (ii) endorsed (expressing agreement with stereotypes/prejudice/discrimination); (iii) anticipated (expecting an experience of prejudice/discrimination); (iv) received (overt experiences of rejection or devaluation); or (v) enacted (exhibiting discriminatory behaviours).

The action-oriented view considers who (or what) gives or receives the stigma. From this perspective distinctions are made between (i) public stigma (stereotypes, prejudice, and discrimination as endorsed by the general population); (ii) structural stigma (prejudice and discrimination through laws, policies, and constitutional practices); (iii) courtesy stigma (stereotypes, prejudice, and discrimination acquired through a connection with a stigmatized group/person); (iv) provider-based stigma (prejudice and discrimination by occupational groups designated to provide assistance to stigmatized groups); and (v) self-stigma (when people who belong to a stigmatized group legitimize publicly held stereotypes and prejudice, and internalize these by applying them to themselves).

These variants of stigma have been examined in a number of studies. For example, work has been conducted to examine the prevalence, severity, and nature of anticipated and experienced stigma amongst people with schizophrenia [14] and depression [15], processes associated with self-stigma [16], and structural influences of how stigma influences health [17].

Rationale for anti-stigma interventions

Stigma and discrimination are, unfortunately, common experiences among people living with a mental illness, and their consequences of these processes can lead to loss of opportunities across many domains of a person's life. For example, stigma and discrimination can function as a barrier to accessing mental health services [18, 19], and make people forego life goals [16]. Discrimination is also important not only because of the impact of experienced unfair treatment and attitudes, but also because already anticipated

concerns regarding stigma and discrimination can serve to limit people's life changes and opportunities. The consequences of experienced and anticipated discrimination in combination are severe: poor access to physical health care [20]; reduced life expectancy [21, 22]; exclusion from higher education [23, 24] and employment [25]; increased risk of contact with criminal justice systems; victimization [26]; and poverty and homelessness.

For many people, the negative consequences of stigma and discrimination have been described as worse than the experience of the mental illness in itself [27]. It is therefore a major public health concern to challenge and aim to reduce the negative social responses to mental illness. Next, this chapter discusses strategies used for such efforts and evidence regarding their effectiveness.

Anti-stigma strategies

Anti-stigma strategies are recognized to utilize a range of different approaches to achieve their aims. These approaches have been categorized, for example, in terms of education (replacing myths about mental illness with accurate knowledge and conceptions), contact (using direct or indirect interactions with people who have a mental illness to challenge stigmatizing attitudes), and protest (attempts to suppress stigmatizing attitudes and representations of mental illness) [28]. Anti-stigma interventions have frequently utilized, in particular, the first two strategies: education and contact.

Early anti-stigma efforts, on both a smaller and larger scale, often used educational approaches. For example, work in the 1950s by Cumming and Cumming in Canada [29] attempted to reduce stigma through providing mental health education via group discussions and films. Also in the UK, the 'Defeat Depression' campaign in the early 1990s aimed to reduce stigma through provision information on depressive illness for public and professional use (e.g. using fact sheets) and public-awareness campaigns [30]. Stigma reduction among health professionals also often relies on educational approaches such as training workshops [31]. Educational approaches are frequently used in mental health literacy work; that is, efforts to improve knowledge and beliefs about mental disorders, to aid the recognition, management, or prevention of mental illness [32–34].

Over time, the use of anti-stigma strategies based on inter-group contact has increased, especially following a meta-analysis by Corrigan et al. in 2012 [35], which highlighted the effectiveness of contact-based interventions. This applies both to tailored interventions for key target groups such as health professionals [36] and police [37], and to social marketing campaigns for the general public, which provide virtual contact through various media [38]. While contact-based education has become the most popular method for work with target groups, the evidence for its long-term impact is limited [39] and there is evidence that education is relatively more effective for young people [35] (discussed further in the 'Evidence from systematic reviews' subsection).

To try to increase the effectiveness of contact-based anti-stigma strategies it could be argued that closer attention should be paid to existing literature on inter-group contact by some of those doing this work. For example, Knaak et al. [36] identified six ingredients for contact-based education with health professionals (discussed further in the 'Healthcare professionals' subsection), without relating these to the ingredients previously identified by inter-group contact theory. In contrast, another study [40] examined changing negative attitudes among students towards a confederate classified as a 'former mental patient', with an approach explicitly informed by theory on inter-group attitudes and contact; namely, the 'Contact Hypothesis' [41]. This proposes that for contact between members of in- and out-groups to lead to favourable outcomes for the out-group member, the two groups need to be afforded equal status during the interaction, and the interaction needs to involve a mutual goal. By following these principles, and incorporating other conditions identified in existing literature as necessary for successful inter-group contact (e.g. the opportunity to get to know the out-group member during the interaction, interaction disconfirming negative stereotypes, active cooperation, interaction including a guiding structure), the study found that after cooperative contact activities initially prejudiced students not only described the 'mental patient' confederate more positively, but these improvements also generalized beyond this specific individual to the out-group overall.

Leading inter-group contact researchers in the UK have discussed the application of inter-group contact theory to mental health-related stigma [42]. This work examined the influence of different types of imagined contact with people with schizophrenia, and concluded that with this kind of challenging out-group (people affected by severe mental illness) imagined contact might, in fact, have a detrimental effect and increase inter-group anxiety unless it was purposefully structured to reflect a positive imagined contact experience. When designing anti-stigma interventions it is therefore important to consider what factors mediate the effectiveness of inter-group contact-based strategies. A meta-analysis of over 500 studies confirmed that contact can diminish prejudice through resulting in reduced anxiety about inter-group contact, and increased empathy and perspective-taking. A further key factor was enhanced knowledge regarding the out-group; however, the mediational value of this influence was weaker than that of reduced anxiety and increased empathy [43].

National anti-stigma programmes

Some anti-stigma efforts have been conducted at a national level [44]. Examples of such work include the 'Time to Change' programme in England (launched in 2008), and 'Opening Minds' in Canada (launched in 2009) [45]. Critically, systematic academic evaluation has been carried out in relation to both programmes. This is important as it helps us understand the extent to which these programmes have been successful. Also, in view of differences between Time to Change and Opening Minds, comparing their findings provides an opportunity for identifying active ingredients and best practices regarding stigma-reduction efforts.

Both programmes were systematic efforts formulated around a theoretical conceptualization of stigma. However, they adhered to different frameworks. Namely, whereas the Time to Change programme took a public health perspective on stigma, defining it in terms of problems relating to knowledge, attitudes, and behaviours [1, 9], the Opening Minds programme used the sociological framework where stigma is considered reflective of the co-occurrence of labelling, stereotyping, separation, status loss, and discrimination [10, 11]. Both programmes built on evidence-based approaches to stigma-reduction, with an emphasis on contact-based education strategies. There were, however, differences in how these strategies were delivered. Time to Change primarily aimed to target the general population via a large-scale mass media social marketing

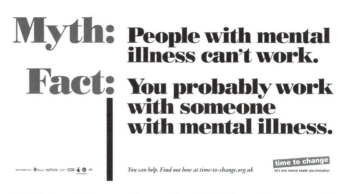

Fig. 44.1 Example of mass media material used within Time to Change, targeted at the general public.
Source: Reproduced with permission from the Time to Change programme, run by the charities Mind and Rethink Mental Illness.

campaigning. The initial focus was on education-based 'myth busting'—see Fig. 44.1 for an example—followed by a focus on reducing prejudice and changing behaviours. Additionally, Time to Change involved local initiatives and work with target groups such as medical students and employers [46, 47]. In contrast, Opening Minds did not include a mass-media element, but solely focused on intensive, targeted work with specific target groups across the country—young people, healthcare providers, the news media, and the workforce—through grassroots input and community programmes [48].

The results of these evaluations indicate that both programmes have been successful in reducing stigma, which demonstrates that there are many ways to structure and deliver effective anti-stigma interventions. In England, following Time to Change, benefits were observed in terms of population-level improvements in stigma-related knowledge, attitudes, social distance, and reported contact with people with mental illness, albeit some of these effects emerged slowly [49, 50]. Positive changes were also evident in mental health service users' reduced reporting of experiences of discrimination [51]. Population-level changes were not achievable in Canada as the programme was conducted at a local level. Evaluation of these local efforts did, however, indicate positive changes. For example, interventions focusing on high-school students were generally successful in improving students' behavioural intentions towards people with a mental illness [52], and, similarly, programmes among healthcare providers generally produced positive results in terms of their attitudes [53]. The goal within Opening Minds is to replicate successful programmes nationally; this work currently involves a national scale-up with the efforts focusing on young people. In terms of future work, these evaluations indicate that in both England and Canada there were gender-based differences in responses to the anti-stigma programmes, with men reporting less contact with people with a mental illness than women. As this kind of contact is important for improved stigma-reduction outcomes, future efforts might benefit from gender-based approaches [45]. Also, interventions aiming to achieve changes at a structural level are needed, as is further work around how mental illness is reported in the media so that unhelpful stereotypes are not perpetuated.

Regarding identifying mechanisms of successful stigma change, albeit Time to Change included smaller efforts with a local or target focus, the intended population-level exposure to the mass-media elements of the programme makes it impossible to examine the impact of these components separately. In contrast, Opening Minds built on community-based efforts only, which were all based on contact-based education strategies but were heterogeneous in nature [45]. In view of this variability, the evaluation of the programme has enabled the identification of how to tailor effectively stigma-interventions for different populations [53] and what the effective programme ingredients are [36]. These findings are discussed in the 'Stigma reduction within key target groups' subsection of this chapter.

Evidence for the effectiveness of anti-stigma interventions

In addition to the examples of Time to Change and Opening Minds, other work has also been conducted to reduce stigma. This section provides an overview of the evidence regarding the effectiveness of anti-stigma interventions from studies that have examined population-level stigma reduction; systematic reviews that have synthesized such evidence; evidence on stigma-reduction efforts targeting particular groups of people; and what can be concluded based on these findings.

Population-level stigma reduction

The effect of anti-stigma interventions targeting the general public has been assessed through controlled interventions, repeated cross-sectional surveys and longitudinal panel studies. For example, when evaluating the impact of mass-media-based anti-stigma programmes in Norway and England, the former, which focused on mental illnesses generally, was found to result in moderate improvements in knowledge and attitudes [54], whereas the latter focused on depression specifically, and resulted in changes in attitudes only [55]. A subsequent anti-stigma programme in England had a broader focus on a range of mental illnesses, and this was found to result in modest improvement in knowledge but no changes in attitudes [56]. A number of studies have examined the effectiveness mental health first aid—that is, psychoeducational efforts aiming to increase mental health literacy, improve attitudes, and stimulate helping behaviours—delivered to whole populations in Australia. The evaluation of this work consistently showed improved attitudes but weaker evidence for achieving improved knowledge [33, 57–60]. Population-level awareness campaigns have likewise been conducted in Austria and Germany, and were found to result in moderate benefits in terms of improved attitudes but no changes in knowledge [61]. 'Beyondblue' was a depression-specific programme in Australia, and it was found to result in improved public attitude and knowledge [62]. Additionally, greater effects were observed following greater exposure to the programme. The 'Like Minds, Like Mine' anti-stigma programme in New Zealand resulted in reduced overall levels of discrimination [63], and there have also been indications of improved knowledge and attitudes following this work. 'See Me' is another national programme aiming to end mental health-related stigma and discrimination, running in Scotland. When the findings of cross-sectional population surveys of public attitudes towards people with mental illness between 1994 and 2003 were compared between Scotland and England (where no comparable programme was underway), attitudes in England were significantly deteriorating, whereas no comparable pattern was noted in Scotland, where attitudes remained largely unchanged

[64]. Another example to mention is the national-level 'Hjärnkoll' programme in Sweden, which started in 2010. The evaluation of this work indicates that, by 2014, its social contact-based strategy had achieved a positive impact on mental health literacy, attitudes, and intended social contact with people with mental illness [65].

Evidence from systematic reviews

In addition to individual studies evaluating the effectiveness of anti-stigma interventions, this evidence has also been examined in systematic literature reviews. These involve a comprehensive, systematic search process to identify studies on a given topic, after which their findings are synthesized for a robust overview of the evidence-base. Next, this chapter outlines the results from four such reviews. Each explored different research questions regarding the effectiveness of anti-stigma strategies, and through considering their findings it is possible to gather a broad overview of evidence in this area.

Corrigan et al. [35] conducted a systematic review to examine the effectiveness of interventions aiming to reduce public stigma. Interventions were classified based on whether they aimed to reduce stigma through one of three strategies: social activism or protest, education of the public, or contact with people who have a mental illness. Overall, 72 studies (involving 38,364 people from 14 countries) were identified for inclusion in the review. The findings of these studies were pooled statistically in a meta-analysis, which revealed that interventions based on education and contact reduced stigma (in terms of improved attitudes and behavioural intentions). Additionally, among adults, contact-based interventions were more effective than education, whereas among adolescents, this pattern was reversed and education-based strategies were better. Furthermore, in relation to contact, face-to-face interactions had a greater effect than contact mediated by videotape. Protest-based intervention strategies were not found to change levels of stigma.

Further evidence on anti-stigma efforts is provided by a systematic review by Clement et al. [38]. The focus here was on mass media interventions specifically; that is, whether campaigns delivered via means such as newspapers, billboards, leaflets, DVDs, television, radio, cinema, and the Internet produced changes in either people's level of prejudice (stigmatizing attitudes) or discrimination (unfair treatment). Twenty-two studies (involving 4490 people) were identified for inclusion in the review. The findings were combined primarily through a narrative text-based summary and explanation, as the studies' heterogeneity prevented statistical synthesis of the results. Nineteen trials examined prejudice outcomes; overall, the findings of these indicated that mass-media-based anti-stigma interventions might lead to small-to-medium-sized reductions in prejudice. There were insufficient data to determine whether comparable effects could be achieved for discrimination; the five trials that examined discrimination outcomes reported mixed findings. It was also concluded that although it would have been useful to examine the cost-effectiveness of mass-media interventions, such assessments were not feasible owing to cost data rarely being available.

The systematic review by Griffiths et al. [66] used the statistical meta-analysis approach to examine the effectiveness of anti-stigma programmes in terms of different kinds of stigma, and different mental health conditions. Thirty-four relevant studies were identified, with the majority evaluating interventions focused not only on reducing personal stigma or social distance (19 articles;

involving 6318 people), but also perceived stigma (six articles, involving 3042 people), and self-stigma (three articles, involving 238 people). Small but significant reductions were observed following interventions targeting personal stigma or social distance across all mental disorders, and also specifically in relation to depression, psychosis, and generic mental illness. Reductions in personal stigma were achieved, for example, through education-based interventions and strategies involving contact with service users. There were too few studies to examine the effectiveness of contact alone. Interventions delivered over the Internet were found to be at least as effective in reducing personal stigma as programmes delivered face-to-face. In contrast to these findings regarding the effectiveness of personal stigma reduction, there was no evidence supporting the effectiveness of interventions targeting perceived stigma or self-stigma.

Finally, the systematic review by Mehta et al. [39] aimed to provide evidence regarding medium- and long-term effectiveness of anti-stigma efforts, and interventions in low- and middle-income countries (LAMICs), as such insights had been noted as lacking [35, 38]. Eighty relevant studies were identified; most ($n = 72$; involving 42,653 people) provided data on medium- and long-term effectiveness, whereas comparatively few studies ($n = 11$; involving 1967 people) considered evidence from LAMICs. The variability in the included studies prevented statistical pooling of the evidence. Rather, a text-based narrative synthesis was provided, structured around changes in stigma in terms of knowledge, attitudes, or behaviour. Regarding evidence on follow-up effects of anti-stigma interventions, where effect sizes could be calculated, these indicated a medium effect for increased knowledge and a small reduction in stigmatizing attitudes. Also, the one study for which effect sizes were available for behavioural outcomes indicated a small reduction. Overall, however, a comparable number of significant and non-significant findings were reported for changes in each of knowledge and attitudes, and for behavioural outcomes more non-significant outcomes were reported than significant findings. Regarding stigma reduction in LAMICs, the studies examining this were varied in design and target populations. The effect size could only be calculated for one study, where a psychoeducation programme was found to result in a large effect in reducing stigmatizing attitudes [67]. When examining overall patterns of significant findings, all but one of the 12 assessments of attitude outcomes indicated a significant reduction following the interventions, whereas neither of the studies considering knowledge-related outcomes reported any evidence of change. No studies examined behavioural outcomes.

Overall, regarding evidence from systematic reviews, a recent narrative review [68] summarized what is known globally from systematic reviews on effective anti-stigma interventions. It concluded that at a population level short-term improvements in attitudes are generally observed, with some evidence also for improved knowledge, and some group-level interventions for people with mental illness show promise and should be examined further. It was noted that studies in the field are generally heterogeneous and commonly have methodological limitations (e.g. weak study designs, small samples). Notably, LAMIC data are missing, and long-term follow-up data and insights into how improvements can be sustained are needed, as are studies considering service-user perspectives and discrimination and behaviour change. It was also reported that there is evidence for short-term attitudinal improvement following anti-stigma interventions focused on specific target groups,

although care should be taken to not over-generalize findings from one target group to another. Next, this chapter discusses such efforts among key target groups in further detail.

Stigma reduction within key target groups

Evidence regarding the effectiveness of anti-stigma efforts is also available from studies considering key target groups. This is of interest, as focusing on stigma-reduction within specific groups can constitute a powerful approach to advancing the life opportunities for people with mental illness [1, 69].

Next this chapter outlines evidence regarding stigma reduction efforts within key target groups, identified as important owing to their high levels of contact with service users (healthcare professionals), position of power (law enforcement officers), or potential for changing the future (students and young people) [69].

Healthcare professionals

Evidence regarding anti-stigma efforts among healthcare professionals has been discussed, for example by Henderson et al. [31]. Their review on stigma in healthcare settings outlined the findings of studies that had assessed whether stigma and discrimination can be decreased in a healthcare context.

The review identified 16 intervention studies that had examined stigma reduction in relation to mental health generally or specific mental health conditions (e.g. borderline personality disorder, substance misuse) among various groups of healthcare and mental healthcare professionals. Most interventions were educational in nature, and these commonly examined attitudinal outcomes, which were generally reported to have improved following participation in the intervention. Some studies also reported improved knowledge and understanding amongst the healthcare staff, and also some outcomes reflecting positive changes in behavioural intentions and clinical competence were reported. When follow-up assessments were conducted these generally indicated that the positive changes had been sustained (e.g. [70, 71]); however, only a few studies had examined this.

Two further studies had examined stigma-reduction in relation to mental illness in general. Both were Internet-based, and appeared successful. In the first, significantly lowered scores for social distance were reported amongst Turkish psychiatrists randomly assigned to receive an instructional email about stigma compared with controls who received a questionnaire on social distance [72]. However, this study did not include any baseline measures, and the findings need to be interpreted in view of this methodological weakness. The other intervention comprised Internet-based education on mental illness to professionals working in long-term care facilities in USA, following which significant positive differences were found for all outcomes including measures of knowledge, attitudes (stereotype endorsement), empathy, self-efficacy, and intentions [73].

More recent evidence on stigma-reduction amongst healthcare providers is also available from work conducted within Canada's Opening Minds anti-stigma initiative [74]. The results of 37 contact-based education projects for healthcare providers within this programme were examined statistically and through qualitative methods, to identify the key ingredients of anti-stigma programs in this context [36]. These are outlined in Box 44.1; based on this work, future anti-stigma interventions for healthcare providers

Adapted from Can J Psychiatry, 59(10 Suppl 1), Knaak, S., Modgill, G., & Patten, S. B, Key Ingredients of Anti-Stigma Programs for Health Care Providers: A Data Synthesis of Evaluative Studies. S19–S26, Copyright (2014), with permission from SAGE Publications.

Anti-stigma ingredient

1. The programme should include social contact in the form of a personal testimony from a trained speaker who has lived experience of mental illness.

2. The programme should employ multiple forms or points of social contact (e.g. a presentation from a live speaker and a video presentation, multiple first-voice speakers, multiple points of social contact between programme participants, and people with lived experience of mental illness).

3. The programme should focus on behaviour change by teaching skills that help healthcare providers know what to say and what to do.

4. The programme should engage in myth-busting.

5. The programme should use an enthusiastic facilitator or instructor who models a person-centred approach (i.e. a person-first perspective as opposed to a pathology-first perspective) to set the tone and guide programme messaging.

6. The program should emphasize and demonstrate recovery as a key part of its messaging.

should include multiple forms of social contact and an emphasis on recovery.

Police officers

Criminal justice professionals are identified as another key group for stigma reduction interventions [69]. The deinstitutionalization of mental health services has led to a significant increase in contact between the police and those with mental illness, and it has been argued that police officers should be provided with education and training to enable them to interact adaptively and with good outcomes with people with mental illness. Not many studies have been conducted in this area, but evidence from two such interventions are summarized.

Firstly, Pinfold et al. [75] evaluated a training intervention with the police force in England. Police officers' ($n = 109$) knowledge, attitudes, and behavioural intentions in relation to mental illness were assessed before and after attending two educational workshops delivered by service users, carers, and people working in the field of mental health. The results indicated that the intervention had produced some improvements in reported attitudes, but the stereotype linking people with mental health problems with violent behaviour was not successfully challenged. The programme goals relating to improving officers' awareness of issues relating to mental health were more successful than goals to influence police officers' reported behavioural intentions. However, objective changes in perceived knowledge were not detected. Additionally, a third of the participants reported positive impacts on police work, particularly improvements

in communication between officers and persons with mental health problems.

Secondly, Hansson and Markström [37] examined the effectiveness of an anti-stigma intervention in a police officer training programme in Sweden, through a controlled pre-post intervention study design with a comparison group and 6-month follow-up of the intervention group. It was found that the anti-stigma intervention was effective in improving police officers' attitudes, mental health literacy, and intentional behaviours. Among the intervention group, improvements were observed in the overall attitude score, and also the 'open-minded' and 'pro-integration' attitude subscales. Also, intentional behaviours had improved (willingness to work with people with mental illness), as had four out of six items assessing mental health literacy. Moreover, these changes were generally still present 6 months later: at follow-up, the intervention group still had improved attitudes in both overall score and in the subscales versus baseline. Also intentional behaviours had improved in terms of an increased willingness to live or work with a person with mental health problems. Mental health literacy had improved for three out of six items. This intervention was well received by the trainees, and some of its key elements have been retained in the regional routine police training programme.

Students

One key target group is young people, including university and college students. A variety of interventions have been developed to reduce mental health-related stigma among such student groups. Their overall effect was examined in a systematic review, conducted by Yamaguchi et al. [76]. Thirty-five relevant studies (involving 4257 people) were identified, considering a range of interventions including social contact with a person with mental health problems, education via text, lecture, film, or role play. A narrative synthesis of these results indicated that live or video-based social contact with people with mental health problems were the most effective interventions in improving attitudes and reducing desire for social distance. Evidence from one study also suggested that a lecture providing treatment information might enhance students' attitudes towards the use of services.

Conclusions

Intervening to reduce stigma and discrimination requires a long-term and sustained commitment [77]. However, the need to improve the evaluation methods and the interventions themselves is an urgent one. Overall, anti-stigma interventions appear to result in small-to-moderate sized effects (as assessed using Cohen's interpretation [78]), and strategies based on contact and first-person narratives appear most effective. At the population level, the available evidence points towards anti-stigma interventions resulting in improved attitudes, at least in the short term. There is also some evidence for improvements in knowledge. For anti-stigma efforts among specific target groups, interventions based on contact likewise seem to result in short-term benefits in terms of improved attitudes, but there is less evidence for achieving changes in knowledge. However, further research is needed to better understand how these effects are mediated, and the evidence is small regarding the effectiveness of anti-stigma strategies in terms of achieving actual behaviour change, despite the salience of this aspect of stigma for stigmatized groups. Indeed, few studies have examined the effectiveness of anti-stigma efforts from the perspective of members of stigmatized groups such as mental health service users.

The research that has examined the effectiveness of anti-stigma interventions has been highly heterogeneous, both in terms of methods and focus of the studies, reflecting the variety of stigma theories and definitions. This variability has complicated efforts to synthesize the evidence. Additionally, the methodological quality of studies is variable. The risk of bias in many studies is thus currently unclear, and further research should include randomized designs for interventions tailored to specific groups; improved reporting of study procedures; validated and appropriate outcome measures; better controlling for confounding factors and potential social desirability bias; increased sample sizes; better sampling procedures to increase representativeness; and follow-up data collection beyond the immediate end of the intervention period. With respect to gaps in research, the most glaring is that regarding the effectiveness of anti-stigma efforts in LAMICs.

It is not usually possible to conduct randomized studies of population-based interventions such as national anti-stigma campaigns. However, other quasi-experimental designs should be considered in order to be more confident that change is attributable to the campaign rather than to secular changes. In the absence of such designs, the use of repeated surveys can be used not just to assess changes in outcomes over time, but to examine whether the outcomes are associated with campaign awareness [79, 80] and to provide feedback in order to improve the intervention. As it seems that short-term interventions often only have a short-term impact, the implication is that we need to study longer-term interventions and to use the interim process and outcome data to improve the interventions along the way.

Intervention development could make greater use of the relevant evidence base such as that on inter-group contact to reduce prejudice, and could expand this field, for example by increasing the number of studies on virtual contact. Care is needed in matching the approach of the intervention to the outcome measures selected; for example, a rights-based intervention will require different outcomes to one using inter-group contact. Process evaluation to assess the context, implementation, and mechanisms of action [81] of theory-based interventions would facilitate the delivery of more effective interventions in future. An example is the process model developed by Knaak et al. [82].

Interventions for target groups could be better tailored by a number of means. Firstly, preparatory work can increase the understanding of the target group and the context of their contact with the stigmatized group, for example using ethnography to inform intervention design. Secondly, greater attention should be paid to the influences of structural and organizational level discrimination on individual-level interactions and the experience of the stigmatized group members. The many directions which can be taken by anti-stigma research make its evaluation an exciting and challenging field.

References

1. Thornicroft G. *Shunned: Discrimination Against People With Mental Illness.* Oxford: Oxford University Press, 2006.
2. Thornicroft G, Evans-Lacko S, Henderson C. Stigma and discrimination. In: Davies S (ed.). *Annual Report of the Chief Medical Officer 2013. Public mental Health Priorities: Investing in the Evidence.* London: Department of Health, 2014.
3. Link BG, Phelan JC. Stigma and its public health implications. *Lancet* 2006; 367: 528–529.
4. Department of Health. No health without mental health. Available at: https://www.gov.uk/government/uploads/system/uploads/attachment_data/file/213761/dh_124058.pdf (2011, accessed 20 June 2016).
5. World Health Organization (WHO). *Mental Health Action Plan 2013–2020.* Geneva: WHO.
6. Corrigan PW, O'Shaughnessy JR. Changing mental illness stigma as it exists in the real world. *Aust Psychol* 2007; 42: 90–97.
7. Goffman E. *Stigma: Notes on the Management of Spoiled Identity.* New York: Simon & Schuster, 1963.
8. Corrigan PW. Mental health stigma as social attribution: implications for research mehtods and attitude change. *Clin Psychol Sci Pract* 2000; 7: 48–67.
9. Thornicroft G, Rose D, Kassam A, et al. Stigma: ignorance, prejudice or discrimination? *Br J Psychiatry* 2007; 190: 192–193.
10. Link BG, Phelan J. Conceptualizing stigma. *Annu Rev Sociol* 2001; 27: 363–385.
11. Link BG, Yang LH, Phelan JC, et al. Measuring mental illness stigma. *Schizophr Bull* 2004; 30: 511–541.
12. Pescosolido BA, Martin JK. The stigma complex. *Annu Rev Sociol* 2015; 41: 87–116.
13. Corrigan PW, Shapiro JR. Measuring the impact of programs that challenge the public stigma of mental illness. *Clin Psychol Rev* 2010; 30: 907–922.
14. Thornicroft G, Brohan E, Rose D, et al. Global pattern of experienced and anticipated discrimination against people with schizophrenia: a cross-sectional survey. *Lancet* 2009; 373: 408–415.
15. Lasalvia A, Zoppei S, Van Bortel T, et al. Global pattern of experienced and anticipated discrimination reported by people with major depressive disorder: a cross-sectional survey. *Lancet* 2013; 381: 55–62.
16. Corrigan PW, Larson JE, Rüsch N. Self-stigma and the 'why try' effect: impact on life goals and evidence-based practices. *World Psychiatry* 2009; 8: 75–81.
17. Hatzenbuehler ML, Phelan JC, Link BG. Stigma as a fundamental cause of population health inequalities. *Am J Public Health* 2013; 103: 813–821.
18. Clement S, Schauman O, Graham T, et al. What is the impact of mental health-related stigma on help-seeking? A systematic review of quantitative and qualitative studies. *Psychol Med* 2015; 45: 11–27.
19. Corrigan PW, Druss BG, Perlick DA. The impact of mental illness stigma on seeking and participating in mental health care. *Psychol Sci Public Interes* 2014; 15: 37–70.
20. Mai Q, Holman CDJ, Sanfilippo FM, et al. Mental illness related disparities in diabetes prevalence, quality of care and outcomes: a population-based longitudinal study. *BMC Med* 2011; 9: 118.
21. Laursen TM, Munk-Olsen T, Nordentoft M, et al. Increased mortality among patients admitted with major psychiatric disorders: a register-based study comparing mortality in unipolar depressive disorder, bipolar affective disorder, schizoaffective disorder, and schizophrenia. *J Clin Psychiatry* 2007; 68: 899–907.
22. Gissler M, Laursen TM, Oesby U, et al. Patterns in mortality among people with severe mental disorders across birth cohorts: a register-based study of Denmark and Finland in 1982–2006. *BMC Public Health* 2013; 13: 834.
23. Suhrcke M, de Paz Nieves C. *The Impact of Health and Health Behaviors on Educational Outcomes in High-income Countries: A Review of the Evidence.* Copenhagen: WHO Regional Office for Europe, 2011.
24. Lee S, Tsang A, Breslau J, et al. Mental disorders and termination of education in high-income and low and middle-income countries: epidemiological study. *Br J Psychiatry* 2009; 194: 411–417.
25. Social Exclusion Unit. Mental Health and Social Exclusion. Available at: http://www.nfao.org/Useful_Websites/MH_Social_Exclusion_report_summary.pdf (2004, accessed 22 April 2013).

26. Clement S, Brohan E, Sayce L, et al. Disability hate crime and targeted violence and hostility: a mental health and discrimination perspective. *J Ment Health* 2011; 20: 219–225.

27. Thornicroft G, Mehta N, Clement S, et al. Evidence for effective interventions to reduce mental-health-related stigma and discrimination. *Lancet* 2015; 387: 1123–1132.

28. Corrigan PW, River LP, Lundin RK, et al. Three strategies for changing attributions about severe mental illness. *Schizophr Bull* 2001; 27: 187–195.

29. Cumming E, Cumming J. *Closed Ranks: An Experiment in Mental Health Education*. Cambridge, MA: Harvard University Press, 1957.

30. Priest RG. A new initiative on depression. *Br J Gen Pract* 1991; 41: 487.

31. Henderson C, Noblett J, Parke H, et al. Mental health-related stigma in health care and mental health-care settings. *Lancet* 2014; 1: 467–482.

32. Jorm AF. Mental health literacy: empowering the community to take action for better mental health. *Am Psychol* 2012; 67: 231–243.

33. Kitchener BA, Jorm AF. Mental health first aid training in a workplace setting: a randomized controlled trial [ISRCTN13249129]. *BMC Psychiatry* 2004; 4: 23.

34. Jorm AF, Kitchener BA, Fischer J-A, et al. Mental Health first aid training by e-learning: a randomized controlled trial. *Aust N Z J Psychiatry* 2010; 44: 1072–1081.

35. Corrigan PW, Morris S, Michaels P, et al. Challenging the public stigma of mental illness: a meta-analysis of outcome studies. *Psychiatr Serv* 2012; 63: 963–973.

36. Knaak S, Modgill G, Patten SB. Key ingredients of anti-stigma programs for health care providers: a data synthesis of evaluative studies. *Can J Psychiatry* 2014; 59: S19–S26.

37. Hansson L, Markström U. The effectiveness of an anti-stigma intervention in a basic police officer training programme: a controlled study. *BMC Psychiatry* 2014; 14: 55.

38. Clement S, Lassman F, Barley E, et al. Mass media interventions for reducing mental health-related stigma. *Cochrane Database Syst Rev*; 2013; 7: CD009453.

39. Mehta N, Clement S, Marcus E, et al. Evidence for effective interventions to reduce mental health-related stigma and discrimination in the medium and long term: systematic review. *Br J Psychiatry* 2015; 207: 377–384.

40. Desforges DM, Lord CG, Ramsey SL, et al. Effects of structured cooperative contact on changing negative attitudes toward stigmatized social groups. *J Pers Soc Psychol* 1991; 60: 531–544.

41. Allport GW. *The Nature of Prejudice*. Reading, MA: Addison-Wesley, 1954.

42. West K, Holmes E, Hewstone M. Enhancing imagined contact to reduce prejudice against people with schizophrenia. *Gr Process Intergr Relations* 2011; 14: 407–428.

43. Pettigrew TF, Tropp LR. How does intergroup contact reduce prejudice? Meta-analytic tests of three mediators. *Eur J Soc Psychol* 2008; 38: 922–934.

44. Borschmann R, Greenberg N, Jones N, et al. Campaigns to reduce mental illness stigma in Europe: a scoping review. *Die Psychiatr* 2014; 11: 43–50.

45. Henderson C, Stuart H, Hansson L. Lessons from the results of three national antistigma programmes. *Acta Psychiatr Scand* 2016; 134: S3–S5.

46. Friedrich B, Evans-Lacko S, London J, et al. Anti-stigma training for medical students: The Education Not Discrimination project. *Br J Psychiatry* 2013; 202: s89–s95.

47. Henderson C, Williams P, Little K, et al. Mental health problems in the workplace: changes in employers' knowledge, attitudes and practices in England 2006-2010. *Br J Psychiatry* 2013; 202: s70–s77.

48. Stuart H, Chen S-P, Christie R, et al. Opening Minds in Canada: background and rationale. *Can J Psychiatry* 2014; 59: S8–S12.

49. Evans-Lacko S, Malcolm E, West K, et al. Influence of Time to Change's social marketing interventions on stigma in England 2009-2011. *Br J Psychiatry Suppl* 2013; 202: s77–s88.

50. Henderson C, Robinson E, Evans-Lacko S, et al. Public knowledge, attitudes, social distance and reported contact regarding people with mental illness 2009–2015. *Acta Psychiatr Scand* 2016; 134: S23–S33.

51. Corker E, Hamilton S, Robinson E, et al. Viewpoint survey of mental health service users' experiences of discrimination in England 2008–2014. *Acta Psychiatr Scand* 2016; 134: S6–S13.

52. Koller M, Stuart H. Reducing stigma in high school youth. *Acta Psychiatr Scand* 2016; 134: S63–S70.

53. Knaak S, Patten S. A grounded theory model for reducing stigma in health professionals in Canada. *Acta Psychiatr Scand* 2016; 134: S53–S62.

54. Søgaard AJ, Fønnebø V. The Norwegian Mental Health Campaign in 1992. Part II: changes in knowledge and attitudes. *Health Educ Res* 1995; 10: 267–278.

55. Paykel ES, Hart D, Priest RG. Changes in public attitudes to depression during the Defeat Depression Campaign. *Br J Psychiatry* 1998; 173: 519–22.

56. Crisp AH (ed). *Every Family in the Land. Understanding Prejudice and Discrimination Against People With Mental Illness*, revised ed. London: The Royal Society of Medicine Press, 2004.

57. Jorm AF, Kitchener BA, Sawyer MG, et al. Mental health first aid training for high school teachers: a cluster randomized trial. *BMC Psychiatry* 2010; 10: 51.

58. Jorm AF, Kitchener BA, O'Kearney R, et al. Mental health first aid training of the public in a rural area: a cluster randomized trial [ISRCTN53887541]. *BMC Psychiatry* 2004; 4: 33.

59. Gulliver A, Griffiths KM, Christensen H, et al. Internet-based interventions to promote mental health help-seeking in elite athletes: an exploratory randomized controlled trial. *J Med Internet Res* 2012; 14: e69.

60. Kitchener BA, Jorm AF. Mental health first aid training for the public: evaluation of effects on knowledge, attitudes and helping behavior. *BMC Psychiatry* 2002; 2: 10.

61. Gaebel W, Zäske H, Baumann AE, et al. Evaluation of the German WPA 'Program against stigma and discrimination because of schizophrenia—Open the Doors': results from representative telephone surveys before and after three years of antistigma interventions. *Schizophr Res* 2008; 98: 184–193.

62. Jorm AF, Christensen H, Griffiths KM. The impact of beyondblue: the national depression initiative on the Australian public's recognition of depression and beliefs about treatments. *Aust N Z J Psychiatry* 2005; 39: 248–254.

63. Thornicroft C, Wyllie A, Thornicroft G, et al. Impact of the 'Like Minds, Like Mine' anti-stigma and discrimination campaign in New Zealand on anticipated and experienced discrimination. *Aust N Z J Psychiatry* 2014; 48: 360–370.

64. Mehta N, Kassam A, Leese M, et al. Public attitudes towards people with mental illness in England and Scotland, 1994–2003. *Br J Psychiatry* 2009; 194: 278–284.

65. Hansson L, Stjernswärd S, Svensson B. Changes in attitudes, intended behaviour, and mental health literacy in the Swedish population 2009–2014: an evaluation of a national antistigma programme. *Acta Psychiatr Scand* 2016; 134: S71–S79.

66. Griffiths KM, Carron-Arthur B, Parsons A, et al. Effectiveness of programs for reducing the stigma associated with mental disorders. A meta-analysis of randomized controlled trials. *World Psychiatry* 2014; 13: 161–175.

67. Gutiérrez-Maldonado J, Caqueo-Urízar A, Ferrer-García M. Effects of a psychoeducational intervention program on the attitudes and health perceptions of relatives of patients with schizophrenia. *Soc Psychiatry Psychiatr Epidemiol* 2009; 44: 343–348.

68. Thornicroft G, Mehta N, Clement S, et al. Evidence for effective interventions to reduce mental-health-related stigma and discrimination. *Lancet* 2016; 387: 1123–1132.

69. Corrigan PW. Target-specific stigma change: a strategy for impacting mental illness stigma. *Psychiatr Rehabil J* 2004; 28: 113–121.

70. Patterson P, Whittington R, Bogg J. Measuring nurse attitudes towards deliberate self-harm: The Self-Harm Antipathy Scale (SHAS). *J Psychiatr Ment Health Nurs* 2007; 14: 438–445.

71. Graham AL, Julian J, Meadows G. Improving responses to depression and related disorders: evaluation of a innovative, general, mental health care workers training program. *Int J Ment Health Syst* 2010; 4: 25.

72. Bayar MR, Poyraz BC, Aksoy-Poyraz C, et al. Reducing mental illness stigma in mental health professionals using a web-based approach. *Isr J Psychiatry Relat Sci* 2009; 46: 226–230.

73. Irvine BA, Billow MB, Bourgeois M, et al. Mental illness training for long term care staff. *J Am Med Dir Assoc* 2012; 13: 81.e7-81.e13.

74. Modgill G, Patten SB, Knaak S, et al. Opening Minds Stigma Scale for Health Care Providers (OMS-HC): examination of psychometric properties and responsiveness. *BMC Psychiatry* 2014; 14: 120.

75. Pinfold V, Huxley P, Thornicroft G, et al. Reducing psychiatric stigma and discrimination—evaluating an educational intervention with the police force in England. *Soc Psychiatry Psychiatr Epidemiol* 2003; 38: 337–344.

76. Yamaguchi S, Wu S-I, Biswas M, et al. Effects of short-term interventions to reduce mental health-related stigma in university or college students: a systematic review. *J Nerv Ment Dis* 2013; 201: 490–503.

77. Sartorius N. Short-lived campaigns are not enough. *Nature* 2010; 468: 163–165.

78. Cohen J. *Statistical Power Analysis for the Behavioral Sciences.* New York: Erlbaum, 1988.

79. Sampogna G, Bakolis I, Robinson E, et al. Experience of the Time to Change programme in England as predictor of mental health service users' stigma coping strategies. *Epidemiol Psychiatr Sci* 2017; 26: 517–525.

80. Sampogna G, Bakolis I, Evans-Lacko S, et al. The impact of social marketing campaigns on reducing mental health stigma: results from the 2009–2014 Time to Change programme. *Eur Psychiatry* 2017; 40: 116–122.

81. Moore G, Audrey S, Barker M, et al. Process evaluation of complex interventions. UK Medical Research Council (MRC) guidance. Available at: https://www.mrc.ac.uk/documents/pdf/mrc-phsrn-process-evaluation-guidance-final/ (accessed 16 March 2018).

82. Knaak S, Patten SB. Building and Delivering Successful Anti-Stigma Programs for Healthcare Workers. Available at: http://www.mentalhealthcommission.ca/sites/default/files/qualitative_model_report_feb_2015_0.pdf (2014, accessed 30 August 2016).

CHAPTER 45

Managing stress

Susan L. Fletcher, Sandra K. Davidson, and Jane M. Gunn

Introduction

We experience stress when we perceive a mismatch between the demands placed upon us and our ability to cope with those demands [1, 2]. We interpret this mismatch as a threat to our well-being, which, in turn, triggers a coordinated physiological response involving the autonomic, neuroendocrine, metabolic, and immune system [3, 4]. Our heart rate increases and blood rushes to our muscles in preparation to fight the threat or flee from it. From an evolutionary perspective, this was a very effective survival mechanism. When unexpectedly confronted by an angry woolly mammoth this sudden surge in hormones enabled our ancestors to fight off the beast or make a quick escape and live for another day. In today's world, stress still has a positive role to play. It keeps us focused and motivated, enhances resilience, and can even improve our immune function [5]. However, when episodes of stress are too frequent or stress is chronic it has a negative impact on our psychological, biological, and social well-being.

What is stress?

At its most basic level, the stress response can be defined as an activation of the sympathetic nervous system. The reader is probably familiar with the fight or flight response, which activates immediate physiological changes, including, but not limited to, pupil dilation, increased heart rate, sweating, and slowed digestion. These acute effects of stress responses are hard-wired and involuntary, and we have all experienced them at one time or another. But dig a little deeper and describing the nature of the stress response is a surprisingly complex task.

Reactions to stress include psychological, physical, and behavioural responses, with relatively little coordination between these domains. For example, a review by Campbell and Ehlert [6] showed that physiological responses and perceived emotional stress corresponded only around a quarter of the time.

Because stress is not currently listed in diagnostic manuals (Box 45.1), there is no defined list of symptoms against which to check one's own stress response, although several symptom inventories have been developed [7]. Nonetheless, in any given month the vast majority of adults report experiencing at least one symptom that they attribute to stress [1]; see Fig. 45.1 for some commonly reported symptoms.

Models of stress

Over the last century, researchers have developed an inordinate number of models of stress—far too many to cover in this chapter.

This is to say nothing of the many broader psychosocial theories one could turn to understand stress, including Bandura's social learning theory and Maslow's hierarchy of needs. Nevertheless, we will endeavour to describe briefly some of the key models of stress, and refer the interested reader to more comprehensive texts on the subject [8–11].

Early models of stress include the Yerkes–Dodson law, which suggests that we need some stress to function effectively (Fig. 45.2); the fight–flight response (or, more recently, the fight–flight–freeze response), which describes the physiological response to acute stress; and the general adaptation syndrome, which extended our understanding of how the body responds to prolonged stress.

These early models were criticized on several fronts, including the simplistic assumption that stressors are always objective, occurring outside the individual, and that stress reactions are an unavoidable passive response [8]. These models suggest little can be done to manage stress other than remove its source. Contemporary models of stress, which include transactional models [2], event-perception models [12], the Conservation of Resources theory [13], and proactive coping theories [14, 15], are more hopeful. They share the central idea that stress arises as a result of an interaction between external demands and internal vulnerabilities, i.e. a mismatch between the perceived threat and the perceived ability to deal with it [3]. These models hypothesize that we can minimize this mismatch, and therefore reduce stress, by reducing our appraisal of threat and increasing our appraisal of our ability to deal with the threat.

The size of the problem

Population-based surveys of the prevalence of stress are relatively recent. More commonly, research has examined specific types of stress in response to specific types of stressors, for example physiological reactivity to public speaking. Consequently, we are only just beginning to understand how much of an issue stress really is.

Although media reports and popular opinion may suggest that our stress levels are continually increasing, population-based surveys from the USA and Australia indicate that average stress over recent years has actually been relatively stable, perhaps even decreasing slightly [1, 21]. In the latest survey conducted by the American Psychological Association, a quarter of American adults reported that they had experienced moderate-to-severe stress in the past 12 months (and stress is just as common in children; see Box 45.2). In Australia, 35% of adults report significant psychological distress, whereas in the UK stress accounts for 35% of all work-related cases of ill health [22]. In Sweden, 13% of employees report burnout resulting from persistent stress [23].

Box 45.1 Stress: not depression or anxiety

One criticism of the construct of stress is that it is not unique, but simply another way of referring to depression and anxiety. There is certainly evidence to support the idea that the three states are not discrete constructs. Depression and anxiety are known as internalizing mental health disorders, as they can be represented by a superordinate 'internalizing' dimension that reflects a propensity to express distress inwardly [16]. To date, the relationship between stress and the internalizing dimension has not been directly investigated. However, stress, like anxiety and depression, is strongly associated with personality traits that are considered reliable indicators of the internalizing dimension of mental health disorder [17, 18].

Although there are obvious similarities between stress and the internalizing disorders, there is also a counterargument that stress is a unique construct that is demonstrated by its association with 'externalizing' behaviours such as aggression and substance use. This relationship provides some support for the argument that stress and depression/anxiety are not synonymous. Further supporting this argument is the finding that people who score highly on measures of stress do not necessarily report high levels of depression or anxiety, and vice versa. Indeed, the Depression, Anxiety, and Stress Scale was developed on exactly this premise and has shown repeatedly that, while related, the three constructs are distinct [19, 20]. Specifically, there is a 40–46% overlap between stress and depression and anxiety, respectively, leaving most of the variation in stress scores independent.

In the final analysis, for many individuals and health professionals the difference between stress and related conditions is an academic one; the presence of distress and the need for intervention is the important issue. For people concerned about the stigma of mental health disorders, being 'stressed' may be a 'safe' way of expressing internal turmoil. However, in some health systems, notably the USA, where a formal psychiatric diagnosis is required to access treatment, this distinction is important. Stress, while a significant personal and public health issue, has not yet made it into the *Diagnostic and Statistical Manual of Mental Disorders* (DSM) or the *International Classification of Diseases* (ICD), and thus does not confer the same status (for better or worse) as its formally recognized cousins.

One of the difficulties in conducting epidemiological research is that stress is poorly defined, and it is possible that study participants respond to survey questions quite differently, depending on their individual interpretation of what is meant by 'stress'. However, ultimately we would argue that this has little effect on the public health implications of these data; if people say they are stressed, they are, and we should aim to intervene accordingly.

The impact of stress

In the short-term, even though stress is unpleasant, once the stressor disappears, the symptoms usually do too, with no long-lasting effects. However, in the face of chronic, very intense, or unpredictable stressors, our health almost inevitably suffers [29]. Unfortunately, many people do experience chronic stress.

Up to a third of adults in nationally representative surveys report that stress has a strong impact on their physical and mental health [1, 21]. Chronic stress is associated with both morbidity and mortality. One mechanism by which stress may impact on mortality is by decreasing heart rate variability; this effect persists even after controlling for behavioural and demographic risk factors for cardiovascular-related mortality such as smoking, body mass index, and age [30]. Chronic stress may also increase mortality risk by suppressing the immune response and decreasing resistance to infection and even certain types of cancer [31]. More recently, research has shown that chronic stress is associated with shortened telomeres [32, 33]. Telomeres act as protective caps on the end of chromosomes and help reduce the chromosomes' deterioration. Telomere length is an indicator of cellular age. Chronic psychological stress appears to exacerbate shortening of telomeres, effectively increasing the rate of cellular ageing.

Mental health problems and substance use disorders are a common consequence of chronic stress. One recent study found that up to 80% of depressive episodes occur within months of a major stressful event [34]. Another study found that almost half of all new cases of anxiety and depression stemmed from high levels of work stress [35]. In addition, epidemiological data show that as the number of recent stressful life events increases, so too does the likelihood of problematic drinking and full-blown alcohol use disorder [36].

The likelihood of experiencing a poor mental health outcome varies partially as a function of the nature of the stressor. For example, interpersonal events, such as relationship breakdown or conflict with others, are more likely to trigger a stress response than non-interpersonal stressors [37, 38]. There is also a general trend for a dose–response relationship; that is, the more severe the stressor, the more stress experienced.

However, it is important to note that, even in the face of the most confronting stressors, chronic and severe stress responses occur relatively infrequently. For example, although both men and women rate rape as one of life's most stressful/traumatic experiences, the development of chronic post-traumatic stress disorder after rape tends to be the exception rather than the rule (Box 45.3) [39, 40]. Thus, it is important to remember that mental health problems are neither a usual, nor an inevitable, consequence of stress.

The good news

Despite the potential negative effects of chronic stress, short-term stress has many benefits. It keeps us focused and motivated, enhances resilience, and can even improve our immune function [5]. In addition, there is growing evidence that acute stress may promote pro-social behaviour such as increased levels of trust, trustworthiness, and sharing. Although the exact nature of this 'tend-and-befriend' response is unclear it may be an effective stress buffering strategy. The tend-and-befriend response was initially thought to apply only to women [41], but recent findings suggest than men also experience an improvement in empathy, trust, and sharing behaviour when under stress [41–43]. By establishing the circumstances under which stress encourages prosocial behaviour in men and women, we may be able to develop intervention approaches to capitalize on this tendency when appropriate, bearing in mind the fact that prosocial behaviour is not always the optimal response.

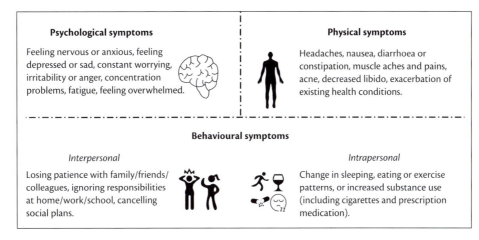

Psychological symptoms	Physical symptoms
Feeling nervous or anxious, feeling depressed or sad, constant worrying, irritability or anger, concentration problems, fatigue, feeling overwhelmed.	Headaches, nausea, diarrhoea or constipation, muscle aches and pains, acne, decreased libido, exacerbation of existing health conditions.

Behavioural symptoms

Interpersonal	*Intrapersonal*
Losing patience with family/friends/colleagues, ignoring responsibilities at home/work/school, cancelling social plans.	Change in sleeping, eating or exercise patterns, or increased substance use (including cigarettes and prescription medication).

Fig. 45.1 Common symptoms of stress.

An interesting line of emerging research is the potential for chronic stress to also have some positive health effects. Its role in suppressing immune responses is theorized to have benefits in autoimmune disease and there is some evidence from animal studies that this is the case. Further research is required to tease out the mechanisms underpinning this effect and the conditions under which it may be replicated without the requirement for autoimmune disease patients to experience chronic stress [31].

Causes of stress

Stress can be caused by an almost infinite number of stressors, which vary in nature, intensity, duration, and the degree to which they can be predicted or controlled. Stressors can be psychological or physiological; real or imagined. Some of the most powerful stressors are psychological in nature and are based on an anticipated threat rather than actual threat [4]. Stressors range from very mild (being stuck in traffic; these stressors are also known as 'daily hassles') to very severe (losing your house in a natural disaster). They may be acute (giving a presentation), repeated (struggling to make monthly mortgage payments), or chronic (living in poverty).

As shown in Fig. 45.3, stressors can be considered along two axes: severity and chronicity. Two stressors may occupy the same space on one dimension but be quite distinct on another; a car accident and job interview are both acute stressors but vastly different in severity. Further, the nature of a stressor can change over time; depending on the frequency and type of daily hassles, their cumulative impact may be better categorized as that of a chronic stressor [44].

The leading sources of stress among adults are remarkably consistent across countries and over time. National surveys in the USA and Australia show that financial issues cause people the most stress, with work (see Box 45.4), family issues, and personal health issues not far behind [1, 21].

Sources of stress are also reasonably consistent across demographic groups, with some noteworthy differences. For example, while money is the top source of stress, regardless of gender [1], women are more likely than men to report issues relating to personal finances, family, health of self and others, maintaining a healthy lifestyle, relationships, and friendship as sources of stress, whereas men are more likely to see the current political climate as a significant stressor [21].

Perhaps not surprisingly, money and work-related stress have an inverse relationship with age, with older people less likely to cite these factors as a source of stress [1, 21]. In Australia, four out of five adults aged between 18 and 36 years report that work is a major source of stress compared with just two out of five adults aged 70 years or older. In contrast, older adults report being stressed by health issues more often than their younger counterparts [21].

For minority groups, including racial/ethnic minorities and people living with a disability, the main sources of stress are similar to the general population; however, the impact of these stressors is more severe. Non-white people are also more likely to report discrimination as a source of stress (e.g. 40% of black people vs 14% of white people) [1]. Finally, and not unexpectedly, financial concerns are a greater source of stress for low-income adults [21, 45].

Risk factors

It's difficult to paint a clear picture of who is most likely to experience stress as there are an almost infinite number of risk factors. Characteristics of the stressor itself, the individual experiencing it (including genes, neurobiology, cognitive processes, temperament, sociodemographic characteristics, etc.), and the environment can all increase the likelihood of a stress response. In addition to the unique effect of each risk factor, multiple risk factors interact with each other, making it difficult to predict who will experience what level of stress.

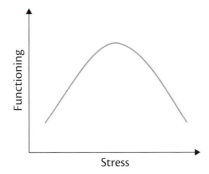

Fig. 45.2 Yerkes–Dodson curve.

Box 45.2 Stress and children

Being stressed is not confined to adults. Research shows that many children and adolescents report significant levels of stress. In fact, American teenagers rate their stress at 5.8 out of 10, whereas American adults rate their stress at 5.1 out of 10 [24].

There appears to be substantial discrepancy between the level of stress children report experiencing and their parent's perception of the level of stress experienced by their child. One study showed that 20% of children aged 8–17 years reported experiencing stress (defined as worrying a lot about things in their lives), yet only 8% of parents thought their child experienced stress [25]. Parents tend to think that children worry more about their relationship with family members than they actually do, whereas children are more stressed about school than parents think they are. Almost a third (29%) of teenagers report that their future after high school is a major source of stress, but only 5% of parents think their child is worried about this. Children also worry more about adult issues than parents expect, with one in three children reporting stress related to family finances [26].

This finding can be considered part of a larger problem of the transmission of stress across generations. Children who believe their parents are always stressed report more stress themselves. Nine out of 10 children say they can recognize when their parents are stressed, pointing to signs such as their parents yelling, arguing, telling the child about their problems, or being too busy to spend time with them [25]. Children experience a range of negative emotions when their parents are stressed, including being sad or worried (39%), frustrated (33%), or scared (13%).

Common symptoms of stress reported by children are similar to those experienced by adults and include headaches, difficulty sleeping, eating too much or little, or having an upset stomach. Once they reach their teenage years, this list expands to include snapping at classmates, neglecting responsibilities, procrastination, and cancelling social plans. The effects of stress on the adolescent brain are still being discovered, but it is likely that the developing brain is more sensitive to stress and stress hormones [27]. This may result in deviations from the path of normal development, although exactly how and when remains to be determined.

Young people often engage in sedentary activities to manage their stress, such as listening to music, playing video games, and watching TV [24]. Yet evidence suggests that physical activity, rather than sedentary activity, is a more effective stress management strategy. Research has shown that in children as young as 8 years of age, physical activity is associated with lower physiological reactivity to stressful events and better mental health [28]. Together, these findings suggest that there is a need to work with young people to help them find more positive ways of managing their stress [25].

Box 45.3 Stress and the *Diagnostic and Statistical Manual of Mental Disorders, 5th Edition* (DSM-5)

As discussed earlier, stress can trigger the development or recurrence of a wide range of mental health problems. In the DSM-5 there is also a new category of diagnosis called 'Trauma- and stressor-related disorders', which specifically recognize the pathogenic effects of major stressors on a person's mental health. Diagnoses in this category include:

- Acute stress disorder: diagnosed 3 days–1 month after a traumatic event (i.e. experiencing or witnessing an event involving actual or threatened death, serious injury, or sexual violence). Requires the presence of at least 9 of a possible 14 symptoms.

- Post-traumatic stress disorder: diagnosed 1 month or more after a traumatic event. Requires at least seven symptoms from four clusters.

- Adjustment disorder: diagnosed after experiencing a major stressor not meeting the criteria for 'traumatic'. Requires the development of emotional/behavioural symptoms within 3 months of the onset of the stressor, and the remission of symptoms within 6 months of the conclusion of the stressor or its consequences.

- Reactive attachment disorder and disinhibited social engagement disorder: diagnosed in children with a consistent pattern of withdrawn behaviour toward caregivers and social and emotional disturbance (reactive); or children who actively approach and interact with unfamiliar adults (disinhibited) after experiencing a pattern of insufficient care.

minority in other English-speaking countries, and the extent to which these risk factors apply globally is unclear.

Demographics

At the population level, several demographic characteristics are associated with an increased likelihood of experiencing stress. For example, studies consistently show that stress decreases with age

We explore some of the more consistent findings with regard to risk factors for stress in the following subsections. However, it is important to reiterate that despite the significance of these factors at a population level, our ability to predict accurately which individuals will be affected by stress (and when and how) is extremely limited. Further, the studies were conducted primarily in the USA, with a

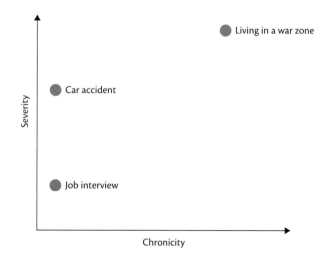

Fig. 45.3 The nature of stressors.

Popular opinion suggests that our jobs are causing us more stress than ever. This is often attributed to the increased prevalence of technology, which makes it difficult to switch off, and the increasingly competitive job market, which makes us fearful to do so. However, the results on job stress are somewhat equivocal, and vary depending on geographical location. For example, a national survey in Australia showed that the average rating of job stress has increased over the last few years [21], whereas in the UK, job stress has remained largely stable [22].

The two major sources of work stress are workload pressure (e.g. tight deadlines; too much responsibility) and lack of managerial support [22]. There is evidence that self-efficacy, i.e. an individual's belief that he or she can cope with demands, is a good indicator of his or her potential to be affected by stress at work. Fida et al. [46] showed that individuals who rate highly their ability to manage negative emotions are less likely to react negatively to work-related stressors. Self-efficacy also mitigates the stress associated with frequent interruptions (e.g. email alerts and instant messages) while performing computer-based tasks [47].

Importantly, the impact of work-related stress is not confined to the individual experiencing it. Work stress is a major contributor to work absenteeism and presenteeism worldwide, at a significant cost to the global economy (between 2% and 4% of gross national product [48, 49]).

among adults [1, 21, 50]. The cross-sectional nature of much of this research makes true comparisons of stress over time problematic and introduces the potential for cohort effects. However, a study by Vasunilashorn et al. [51] addresses this issue by using a longitudinal data set, with the same individuals assessed three times between 1999 and 2007. In this nationally representative, longitudinal study of older adults in Taiwan, perceived stress declined over time, providing support for the finding from cross-sectional studies that the interaction between age and stress is a true age effect rather than generational differences. It is also worth noting that while perceived stress decreases with age, exposure to stressors showed the reverse pattern, highlighting the importance of distinguishing between the two.

Another risk factor for stress is gender. Women typically report more stress than men [1, 21, 22, 50]. This supports the suggested link between stress and the internalizing psychiatric disorders (depression and anxiety), which are consistently demonstrated to affect women at around twice the rate of men [52].

In general, minority demographic groups report higher levels of stress, with both average stress levels and the proportion of individuals experiencing extreme stress higher in adults with a disability, racial and ethnic minorities, and those who identify as lesbian, gay, bisexual, or transgender (LGBT) [1]. Experiencing discrimination is associated with higher stress, and, for many, results in a chronic state of hypervigilance and behaviour change.

Low socio-economic status (SES) is also consistently identified as a risk factor for stress [21, 45, 53–55]. A range of factors are thought to account for the discrepancy in reported stress between people in higher and lower SES groups. It is well established that people living in disadvantaged areas have increased exposure to social and environmental conditions that trigger a stress response, including overcrowding, unemployment, conflict, crime, excessive noise, discrimination, and uncertainty [55–57]. It is also believed that the subjective experience of disadvantage relative to other people in the same community is a source of chronic stress [58]. The negative effect of relative deprivation may be exacerbated by stress-related coping responses (e.g. more smoking, heavier drinking), as well as invidious social comparisons [59]. The effects of chronic stress arising from low SES accumulate over time, but, worryingly, the biological manifestations of stressful living conditions can be seen in children as young as 4 years of age [60].

Does stress promote stress?

Stress and stressors can operate in a mutually reinforcing pattern. Results of a longitudinal study of 15–20 year olds suggest that past exposure to acute stressors (including early life adversity) is a risk factor for future exposure to acute stressors, whereas a history of high levels of perceived stress predicted high levels of perceived stress in the future [61]. In addition, high levels of perceived stress at age 15 years predicted experiencing acute stressors at age 20 years, indicating a bidirectional relationship between the two [61].

Chronic stress also affects our ability to deal with acute stressors, and, once again, the relationship is complex. Several studies have shown that regular exposure to low-level daily stressors lowers resilience to major stressors, making individuals more vulnerable to poor outcomes (e.g. routine work stress in police officers predicts the development of post-traumatic stress symptoms after a traumatic event, often more strongly than trauma exposure itself [62]). However, there is evidence that a moderate level of chronic stress is beneficial as it allows us to develop coping skills, which enhance our resilience in the face of mild, acute stress [63]. Therefore, we return to the idea that some stress is beneficial, but unrelenting chronic stress or an extremely severe acute stressor can impair our ability to function effectively.

Intrapersonal factors

Mental health problems are not only a consequence of stress, but can also increase the likelihood of being exposed to a stressor. This effect is most well documented for depression, where both personal and family history of mental illness predict exposure to stressful life events and experiencing a chronic stress response [61, 64]. There is also some evidence that anxiety plays a role in determining stressor exposure [65].

Similarly, for many people, drinking alcohol is a way of coping with stress. A study by Jones et al. [66] suggests that regular alcohol consumption is associated with diminished physiological (but not psychological) responses to mental stress. However, other research indicates that episodic evening drinking, to cope with the day's stress, is associated with more intense reactions to stressors the following day [67]. Therefore, alcohol appears to be both a risk and protective factor against the experience of stress, depending on how much and how often it is consumed.

Finally, personality traits (particularly neuroticism) predict both exposure to major stressors and the subsequent expression of a stress response [64, 68, 69]. Pessimism, a construct related to but distinct from neuroticism, appears to increase physiological stress responses in the face of perceived stress, whereas people who are optimistic by nature are protected against drastic changes in their physiological arousal when they experience higher-than-usual stress [70].

Preventing and managing stress

Interventions targeting stress can be categorized as primary, secondary, or tertiary interventions [71, 72]. As shown in Fig. 45.4, primary interventions aim to prevent stress from occurring, whereas secondary and tertiary interventions aim to manage stress once it has occurred [73].

Overall, there are few robust evaluations of interventions to reduce stress compared with studies investigating the prevalence, causes, and consequences of stress [71]. In this section, we describe different types of interventions for managing stress, and where data are available we provide a summary of the evidence on the effectiveness of different interventions.

Primary prevention

Organizational interventions in the workplace

Governments and organizations are increasingly aware of the negative impact work-related stress has on employee health and productivity, and this has led to a proliferation of workplace interventions to reduce stress among employees [48, 49, 73, 74]. A significant number of these involve primary interventions that aim to reduce stress by modifying elements of the work environment or the characteristics of the work requirements. By far, the most common strategy used in workplace stress reduction interventions is job redesign or restructuring [73]. This is followed (in order) by increasing participation and autonomy; incorporating training and education; implementing co-worker support groups;

modifying physical and environmental characteristics; improving communication; and resolving role issues [73].

A recent Cochrane review of interventions aimed at preventing psychological stress in healthcare workers concluded that of the range of organizational interventions tested (e.g. changing working conditions, organizing support, changing care, increasing communication skills, and changing work schedules), only changing work schedules, specifically from being continuous to incorporating weekend breaks, or changing from a 4-week to a 2-week schedule, was found to be effective. None of the other interventions were more effective than no intervention or an alternative intervention [75].

Another Cochrane review, this time examining the effectiveness of organizational interventions for reducing work-related stress in teachers, identified only four primary prevention interventions. Intervention components included work changes (e.g. re-designing work, establishing flexible work schedules, and redesigning the work environment); coaching support; individual training; and a multi-component intervention comprising bonus pay, job promotion opportunities, and mentoring [76]. Unfortunately, incomplete reporting of intervention components and outcomes, together with high attrition among participants, meant that the quality of evidence was low for all studies. Currently, there is weak evidence that re-designing the way teachers work may lead to improvements in their well-being and retention rates [76].

Overall, evidence for the effectiveness of workplace interventions for reducing employee stress is limited [73, 75, 76]. Further research using robust evaluation methods are needed to identify which elements of primary stress reduction interventions are most effective and for whom.

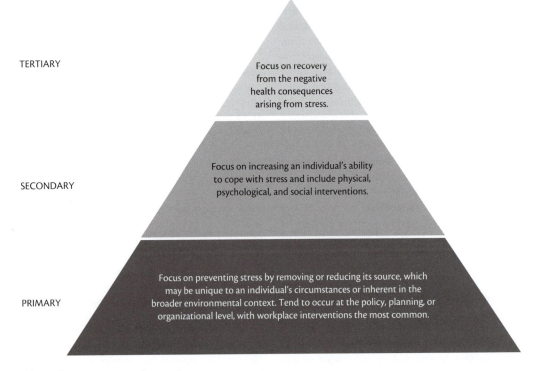

Fig. 45.4 Nature and focus of stress-management interventions.

Exposure to natural stimuli

A potentially promising primary intervention for preventing stress is exposure to natural environments [77]. Exposure to green spaces is hypothesized to prevent stress because natural environments elicit different patterns of psychological and physiological responses, particularly with regard to the parasympathetic nervous system, than urban and built environments [78–80].

Studies conducted in the workplace [81, 82], community [83], and hospital settings [84] have shown that when people are surrounded by green spaces they have lower levels of physiological and psychological stress than when they are surrounded by the built environment. In the community, exposure to the natural environment may include the presence of trees, parks, and other natural areas, whereas in the workplace or hospital setting exposure to the natural environment might include visual or physical access to gardens or other greenery [82].

Secondary prevention

Unhealthy stress management

People use a wide array of strategies to manage their stress which, to some extent, reflects individual differences in lifestyle and coping methods [21, 85]. Notably, some of the strategies known to be unhelpful (e.g. alcohol and substance use) because of their potential to inhibit helpful coping strategies [67] are rated as very effective among the people who use them [21]. Consistent with epidemiological studies showing that people living in low SES environments are more likely to engage in unhealthy behaviours [86], 25% of low-income Americans say they smoke to combat stress and 20% say they use alcohol [24] versus 6% and 7%, respectively, of more affluent Americans.

Relaxation

Many activities can promote the body's natural relaxation response, which is characterized by slower breathing, lower blood pressure, and a subjective feeling of well-being [87]. The scientific literature is full of studies examining the effect of relaxation activities on a range of health conditions [1, 21, 87]. However, the relaxation activities people report doing and the relaxation techniques scientists study are quite different.

The most common things people report doing to manage their stress are passive relaxation activities such as listening to music, going online, watching TV or movies, and reading [1, 21]. People who use passive relaxation techniques rate them as the most effective strategy in managing stress [21]. In contrast, the relaxation techniques examined in the scientific literature are typically active relaxation exercises (e.g. progressive muscle relaxation, guided imagery, biofeedback, self-hypnosis, deep breathing and massage [75, 87]), most of which require consistent practice in order to for the potential benefits to be realized.

Few studies of active relaxation have examined stress as a primary outcome, tending instead to investigate its effect on a condition like anxiety, depression, or chronic pain. However, there is some evidence to indicate that relaxation techniques are beneficial in reducing the acute physical symptoms of stress (e.g. blood pressure) and improving conditions affected by stress (e.g. insomnia) [88, 89]. In addition, Smith et al. [90] found that yoga and a 10-week, 1 hour a week progressive muscle relaxation course were equally effective in reducing stress, and four of six studies in a large

review by Ruotsalainen et al. [75] found that massage was more effective in reducing stress than no intervention.

Exercise

Physical activity is one of the most common strategies people use to manage stress. Almost half (47%) of American adults and 69% of Australian adults attempt to manage their stress by exercising, walking, meditation or yoga, and playing sports [1, 91].

Most people who use physical activity to manage stress believe it is at least moderately effective in achieving this goal [91]. Population-based studies show that individuals who exercise 2–3 times a week have significantly lower levels of perceived stress than people who do no exercise [92], whereas Swedish researchers found that exercising 1–2 times per week was beneficial in preventing stress-related burnout [93].

The psychological mechanisms linking exercise with reduced stress may include positive feedback from others, increased sense of mastery and self-worth, and distraction from daily hassles [94, 95]. Regular exercisers also report increased social contact and community integration [92].

Social support

It is increasingly recognized that having adequate social support is one of the strongest predictors of good physical and mental health [96–100]. The perception that you are loved, cared for, and listened to by people you trust can reduce the impact of life stressors [1, 101–103]. In Australia, 83% of adults report spending time with family or friends to reduce stress [91], whereas over a third (35%) of American adults manage stress by spending time with family [1]. Among people who draw on social support to manage stress, 84% rate it to be at least moderately effective [91].

Meditation and mindfulness

Meditation and mindfulness-based stress reduction has grown in popularity over recent decades and is used by a small, but increasing, proportion of the population to help manage stress [1, 104, 105]. Meditation emphasizes mindfulness, concentration, and automatic self-transcendence, whereas mindfulness-based stress reduction emphasizes training in present-focused awareness. Many studies have investigated the effect of these techniques on stress and general psychological distress; however, relatively few are high-quality, randomized controlled trials from which good evidence can be extracted. Earlier meta-analyses are likely to have overestimated the effect of mindfulness on reducing stress by including quasi-experimental, non-randomized, and observational studies [106]. A recent meta-analysis, which included only randomized controlled trials with adequate placebo, concluded that mindfulness-based meditation programmes have a small but positive effect on reducing psychological stress [104, 107]. Currently, there is insufficient evidence that mediation programmes influence health-related behaviours affected by stress (e.g. sleep, substance use) [104].

Cognitive–behavioural therapy for stress

Cognitive behavioural therapy (CBT) teaches individuals to identify and change maladaptive thoughts and behaviours that contribute to, and help maintain, distress [108]. CBT for stress can be part of a primary, secondary, or tertiary intervention depending on when and where it is delivered and who delivers it. CBT is an essential tool for mental health professionals who work with individuals seeking to recover from the harmful effects of stress (i.e. a tertiary intervention). However, because the core aim of CBT is to improve the way an individual interprets and responds to stressors, we have included it in this section on secondary prevention.

Several meta-analyses have examined whether CBT delivered in the workplace can prevent and reduce stress among employees [75, 109–111]. These interventions are typically group-based and teach core CBT strategies, including identifying negative thoughts; challenging maladaptive beliefs and attitudes; and improving one's behavioural response to stressors. Overall, the evidence suggests that workplace CBT interventions are effective in reducing stress, at least compared with no intervention [109]. However, CBT does not appear to be more effective than other workplace interventions, such as job redesign [75].

Tertiary interventions

Employee-assistance programmes

Employee-assistance programmes (EAPs) are workplace-based interventions that were originally designed for employees with substance use issues but have extended to address other issues that affect employees, including stress [112]. In many organizations, EAPs are the first stage of tertiary treatment, offering short-term counselling and, where necessary, referral to an external health professional [112, 113]. Overall, the limited evidence available suggests that EAPs have a positive impact on the emotional well-being of employees and that employees perceive EAPs to be a valuable workplace resource [114].

Mental health professionals

The perception that mental health professionals are a valuable resource in managing stress is gathering strength. The most recent American survey found that 45% of adults believed that psychologists could help with managing stress versus 31% in the previous year [1]. A smaller but still sizeable proportion of adults (around 13% of Australians in 2014) actually seek help [21]. It remains to be seen whether the proportion of people seeking care from health professionals increases as the evidence for effective primary and secondary management strategies grows.

Conclusions

In this chapter we have provided an overview of what stress is, how common it is, the factors associated with developing stress and interventions that might be useful in managing stress. As we have noted throughout the chapter, stress is an inevitable part of living; to experience stress is to know one is alive. Stress can have a positive impact on well-being; however, when stress is overwhelming it can be as disabling as anxiety or depression—two closely aligned problems that have received a great deal more public attention. With regard to the negative impact of stress, it is difficult to know exactly where the tipping point is for a particular individual. Future research aimed at understanding the factors and mechanisms that tip positive stress responses into negative stress responses will assist us in being able to prevent the adverse consequences associated with stress. It is likely we will find complex gene–environment interactions at the heart of this puzzle. On the basis of current evidence, routinely using exercise and mindfulness-based practices for stress management appears to offer more positives than negatives

and should be encouraged and maintained, from early life through to aged care.

References

1. American Psychological Association (APA). *Stress in America: The Impact of Discrimination.* Washington, DC: APA, 2016.
2. Lazarus RS, Folkman S. *Stress, Appraisal, and Coping.* New York: Springer, 1984.
3. Hancock PA, Szalma JL (eds). *Performance Under Stress.* Hampshire: Ashgate Publishing, 2008.
4. Lupien SJ, McEwen BS, Gunnar MR, Heim C. Effects of stress throughout the lifespan on the brain, behaviour and cognition. *Nat Rev Neurosci* 2009; 10: 434–445.
5. Segerstrom SC, Miller GE. Psychological stress and the human immune system: a meta-analytic study of 30 years of inquiry. *Psychol Bull* 2004; 130: 601–630.
6. Campbell J, Ehlert U. Acute psychosocial stress: does the emotional stress response correspond with physiological responses? *Psychoneuroendocrinology* 2012; 37: 1111–1134.
7. Carlson LE, Thomas BC. Development of the Calgary Symptoms of Stress Inventory (C-SOSI). *Int J Behav Med* 2007; 14: 249–256.
8. Devonport T. *Managing Stress: From Theory to Application.* New York: Nova Publishers, 2011.
9. Krohne HW. Stress and coping theories. In: Smelser NJ, Baltes PB (eds). *The International Encyclopedia of the Social and Behavioural Sciences.* Oxford: Elsevier, 2001, pp. 15163–15170.
10. Mark GM, Smith AP. Stress models: a review and suggested new direction. *Occup Health Psychol* 2008; 3: 111–144.
11. Palmer S, Gyllensten K (eds). *Psychological Stress, Resilience and Wellbeing.* London: SAGE, 2015.
12. Spielberger CD (ed.). *Anxiety: Current Trends in Theory and Research.* New York: Academic Press, 1972.
13. Hobfoll SE. Conservation of resources: a new attempt at conceptualizing stress. *Am Psychol* 1989; 44: 513–524.
14. Aspinwall LG, Taylor SE. A stitch in time: self-regulation and proactive coping. *Psychol Bull* 1997; 121: 417–436.
15. Schwarzer R, Taubert S. Tenacious goal pursuits and striving toward personal growth: proactive coping. In: Frydenberg E (ed.). *Beyond Coping: Meeting Goals, Visions and Challenges.* London: Oxford University Press, 2002, pp. 19–35.
16. Krueger RF. The structure of common mental disorders. *Arch Gen Psychiat* 1999; 56: 921–926.
17. Uliaszek AA, Zinbarg RE, Mineka S, et al. The role of neuroticism and extraversion in the stress-anxiety and stress-depression relationships. *Anxiety Stress Coping* 2010; 23: 363–381.
18. Watson D. Intraindividual and interindividual analyses of positive and negative affect: their relation to health complaints, perceived stress, and daily activities. *J Person Soc Psychol* 1988; 54: 1020–1030.
19. Henry JD, Crawford JR. The short-form version of the Depression Anxiety Stress Scales (DASS-21): construct validity and normative data in a large non-clinical sample. *Br J Clin Psychol* 2005; 44: 227–239.
20. Lovibond PF, Lovibond SH. The structure of negative emotional states—Comparison of the Depression Anxiety Stress Scales (DASS) with the Beck Depression and Anxiety Inventories. *Behav Res Ther* 1995; 33: 335–343.
21. Australian Psychological Society (APS). *Stress and Wellbeing in Australia Survey 2014.* Melbourne: APS, 2014.
22. Health and Safety Executive. Work related stress, anxiety and depression statistics in Great Britain 2015. Available at: www.hse.gov.uk/statistics/ (accessed 16 March 2018).
23. Norlund S, Reuterwall C, Hoog J, Lindahl B, Janlert U, Birgander LS. Burnout, working conditions and gender: results from the northern Sweden MONICA Study. *BMC Public Health* 2010;10.
24. American Psychological Association (APA). *Stress in America: Are Teens Adopting Adults' Stress Habits?* Washington, DC: APA, 2014.

25. American Psychological Association (APA). *Stress in America Findings.* Washington, DC: APA, 2010.

26. American Psychological Association (APA). *Stress in America 2009.* Washington, DC: APA, 2009.

27. Conrad CD (ed.). *The Handbook of Stress: Neuropsychological Effects on the Brain.* Chichester: Wiley-Blackwell, 2011.

28. Martikainen S, Pesonen AK, Lahti J, et al. Higher levels of physical activity are associated with lower hypothalamic-pituitary-adrenocortical axis reactivity to psychosocial stress in children. *J Clin Endocr Metab* 2013; 98: E619–E27.

29. McEwen BS. Protection and damage from acute and chronic stress: allostasis and allostatic overload and relevance to the pathophysiology of psychiatric disorders. *Ann N Y Acad Sci* 2004; 1032: 1–7.

30. Lampert R, Tuit K, Hong KI, Donovan T, Lee F, Sinha R. Cumulative stress and autonomic dysregulation in a community sample. *Stress* 2016; 19: 269–279.

31. Dhabhar FS. Effects of stress on immune function: the good, the bad, and the beautiful. *Immunol Res* 2014; 58: 193–210.

32. O'Donovan A, Tomiyama AJ, Lin J, et al. Stress appraisals and cellular aging: a key role for anticipatory threat in the relationship between psychological stress and telomere length. *Brain Behav Immun* 2012; 26: 573–579.

33. Prather AA, Gurfein B, Moran P, et al. Tired telomeres: poor global sleep quality, perceived stress, and telomere length in immune cell subsets in obese men and women. *Brain Behav Immun* 2015; 47: 155–162.

34. Hammen C. Depression and stressful environments: Identifying gaps in conceptualization and measurement. *Anxiety Stress Coping* 2016; 29: 335–351.

35. Melchior M, Caspi A, Milne BJ, Danese A, Poulton R, Moffitt TE. Work stress precipitates depression and anxiety in young, working women and men. *Psychol Med* 2007; 37: 1119–1129.

36. Keyes KM, Hatzenbuehler ML, Grant BF, Hasin DS. Stress and alcohol: epidemiologic evidence. *Alcohol Res* 2012; 34: 391–400.

37. Forbes D, Fletcher S, Parslow R, et al. Trauma at the hands of another: Longitudinal study of differences in the posttraumatic stress disorder symptom profile following interpersonal compared with noninterpersonal trauma. *J Clin Psychiatry* 2012; 73: 372–6.

38. Vrshek-Schallhorn S, Stroud CB, Mineka S, et al. Chronic and episodic interpersonal stress as statistically unique predictors of depression in two samples of emerging adults. *J Abnorm Psychol* 2015; 124: 918–932.

39. Creamer M, Burgess P, McFarlane AC. Post-traumatic stress disorder: findings from the Australian National Survey of Mental Health and Well-being. *Psychol Med* 2001; 31: 1237–1247.

40. Kessler RC, Sonnega A, Bromet E, Hughes M, Nelson CB. Posttraumatic stress disorder in the National Comorbidity Survey. *Arch Gen Psychiat* 1995; 52: 1048–1060.

41. Tomova L, von Dawans B, Heinrichs M, Silani G, Lamm C. Is stress affecting our ability to tune into others? Evidence for gender differences in the effects of stress on self-other distinction. *Psychoneuroendocrinology* 2014; 43: 95–104.

42. von Dawans B, Fishbacher U, Kirschbaum C, Fehr E, Heinrichs M. The social dimension of stress reactivity: Acute stress increases prosocial behavior in humans. *Psychol Sci* 2012; 23: 651–660.

43. Wolf OT, Schulte JM, Drimalla H, Hamacher-Dang TC, Knoch D, Dziobek I. Enhanced emotional empathy after psychosocial stress in young healthy men. *Stress* 2015; 18: 631–637.

44. Selye H. The evolution of the stress concept. *Am Sci* 1973; 61: 692–699.

45. American Psychological Association (APA). *Stress in America: Paying With Our Health.* Washington, DC: APA, 2015.

46. Fida R, Paciello M, Tramontano C, Barbaranelli C, Farnese ML. 'Yes, I Can': the protective role of personal self-efficacy in hindering counterproductive work behavior under stressful conditions. *Anxiety Stress Coping* 2015; 28: 479–499.

47. Tams S, Thatcher J, Grover V, Pak R. Selective attention as a protagonist in contemporary workplace stress: implications for the interruption age. *Anxiety Stress Coping* 2015; 28: 663–686.

48. Medibank Private. *The Cost of Workplace Stress in Australia.* Canberra: Medibank Private, 2008.

49. World Health Organization (WHO). *PRIMA-EF: Guidance on the European Framework for Psychosocial Risk Management: A Resource for Employers and Worker Representatives.* Geneva: WHO, 2008.

50. Cohen S, Janicki-Deverts D. Who's stressed? Distributions of psychological stress in the United States in probability samples from 1983, 2006, and 2009. *J Appl Soc Psychol* 2012; 42: 1320–1334.

51. Vasunilashorn S, Lynch SM, Glei DA, Weinstein M, Goldman N. Exposure to stressors and trajectories of perceived stress among older adults. *J Gerontol B Psychol Sci Soc Sci* 2015; 70: 329–337.

52. Eaton NR, Keyes KM, Krueger RF, et al. An invariant dimensional liability model of gender differences in mental disorder prevalence: evidence from a national sample. *J Abnorm Psychol* 2012; 121: 282–288.

53. Adler NE, Rehkopf DH. U.S. disparities in health: descriptions, causes, and mechanisms. *Annu Rev Public Health* 2008; 29: 235–252.

54. Cohen S, Schwartz JE, Epele E, Kirschbaum C, Sydney S, Seeman T. Socioeconomic status, race, and diurnal cortisol decline in the Coronary Artery Risk Development in Young Adults (CARDIA) study. *Psychosom Med* 2006; 68: 41–50.

55. Wilkinson R, Marmot M. *Social Determinants of Health: The Solid Facts.* Copenhagen: World Health Organization, 2003.

56. Baum A, Garofalo JP, Yali AM. Socioeconomic status and chronic stress. Does stress account for SES effects on health? *Ann N Y Acad Sci* 1999; 896: 131–144.

57. Kuruvilla A, Jacob KS. Poverty, social stress & mental health. *Indian J Med Res* 2007; 126: 273–278.

58. Marmot M. Status syndrome. *Significance* 2004; 1: 150–154.

59. Kopp MS, Skrabski A, Szekely A, Stauder A, Williams R. Chronic stress and social changes: socioeconomic determination of chronic stress. *Ann N Y Acad Sci* 2007; 1113: 325–338.

60. Vliegenthart J, Noppe G, van Rossum EFC, Koper JW, Raat H, van den Akker ELT. Socioeconomic status in children is associated with hair cortisol levels as a biological measure of chronic stress. *Psychoneuroendocrinology* 2016; 65: 9–14.

61. Hammen C, Brennan PA, Le Brocque R. Youth depression and early childrearing: stress generation and intergenerational transmission of depression. *J Consult Clin Psych* 2011; 79: 353–363.

62. Liberman AM, Best SR, Metzler TJ, Fagan JA, Weiss DS, Marmar CR. Routine occupational stress and psychological distress in police. *Policing* 2002; 25: 421–439.

63. Seery MD, Leo RJ, Lupien SP, Kondrak CL, Almonte JL. An upside to adversity? Moderate cumulative lifetime adversity is associated with resilient responses in the face of controlled stressors. *Psychol Sci* 2013; 24: 1181–1189.

64. Liu RT, Alloy LB. Stress generation in depression: a systematic review of the empirical literature and recommendations for future study. *Clin Psychol Rev* 2010; 30: 582–593.

65. Phillips AC, Carroll D, Der G. Negative life events and symptoms of depression and anxiety: Stress causation and/or stress generation. *Anxiety Stress Coping* 2015; 28: 357–371.

66. Jones A, McMillan MR, Jones RW, et al. Habitual alcohol consumption is associated with lower cardiovascular stress responses—a novel explanation for the known cardiovascular benefits of alcohol? *Stress* 2013; 16: 369–376.

67. Armeli S, O'Hara RE, Covault J, Scott DM, Tennen H. Episode-specific drinking-to-cope motivation and next-day stress-reactivity. *Anxiety Stress Coping* 2016; 29: 673–684.

68. Fletcher S. *Personality and the Trajectory of Posttraumatic Psychopathology.* Melbourne: University of Melbourne, 2015.

69. Bibbey A, Carroll D, Roseboom TJ, Phillips AC, de Rooij SR. Personality and physiological reactions to acute psychological stress. *Int J Psychophysiol* 2013; 90: 28–36.

70. Jobin J, Wrosch C, Scheier MF. Associations between dispositional optimism and diurnal cortisol in a community sample: when stress is perceived as higher than normal. *Health Psychol* 2014; 33: 382–391.

71. Probst TM. Conducting effective stress intervention research: strategies for achieving an elusive goal. *Stress Health* 2013; 29: 1–4.

72. Harvey SB, Joyce S, Modini M, et al. *Work and Depression/ Anxiety Disorders—A Systematic Review of Reviews*. New South Wales: University of New South Wales, 2012.

73. Bergeman L, Corabian P, Harstall C. *Effectiveness of Organizational Interventions for the Prevention of Workplace Stress*. Edmonton: Institute of Health Economics, 2009.

74. National Health Service Employers. *Guidance on Prevention and Management of Stress at Work*. London: National Health Service, 2014.

75. Ruotsalainen JH, Verbeek JH, Marine A, Serra C. Preventing occupational stress in healthcare workers. *Cochrane Database Syst Rev* 2015; 4: CD002892.

76. Naghieh A, Montgomery P, Bonell CP, Thompson M, Aber JL. Organisational interventions for improving wellbeing and reducing work-related stress in teachers. *Cochrane Database Syst Rev* 2015; 4: CD10306.

77. Maller C, Townsend M, Pryor A, Brown P, St Leger L. Healthy nature healthy people: 'Contact with nature' as an upstream health promotion intervention for populations. *Health Promot Int* 2006; 21: 45–54.

78. Berto R. The role of nature in coping with psycho-physiological stress: a literature review on restorativeness. *Behav Sci* 2014; 4: 394.

79. Ulrich RS. Natural versus urban scenes: some psychophysiological effects. *Environ Behav* 1981; 13: 523–556.

80. Ulrich RS, Simons RF, Losito BD, Fiorito E, Miles MA, Zelson M. Stress recovery during exposure to natural and urban environments. Journal of *Environ Psychol* 1991; 11: 201–230.

81. Beil K, Hanes D. The influence of urban natural and built environments on physiological and psychological measures of stress—a pilot study. *Int J Environ Res Public Health* 2013; 10: 1250–1267.

82. Lottrup L, Grahn P, Stigsdotter UK. Workplace greenery and perceived level of stress: Benefits of access to a green outdoor environment at the workplace. *Landscape Urban Plan* 2013; 110: 5–11.

83. Roe JJ, Thompson CW, Aspinall PA, et al. Green space and stress: evidence from cortisol measures in deprived urban communities. *Int J Environ Res Public Health* 2013; 10: 4086–4103.

84. Beukeboom CJ, Langeveld D, Tanja-Dijkstra K. Stress-reducing effects of real and artificial nature in a hospital waiting room. *J Altern Complement Med* 2012; 18: 329–333.

85. Carr D, Umberson D. The social psychology of stress, health, and coping. In: DeLamater J, Ward A (eds). *Handbook of Social Psychology*. New York: Springer, 2013, pp. 465–487.

86. Pampel FC, Krueger PM, Denney JT. Socioeconomic disparities in health behaviours. *Annu Rev Sociol* 2010; 36: 349–370.

87. National Institutes of Health. *Relaxation Techniques*. Bethesda, MD: National Center for Complementary and Integrative Health, 2014.

88. Dusek JA, Hibberd PL, Buczynski B, et al. Stress management versus lifestyle modification on systolic hypertension and medication elimination: a randomized trial. *J Altern Complement Med* 2008; 14: 129–138.

89. Morin CM, Bootzin RR, Buysse DJ, Edinger JD, Espie CA, Lichstein KL. Psychological And behavioral treatment of insomnia: update of the recent evidence (1998–2004). *Sleep* 2006; 29: 1398–1414.

90. Smith C, Hancock H, Blake-Mortimer J, Eckert K. A randomised comparative trial of yoga and relaxation to reduce stress and anxiety. *Complement Ther Med* 2007; 15: 77–83.

91. Australian Psychological Society. Stress & wellbeing: how Australians are coping with life 2015. Available from: https://trove.nla.gov.au/work/199785951?q&versionId=219017795 (accessed 16 March 2018).

92. Hassmén P, Koivula N, Uutela A. Physical exercise and psychological well-being: a population study in Finland. *Prev Med* 2000; 30: 17–25.

93. Lindegård A, Jonsdottir IH, Börjesson M, Lindwall M, Gerber M. Changes in mental health in compliers and non-compliers with physical activity recommendations in patients with stress-related exhaustion. *BMC Psychiatry* 2015; 15: 1–10.

94. Mirza I, Pit SW. Exercise for positive mental health outcomes in adults. *Cochrane Database Syst Rev* 2006; 1: CD005615.

95. Stathopoulou G, Powers MB, Berry AC, Smits JAJ, Otto MW. Exercise interventions for mental health: a quantitative and qualitative review. *Clin Psychol* 2006; 13: 179–193.

96. Davidson SK, Dowrick CF, Gunn JM. Impact of functional and structural social relationships on two year depression outcomes: a multivariate analysis. *J Affect Disord* 2016; 193: 274–281.

97. Coyne JC, Downey G. Social factors and psychopathology: stress, social support, and coping processes. *Annu Rev Psychol* 1991; 42: 401–425.

98. Holt-Lunstad J, Smith TB, Layton JB. Social relationships and mortality risk: a meta-analytic review. *PLOS Med* 2010; 7: e1000316.

99. Thoits PA. Mechanisms linking social ties and support to physical and mental health. *J Health Soc Behav* 2011; 52: 145–161.

100. Ozbay F, Johnson DC, Dimoulas E, Morgan CA, Charney D, Southwick S. Social support and resilience to stress: from neurobiology to clinical practice. *Psychiatry* 2007; 4: 35–40.

101. Cohen S. Social relationships and health. *Am Psychol* 2004; 59: 676–684.

102. Umberson D, Montez JK. Social relationships and health: a flashpoint for health policy. *J Health Soc Behav* 2010; 51(1 suppl.): S54–S66.

103. Cohen S, Wills TA. Stress, social support, and the buffering hypothesis. *Psychol Bull* 1985; 98: 310–357.

104. Goyal M, Singh S, Sibinga EMS, et al. Meditation programs for psychological stress and well-being: A systematic review and meta-analysis. *JAMA Intern Med* 2014; 174: 357–368.

105. Chiesa A, Serretti A. Mindfulness-based stress reduction for stress management in healthy people: a review and meta-analysis. *J Altern Complement Med* 2009; 15: 593–600.

106. Coronado-Montoya S, Levis AW, Kwakkenbos L, Steele RJ, Turner EH, Thombs BD. Reporting of positive results in randomized controlled trials of mindfulness-based mental health interventions. *PLOS ONE* 2016; 11: e0153220.

107. Bohlmeijer E, Prenger R, Taal E, Cuijpers P. The effects of mindfulness-based stress reduction therapy on mental health of adults with a chronic medical disease: a meta-analysis. *J Psychosom Res* 2010; 68: 539–544.

108. Beck JS. *Cognitive Behavior Therapy: Basics and Beyond*, 2nd ed. New York: The Guilford Press, 2011.

109. Hofmann SG, Asnaani A, Vonk IJJ, Sawyer AT, Fang A. The efficacy of cognitive behavioral therapy: a review of meta-analyses. *Cogn Ther Res* 2012; 36: 427–440.

110. Richardson KM, Rothstein HR. Effects of occupational stress management intervention programs: a meta-analysis. *J Occup Health Psychol* 2008; 13: 69–93.

111. van der Klink JJL, Blonk RWB, Schene AH., van Dijk FJH. The benefits of interventions for work-related stress. *Am J Public Health* 2001; 91: 270–276.

112. Levy Merrick ES, Volpe-Vartanian J, Horgan CM, McCann B. Revisiting employee assistance programs and substance use problems in the workplace: Key issues and a research agenda. *Psychiatr Serv* 2007; 58: 1262–1264.

113. Azzone V, McCann B, Merrick EL, Hiatt D, Hodgkin D, Horgan C. Workplace stress, organizational factors and EAP utilization. *J Workplace Behav Health* 2009; 24: 344–356.

114. Kirk AK, Brown DF. Employee assistance programs: a review of the management of stress and wellbeing through workplace counselling and consulting. *Aust Psychol* 2003; 38: 138–143.

CHAPTER 46

Psychological intervention as a measure for promoting public mental health
Is it a white elephant?

Roger M. K. Ng and Che Kin Lee

Mental disorder as a global issue

The first 17 World Mental Health surveys conducted in 28 countries throughout the world have shown that mental disorders are highly prevalent, with an inter-quartile range of 12-month *Diagnostic and Statistical Manual of Mental Disorders*, 4th Editon, disorder prevalence estimated as around 9.8–19.1% [1]. Furthermore, many mental disorders were found to have their time of onset during childhood or adolescent periods. As such, these disorders would have a significant adverse impact on the trajectory of the subsequent development of these individuals. Mental disorders were also associated with marked role impairment and substantial years of life lost due to premature morbidity and years lived with disability [2]. Therefore, provision of timely evidence-based interventions to prevent the onset, halt the progression, and minimize the development of co-morbidities and treatment-resistant symptoms will be of immense benefit to the improvement of global mental health.

Given the high prevalence of mental disorders around the globe and the limited amount of resources allocated to public mental health services, it is important to invest scarce resources in effective interventions for mental disorders that are not only most prevalent, but also that exact high individual and societal costs. Anxiety disorders were consistently found to be the most prevalent class of mental disorders [3], followed by mood disorders (namely depressive disorders) [4]. Depressive and anxiety disorders accounted for 40.5% and 14.6% of disability-adjusted life years caused by mental and substance use disorders, respectively [2]. The other two commonly occurring classes of disorders are externalizing disorders (attention deficit hyperactivity disorder, oppositional defiant disorder, conduct disorder, and intermittent explosive disorder) and substance use disorders (alcohol and illicit drug abuse and dependence). From a public health perspective, allocating valuable resources to treatment of these disorders therefore appears to be most cost-effective.

Apart from providing timely evidence-based interventions for these full-blown mental disorders, another important consideration from the public health perspective is that clinically significant subthreshold manifestations of these disorders are more prevalent than the full-blown disorders themselves [5]. Furthermore, sub-threshold bipolar disorders [6] and sub-threshold anxiety and depressive disorders [7] were associated with significant role impairment and heightened risks of conversion to full-blown disorders. Early intervention of such sub-threshold disorders would therefore lead to a reduction in role impairment and subsequent conversion to full-blown disorders.

The third pertinent question from the public health perspective is whether such interventions are acceptable and feasible in low- and middle-income countries (LAMICs). Previous studies have consistently found that indicators of poverty were strongly associated with the development of common mental disorders (CMD), the most consistent association being with low levels of education [8]. It has been consistently shown that CMD are prevalent but undertreated in LAMICs [9]. Furthermore, psychosocial interventions were beneficial for cognitive development and improved educational outcomes in disadvantaged children, which, in turn, led to positive impacts on mental health [8]. Psychosocial interventions in the form of short-term structured psychotherapy delivered at primary care level are also effective in inducing remission of CMD in these countries [8, 10]. Therefore, the core question is how such evidence-based psychosocial interventions can become available in these countries. Given the lack of trained experts and mental health facilities in many of these countries, wide dissemination of effective psychological interventions would imply training local health counsellors in delivering brief manual-based interventions with minimal supervision. A recent successful example is that brief manual-based problem-solving therapy delivered by lay health workers under weekly group supervision by a general nurse with training in counselling was effective in treating anxiety and depression in primary care clinics in Zimbabwe [11]. In areas where experienced clinicians are not available or accessible, peer supervision among local health counsellors may possibly be a viable alternative. Yet, this model of peer supervision warrants further research.

This chapter will examine the current evidence of psychological interventions in the treatment of CMD and substance misuse at the primary care level, as well as in the prevention of CMD applied universally or to target at-risk populations.

Psychological interventions of common mental disorders in primary care

While antidepressants have been found to be efficacious in the treatment of anxiety and depressive disorders, there are still questions about their efficacy and risk–benefit balance in specific groups of patients [12]. Among all different types of brief psychological interventions for primary care patients with depression and anxiety, most studies were of cognitive–behavioural therapy (CBT) [13]. Both antidepressants and CBT have been found to be equally efficacious in the treatment of primary care patients with mild depression [14]. Furthermore, when primary care patients have poor responses to antidepressants, CBT has been found to be an effective adjunct to pharmacotherapy [15]. Preventive CBT delivered during the remission phase was also superior to antidepressants and usual care in preventing subsequent relapse and recurrence of depressive disorders [16]. Apart from its efficacy in depression, there is increasing evidence that primary care patients with panic disorders [17] and multiple anxiety disorders [18] can benefit from a combination of medications and CBT. What is encouraging is that CBT-naïve and mid-level community mental health workers could also deliver effective protocol-driven CBT after brief training [17, 18]. Behavioural activation (BA), a simpler psychological treatment based on CBT principles, delivered by junior mental health workers, is shown to be a type of psychological therapy for depression with a similar efficacy to CBT [19]. The junior mental health workers recruited in the trial were graduates who had no mental health qualifications or formal training in psychological interventions. They received 5 days of training in BA followed by a 60-minute clinical supervision fortnightly from psychological therapists clinically experienced in BA. As such, BA can be a cost-effective psychological treatment for adults with depression and will potentially lead to a great impact on treatment of depression from a public health perspective.

Despite the evidence, CBT and BA might be difficult to access for various personal and geographical reasons. To address this accessibility problem, studies have attempted to explore the delivery of CBT using modern communication technology. Telephone-administered CBT has been found to have similar efficacy but lower rates of attrition than face-to-face CBT for primary care patients with mild-to-moderate depression [20]. A computerized eight-session CBT programme conducted and supported in the primary care office has also been found to be an effective and acceptable treatment for patients with depression or anxiety of mild-to-moderate severity [21]. CBT administered online by a CBT therapist with or without medications has been found to be more efficacious than usual treatment for depression [22]. Internet-based structured modular CBT programmes with time-limited support by a clinician has also been found to be effective for patients with anxiety disorders [23], depressive disorders [24, 25], and mixed depressive and anxiety disorders [23, 26]. The amount of time spent by the clinician in such Internet-based CBT programmes monitoring and responding to changes in online outcome ratings was minimal [26]. Two meta-analyses have even suggested that

Internet-based CBT reduced symptoms in both depression and anxiety even without therapist input [27, 28]. However, a word of caution: Internet-based CBT without any clinical support may not be beneficial to people with untreated, full-blown depression in the community [29]. Besides, the median adherence rate of 56% to the clinician-assisted Internet-based CBT is disappointingly low [30]. Further research is thus needed to improve adherence rates to Internet-based programmes and to enhance the efficacy of CBT with limited or no therapist input. Furthermore, the efficacy of these Internet-based CBT was researched in Western countries and their efficacy in developing countries awaits further investigation.

In LAMICs where availability of and accessibility to portable devices and Internet services are limited, CBT needs to be provided by face-to-face interventions. It is encouraging to see that brief, protocol-driven psychological interventions (generic counselling with or without cognitive–behavioural strategies) by trained lay health counsellors have been proven to be effective and feasible for anxiety and depression [31]. Research experience suggests that these lay therapists with no mental health background should preferably be young, female adults, gender-matched with the patient groups, trained in therapy skills rather than theory, and supported with a well-defined, structured supervisory protocol by a skilled mental health professional [32]. Given that BA may be a simpler psychological treatment than CBT for depression [19], whether this intervention can be adapted and disseminated to these countries with low resources will be an urgent and important public health research topic.

While the aforementioned studies suggest that CBT is most researched and therefore recommended as the first-line intervention for the conditions discussed, a recent meta-analyses has reported that other brief psychological therapies (i.e. counselling and problem-solving therapy) have a similar efficacy to CBT for the treatment of CMD in primary care settings [13]. A five-session online course of problem-solving therapy (PST) produced a faster improvement in depressive and anxiety symptoms than an eight-session online course of CBT [25], suggesting short-term PST-based intervention being a valuable alternative to CBT. Similarly, patients with HIV with depression in Zimbabwe reported a significant reduction in symptoms after a six-session course of PST delivered by lay health workers under the supervision of a general nurse with training in counseling [11]. Generic counselling also has a similar efficacy to antidepressants for patients with mild-to-moderate depression in primary care in the UK, although antidepressants have a shorter time to remission [33]. Interpersonal therapy (IPT) with or without antidepressants delivered by trained lay health counsellors was also more effective than usual primary care for CMD in India [31]. This collaborative stepped-care model involving trained lay health counsellors providing first-line IPT and secondary referral to mental health specialists for severe or treatment-resistant cases addresses the issue of lack of specialist resources in remote or poor regions [31]. In summary, time-limited, protocol-driven, structured psychotherapy appears to be a promising psychological intervention for people with CMD in countries with different levels of income.

Psychological interventions of drug misuse at primary care and community level

As mentioned in the introductory section, substance and alcohol abuse are also highly prevalent mental disorders in the community.

In the past two decades, there has been a surge of interest in using contingency management based on behavioural principles to reduce the frequency of drug abuse in the community. Higgins et al. [34] found that patients who received behaviour therapy plus contingent vouchers exchangeable for retail goods and services upon submission of cocaine-free urine specimens were more likely to achieve cocaine abstinence than those on behaviour therapy alone during treatment and at the 6-month post-treatment follow-up. Furthermore, patients who obtained vouchers contingent upon abstinence had a higher abstinence rate than those who were given vouchers regardless of urine specimen results, thereby demonstrating the efficacy of contingent reinforcement [35]. While some patients might not benefit from standalone psychological interventions, a recent systematic review has supported the value of providing adjunct psychological interventions (predominantly contingency management and CBT) for the treatment of opioid addictions [36].

Substance and alcohol misuse are also highly co-morbid with CMD and worsen the prognosis of depression. A randomized controlled trial (RCT) compared the efficacy of CBT versus brief intervention in treating co-morbid depression and alcohol/cannabis misuse [37]. All participants received a brief intervention (one-session manualized intervention with brief advice to reduce alcohol/cannabis misuse and self-help materials for these problems) followed by random allocation to either nine sessions of motivational interviewing (MI) and CBT or no further treatment (brief intervention) for 3 months. Participants in the MI/CBT arm were further randomized to either 'live' therapy (i.e. delivered by a psychologist in person) or computer-based programme (with brief 10–15-minute weekly psychologist input; SHADE program). Participants in the MI/CBT programme had lower levels of depression than those in brief intervention alone, with those in the live-therapy group having a strong short-term benefit eventually caught up by the SHADE program at the 12-month follow-up. However, alcohol misuse responded well to brief intervention alone, whereas cannabis misuse responded better to MI/CBT than brief intervention alone. Furthermore, those in the computer-based programme had a better outcome in cannabis misuse than those in the live-therapy group. The current results suggest that computer-based intervention is a cost-effective treatment for co-morbid depression and cannabis misuse. As computer-based programme minimizes the therapist's contact time and fits well with the youth culture, on-line computer-based CBT should be further explored as a promising treatment of depression with associated co-morbidities of drug and alcohol misuse in young populations.

Universal approaches to preventing psychiatric disorders

The aforementioned evidence shows that short-term psychological interventions for full-blown CMD lead to enhanced recovery. A logical question to follow is to understand whether psychological interventions are effective for preventing the development of CMD. The usual goals of prevention programmes are to enhance well-being, reduce current sub-threshold levels of symptomatology, and improve future coping. These programmes can be provided to all individuals in a specified population (universal prevention), regardless of risk status, or toward individuals who are identified as having an increased vulnerability for a disorder based on some individual

assessment but who are currently asymptomatic (indicated prevention) or targeted towards sub-populations identified as being at elevated risk for a disorder (selective prevention) [38].

Given that CMD usually develop in late childhood and early adolescence [39], it is not surprising that most preventive psychological intervention programmes were provided to children and adolescents. As schools provide a convenient and accessible location for delivering prevention programmes, most of these programmes were delivered by trained teachers or researchers in school. A universal prevention study with high-school students showed that teaching classes based on cognitive and interpersonal models were effective in reducing depressive symptoms [40]. However, another pragmatic cluster-based RCT found that classroom-based CBT incorporated into the school curriculum was not effective in reducing depressive symptoms in younger adolescents (aged 12–16 years) when compared with a time-matched attention control group and usual school class group [41]. The classroom-based CBT group might even have had higher depressive symptoms than the other two groups at the 12-month follow-up [41]. The possibility of worse outcome after school-based programmes has also been found for attention deficit hyperactivity disorder [42]. Given that trained school teachers were found to be less effective than trained graduates and health professionals in providing mental health programmes [43], failure of delivery of effective prevention programmes to school adolescents might explain the current non-significant findings. Besides, the delivery of classroom-based CBT might need to be age- and phase-specific, with the content and mode of delivery of the programmes adapted to different psychological and social needs at different ages and school levels. The involvement of parents and families might be essential for CBT targeting young school children.

Universal approaches have also been used in the prevention of anxiety among children as young as preschool and through middle-school. A universal programme consisting of six sessions of training parents in building positive expectations and of social competency in children has been found to be effective in reducing child internalizing and externalizing problems via teacher report [44]. A 10-session family-group CBT programme routinely implemented as part of the school curriculum—the FRIENDS programme—has been found to be effective as a universal prevention in reducing anxiety and depression in children in grades 6 and 9 [45]. The reduction in anxiety was maintained at subsequent follow-ups at 12, 24, and 36 months [46]. A replication trial of the FRIENDS programme was conducted for children aged 9–12 years in 14 schools in Germany [47]. Children in the FRIENDS programme had significantly fewer anxiety and depressive symptoms, as well as lower perfectionism scores, than children in the control group at the 12-month follow-up. Younger children (9–10 years of age) experienced immediate improvement upon completion of the programme, but older children (11–12 years of age) only exhibited improvement at the 6- and 12-month follow-ups. Another 12-week CBT intervention programme led either by teachers or psychologists was reported to be effective in reducing symptoms of anxiety in children aged 10–12 years [48]. It is worth noting that most universal interventions for children with anxiety have shown that the impact is greatest on girls and those aged 11 and 12 years [49]. The differential effects of CBT on the prevention of anxiety and depressive symptoms in school-based programmes might reflect the fact that such programmes may work better for children than adolescents and for anxiety rather than depressive symptoms. The involvement of family members for younger children and adolescents may also be key factors of success of the programmes.

Besides targeting prevention of anxiety and depression, universal prevention programmes based on social information processing approaches for prevention of violence and aggression in schools were also developed. The studies show an encouraging 25–30% reduction in the base rate of aggressive problems in an average school [50, 51]. Some of these programmes also have the additional benefits of reducing the early initiation of alcohol use and progression of alcohol use in adolescents [52]. Most of these programmes focus on teaching knowledge about violence and aggression, enhancing empathy skills, and modifying disruptive and antisocial behaviours by changing cognitive and affective mechanisms (i.e. cognitive shift and emotional-regulation skills) linked with such behaviours, as well as social skills training for enhancing the repertoire of pro-social behaviours [51].

Universal prevention programmes have also been developed for preventing alcohol misuse [52]. Family-focused interventions delivered in the preschool years were found to reduce aggressive behaviours that might subsequently reduce alcohol use. Such family-based interventions have focused mainly on developing healthy parent–child relationships, building children's social and cognitive competence for school life [53, 54]. Small group and home-based family interventions targeting young people aged 10–15 years have also been shown to delay the initiation of alcohol use [55]. Unlike family intervention for younger children, these interventions for young people focused on parent–child bonding, effective parental discipline, and parental involvement in youth activities. Furthermore, school-based interventions that emphasize coaching of life skills and emotional-regulation skills, peer-refusal skills, education on the risks of drinking, and focus on positive relationships have also been found to be effective in reducing early initiation of alcohol use in early adolescence [56]. It is also worth noting that multi-component interventions that address different life domains (e.g. school, family, peer relationships, etc.) may be more promising than single-component interventions [52].

Apart from alcohol misuse, drug misuse is another major problem among children and adolescents. Universal school-based drug abuse curricula were designed for classroom delivery in junior and middle-high schools. A meta-analysis of 29 RCTs evaluating efficacy of universal, school-based drug prevention programmes in reducing marijuana and other illicit drug misuse found that skills-based interventions are more effective than affective or knowledge-based interventions [57]. The skills taught to the students included assertiveness in resisting peer pressure to take drugs and social skills to improve self-esteem and decision-making. As pointed out by Flynn et al. [58], most studies with positive results were conducted by the programme developers under stringent research conditions with multiple outcome measures, thereby casting doubt about its generalizability to other non-research settings. In order to address this limitation, Flynn et al. [58] conducted a recent meta-analysis that identified studies of school-based prevention conducted by independent researchers. Only six RCTs were identified and the meta-analysis revealed that these programmes failed to reduce drug misuse among junior and middle-high-school students in the USA [58]. Such conflicting findings have highlighted the need of

more independent, large-scale research across different settings in order to understand the value of universal prevention programmes for drug misuse in young population.

While universal prevention programmes targeting illicit drug misuse may have conflicting results, programmes targeting tobacco use in adolescents have been found to be more encouraging. Multiple reviews have supported the efficacy of universal school-based prevention programme on tobacco use for junior- to middle-grade school children [59]. A recent meta-analysis of behavioural interventions (education, counselling, MI) of smoking in school-aged children and adolescents shows that intervention participants were 18% less likely to report having started smoking relative to controls. For smoking cessation, intervention participants were 34% more likely to report having quit smoking relative to controls [60]. With the explosive use of the Internet, there might be a potential to utilize new social media to implement smoking prevention programmes. An ad hoc smoking prevention lecture to high-school students that incorporated elements of Facebook-integrated education programmes was delivered to 225 students aged 15 and 18 years. The results showed that 15.9% of students had posted anti-smoking messages within a 72-hour period, which were spread via news feeds to their 20,095 Facebook friends [61]. Although the study did not evaluate the behavioural outcome of the students or their Facebook friends, the study highlighted the potential penetrative power of social media in reaching target populations for public health prevention purposes.

One possible confounder that determines success of a school-based programme is its level of partnership with other community-based agencies like youth-serving community groups and governmental bodies. Inter-agency partnership programmes have been found to be successful in lowering rates of early drug and alcohol use in school children [52, 62]. Such multi-agency universal approaches offer non-stigmatizing interventions to all students, involve low-cost strategies, and target a single problem that might ramify into a vast array of disorders or dysfunctions if left untreated. However, such approaches also require support from multiple authorities, including school administrations, education boards, parent groups, and so on. Furthermore, the relatively low dose of preventive intervention might not be effective to alter the developmental trajectory of children at risk of developing subsequent psychiatric disorders [63]. Therefore, further high-quality research on universal programmes of prevention of mental disorders that involve relevant stakeholders in the family and the community are urgently called for.

Indicated preventive approaches in the conversion of sub-threshold symptoms into full-blown disorders

Sub-threshold disorders are important targets of indicated prevention as they are associated with similar levels of psychosocial impairment as full-blown clinical disorders and with increased risks of developing full-blown disorders [7]. A recent review has supported a dimensional view of depressive disorders in children and adolescents suggesting sub-threshold depression to be a precursor to major depressive disorder [64]. Furthermore, 10–20% of people with minor depression develop full major depression within

3 years [65]. A history of anxiety disorder and sub-threshold anxiety symptoms also independently predicts the onset of full-blown anxiety within 2 years [66]. Apart from CMD like depression, 17–38% of people with problem drinking will escalate their drinking to alcohol use disorder within 5 years [67]. The early recognition and prompt resolution of sub-threshold symptoms should therefore be regarded as an important preventive approach of full-blown disorders.

There is accumulating evidence that CBT is effective in reducing sub-threshold anxiety and depressive symptoms in children and adolescents [39]. A recent meta-analysis found that individual CBT was more effective than waiting list or active controls group in reducing sub-threshold and threshold levels of anxiety symptoms in children and adolescents, although the effect size was larger for adolescents than children [68]. For sub-threshold anxiety in children, school-based interventions using CBT approaches with or without parental training were examined. Second- to fifth-grade school children were first screened for anxiety symptoms of mild grade. They were then randomized to one of the three arms: (i) child group CBT; (ii) child group CBT plus concurrent parent training group; and (iii) no treatment control [69]. All groups met for nine weekly, 60-minute sessions. Booster sessions were conducted at 1 and 3 months post-treatment. Each child group was led by three therapists and 1–2 therapists for the parent group. Each group had a primary therapist experienced in CBT. Both active CBT interventions were more effective than no treatment in reducing child anxiety symptoms.

A group conducted a RCT comparing primary care doctor MI (5–10 minutes) plus an Internet CBT programme versus brief advice (1–2 minutes) plus an Internet CBT programme for treatment of sub-threshold depressive symptoms in adolescents aged 14–21 years [70]. The proportion of adolescents having clinically significant depressive symptoms declined significantly in both groups post-treatment, but fewer adolescents in the MI group developed a subsequent depressive episode over 12 weeks [70]. In taking advantage of the popular subculture of online media for communication among adolescents, another Dutch research group developed an online closed chat group CBT programme ('Master Your Mood' (MYM)) for adolescents with sub-threshold depressive symptoms. The facilitators were trained mental health professionals who provided the course materials adapted from standard CBT protocol as homework and orchestrated the closed chat group of a maximum of six adolescents [71]. The MYM group had lower levels of depressive and anxiety symptoms, as well as a higher sense of mastery than the waiting control group over a period of 3 months [72]. In comparison with an individual eight-session CBT-based online self-help intervention with professional support for adults, the facilitated six-session MYM course entailed less supervision time per participant (eight-session online CBT (160 minutes) vs. six-session MYM (135 minutes)). Furthermore, the effect size of MYM was larger than the eight-session online CBT. Given that many young people with sub-threshold symptoms might be reluctant to seek formal mental health care for fear of stigma, brief therapist-assisted therapy conducted via Internet media might be a promising approach that warrants intensive research.

Internet-based CBT has also been extended for use in young people with sub-threshold depression and co-morbid problem drinking. Young people aged 18–25 years were randomized to either the DEAL project (DEpression-ALcohol project) or the HealthWatch control programme [73]. The DEAL project consisted of four 1-hour modules to be completed over a 4-week period. The content of the modules was similar to the SHADE programme for treatment of threshold depressive and addictive disorders (see the section 'Psychological interventions of common mental disorders in primary care') [37]. HealthWatch is a 12-module attention-control condition that provides the participants with information about various health concerns and invites them to complete various surveys. The information concerns environmental changes, mental and physical activity, and relationships. There were significantly greater reductions in depressive symptoms and drinking in the DEAL group compared with the HealthWatch group at post-treatment. Positive outcomes were also maintained in the DEAL group at the 3- and 6-month follow-ups. However, between-group differences disappeared at later time points. This study has suggested that a briefer, unguided, and exclusively online CBT intervention (DEAL) might lead to significant reductions in symptoms. However, it also highlights that young people motivated to seek help for their sub-threshold symptoms might experience symptom reduction by being prompted for self-reflection by the online questionnaires [73], or by being actively distracted from depressive rumination by the online materials discussed in the HealthWatch control programme. Given their value in reaching a large target group of young people with sub-threshold depressive symptoms and problem drinking, Internet-based CBT programmes warrant further research in non-Western countries to assess its generalizability to other countries.

Apart from its preventive value in depression and anxiety for children and adolescents, psychological treatments have been found to reduce the severity of depressive symptomatology among adults with sub-threshold depression in the short term and, to a lesser extent, in the long term [74]. Furthermore, there was also a trend indicating reduced incidence of major depression during subsequent follow-up [74]. What is also encouraging is that Internet-based CBT was found to be similar in efficacy to group CBT but more effective than a waiting list control condition in the treatment of sub-threshold depression among people over 50 years of age [75]. The improvement was maintained at the 12-month follow-up [76]. Given that elderly patients may have geographical and mobility barriers, as well as multiple medical appointments for other co-morbid physical problems, evidence-based Internet interventions at home or in elderly care centres will definitely enhance the accessibility and acceptability of CBT for elderly patients in countries with good access to the Internet.

These results suggest that early identification and prompt psychological interventions delivered in person or online are effective in preventing the progression of sub-threshold symptoms to full-blown disorders. What is also important from a public health perspective is that the dose and complexity of therapy required to achieve a significant impact on sub-threshold disorders appears to be lower than that for full-blown ones. This will imply that such interventions might be more easily disseminated to countries with limited access to expert therapists. Future research should explore the effectiveness of these psychological interventions in LAMICs.

Selective preventive approaches to vulnerable sub-populations using psychological interventions

Inhibition and social withdrawal were established risk factors for later anxiety disorders in preschool children. Parents of children identified to have a large number of withdrawn/inhibited behaviours were randomized to receive either six group sessions of CBT or no intervention. The children of parents in the CBT group were found to have a lower incidence of anxiety disorders than the control group at the 12-month follow-up [77]. A recent cluster RCT of school-based, brief personality-targeted interventions for ninth-grade students with high personality risk factors for substance abuse showed that there was a significant reduction in incidence rates of problem drinking and binge drinking [78]. There are four different two-session interventions targeting the four personality risk dimensions, namely anxiety sensitivity, hopelessness, impulsivity, and sensation seeking. The interventions not only incorporated components from motivational enhancement therapy and CBT for depression, anxiety, and impulsivity, but also adapted to target personality traits rather than problems. The trainee teachers were introduced about the psycho-educational, motivational, and cognitive-behavioural components of the intervention package in a 2–3-day training workshop. These trainees also received a minimum of 4 hours of supervision and feedback in running through a full intervention package. Eighty-four per cent of the trainee teachers successfully completed the training and qualified as trial facilitators, suggesting the feasibility of training for the teachers. Eighty-three per cent of high-risk students in intervention schools received an intervention, suggesting that the intervention could be assimilated into school routines without a major impact on school academic programmes [78].

Peripartum period in women represents another risky time point in developing CMD, especially depression. Given the common occurrence of depression and its impact on pregnant and postpartum women and their children, the US Preventive Services Task Force has recently recommended screening for depression in pregnant and postpartum women [79]. For antenatal periods, women on public assistance who received nurse-led group IPT during pregnancy were found to be less likely to develop depression and use mental health services at 6 and 12 months postpartum [80]. For postpartum periods, a recent cluster RCT shows that health visitors trained in delivering brief sessions based on CBT or person-centred principles were effective in preventing the onset of postpartum depression 6–18 months postnatally among non-depressed women [81]. Given maternal time constraints immediately after delivery and mothers' fears of being judged, being labelled as mentally ill, and having their infants taken away, depressed mother had low acceptability and access to conventional mental health care. An alternative is to provide psychological therapy away from conventional mental health service centres. It is encouraging to note that eight weekly sessions of telephone-administered IPT administered by nurse-midwives were found to be effective in reducing depressive symptoms when compared with the treatment as usual group [82]. There is also some preliminary evidence that computer- or web-based interventions delivered in the postpartum period were also effective in reducing depressive symptoms at either post-treatment

or follow-up (3–12 months after study completion) [83]. These online interventions were mostly based on CBT principles of cognitive reappraisal and behavioural activation, conducted either weekly or biweekly for around 6–12 weeks, and supplemented by online or telephone support by therapists with or without peers. Although these two online programmes have been used to reduce depressive symptoms in postpartum women rather than for the prevention of the onset of depression, such online programmes warrant further research as selective prevention interventions given the widespread use of online media in the childbearing population. However, the major challenge is that the attrition rates within the studies were high (13–65%). Further high-quality studies are urgently needed to investigate the acceptability and efficacy of this potentially promising treatment for postpartum women. How these evidence-based prevention programmes can be adapted to benefit pregnant and postpartum women in low-income countries should also be examined in future.

Another vulnerable group for mental ill health is the refugee population. As of 2014, there were an estimated 14 million refugees [84]. The number of refugees has been rising since 2005 as a result of new and continuing conflicts in the Middle East and Northeast Africa [84]. Although many refugees demonstrate certain degrees of resilience and adaptability to new environment, their pre-migration traumatic experiences and challenging circumstances associated with resettlement cause substantial psychological distress for these refugees, especially young people [85]. There is good evidence of a dose–response relationship between cumulative war trauma and torture and development and maintenance of post-traumatic stress disorder (PTSD) [86]. Furthermore, preparedness for torture, social and family support, and religious beliefs are protective against PTSD following war trauma and torture [86]. Refugees and victims of war trauma thus represent an important vulnerable group for selective prevention of psychiatric disorders.

It is important to note that 51% of refugees are younger than 18 years of age [84]. The young refugees therefore represent a particularly vulnerable group as many of them are separated from their families and exposed to exploitation, trafficking, and abuse. For refugee children and adolescents forcibly displaced to high-income countries, stable settlement and social support in the host country have a positive effect on the child's psychological functioning [87]. The provision of a safe, sheltered environment, good social network, and religious support are thus important measures to maintain mental health among these vulnerable people [87]. Nevertheless, many refugee children might still display mental health problems after settlement in the host countries and require selective prevention programmes. Given that many children will attend school and receive education in host countries, schools are very often the first and primary social institutions of socialization within which refugee students interact with others [88]. Schools are thus uniquely positioned as primary service sites for screening and preventing psychiatric disorders among these vulnerable children. The school environment is also readily accessible and reduces stigma associated with treatment. A recent meta-analysis supports that expressive therapies in the form of art and music, trauma-focused CBT, and multi-tiered therapy consisting of psycho-education, skills-building, and trauma-focused CBT for students referred by teachers were all effective therapies for refugee school children in preventing onset of PTSD [89]. However, it is important to highlight that current evidence does not support routine implementation of any type of psychological interventions to all individuals after trauma [90].

However, trauma-focused CBT for recent adult survivors of significant trauma with definite post-traumatic symptoms have been demonstrated to be beneficial. These survivors were frequently diagnosed as suffering from acute stress disorder, a diagnosis associated with increased risks of developing PTSD. Early intervention of patients with trauma-related acute stress disorder was effective in preventing the subsequent onset of PTSD, a disabling disorder that runs a chronic course if left untreated [90]. As such, this trauma-focused CBT intervention is better regarded as an indicated prevention of conversion of sub-threshold symptoms into full-blown clinical disorders. Although such prevention programmes appear to be effective, it is important to adapt such trauma-focused therapies for different cultures and for delivery by therapists with limited training and supervision. Furthermore, there has been evidence that different components of CBT might be effective for PTSD related to different types of trauma (e.g. trauma-focused CBT for victims of road traffic accidents and prolonged exposure for victims of sexual trauma) [91]. In summary, selective prevention for refugees should only be restricted to vulnerable children in schools, but should not be provided routinely to adult refugees without sub-threshold or threshold traumatic or mood symptoms.

Conclusions

CMD are prevalent in countries of all income levels and exact tremendous direct and indirect costs to society. As the vast majority of sufferers do not have access to mental health care provided by trained mental health professionals, the provision of prevention and treatment programmes need to be delivered by lay health workers or even peer volunteers. In order to maximize cost-effectiveness of such prevention and treatment programmes, these programmes need to be evidence-based, time-limited, readily delivered by lay workers with minimal training and supervision, and culturally relevant and acceptable. Psychological interventions, especially short-term manualized and structured CBT, appear to be applicable and adaptable in various settings for different age groups. The major challenge is how effective components of CBT can be dismantled and delivered by lay health workers or peer volunteers to a large population of people. The COBRA study on the effectiveness of behavioural activation, a key component of CBT, delivered by junior mental health workers for depression is an example of how this challenge may be overcome [19]. Further research is much needed to identify more psychological interventions that can be widely disseminated in LAMICs. The use of Internet and social media for the delivery of interventions is a promising new approach for patients with concerns about stigma associated with treatment and with poor access to mental health care. Online or telephone supervision of inexperienced therapists by distant expert therapists is also a novel application of modern technology to support the dissemination of effective psychological interventions to remote regions. With increasing availability and accessibility of Internet services and smartphones in different parts of the world, this treatment and training modality will have great potential of application to future public mental health.

References

1. Kessler KC, Angermeyer M, Anthony JC, et al. Lifetime prevalence and age-of-onset distributions of mental disorders in the World Health Organization's World Mental Health Survey Initiative. *World Psychiatry* 2007; 6: 168–176.
2. Whiteford HA, Degenhardt L, Rehm J, et al. Global burden of disease attributable to mental and substance use disorders: findings from the Global Burden of Disease Study 2010. *Lancet* 2013; 382: 1575–1586.
3. Kessler RC, Chiu WT, Demler O, Walters EE. Prevalence, severity, and comorbidity of 12-month DSM-IV disorders in the National Comorbidity Survey Replication. *Arch Gen Psychiatry* 2005; 62: 617–627.
4. Kessler RC, Berglund P, Demler O, et al. The epidemiology of major depressive disorder: results from the National Comorbidity Survey Replication (NCS-R). *JAMA* 2003; 289: 3095–3105.
5. Brown TA, Barlow DH. Dimensional versus categorical classification of mental disorders in the fifth edition of the Diagnostic and Statistical Manual of Mental Disorders and beyond: comment on the special section. *J Abnorm Psychol* 2005; 114: 551–556.
6. Merikangas KR, Jin R, He JP, et al. Prevalence and correlates of bipolar spectrum disorder in the Mental Health Survey Initiative. *Arch Gen Psychiatry* 2011; 68: 241–251.
7. Fergusson DM. Horwood J, Ridder EM, Beautrais AL. Subthreshold depression in adolescence and mental health outcomes in adulthood. *Arch Gen Psychiatry* 2005; 62: 66–72.
8. Patel V, Kleinman A. Poverty and common mental disorders in developing countries. *Bull World Health Organ* 2003; 81: 609–615.
9. Lund C, Breen A. Flisher AJ, et al. Poverty and common mental disorders in low and middle income countries. *Soc Sci Med* 2010; 71: 517–528.
10. Sumathipala A, Hewege S, Hanwella R, Mann AH. Randomized controlled trial of cognitive behaviour therapy for repeated consultations for medically unexplained complaints: a feasibility study in Sri Lanka. *Psychol Med* 2000; 30: 747–757.
11. Chibanda D, Mesu P, Kajawu L, Cowan F, Araya R, Abas MA. Problem-solving therapy for depression and common mental disorders in Zimbabwe: piloting a task shifting primary mental health care intervention in a population with a high prevalence of people living with HIV. *BMC Public Health* 2011; 11: 828.
12. Kirsch I, Deacon BJ, Huedo-Medina TB, Scoboria A, Moore TJ, Johnson BT. Initial severity and antidepressant benefits: a meta-analysis of data submitted to the Food and Drug Administration. *PLOS Med* 2008; 5: e45.
13. Cape J, Whittington C, Buszewicz M, Wallace P, Underwood L. Brief psychological therapies for anxiety and depression in primary care: meta-analysis and meta-regression. *BMC Med* 2010; 8: 38.
14. Hegerl U, Hautzinger M, Mergl R, et al. Effects of pharmacotherapy and psychotherapy in depressed primary-care patients: a randomized, controlled trial including a patients' choice arm. *Int J Neuropsychopharmacol* 2010; 13: 31–44.
15. Wiles N, Thomas L, Abel A, et al. Cognitive-behavioural therapy as an adjunct to pharmacotherapy for primary care based patients with treatment-resistant depression: results of CoBalT randomised controlled trial. *Lancet* 2013; 381: 375–384.
16. Biesheuvel-Leliefeld KE, Kok GD, Bockting CL, et al. Effectiveness of psychological interventions in preventing recurrence of depressive disorder: meta-analysis and meta-regression. *J Affect Disord* 2015; 174: 400–410.
17. Roy-Byrne PP, Craske MG, Stein MB, et al. A randomized effectiveness trial of cognitive-behavioural therapy and medication for primary care panic disorder. *Arch Gen Psychiatry* 2005; 62: 290–298.
18. Roy-Byrne P, Craske MG, Sullivan G, et al. Delivery of evidence-based treatment for multiple anxiety disorders in primary care. A randomized controlled trial. *JAMA* 2010; 303: 1921–1928.
19. Richards DA, Ekers D, McMillan D, et al. Cost and outcome of behavioural activation versus cognitive behaviour therapy for

depression (COBRA): a randomised, controlled, non-inferiority trial. *Lancet* 2016; 388: 871–880.

20. Mohr DC, Ho J, Duffecy J, et al. Effect of telephone-administered vs face-to-face cognitive behavioural therapy on adherence to therapy and depression outcomes among primary care patients. *JAMA* 2012; 307: 2278–2285.

21. Proudfoot J, Ryden C, Everitt B, et al. Clinical efficacy of computerised cognitive-behavioural therapy for anxiety and depression in primary care: randomised controlled trial. *Br J Psychiatry* 2004; 185: 46–54.

22. Kessler D, Lewis G, Kaur S, et al. Therapist-delivered internet psychotherapy for depression in primary care: a randomised controlled trial. *Lancet* 2009; 374: 628–634.

23. Titov N, Dear BF, Schwencke G, et al. Transdiagnostic Internet treatment for anxiety and depression: a randomized controlled trial. *Behav Res Ther* 2011; 49: 441–452.

24. Titov N. Internet-delivered psychotherapy for depression in adults. *Curr Opin Psychiatry* 2011; 24: 18–23.

25. Warmerdam L, van Straten A, Twisk J, Riper H, Cuijpers P. Internet-based treatment for adults with depressive symptoms: randomized controlled trial. *J Med Internet Res* 2008; 10: e44.

26. Newby JM, Mackenzie A, Williams AD, et al. Internet cognitive behavioural therapy for mixed anxiety and depression: a randomized controlled trial and evidence of effectiveness in primary care. *Psychol Med* 2013; 43: 2635–2648.

27. Christensen H, Griffiths KM, MacKinnon AJ, Brittliffe K. Online randomized controlled trial of brief and full cognitive behaviour therapy for depression. *Psychol Med* 2006; 36: 1737–1746.

28. Griffiths KM, Farrer L, Christensen H. The efficacy of internet interventions for depression and anxiety disorders: a review of randomised controlled trials. *Med J Aust* 2010; 192: S4–S11.

29. De Graaf LE, Gerhards SA, Arntz A, et al. Clinical effectiveness of online computerised cognitive-behavioural therapy without support for depression in primary care: randomised trial. *Br J Psychiatry* 2009; 195: 73–80.

30. Waller R, Gilbody S. Barriers to the uptake of computerized cognitive behavioural therapy: a systematic review of the quantitative and qualitative evidence. *Psychol Med* 2009; 39: 705–712.

31. Patel V, Weiss HA, Chowdhary N, et al. Effectiveness of an intervention led by lay health counsellors for depressive and anxiety disorders in primary care in Goa, India (MANAS): a cluster randomised control trial. *Lancet* 2010; 376: 2086–2095.

32. Patel V, Chowdhary N, Rahman A, Verdeli H. Improving access to psychological treatments: lessons from developing countries. *Behav Res Ther* 2011; 49: 523–528.

33. Bedi N, Lee A, Harrison G, et al. Assessing effectiveness of treatment of depression in primary care. *Br J Psychiatry* 2011; 177: 312–318.

34. Higgins ST, Badger GJ, Budney AJ. Initial abstinence and success in achieving longer term cocaine abstinence. *Exp Clin Psychopharmacol* 2000; 8: 377–386.

35. Higgin ST, Wong CJ, Badger GJ, Ogden DE, Dantona RL. Contingent reinforcement increases cocaine abstinence during outpatient treatment and 1 year of follow-up. *J Consult Clin Psychol* 2000; 68: 64–72.

36. Dugosh K, Abraham A, Seymour B, McLoyd K, Chalk M, Festinger D. A systematic review on the use of psychosocial interventions in conjunction with medications for the treatment of opioid addiction. *J Addict Med* 2016; 10: 93–103.

37. Kay-Lambkin FJ, Baker AL, Lewin TJ, Carr VJ. Computer-based psychological treatment for comorbid depression and problematic alcohol and/or cannabis use: a randomized controlled trial of clinical efficacy. *Addiction* 2009; 104: 378–388.

38. Gordon RS, Jr. An operational classification of disease prevention. *Public Health Rep* 1983; 98: 107–109.

39. Bertha EA, Balazs J. Subthreshold depression in adolescence: a systematic review. *Eur Child Adolesc Psychiatry* 2013; 22: 589–603.

40. Horowitz J L, Garber J, Ciesia JA, Young JF, Mufson L. Prevention of depressive symptoms in adolescents: a randomized trial of cognitive-behavioral and interpersonal prevention programs. *J Consult Clin Psychol* 2007; 75: 693–706.

41. Stallard P, Sayal K, Phillips R, et al. Classroom based cognitive behavioural therapy in reducing symptoms of depression in high risk adolescents: pragmatic cluster randomised controlled trial. *BMJ* 2012; 345: e6058.

42. Sayal K, Owen V, White K, Merrell C, Tymms P, Taylor E. The impact of early school-based screening and intervention programs for ADHD on children's outcomes and access to services—follow up of a school-based trial at age 10 years. *Arch Pediatr Adolesc Med* 2010; 164: 462–469.

43. Calear AL, Christensen H. Systematic review of school-based prevention and early intervention programs for depression. *J Adolesc* 2010; 33: 429–438.

44. Dadds MR, Roth JH. Prevention of anxiety disorders: Results of a universal trial with young children. *J Child Fam Stud* 2008; 17: 320–335.

45. Lowry-Webster HM, Barrett PM, Dadds MR. A universal prevention trial of anxiety and depressive symptomatology in childhood: preliminary data from an Australian study. *Behav Change* 2001; 18: 36–50.

46. Barratt PM, Farrell LJ, Ollendick TH, Dadds M. Long-term outcomes of an Australian universal prevention trial of anxiety and depression symptoms in children and youth: an evaluation of the Friends Program. *J Clin Child Adolesc Psychol* 2006; 35: 403–411.

47. Essau CA, Conradt J, Sasagawa S, Ollendick TH. Prevention of anxiety symptoms in children: Results from a universal school-based trial. *Behav Ther* 2012; 43: 450–464.

48. Barratt P, Turner C. Prevention of anxiety symptoms in primary school children: preliminary results from a universal school-based trial. *Br J Clin Psychol* 2001; 40: 399–410.

49. Neil NL, Christensen H. Australian school-based prevention and early intervention programs for anxiety and depression: a systematic review. *Med J Aust* 2007; 186: 305–308.

50. Wilson SJ, Lipsey MW. Effectiveness of school-based intervention programs on aggressive behavior: update of a meta-analysis. *Am J Prev Med* 2007; 33: S130–S143.

51. Hahn R, Fuqua-Whitley D, Wethington H, et al. Effectiveness of universal school-based programs to prevent violent and aggressive behavior: a systematic review. *Am J Prev Med* 2007; 33: S114–S129.

52. Spoth RL, Greenberg MT, Turrisi R. Preventive interventions addressing underage drinking: state of evidence and steps toward public health impact. *Pediatrics* 2008; 121(Suppl. 4): S311–S336.

53. Shure MB, Spivack G. Interpersonal problem solving in children: a cognitive approach to prevention. *Am J Commun Psychol* 1982; 10: 341–356.

54. Kratchowill TR, McDonald L, Levin JR, Young Bear-Tibbets H, Demaray MK. Families and Schools Together: an experimental analysis of a parent-mediated multi-family group program for American Indian children. *J School Psychol* 2004; 42: 359–383.

55. Spoth R, Randall GK, Shin C, Redmond C. Randomized study of combined universal family and school preventive interventions: patterns of long-term effects on initiation, regular use, and weekly drunkenness. *Psychol Addict Behav* 2005; 19: 372–381.

56. Hecht ML, Marsiglia FF, Elek E, et al. Culturally grounded substance use prevention: an evaluation of the Keepin' it R.E.A.L. curriculum. *Prev Sci* 2003; 4: 233–248.

57. Faggiano F, Vigna-Taglianti FD, Versino E, Zambon A, Borraccino A, Lemma P. School-based prevention for illicit drug use: a systematic review. *Prev Med* 2008; 46: 385–396.

58. Flynn AB, Falco M, Hocini S. Independent evaluation of middle school-based drug prevention curricula. *JAMA Pediatr* 2015; 169: 1046–1052.

59. Dobbins M, DeCorby K, Manske S, Goldblatt, E. Effective practices for school-based tobacco use prevention. *Prev Med* 2008; 46: 289–297.

60. Peirson L, Ali MU, Kenny M, Raina P, Sherifali D. Interventions for prevention and treatment of tobacco smoking in school-aged children

and adolescents: a systematic review and meta-analysis. *Prev Med* 2016; 85: 20–31.

61. Kousolis AA, Kympouropoulos SP, Pouli DK, Economopoulos KP, Vardavas CI. From the Classroom to Facebook. A fresh new approach for youth tobacco prevention. *Am J Health Promot* 2016; 30: 390–393.

62. Feinberg ME, Jones DJ, Greenberg MT, Osgood WO, Bontempo D. Effects of the Communities That Care Model in Pennsylvania on change in youth risk and problem behaviors. *Prev Sci* 2010; 11: 163–171.

63. Greenberg MT. School-based prevention: current status and future challenges. *Effect Educ* 2010; 2: 27–52.

64. Wesselhoeft R, Sorensen MJ, Heiervang ER, Bilenberg N. Subthreshold depression in children and adolescents—a systematic review. *J Affect Disord* 2013; 151: 7–22.

65. Cuijpers P, Smit F. Subthreshold depression as a risk indicator for major depressive disorder: a systematic review of prospective studies. *Acta Psychiatr Scand* 2004; 109: 325–331.

66. Karsten J, Hartman CA, Smit JH, et al. Psychiatric history and subthreshold symptoms as predictors of occurrence of depressive or anxiety disorder within 2 years. *Br J Psychiatry* 2011; 198: 206–212.

67. Eng MY, Schuckit MA, Smith TL. A five-year prospective study of diagnostic orphans for alcohol use disorders. *J Stud Alcohol* 2003; 64: 227–234.

68. Reynolds S, Wilson C, Austin J, Hooper L. Effects of psychotherapy for anxiety in children and adolescents: a meta-analytic review. *Clin Psychol Rev* 2012; 32: 251–262.

69. Bernstein GA, Layne AE, Egan EA, Tennison MA. School-based interventions for anxious children. *J Am Acad Child Adolesc Psychiatry* 2005; 44: 1118–1127.

70. Van Voorhees BW, Fogel J, Reinecke MA, et al. Randomized clinical trial of an internet-based depression prevention program for adolescents (Project CATCH-IT) in primary care: 12-week outcomes. *J Dev Behav Pediatr* 2009; 30: 23–37.

71. Gerrits RS, van der Zanden AP, Visscher RE, Conijn BP. Master your mood online: a preventive chat group intervention for adolescents. *Aust E J Adv Ment Health* 2007; 6: 1–11.

72. Van der Zanden, Kramer J, Gerrits R, Cuijpers P. Effectiveness of an online group course for depression in adolescents and young adults: a randomized trial. *J Med Internet Res* 2012; 14: e86.

73. Deady M, Mills KL, Teesson M, Kay-Lambkin F. An online intervention for co-occurring depression and problematic alcohol use in young people: primary outcomes from a randomized controlled trial. *J Med Internet Res* 2016; 18: e71.

74. Cuijpers P, Smit F, Van Straten A. Psychological treatments of subthreshold depression: a meta-analytic review. *Acta Psychiatr Scand* 2007; 115: 434–441.

75. Spek V, Nyklicek I, Smits N, et al. Internet-based cognitive behavioural therapy for subthreshold depression in people over 50 years old: a randomized controlled trial. *Psychol Med* 2007; 37: 1797–1806.

76. Spek V, Cuijpers P, Nyklicek I, et al. One-year follow-up results of a randomized controlled clinical trial on internet-based cognitive behavioural therapy for sub-threshold depression in people over 50 years old. *Psychol Med* 2008; 38: 635–639.

77. Rapee RM, Kennedy S, Ingram M, Edwards S, Sweeney L. Prevention and early intervention of anxiety disorders in inhibited preschool children. *J Consult Clin Psychol* 2005; 73: 488–497.

78. Conrod PJ, O'Leary-Barrett M, Newton N, et al. Effectiveness of a selective, personality-targeted prevention program for adolescent alcohol use and misuse: a cluster randomized controlled trial. *JAMA Psychiatry* 2013; 70: 334–342.

79. Siu AL, Bibbons-Domingo K, Grossman DC, et al. Screening for depression in adults: US Preventive Services Task Force recommendation statement. *JAMA* 2016; 315: 380–387.

80. Zlotnick C, Tzilos G, Miller I, Seifer R, Stout R. Randomized controlled trial to prevent postpartum depression in mothers on public assistance. *J Affect Disord* 2016; 189: 263–268.

81. Brugha TS, Morell CJ, Slade P, Walters SJ. Universal prevention of depression in women postnatally: cluster randomized trial evidence in primary care. *Psychol Med* 2011; 41: 739–748.

82. Posmontier B, Neugebauer R, Stuart S, Chittams J, Shaughnessy R. Telephone-administered interpersonal psychotherapy by nurse-midwives for postpartum depression. *J Midwifery Womens Health* 2016; 61: 456–466.

83. Lee EW, Denison FC, Hor K, Reynolds RM. Web-based interventions for prevention and treatment of perinatal mood disorders: a systematic review. *BMC Pregnancy Childbirth* 2016; 16: 38.

84. Lindert J, Carta MG, Schafer I, Mollica RF. Refugees mental health—a public mental health challenge. *Eur J Public Health* 2016; 26: 374–375.

85. Bronstein I, Montgomery P. Psychological distress in refugee children: a systematic review. *Clin Child Fam Psychol Rev* 2011; 14: 44–56.

86. Johnson H, Thompson A. The development and maintenance of post-traumatic stress disorder (PTSD) in civilian adult survivors of war trauma and torture: a review. *Clin Psychol Rev* 2008; 28: 36–47.

87. Fazel M, Reed RV, Panter-Brick C, Stein A. Mental health of displaced and refugee children and adolescents resettled in high income countries: risk and protective factors. *Lancet* 2012; 379: 266–282.

88. Wilkinson L. Factors influencing the academic success of refugee youth in Canada. *J Youth Stud* 2002; 5: 173–193.

89. Sullivan AL, Simonson GR. A systematic review of school-based social-emotional interventions for refugee and war-traumatized youth. *Rev Educ Res* 2016; 86: 503–530.

90. Roberts NP, Kitchiner NJ, Kenardy J, Bisson JI. Multiple session early psychological interventions for the prevention of post-traumatic stress disorder. *Cochrane Database Syst Rev* 2009; 3: CD06869.

91. Qi W, Gevonden M, Shalev A. Prevention of post-traumatic stress disorder after trauma: current evidence and future directions. *Curr Psychiatry Rep* 2016; 18: 1–11.

CHAPTER 47

Diet, environment, and mental health

Ursula Werneke and Ingvar A. Bergdahl

Introduction

While there is no doubt that dietary and environmental factors interact with mental health, the relationship between these factors remains complex. The notion that the way we eat affects the way we feel is immensely popular, as evidenced by the countless books, websites, and other media contributions. But the interaction between diet and mental health is bidirectional. Dietary choices may affect mental health, and mental health may affect dietary choices. Sometimes, it is possible to identify a *specific* nutritional deficiency as *the* precipitant of a mental health problem. But, more often, diet is just one of *many* factors affecting mental health. In such cases, even if we identify a nutritional deficiency, we cannot take for granted that replacement of the missing substance will always lead to improvement of the mental state. Nor can we take it for granted that supplementation of nutraceuticals does not ever have any adverse effects. The interaction between environmental factors and mental health is equally complex. Only occasionally is it possible to identify an environmental toxin as a culprit of mental ill health. But, at the same time, the environment affects populations as a whole. In the first part of this chapter, we look at nutritional deficiencies that can give rise to mental ill health. Then, we explore diets and 'superfoods' people might try to improve their mental health. We also look at some interactions between foodstuffs and psychotropic medicines. In the final part of this chapter, we review environmental toxins that may affect mental health.

Nutritional deficiencies and mental health

A healthy, well-balanced diet should provide us with all essential food components. Yet, nutritional deficiencies arise, where access to food is restricted, or essential food components are lacking. Currently, about 800 million people remain undernourished worldwide. The vast majority of these live in developing countries, where about 13% of the population is undernourished. Up to one-third of children in developing countries and one-quarter of all children worldwide are stunted in development. At the same time, 1.9 billion adults are overweight and 600 million are obese. For the first time in history, overweight kills more people than underweight. Hence, in higher-income countries, nutritional deficiencies are more likely to be caused by adherence to one-sided unbalanced diets. Alcohol and amphetamine-type drug use can also significantly reduce food intake or shift it towards carbohydrates. Additionally,

alcohol interferes with B vitamins, leading to specific nutritional deficiencies. Eating disorders and consuming diseases, such as cancer or HIV, can lead to starvation in higher-income countries. Bariatric surgery, associated with malabsorption, can also result in significant nutritional deficits.

It has become increasingly clear that nutrition affects mental health in both higher- and lower-income countries. At the same time, treatment outcomes of mental health problems remain suboptimal. Possibly, nutrition is one of the missing links accounting for the immense global burden of mental ill health. However, only recently has the impact of nutritional factors on mental health attracted more attention [1].

Nutrition and the brain

Nutritional factors impact on the brain in various ways. Firstly, nutrition provides the essential building blocks for the grey and white matter. Here, lipids are particularly important—the brain is essentially a fatty organ. The lipid content varies between the different anatomical structures. Myelin contains about 80% lipids, white matter up to 66%, and grey matter up to 40%. At the cellular level, sphingolipids, cholesterol, and phospholipids are the main constituents of cell membranes. They play a key role in maintaining cellular integrity, neuroplasticity, and facilitating information transmission. This makes lipids a main target for the prevention of psychiatric disorders. From a mental health point of view, propagation of low fat and low cholesterol diets may thus be undesirable. A recent systematic review found that dietary interventions improving depression outcomes were less likely to recommend leaner meat products or a low-cholesterol diet [2].

The brain has the highest metabolic rate of all organs. It takes up about 2% of the human body mass but nearly 20% of daily energy consumption. The brain preferentially uses glucose. When glucose is limited the brain is served first. It is virtually impossible to starve the brain under physiological, i.e. non-diabetic, conditions. But even small fluctuations in energy level can affect reason and judgement. A study exploring the impact of 'what the judge ate for breakfast' showed that the amount of favourable parole decisions was 65% at the beginning of a session, gradually dropping to zero during the session, and jumping up to 65% again after the next food break [3]. During starvation, the brain switches to ketone bodies within 72 hours. These can supply about 60% of the cerebral energy requirements. The remainder is met through glycogenesis. Ketone bodies may increase metabolic efficiency. Diet-inducing mild ketosis have been implicated for the treatment of some neurodevelopmental and neurodegenerative diseases [4]. A regular energy supply is necessary for the brain to function properly. Cognition and mood may be affected early if energy requirements are not met. Finally, vitamins and minerals are involved in pre- and postnatal brain development. They facilitate neurogenesis, proliferation, and differentiation of nerve cells; manufacture and functioning of cell membranes, myelin sheaths, and neurotransmitters; energy utilization; and antioxidant and anti-inflammatory effects.

Nutrition and mental health: a neurodevelopmental perspective

The neural stem starts forming from the second gestational week. The neural tube forms in the third and closes in the fourth gestational week. In the fetal development phase, neurogenesis prevails. Postnatally, myelination dominates, shifting the relative balance between grey and white matter. The 'rewiring' of the brain continues in adolescence, where brain plasticity still overrides brain stability. In adulthood, the brain becomes more stable. But it still retains some plastic capacity. This, to some extent, allows neuro-regeneration [5, 6]. The neurodevelopmental timeline highlights the importance of adequate nutrition during maternity and early child development. Then, the foundations for brain connectivity are laid. Intuitively, we might assume that nutritional problems at these earlier neurodevelopmental phases would lead to more irreversible damage than deficiencies later in life. For instance, serotonergic neurons develop in the second gestational week [5]. Discrete problems at this early stage could account for disorders related to serotonin in later life.

Still, nutritional factors may be more important in adolescence than hitherto assumed. Adolescence is a critical period for the development of dopaminergic systems. The timeline also emphasizes the importance of adequate nutrition throughout life. The 'rewiring' of the brain never stops, even if the balance in adulthood is shifted from brain plasticity to brain stability. Folic acid is required early in gestation for the correct development and closure of the neural tube. Otherwise, we know relatively little about the specific role of particular nutrients and potentially critical periods for nutritional deficiencies. We can assume that the earlier nutritional deficiencies occur, the more pervasive are the adverse effects on neurodevelopment. But we do not know how far cerebral repair mechanisms—generally and individually—can repair nutritionally related neuronal damage.

The significance of maternal and early-life nutrition for brain development, subsequent mental health, and social functioning has been studied in the context of periods of famine [1]. Two such tragic 'natural experiments' are the Dutch hunger winter 1944–45 and the Chinese famine 1959–61. Results from the Dutch hunger winter cohort suggest an increased risk of schizophrenia and affective disorders, linked to nutritional deficits during the first trimester of pregnancy [7, 8]. Major depression was significantly associated with nutritional deprivation in the third and non-significantly in the second trimester [9]. Initial results from the Chinese famine showed an association between nutritional deprivation in early pregnancy and an increased risk of schizophrenia. A more recent study showed an association between famine and subsequent

schizophrenia in the urban, but not in the rural, Chinese population. Possibly, this is explained by a higher infant mortality in the rural population during the famine [10]. The overall evidence suggests that there is some association between malnutrition and later adverse mental health outcomes. We do not yet understand the nature and degree of such an association. Observed effects may be subject to many confounders.

Omega-3 fatty acids

Chemically, the name omega-3 indicates an unsaturated fatty acid with the first double bond between the third and the fourth carbon atom. Omega-3 fatty acids are also called n-3 fatty acids or ω-3 fatty acids. Omega-3 with two or more double bonds are polyunsaturated fatty acids. Sometimes, they are also called highly unsaturated fatty acids. From a mental health point of view, the most important omega-3 fatty acids are two long-chain acids, eicosapentaenoic acid (EPA) and docosahexaenoic acid (DHA). EPA is an omega-3 fatty acid with 20 carbon atoms, five double bounds, and the first double bond inserted at the third carbon atom (i.e. C20:5n-3). DHA is an omega-3 fatty acid with 22 carbon atoms, six double bounds, and the first double bond inserted at the third carbon atom (i.e. C22:6n-3). The main source of EPA and DHA in human diet is fish. Oily fish, such as mackerel, salmon, and sardines, are particularly rich in EPA and DHA. To a small extent, humans can synthesize EPA from the shorter-chain alpha-linolenic acid and convert EPA into DHA. Depending on maternal omega-3 intake, EPA and DHA are also present in breast milk. Omega-3 fatty acids are thought to carry numerous health benefits in relation to cardiac and mental health. Mental health benefits may stem from the neurotrophic, anti-inflammatory, and anticoagulant properties. Omega-3 fatty acids have been subject to intensive research summarized in several systematic reviews and meta-analyses. In the mental health field, most of the work concerns mood disorders, psychosis, and dementia.

Omega-3 fatty acids have emerged as a treatment of major depression. Augmentation therapy seems more effective than monotherapy. Yet, a recent Cochrane review concluded that the evidence remained inconclusive. Studies were heterogeneous and yielded conflicting results [11]. Since then, three further meta-analyses have appeared, endorsing the effects of omega-3 fatty acids in the treatment of depression. Again, addition to standard antidepressant therapy showed more promise than monotherapy. These studies also suggested that EPA but not DHA might be the effective agent [12]. The effect of omega-3 fatty acids may even extend to the treatment of bipolar depression but not to the *prevention* of major depression. At present, the evidence remains inconclusive [13, 14].

Omega-3 fatty acids have also been implicated for the treatment of schizophrenia, but the evidence remains inconclusive. The effect of omega-3 fatty acids may be confined to the early stages of schizophrenia or the prevention of progression from prodromal to open psychotic states [15, 16]. The evidence regarding prevention of dementia with omega-3 fatty acids and attention deficit hyperactivity disorder (ADHD) remains conflicting.

In view of the potential health benefits of omega-3 fatty acids, the National Health Service of England and Wales recommends intake of at least two portions (140 g/portion) of fish a week. One of these should be oily. Owing to the risk of contamination with environmental pollutants, the general population should not eat more than four portions of oily fish per week. Women who are planning pregnancy, are pregnant, or breastfeeding should not eat more than two portions of oily fish per week [17]. Omega-3 fatty acid supplements are generally considered safe. In individuals with depression or at risk of psychosis, benefits of fish oil supplementation may outweigh the risks. One gram per day usually suffices, and higher doses may not yield additional benefits. Fish oil contains vitamin A in varying amounts, which may not always be stated clearly on the label. As a rule of thumb, liver-based fish oils, such as cod liver oil, contain more vitamin A than other fish oils. The total intake of vitamin A, from supplements and diet combined, should not exceed 1.5 mg per day. Pregnant women should avoid supplements containing vitamin A altogether because of its potentially teratogenic effects [17].

Vitamins and minerals

Vitamins and minerals are essential for the normal functioning of body and brain. An ancient Greek legend of iron treatment is probably the first account of a mineral being used therapeutically. In this account, a Greek king was cured of infertility by wine, which had rust scrapings added [18]. In the seventeenth century, iron was used for the treatment of 'chlorosis', which was thought to be a type of 'hysteria', now known to be iron-deficiency anaemia. At the beginning of the eighteenth century, iron was recognized as a constituent of blood [18]. Another relatively early example of the therapeutic use of minerals is iodine. In the late nineteenth century, two German scientists discovered that thyroid extract obtained from sheep glands contained iodine. This was first administered therapeutically in 1896 [18]. The understanding of the significance of vitamins for mental health began with the discovery of thiamine (vitamin B1). In 1886, the Dutch government had sent two doctors to Sumatra and Java to investigate the high occurrence of beriberi in their soldiers and prisoners. The cause of beriberi was first assumed either infectious or toxic. It then emerged that beriberi only affected people eating highly polished white rice but not others, who were eating unmilled brown rice. An 'antineuritic' substance, protecting the nervous system from inflammation, was postulated. This was subsequently identified as thiamine [18].

Vitamins

Vitamins are substances the human organism requires but cannot synthesize itself. Vitamins A, D, E, and K are fat-soluble. B-group vitamins and vitamin C are water-soluble. Health problems can arise from under- or oversupply of vitamins. Undersupply generally occurs in the context of reduced food intake or—in its extreme form—starvation, selective food intake, malabsorption, or harmful use of alcohol. Additionally, deficiencies in fat-soluble vitamins can occur in the context of low-fat diets. Oversupply is often due to increased supplement use. Excess water-soluble vitamins are mostly excreted with urine. This makes toxic states due to water-soluble vitamins rare. The exception is vitamin B6, which, in excess, can lead to neuropathy. Oversupply of fat-soluble vitamins can lead to accumulation in tissues. It is important to observe safe upper limits, particularly for vitamin A. *All* vitamins in deficiency or excess can give rise not only to physical health, but also mental health problems (Table 47.1) [19–31]. Most commonly, folic acid, vitamin B12, and vitamin D deficiencies are associated with mental health problems.

Folic acid and vitamin B12

Folic acid and vitamin B12 are key methyl donors and play fundamental roles in the synthesis of neurotransmitters and DNA. Methylation of DNA controls the activation of genes to start or stop transcription [28]. Folic acid and vitamin B12 are required to methylate homocysteine to methionine. Methionine is then converted to S-adenosyl methionine (SAMe). It follows that elevated levels of homocysteine can indicate folic acid or vitamin B12 deficiency. SAMe is a methyl donor in its own right, involved in the synthesis of phosphatidylcholine, a major compound of cell membranes. SAMe also transfers methyl to monoamines, such as serotonin, melatonin, noradrenaline, and dopamine. SAMe is available as a complementary medicine. Preliminary evidence suggests antidepressant effects. However, SAMe is best administered parenterally. Taken orally, it may not be absorbed sufficiently. The evidence for the antidepressant effects of folic acid and vitamin B12 is less clear cut. Folic acid replacement can mask vitamin 12 deficiency. Hence, it is important to determine the levels of both folic acid and vitamin B12 before initiating substitution. Folic acid is crucial for neural tube and early brain development (Table 47.1). Women who are or wish to become pregnant should take a supplement of 0.4 mg (400 µg) of folic acid from the day of stopping contraception to the twelfth week of pregnancy. Women with a family history of neural tube defects should take 5 mg of folic acid until twelfth week of pregnancy [17].

Vitamin D

Vitamin D is found in relatively few foods, such as fortified cereals and fats, dairy, and animal products. It is mainly produced by the skin under the influence of ultraviolet (UV) light. Vitamin D deficiency may arise from a lack of exposure to sunlight, such as in the winter months of Northern latitudes, life in institutionalized or homebound settings, and when wearing clothing that covers the whole body. People with darker skin also produce less vitamin D. If access to UV light is restricted, vitamin D needs to be taken in from food.

Vitamin D has numerous neuroprotective and neurotrophic functions. It acts as an antioxidant, modulates dopamine and noradrenaline, and facilitates calcium signalling. Vitamin D also has anti-inflammatory properties. Yet, little is known about the actual impact of vitamin D deficiency on brain development and function [21]. Vitamin D deficiency may be associated with schizophrenia, but figures vary widely. In one meta-analysis, severe vitamin D deficiency was found in 8–95% of all individuals with psychosis [32]. Intriguingly, one study identified both neonatal vitamin D deficiency and excess as risk factors for schizophrenia in later life [33]. The association between low vitamin D levels and depression remains equally inconsistent [34]. Intervention trials show conflicting results [21, 22]. From a public health point of view, the verdict on vitamin D supplementation is still out.

Vitamin B1

Vitamin B1 (thiamine) is one example of a *specific* vitamin deficiency that warrants substitution. Vitamin B1 exerts key functions in the metabolism of carbohydrates and branched amino acids. It contributes to neurotransmitters, nucleotides, and myelin synthesis. Vitamin B1 may also be involved in the regulation of the immune and anti-inflammatory responses [26, 35]. Chronic

Table 47.1 Vitamins and their relevance to mental health

Vitamin	Impact in terms of availability or action of other vitamins or nutrients with potential CNS relevance	CNS implications	Special situations where deficiencies can occur	Implications of deficiency for neurodevelopment	Potential contribution of deficiency to mental health problems in adulthood	Supplementation for treatment of mental health problems
All			Conditions associated with starvation and malabsorption			
Vitamin A (retinol)/ β-carotene (provitamin A) [19, 20]	*Deficiency* ↓ Iron; ↓ DHA *Excess* ↓ Vitamin C; ↓ thyroid; hormone; ↓ vitamin K	Regulation of neural plasticity in hippocampus, olfactory bulb, and hypothalamus; alters glutamatergic and dopaminergic neurotransmission?	Bariatric surgery; alcohol misuse, alcohol can act as a vitamin A antagonist; chronic liver disease; HIV; opportunistic infections	Leading cause of preventable blindness in young children in the developing world; ↑ risk of hydrocephalus arising from neural tube defects?	Not well established, may affect the circadian rhythm; ↓ ability to sense flavours may lead to ↓ food intake; potentially contributes to depression, stress, memory impairment, AD, ASD, and schizophrenia	Only explored in the context of eye disease *CAUTION: high-dose vitamin A is teratogenic and can lead to severe neural tube defects*
Vitamin D (vitamin D3/ cholecalciferol) [12, 21, 22]	*Deficiency* ↓ Calcium *Excess* ↑ Calcium	Neuroprotective and neurotrophic; antioxidant; ↑ availability of DA and NA; modulates Ca signalling	Lack of exposure to sunlight such as in homebound or institutionalized life circumstances, full-body clothing, refugee situations	↑Risk of schizophrenia in conjunction with other risk factors	Depression; SAD? Cognitive impairment, dementia	Depression: conflicting evidence from meta-analyses; psychosis: not explored
Vitamin E (α-tocopherol) [23, 24]	*Excess* ↓ Vitamin K	Normal maintenance of biomembranes; neuroprotective; antioxidant		Unclear	No specific condition identified; oxidative damage has been implicated in the development of movement disorders such as tardive dyskinesia	Tardive dyskinesia: insufficient evidence; if any effect, limited to slowing rather than preventing tardive dyskinesia
Vitamin K (vitamin K1: phylloquinone; vitamin K2 varieties: menaquinones) [25]		Neuroprotective, anti-inflammatory; anti-apoptotic; angiogenic; sphingolipid metabolism	Treatment with warfarin or phenytoin; chronic alcoholism, FAS	Warfarin (a vitamin K antagonist) embryopathy associated with optic atrophy, blindness, microcephaly, cerebral ventricle dilatation, mental retardation	↓ Cognitive performance	Prevention of vitamin K deficiency bleeding in newborns; otherwise not systematically explored
Vitamin B1 (thiamine) [26]	Glucose and carbohydrate intake ↑ requirement	Cerebral energy metabolism, synthesis of nucleic acids; neurotransmitters, myelin, and ATP; protection from oxidative stress; medication of nerve membrane function; ↑ glutamate	Chronic alcoholism; mental disorders associated with poor nutritional intake, including anorexia nervosa and schizophrenia; bariatric surgery; hyperemesis gravidarum; accelerated metabolism such as in thyreotoxicosis and consuming diseases	Psychomotor abnormalities	Wernicke's encephalopathy, beriberi; may manifest with acute confusion, cognitive impairment, ataxia, and eye movement abnormalities; ↑ Korsakoff syndrome with anterograde amnesia, if Wernicke's encephalopathy remains untreated	Treatment and prophylaxis of Wernicke's encephalopathy and beriberi; *Simultaneous administration of magnesium may ↑ treatment effect*

Table 47.1 Continued

Vitamin	Impact in terms of availability or action of other vitamins or nutrients with potential CNS relevance	CNS implications	Special situations where deficiencies can occur	Implications of deficiency for neurodevelopment	Potential contribution of deficiency to mental health problems in adulthood	Supplementation for treatment of mental health problems
Vitamin B2 (riboflavin) [27, 28]	Involved in the metabolism of niacin vitamin B6, folate, vitamin B12, and tryptophan; *Deficiency* ↓ iron; ↓ zinc; ↓ calcium	Lipid metabolism; maintains stability of cell membranes; cofactor in the folate cycle effecting the methylation of homocysteine to methionine; antioxidant; ↑ availability of other antioxidants such as gluthathione; involved in mitochondrial function; ↑ iron absorption, regulation of thyroid hormone	In neonates receiving phototherapy for jaundice	Unclear	Unspecific; fatigue; personality change	Not explored in the mental health context
Niacin (vitamin B3 in two forms: nicotinic acid and nicotinamide) [19, 29]		Facilitates via NAD and/or NADP glucose and fat metabolism and synthesis and processing of lipids and steroids; involved in phospholipid signalling	Hartnup disease; chronic alcohol misuse	Unclear	Pellagra with depression, fatigue, insomnia, and memory and visual impairment; psychosis in a subgroup of individuals; niacin 1 receptor upregulated in Parkinson's disease and downregulated in schizophrenia	Treatment of pellagra
Panthothenic acid (vitamin B5) [19]		Provides acetyl and succinyl CoA to a multitude of chemical reactions		Inborn errors of acetyl CoA synthesis	Fatigue; insomnia; apathy; irritability; restlessness	Not explored
Vitamin B6 (pyridoxine) [19, 28]	Requires riboflavin, zinc, and magnesium to unfold its physiological actions *Deficiency* ↓ niacin; ↓ vitamin B12	Methyl donor (one-carbon cycle); cofactor in the conversion of homocysteine to cysteine amino acid metabolism; modification of steroid hormones, manufacture and/or metabolism of serotonin, NA, DA, GABA, and glutamate		Seizures; mental retardation; death	Depression, irritability; 'loss of sense of responsibility'	Pyridoxine-dependent epilepsy; cognitive impairment: no clear evidence; otherwise not explored *CAUTION: overconsumption can lead to nerve damage*

(Continued)

Table 47.1 Continued

Vitamin	Impact in terms of availability or action of other vitamins or nutrients with potential CNS relevance	CNS implications	Special situations where deficiencies can occur	Implications of deficiency for neurodevelopment	Potential contribution of deficiency to mental health problems in adulthood	Supplementation for treatment of mental health problems
Vitamin B12 (cobalamin) [19, 28, 30]	*Deficiency:* ↑ homocysteine	Methyl donor (one-carbon cycle); involved in the methylation of many substances, including neurotransmitters, phospholipids, and DNA; cofactor in the folate cycle effecting the methylation of homocysteine to methionine	Alcohol misuse; gastric atrophy; vegan diet; anti-acid agents, e.g. histamine 2 antagonists and proton pump inhibitors	↑ Risk of brain atrophy; neural tube defects; infantile tremor syndrome	Depression; psychosis; cognitive impairment; dementia, dependent and independent of homocysteine	Treatment of pernicious anaemia; depression: conflicting results; cognitive impairment: inconclusive for treatment, irrespective of homocysteine level
Folate (folic acid, vitamin B9) [12, 19, 28]	Synergistic with vitamin B12 via methionine synthase *Deficiency* ↑ homocysteine; *Excess* ↑ zinc?	Methyl donor (one-carbon cycle), methylation of homocysteine to methionine; neural tube and spine development; synthesis of serotonin, NA and DA	Treatment with anti-epileptics, e.g. sodium valproate	Neural tube defects	Depression; cognitive impairment, dementia dependent and independent of ↑ homocysteine	Prevention of neural tube effects; depression: inconclusive evidence, metabolites, e.g. methylfolate and S-adenosyl methionine (SAMe) may be more effective; cognitive impairment: inconclusive irrespective of homocysteine level
Biotin (vitamin B7 vitamin H) [19]		Glucose metabolism	Total parenteral nutrition; consumption of large amounts of raw egg white ('egg white injury')	Lethargy	Anorexia; hallucinations; depression; somnolence	Not explored
Choline (grouped with B vitamins, although humans can synthesize in small amounts [28, 31]		Methylation of homocysteine to methionine via betaine; synthesis of phospholipids, including sphingomyelin, maturation of GABA synapses		Neural tube defects	Cognitive/memory impairment	Developmental outcomes and prevention of mental illness for children affected by FAS: preliminary conflicting evidence
Vitamin C (ascorbic acid) [12, 19]	↓ Vitamin B12 alters absorption of metal irons	Antioxidant		Unclear	Fatigue; weakness; depression	Inconclusive evidence regarding treatment of depression; no clear evidence of efficacy for the treatment of cognitive impairment

Note: CNS: central nervous system; DHA: docosahexaenoic acid; AD: Alzheimer's disease; ASD: autism spectrum disorder; DA: dopamine; NA: noradrenaline; SAD: seasonal affective disorder; FAS: fetal alcohol syndrome; ATP: adenosine triphosphate; NAD: nicotinamide adenine dinucleotide; NADP: nicotinamide adenine dinucleotide phosphate; GABA: gamma-aminobutyric acid.

vitamin B1 deficiency gives rise to beriberi and acute vitamin B1 deficiency to Wernicke's encephalopathy.

Beriberi can manifest itself in various forms. Dry beriberi mainly affects the peripheral nerves, leading to a symmetrical neuropathy with hyporeflexia. Wet beriberi affects the heart and cardiovascular system, commonly associated with oedema. The worldwide prevalence of beriberi fluctuates. Most commonly, beriberi occurs in low- and middle-income countries, in which populations rely on polished white rice or other processed carbohydrate staples. Such staples have the outer shell (bran) removed and/or are not fortified with vitamin B1. Refugee populations with limited access to food may also have low vitamin B1 intakes. As vitamin B1 levels depend on carbohydrate intake, individuals with an excessive intake of sweet drinks may also be at risk. Finally, heavy ingestion of foodstuffs that counteract vitamin B1 can cause vitamin B1 deficiency. Such foodstuffs include betel nuts, tea leaves, and coffee. Some fish and shellfish host bacteria that contain thiaminases, which break down vitamin B1. Gastroenteritis leading to diarrhoea and vomiting can aggravate an already compromised nutritional status. The amount of vitamin B1 in breast milk varies. Newborn babies from deprived populations, only relying on breast milk, may be at risk of vitamin B1 deficiency [35].

Wernicke's encephalopathy is an acute and potentially life-threatening complication of vitamin B1 deficiency. Wernicke's encephalopathy occurs most commonly in the context of chronic alcohol abuse. However, in principle, Wernicke's encephalopathy can occur in any condition linked to starvation or malabsorption. Such conditions include bariatric surgery, consuming diseases, hyperemesis gravidarum, and anorexia nervosa [26]. The 'typical' clinical triad of mental status changes, ataxia, and ocular abnormalities only occurs in a minority of patients. Hence, the condition is often unrecognized and prevalence figures vary widely. In alcohol-related conditions, it may rise to more than 10% [26]. Alcohol is such a strong risk factor for Wernicke's encephalopathy because chronic alcohol intake is not only associated with a reduced food intake. Increased intake of carbohydrates and a decrease of vitamin B1 absorption are further causes.

In developing countries, prevention of alcohol misuse is the most pressing priority for the prevention of Wernicke's encephalopathy. Untreated, Wernicke's encephalopathy can lead to death or Korsakoff syndrome, associated with severe irreversible anterograde and retrograde amnesia. Thus, all individuals at risk of Wernicke's encephalopathy should receive prophylaxis with vitamin B1. The higher the risk, the more indicated is parenteral prophylaxis. If Wernicke's encephalopathy is suspected, assertive treatment with high doses of intravenous vitamin B1 is required. Importantly, harmful use of alcohol can also lead to an increased risk of deficiencies of other B vitamins. Such deficiencies need correction at the same time. Magnesium is a cofactor in the conversion of vitamin B1 to its biologically active form. As chronic alcohol misuse can lead to magnesium deficiency, it makes sense to add magnesium to vitamin B1 prophylaxis and treatment of Wernicke's encephalopathy. Magnesium deficiency may account for treatment failures of vitamin B1. At present, international treatment recommendations vary regarding the use and dosing of magnesium in this context.

Key minerals for mental health

Mineral deficiencies can also give rise to mental health problems. Particularly implicated are calcium, iron, and iodine, all of which are routinely measured in clinical practice (Table 47.2) [19, 36–41]. Calcium deficiency *and* excess can lead to altered mental states. Calcium deficiency most commonly occurs in the context of malignancies or hypoparathyroidism. Reduced levels of vitamin D can facilitate calcium deficiency. About 10–42% of patients treated with lithium develop some degree of hypercalcaemia. Possibly, lithium shifts the set point for parathyroid hormone. But not all individuals with lithium-associated hypercalcaemia have hyperparathyroidism. The exact mechanism of lithium-associated hypercalcaemia remains unclear. Iron deficiency is linked to blood loss. This can lead to fatigue and depression. Physiologically, iron deficiency occurs in the context of menstrual bleeds. Any unexplained iron deficiency warrants medical investigation to detect the underlying cause. In such cases, supplementation of iron without medical evaluation is not acceptable. Iron excess has been implicated in the pathophysiology of various neurodegenerative disorders. Iodine deficiency is a cause of hypothyroidism, which can affect mental health. The deficiency is most common to remote inland areas with limited access to seafood. Adding iodine to foodstuffs, such as table salt, can prevent iron deficiency.

Copper, magnesium, selenium, and zinc can also adversely affect mental health. These minerals are not routinely screened. They should be considered if mental health problems persist but no explanation can be found (Table 47.2). The most well-known condition related to copper is Wilson's disease, which is associated with psychiatric symptoms, movement disorder, and liver disease. In Wilson's disease, tissues accumulate copper to pathological levels. This is *not* the consequence of excess copper intake, but due to a genetic mutation of the copper transport proteins. Wilson's disease is an autosomal recessive disorder with prevalence estimates ranging from 1 in 10,000–30,000 live births. About 1 in 90 persons may carry the mutation. In isolated communities with consanguinity, the prevalence may be much higher [42]. Magnesium is a cofactor to many biochemical reactions in the body. We have already explored this in the context of vitamin B1 deficiency. Surveys from the USA indicate that about half of the population may have an insufficient magnesium intake [43]. Magnesium deficiencies are difficult to spot because 99% of the body's magnesium is intracellular. Thus, normal magnesium levels do not exclude deficiency. Selenium is an antioxidant with neuroprotective properties. Selenium also facilitates several neurotransmitters. Depending on the selenium contents in plants, selenium intake is highly variable between countries and within countries between regions [39]. Zinc has been implicated in a plethora of neurodegenerative disorders, including Alzheimer's disease, Parkinson's disease, and Huntington's disease. Zinc deficiency can also affect mood and appetite. Zinc is mainly found in animal products. Consequently, poverty increases vulnerability. Zinc deficiency is a major public health concern in low-income countries with limited access to proteins. Currently, about 17% of the world population is at risk of zinc deficiency [44]. The public mental health significance of zinc deficiency is most likely underestimated at present.

Table 47.2 Minerals and their relevance to mental health

Mineral	Impact in terms of availability or action of other vitamins or nutrients with potential CNS relevance	CNS implications	Special situations where abnormalities can occur	Implications of deficiency for neurodevelopment	Potential contribution of abnormalities to mental health problems in adulthood	Supplementation for treatment of mental health problems
All			Conditions associated with starvation, malabsorption, or overconsumption			
Calcium [19, 36]	Magnesium excess ↓ zinc; ↓ iron	Key role in cellular signal transmission; voltage-gated calcium channels control neurotransmitter release, muscle contraction, and cell excitability	*Deficiency:* ↓ vitamin D; hypo- and pseudohypoparathyroidism; remineralization of the bone after parathyroidectomy (hungry bone syndrome); ↓ magnesium; renal disease; malignancies *Rarer causes:* acute rhabdomyolysis; acute pancreatitis; ehylene glycol poisoning; bone marrow transplantation *Excess:* primary hyperparathyroidism; malignancy *Rarer causes:* sarcoidosis, tuberculosis, some tumours, e.g. lymphomas; lithium treatment; thiazide treatment; thyrotoxicosis; recovery from rhabdomyolysis; acute renal failure—diuretic phase; milk alkali syndrome	Unclear	*Deficiency:* depression, cognitive impairment, fatigue, seizures; *Excess:* fatigue, lethargy, weakness, confusion	Mood disorders: not explored; premenstrual syndrome: some evidence but unclear if equally effective as SSRIs or oral contraceptives
Copper [19, 36]	*Excess* ↓ zinc	Cofactor in many enzymatic reactions, including synthesis of DA and NA	*Deficiency:* overconsumption of zinc; bariatric surgery; Menke's disease (kinky hair disease) *Excess:* Wilson's disease (hepatolenticular degeneration); Indian childhood cirrhosis; *CAUTION:* *accumulation of copper in tissues but low serum copper levels*	Developmental delay; seizures	*Deficiency:* cognitive deficits *Excess:* encephalopathy, cognitive impairment, dysexecutive syndrome, mood swings, psychosis *Watch out for concomitant movement disorders and liver disease*	Treatment specific to the particular cause of deficiency or excess

Table 47.2 Continued

Mineral	Impact in terms of availability or action of other vitamins or nutrients with potential CNS relevance	CNS implications	Special situations where abnormalities can occur	Implications of deficiency for neurodevelopment	Potential contribution of abnormalities to mental health problems in adulthood	Supplementation for treatment of mental health problems
Iodine [19]	Selenium	Essential constituent of the thyroid hormones T4 and T3	*Deficiency:* autoimmune thyroid disease; lithium treatment	Developmental delay (cretinism)	*Deficiency:* hypothyroidism (myxoedema) with depression, lethargy, and cognitive impairment) *Excess:* hyperthyroidism	Treatment specific to the particular cause of deficiency or excess
Iron [19, 37]	*Excess:* ↓ copper; ↓ zinc	Major redox system in the body as part of haem proteins found in haemoglobin, myoglobin, and cytochromes	*Deficiency:* menstrual bleeds; pathological blood loss, e.g. in the context of acute trauma; GI bleeds	Neurodevelopmental problems affecting mood and learning ability; implicated in ADHD	*Deficiency:* fatigue, depression; restless legs syndrome (Willis-Ekbom disease) *Excess:* fatigue; brain iron accumulation implicated in neurodegenerative conditions with cognitive impairment and/or movement disorder	Treatment specific to the particular cause of deficiency or excess; ADHD: inconclusive evidence; *CAUTION: iron deficiency not associated with menstrual bleeds requires investigation and not just iron supplementation*
Magnesium [19, 38]	Calcium; vitamin D	Cofactor in many enzyme systems required for protein synthesis, energy generation, cell metabolism, and cell division; facilitates actions of vitamin D and PTH	*Deficiency:* chronic alcoholism; prolonged IV fluids; treatment with diuretics, aminoglycosides, or cisplatin	Unclear	May lead to hypocalcaemia	Neuroprotection for preterm infants; neuroprotection in adults: inconclusive evidence, fibromyalgia: preliminary evidence
Selenium [39]	Iodine	Antioxidant; neuroprotective; facilitates thyroid function, e.g. required for the conversion from T4 to T3, facilitates neurotransmission of GABA, glutamate, DA, and acetylcholine	*Deficiency:* total parenteral nutrition	Unclear	Depression; cognitive impairment; implicated in neurodegenerative diseases and movement disorders	Depression: conflicting evidence
Zinc [28, 40, 41]	*Excess* ↓ copper	Part of > 200 metalloenzymes; methylation of homocysteine to methionine via the methionine cycle involving betaine; ↓ glutamate, ↑ GABA; modulates synaptic activity and neuronal plasticity	*Deficiency:* burns; liver and renal disease; inflammatory GI, e.g. Crohn's disease; anorexia nervosa; anabolic steroids; sickle cell anaemia; acrodematitis enteropathica	Developmental delay, growth retardation; intellectual impairment; implicated in ADHD	*Deficiency:* depression and bipolar disorder; cognitive impairment; implicated in several neurodegenerative conditions; maintains appetite loss in anorexia nervosa	Anorexia nervosa: preliminary evidence; depression: preliminary evidence; ADHD: inconclusive evidence

Note: CNS: central nervous system; DA: dopamine; NA: noradrenaline; SSRI: selective serotonin reuptake inhibitor; T4: thyroxine; T3: triiodothyronine; GI: gastrointestinal, ADHD: attention deficit hyperactivity disorder; PTH: parathyroid hormone; IV: intravenous; GABA: gamma-aminobutyric acid.

Diets for mental health

Promoting diets for mental health is extremely popular, as can be judged by the representation of the topic on the Internet. Searching 'food for mood' on the search engine Google yielded 29,800,000 hits on 19 March 2018. 'Eating yourself happy' yielded 68,900,000 results on the same day. Very little is known about the effectiveness of dietary interventions for mental health. We have already seen that the association of specific vitamin and mineral deficiencies with mental health problems does not automatically translate into improvements of mental health, when the missing agent is substituted. Diets are a way to address several nutritional deficits at the same time. Eating more fish, adhering to a Mediterranean diet, and adding vitamin B supplements may all improve mood and cognition. Yet, the evidence remains limited and conflicting (Table 47.3) [45–53]. Larger trials are underway to investigate this question [1].

Diets for neurodevelopmental disorders

The use of diets for treating brain-related disorders goes back over 2000 years. In 500 BC, dietary regimens and fasting were used to treat epilepsy. In the 1920s, the ketogenic diet was introduced as an effective treatment of some forms of childhood epilepsy. With the advent of modern anti-epileptic drugs in the 1940s, the ketogenic diet declined in significance. Only in recent years has the interest in this diet been revived. The interest has expanded to the general question of the utility of dietary approaches for the treatment or prevention of neurodevelopmental disorders, such as ADHD and autistic spectrum disorders. All such diets aim at restricting or eliminating food components purported to harm the developing brain (Table 47.4) [4, 54, 55]. For most diets, the evidence is limited and conflicting. But there are two intriguing studies. The Raine cohort from Western Australia tested the association between a Western-style diet and ADHD versus a 'healthy' diet. The Western-style diet had a higher intake of total fat, saturated fat, refined sugars, and sodium, and a lower intake of omega-3 fatty acids, fibre, and folate. The 'healthy' diet had a higher intake of omega-3 fatty acids, fibre, and folate, and lower intake of total fat, saturated fat, refined sugars, and sodium. The study followed the dietary patterns of 1799 children from birth to the age of 14 years. In this cohort, the risk of ADHD was double in individuals with a higher intake of a Western-style diet [56]. Another trial among young adults in a UK prison showed that combined supplementation with a multi-vitamin/mineral and an omega 3/6 fatty acid preparation led to a significant reduction in antisocial behaviour [57].

At present, clinicians may find it difficult to recommend specific dietary approaches beyond a 'healthy' dietary pattern. Yet, parents are faced with a lack of effective treatments. Desperate not to miss a window of opportunity in their children's neurodevelopment, they may wish to try such diets. Ultimately, clinicians have to strike a balance between potential risks and benefits.

Superfoods

For some health problems, when there is a clearly identified deficiency, it makes sense to increase foods rich in the missing ingredient or use supplements. We have looked at this in the context of minerals and vitamins. However, improving mental health through superfoods is difficult. For instance, depression is associated with a lack of serotonin. But eating foods containing high amounts of the precursor L-tryptophan, such as bananas or turkey, does not cure depression [58]. Chocolate contains polyphenols that may act on gamma-aminobutyric acid. Chocolate also contains adenosine, traditionally credited with mood-lifting properties. An increased sense of calmness and contentedness has recently been demonstrated for people without mental health problems [59]. But, overall, the clinical evidence for individuals suffering from major depression remains limited. To make cocoa products palatable, considerable amounts of sugar and fat are required. Eaten in substantial amounts, this adds more calories to the diet. Dopamine is another potential target. Observational studies have credited coffee, tea, and cocoa with antidepressant properties. It remains unclear which constituents mediate the antidepressant effect, but caffeine seems a key ingredient. Caffeine has synergistic effects with noradrenaline. Caffeine also elevates dopamine concentrations by binding through adenosine receptors [60]. Foods containing tyrosine are widely promoted as dopamine boosters. Yet, there is no evidence available that focusing on foods containing high amounts of the dopamine precursor tyrosine, such as meats, fish eggs, wholegrain cereals, and bananas, has significant stimulant effects. 'Eating yourself happy', although intuitively appealing, remains a concept difficult to prove.

Interactions between foodstuffs and psychotropic medications

Under some circumstances, foodstuffs and psychotropic drugs can interact. The most notable example is the interaction of tyramine-containing foods with irreversible monoamino-oxidase inhibitors. Such combinations increase the risk of hypertensive crisis. This interaction is known as the 'cheese reaction' as most cheeses contain substantial amounts of tyramine. Another example of a food–drug interaction is grapefruit or grapefruit juice, which, via cytochrome P450 (CYP)3A inhibition, increases the plasma levels of drugs that are substrates. Although not a foodstuff, it is important to highlight tobacco smoke as a potent CYP1 inducer. Smoking may lower the plasma levels of respective substrates, such as clozapine. Foodstuffs that change the water balance can interfere with lithium. This can occur if the intake varies substantially from what is usually consumed. Owing to its diuretic properties, coffee can potentially interact with lithium. The sodium ions in table salt can directly compete with lithium ions. Rarely do psychotropic treatments require dietary adjustments. Yet, potential food–drug interactions should be considered if unexpected medical or psychiatric symptoms occur and no other explanation can be found.

Mental health and the environment

Several examples exist of environmental agents causing mental health problems. A classic example is mercury intoxication of hatmakers, from which the saying 'mad as a hatter' stems. Other environmental factors, such as lead, can subclinically affect the mental health of major parts of a population. One extreme example is the interactions between toxic exposures and stress reactions linked to disaster and war scenarios [61]. In this section, we will focus on substances that may affect mental health following exposure from the general environment, including

Table 47.3 Dietary approaches and risk depression and cognitive impairment: the recent evidence

	Diet	Meta-analysis: pooled RR for observational studies (95% CI)	RR for RCTs	Significant change in risk
Depression				
Li et al., 2016 [45]	Fish	0.83 (0.74–0.93)		↓
Lai et al., 2015 [46]	'Healthy'	0.84 (0.76–0.92)		↓
	Western	1.17 (0.97–1.41)		–
Sánchez-Villega et al., 2013 [47]	Mediterranean + nuts		0.78 (0.55–1.10)	–
	As above in individuals with DM2 only		0.59 (0.36–0.98)	↓
Psaltopoulou et al., 2013 [48]	Mediterranean diet	0.68 (0.54–0.86)		↓
Cognitive impairment/dementia*				
Zhang et al., 2016 [49]	Fish (one serving/week increment)	0.95 (0.90–0.99) Dementia		↓
		0.93 (0.90–0.95) AD		↓
Cao et al., 2015 [50]	Unsaturated fatty acids	0.84 (0.74–0.95)		↓
	Antioxidants (vitamin E, vitamin C, or flavonoids)	0.87 (0.77–0.98)		↓
	Vitamin B	0.72 (0.54–0.96)		↓
	Mediterranean diet	0.69 (0.57–0.84)		↓
	Fish	0.79 (0.59–1.06)		–
	Fruit and vegetable	0.46 (0.16–1.32)		–
	Alcohol	0.74 (0.55–1.01)		–
	Aluminium	2.24 (1.49–3.37)		↑
	Smoking	1.43 (1.15–1.77)		↑
	Vitamin D	1.52 (1.17–1.98)		↑
Wu et al., 2015 [51]	Fish (high vs low)	36% (8–56%) ↓ risk of AD		↓
Xu et al., 2015 [52]	Healthy, including Mediterranean	0.43 (0.24–0.63)		↓
	Fish	0.70 (0.47–0.93)		↓
	Coffee/caffeine containing drinks	0.54 (0.39–0.69)		↓
	Alcohol: light to moderate vs never	0.76 (0.57–0.95)		↓
	Alcohol: high vs low/never	0.96 (0.18–1.74)		–
Valls-Pedret et al., 2015 [53]	Mediterranean diet + extra virgin olive oil			
	Change in memory scores*		0.04 (−0.09 to 0.18)	
	Change in frontal cognition scores*		0.23 (0.03–0.43]	↓
	Change in global cognition scores*		0.05 (−0.11 to0.21)	–
	Mediterranean diet + nuts			–
	Change in memory scores*		0.09 (−0.05 to 0.23)	–
	Change in frontal cognition scores*		0.03 (− 0.25 to 0.31)	–
	Change in global cognition scores*		−0.05 (−0.27 to 0.18)	–
Psaltopoulou et al., 2013 [48]	Mediterranean diet	0.60 (0.43–0.83)		↓

Note: RR: relative risk; CI: confidence interval; RCT: randomized controlled trial; DM2: type 2 diabetes mellitus; AD: Alzheimer's disease. *Fully adjusted models for a variety of group characteristics and follow-up time.

Table 47.4 Diets used for the treatment of autism spectrum disorders (ASD) and attention deficit hyperactivity disorder (ADHD)

Diet	Purported mechanism of action	Foods/drinks eliminated/restricted	Effect (95% CI)	Potential safety concerns
ADHD				
Oligo-antigenic (hypoallergenic/elimination diet) [54]	Hypersensitivity reaction to allergens	Items known to cause food allergies	Meta-analysis: standardized mean difference pre-/post-treatment change; all trials: 1.48 (0.85–2.36); observer-blinded trials only: 0.51 (−0.02 to 1.54)	
Food colour elimination, including Feingold diet (additive and salicylate-free diet) [54]	Hypersensitivity reaction to allergens	Items containing synthetic food colours, particularly red and orange; artificial sweeteners, e.g. aspartame; preservatives; salicylate	Meta-analysis: standardized mean difference pre-/post-treatment change; all trials: 0.32 (0.06–0.58) observer-blinded trials only: 0.42 (0.13–0.70).	
Elimination of sugar [55]	Sugar affecting cognition and behaviour possible in subgroups of children	Items containing free sugar	No evidence available	
ASD				
Gluten-casein free diet [55]	'Opioid excess' theory. Purports incomplete breakdown of gluten and casein in the gut lead to the formation of opioid-like peptides that cause neurobehavioural symptoms. Such peptides are assumed to be released through a leaky gut	Items containing gluten or casein	Meta-analysis unclear, only two small studies available	Bone loss, ensure adequate vitamin D, calcium, and protein intake
Ketogenic (high-fat, low-carbohydrate) diet [4]	Effective as a treatment for epilepsy (particularly myoclonic epilepsy) and observed to improve attention and behaviour. Targets mitochondrial dysfunction and hence deficient energy utilization, deficient glucose oxidation in the brain, also GABA?	Items containing carbohydrates; requires high fat intake at the same time	Preliminary evidence of effect based on one small trial	May ↓ growth and ↑ cholesterol

Note: CI: confidence interval; GABA: gamma-aminobutyric acid.

some aspects of occupational exposure to toxic substances. We will not deal with aspects of the physical environment, such as noise, daylight, and city planning, and mention electromagnetic fields only briefly.

Examples of environmental hazards

The detrimental effect of lead on the developing brain remains highly relevant to public mental health. The effect may be subtle for each individual child. But, at the population level, the aggregate effect is substantial [62]. Following the discontinuation of leaded petrol, lead concentrations in blood fell across populations worldwide. Thus, preventive interventions targeted at environmental toxins *can* have a huge public mental health impact. However, lead exposure from paint or contaminated drinking water still poses a hazard to children in parts of the world, including wealthy countries, such as the USA.

People living in contaminated areas, for example near agricultural or industrial sites, may become exposed to environmental toxins. This occurs most commonly—but not exclusively—in high-poverty neighbourhoods, for instance in the vicinity of banana plantations and metal smelters. Such exposures are often preventable and, from the public health perspective, it is important to identify areas where undue exposures occur.

Clinical assessment of environmental factors

Screening for environmental substances in, for example, blood or urine is sometimes used to identify populations or individuals with undue exposure. We have already mentioned the example of children in areas with a risk of lead exposure. In contrast, none of the general psychiatric diagnoses warrants screening for an environmental substance in a patient, unless there are indications of intoxication or a specific environmental or occupational exposure.

In order to find such indications, it is important to consider occupation when taking the patient's history. When suspicions of a relevant exposure appear, these should be investigated further, for instance by consulting the occupational health literature or referring to an occupational health clinic [63, 64]. Mental health problems following occupational exposures include Parkinson-like symptoms, often coupled with depression, from manganese in the hard-metal industry. Organic solvents can affect cognitive function. Exposure to pesticides, mercury, and lead can lead to mood alterations. Assessment of exposure in the workplace may require the professional expertise of an occupational health clinic.

Environmental public health interventions

At the population level, actions have been taken to decrease environmental exposures to substances that affect mental health. Although controversial at the time, many of these are today believed to have significantly improved public mental health.

Within occupational medicine, one example from the 1980s is the phase out of paints based on organic solvents. Until the 1990s, several decades of exposure to organic solvents generated a continuous inflow of cognitively impaired patients to occupational health clinics, for example in Scandinavian countries. These patients were usually former painters. Scandinavian painters were particularly affected because they tended to have low job mobility. This means that they remained painters and were exposed to organic solvents throughout their working life. The inflow of these patients stopped almost completely following the replacement of organic solvent paints with water-based paints.

The results of interventions in the external environment are not easy to perceive at individual level. We have already mentioned the benefit of a worldwide decrease in lead exposure. Exposure to methylmercury and polychlorinated biphenyl is another example. This occurs in communities that consume contaminated fish, such as whale in the Faroe Islands, and among Inuit populations. Reduction of exposure to such toxins is considered an important public health improvement, even if reduction of the incidence of clinical cases is not easily observed. An average gain of few points on the IQ scale across a population is only of marginal impact to an individual. Yet, it causes a population-based IQ shift of public health dimensions [62].

Environmental substances and mental health: Cause or association?

A number of environmental pollutants have been associated with loss of cognitive function or disorders of neurological or neurodegenerative nature (Table 47.5) [62, 65–77]. Substances vary largely in regard to public health impact and contribution of aetiology to mental health problems. For many substances we do not know if observed associations are causal or not. Bellinger [78] applied a population-based approach to estimate the contributions of environmental and other risk factors to the neurodevelopment of 0–5-year-old US children. In this population of 25.5 million children, lead exposure was estimated to cause a loss of 23 million IQ points. This was less than the loss caused by preterm birth (34 million) but more than ADHD (19 million), iron deficiency (9 million), and postnatal brain injury (6 million). The dose–response curve for lead is relatively well described after several decades of ambitious epidemiological research. In the same study [78], the effect of organophosphate pesticides was estimated to cause a 17 million IQ points loss. But it is much more difficult to attribute causally this IQ loss to organophosphate pesticides. The dose–response relationship has been examined in only two relatively recent studies, leaving considerable uncertainty both about causation and the shape of any dose–response association. The uncertainty is greatest for low levels of exposure, which is found most commonly.

When deriving causation from epidemiological findings, confounding is always a critical issue. Confounding produces false associations, for example if an exposure is most common among children with poor access to intellectual stimulation. Confounding can also hide associations, for instance if an exposure is instead most common among children with a social and educational advantage. Publication bias can also affect the assessment of newly discovered risks, which may become over-reported. Studies that observe an association may have a larger probability of being published than those rejecting an association, especially if the association has never been observed before. Among the factors listed in Table 47.5, lead and methylmercury have been thoroughly studied for decades. Air pollutants, arsenic, cadmium, organophosphates, and organic product chemicals have only more recently given rise to concerns about public and mental health implications. Manganese takes a middle place in this sense.

Several other environmental factors have been studied and intensely discussed in relation to mental health. However, there is only little or no evidence that they cause specific mental health problems. Several well-designed studies are available that should have captured potential detrimental effects. There is a lack of evidence regarding adverse effects on cognitive function in humans from radio frequent fields from mobile phones, base stations, or Wi-Fi hotspots. Meta-analyses and provocation studies do not support the assumption that electromagnetic fields can cause intolerance reactions [79]. Similarly, there is no evidence for concluding that the low exposure to inorganic mercury from normal amalgam tooth fillings causes adverse psychiatric effects [80]. However, some caution may be warranted for pregnant women and in situations in which very extreme wear occurs. Examples for these are bruxism, extreme exposure of the amalgam surface to acidic foods or drinks, or extreme chewing habits.

There remains uncertainty about whether all of the substances listed in Table 47.5 really do affect mental health. While this must be acknowledged, it must also be noted that our ability to identify which substances are safe, and which are not, is limited [76]. Epidemiology is a blunt tool that relies on observations in real life. Estimating a mother's exposure during a 9-month pregnancy or child's exposure during the first years of life is difficult for most substances. Even more difficult is exposure assessment over a whole lifespan for studies of neurodegenerative effects in old age. These limitations, and the evidence that environmental factors apparently mostly have small effects in many individuals, make it difficult to arrive at firm conclusion about the impact of environmental factors on mental health. At present, public mental health would benefit from some societal caution concerning chemicals and other environmental factors that potentially have neurodevelopmental or neurodegenerative effects.

Table 47.5 Environmental substances and their relevance to mental health

Substance	Exposure	Potential mechanisms of CNS impact	Potential neurodevelopmental effects	Potential mental effects in adults	Mental public health impact
Air pollution [65]	Traffic, combustion, industry, abrasive processes	Inflammatory and vascular effects; may affect neurodevelopment and the adult brain	In recent studies, exposure *in utero*: impaired IQ and learning in children. Postnatal exposure: memory impairments	In recent studies, impaired cognitive function in adults, e.g. memory and execution, also with dementia	Insufficient evidence for a causal association. A causal association would have significant public health impact, as exposure very common
Arsenic [66]	Drinking water in certain areas, rice	Uncertain. Direct toxic properties; possibly, epigenetic effects on methylation patterns	In recent studies, children's IQ inversely associated with arsenic exposure; associations stronger with *current* than with previous or *in utero* exposure	No strong indications	Insufficient evidence for a causal association. Exposure affects hundreds of millions of people worldwide: in Bangladesh but also, e.g., in Argentina, and the USA
Cadmium [67, 68]	Smoking, food, mainly cereals and vegetables	Very little known, oxidative stress may be involved	In recent studies, inverse associations between cadmium exposure and IQ and other cognitive measures; results less consistent for behavioural disturbance	Limited evidence; possibly involvement in neurodegeneration [69]	Suggestive evidence of an association between cognition and prenatal or childhood exposure. Insufficient evidence to assess public health impact
Lead [62, 70, 71]	Lead paint, occupational exposure, lead-glazed ceramics, some Ayurveda preparations, water contaminated by lead pipes or lead-containing brass, proximity to lead-emitting industry, dust, food, e.g. liver	Affects neural signalling by interfering with calcium, ↓ signal velocity; interferes with synaptogenesis and myelination in early childhood	Intoxication may cause encephalopathy; associations between cognition (IQ) and post- or prenatal exposure; associations with behavioural impairments, e.g. ADHD and criminality in several studies	Intoxications from, e.g., occupational exposure or use of lead-glazed ceramics cause ↓ libido, hostility, depression, and other psychiatric symptoms; associations between lead exposure and neurodegenerative disorders, e.g. ALS, AD, and PD	Cognitive loss for today's children due to lead: ~0.5–1 IQ points, on average; possibly some impact on behaviour; uncertain whether loss of cognitive function and/or neurodegenerative effects occur at older age
Manganese [72]	Occupational airborne exposure, food, tea, drinking water, airborne dust	Affects dopamine transport and receptors; essential for several functions, including prenatal and neonatal development. Inhaled and ingested manganese appear to have different toxicity	Inverse associations with IQ or other mental development indices in several small studies	Occupational airborne exposure can cause manganism with mood changes and symptoms resembling PD; non-occupational environmental exposure↑ frequency of signs of parkinsonism	Scattered evidence; may have an impact on children's cognitive development and adult Parkinson-like symptoms in areas with exposure from, e.g., industrial processes, drinking water, or fuel additives
Methylmercury [62, 73]	Fish, especially large and/or predatory species or from contaminated waters	Affects synaptogenesis and the proliferation and migration of neurons. ↑ cellular oxidative stress	Very high exposure *in utero* may cause cerebral palsy and severe developmental retardation; associations in populations with high intake of fish or whale between impaired cognitive function in children and postnatal methylmercury exposure	The major neurological effects in adults are not mental health related	May affect cognitive performance in populations with high consumption of contaminated fish or meat from marine mammals

Table 47.5 Continued

Substance	Exposure	Potential mechanisms of CNS impact	Potential neurodevelopmental effects	Potential mental effects in adults	Mental public health impact
Organo-halogens that are persistent organic pollutants [74]	PCB: fatty food of animal origin, e.g. fish, meat, dairy products; environmental exposure. PBDE: products with flame retardants, dust DDT and DDE: local contamination in agricultural areas, fatty food of animal origin, vegetables grown in treated areas	Potentially, interference with thyroid hormone signalling in the developing brain, and effects on neurotransmitter systems	PCB: associations with neurodevelopmental outcomes in several studies, but results not fully consistent PBDE: few but more consistent results pointing at poorer development and lower IQ DDT and DDE: associations with poorer outcome in some studies, but results inconsistent	Limited evidence. Possibly, depression following high occupational exposure to PCB [75]	Not possible to asses impact
Organophoshates, e.g. the pesticide chlorpyrifos [76]	Acute intoxication in children occurs in areas with insufficiently controlled use; exposure occurs after local contamination in agricultural areas and domestic use; low-grade exposure through food	Inhibits cholinesterase, altering acetylcholine levels, which may affect synapse formation	In recent studies, associations between *in utero* exposure and neurobehavioural deficits and head circumference	Numerous intoxications worldwide, often after occupational exposure	Studies few and relatively recent. If associations causal and dose–response related at low levels, then significant public health impact possible, as exposure is common
Product chemicals with endocrine disrupting properties [74]	Bisphenol A: canned food [77], other food or water from polycarbonate or epoxy containers or piping; phtalates: plasticizers in, e.g., PVC in housing, e.g., floor mats or products	Bisphenol A is an oestrogen-mimicking substance; uncertain mechanisms regarding potential neurobehavioral effects are uncertain; phtalates have androgenic properties with uncertain effect on neurodevelopment; possibly, thyroid hormone-related effects have an impact	Bisphenol A: some but not consistent associations with child behaviour; phtalates: associations with development and behaviour reported; results somewhat inconsistent, maybe because of sex-specific effects	Only few cross-sectional studies	Impossible to assess

Note: CNS: central nervous system; ADHD: attention deficit hyperactivity disorder; ALS: amyotrophic lateral sclerosis; AD: Alzheimer's disease; PD: Parkinson's disease; PCB: polychlorinated biphenyl; PBDE: polybrominated diphenyl ethers; DDT: dichlorodiphenyltrichloroethane; DDE: dichlorodiphenyldichloroethylene; PVC: polyvinyl chloride.

References

1. Sarris J, Logan AC, Akbaraly TN. Nutritional medicine as mainstream in psychiatry. *Lancet Psychiatry* 2015; 2: 271–274.
2. Opie RS, O'Neil A, Itsiopoulos C, Jacka FN. The impact of whole-of-diet interventions on depression and anxiety: a systematic review of randomised controlled trials. *Public Health Nutr* 2015; 18: 2074–2093.
3. Danziger S, Levav J, Avnaim-Pesso L. Extraneous factors in judicial decisions. *Proc Natl Acad Sci U S A* 2011; 108: 6889–6892.
4. Evangeliou A, Vlachonikolis I, Mihailidou H, et al. Application of a ketogenic diet in children with autistic behavior: pilot study. *J Child Neurol* 2003; 18: 113–118.
5. Gaspar P, Cases O, Maroteaux L. The developmental role of serotonin: news from mouse molecular genetics. *Nat Rev Neurosci* 2003; 4: 1002–1012.
6. Stiles J, Jernigan TL. The basics of brain development. *Neuropsychol Rev* 2010; 20: 327–348.
7. Susser E, Neugebauer R, Hoek HW, Brown AS, Lin S, Labovitz D. Schizophrenia after prenatal famine. Further evidence. *Arch Gen Psychiatry* 1996; 53: 25–31.
8. Franzek EJ, Sprangers N, Janssens AC, Van Duijn CM, Van De Wetering BJ. Prenatal exposure to the 1944–45 Dutch 'hunger winter' and addiction later in life. *Addiction* 2008; 103: 433–438.
9. Brown AS, van Os J, Driessens C, Hoek HW, Susser ES. Further evidence of relation between prenatal famine and major affective disorder. *Am J Psychiatry* 2000; 157: 190–195.
10. Song S, Wang W, Hu P. Famine, death, and madness: schizophrenia in early adulthood after prenatal exposure to the Chinese Great Leap Forward Famine. *Soc Sci Med* 2009; 68: 1315–1321.
11. Appleton KM, Sallis HM, Perry R, Ness AR, Churchill R. Omega-3 fatty acids for depression in adults. *Cochrane Database Syst Rev* 2015; 11: CD004692.
12. Sarris J, Murphy J, Mischoulon D, et al. Adjunctive nutraceuticals for depression: a systematic review and meta-analyses. *Am J Psychiatry* 2016; 173: 575–587.

13. Rosenblat JD, Kakar R, Berk M, et al. Anti-inflammatory agents in the treatment of bipolar depression: a systematic review and meta-analysis. *Bipolar Disord* 2016; 18: 89–101.

14. Hallahan B, Ryan T, Hibbeln JR, Murray IT, et al. Efficacy of omega-3 highly unsaturated fatty acids in the treatment of depression. *Br J Psychiatry* 2016; 209: 192–201.

15. Amminger GP, Schäfer MR, Schlögelhofer M, Klier CM, McGorry PD. Longer-term outcome in the prevention of psychotic disorders by the Vienna omega-3 study. *Nat Commun* 2015; 6: 7934.

16. Chen AT, Chibnall JT, Nasrallah HA. A meta-analysis of placebo-controlled trials of omega-3 fatty acid augmentation in schizophrenia: possible stage-specific effects. *Ann Clin Psychiatry* 2015; 27, 289–296.

17. NHS Choices. Health A-Z. Available at: http://www.nhs.uk/pages/home.aspx (accessed 16 June 2017).

18. Sneader W. *Drug Discovery—a history*. Chichester: John Wiley & Sons, 2005.

19. Food Standards Agency. Expert Group on Vitamins and Minerals (2003) Safe Upper Levels for Vitamins and Minerals. Available at: https://cot.food.gov.uk/committee/committee-on-toxicity/cotreports/cotjointreps/evmreport (accessed 16 June 2017).

20. Shearer KD, Stoney PN, Morgan PJ, McCaffery PJ. A vitamin for the brain. *Trends Neurosci* 2012; 35: 733–741.

21. Cui X, Gooch H, Groves NJ, et al. Vitamin D and the brain: key questions for future research. *J Steroid Biochem Mol Biol* 2015; 148: 305–309.

22. Parker G, Brotchie H. 'D'for depression: any role for vitamin D? 'Food for Thought' II. *Acta Psychiatr Scand* 2011; 124: 243–249.

23. Bhidayasiri R, Fahn S, Weiner WJ, Gronseth GS, Sullivan KL, Zesiewicz. A. Evidence-based guideline: treatment of tardive syndromes: report of the Guideline Development Subcommittee of the American Academy of Neurology. *Neurology* 2013; 81: 463–469.

24. Soares-Weiser K, Maayan N, McGrath J. Vitamin E for neuroleptic-induced tardive dyskinesia. *Cochrane Database Syst Rev* 2011; 2: CD000209.

25. Ferland G. Vitamin K and brain function. *Semin Thromb Hemost* 2013; 39: 849–855.

26. Sechi G, Serra A. Wernicke's encephalopathy: new clinical settings and recent advances in diagnosis and management. *Lancet Neurol* 2007; 6: 442–455.

27. Thakur K, Tomar SK, Singh AK, Mandal S, Arora S. Riboflavin and health: a review of recent human research *Crit Rev Food Sci Nutr* 2016; 53: 3650–3660.

28. Glier MB, Green TJ, Devlin AM. Methyl nutrients, DNA methylation, and cardiovascular disease. *Mol Nutr Food Res* 2014; 58: 172–182.

29. Yao JK, Dougherty GG Jr, Gautier CH, et al. Prevalence and specificity of the abnormal niacin response: a potential endophenotype marker in schizophrenia. *Schizophr Bull* 2016; 42: 369–76.

30. Rathod R, Kale A, Joshi S. Novel insights into the effect of vitamin B$_{12}$ and omega-3 fatty acids on brain function. *J Biomed Sci* 2016; 23: 17.

31. Ross RG, Hunter SK, Hoffman MC, et al. Perinatal phosphatidylcholine supplementation and early childhood behavior problems: evidence for CHRNA7 moderation. *Am J Psychiatry* 2016; 173: 509–516.

32. Belvederi Murri M, Respino M, Masotti M, et al. Vitamin D and psychosis: mini meta-analysis. *Schizophr Res* 2013; 150: 235–239.

33. McGrath JJ, Eyles DW, Pedersen CB, et al. Neonatal vitamin D status and risk of schizophrenia: a population-based case-control study. *Arch Gen Psychiatry* 2010; 67: 889–894.

34. Anglin RE, Samaan Z, Walter SD, McDonald SD. Vitamin D deficiency and depression in adults: systematic review and meta-analysis. *Br J Psychiatry* 2013; 202: 100–107.

35. Hiffler L, Rakotoambinina B, Lafferty N, Martinez Garcia D. Thiamine Deficiency in Tropical Pediatrics: New Insights into a Neglected but Vital Metabolic Challenge. *Front Nutr* 2016; 3: 16.

36. Gaw A, Murphy MJ, Srivastava R, Cowan RA, O'Reilly DStJ. *Clinical Biochemistry*. Edinburgh: Churchill Livingstone Elsevier, 2013.

37. Bakoyiannis I, Gkioka E, Daskalopoulou A, Korou LM, Perrea D, Pergialiotis V. An explanation of the pathophysiology of adverse neurodevelopmental outcomes in iron deficiency. *Rev Neurosci* 2015; 26: 479–488.

38. Zeng X, Xue Y, Tian Q, Sun R, An R. Effects and safety of magnesium sulfate on neuroprotection: a meta-analysis based on PRISMA guidelines. *Medicine (Baltimore)* 2016; 95: e2451.

39. Rayman MP. Selenium and human health. *Lancet* 2012; 379: 1256–1268.

40. Prakash A, Bharti K, Majeed AB. Zinc: indications in brain disorders. *Fundam Clin Pharmacol* 2015; 29: 131–149.

41. Lai J, Moxey A, Nowak G, Vashum K, Bailey K, McEvoy M. The efficacy of zinc supplementation in depression: systematic review of randomised controlled trials. *J Affect Disord* 2012; 136: e31–e39.

42. Schilsky ML. Wilson's disease: Epidemiology and pathogenesis. Available at: https://www.uptodate.com/contents/wilson-disease-epidemiology-and-pathogenesis (accessed 16 June 2016).

43. Rosanoff A, Weaver CM, Rude RK. Suboptimal magnesium status in the United States: are the health consequences underestimated? *Nutr Rev* 2012; 70: 153–164.

44. Wessells KR, Brown KH. Estimating the global prevalence of zinc deficiency: results based on zinc availability in national food supplies and the prevalence of stunting. *PLOS ONE* 2012; 7: e50568.

45. Li F, Liu X, Zhang D. Fish consumption and risk of depression: a meta-analysis. *J Epidemiol Commun Health* 2016; 70: 299–304.

46. Lai JS, Hiles S, Bisquera A, Hure AJ, McEvoy M, Attia J. A systematic review and meta-analysis of dietary patterns and depression in community-dwelling adults. *Am J Clin Nutr* 2014; 99: 181–197.

47. Sánchez-Villegas A, Martínez-González MA, Estruch R, et al. Mediterranean dietary pattern and depression: the PREDIMED randomized trial. *BMC Med* 2013; 11: 208.

48. Psaltopoulou T, Sergentanis TN, Panagiotakos DB, Sergentanis IN, Kosti R, Scarmeas N. Mediterranean diet, stroke, cognitive impairment, and depression: a meta-analysis. *Ann Neurol* 2013; 74: 580–591.

49. Zhang Y, Chen J, Qiu J, Li Y, Wang J, Jiao J. Intakes of fish and polyunsaturated fatty acids and mild-to-severe cognitive impairment risks: a dose-response meta-analysis of 21 cohort studies. *Am J Clin Nutr* 2016; 103: 330–340.

50. Cao L, Tan L, Wang HF, et al. Dietary patterns and risk of dementia: a systematic review and meta-analysis of cohort studies. *Mol Neurobiol* 2015; 53: 6144–6154.

51. Wu S, Ding Y, Wu F, Li R, Hou J, Mao P. Omega-3 fatty acids intake and risks of dementia and Alzheimer's disease: a meta-analysis. *Neurosci Biobehav Rev* 2015; 48: 1–9.

52. Xu W, Tan L, Wang HF, et al. Meta-analysis of modifiable risk factors for Alzheimer's disease. *J Neurol Neurosurg Psychiatry* 2015; 86: 1299–1306.

53. Valls-Pedret C, Sala-Vila A, Serra-Mir M, et al. Mediterranean Diet and Age-Related Cognitive Decline: A Randomized Clinical Trial. *J Am Med Assoc Intern Med* 2015; 175: 1094–1103.

54. Sonuga-Barke EJ, Brandeis D, Cortese S, et al. Nonpharmacological interventions for ADHD: systematic review and meta-analyses of randomized controlled trials of dietary and psychological treatments. *Am J Psychiatry* 2013; 170: 275–289.

55. Millward C, Ferriter M, Calver S, Connell-Jones G. Gluten- and casein-free diets for autistic spectrum disorder. *Cochrane Database Syst Rev* 2008; 2: CD003498.

56. Howard AL, Robinson M, Smith GJ, Ambrosini GL, Piek JP, Oddy WH. ADHD is associated with a 'Western' dietary pattern in adolescents. *J Attention Disord* 2008; 15: 403–411.

57. Gesch CB, Hammond SM, Hampson SE, Eves A, Crowder MJ. Influence of supplementary vitamins, minerals and essential fatty acids on the antisocial behaviour of young adult prisoners. randomised, placebo-controlled trial. *Br J Psychiatry* 2002; 181: 22–28.

58. Young SN. How to increase serotonin in the human brain without drugs. *J Psychiatry Neurosci* 2007; 32: 394–399.

59. Pase MP, Scholey AB, Pipingas A, et al. Cocoa polyphenols enhance positive mood states but not cognitive performance: a randomized, placebo-controlled trial. *J Psychopharmacol* 2013; 27: 451–458.

60. García-Blanco T, Dávalos A, Visioli F. Tea, cocoa, coffee, and affective disorders: vicious or virtuous cycle? *J Affect Disord* 2017; 224: 61–68.

61. Brown JS, Jr. Psychiatric issues in toxic exposures. *Psychiatr Clin North Am* 2007; 30: 837–854.

62. Lanphear BP. The impact of toxins on the developing brain. *Annu Rev Public Health* 2015; 36: 211–230.

63. Rosenberg NL. *Occupational and Environmental Neurology.* Oxford: Butterworth-Heinemann, 1995.

64. Rosenstock L, Cullen MR, Brodkin CA, Redlich CA. *Textbook of Clinical Occupational and Environmental Medicine.* Oxford: Elsevier Saunders, 2005.

65. Clifford A, Lang L, Chen R, Anstey KJ, Seaton A. Exposure to air pollution and cognitive functioning across the life course—a systematic literature review. *Environ Res* 2016; 147: 383–398.

66. Tsuji JS, Garry MR, Perez V, Chang ET. Low-level arsenic exposure and developmental neurotoxicity in children: a systematic review and risk assessment. *Toxicology* 2015; 337: 91–107.

67. European Food Safety Authority. Scientific opinion of the panel on contaminants in the food chain on a request from the European Commission on cadmium in food. *The EFSA Journal* 2009; 980: 1–139.

68. Sanders AP, Henn BC, Wright RO. Perinatal and childhood exposure to cadmium, manganese, and metal mixtures and effects on cognition and behavior: a review of recent literature. *Curr Environ Health Rep* 2015; 3: 284–294.

69. Ciesielski T, Bellinger DC, Schwartz J, Hauser R, Wright RO. Associations between cadmium exposure and neurocognitive test scores in a cross-sectional study of US adults. *Environ Health* 2013; 12: 13.

70. Skerfving S, Bergdahl IA. Lead. In: Nordberg GF, Fowler BA, Nordberg M (eds). *Handbook on the Toxicology of Metals.* Cambridge, MA: Academic Press, 2015, pp. 911–967.

71. Chin-Chan M, Navarro-Yepes J, Quintanilla-Vega B. Environmental pollutants as risk factors for neurodegenerative disorders: Alzheimer and Parkinson diseases. *Front Cell Neurosci* 2015; 9: 124.

72. Lucchini RG, Aschner M, Kim Y, Šarić M. Manganese. In: Nordberg GF, Fowler BA, Nordberg M (eds). *Handbook on the Toxicology of Metals.* Cambridge, MA: Academic Press, 2015, pp. 975–1011.

73. European Food Safety Authority Panel on Contaminants in the Food Chain (CONTAM). Scientific Opinion on the risk for public health related to the presence of mercury and methylmercury in food. *EFSA J* 2012; 10: 2985.

74. Berghuis SA, Bos AF, Sauer PJJ, Roze E. Developmental neurotoxicity of persistent organic pollutants: an update on childhood outcome. *Arch Toxicol* 2015; 89: 687–709.

75. Gaum PM, Esser A, Schettgen T, Gube M, Kraus T, Lang J. Prevalence and incidence rates of mental syndromes after occupational exposure to polychlorinated biphenyls. *Int J Hyg Environ Health* 2014; 217: 765–774.

76. Grandjean P, Landrigan PJ. Neurobehavioural effects of developmental toxicity. *Lancet Neurol* 2014; 13: 330–338.

77. Hartle JC, Navas-Acien A, Lawrence RS. The consumption of canned food and beverages and urinary Bisphenol A concentrations in NHANES 2003-2008. *Environ Res* 2016; 150: 375–382.

78. Bellinger DC. A strategy for comparing the contributions of environmental chemicals and other risk factors to neurodevelopment of children. *Environ Health Perspect* 2012; 120: 501–507.

79. Scientific Committee on Emerging and Newly Identified Health Risks. Opinon on potential health effects of exposure to electromagnetic fields. *Bioelectromagnetics* 2015; 36: 480–484.

80. U.S. Food & Drug Administration. White Paper: FDA Update/Review of Potential Adverse Health Risks Associated with Exposure to Mercury in Dental Amalgam. Available at: https://www.fda.gov/MedicalDevices/ProductsandMedicalProcedures/DentalProducts/DentalAmalgam/ucm171117.htm (accessed 19 March 2018).

CHAPTER 48

Mental health and its social determinants
Some experiences of the Self-Employed Women's Association (SEWA) in India

Mirai Chatterjee

Leela's story and that of millions of informal workers

Leela is an old-clothes vendor who has struggled with depression for years. She is poor and self-employed, like millions of others engaged in the informal economy in India. Informal workers—manual labourers, small and marginal farmers, construction workers, street vendors, small producers, and home-based workers—account for over 93% of the Indian workforce. They lead precarious lives, eking out a living as best as they can, sometimes by engaging in multiple economic activities for survival. Their lives are a quest for some measure of work and income security, and social security, including health care.

Leela's mother, Laxmi, was a member of a union—the Self-Employed Women's Association (SEWA) in Ahmedabad, India. Leela learned her trade from her mother—buying old clothes from middle-class women in exchange for cash or utensils. She mends the old clothes, washes and irons them, and then sells them at the Sunday bazaar at the riverfront. Her mother stopped her schooling and married her at a young age to another street vendor. She had two children. Her marriage did not last. Her husband was a heavy drinker and spent all their hard-earned money on alcohol and other women. Leela was heartbroken but did all she could to raise her young children. One day, her husband announced that he was divorcing her. Their's was an arranged marriage under customary Hindu tradition and not under the civil code, which gives women equal rights. The dissolution of the marriage was pronounced by her Vaghari caste Panch, a Committee of Elders, all of whom were men. Not only did she get no alimony or compensation of any kind, but also her two children were taken from her. Leela was grief-stricken and wept for days and did not eat. Soon she slipped into depression. Her mother said she was often violent, striking out at anyone who passed by. Her neighbours and family locked her up in a little hut, saying she had become possessed. Food was given periodically, but she was not allowed to leave the hut. That was when we met her.

Dishevelled and distraught, having not eaten or bathed in days, Leela was alone and abandoned. SEWA's health workers, also informal women workers, organized several meetings with her family and neighbours, and all agreed to release Leela from the hut. Gently, we bathed her, combed her hair, and fed her. We then made sure she came to our health centre every day. Slowly, she began to play with the children that were around and helped in giving medicines to women. She began to put on some weight and started selling old clothes again, earning a living. She began seeing a doctor at the government hospital who treated her for depression. He advised that, above all, we continue supporting her through SEWA.

Over the four decades since we have been organizing poor women like Leela into unions and then cooperatives, we have met many women like her, who have struggled with depression and other mental illnesses. Informal women workers struggle against poverty and also gender discrimination in a still-traditional and deeply patriarchal society. Time and again we have approached the caste and religious committees who preside over all social and cultural issues, and are told that this is how it has always been. Only recently, after our SEWA sisters developed as strong leaders in their communities, have these caste committees begun to include women as elders, with some role in decision-making on marital disputes and other matters.

SEWA was formed as part of the labour movement to promote women's rights as workers and economic actors. It has been organizing women for full employment at the household level, including work and income security, food security, and social security. The latter includes, at the least, health care, child care, insurance, housing with basic amenities like a tap and toilet in every home, and pension. We have learned that full employment alone—this holistic and integrated approach to basic needs and survival—is what will eventually lead our sisters out of poverty and vulnerability, and towards self-reliance. Self-reliance includes both financial viability of a woman's economic activity or work, and decision-making and control over her life.

We had no mental health professionals on our team. What we did have was the SEWA sisterhood, and our daily experiences of working shoulder-to-shoulder with poor women. We also had faith in their abilities to lead their families out of poverty. The process is a constant struggle—there are ups and downs, like life itself, but the downs are exacerbated by vulnerability and gender discrimination at every step.

What we did

Perhaps SEWA's biggest contribution was to build the sisterhood. Scattered and isolated in their homes, women cannot emerge from poverty or work out solutions alone. We have been able to organize and unite women across caste, class, religious, linguistic, and geographical lines, building a union and movement of almost 1.5 million workers across 15 states in India. Just this act itself seems to be a source of strength and comfort to women. We often hear our SEWA sisters say 'Our SEWA is like our mother's home'— the ultimate compliment as far as Indian women are concerned, as it harks back to happier and carefree times as young girls in their family home, as opposed to their husbands' and in-laws' households.

Furthermore, SEWA has been organizing women around issues of livelihood (work and income security) and social security (health care, child care, insurance, pension, and housing with basic amenities like a tap and toilet in every home). We have learned that economic empowerment contributes to women's overall well-being, including their mental health. Often our SEWA sisters say, 'now, at long last, we have secure livelihoods, and enough to eat, feed, and educate our children. We have peace of mind'. From a situation of dependence on husbands, brothers, and fathers, women, for the first time, have their own incomes, and their own bank accounts, insurance, and pension, among other support services. While the impact of all of this from the point of view of mental health has not been studied, the impact on their overall self-reliance is evident. Thousands of women have taken themselves and their families out of poverty and towards financial self-reliance. They also begin to take decisions in all spheres of their lives, including hard decisions concerning their spouses and the violence that they have borne for years.

One such SEWA sister is Saira. Abandoned by her mother, she was raised by an aunt, and faced deprivation and struggle at every step. We met Saira during the violence in the aftermath of the destruction of the Babri Mosque in North India in 1992. There was rioting and communal violence between Hindus and Muslims across the country, including in Ahmedabad, the city where SEWA was established. Saira's home was destroyed in the violence, and, as part of SEWA's relief and rehabilitation efforts, we were able to provide her with a sewing machine, to sew, earn a living, and begin rebuilding her life. We learned then that Saira was a young woman of immense courage. Her husband was a gambler and used up whatever little he earned, and also Saira's daily earnings. They had two young children who Saira provided for, as best as she could.

Soon Saira was chosen by local SEWA members as the health worker for her community. Not only was she a fast learner, grasping the basics of primary health care with great interest, but she also proved to be an excellent health educator. She was compassionate and caring, having understood deprivation and suffering from an early age. She began to care for the women in the relief camps, helping them to heal by linking them with counsellors, doctors, and, importantly, by joining SEWA for support and solidarity.

Once she obtained a steady income from both her health work at SEWA and sewing, her husband's pressure for money for gambling increased. When she resisted, he was violent. She opened her own bank account in SEWA Bank, a women's cooperative bank in which she quickly became a shareholder, and quietly took out a loan to buy herself a separate house. She paid her loan instalments regularly from her own earnings, and ensured, with SEWA's help, that the house was in her name only. For the first time in her life, apart from her sewing machine, she had an asset of her own. He husband continued pressurizing her and one time when she was in health training, he sold off her sewing machine so that he could gamble. That was the last straw for Saira. She asked him to leave. With her own house, she was able to take this action, which few informal women workers are able to do.

There are many other examples and stories of SEWA sisters who have slowly strengthened or developed their own livelihoods, obtained a regular income, and built up assets. Having regular work and their own steady source of income, then building up their assets in their own name is key for economic empowerment and self-reliance of women like Saira. It not only helps them develop independence and autonomy, but also creates options for life choices that were just not available earlier.

Another key to securing women's mental health and overall well-being has been providing them with basic services, which they need for economic empowerment. Banking is one such service, and the first to be developed by SEWA. In fact, one of the earliest demands of SEWA members was access to financial services. They told us that they could not emerge from poverty if they were indebted to moneylenders, large merchants, and landlords. They were paying interest rates of 60% per annum and therefore could hardly escape from the vicious cycle of poverty and indebtedness. Many were in exploitative debt-bondage situations for generations. One such family was that of Samuben, a landless agricultural labourer whose husband was in debt bondage to a landlord, paying off debts incurred by his father. Although bonded labour is forbidden by law in India, we have, over the years, come across new and hidden forms of bondage. When Samuben joined SEWA, she and her three young sons had to struggle to eat even one meal a day. They lived in a one-room mud hut that collapsed during the monsoons. Samuben was the only semi-literate woman in her village, Gokulpura, and was chosen to be a SEWA health worker. She was diligent and active, winning the trust of all. With her now regular income, she not only served others, but began to save regularly, opened her bank account, and took out a loan to free her husband from debt bondage. Once freed, he began to work as a construction labourer and, with two sources of income, Samuben and her family slowly emerged from poverty, literally before our eyes. She took another loan to build a solid house, got scholarships to educate her sons with SEWA's support, and finally had enough to eat. She also formed a saving and credit self-help group in her village and helped SEWA Bank to extend its financial services to rural women like herself. Not surprisingly, she was elected leader of her village's self-help group, and was then elected to her village panchayat, the local self-government structure in India's rural areas.

SEWA Bank has, over the 44 years of its existence, supported thousands of urban and rural informal women workers in asset-building. This has included developing their businesses, repairing a leaking roof, paying off debts to moneylenders and others, and reclaiming mortgaged land and machines. In the latter, SEWA Bank has insisted that the land and other assets should be in women's names, or at least that titles be jointly held with spouses.

Another essential service developed for, by, and with women is child care or day care. Most of our members are mothers, in addition to working both inside and outside the home. Naturally, they are concerned about their children's well-being. Throughout the years, we have heard our SEWA sisters say: 'We have lived hard lives but hope for a better future for our children. We want to educate them and help them earn a decent living'.

We also saw them struggle to earn and take care of their young children as best as they could. Hence, SEWA started crèches for infants and young children of our members, according to their hours of work, and at locations that were suitable to them. We trained some of them to be the crèche workers in the centres we set up. The children obtained comprehensive and holistic care, including freshly cooked food, regular health check-ups, age-appropriate early childhood education, and experience of the joy of learning. This not only resulted in the children's healthy growth and development, but it also resulted in significant income increases of the mothers. In one study of agricultural workers and their children, we learned that women's income went up by at least 50% when they had access to SEWA's crèches. The mothers also reported 'peace of mind'.

As the number of childcare centres increased, we decided to form a cooperative of the crèche workers and mothers, called Sangini. This brought women together on a common platform to work collectively for their children and in a manner that would be sustainable in the long term.

Following close on the heels of our childcare service was health care. SEWA's healthcare cooperative is called Lok Swasthya SEWA Mandli (or 'LSM'). Through SEWA Bank's depositors—all informal workers—we learned that women saved regularly, but their deposits were quickly used up during illness or other family crises. We also learned that sickness was the top reason for taking out loans and defaulting on them. This forced us to set up a community-based health programme with our SEWA sisters as the barefoot doctors of their own communities. As our health workers, such as Saira and Samuben, developed their knowledge and skills in health work, and when we had a critical mass of 50 health workers, we registered our own health cooperative. The first of its kind, we had to convince the registrar of the government's cooperative department that such a cooperative was, indeed, feasible and could be viable. Fortunately, we had the earlier experience of SEWA Bank, by then a well-functioning and profitable cooperative, to make our case.

The cooperative structure has, throughout SEWA's history, served to bind informal women together. The union is generally the first point of contact for SEWA members, but it is in the cooperative where they interact and work closely together every day on common issues like banking, health care, or child care. In the union, they feel linked to thousands of other women like themselves and it gives them a collective strength, and a feeling of unity, solidarity, and power. In cooperatives they are themselves are the users, managers, and owners of their own organization, as they are shareholders. This means that each of them contributes from their hard-earned resources toward the share capital, and pays for an individual share, entitling them to vote on all matters pertaining to their cooperative. Further, in the cooperative, they collectively pursue their economic activity or service, obtaining productive work and income, and also a share of the surplus or profits generated, through dividends on their shares. The cooperatives are thus an alternative source of employment and constructive action for, by, and with workers. We

have found this joint strategy of unions and cooperatives to be very useful in organizing workers for their economic empowerment, self-esteem, and self-reliance.

In the health cooperative, women were trained as health workers to provide primary health care, including health education, referral care, generic medicines, and, later, some counselling. They provided these services to other informal workers and their families. Over three decades ago, when SEWA first started its health work, primary health care or public health services were scarcely available. SEWA health workers would go door-to-door explaining how to stay healthy, what women could eat locally, how to control tuberculosis, and would then provide some essential medicines. It was then that we learned from women about how 'their bodies were their only assets', and also how little knowledge and control they had over their own bodies. This was especially true of reproductive and sexual health, including contraception. On one hand, they explained, they needed to be healthy to work and earn. On the other, they were frequently sick. They also had repeated childbirth, itself a risk. They often did not want to have more children, but this was not a choice for them, decided by husbands and other family members, especially if they had no male child.

In our first health education session, Sumanben, a street vendor and grandmother with six of her own children, said she had no knowledge of reproductive physiology and that the training was an eye-opener. She also explained that women like her had to have 4–6 children so that 2–3 survived. Fortunately, there have been marked declines in child and infant mortality rates over the past three decades, but the anxiety felt by thousands of women with regard to their children's well-being continues to add to their already vulnerable lives.

Yet another service that has provided both solidarity and support to women is SEWA's insurance, now provided through a national cooperative, VimoSEWA. From both SEWA Bank's and Lok Swasthya SEWA health cooperative's experiences, we saw how sickness and other contingencies like accidents, natural and human-made disasters, like communal violence, and even death of spouse or other family member resulted not only in suffering, but also in a downward spiral in the family's economic status. These crises were frequent, and generally affected the poorest and weakest most severely, such as single mothers, widows, and disabled women.

Our members told us that they had to go to family members and neighbours in such times of crisis, and also to moneylenders and landlords, from whom they borrowed at high interest rates to tide them over during the crises. It was then that they asked if SEWA could provide insurance. While insurance companies at that time were all nationalized, there was very little outreach by them to poor women or low-income households. In fact, when we approached them for services, they said 'women are bad risk' and were uninsurable. In the early 1990s, when SEWA's membership had grown to 50,000, two insurance companies agreed to work with us—one, the Life Insurance Corporation, to provide natural death coverage, and the other, the United India Insurance Company, for health and accident coverage. From 7000 insured members in Ahmedabad in 1992, today SEWA Insurance, now a cooperative called VimoSEWA, has over 100,000 insured women in five Indian states. Every year, millions of rupees worth of claims for health, accident, and death reach women and their families. In 2015, 11 million rupees' worth of claim payments went to 1900 women and their family members. This is not only a significant economic support in their hour of need, but also the women tell us that they feel they are not alone. We frequently hear them say, 'We cannot get our loved ones back, but at least we are not alone and the money helps us face the challenges that lie ahead'. Thus, VimoSEWA serves, like the other services, as the glue that strengthens and maintains the SEWA solidarity and sisterhood.

Perhaps nothing exemplifies the solidarity and sisterhood more than the collective action taken during disasters. Unfortunately, over the years, we have seen the impact of disasters—both human-made and natural—on our members and their families. Already poor and vulnerable, such disasters—for example, the earthquake of 2001, cyclones, torrential rains and floods, droughts, and communal violence—push women deeper into poverty and indebtedness. In addition, there are the severe mental health consequences and impacts of the disasters that women have lived through. Our approach to dealing with disasters has involved immediate relief, and, later, long-term rehabilitation.

One of the things that seem to have a lasting impact is that SEWA teams immediately go out to the affected areas, meeting with women and their families, assessing impact and damage through careful surveys and on-the-spot evaluations. Just acknowledging their pain and suffering is a support. On numerous such occasions, our SEWA sisters say, 'You risked your own lives just to see whether we are alive. That itself gives us strength to face this calamity'. When unprecedented communal violence spread in 2002 in Gujarat, relief teams consisting of both Hindus and Muslims went to all the affected areas. We provided medical care, conducted surveys of losses for insurance, and gave tools and means of livelihood, like sewing machines, to women in the camps where thousands had taken shelter. They told us later that earning some much-needed money gave them the will to live and rebuild. Women also became involved in cooking and feeding others in the camps, and through serving others, began to deal with their own pain and loss.

We were also able to identify and work with the widows and orphans to ensure that they got their compensation packages and to bring them in to the SEWA family. Some of these women rose to become leaders in the SEWA movement; others became health workers, like Saira, childcare workers, and insurance promoters. During disasters, like the communal violence of 2002, our membership rose significantly, as many women who obtained some support came into the SEWA fold.

This was true also during the worst earthquake that we experienced in 2001. As we joined others from across India and the world to support both our members and those who were not, we came into contact with women in the remote villages of our state. The first thing they asked for was not food but work. 'Give us work. Any work, so that we can earn and begin to rebuild our lives'. It is then that we understood that livelihoods were not only the lifeline for survival of the poor, but also served as therapy in times of disaster and trauma.

We also set up support services after such disasters. Within a month of both the earthquake and the violence of 2002, we were able to survey all the damage, make assessments with the insurance companies, and pay out claims to women and their families, providing them with some money to rebuild their homes and their lives. After both these disasters, at our members' request, we set up childcare centres in tents, as there were no buildings left after the earthquake. We provided books, toys, and games so that children of all ages were engaged and could slowly emerge from the trauma of

all that they had been through. Our members later told us that this was a huge support, as it kept their children busy, and enabled them to earn and build their homes again.

Similarly, during the violence, we ran childcare centres in the relief camps where various activities were carried out with children of all ages. We also had doctors from the public hospitals conduct regular check-ups. All the centres we set up are still running today, and have become the focal point for health, child development, and peace action in their communities. Parents meet every month to not only discuss their children's progress, but also to take up community action like cleanliness campaigns or celebrate each other's religious festivals.

Several young women involved in these activities have developed into strong community leaders. Rehana was a tea seller and her little shop was destroyed in the violence. She found a new vocation as a childcare worker and over just a few years became adept at this and also developed as a strong leader in her neighbourhood. She was elected to the board of the childcare cooperative, and later went to Ethiopia to help women there build up their own childcare centres. She has become a role model for young women in her community.

One aspect of these disasters that was new to us was trauma counselling. Whether during the earthquake, floods, cyclones, or the violence, it was clear to us that we needed to learn how to counsel our sisters who had been through so much. Fortunately, mental health professionals from the National Institute of Mental Health and Neurological Sciences (NIMHANS), in Bengaluru, assisted us. Dr Shekhar and his team trained our health workers, childcare workers, and other grassroots-level leaders to be the barefoot counsellors of their neighbourhoods. Slowly, those who had suffered so much loss began speaking about their grief and all that they had witnessed. This was our first intervention on mental health at SEWA, and we resolved to take this forward as part of our primary healthcare work.

One incident of solidarity and healing stands out among many. It happened after the communal violence of 2002, when we first entered curfew-bound areas. We were relieved to see each other alive and well, and gathered in the middle of the street, a group of 10 of us, hugging each other and weeping for what had befallen us and our city. As we stood with our arms around each other, men from the area collected, watching the scene of sisterhood and solidarity in silence. These were dangerous times, when women were not safe. Yet there was no danger in the air, only reconciliation and solidarity. Later, women from that area told us that their men said this was a first—women of all communities empathizing with each other like sisters. They felt it did much to heal their own pain and that of their community.

Another intervention was that of taking the widows of the violence into the SEWA family. The then prime minister of India had specifically asked that SEWA help the widows, whom we called 'Shantas' or 'Women of Peace'. All the Shantas obtained financial compensation for their losses and to rebuild through livelihoods. Their children also obtained funds, which we helped them put in long-term fixed-deposit accounts in their own names. It was not easy for the Shantas to navigate all that was required of them to obtain the funds. Also, family members suddenly showed up and insisted that they would manage their finances. We had to protect them from this and more. But, most of all, they could not forget all they had seen and the deaths of their husbands. Shahnaz was a young widow with four children who witnessed her husband being shot. She became an insurance promoter with VimoSEWA, SEWA's insurance cooperative, for a while but slipped into a deep depression and even experienced seizures. She could not work and was on treatment for years. We still keep in touch with her and try to support her as best as we can. There were many others who also suffered from varying degrees of depression and insomnia. Still, we did our best to include Shantas in all aspects of SEWA and the SEWA movement, and today many of them can stand on their own feet and are educating their children.

Taking up mental health issues at SEWA

Although solidarity and the SEWA sisterhood undoubtedly provided some support and solace to women, we realized that this was not enough. We had to learn more about mental health, and then engage with professionals to provide some support, at least at the primary care level. We began to explore how we might meet the challenge of mental health. One opportunity presented itself. Over the years, we have had the good fortune of having talented young interns at SEWA. One such intern, Dr Ronak Patel, came to us as a new graduate from Harvard Medical School. In the course of his time with us, he helped us conduct a survey on mental health. We were shocked to find fairly high levels of depression and other mental illness in our survey. In total, 840 women participated in the survey, 88% of them from urban areas, and the remaining from rural areas. We found that women had no knowledge about depression or mental health-related issues, and most were not even able to identify the symptoms.

In order to address these issues we undertook community-based campaigns to create awareness about mental health among our members. We found the response of our SEWA sisters to be more than we expected. Women began openly sharing their problems with our health workers and trainers, and discussed how these could be dealt with. In the process of our campaigns, we realized that there was a need to identify women who could provide counselling at the community level. Hence, we trained a team of our health workers to detect the early signs and symptoms of depression and other mental illnesses, and also to provide some basic counselling. Local women were not only able to provide these services, as they enjoyed the trust of their own communities, but they also worked hard to spread awareness against the social stigma of mental health. This helped in both early detection and also in encouraging women and others to seek further care and treatment.

We have learned that creating an understanding of mental health is a very important step in developing an atmosphere that encourages women and young girls to come forward and seek professional help. In addition, the presence of community-based women counsellors as the first point of contact is helpful, as they can do the screening before referring to higher levels of care. We also observed that at the local level, the doctors and other staff in primary health centres (PHCs) or urban health centres (UHC) do not have the orientation to mental illness nor do they have the necessary training to assess and diagnose people.

Organizing health camps for the early detection of mental illnesses has helped us to detect and then refer women and their family members to local health facilities. The community-based counsellors can play a proactive role in mobilizing women and young girls for these camps. Health personnel from the PHCs or UHCs then provide the necessary services in the camps. SEWA health workers then did the follow-up, through regular home visits, and ensuring that treatment schedules were followed.

Our interactions with health service providers also brought out the fact that there is a need to organize workshops for health personnel in PHCs and UHCs, in order to sensitize them to mental health issues.

Soon we extended our work to adolescent girls and boys, and young women and men. Lack of timely and relevant information, low socio-economic status, lack of educational opportunities, traditional practices such as early marriage, and, more recently, prenatal sex determination, all added to their vulnerability, especially of girls and young women. Providing them with knowledge and skills was the first step towards awareness. This then led to action to address their issues. It is in the adolescent and young adult years that they require support, direction, and some possible answers to their many doubts and questions—about their changing bodies, their new relationships, and with the opposite sex, about career options and employment opportunities, and their place in the changing world of today.

We initiated a programme to work with young people to address gender-based discrimination and violence. We organized small group discussions in safe spaces, provided counselling, and encouraged collective action in their communities. In addition, we organized health and sex education. We found that after our education sessions, in which issues related to gender violence and discrimination were discussed, girls started to speak out on issues once considered to be taboo, including sexual abuse by family members. We also introduced ideas of gender equality and, slowly, both girls and boys realized that domestic violence is not 'normal'.

To continue our work with young people, we organized them into 'mandals' or collectives of about 15 persons. Eighty such mandals were formed, and through these we were able to reach out to many young people. Our community-based counsellors played a key role in both setting up the mandals and keeping them going. The issues for which the adolescent girls came for counselling included reproductive and sexual health problems, and also social issues like not being allowed to finish schooling, and early marriage. The adolescent boys also shared their issues, including not being able to concentrate on their studies owing to the pressure of family responsibilities. These issues were identified by the mandal members themselves, and brought to the notice of the counsellors. Where required, the counsellors then referred people to further care.

Young people, especially women and young girls in both urban and rural areas, face many challenges and are left with few ways to speak of the pressures and problems they face on a daily basis. From our field-level experiences, we have seen that they need someone at the local level whom they can trust, preferably from their own community—a trained counsellor. It is also important to provide spaces for adolescents and young women via their mandals or collectives where they can share their problems and obtain support.

Meanwhile, at SEWA's main office we began a counselling centre for our members. Fortunately, we had Dr Renuka Patwa, a gynaecologist and long-time colleague, to help us set up for this. She is trusted by SEWA members because of her long years of service to SEWA, and women told her openly about all their mental health issues. She then helped us refer to psychiatrists when needed. This opened a veritable floodgate of issues. We learned about childhood sexual abuse among our SEWA sisters, depression, and untreated schizophrenia, among other issues. Several of our members' children were suicidal and we were able to take early action. Women also spoke of sexual harassment in the workplace, and how this caused mental health problems. In particular, we learned that contractors and foremen at construction sites sexually harassed women workers, offering them work only if they provided sexual favours. We had several meetings with construction workers and formed support groups so that they could collectively resist such exploitation. Now we rarely hear of this kind of harassment among our members.

Slowly, mental health is becoming an action point for the SEWA movement. Learning from the experiences in Gujarat, where the SEWA movement began, other SEWAs—in Delhi, for example, are taking the help of local mental health experts to train grassroots leaders as barefoot counsellors. Workshops have been organized with the help of psychiatrists, enabling SEWA sisters in other states to recognize early signs and symptoms, and understand mental health.

Moving forward on mental health

While SEWA has always favoured an integrated and holistic approach to women's well-being, we realize that this is not enough. We have seen how basic work, income, and food and social security leads women towards self-reliance, and they repeatedly tell us, 'now we can live in peace'. Poverty and gender discrimination are themselves stressors that SEWA seeks to reduce through collective action. However, women need more support for the mental health problems that they themselves or their family members face. Alcoholism among their men-folk, for example, is a major source of stress. Sometimes all they go through seems to lead them into further into depression. We try our best to support them through the SEWA sisterhood.

One of the major issues we face is the lack of attention paid to mental health at the policy level. In fact, there has been little focus on public health since India's independence in 1947, although the leaders of our freedom movement, including Mahatma Gandhi and Pandit Nehru, emphasized it in pre-independence national agenda and plans. There have been very low investments in public

health—expenditure on it currently is barely 1.1% of gross domestic product. Mental health has been one of the worst sufferers, although it is acknowledged as a major cause of illness, especially among women in India. Even today, the latest National Health Policy 2017 yet to be implemented, has barely a paragraph or two on this vital area of our citizen's health. It is acknowledged as a need, but there is little by way of concrete recommendations for action.

Our own experience at SEWA points to the need for major changes in mental health policy and implementation, with attention paid to primary care, referral services, and also on the social determinants of mental health. This aspect of our people's health and well-being needs special attention and investment. It also needs to be integrated with primary health care, another underfunded area of public health. Policymakers and legislators in India, with the support of civil society and local people, will have to develop ways in which the social determinants of mental health can be addressed, and with people, especially women, at the centre of all our efforts.

At the same time, our work and that of other community-based and non-governmental organizations points to the need for front-line workers, preferably women, as counsellors and also health workers to detect and screen for mental illness in a timely and sensitive manner. We will have to train them not only in mental health, but also in ways to counter the stigma and silence that shrouds mental health in India. We have found women at the grassroots level to be committed mental health workers and leaders, in general. They are the key to effective and low-cost mental health prevention and screening. They must be supported by regular training, incentives to keep them active and committed, and by referral care at facilities offering tertiary care.

Perhaps above all, the SEWA experience points to the need to organize the poor and vulnerable, especially women in our society, enabling them to act in the interests of their own well-being and mental health. Through the collective strength and enhanced bargaining power that comes from organizing into membership-based organizations like unions, cooperatives, self-help groups, and their federations, women will find the solidarity and sisterhood that they need to both emerge from poverty and to have some measure of health security.

CHAPTER 49

Intimate partner violence

Carmen Wong, Wai Ching Ng, Hua Zhong, and Anne Scully-Hill

Introduction

Domestic violence (DV), spouse abuse, and wife battering, are different forms of naming IPV of different degrees and kinds of intimate partner relationship. The World Health Organization (WHO) adopted IPV as a general broader term to cover almost all types of intimate partners and refers to any action that causes physical, sexual, and psychological harm to those in the relationship [1]. This term includes 'behavior within an intimate relationship that causes or has the potential to cause physical, sexual, or psychological harm, including acts of physical aggression, sexual coercion, psychological abuse, and controlling behaviors' [2].[1]

The prevalence of domestic violence across countries

The definition and measurement of DV vary in different institutions and cultural backgrounds for different purposes and contexts; thus, it is difficult to estimate and compare the prevalence and incidence of DV in different societies inside countries [3]. Some scholars support the prevalence of DV to be calculated on the basis of population-based surveys by asking respondents' (both men and women) experience of aggressive acts, whereas others tend to survey/interview clinical/shelter samples of victims and/or perpetrators of DV [4, 5].

In fact, both methods have limitations: surveying community samples may ignore the serious cases of women being battered by men as those serious cases are rarely seen in the general public [4]; the clinical/shelter samples are usually small and biased to generalize the overall rates of DV [6]. Moreover, both methods face the problem of under-reporting as victims, especially female victims, are often reluctant to disclose their experience and seek outsiders' help, owing to social norms, legal, and safety concerns [7–9]. The prevalence of DV can vary according to reporting methods,

for example in the USA results report 6.3% of DV in a healthcare survey versus 55% in women visiting primary care clinic [10].

In many developed societies, there are sufficient resources to conduct nationally representative surveys to estimate the overall prevalence of DV. Using the USA as an example, previous studies have shown consistent findings that the rates of DV for men and women are, in fact, similar and there is also little gender difference in terms of the perpetration rates. Based on the US National Family Violence Survey [6], the national prevalence of assaults by men were 122 per 1000 couples versus 124 per 1000 couples for assaults by women; even for serious assaults, the gender-specific rates are 50 per 1000 couples (by men) versus 46 per 1000 couples (by women). In terms of perpetration rates, it is 25–40% for men and 36–50% for women after comparing three large-scale community surveys [11]. These large-scale surveys cannot catch the most serious male-to-female family violence cases. To be complimentary, some studies have tried to use arrest rates of DV in the USA to indicate the prevalence of serious battering cases and they found that the male arrest rate for partner violence is seven times higher than the female arrest rate [7]. However, the official arrest statistics have been criticized owing to their dependence on citizens' reporting behaviours and police reactions toward different genders [12]. By focusing on women and using more detailed measures on male-perpetrated family violence,[2] some surveys provide a rough estimation of the national prevalence of male-to-female partner abuse: about 8% of women in the USA experience DV per year and 3% of US women were seriously assaulted by their partners [13].

In other parts of the world, especially developing countries, it is difficult to conduct large-scale and representative surveys to estimate the national-level prevalence of DV. For instance, a solid study has reviewed all the available data sources and finally concluded that no Latin American country has all the information required to understand the situations of DV [14]. But there is a certain consensus that male-to-female DV is more prevalent in developing societies. Using official data collected from different countries, the

---

[1] Acts of physical violence: slapping, hitting, kicking, and beating. Sexual violence: forced sexual intercourse and other forms of sexual coercion. Emotional (psychological) abuse: insults, belittling, constant humiliation, intimidation (e.g. destroying things), threats of harm, threats to take away children. Controlling behaviours: isolating a person from family and friends; monitoring their movements; and restricting access to financial resources, employment, education or medical care (WHO, 2010).

[2] IPV or DV is a subtype of family violence. Family violence is 'any form of maltreatment-including physical, sexual, and emotional (inclusive of both verbal and psychological abuse), as well as neglect- perpetrated or witnessed by one or more members of a family and / or intimate relationship upon one of more other members of that family or relationship'. Therefore, family violence include IPV, child abuse and sibling abuse, elderly abuse within the family relationship

United Nations' (UN) statistics have indicated that, globally, two in three victims of intimate partner/family-related homicide are women [15]. Meanwhile, the prevalence of male-to-female IPV varies as a result of different research methods, for example the reported percentage of women who have experienced IPV at least once in their lifetime has been reported to be 13–46% in Europe, 7–32% in North America, 17–68% in Oceania, 6–67% in Asia, 6–64% in Africa, and 14–38% in Latin America and the Caribbean, and the prevalence rate can vary greatly even in the same area. The type of abuse may also vary, with a reported 13–61% of women having suffered physical violence; 6–59% of women having encountered sexual violence; and 20–75% of women having experienced emotional abuse by a partner [16].

Explanatory models of domestic violence

Prior research explaining variations of DV across countries largely focus on the macro social factors related to gender inequality. Factors affecting the variations of DV in different societies are broadly summarized in the following subsections.

Patriarchal system

Women in traditional societies are at greater risk of being assaulted by their partners because they have lower social status. Men devalue women and mistreat them in a variety of ways. As a result, women who live in countries with more stereotypical attitudes toward women's roles should have higher risks of DV. That is why, in general, women in developing countries suffer more from DV than their counterparts in developed countries. Such explanations have also been identified in specific empirical studies of DV in China, Vietnam, Bangladesh, the South Pacific region, Uganda, and Iran [8, 17–21].

Economic disadvantages of women

Although some women in the world, especially middle- and upper-class women in developed societies, have gained more economic opportunities so that they may have more equal status in their families and experience less DV, others have become more vulnerable to stressful economic circumstances brought about by recent social changes [22]. This explanation is in line with the marginalization perspective on women and development in their common assumption that females are marginalized by development-related processes [23–25]. As these scholars speculated, female economic vulnerability (some scholars call it 'feminization of poverty') can come from several factors that accompany development. Structural factors associated with income inequality between men and women include segregation of females into low-status and low-wage jobs, and the resulting unequal income distribution between men and women. Increased rates of divorce, illegitimacy, and father-absent households also lead to a loss of income for women. Women in some countries also disproportionately bear the burden of globalization (i.e. sex tourism and international human trafficking of women/young girls). In both developed and developing countries, scholars have found solid evidence to support this economic explanation. For instance, in the USA, women living in poor communities with residential instability and concentrated disadvantages are more likely to experience DV [26]; in Jordan, a typical Islamic society with high level of gender inequality, scholars have found that women's labour force participation could reduce their risks of

experiencing DV [27]; in South Asia and the South Pacific Region, the high prevalence of DV is also related to the economic dependence of women on men [19, 28].

The effects of culture/religion

Although the oppression of women in the patriarchal system is relatively universal in the world, some societies have more distinct cultural components and religions that further devalue women's social status and increase their risks of suffering DV. In China, according to the long-lasting Confucian beliefs, women are expected to be good daughters, wives, and mothers. To safeguard their reputation and save 'face', many Chinese women have to tolerate DV and do not disclose their experience [8, 29]. In South Asia, the major cause of DV is the solicitation of dowry [28, 30]. Prior studies also showed that religions like Islam and Hindu increase and reinforce the traditional gender hierarchy so that there are more battered women in these societies [9, 21].

Negative effects of immigration

Scholars in the field of immigration have identified that international immigrants, owing to lack of resources and systematic exclusion in receiving societies [31, 32], are more likely to be victimized [33, 34]. For similar reasons, female immigrants are also more likely to experience DV than their local counterparts [35–37]. A typical pattern of immigration is that people from a less developed society move into a more developed society. To pursue a better quality of life, a great proportion of such female immigrants marry local men, as is the situation in Hong Kong. The significant cultural difference and unequal socio-economic status between husbands and wives would increase the conflicts within these families. The husbands may then exert violence as their wives have limited resources to protect themselves and also are less likely to be protected by the biased mainstream society [38, 39]. For immigrant families where both husbands and wives come from the same country of origin, scholars find that immigration may increase women's workforce participation and their husbands' social statuses gradually decline, which often threatens the man's traditional dominance and leads to more DV as men attempt to regain control over women [40, 41]. Furthermore, immigrant women experience 'multiple marginalization' in a combination of the impacts of gender, race, and class that deters them from seeking help. Again, limited resources and marginalization in the mainstream society further constrain the ability of these battered female immigrants for resistance.

Physical and mental health consequences of intimate partner violence

Worldwide, studies have investigated the relationship between IPV and public health problems in both women and men, and it is found that IPV can adversely affect a person's physical and mental health [42–49]. Regarding physical health, victims of IPV can suffer from injury [50–53], chronic pain and cardiac disease [54–58], gastrointestinal disorders [59–61], and disability [62–64]. Moreover, meta-analytic studies have indicated that a wide range of mental health issues are associated with IPV, including behavioural disturbances such as eating disorders, sleep disorders, alcohol, and substance abuse, to borderline and antisocial personality and psychosomatic disorders, as well as anxiety disorders such as post-traumatic stress disorder (PTSD), depression, suicidal and self-harming behaviours, and non-affective psychosis [64]. Systematic reviews drawn from cross-sectional studies [65–67] to longitudinal studies [56, 68–70] illustrate a consistent connection between mental disorder and IPV, with a reported '3-fold increased risk of depressive disorders and 7-fold increased risk of post-traumatic stress disorder (PTSD) among victims of domestic violence abuse' [56]. Up to 64% of women victims experience PTSD, 48% experience depression, and 18% attempt or commit suicide [71]. In addition, findings suggest that women with severe mental illness have a higher risk of violence victimization than men [72]. For older adults, it is estimated that 20–30% of adults aged 60 years and older have experienced IPV, with the majority being women and associated with mental health issues of depression and anxiety [73].

Across all diagnostic categories, both men and women with mental health disorders have higher prevalence of, and are more likely to be, victims of IPV [56, 74]. Access to support and inventions can be particularly problematic for victims of IPV with mental ill health and they may contact up to 10 agencies before they are able to get appropriate help and support [75]. This, in part, has been attributed to the predominant use of a medical model by professionals in understanding mental ill health, which focuses on medical and psychological symptoms rather than underlying psychological and social problems, which may enhance disclosure of the situation of DV [76]. Although the victim may have access to clinics or professionals who may offer support, other barriers may prevent disclosure. This may include a lack of rapport [77], time constraints [78], the presence of partners during consultations or a lack of expertise [79], and fear of offending or re-traumatizing victims by the professionals [56, 76]. Male clinicians may also be less likely to ask about DV than female clinicians [80]. Professionals who lack expertise may also blame women for returning to the abuser [81, 82]. This may be more devastating to those victims who have a close continuous therapeutic relationship [77].

Meanwhile, the reluctance to disclose may also be the victim's wish to protect intimate relationships or, in the gendered role, to 'nurture' relationships. In some instances, these women's beliefs are reinforced by their own families, who actively shame or forcibly encourage the women to return to their abusing partner. Women may also blame themselves and be blamed by others for the inability to leave or for inciting the cycle of abuse when returning [81]. Protective factors for IPV may include work and family coherence, which can help disclosure [83].

Long-term impact of intimate partner violence on victim, family, and community, and prevention

IPV may also be defined as a crime against the safety of the family members, an interpersonal issue between the couple, 'their' family problem, and a public health concern. IPV can affect the well-being of individuals, family, and communities involved, as well as children who witness the abuse. The impact may vary in individuals of distinct eco-socio-physio-ethical-spiritual backgrounds, experience of seeking social support, and utilization of community resources. The negative consequences of IPV can be lifelong and interact in a recycle of violence, passed from individual to community then from generation to generation. Therefore, the society as a whole

has a responsibility and should exert efforts to end IPV. Meanwhile, the way in which a community responds to, or intervenes in, IPV depends on how a society views the nature of IPV.

Battered wives reported difficulties in the process of leaving the abuser. Globally, at least one out of seven homicides and more than one-third of female homicides are perpetrated by an intimate partner [84]. The prior concern of IPV intervention is the safety of the battered victims and their children through law reform, police intervention, legal aid, and legal protection, and specialized social service units for family and child protection provide a package of crisis intervention, statutory protection, and treatment to victims of IPV and their family members.

In 2002, the WHO proposed a public health approach in combating IPV. Public health interventions are traditionally characterized in terms of three levels of prevention: primary, secondary, and tertiary. The primary prevention aims to prevent IPV before it occurs, such as via community education; the secondary prevention focuses on the more immediate responses to violence, such as pre-hospital care, or emergency service or medical follow-up. The tertiary prevention focuses on long-term care in the wake of violence, such as rehabilitation and re-integration, and attempts to lessen trauma or reduce the associated long-term disability. This includes universal interventions with the general population, selected interventions with high-risk groups, and indicated interventions in demonstrated violent behaviour. IPV interventions and prevention require a multi-level approach to involve individual, relationship, community-based efforts and of the larger social and cultural environment in order to promote a bias free, supportive, and protective environment for victims of DV. New guidelines from the WHO recommended addressing the needs of patients through the partnership of primary care and mental health services with IPV services [85].

A central mechanism composed of representatives from related government officials and non-governmental organization service providers is essential in both responding and mapping out strategies and approaches to address the problem on DV. Additionally, a multi-disciplinary procedural guide for handling IPV is indispensable to facilitate the multi-professional collaborative intervention in cases of DV. There is increased focus on family and psychological support, for example shelters for women that render hospitality to battered wives and their children; victim support programmes for legal protection, crisis intervention, counselling, and physical needs. In addition, gender-sensitive training for related professionals is critical in raising awareness of predominant prejudices surrounding DV in society.

Interventions in a dynamic process of change

The most challenging aspects in the prevention and intervention of IPV are victims' reluctance to disclose, seek help, and acknowledge IPV, as attributed to male dominance, in both the public and private sectors. In addition, gender role stereotyping in the patriarchal society may cultivate the general acceptance of violence against women and can promote the preservation of family reputation at the cost of the victim's suffering.

The decision-making of victims of IPV in seeking change is a complex process. The Transtheoretical Model of Behavior Change (TM), first developed by Prochaska [86] and published by

Dienemann et al. [87], can be used to describe the five stages applicable to IPV [88].

To simplify, the victim may consider or implement changes along a continuum of stages from (1) precontemplation (the victim is not aware of or is minimizing the problem and remains committed to the relationship) to (2) contemplation (acknowledging the problem and considering changes) to (3) preparation (making plans for change) to (4) action (following the plan made, e.g. breaks away or negotiates power); to (5) maintenance (keeping the new actions as part of daily activities, e.g. establishes a new life). However, the actions of victims are characterized using terms such as 'recycling', 'returning' and 'relapse' [89]. It clearly indicates that the victim of IPV struggles back and forth in the changing process and it takes time for the abused to identify and acknowledge the abusive relationship, recognizing what is necessary and having the courage, and being decisive, to extricate themselves from the abusive but intimate relationship.

Comparatively, interventions with victims at different stages may require different types of interventions from identifying abuse and risks, providing information and support, and developing safety plans to anticipating signs of 'returning', and so on. Risk-assessment tools have been developed to screen for victims of IPV in hospitals and in police stations, and by social services, which also help the affected person to acknowledge the risk of IPV that they are facing. Multidisciplinary handling procedural guidelines and multidisciplinary intervention service teams can be established for handling crises and providing comprehensive care to and intervention for IPV victims.

The major dilemma for victims of IPV is whether to leave the relationship permanently and start a new life [90–93]. The struggle can be explained by the sufficiency of legal and social support [94, 95], financial resources [96], and of better parenting for children [92]. The basic needs are always prioritized, such as financial support, housing assistance, children's education, and the guarantee of personal safety. Resources are essential in the decision-making process and as providing means for victims to carry out their choices [97]. Safety plans and escape plans will be worked out in collaboration with the battered partner to outline specific safety and escape strategies that victims can use in a wide range of abusive situations for safeguarding victims of IPV and their children who remain in the abusive relationship [98]. Besides, the collaborative working relationship between criminal justice and community service is important in fulfilling the legal, physical, psychological, sociocultural, financial, and practical needs of victims of IPV [99].

Dyadic interventions

IPV is a spouse-abuse problem and can concurrently be a parent–child issue. In total, 30–70% of DV cases co-occur with child abuse and maltreatment [100, 101]. Children exposed to their parents' abusive and violent relationship can also be negatively affected [102]. Almost 50% of children exposed to IPV developed post-traumatic stress symptoms and are at increased risk for depression [103]. Hence, involving child protection services and the child's perspective in the safety plan are necessary in order to ensure that the needs of children at different ages are effectively considered and addressed [104].

Studies find that the pattern of IPV is replicated in other relationships, families, and communities so that IPV not only damages the victims, but also impacts negatively on their other relationships. For example, children are affected in the mother–child relationship [105, 106]. Mothers exposed to IPV have experienced explosive anger and are associated with a pattern of harsh parenting [107]. Parental conflict has been found to influence negatively children's academic, behavioural, and social-emotional performance [108]. IPV diminished parental capacity as a result of lower self-worth and competencies, and increased children's social disruptive behaviour, which, in turn, may be destructive to the mother–child relationship [101]. Abused women may also have generally poor relationships with their children [109].

Therefore, the parent–child relationship is a primary concern of treatment. The dyadic-focused interventions such as child–parent psychotherapy for family violence and parent–child interaction therapy are found to be effective and should be employed to utilize the mother–child relationship as a change mechanism [101]. Evidence shows that both the parent–child relationship and the parenting skill of participants can benefit from child–parent relationship training [110].

Regardless of the victim's decision to remain with the abuser or start a new life on their own or with their children, individual and relational recovery are the main concerns during the aftermath of IPV. Such recovery may be confounded by concurrent moderate-to-severe physical injuries and mental illness that can bring lifelong impairment and/or disability [90, 93, 111–113].

A supportive social network is a crucial element in the recovery of victims of IPV [114, 115]. Spiritual factors, for example religion, can be helpful in the recovery from the trauma of DV [114, 116–118]. Also, self-efficacy was found to be positively correlated with recovery from DV [119]. Significant improvements were found in children and parents who participated in community-based group intervention programme for children and adults exposed to family violence [120].

Fainsilber et al. [103] found an indirect relationship between the parent's emotional socialization and child adjustment. The study result affirmed the impact of the parent's response to the child's emotion in fostering the healthy development of emotion resilience abilities in the child and protecting them from developing post-traumatic stress disorder and depression [101]. Thus, efforts should focus on parental awareness, acceptance, and coaching of children's emotions. The emotion-coaching intervention programme should aim at teaching parents specific ways to talk to their children about emotion and addressing their beliefs and attitudes about emotion [121]. Meanwhile, the mindfulness-based parenting intervention is helpful in reducing negative mother–child interaction by decreasing the mother's emotional response and increasing their awareness of their own emotions [103].

Engagements with perpetrators are necessary as many victims do not want to leave the abusive relationship. This may encompass inclusion of perpetrators in assessments and referring them to batterer or anger-management programmes, counselling, and related services such as substance or alcohol abuse programmes [122]. Community-based research indicated that continuing contact between the father and the child has both positive and negative impacts on child adjustment. The ability of the father to talk about emotion with their child may be a protective factor in preventing the child from condition of social isolation, withdrawal, and loneliness [121].

Community and primary care interventions

Community-level education can have an indirect relation to IPV [123]. Anti-IPV education in schools and communities against IPV and promoting mutual respect within a couple's relationship is significant in asserting the rights of IPV victims, raising the awareness of public concern in combating IPV and establishing a supportive ecology to facilitate and encourage the victim of IPV to leave the abusive relationship.

In primary care, recovery intervention may include psychological interventions (e.g. cognitive–behavioural therapy techniques, Acceptance and Commitment Therapy, mindfulness or relaxation therapies, advocacy and empowerment interventions, child and mother interventions, holistic healing, targeted perpetrator or victim programmes), as well as specific programmes for those with sexual violence and trauma [46]. The need to enhance psychological skills training has been highlighted and particularly for non-specialist support workers in advocacy agencies [46, 124, 125].

Studies found that mental disorders in late adolescent are a risk factor both for men and women involved in IPV [126]. Empirical findings indicate that the childhood adolescence risk factor can predict DV perpetration and victimization in adulthood [127, 128]. More recent IPV interventions adopt a developmental perspective, which explores family risks for IPV and designs interventions tailored to an individual's level of development risk for IPV [125].

Policy and legal efforts to protect victims of intimate partner violence

Historically, legal intervention in the family sphere has been limited and so before the middle of the twentieth century there were few specialist laws on DV. However, with the rise of the women's movement in the West from the 1960s onwards, legislatures and courts began to address 'domestic violence' as a specific phenomenon requiring specialist legal intervention.

Given that statistics around the world consistently show that women and girls form the overwhelming majority of victims of IPV [129], the approach of policymakers from jurisdiction to jurisdiction will often depend upon the status of women in the given population and the extent to which the family and domestic realm are viewed as a private domain immune from public scrutiny and sanction [130]. Policies addressing IPV have been adopted around the world and range from the broad and multidisciplinary, including legal, educational, and social welfare policies to a far less interventionist approach.[3]

As the majority of victims of IPV are women and girls, a significant proportion of the laws addressed are framed as responses to 'IPV against women and girls'. This is in no way intended to diminish or ignore the suffering of male victims of IPV. The following illustrations provide a limited snapshot into the issues around policies and laws relating to IPV.

A general normative statement

A starting point for policymakers is often to adopt a normative statement as to the fundamentally unacceptable nature of IPV. For example, internationally, the Committee to the UN Convention on the Elimination of All forms of Discrimination against Women (CEDAW)[4] has noted in General Comment no. 19 that '[f]amily violence is one of the most insidious forms of violence against women. It is prevalent in all societies'. Regionally, declarations of commitment to the eradication of DV include, amongst others,[5] the ASEAN declaration that 'violence against women and violence against children ... must be eliminated as they impair human rights and fundamental freedoms of women and children'. The Council of Europe has established the 'Convention on preventing and combating violence against women and domestic violence', which 'condemn[s] all forms of violence against women and domestic violence', making key statements about the detrimental nature and broad scope of IPV [131].

Nationally, Barack Obama, then president of the USA, announced: 'Too many individuals, regardless of age, ability, sex, sexual orientation, gender identity, circumstance, or race, face the pain and fear of domestic violence ... we shine a light on this violation of the basic human right to be free from violence and abuse ... '.[6] In Hong Kong, the Chief Executive said in his 2005–06 Policy Address: 'The Government does not tolerate domestic violence ... We will also pursue the perpetrators of violence and bring them to justice ...' [132]. District and provincial legislatures have also set a general normative standard within their own regional legislation.[7]

These broad normative statements serve educative and symbolic purposes by condemning IPV and affirming a jurisdictional intention to eradicate it [133], usually by enacting legislation.

Policies on interpersonal violence enacted into law

In some jurisdictions the law has historically not intervened in 'family' matters, especially with regard to IPV.[8] Elsewhere, the law

[3] See United Nations Economic and Social Affairs (2015). *The World's Women 2015, Trends and Statistics*, p. 160: 'At least 119 countries have passed laws on domestic violence ... and 52 have laws on marital rape. However, even when laws exist, this does not mean they are always compliant with international standards and recommendations or implemented'.

[4] In the 188 States that are Parties to the Convention on the Elimination of Discrimination Against Women (CEDAW), the government of each State is required to adopt measures to achieve the eradication of violence against women. In the further 99 States that are signatories to the Convention. while they are not legally bound by the Treaty they are to politically support the aims of the Convention. See: http://www.un.org/womenwatch/daw/cedaw/
[5] For a comprehensive survey of regional and international instruments, see the United Nations' 'Background Paper for the Expert Group Meeting on Good Practices in Legislation on Violence Against Women' EGM/GPLVAW/2008/BP.01 (7 May 2008) at pp. 3–8.
[6] https://www.whitehouse.gov/the-press-office/2016/10/01/presidential-proclamation-national-domestic-violence-awareness-month (accessed on 20 October 2016). See also 4.41302 Violence Against Women and Department of Justice Reauthorization Act of 2005 (USA).
[7] See, e.g., the legislation passed at state level in Victoria, Australia: the preamble to the Family Violence Protection Act 2008 states that 'non-violence is a fundamental social value; family violence is a violation of human rights; family violence is not acceptable in any community or culture; and the justice system should respect the views of victims of family violence'.
[8] Today in Russia there is no specific legislation to address domestic violence, although the criminal law will apply to a domestic assault as to an assault carried out in any other environment. See: A Landscape Analysis of Domestic Violence Laws (2013) Trust Law Connect at p. 269; see http://www.trust.org/publications/i/?id=fe9c538d-96ae-41c6-9dc8-148f793248fb (accessed 20 October 2016).

has developed to offer different forms of justice and protection for those subjected to IPV.

1. *Defining IPV or DV in law*: In some jurisdictions, even though IPV may be a criminal offence or may be subject to special civil law remedies, such as restraining orders, there may not be an express legal definition of 'DV' or 'IPV'. This may be because DV/IPV is considered a physical assault like any other.[9] And no separate definition is necessary. Alternatively, where DV/IPV is recognized as a specific form of harm, the definition may be left open so that the courts can develop its meaning incrementally.[10] Where a definition is adopted in law, this may be limited to physical and maybe sexual or psychological violence.[11] Alternatively, a broader definition may be adopted to achieve legal certainty and to serve an educational purpose. For example, New Zealand's Domestic Violence Act 1995, sections 3 and 4, defines DV as: 'physical abuse; sexual abuse; psychological abuse, including, but not limited to, intimidation, harassment, damage to property, threats of physical abuse, sexual abuse, or psychological abuse, financial or economic abuse (for example, denying or limiting access to financial resources, or preventing or restricting employment opportunities or access to education) and, in relation to a child, a person psychologically abuses a child if that person causes or allows the child to see or hear the physical, sexual, or psychological abuse of a person with whom the child has a domestic relationship; or puts the child, or allows the child to be put, at real risk of seeing or hearing that abuse occurring'.[12]

Other jurisdictions have added incrementally to their definitions of DV/IPV. For example, English law has recently introduced an offence of 'coercive and controlling behaviour' in domestic or intimate relationships.[13] Jurisdictions may also adopt working definitions, not enshrined in law, in order to guide and educate stakeholders.[14]

2. *Legal definition of 'eligible relationship'*: Laws relating to DV/IPV may apply to either a narrow or wide range of relationships: from spousal or spousal-like cohabitation relationships[15] to 'family members'[16] to the broadest possible range of 'intimate' and 'family' relationships. The South African Domestic Violence Act presents an example of a very broad range of 'domestic relationships'. These include parties, heterosexual or homosexual, who 'currently live or have lived together in a relationship of a marital nature and even if they are not married to each other or are unable to marry each other. The parties may be dating, engaged or in a customary relationship or an actual or perceived romantic, intimate or sexual relationship over any period of time, or where they share or have recently shared the same residence' [134].[17] Legal protection from DV is increasingly being extended to same-sex couples.[18] However, this is not universal.[19]

3. *DV directed towards or witnessed by children*: Most jurisdictions have laws to protect children from physical or emotional abuse directed at them.[20] However, research shows the psychological and emotional damage done to children not only from being directly subject to DV, but also by witnessing DV/IPV experienced by a loved one [135]. Consequently, some jurisdictions have enacted laws to address this also.[21]

4. *Criminal law*: Jurisdictions may treat DV/IPV as a specific criminal offence or as an offence like any other assault. If the latter, the domestic setting of the assault may be admitted as an aggravating factor attracting a more severe penalty.[22] In criminal law, the party prosecuting the accused is the State and not the victim. However, the burden to report a crime, to support a prosecution, and to provide evidence at trial is on the victim. Given the nature of the relationship between a perpetrator and victim of IPV, often the victim will feel psychologically or emotionally unable to take any of these steps, having 'learned helplessness' as a result of the abuser's controlling or violent behaviour [136]. The victim may also, entirely rationally, fear for their safety if they speak out about the abuse. Historically, this dilemma has led to

---

[9] As was the case in England for a time and still is in Hong Kong.

[10] As was decided in Hong Kong when the reform of the laws on domestic violence was considered in 2007; see LC Paper No. CB(2)330/07-08(01).

[11] For example, see Japan's Act on the Prevention of Spousal Violence and Protection of Victims, which defines domestic violence as 'bodily harm by one spouse (illegal attacks threatening the other's life or body) or the words and deeds of one spouse that cause equivalent psychological or physical harm to the other'.

[12] Reproduced from New Zealand Legislation, Domestic Violence Act 1995, Crown Copyright.

[13] Serious Crime Act 2015 s.76.

[14] The UK non-legal definition: 'any incident or pattern of incidents of controlling, coercive, threatening behaviour, violence or abuse between those aged 16 or over who are, or have been, intimate partners or family members regardless of gender or sexuality. The abuse can encompass, but is not limited to: psychological, physical, sexual, financial'. See: https://www.gov.uk/guidance/domestic-violence-and-abuse (accessed 20 October 2016).

[15] China's recent Domestic Violence Law 2015 relates to family members and cohabitation relationships but seems not to include same-sex couples nor former cohabiting couples: https://www.theguardian.com/world/2015/dec/27/china-passes-first-domestic-violence-law (accessed 20 October 2016).

[16] See Singapore's Women's Charter, s.64.

[17] Reproduced from Thomson Reuters Foundation, A Landscape Analysis of Domestic Violence Laws, Copyright (2013), with permission from Thomson Reuters Foundation.

[18] Hong Kong's 2009 reform included same-sex couples in its Domestic and Cohabitation Relationship Violence Ordinance (Cap 189): s. 3B.

[19] Singapore's Women's Charter provisions apply to 'family members'. Same-sex relationships are not recognized under Singapore law: Prime Minister Lee Hsien Loong has said 'The family is the basic building block of this society. And by family in Singapore we mean one man, one woman, marrying, having children and bringing up children within that framework of a stable family unit'. Hansard, 23 October 2007.

[20] All States parties that have signed and ratified the United Nations Convention on the Rights of the Child should enact such laws. Only two countries, the USA and South Sudan, have not ratified the Convention.

[21] See the state-level legislation for the State of Victoria, Australia: Family Violence Protection Act 2008 s.5(b)(1)(b); also see s.31 Children Act 1989 (UK) amended in 2002 expanding the definition of harm done to a child to include 'impairment suffered from seeing or hearing the ill-treatment of another'.

[22] For example, the French Criminal Code s.222-3 and s.222-8 provides that where the victim of an intentional and unintentional killing is the perpetrator's spouse or partner, this is an aggravating circumstance. In the UK, the Sentencing Council's 'Overarching Principles: Domestic Violence Definitive Guideline' (2006) states that the domestic setting may be an aggravating factor: http://www.sentencingcouncil.org.uk/wp-content/uploads/web_domestic_violence.pdf at pp. 3–5.

low rates of arrest, prosecution, and conviction of perpetrators.[23] To address this, multiple jurisdictions have introduced mandatory or preferred arrest policies so that the burden is taken off the victim and placed on the state. 'A mandatory arrest law states that an officer must make an arrest if (s)he finds probable cause to believe that an offence has been committed, a preferred arrest law instructs the responding officer that arrest is the preferred response' [137].

Hirschel et al. conducted research in 19 American states on the impact of adopting mandatory or preferred arrest laws. They found the new laws resulted in higher rates of arrest not only in physical violence cases, but also in intimidation cases.[24] However, the risk is that mandatory arrest policies result in both parties being arrested and thus overall higher arrest rates. Some states have introduced 'the primary aggressor rule' to ensure that the arrest laws are not applied mechanistically and that the victim is not further traumatized by being arrested.[25] Research from New Zealand shows that mandatory/preferred arrest laws achieve best results when coupled with a multidisciplinary approach to DV/IPV. This approach requires that, subsequent to an arrest being made, perpetrators, as well as victims, are referred to social service agencies for support and therapeutic intervention [138].

5. *Civil law*: Unlike the criminal law, in civil law the parties to the case are not the State against the accused but are the claimant 'victim' against the alleged perpetrator. The victim can seek non-criminal measures in the form of court orders against the perpetrator to prevent further abuse. These include restraining orders prohibiting the abuser from making any contact with the victim, occupation rights to the family home, and/or the exclusion of the perpetrator from the family home.[26] The victim may also make a civil claim for compensation for harm done. Bringing a civil law case requires the victim to pursue her own claim against the abuser and, consequently, support from social welfare agencies or third parties will often be necessary [139].

6. *Crossover interventions*: It is now possible in many jurisdictions for a court to require a perpetrator to attend therapy of some kind in order to address the emotional or psychological issues underlying the violence. In some jurisdictions, this may be an aspect of criminal sentencing, whereas in others it falls within the scope of a civil remedy, often attached to a restraining order. Therapeutic interventions have developed over time, since the first American programme was introduced in 1977.[27] In 2008 Hong Kong conferred power on its judges to order attendance at a 'Batterer Intervention Programme' in cases where the abuser was subject to a non-molestation order.[28] Therapeutic interventions can be attractive adjuncts or alternatives to imprisonment for a number of reasons: while a custodial sentence means that the victim is safe as long as the abuser is in prison, they may not be safe when the abuser is released; without counselling the abuser while in prison, nothing will have been done to address the underlying cause of the DV/IPV; and, if the abuser is the family's main breadwinner, the family may consequently lose their financial security and even their home [140]. [29] Similarly, with court orders restraining the abuser from contacting the victim, these orders alone do not address the root cause of the DV/IPV and so the abuse may continue.

7. *Training for justice system personnel:* Past research has shown that criminal laws against DV/IPV are most effective when implemented by specially trained personnel. Police, as first-responders, have been the focus of various training initiatives, with often positive results. In Slovenia '[t]he police force is one of the institutions that has contributed significantly to changing attitudes towards domestic violence in recent years'.[30] Albania's Law on Measures against Violence in Family Relations contains requirements for police training. A detailed 'Police Protocol on Domestic Violence Cases' trains police officers by linking police responsibilities to specific clauses of the new law, helping police understand that their investigative duties are not optional, but mandated by law [141]. This should help overcome earlier police attitudes that DV/IPV cases are not 'crime-fighting' but 'social work' and thus not 'real' police work [142]. However, experience in the UK, where there are specialized domestic violence officers (DVOs) within police forces, has been mixed. Research has shown that officers who specialize in domestic violence cases are able to become more knowledgeable about the issues and can serve as a "focal point for inter-agency work" but DVOs also reported that their work was not taken seriously within the force [143].

A number of jurisdictions have also required specialist training for judges hearing DV/IPV cases. Australia has just adopted a *National Domestic and Family Violence Bench Book* to offer guidance to judges dealing with family and domestic violence cases [144].

According to the UN statistics, 119 countries have passed laws against DV/IPV. Those societies with established legal protections for victims of DV and mature treatment programmes for perpetrators are expected to have lower risks of DV/IPV. Conversely, in China, where laws against DV were formally passed in 2015, a survey of criminal justice officials in China reflects that the majority of them still consider DV as a family issue and they also know very little about women's rights [145]. It may take a long period of time for the changing of attitudes among law enforcement practitioners. In Latin America, although

[23] Edwards SSM. *Policing Domestic Violence: Women, the Law and the State* London: SAGE Publications, 1989.

[24] Hirschel D, Buzawa E, Pattavina A, Faggiani D. Domestic violence and mandatory arrest laws: to what extent do they influence police arrest decisions. *J Crim Law Criminol* 2007; 98: 255–298 at pp. 293–296.

[25] See Hirschel et al. (2007) in Note 24 at pp. 296–297.

[26] For a comparison of six Asia/Asia-Pacific jurisdictions' protection orders see Chan W-C. 'A review of civil protection orders in six jurisdictions'. *Statute Law Rev* 2017; 38: 1–22,

[27] See http://www.emergedv.com (accessed 20 October 2016); on therapeutic programmes in the USA generally, see http://www.stopvaw.org/Influential_US_Batterers_Intervention_Programs.html (accessed 20 October 2016).

[28] Domestic & Cohabitation Relationships Violence Ordinance (Cap 189): sections 3, 3A and 3B.

[29] Erez E. Domestic violence and the criminal justice system: an overview. *Online J Issues Nurs* 2002; 7: Manuscript 3.

[30] International Helsinki Federation for Human Rights, Women 2000: An Investigation into the Status of Women's Rights in Central and South-Eastern Europe and the Newly Independent States 421 (2000).

many countries such as Brazil, Chile, Colombia, Costa Rica, and Mexico have made great progress in making laws against interpersonal violence, they face a lot of barriers, including the weak commitment by courts and police (similar to China), low budgets for law enforcement, and lack of cooperation between private and public organizations [146].

In terms of cultural awareness, and in response to the underutilization of mainstream social services by ethnic minority women, the introduction of social policy measures and structural accommodations are needed to eliminate barriers to seeking assistance. These measures would include developing proactive criminal justice systems that reach out to victims [147], collaboration between relevant professionals and religious institutions, universal screening for effective early identification of women experiencing DV/IPV [148], and providing culturally appropriate, sensitive intervention, and linguistic assistance in law enforcement, legal proceedings, and emergency services [149].

Conclusions

There are limitations in research methodology to ascertain the prevalence of IPV. However, IPV is worldwide and present across developing and developed countries. Several explanatory models have been postulated and relate to patriarchy, culture, and interacting factors. IPV has physical and mental health sequelae, and violence can perpetuate within families and communities. The implementation of treatment and intervention can be difficult as IPV is deeply rooted in multiple contexts, both internal and external. Thus, a multi-level and integrated approach to assessment and intervention regarding IPV are recommended. Recent guidance and studies show that relational recovery for the victim and family is paramount. Perpetrator engagement and victim safety is important. To tackle IPV, efforts necessitate individual, professional, and community reflection on gender sensitivity and multidisciplinary collaboration in local and national arenas. Moreover, there needs to be concurrent progress in policies and laws, and the need for interdisciplinary efforts across legal, educational, medical, and social capacities to effect change and to meet the needs of victims of IPV worldwide.

References

1. World Health Organization (WHO), Pan American Health Organization (PAHO). *Intimate Partner Violence*. Geneva, WHO, 2012.
2. World Health Organization (WHO)/London School of Hygiene and Tropical Medicine. *Preventing Intimate Partner and Sexual Violence Against Women: Taking Action and Generating Evidence*. Geneva: WHO, 2010.
3. Loseke D, Gelles R, Cavanaugh M. *Current Controversies on Family Violence*. Thousand Oaks, CA: SAGE, 2005.
4. Johnson M. Patriarchal terrorism and common couple violence: two forms of violence against women. *J Marriage Fam* 1995; 57: 283.
5. Archer J. Sex differences in aggression between heterosexual partners: A meta-analytic review. *Psychol Bull* 2000; 126: 651–680.
6. Tolan P, Gorman-Smith D, Henry D. Family violence. *Annu Rev Psychol* 2006; 57: 557–583.
7. Loseke D, Kurz D. Men's violence toward women is the serious social problem. In: Loseke DR, Gelles R, Cavanaugh MM (eds). *Current Controversies on Family Violence*. Thousand Oaks, CA: SAGE, 2005, pp. 79–96.
8. Thurston W, Tam D, Dawson M, Jackson M, Kwok S. The intersection of gender and other social institutions in constructing gender-based violence in Guangzhou China. *J Interper Violence* 2016; 31: 694–714.
9. Panchanadeswaran S. The voices of battered women in India. *Violence Against Women* 2005; 11: 736–758.
10. Hathaway J, Mucci L, Silverman J, Brooks D, Mathews R, Pavlos C. Health status and health care use of Massachusetts women reporting partner abuse. *Am J Prev Med* 2000; 19: 302–307.
11. Moffitt T, Caspi A. *Findings About Partner Violence from Dunedin Multidisciplinary Health and Development Study. Report NCJ 170018.* Washington, DC: U.S. Department of Justice, Office of Justice Programs, National Institution of Justice, 1999.
12. Steffensmeier D, Schwartz J, Zhong H, Ackerman J. An assessment of recent trends in girls' violence using diverse longitudinal sources: is the gender gap closing? *Criminology* 2005; 43: 355–406.
13. Jordan C, Campbell R, Follingstad D. Violence and women's mental health: the impact of physical, sexual, and psychological aggression. *Annu Rev Clin Psychol* 2010; 6: 607–628.
14. Fries V. *Estudio de la Informacíon Sobre la Violencia Contra la Mujer en America Latina y el Caribe. Serie Mujer y Desarrollo 99.* Santiago de Chile: CEPAL, 2010.
15. United Nations Statistics Division. The world's women 2015. Available at: https://unstats.un.org/unsd/gender/worldswomen.html (accessed 19 March 2018).
16. World Health Organization (WHO). *WHO Multi-country Study on Women's Health and Domestic Violence Against Women: Initial Results on Prevalence, Health Outcomes and Women's Responses.* Geneva: WHO, 2005.
17. Trinh O, Oh J, Choi S, To K, Do D. Changes and socioeconomic factors associated with attitudes towards domestic violence among Vietnamese women aged 15–49: findings from the Multiple Indicator Cluster Surveys, 2006–2011. *Glob Health Action* 2016; 9: 10.3402/gha.v9.29577.
18. Panchanadeswaran S. The voices of battered women in India. *Violence Against Women* 2005; 11: 736–758.
19. Taylor C. Domestic violence and its prevalence in small island developing states—South Pacific Region. *Pac J Reprod Health* 2016; 1.
20. Tsai A, Wolfe W, Kumbakumba E, et al. Prospective study of the mental health consequences of sexual violence among women living with HIV in rural Uganda. *J Interpers Violence* 2015; 31: 1531–1553.
21. Kargar Jahromi M, Jamali S, Koshkaki A, Javadpour S. Prevalence and risk factors of domestic violence against women by their husbands in Iran. *Global J Health Sci* 2015; 8: 175.
22. Schwartz J. Family structure as a source of female and male homicide in the United States. *Homicide Stud* 2006; 10: 253–278.
23. Moghadam V. *The Feminization of Poverty? Notes on a Concept and Trends.* Normal, IL: Illinois State University, 1997.
24. Chow E. Gender matters studying globalization and social change in the 21st century. *Int Sociol* 2003; 18: 443–460.
25. Koczberski G. Women in development: a critical analysis. *Third World Q* 1998; 19: 395–410.
26. Morgan R, Jasinski J. Tracking violence: using structural-level characteristics in the analysis of domestic violence in Chicago and the state of Illinois. *Crime Delinquency* 2016; 63: 391–411.
27. Lenze J, Klasen S. Does women's labor force participation reduce domestic violence? Evidence from Jordan. *Fem Econ* 2016; 1: 1–29.
28. Young K, Hassan S. An assessment of the prevalence, perceived significance, and response to dowry solicitation and domestic violence in Bangladesh. *J Interpers Violence* 2016 (Epub ahead of print).
29. Wan G. *Female Violent Offending in China: A Socialist Feminist Perspective.* Guelph: University of Guelph, 2012.
30. Khan A, Hussain R. Violence against women in Pakistan: perceptions and experiences of domestic violence. *Asian Stud Rev* 2008; 32: 239–253.
31. Portes A. Immigration theory for a new century: some problems and opportunities. *Int Migr Rev* 1997; 31: 799.
32. Gore C. Introduction: markets, citizenship and social exclusion. In: Rodgers G, Gore C, Figueiredo JB (eds). *Social Exclusion: Rhetoric, Reality, Responses.* Geneva: International Institute for Labour Studies, 1995, pp. 1–40.

33. Sulkowski M, Bauman S, Wright S, Nixon C, Davis S. Peer victimization in youth from immigrant and non-immigrant US families. *School Psychol Int* 2014; 35: 649–669.

34. Le T, Wallen J. Risks of non-familial violent physical and emotional victimization in four Asian ethnic groups. *J Immigr Minor Health* 2007; 11: 174–187.

35. Um M, Kim H, Palinkas L. Correlates of domestic violence victimization among North Korean refugee women in South Korea. *J Interpers Violence* 2016 (Epub ahead of print).

36. Raj A, Silverman J. Immigrant South Asian women at greater risk for injury from intimate partner violence. *Am J Public Health* 2003; 93: 435–437.

37. Lee Y, Hadeed L. Intimate partner violence among Asian immigrant communities: health/mental health consequences, help-seeking behaviors, and service utilization. *Trauma Violence Abuse* 2009; 10: 143–170.

38. Cheung A, Choi S. Non-traditional wives with traditional husbands: gender ideology and husband-to-wife physical violence in Chinese society. *Violence Against Women* 2016; 22: 1704–1724.

39. Leung L. Deconstructing the myths about intimate partner violence: a critical discourse analysis of news reporting in Hong Kong. *J Interpers Violence* 2016 (Epub ahead of print).

40. Menjívar C, Salcido O. Immigrant women and domestic violence: common experiences in different countries. *Gender Soc* 2002; 16: 898–920.

41. Yick A. Feminist theory and status inconsistency theory: application to domestic violence in Chinese immigrant familes. *Violence Against Women* 2001; 7: 545–562.

42. Buller A, Devries K, Howard L, Bacchus L. Associations between intimate partner violence and health among men who have sex with men: a systematic review and meta-analysis. *PLOS Med* 2014; 11: e1001609.

43. Hester M, Ferrari G, Jones S, et al. Occurrence and impact of negative behaviour, including domestic violence and abuse, in men attending UK primary care health clinics: a cross-sectional survey. *BMJ Open* 2015; 5: e007141–e007141.

44. Jonas S, Khalifeh H, Bebbington P, et al. Gender differences in intimate partner violence and psychiatric disorders in England: results from the 2007 adult psychiatric morbidity survey. *Epidemiol Psychiatr Sci* 2014; 23: 189–199.

45. Beydoun H, Williams M, Beydoun M, Eid S, Zonderman A. Relationship of physical intimate partner violence with mental health diagnoses in the nationwide emergency department sample. *J Womens Health (Larchmt)* 2017; 26: 141–151.

46. Trevillion K, Corker E, Capron L, Oram S. Improving mental health service responses to domestic violence and abuse. *Int Rev Psychiatry* 2016; 28: 423–432.

47. Ferrari G, Agnew-Davies R, Bailey J, et al. Domestic violence and mental health: a cross-sectional survey of women seeking help from domestic violence support services. *Glob Health Action* 2016; 9: 29890.

48. Knight L, Hester M. Domestic violence and mental health in older adults. *Int Rev Psychiatry* 2016; 28: 464–474.

49. Iverson K, Vogt D, Dichter M, et al. Intimate partner violence and current mental health needs among female veterans. *J Am Board Fam Med* 2015; 28: 772–776.

50. St. Ivany A, Schminkey D. Intimate partner violence and traumatic brain injury. *Fam Commun Health* 2016; 39: 129–137.

51. Walton-Moss B, Manganello J, Frye V, Campbell J. Risk factors for intimate partner violence and associated injury among urban women. *J Commun Health* 2005; 30: 377–389.

52. Wu V, Huff H, Bhandari M. Pattern of physical injury associated with intimate partner violence in women presenting to the emergency department: a systematic review and meta-analysis. *Trauma, Violence Abuse* 2010; 11: 71–82.

53. Tjaden P, Thoennes N. *Prevalence, Incidence, and Consequences of Violence Against Women.* Washington, DC: U.S. Dept. of Justice, Office of Justice Programs, National Institute of Justice, 1998.

54. World Report on Violence and Health. *NSW Public Health Bull* 2002; 13: 190.

55. Stewart D, MacMillan H, Wathen C. Intimate partner violence. *Can J Psychiatry* 2013; 58: 1–15.

56. Trevillion K, Oram S, Feder G, Howard L. Experiences of domestic violence and mental disorders: a systematic review and meta-analysis. *PLOS ONE* 2012; 7: e51740.

57. World Health Organization. Global and regional estimates of violence against women: prevalence and health effects of intimate partner violence and non-partner sexual violence. Available at: http://www.who.int/reproductivehealth/publications/violence/9789241564625/en/ (2013, accessed 20 March 2018).

58. World Health Organization/ London School of Hygiene and Tropical Medicine. Preventing intimate partner and sexual violence against women: taking action and generating evidence. Available at: http://www.who.int/reproductivehealth/publications/violence/9789241564007/en/ (2010, accessed 20 March 2018).

59. Bonomi A. Medical and psychosocial diagnoses in women with a history of intimate partner violence. *Arch Intern Med* 2009; 169: 1692.

60. Campbell J. Health consequences of intimate partner violence. *Lancet* 2002; 359: 1331–1336.

61. Wong J, Mellor D. Intimate partner violence and women's health and wellbeing: Impacts, risk factors and responses. *Contemp Nurse* 2014; 46: 170–179.

62. Breiding M, Armour B. The association between disability and intimate partner violence in the United States. *Ann Epidemiol* 2015; 25: 455–457.

63. Hahn J, McCormick M, Silverman J, Robinson E, Koenen K. Examining the impact of disability status on intimate partner violence victimization in a population sample. *J Interpers Violence* 2014; 29: 3063–3085.

64. Wathen C, MacGregor J, MacQuarrie B. Relationships among intimate partner violence, work, and health. *J Interpers Violence* 2016 (Epub ahead of print).

65. Du Mont J, Forte T. Intimate partner violence among women with mental health-related activity limitations: a Canadian population based study. *BMC Public Health* 2014; 14: 51.

66. Jones L, Hughes M, Unterstaller U. Post-traumatic stress disorder (PTSD) in victims of domestic violence: a review of the research. *Trauma Violence Abuse* 2001; 2: 99–119.

67. Golding M. Intimate partner violence as a risk factor for mental disorders: A meta-analysis. *J Fam Violence* 1999; 14: 99–132.

68. Howard L, Oram S, Galley H, Trevillion K, Feder G. Domestic violence and perinatal mental disorders: a systematic review and meta-analysis. *PLOS Med* 2013; 10: e1001452.

69. Dekel R, Solomon Z. Marital relations among former prisoners of war: contribution of posttraumatic stress disorder, aggression, and sexual satisfaction. *J Fam Psychol* 2006; 20: 709–712.

70. Devries K, Mak J, Bacchus L, et al. Intimate partner violence and incident depressive symptoms and suicide attempts: a systematic review of longitudinal studies. *PLOS Med* 2013; 10: e1001439.

71. Itzin C. *Tackling the Health and Mental Health Effects of Domestic and Sexual Violence and Abuse.* London: DH Publications, 2006.

72. Khalifeh H, Dean K. Gender and violence against people with severe mental illness. *Int Rev Psychiatry* 2010; 22: 535–546.

73. Fisher B, Regan S. The extent and frequency of abuse in the lives of older women and their relationship with health outcomes. *Gerontologist* 2006; 46: 200–209.

74. Coid J, Petruckevitch A, Chung W, Richardson J, Moorey S, Feder G. Abusive experiences and psychiatric morbidity in women primary care attenders. *Br J Psychiatry* 2003; 183: 332–339.

75. Humphreys C. Mental health and domestic violence: 'I call it symptoms of abuse'. *Br J Soc Work* 2003; 33: 209–226.

76. Rose D, Trevillion K, Woodall A, Morgan C, Feder G, Howard L. Barriers and facilitators of disclosures of domestic violence by mental health service users: qualitative study. *Br J Psychiatry* 2011; 198: 189–194.

77. Currier GW, Barthauer LM, Begier E, Bruce ML. Training and experience of psychiatric residents in identifying domestic violence. *Psychiatr Serv* 1996; 47: 529–530.

78. Hamberger KL, Phelan MB. Spousal abuse in psychiatric and mental health settings. In: *Domestic Violence Screening and Intervention in Medical and Mental Health Care Settings*. New York: Springer, 2004.

79. Klap R, Tang L, Wells K, Starks S, Rodriguez M. Screening for domestic violence among adult women in the United States. *J Gen Intern Med* 2007; 22: 579–584.

80. Nyame S, Howard LM, Feder G, Trevillion K. A survey of mental health professionals' knowledge, atti- tudes and preparedness to respond to domestic violence. *J Ment Health* 2013; 22: 536–543.

81. Ramon S, Vakalopoulou A, Lloyd M, Rollè L, Roszcynskya-Michta J, Videmšek P. Understanding the connections between intimate partner domestic violence and mental health within the European context: implications for innovative practice. *Dialogue Prax* 2015; 4: 1–21.

82. Salyers MP, Evans LJ, Bond GR, Meyer PS. Barriers to assessment and treatment of posttraumatic stress disorder and other trauma-related problems in peo- ple with severe mental illness: clinician perspectives. *Commun Ment Health J* 2004; 40: 17–31.

83. Hegarty K, Tarzia L, Hooker L, Taft A. Interventions to support recovery after domestic and sexual violence in primary care. *Int Rev Psychiatry* 2016; 28: 519–532.

84. Stöckl H, Devries K, Rotstein A, et al. The global prevalence of intimate partner homicide: a systematic review. *Lancet* 2013; 382: 859–865.

85. Krug E. *World Report on Violence and Health*. Geneva: WHO, 2002.

86. Prochaska J. *Systems of Psychotherapy: A Transtheoretical Analysis*. Homewood, IL: Dorsey, 1979.

87. Dienemann J, Campbell J, Landenburger K, Curry M. The domestic violence survivor assessment: a tool for counseling women in intimate partner violence relationships. *Patient Educ Couns* 2002; 46: 221–228.

88. Dienemann J, Neese J, Lowry S. Psychometric properties of the domestic violence survivor assessment. *Arch Psychiatr Nurs* 2009; 23: 111–118.

89. Frasier P, Slatt L, Kowlowitz V, Glowa P. Using the stages of change model to counsel victims of intimate partner violence. *Patient Educ Counsel* 2001; 43: 211–217.

90. Johnston-McCabe P, Levi-Minzi M, Van Hasselt V, Vanderbeek A. Domestic violence and social support in a clinical sample of deaf and hard of hearing women. *J Fam Violence* 2010; 26: 63–69.

91. Labronici L. Resilience in women victims of domestic violence: a phenomenological view. *Text Context Nurs* 2012; 21: 625–632.

92. Halket M, Gormley K, Mello N, Rosenthal L, Mirkin M. Stay with or leave the abuser? The effects of domestic violence victim's decision on attributions made by young adults. *J Fam Violence* 2014; 29: 35–49.

93. Wong J, Mellor D. Intimate partner violence and women's health and wellbeing: Impacts, risk factors and responses. *Contemp Nurse* 2014; 46: 170–179.

94. Burman E, Chantler K. Domestic violence and minoritisation: legal and policy barriers facing minoritized women leaving violent relationships. *Int J Law Psychiatry* 2005; 28: 59–74.

95. Paat Y. Risk and resilience of immigrant women in intimate partner violence. *J Hum Behav Soc Environ* 2014; 24: 725–740.

96. Baker C, Billhardt K, Warren J, Rollins C, Glass N. Domestic violence, housing instability, and homelessness: a review of housing policies and program practices for meeting the needs of survivors. *Aggress Violent Behav* 2010; 15: 430–439.

97. Rolling E, Brosi S. A multi-leveled and integrated approach to assessment and intervention of intimate partner violence. *J Fam Violence* 2010; 25: 229–236.

98. Murray C, Horton G, Johnson C, et al. Domestic violence service providers' perceptions of safety planning: a focus group study. *J Fam Violence* 2015; 30: 381–392.

99. Tam D, Tutty L, Zhuang Z, Paz E. Racial minority women and criminal justice responses to domestic violence. *J Fam Violence* 2016; 31: 527–538.

100. Rumm P, Cummings P, Krauss M, Bell M, Rivara F. Identified spouse abuse as a risk factor for child abuse. *Child Abuse Negl* 2000; 24: 1375–1381.

101. Borrego J, Gutow M, Reicher S, Barker C. Parent–child interaction therapy with domestic violence populations. *J Fam Violence* 2008; 23: 495–505.

102. Vameghi M, Feizzadeh A, Mirabzadeh A, Feizzadeh G. Exposure to domestic violence between parents: a perspective from Tehran, Iran. *J Interpers Violence* 2010; 25: 1006–1021.

103. Fainsilber-Katz L, Stettler N, Gurtovenko K. Traumatic stress symptoms in children exposed to intimate partner violence: the role of parent emotion socialization and children's emotion regulation abilities. *Soc Dev* 2015; 25: 47–65.

104. Horton E, Murray C, Garr B, Notestine L, Flasch P, Johnson C. Provider perceptions of safety planning with children impacted by intimate partner violence. *Child Youth Servi Rev* 2014; 42: 67–73.

105. Humphreys C, Thiara R, Mullender A, Skamballis A. 'Talking to mum'. *J Soc Work* 2006; 6: 53–63.

106. Stanley N, Miller P, Richardson Foster H, Thomson G. A stop-start response: social services' interventions with children and families notified following domestic violence incidents. *Br J Soc Work* 2011; 41: 296–313.

107. Rees S, Thorpe R, Tol W, Fonseca M, Silove D. Testing a cycle of family violence model in conflict-affected, low-income countries: a qualitative study from Timor-Leste. *Soc Sci Med* 2015; 130: 284–291.

108. Riggio H. Parental marital conflict and divorce, parent-child relationships, social support, and relationship anxiety in young adulthood. *Pers Relationsh* 2004; 11: 99–114.

109. McNeal C, Amato P. Parents' marital violence: long-term consequences for children. *J Fam Issues* 1998; 19: 123–139.

110. Kinsworthy S, Garza Y. Filial therapy with victims of family violence: a phenomenological study. *J Fam Violence* 2010; 25: 423–429.

111. Campbell J. Health consequences of intimate partner violence. *Lancet* 2002; 359: 1331–1336.

112. Bonomi A. Medical and psychosocial diagnoses in women with a history of intimate partner violence. *Arch Intern Med* 2009; 169: 1692.

113. Wong F, DiGangi J, Young D, Huang Z, Smith B, John D. Intimate partner violence, depression, and alcohol use among a sample of foreign-born Southeast Asian women in an urban setting in the United States. *J Interpers Violence* 2010; 26: 211–229.

114. Collis S. The analysis of young people's experiences of domestic violence: spiritual and emotional journeys through suffering. *Int J Child Spirit* 2009; 14: 339–353.

115. Labronici L. Resilience in women victims of domestic violence: a phenomenological view. *Text Context Nurs*. 2012; 21: 625–632.

116. Yick A. A metasynthesis of qualitative findings on the role of spirituality and religiosity among culturally diverse domestic violence survivors. *Qual Health Res* 2008; 18: 1289–1306.

117. Benavides L. A phenomenological study of spirituality as a protective factor for adolescents exposed to domestic violence. *J Soc Serv Res* 2012; 38: 165–174.

118. Lanz P, Guevara L, Poo M, Smeke E, Gallego M. Association between coping behaviors, domestic violence and depression in parents of children with Down's syndrome. *Br J Appl Sci Technol* 2015; 6: 8–14.

119. DeCou C, Lynch S, Cole T, Kaplan S. Coping self-efficacy moderates the association between severity of partner violence and PTSD symptoms among incarcerated women. *J Trauma Stress* 2015; 28: 465–468.

120. Becker K, Mathis G, Mueller C, Issari K, Atta S. Community-based treatment outcomes for parents and children exposed to domestic violence. *J Emotion Abuse* 2008; 8: 187–204.

121. Katz L. Windecker-Nelson B. Domestic violence, emotion coaching, and child adjustment. *J Fam Psychol* 2006; 20: 56–67.

122. Stanley N, Miller P, Richardson Foster H, Thomson G. A stop-start response: social services' interventions with children and families notified following domestic violence incidents. *Br J Soc Work* 2011; 41: 296–313.

123. Vander-Ende K, Yount K, Dynes M, Sibley L. Community-level correlates of intimate partner violence against women globally: a systematic review. *Soc Sci Med* 2012; 75: 1143–1155.

124. National Institute of Health and Care Excellence. PH50: Domestic violence and abuse: multi-agency working. Available at: https://www.nice.org.uk/guidance/ph50/resources/domestic-violence-and-abuse-multiagency-working-pdf-1996411687621 (2014, accessed 20 March 2018).

125. National Center on Domestic Violence, Trauma & Mental Health. NCDVTMH Review of Trauma-Specific Treatment in the Context of Domestic Violence. Available at: http://www.nationalcenterdvtraumamh.org/publications-products/ncdvtmh-review-of-trauma-specific-treatment-in-the-context-of-domestic-violence/ (2016, accessed 8 December 2016).

126. Ehrensaft M. Intimate partner violence: persistence of myths and implications for intervention. *Child Youth Serv Rev* 2008; 30: 276–286.

127. World Health Organization. Repsonding to intimate partner violence and sexual violence against women. Available at: http://www.who.int/reproductivehealth/publications/violence/9789241548595/en/ (2013, accessed 20 March 2018).

128. Costa B, Kaestle C, Walker A, et al. Longitudinal predictors of domestic violence perpetration and victimization: a systematic review. *Aggress Violent Behav* 2015; 24: 261–272.

129. World Health Organization. Violence against women. Available at: http://www.who.int/mediacentre/factsheets/fs239/en (2016, accessed 20 March 2018).

130. Russell D. *Violence Against Wives: A Case Against the Patriarchy.* New York: Free Press, 1979.

131. Council of Europe. Council of Europe Convention on preventing and combating violence against women and domestic violence. Available at: http://www.coe.int/en/web/conventions/full-list/-/conventions/rms/090000168008482e (2016, accessed 24 November 2016).

132. Women's Commission. The Women's Commission Report: Women's Safety in Hong Kong: Eliminating Domestic Violence. Available at: http://www.women.gov.hk/download/empowerment/women_safety_report.pdf (2016, accessed 20 March 2018).

133. Global Rights for Women. International, Regional and National Legal Frameworks—Global Rights for Women. Available at: http://globalrightsforwomen.org/resources-for-legal-reform/legal-framework/ (2016, accessed 20 March 2018).

134. Thomson Reuters Foundation. A Landscape Analysis of Domestic Violence Laws (Chinese version). Available at: http://www.trust.org/publications/i/?id=fe9c538d-96ae-41c6-9dc8-148f793248fb (2014, accessed 24 November 2016).

135. Kimball E. Edleson revisited: reviewing children's witnessing of domestic violence 15 years later. *J Fam Violence* 2016; 31: 625–637.

136. Walker L. *The Battered Woman.* New York: Harper & Row, 1979.

137. Hirschel D, Buzawa E, Pattavina A, Faggiani D. Domestic violence and mandatory arrest laws: to what extent do they influence police arrest decisions. *J Crim Law Criminol* 2007; 98: 255–298.

138. Ministry of Social Development. Domestic Violence and Pro-Arrest Policy. Available at: https://www.msd.govt.nz/about-msd-and-our-work/publications-resources/journals-and-magazines/social-policy-journal/spj33/33-domestic-violence-and-pro-arrest-policy-p1-14.html (2008, accessed 20 March 2018).

139. Barrow A, Scully-Hill A. Failing to implement CEDAW in Hong Kong: why isn't anyone using the domestic and cohabitation relationships violence ordinance? *Int J Law Policy Fam* 2016; 30: 50–78.

140. Erez E. Domestic violence and the criminal justice system: an overview. *Online J Issues Nurs* 2002; 7: 4.

141. UN Women. Police training. Available at: http://www.endvawnow.org/en/articles/137-police-training.html?next=138 (accessed 20 March 2018).

142. Balenovich J, Grossi E, Hughes T. Toward a balanced approach: defining police roles in responding to domestic violence. *Am J Crim Justice* 2008; 33: 19–31.

143. Plotnikoff J, Woolfson R. *Policing Domestic Violence.* London: Home Office, Policing and Reducing Crime Unit, Research, Development and Statistics Directorate, 1998.

144. TC Beirne School of Law. Domestic violence benchbook. Available at: https://law.uq.edu.au/project/domestic-violence-benchbook (accessed 20 March 2018).

145. Zhong H. Victim protection in domestic violence: current situations and future development in China. In: Zhang H, Huang Y, Zhao R (eds). *Studies on Victim Protections.* Beijing: China Court Press, 2017.

146. García B, de Oliveira O. Family changes and public policies in Latin America. *Annu Rev Sociol* 2011; 37: 593–611.

147. Tam D, Tutty L, Zhuang Z, Paz E. Racial minority women and criminal justice responses to domestic violence. *J Fam Violence* 2015; 31: 527–538.

148. Nelson H, Bougatsos C, Blazina I. Screening women for intimate partner violence: a systematic review to update the U.S. Preventive Services Task Force Recommendation. *Ann Intern Med* 2012; 156: 796.

149. Lee Y. Hadeed L. Intimate partner violence among Asian immigrant communities: health/mental health consequences, help-seeking behaviors, and service utilization. *Trauma Violence Abuse* 2009; 10: 143–170.

CHAPTER 50

Poverty and interpersonal violence

Supraja T. A, D. Padmavathy, and Prabha S. Chandra

Defining interpersonal violence

The World Report on Violence and Health presents a typology of violence that, while not uniformly accepted, can be a useful way in which to understand the contexts in which violence occurs and the interactions between types of violence [1]. This typology distinguishes four modes in which violence may be inflicted: physical; sexual; psychological attack; deprivation. It further divides the general definition of violence into three subtypes according to the victim–perpetrator relationship.

- **Self-directed violence** refers to violence in which the perpetrator and the victim are the same individual and is subdivided into *self-abuse* and *suicide*.

- **Interpersonal violence** refers to violence between individuals, and is subdivided into *family and intimate partner violence* and *community violence*. The former category includes child maltreatment, intimate partner violence, and elder abuse, whereas the latter is broken down into *acquaintance* and *stranger* violence and includes youth violence, assault by strangers, violence related to property crimes, and violence in workplaces and other institutions.

- **Collective violence** refers to violence committed by larger groups of individuals and can be subdivided into social, political, and economic violence.

Interpersonal violence occurs when one person uses power and control over another through physical, sexual, or emotional threats or actions, economic control, isolation, or other kinds of coercive behaviour [1].

Different types of interpersonal violence

Abuse is any behaviour toward another person that is physically violent or involves emotional coercion, or both, and one person is in a position of authority.

Bullying is a type of harassment that can be either verbal or physical, or both. It can also take the form of coercion where someone is threatened by another person and, as a result of those threats, the bully's victim feels intimidated and pressured into acting a certain way or doing a certain thing. Bullying can occur in all settings—at school, work, or home, in the neighbourhood, and online [2].

Dating/relationship violence occurs when one intimate or romantic partner tries to maintain power and control over the other through words and actions that are physically and emotionally abusive. Dating violence can take many forms, including physical violence, coercion, threats, intimidation, isolation, and emotional, sexual, or economic abuse. It occurs in both heterosexual and homosexual relationships and can be instigated by either males or females. Women aged 16–24 experience the highest per capita rates of intimate violence—nearly 20 per 1000 women [3]. Some examples of dating violence include hitting, slapping, kicking, punching, strangling, holding down, abandoning in a dangerous place, and forcing or attempting to force unwanted sexual acts.

Sexual violence is any type of sexual activity that a person does not agree to. It includes inappropriate touching; vaginal, anal, or oral penetration; sexual intercourse that a person says no to; rape or attempted rape; sexual harassment; threats; or peeping. Sexual violence can be verbal, visual, or anything that forces a person to join in unwanted sexual contact or attention. Examples of this are voyeurism (when someone watches private sexual acts), exhibitionism (when someone exposes him/herself in public), incest (sexual contact between family members), and sexual harassment [4].

Youth violence refers to aggressive behaviours, including slapping, hitting, kicking, bullying, punching, fist fighting, and knife fighting, as well as robbery, rape, and homicide.

Gang violence refers to acts of aggression and violence and criminal activity committed by a group of peers where the group usually has an identity (e.g. a name, a sign, a neighbourhood). In some neighbourhoods, the pressure to join a gang occurs early and can be very difficult to resist. Members often join to feel a sense of family and community, and to achieve power and respect. On the flip side, members may worry about their own safety and fears of being abused by others in the gang. Gang members include both males and females [5].

Poverty and interpersonal violence

Poverty and interpersonal violence are linked as not just indicators for each other, but also as factors that have similar impacts on both individuals and communities.

There has been consistent increase in the numbers of women and families seeking assistance, and a simultaneous increase has been recorded in the reports of abuse, specifically those that are more violent in nature.

Surveys on women's shelters have reported a rise in the numbers of women seeking help in 78% of shelters, with 58% reporting records of more violent forms of abuse [6].

Over the years media sources have reported not merely individual accounts of abuse related to economic stress or poverty, but also the thematic occurrences of poverty and abuse bidirectionally and the patterns linking them. The relationship between poverty and violence is not a simplistic one, as we see that individuals across socio-economic classes and circumstances experience violence [7]. Poverty exacerbates the occurrence and severity of violence in those already experiencing it.

While poverty does not directly cause violence or abuse, in the human rights context, it is in itself a form of violence that occurs along economic parallels. Extreme poverty is a form of structural violence. Violence and abuse, even in the absence of poverty incur costs; the cost of violence is often the continuation of poverty, economic deprivation, or exploitation [2, 7]. Poverty, in fact, stems from social injustices that emerge from multiple aspects.

The relationship between poverty and domestic violence is bidirectional; that is, poverty incites violence and poverty stems from violence. Hence, being trapped in poverty or violence often implies being trapped in the other [8]. Those trapped in poverty are already at a disadvantage, and the abuse further limits the person and reduces their capacity, independence, and availability and access to resources.

However, it is often difficult to leave a violent relationship as leaving may seem to be a more expensive option. Efforts to leave violent relationships or circumvent abuse often result in the victim incurring heavy costs, and the effects of violent abuse result in legal and health complications creating even further need for intervention and social assistance.

There exists the threat of losing their job, home, health care, or access to income and financial support. When victims make attempts to seek justice through legal channels, they are faced with issues of large fees attached to criminal and civil actions and procedures. Owing to these, attempting to leave abusive relationships can cause further poverty and further threats of abuse [8, 9].

Poverty restricts choices and, when coupled with violence, it destabilizes basic security not just for those in the violent relationship, but for everyone related to them and the larger community where they live.

Combating either poverty or domestic violence would first require acknowledging the relationship between the two and focusing on human rights as a means to redress both. When poverty and abuse are seen as issues of human rights, their underlying causes and potential alleviations are also visible through the same lens [9].

Theories of violence

General systems theory approach

The general systems theory views continuing violence as a systemic product rather than a product of individual behaviour pathology. It specifies the 'positive feedback' processes that produce an upward spiral of violence, the 'negative feedback' or dampening processes that serve to maintain the level of violence within tolerable limits, and the morphogenic processes that change the role structure of the family.

Violence between family members is seen as arising from diverse causes, including normative expectations, personality traits such as aggressiveness, frustrations due to role blockages, and conflicts. It considers that relative to the rate of publicly known or treated violence between family members, the actual occurrence is extremely high and that most violence is either denied or not labelled as deviance.

Stereotyped imagery of family violence is learned in early childhood from parents, siblings, and other children, and is continually re-affirmed through ongoing social interaction.

The probability of continued violence increases when violent persons are rewarded for violent acts if these acts produce the desired results or when the use of violence is contrary to family norms, and creates further 'secondary conflict' over the use of violence to settle the original conflict [10].

Social learning theory

Social learning theory contends that behaviours are learned through observation and imitation of other people's behaviour. Behaviour is subsequently maintained through differential reinforcement, initially by the parent, and then later by others and through automatic reinforcement. A fundamental tenet of this theory is that early parental interactions are particularly salient models from which a child learns a variety of behaviours. In terms of explaining violent behaviour, social learning theory is a potentially parsimonious framework that may significantly contribute to our understanding of dating violence. For instance, the intergenerational transmission of violence hypothesis, which is based on social learning theory, proposes that coercive and aversive interpersonal behaviours are learned through violent interactions in one's family of origin [11]. Parenting skills may play a role along with society's attitudes towards gender, as well as violence (see Chapter 40).

Riggs and O'Leary [12] developed the background situational model, based primarily on social learning and conflict theory. They assert that variables causally related to dating violence can be categorized as background variables, such as violence in the family of origin, which, in turn, promote acceptance of aggression as a strategy for resolving conflicts, and situational variables, such as relationship satisfaction, communication skills, and alcohol use.

Social disorganization theory

Social disorganization theory links concentrated disadvantage, residential stability, and ethnic heterogeneity with variations in social organization and the collective capacity to control local crime. The social disorganization approach suggests that neighbourhood poverty, residential instability, and ethnic heterogeneity decrease the community level capacity to regulate local crime. Poverty diminishes the resources necessary to sustain basic institutions like family, schools, places of worship, and voluntary organizations in urban neighbourhoods. Poverty also contributes to residential instability and ethnic heterogeneity, both of which inhibit the formation of durable relationships, weaken community attachments, and complicate efforts to implement shared goals. In their research, Shaw and McKay [13] found that these structural factors continued to affect crime rates, regardless of ethnic and racial population succession, suggesting that macro-level processes exert effects on crime independent of the characteristics of individuals who make up disadvantaged neighbourhoods [13].

Ecological theory

The ecological theory, while focusing on the individual as the unit of analysis for addressing violence, considers the individual's environment and relationships as being essential in understanding the violent behaviours. The basis of the ecological perspective is that the more precise variables (e.g. individual development) are nested within broader variables (e.g. cultural norms, subcultures). Dutton [14] identifies four levels of systemic social context that bear upon individual behaviour: The *macro-system*, which is composed of broad cultural values, social, and belief systems; the *exo-system*, composed of the groups and institutions (e.g. school, work, and peers) that connect the family to the larger environment; the *micro-system*, which is the family unit and the immediate context that surrounds the individual; and, finally, *ontogenetic* factors, which refers to an individual's personal development. Dutton [14] asserts that factors from all four of these systemic levels come to bear on any given situation of violence. The ecological perspective is consistent with the systems theory focus on the complex and interrelated networks of systems that influence behaviour.

Feminist theory and domestic violence

The feminist theory of violence asserts that although there are numerous types of violence within families (e.g. violence between children, between parents and children, and between spouses), violence against wives is a separate phenomenon with its own causes, correlates, and properties and therefore cannot be viewed through the same lens as other types of family violence [15].

Feminist theory in violence emphasizes gender and power inequality in heterosexual relationships [16]. It views interpersonal violence as a manifestation of prevailing power structures of male dominance and female subservience, and believes that this power inequality leads to violent behaviours in interpersonal relationships.

Feminist theorists assert that the patriarchal domination of women through wife abuse has been maintained through a long cultural history of legally sanctioned male subordination, abuse, and control of women. They state that this history of inequality is still at work in the fundamental fabric of the marriage relationship in terms of gender roles and norms and social sanctioning of male domination. The feminist theories view female-perpetrated violence as the result of self-defensive behaviours and as qualitatively distinct from male perpetration, which is often intended to evoke fear and to oppress the victim [17].

These theorists maintain that gender, rather than the family, should be the central unit of analysis in any interpersonal violence theory, as it is the primary framework that defines the problem. While acknowledging the causal complexity of interpersonal violence, they assert that, despite the complexity, the most fundamental feminist perception is that violence and specifically intimate partner violence cannot be adequately understood unless gender and power are taken into account.

Similar propositions are placed in the context of violence in same-sex relationships, which state that the use of violence in gay and lesbian relationships is more about power rather than gender. While there is power abuse in both heterosexual and gay and lesbian relationships, the source of power differs in that gender is the defining factor in the heterosexual context, whereas power in same-sex relationships may be a function of various elements such as education, class, ethnicity, or an interplay of these factors [18].

Impact of poverty and interpersonal violence

Childhood

Children growing up in poor families are at increased risk for health problems that may persist into adulthood [19–23]. Neighbourhood-level studies have identified established links between poverty and poor physical health in adulthood [24–26]. The few studies that have examined the role of individual level poverty within the context of the community have found that both family and neighbourhood factors need to be considered while examining its relationship with physical and psychological health and well-being [24, 25, 27].

Theoretical models of the impact of early stressful experiences indicate that neglect during childhood may lead to poor physical health by disrupting the stress-response pathways and psychosocial functioning. Furthermore, childhood risk factors of neglect and poverty tend to co-occur and poverty partially accounts for the negative consequences associated with neglect. These factors potentially contribute to the development of risky behaviours in adolescence and adulthood [28].

Children experiencing early family and neighbourhood violence have significantly lower school-age competence and poorer emotional health in elementary school. Symptoms of early trauma may potentially encumber developmental progress [29]. In particular, young children manifesting avoidance and arousal symptoms have a heightened risk for later internalizing symptoms and poorer social competence and those with early arousal have a heightened risk for later externalizing symptoms [30].

Adolescence

The World Health Organization listed interpersonal violence as the fifth leading cause of death amongst adolescents in 2012 [31, 32]. Living in impoverished neighbourhoods is stressful for adolescents and one of the most common associated stressors in such conditions is violence. Impoverished neighbourhoods witness significantly more incidents of violence compared with non-impoverished neighbourhoods [33–35].

Other potential stressors associated with life in poverty include high arrest rates [36], school failure [37], food insecurity [38], and poor physical health [39]. The violence and other stressors in impoverished neighbourhoods have been associated with several negative psychological outcomes, including post-traumatic stress disorder [40] and hopelessness [33].

The association between violence and risky sexual behaviour in adolescents (e.g. multiple sexual partnerships) is established. Sexual violence is prevalent in low socio-economic settings across global communities and the effects of sexual abuse are seen in the form of higher sexual risk and use of substances [41, 42]. These factors contribute to making adolescent sexual violence (including the perpetration and victimization) an important public health concern with implications on sexual and reproductive health.

Old age

Elder abuse affects almost one in six older people (more than 140 million worldwide). The most prevalent subtypes of elder abuse have been identified to be psychological abuse, followed by financial abuse, neglect, physical abuse, and sexual abuse [43]. Psychological

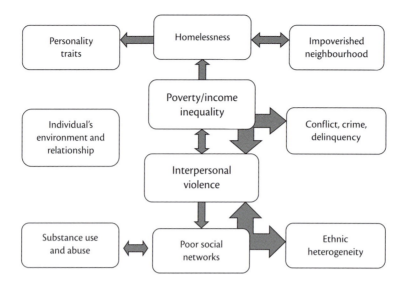

Fig. 50.1 Conceptual framework: poverty and interpersonal violence.

abuse among the elderly can lead to reactions of distress, fear, anxiety, and put them at risk for depression. Physical abuse apart from causing injuries can result in problems with nutrition and hydration, disrupt sleep, cause chronic physical pain, and increase risks of premature death [44, 45]. While these effects of abuse are observable among all elderly persons in general, poverty can accentuate the severity of the same and add the burden of homelessness as ageing puts them at a disadvantage of not being able to earn a sustainable living.

Enhancing the protective factors can potentially reduce the risk of experiencing abuse and neglect. A strong interpersonal network (multiple strong relationships with people of varying social status) and living in a supportive community environment (including agencies/organizations providing resources and services) with high cohesion, community identity, and collective efficacy can serve as potential protective factors to mitigate the effects of poverty and violence among the elderly [46].

Poverty and interpersonal violence

Research studies and meta-analyses over the past two decades have established that there is a robust tendency for violence to be more common in societies where income differences were larger [47, 48]. Poverty strengthens the transactional aspect of the relationship between structural and interpersonal violence as it functions both as the context in which structural violence flourishes, as well as a consequence of it [49]. Poverty creates a specific context in which structural as well as other types of violence can flourish, as poor neighbourhoods are often overcrowded, isolated, and unhygienic. In addition, poor neighbourhoods pose a higher risk for substance use and abuse.

Violence at the structural level places people at increased risk for more violent consequences and influences violence at the sociopolitical and interpersonal levels [49].

In situations of widespread and severe inequality, the urban poor are undervalued and marginalized, and their daily living conditions heighten the potential for the emergence of conflict, crime, or

violence [50]. Increased levels of urban violence are also closely tied to processes of globalization and structural adjustment, as well as political democratization. As the daily living conditions of the urban poor become more precarious (particularly relative to the wealthy), the potential for conflict, crime, or violence escalates [51].

However, while poverty has long been considered a key determinant of urban violence, this relationship has been challenged as being too simplistic. Statistical modelling has shown that income inequality offers more explanatory power than poverty. Income inequality and the unequal distribution of economic opportunities across groups are believed to promote violence as compared with per capita income, which does not appear to have a clear effect [52]. The following framework illustrates the relationship between violence, poverty, and related factors (Fig. 50.1).

Preventive and protective factors for interpersonal violence

The goal of violence prevention is to stop violence before it begins. A four-level social-ecological model for understanding and dealing with violence has been proposed by the Centers for Disease Control and Prevention. The four levels are individual, relationship, community, and societal. Each of these levels functions as a level of influence and also as a key point for prevention [53]. In order to prevent violence, it is important to implement programmes and policies that can reduce risk factors and increase protective factors at each of the different levels in the model.

At the individual level, the protective factors focus on personal characteristics, biological factors, behaviour, and personal experience, and prevention strategies are often designed to promote attitudes, beliefs, and behaviours that ultimately prevent violence. Specific approaches include education and life skills training and some effective strategies comprise school-based programmes that help students develop social, emotional, and behavioural skills to build positive relationships, in-house programmes that teach parents skills for age-appropriate childcare, and so on.

The protective factors at the relationship level focuses on interaction between two or more people. Prevention strategies at this level may include parenting or family-focused prevention programmes, and mentoring and peer programmes designed to reduce conflict, cultivate problem-solving skills, and promote healthy relationships. Some possible strategies include education and family support to promote positive development, mentoring programmes pairing young people with caring adults, workshops for couples that focus on communication strategies, and so on.

The protective factors at community level focus on settings or institutions in which social relationships take place. Prevention strategies at this level are typically designed to affect the social and physical environment—for example, by reducing social isolation, improving economic and housing opportunities in neighbourhoods, as well as the climate, processes, and policies within the workplace settings. Strategies like better physical structures for community living, safe recreational areas for residents, policies to prevent bullying behaviour, and better employment opportunities can be employed.

The protective factors at societal level focus on societal factors that create either a level of acceptance or intolerance for violence. Some of the strategies could be better working conditions and national media to create awareness and change the way people think about violence.

Social–emotional skills such as interpersonal skills and stress management skills act as protective factors for bullying and violence outcomes. Greater interpersonal skills and greater stress-management skills are significantly associated with lower odds of involvement in acts of violence and also with lower levels of physical bullying and relational aggression [54]. High levels of participation in extracurricular activities and positive parent–child relations appeared to function as protective factors, weakening the positive association between exposures to violence and externalizing problems [55].

Interventions

Interventions for persons living in impoverished conditions and experiencing interpersonal violence should be designed based on the life-cycle stage and considering the needs of the target group and the specific impacts on them. Studies that have focused on intervening with these groups have identified certain components that have been found to be effective in working with them. A list of recent studies on intervention for interpersonal violence and/or poverty is given in Table 50.1.

Vulnerable groups

Witnessing or experiencing violence in childhood can be traumatic and result in internalizing or externalizing symptoms in the children. In working with children exposed to violence, multi-family group programmes developed for families facing contemporary social and urban problems have been recommended [56]. Also, cognitive–behavioural interventions for trauma in school settings have been found to be effective in lessening symptoms of depression, as well as psychosocial dysfunction [57].

Children and adolescents who are persistently exposed to violence and poverty tend to express rage, mistrust, and hopelessness in general. Programmes designed for these young people have predominantly included the following essential elements: street outreach and referral; needs and interest assessments; provisions for supportive, personal relationships with adults; availability of role models; peer group discussions; family interventions; neighbourhood projects, and education and job preparedness training [58]. Furthermore, in working with children and adolescents from minority populations, components focusing on the enhancement of ethnic/cultural pride have been found to mediate beneficial behaviour change [59].

The association between violence during pregnancy and poor pregnancy outcomes has been well-established. A cognitive behavioural intervention for the reduction of IPV recurrence during pregnancy and improving pregnancy outcomes during prenatal and postpartum care in mothers reporting interpersonal violence victimization was found to universally reduce certain forms of violence such as slapping, grabbing, pushing, and shoving, and twisting of the arm or hair, as well as to reduce the incidence of poor outcomes, namely very low birthweight and very preterm births [60]. Studies among perinatal women have also found that maternal emotional health showed improvement and maternal depression was reduced following a home-visiting intervention over a 3-year period after their children were born [61].

Structural interventions

Economic empowerment strategies are an important means to poverty alleviation and have also been found to facilitate the reduction of interpersonal violence. Structural interventions for prevention of violence have been tested and found to be feasible and helpful, and inclusion of gender training to socio-economic programming can offer social and health benefits. Evidence of this is provided by the IMAGE study, which was a poverty-focused microfinance-based structural intervention combining gender equity components with economic empowerment programming. This intervention reported increased household economic well-being, social capital, and empowerment and reduced vulnerability to violence [62]. In another randomized controlled trial, an intervention component addressing household gender inequities alongside economic empowerment programming, significantly reduced past-year physical interpersonal violence among women who participated in more than 75% of the programme with their male partner. The intervention also resulted in a reduction of economic abuse and altered attitudes regarding the justification and acceptance of IPV among the women [63].

Conclusions

The interaction between poverty and interpersonal violence is influenced by multiple personal, social, and communal factors. The nature of this interaction and their influences need to be well examined and established for diverse groups in order to develop effective strategies for dealing with them. As structural interventions in the past have shown, interventions aiming at assuaging the impact of either poverty or violence should inevitably include components to address each other. While essential strategies of intervention are increasingly being identified, developing sustainable and replicable intervention models is a priority for engaging with persons facing these challenges.

Table 50.1 Interventions for interpersonal violence (IPV) and/or poverty

Country	Reference	Year	Target group	Aim	Components of intervention
South Africa	Rotheram-Borus et al. [61]	2015	Pregnant women	Examining how risk factors interact and how each of the factors is related to demographic and behavioural contexts that are potential avenues for intervention for violence	Home visitation to provide information about general maternal child health, HIV/TB, alcohol use, and nutrition
Botswana, Namibia, Swaziland	Cameron et al. [64]	2014	Community members	Describing implementation research of an intervention in a complex HIV prevention randomized trial	Population health intervention to reduce gender violence—educational audio docu-drama series discussing with community groups evidence about violence against women, sexual violence, abuse of children, transactional sex, transgenerational sex, choice disability, and HIV risk
Mexico	Falb et al. [65]	2014	Non-pregnant or first trimester women	Assessing the efficacy of an enhanced nurse-delivered screening and counselling programme on past year IPV	Integrated IPV and health screening, supportive care, safety planning and harm reduction counselling, supportive referrals, and booster counselling sessions
USA	Taha et al. [66]	2014	Low-income abused women, recent suicidal attempt	Examining the relative efficacy of a culturally sensitive empowerment group intervention aimed at increasing self-esteem, hopefulness, and effectiveness in obtaining resources	Providing access to health care, increasing connectedness, enhancing social skills, and reducing the residual effects of trauma
Côte d'Ivoire	Gupta et al. [63]	2013	Women and spouse/male family member	To evaluate the incremental impact of adding 'gender dialogue groups' on levels of IPV for women and their partners (aiming to change gender norms) to an economic empowerment programme for women	Household economy, household cash flow, setting financial goals dealing with financial stress, and budgeting and planning
USA	Enriquez et al. [67]	2012	Hispanic teenagers, low income	Pilot testing of a school-based group format intervention, which aimed to enhance interpersonal violence prevention efficacy	Gender specific roles and rites of passage, how teenage violence affects the individual, family, and community. Alternatives to violence: self-control, culture, life and destiny, making commitments/goals

Table 50.1 Continued

Country	Reference	Year	Target group	Aim	Components of intervention
USA	Cleary Bradley and Gottman [68]	2012	Low-income, situationally violent couples	Evaluating a conjoint couple and relationship education programme designed to reduce IPV	Psycho-educational intervention through a skills-based approach focusing on helping couples learn techniques to foster stronger relationships and facilitate conflict management
USA	Zlotnick and Street [69]	2011	Pregnant women	Examining the initial feasibility, acceptability, and effects of an intervention in reducing PTSD and depressive symptoms from pregnancy until 3 months postpartum	Based on interpersonal psychotherapy— evaluation of relationships, disputes/abuse; stress-management skills, cycle of abuse, and making a safety plan; emotional risks of abuse and postpartum depression, PTSD and substance use, management of role transitions; asking for support, resolving interpersonal conflicts, and goal-setting

Note: TB: tuberculosis; PTSD: post-traumatic stress disorder.

References

1. Krug EG, Mercy JA, Dahlberg LL, Zwi AB. Public health The world report on violence and health. *Lancet* 2002; 360: 1083–1088.
2. Grych J, Swan S. Toward a more comprehensive understanding of interpersonal violence: introduction to the special issue on interconnections among different types of violence. *Psychol Violence* 2012; 2: 105–110.
3. Rennison C, Welchans S. Intimate Partner Violence. Available at: http://citeseerx.ist.psu.edu/viewdoc/download?doi=10.1.1.159.2279&rep=rep1&type=pdf (accessed 20 March 2018).
4. Womenshealth.gov. Dating violence and abuse. Available at: https://www.womenshealth.gov/violence-against-women/types-of-violence/dating-violence.html (accessed 26 March 2017).
5. Braga AA, McDevitt J, Pierce GL. Understanding and preventing gang violence: problem analysis and response development in Lowell, Massachusetts. *Police Q* 2006; 9: 20–46.
6. The Mary Kay Foundation. Mary Kay Truth About Abuse survey Report, 2013. Available at: http://content2.marykayintouch.com/Public/MKACF/Documents/2013survey.pdf (accessed 20 March 2018).
7. Krueger AB, Malečková J. Education, poverty and terrorism: is there a causal connection? *J Econ Perspect* 2003; 17: 119–144.
8. The World Bank. *Violence in the City: Understanding and Supporting Community Responses to Urban Violence.* Washington, DC: World Bank, 2010.
9. Verfaillie N. The Connection Between Poverty and Domestic Violence. Available at: http://www.borgenmagazine.com/connection-poverty-domestic-violence/ (accessed 20 March 2018).
10. Straus MA. A general systems theory approach to a theory of violence between family members. *Soc Sci Inf* 1973; 12: 105–125.
11. Shorey RC, Cornelius TL, Bell KM. A critical review of theoretical frameworks for dating violence: comparing the dating and marital fields. *Aggress Violent Behav* 2008; 13: 185–194.
12. Riggs D, O'Leary K. A theoretical model of courtship aggression. In: Good MAP, Stets J (eds). *Violence in Dating Relationships: Emerging Social Issues.* New York: Praeger, 1989, pp. 53–71.
13. Shaw C, McKay H. *Juvenile Delinquency and Urban Areas.* Chicago, IL: University of Chicago Press, 1942.
14. Dutton DG. Nested ecological theory. In: Dutton DG (ed.) *Rethinking Domestic Violence.* Vancouver: UBC Press, 2006, pp. 18–40.
15. Lawson J. Sociological theories of intimate partner violence. *J Hum Behav Soc Environ* 2012; 22: 572–590.
16. Pence E, Paymar M. *Education Groups for Men who Batter: The Duluth Model.* Berlin: Springer, 1993.
17. Herman J. *Trauma and Recovery.* New York: Basic Books, 1997.
18. Perilla JL, Frndak K, Lillard D, East C. A working analysis of women's use of violence in the context of learning, opportunity, and choice. *Violence Against Women* 2003; 9: 10–46.
19. Adler N, Rehkopf D. U. S. disparities in health: descriptions, causes, and mechanisms. *Annu Rev Public Health* 2008; 29: 213–252.
20. Case A, Lubotsky D, Paxson C. Economic status and health in childhood: the origins of the gradient. *Am Econ Rev* 2002; 92: 1308–1334.
21. Cohen S, Janicki-Deverts S, Chen E, Matthews K. Childhood socioeconomic status and adult health. *Ann N Y Acad Sci* 2010; 1186: 37–55.
22. Conroy K, Sandel M, Zuckerman B. Poverty grown up: How childhood socioeconomic status impacts adult health. *J Dev Behav Pediatr* 2010; 31: 154–160.
23. Galobardes B, Lynch J, Davey SG. Childhood socioeconomic circumstances and cause-specific mortality in adulthood: systematic review and interpretation. *Epidemiol Rev* 2004; 26: 7–21.
24. Franzini L, Caughty M, Spears E, Esquer F. Neighborhood economic conditions, social processes and self-rated health in low-income neighborhoods in Texas: a multilevel latent variables model. *Soc Sci Med* 2005; 61: 1135–1150.

25. Moore S, Daniel M, Bockenholt U, et al. Associations among socioeconomic status, perceived neighborhood control, perceived individual control and self-reported health. *J Community Psychol* 2010; 38: 729–741.

26. Wilkinson R, Pickett K. The problems of relative deprivation: why some societies do better than others. *Soc Sci Med* 2007; 65: 1965–1978.

27. Case A, Fertig A, Paxson C. The lasting impact of childhood health and circumstance. *J Health Econ* 2005; 24: 365–389.

28. Repetti R, Taylor S, Seeman T. Risky families: family social environments and the mental and physical health of offspring. *Psychol Bull* 2002; 128: 330–366.

29. Crowe S., Blair R. The development of antisocial behavior: what can we learn from functional neuroimaging studies? *Dev Psychopathol* 2008; 20: 1145–1159.

30. Briggs-Gowan MJ, Carter AS, Ford JD. Parsing the effects violence exposure in early childhood: modeling developmental pathways. *J Pediatr Psychol* 2012; 37: 11–22.

31. World Health Organization. Adolescent health epidemiology. Available at: http://www.who.int/maternal_child_adolescent/epidemiology/adolescence/en/ (accessed 20 March 2018).

32. Otwombe KN, Dietrich J, Sikkema KJ, et al. Exposure to and experiences of violence among adolescents in lower socio-economic groups in Johannesburg, South Africa. *BMC Public Health* 2015; 15: 450.

33. Bolland JM, Bryant CM, Lian BE, McCallum DM, Vazsonyi AT, Barth JM. Development and risk behavior among African American, Caucasian, and mixed-race adolescents living in high poverty inner-city neighborhoods. *Am J Community Psychol* 2007; 40: 230–249.

34. Richters JS, Martinez P. The NIMH community violence project: I. Children as victims and witnesses to violence. *Psychiatry* 1993; 56: 7–21.

35. Umlauf MG, Bolland AC, Bolland KA, Tomek S, Bolland JM. The effects of age, gender, hopelessness, and exposure to violence on sleep disorder symptoms and daytime sleepiness among adolescents in impoverished neighborhoods. *J Youth Adolesc* 2014; 44: 518–542.

36. Warner BD, Coomer BW. Neighborhood drug arrest rates: are they a meaningful indicator of drug activity? A research note. *J Crime Delinq* 2003; 40: 123–138.

37. Ludwig J, Ladd HF, Duncan GJ. Urban poverty and educational outcomes. *Brookings-Wharton Papers on Urban Affairs* 2001; 1: 147–188.

38. Rose D. Economic determinants and dietary consequences of food insecurity in the United States. *J Nutr* 1999; 129: 517S–520S.

39. Newacheck PW, Hung YY, Park MJ, Brindis CD, Irwin CE. Disparities in adolescent health and health care: does socioeconomic status matter? *Health Serv Res* 2003; 38: 1235–1252.

40. Cooley-Quille M, Boyd RC, Frantz E, Walsh J. Emotional and behavioral impact of exposure to community violence in inner-city adolescents. *J Clin child Adolesc Psychol* 2001; 30: 199–206.

41. Merrick J, Kandel I, Omar HA. Adolescence, violence, and public health. *Front Public Health* 2013; 1: 1–2.

42. Richter L, Komarek A, Desmond C, et al. Reported physical and sexual abuse in childhood and adult HIV risk behaviour in three African countries: findings from Project Accept (HPTN-043). *AIDS Behav* 2013; 18: 381–389.

43. Yon Y, Mikton C, Gassoumis Z, Wilber K. Elder abuse prevalence in community settings: a systematic review and meta-analysis. *Lancet Glob Health* 2017; 5: e147–e156.

44. Anetzberger G. *The Clinical Management of Elder Abuse*. New York: Hawthorne Press, 2004.

45. Lindbloom EJ, Brandt J, Hough L, Meadows SE. Elder mistreatment in the nursing home: a systematic review. *J Am Med Dir Assoc* 2007; 8: 610–616.

46. Centers for Disease Control and Prevention. Elder Abuse: Risk and Protective Factors Available at: https://www.cdc.gov/violenceprevention/elderabuse/riskprotectivefactors.html (accessed 20 March 2018).

47. Hsieh C-C, Pugh MD. Poverty, income inequality, and violent crime: a meta-analysis of recent aggregate data studies. *Crim Justice Rev* 1993; 18: 182–202.

48. Pickett KE, Wilkinson RG. Income inequality and health: a causal review. *Soc Sci Med* 2015; 128: 316–326.

49. James SE, Johnson J, Raghavan C, Lemos T, Barakett M, Woolis D. The violent matrix: a study of structural, interpersonal, and intrapersonal violence among a sample of poor women. *Am J Community Psychol* 2003; 31: 129–141.

50. Winton A. Urban violence : a guide to the literature. *Environ Urban* 2004; 16: 165–184.

51. Giddens A. *Sociology*, 6th ed. London: Polity Press, 2011.

52. Muggah R. Researching the urban dilemma: urbanization, poverty and violence. Available at: https://www.idrc.ca/sites/default/files/sp/Images/Researching-the-Urban-Dilemma-Baseline-study.pdf (accessed 20 March 2018).

53. Centers for Disease Control and Prevention. The Social-Ecological Model: A Framework for Violence Prevention. Available at: https://www.cdc.gov/violenceprevention/pdf/sem_framewrk-a.pdf (accessed 20 March 2018).

54. Polan J, Sieving R, McMorris B. Are young adolescents' social and emotional skills protective against involvement in violence and bullying behaviors? *Health Promot Pract* 2013; 14: 599–606.

55. Hardaway C, McLoyd V, Wood D. Exposure to violence and socioemotional adjustment in low-income youth: an examination of protective factors. *Am J Community Psychol* 2014; 49: 112–126.

56. DeVoe ER, Dean K, Traube D, McKay MM. The SURVIVE community project: a family-based intervention to reduce the impact of violence exposures in urban youth. *J Aggress Maltreat Trauma* 2005; 11: 95–116.

57. Chamberlain L. Comprehensive Review of Interventions for Children Exposed to Domestic Violence. Available at: http://promising.futureswithoutviolence.org/files/2012/01/Comprehensive-Review-of-Interventions-for-Children-Exposed-to-Domestic-Violence-FINAL.pdf (accessed 20 March 2018).

58. Greene M. Chronic exposure to violence and poverty: Interventions that work for youth. *Crime Delinq* 1993; 39: 106–124.

59. DiClemente RJ, Wingood GM, Rose E, Sales JM, Crosby RA. Evaluation of an HIV/STD sexual risk-reduction intervention for pregnant African American adolescents attending a prenatal clinic in an urban public hospital: preliminary evidence of efficacy. *J Pediatric Adolesc Gynecol* 2010; 23: 32–38.

60. Kiely M, El-mohandes AAE, El-khorazaty MN, Gantz MG. An integrated intervention to reduce intimate partner violence in pregnancy: a randomized trial. *Obstet Gynecol* 2011; 115: 273–283.

61. Rotheram-Borus MJ, Tomlinson M, Roux I Le, Stein JA. Alcohol use, partner violence, and depression: a cluster randomized controlled trial among urban South African mothers over 3 years. *Am J Prev Med* 2015; 49: 715–725.

62. Pronyk PM, Hargreaves JR, Kim JC, et al. Effect of a structural intervention for the prevention of intimate-partner violence and HIV in rural South Africa: a cluster randomised trial. *Lancet* 2006; 368: 1973–1983.

63. Gupta J, Falb KL, Lehmann H, et al. Gender norms and economic empowerment intervention to reduce intimate partner violence against women in rural Côte d'Ivoire: a randomized controlled pilot study. *BMC Int Health Hum Rights* 2013; 13: 46.

64. Cameron M, Cockcroft A, Waichigo GW, Marokoane N, Laetsang D, Andersson N. From knowledge to action: participant stories of a population health intervention to reduce gender violence and HIV in three southern African countries. *AIDS Care* 2014; 26: 1534–1540.

65. Falb KL, Diaz-Olavarrieta C, Campos PA, et al. Evaluating a health care provider delivered intervention to reduce intimate partner violence and mitigate associated health risks: study protocol for a randomized controlled trial in Mexico City. *BMC Public Health* 2014; 14: 772.

66. Taha F, Zhang H, Snead K, et al. Effects of a culturally informed intervention on abused, suicidal African American women. *Cultur Divers Ethnic Minor Psychol* 2015; 21: 560–570.

67. Enriquez M, Kelly PJ, Cheng AL, Hunter J, Mendez E. An Intervention to address interpersonal violence among low-income midwestern Hispanic-American teens. *J Immigr Minor Health* 2012; 14: 292–299.

68. Cleary Bradley RP, Gottman JM. Reducing situational violence in low-income couples by fostering healthy relationships. *J Marital Fam Ther* 2012; 38(Suppl. 1): 187–198.

69. Zlotnick C, Street D. An interpersonally based intervention for low-income pregant women with intimate partner violence: a pilot study. *Arch Womens Ment Health* 2011; 14: 55–65.

CHAPTER 51

Non-governmental organizations and mental health

Marguerite Regan, Jenny Edwards, and Iris Elliott

Introduction

In the last two decades, the understanding of mental health has expanded from the traditional, biomedical model that dominated historically, to a broader perspective that takes into account the social, environmental, and economic determinants of mental health, human rights and equality.

There is increasing understanding about the interplay and impact of poor mental health on society and the opportunities both to prevent mental health problems from developing and escalating and to recover from mental health problems, as well as how to stay mentally well.

Despite this, mental health is still, for the most part, a neglected issue in countries' public health services and non-governmental organization (NGO) programmes of work. This is unfortunate given how well-placed NGOs are to play a transformative role in improving the lives of people living with mental health problems. They can be central to improving the mental health of communities, particularly those with higher exposure to risk and fewer opportunities to protect and promote their mental health. This is even more pertinent in low- and middle-income countries (LAMICs), where poverty compounds the issue, and there is a lack of mental health clinicians, limited services, and high levels of mental health stigma and discrimination.

In this chapter, we will examine the contribution of NGOs to meeting the mental health needs of individuals, families, and communities.

Definitions and international overview

It can be argued that almost all NGOs have a role within public mental health, as they address the complex challenges of the social, economic, and environmental contexts in which people live and which determine their mental health. Considerable public mental health improvement could be achieved if, for example, non-mental health NGOs purposefully and systematically considered how they could lever their activities to enhance the mental health of the people with whom they work and within the policies for which they advocate. However, the focus of this chapter is on mental health NGOs.

Defining mental health non-governmental organizations

NGOs are formal, independent institutions, which play a vital role in society by building social capital, trust and shared values, and bringing about positive changes.

The United Nations (UN) coined the term 'non-governmental organization' in 1945 to mean a not-for-profit, voluntary citizens' group, which is organized on a local, national, or international level to address issues in support of the public good. However, the term is not used consistently across the world, and the sector is populated by extremely diverse organizations with heterogeneous missions and structures; sometimes making it difficult to distinguish what is and what is not a NGO.

NGOs are part of civil society, with is sometimes referred to as the third sector, alongside other entities such as faith-based organizations, trade unions, think tanks, and other organizations that are neither private nor state run. Civil society organizations are defined by the Organisation for Economic Co-operation and Development to

> include all non-market and non-state organizations outside of the family in which people organize themselves to pursue shared interests in the public domain. Examples include community-based organizations and village associations, environmental groups, women's rights groups, farmers' associations, faith-based organizations, labour unions, co-operatives, professional associations, chambers of commerce, independent research institutes and the not-for-profit media [1].

Although the focus of this chapter is specifically on NGOs, it is important to note that all civil society organizations are relevant to public mental health, and play a key role at local, regional, national, and global levels, given their identity-specific activities that can often target those at great risk of mental health problems, and their role in mobilizing and advocating for change on determinants of mental health.

For the purpose of this chapter, we will be discussing NGOs that encompass the following characteristics:

◆ were not created to generate profit, although they may engage in income generating ventures and use the revenue to deliver their work;

- were formed voluntarily;
- have a formal or institutional status, which distinguishes them from ad hoc groups;
- are independent of government, authorities, for-profit organizations, and political parties (although funding may compromise this independence);
- act in the public sphere to address issues in support of the public good.

The role of mental health non-governmental organizations

NGOs tend to be task-orientated and perform a variety of functions, depending on their particular strengths, in order to support people with mental health problems. These range from supporting individual's needs, plugging service gaps, building capacity, and advocating for policy and investment to providing technical expertise, undertaking research, raising awareness to tackle stigma and discrimination, and campaigning for human rights' protection. Despite differences in approach and function, NGOs working with people with mental health problems tend to share a similar ethos and understanding of mental health that allows them to engage, involve, and support appropriately [2].

Service provision

Most NGOs working in mental health focus on undertaking assessment and providing a diagnosis, supplying interventions and treatments, and providing rehabilitation services in order to fill gaps in state provision. Some do this through hospital-based care, but many NGOs develop outreach and community-based programmes, which often have a preventative and co-productive character aimed at avoiding escalation of issues that would lead to hospital treatment being required. One such example is Clubhouse International, which through its 320 local Clubhouses around the world offer people living with mental health problems access to physical and mental health care and services, as well as housing, employment, and education support, in a safe and supportive community environment.[1]

NGOs often develop multifaceted and integrated intervention approaches, including using support groups, because such peer and self-management modalities are much more efficient to provide than individual treatment when resources are limited, and have proven to be effective, particularly when they resonate with social and cultural norms.

Capacity building

Many parts of the world lack specialist mental health personnel. NGOs address this by building the skills of existing staff and community members through running in-house training, or providing staff and community members with opportunities to undertake external courses and workshops. BasicNeeds, a UK NGO working across Africa and Asia, has developed a social enterprise programme for capacity building of local Ugandan NGOs in areas they cannot reach, supporting them to incorporate mental health work into their work, which they are currently

evaluating to find out if it is as effective and cost-efficient as delivering services directly.[2] The Mental Health Action Trust in India has developed a model of free, comprehensive mental health care involving local partners and volunteers being trained to function as volunteer care workers, known as mental health care coordinators, to increase the mental health care available across Kerala.[3]

There are numerous courses offered online, both free and costed, that NGO staff can access developed by universities and other NGOs. Digital platforms can make an important contribution in the provision of mental health care and support, and capacity building. Coursea offers free online courses developed by universities on a range of mental health topics.[4] A full video training package for using the World Health Organization (WHO) Mental Health Gap Action Programme (mhGAP),[5] designed for non-specialized healthcare professionals by the WHO and International Medical Corps is a good example of cross-organisational collaboration.[6]

Some NGOs build the capacity of people with lived experience of mental health problems, and actively encourage the participation of individuals and communities in the development and delivery of mental health policies, processes, and services. Batyr is an Australian NGO that trains young people to speak about their mental health problems so they can deliver peer-to-peer programmes, reduce stigma, and encourage help seeking.[7] Together is one example of many English charities working alongside people with mental health issues on their journey towards independent and fulfilling lives.[8]

Advocacy

NGOs are often tasked with bringing stakeholders' concerns to government, to assist government in developing policy solutions, and helping to monitor the development and implementation of policies and agreements, especially in relation to human rights. A recent successful advocacy campaign supported heavily by NGOs was the FundaMental SDG campaign, undertaken initially to ensure mental health was represented in the UN post-2015 Sustainable Development Goals (SDGs), and then campaigned for mental health specific objectives (discussed in more detail on page 491) [3].

Change is also pursued by responding to government and authorities' calls for evidence through written consultations or stakeholder engagement, which give NGOs an opportunity to inform the development of policy and practice by sharing their experiences and the experiences of their stakeholders, and bringing relevant research to policymakers' attention.

Advocacy is often most effectively applied at local level when NGOs have an open dialogue with local authorities and elected

---

[1] Clubhouse International: http://clubhouse-intl.org/

[2] BasicNeeds: http://www.basicneeds.org/
[3] Mental Health Action trust (MHAT): http://mhatkerala.org/home.html
[4] Coursera: https://www.coursera.org/
[5] mhGAP aims to scale up services for mental, neurological, and substance use disorders for countries, especially those of low and middle income (http://www.who.int/mental_health/mhgap/en/).
[6] mhGAP training videos can be watched on YouTube: https://www.youtube.com/user/mhGAPtraining
[7] BATYR: http://www.batyr.com.au/
[8] Together UK: http://www.together-uk.org/

representatives to make the case for the introduction of services, changes to the way they operate, raising standards, or to seek practical support for the efforts of the community itself. Citizens, a group of people who have experienced mental health issues, homelessness, addictions, or contact with criminal justice, have developed an evaluation model that involves locals being trained to evaluate services and provide feedback and recommendations to local authorities [4].

Expertise

NGOs are often in a strong and trusted position that allows them to provide analysis and technical expertise to governments and authorities. Their independence of political structures means they are often in place longer than political regimes and can bring a historical perspective to new governing bodies. They are also able to provide locally sourced information and to draw on real-life experience that may be unknown or unavailable to governments. Combined, these factors give some NGOs the authority to exert real influence on the development of policies and programmes by participating in national and international meetings, conferences, and negotiations. In 2015 mental health NGOs including Mind and Rethink provided technical expertise during the development of NHS England's 'Five Year Forward View for Mental Health' [5].

Research

Traditionally, NGOs were primarily involved in service provision and advocacy-related activities, with research seen as an activity restricted to academia. However, some NGOs, such as the UK's Mental Health Foundation, have strong research functions. Established in 1949 its charitable purpose is to develop the mental health evidence base, produce evidence-based public information to promote public awareness, and advocate for innovative supports and services for people with mental health problems and their families. The Foundation has become a leader in involving people with lived experience in research, such as their landmark 'Strategies for Living' programme, which investigated support and strategies found to be helpful in the lives of people with mental health problems, the 'Right Here' programme, which worked with young people, and the Peer Research Collective currently being hosted in Scotland [6]. McPin is a mental health research NGO that focuses on research by experts by experience.[9]

Increasingly, NGOs are participating in or developing action-orientated research programmes to evaluate the effect of their work on mental health, creating a stronger evidence base for advocating to governments and funders to secure further investment in mental health. Often, the research undertaken by NGOs is seen as innovative and ground-breaking [7]. The Charity Evaluation Working Group (CHeW) is an evaluation community of practice and peer support for evaluation and research managers in the third sector that is working to improve the monitoring and evaluation being done by UK NGOs. Survivor Research UK has developed as a virtual collective of people with lived experience of mental health problems, particularly those from black, Asian, and minority ethnic and marginalized groups, who offer consulting services in designing, conducing, and delivering research, evaluation, and training initiatives.[10]

Stigma and discrimination

Stigma and discrimination can be as damaging as the symptoms experienced by someone with a mental health problem.[11] The fear of stigma can prevent help-seeking by people experiencing a crisis or their families; and stigma exposes people and their families to discrimination in their communities, educational settings, and workplaces, and may lead to experiences of abuse and violence such as hate crime. Many mental health NGOs have tackling stigma and discrimination as part of their core remit, given its terrible impact on peoples' mental health, help-seeking behaviours, and ability to reach their full potential and participate within society. Shifting societies' negative and dangerous perceptions of mental health is often done through programmes based on social contact such as See Me in Scotland,[12] and social marketing such as Time to Change in England.[13] Other campaigns use celebrities' experiences of mental health problems to tacking stigma and get conversations starting, such as the Heads Together campaign featuring Prince Harry and Lady Gaga.[14] The Global Anti-Stigma Alliance brings together such campaigns to share innovation, evidence, and resources.[15]

History of mental health NGOs

As previously mentioned, historically NGOs had mental health care, treatment, and rehabilitation as their main priorities, developing adapted models to respond to need and suit the situation. Many mental health NGOs, especially in LAMICs, were founded by psychiatrists, giving their mission a clinical focus, although the approach was often a more holistic one than that taken in conventional mental health settings.

Severe mental health problems, suicide, and substance abuse were key areas of concern for NGOs during the 1980s and 1990s, often driven by prominent media coverage of these issues. More recently, given the expanded knowledge around mental health and prevalence rates of common mental health problems, anxiety and depression are increasingly being identified by NGOs as major threats to quality of life and well-being, which need to be tackled because of their widespread and pervasive impact on population health.

Most mental health NGOs have diversified from the traditional activities they began with, such as providing services, to integrate other activities and functions into their work, including conducting research, or dealing with the social or legal issues related to mental health.

Many NGOs that emerged from the disability rights movements have integrated mental health into their work owing to the significant human rights' violations experienced by people with mental health problems, particularly around deprivation of liberty, coerced and intrusive treatment, and capacity. A key example of this is the British Institute for Human Rights, which has delivered a programme for people with mental health problems and their carers to

---

[9] http://mcpin.org/
[10] Survivor Research UK: http://www.survivor-research.com/

[11] National Consortium on Stigma and Empowerment: http://www.stigmaandempowerment.org/dr-corrigans-lab
[12] See Me Scotland: https://www.seemescotland.org/
[13] Time to Change: http://www.time-to-change.org.uk/
[14] Heads Together: https://www.headstogether.org.uk/
[15] The Global Anti-Stigma Alliance: http://www.time-to-change.org.uk/globalalliance

understand and apply their human rights, and to advocate within national, and international systems [8].

Although it is still not as widespread as one would hope, NGOs working on physical health and disability issues have also started to expand their remit to include mental health. It will be interesting to track the impact of the UN convention on the Rights of Persons with Disabilities regarding intersectionality across different disabilities: physical, sensory, intellectual, and psychosocial. This is key to achieving parity and integration of mental health into public health, as it allows for mental health not to be dealt with in a 'silo' but instead located within a holistic framing of health. An example of this is England's Smoking and Mental Health Partnership, which brings together NGOs that focus on cancer, smoking cessation, and non-communicable diseases with mental health charities, to combat smoking among people with mental health problems. This is a public health priority as smoking rates among people with a mental health problems are more than double that of the general population [9].

There has also been an increasing focus on programmes of work to support families and carers of people affected by mental health problems, for example Siblings Australia[16] and Children of Parents with a Mental Illness.[17] Box 51.1 describes the difference between NGOs that are led by professionals and those run by people with lived experience.

Current policy frameworks and levers

As well as implementing mental health programmes at various levels and reaching remote and neglected groups and populations, NGOs advocate for public health policy too. NGOs have played a key role in driving forward the mental health policy agenda and ensuring it is now a priority for many countries and at an international level.

The last decade has seen a significant shift in the acknowledgement and understanding of mental health as a driver of individual, community, economic, and societal health and success. Here are some of the recent policy developments that NGOs played a role in.

2006: The United Nations Convention on the Rights of Persons with Disability

The UN Convention on the Rights of Persons with Disability (UNCRPD) has created a 'climate of change', with its adoption of a social model of disability [10]. The Convention does not create any new human rights but rather represents a highly engaged, global exercise in the interpretation and framing of existing civil, political, economic, social, and cultural rights by members of the disability movement. UNCRPD includes Article 32 International Cooperation, which drives solidarity by requiring international development programmes to be inclusive and accessible; facilitating and supporting capacity building; facilitating research and access to scientific and technical expertise; and providing technical and economic assistance [11]. The UN keeps a live register of Member States, which have signed and ratified the Convention [11].

Mental health NGOs play an important role in ensuring the implementation of Member States' international, regional, and national human rights commitments, aided by the system of

---

Box 51.1 Professional led versus user led

It is useful to note the distinction between NGOs led by professionals and NGOs where service users and people with lived experience lead the organization. The latter are sometimes referred to as the 'fourth sector', and those involved often also have relevant professional training but became engaged primarily as a result of their personal experience. User/lived experience-led groups are emerging as key drivers of change in some countries by advocating for mental health through voicing their own experiences. They are often best placed to lead transformations in how mental health is viewed and tackled, owing to their personal and collective expertise, commitment to place people with lived experience and carers at the heart of their approach, and motivation to find practical solutions that will work in the local context. Research has shown that service users want other users or people with lived experience as their advocates because they feel that the experience of having a mental health problem may not be fully appreciated by a professional without such personal experience.

The National Survivor User Network (NSUN) is an independent, service user-led charity in England whose mission is 'to create a network which will engage and support the wide diversity of mental health services users and survivors across England to strengthen the user voice'.[1] In Nepal, the National Mental Health Service User Organisation, KOSHISH, provides emergency support for women abandoned by their families because of their mental health problems, and advocate for mental health services. In 2014 they were successful in getting the government to establish a mental health unit (www.koshishnepal.org).

Governments need to recognize the validity of the lived experience/service-user perspective and give it similar weight to clinical opinion. It is important that professional-led organizations support the development of user-led advocacy organizations by supporting them to develop the skills, knowledge, and networks to be effective [34]. This is not to diminish the work done by professional-led NGOs, who highly value the involvement of people with lived experience, families, and other stakeholders in their work.

1 http://www.nsun.org.uk/

National Human Rights Institutions and other human rights architecture.

2013: World Health Organization Mental Health Action Plan

The adoption of the WHO Mental Health Action Plan in 2013 was a game changer for the prioritization of mental health by Member States [12]. The strategy recognized clearly the contribution of NGOs to improving the state of public mental health and called for:

- NGOs to strengthen governance for mental health by helping 'to create more effective and accountable policies, laws and services for mental health in a manner consistent with international and regional human rights instruments' (p. 11);

---

[16] Siblings Australia: http://siblingsaustralia.org.au/
[17] Children of Parents with a Mental Illness: http://www.copmi.net.au/

◆ 'greater collaboration with "informal" mental health providers (including) local nongovernmental organisations' (p. 14);

◆ data collected and submitted by NGOs to be used to supplement and expand the information gathered through mental health systems in relation to the extent of the problem, scale of interventions, and services, as well as health and other outcomes (p. 19);

◆ the establishment of NGO-run community mental health services to be supported (p. 25).

2015: Sustainable Development Goals

On an international development level, mental health was largely omitted from the Millennium Development Goals, which were a set of eight development targets in place from 2000 to 2015 [13]. The development of a post-2015 set of targets by the UN, known as the Sustainable Development Goals (SDGs), was also in danger of neglecting mental health, despite the increased prioritization that had occurred in the intervening years. Campaigners recognized that it required a dedicated target to ensure that mental health is a priority issue for governments.

A global initiative campaigning for the inclusion of mental health in the SDGs, known as 'FundaMentalSDG', emerged, driven primarily by academics and the NGO sector [4]. The consortium gained the support of the UK government, illustrated by a report on Mental Health for Sustainable Development published by the Westminster All Party Parliamentary Group for Global Health. This report recommended that the UK should lobby for the inclusion of the following mental health target within the Health Goal in the SDGs:

> The provision of mental and physical health and social care services for people with mental disorders, in parity with resources for services addressing physical health and working towards universal coverage [14].

Following the success of this campaign, the FundaMentalSDG campaigners then advocated for powerful mental health indicators to be included in the UN action plan, which resulted in one indicator on suicide mortality rate and another on coverage of treatment interventions for substance use disorders [15].

2016: World Bank/World Health Organization Joint Meeting on Mental Health

'Out of the Shadows: Making Mental Health a Global Priority' was a 2-day event co-hosted by The World Bank and the WHO in 2016. Its aim was to move mental health from the margins by engaging finance ministers, multi- and bilateral organizations, the business community, NGOs, and others in a conversation about the urgent investments needed in mental health services, and the expected returns in terms of health, social, and economic benefits. The objectives were: (i) to present the case for investing in mental health; (ii) to identify entry points for renewed action and investment at the country, regional, and global levels, including consideration of financing mechanisms for enhanced financial and social protection, as well as expanded service access; and (iii) to mobilize a global coalition for action for scaled-up implementation [16].

Mapping mental health non-governmental organizations across the world

The extent to which mental health is a key focus for NGOs across the world varies widely between regions. Some NGOs focus solely on mental health and others incorporate it as part of their programmes, but often NGOs do not address it at all because they see it as outside their remit.

The evolving concept of mental health and its intrinsic links to equity, poverty, race, and gender means that the range of NGOs working directly and indirectly on improving mental health of individuals and communities is both wide ranging and diverse. However, because the relationship between social determinants and mental health is not widely known, understood, or tracked in outcomes, the full impact of this work is unknown, unrecognized, and unreported. There is currently no accurate count of how many NGOs include mental health as part of their mission, but the numbers are limited [17].

International networks

Regional and global communities of mental health organizations have begun to emerge in the last decade, enabled largely by advances in technology and increased access to the Internet. The next subsections outline some of the major networks that are active.

The Movement for Global Mental Health

The Movement for Global Mental Health (MGMH) is a network of individuals and organizations that aims to improve services for people living with mental health problems, especially in LAMICs. MGMH emerged from a Call to Action in the first *Lancet* series on global mental health in 2007 [18] and has grown consistently since then to a membership of approximately 200 institutions, a majority of which are NGOs. MGMH enables members to network, share knowledge, join national and international campaigning, and participate in a biannual summit. See http://globalmentalhealth.org

Mental Health and Psychosocial Support Network

The Mental Health and Psychosocial Support Network (MHPSS) is an online platform that enables organizations to share resources and information related to mental health and psychosocial support, both in emergency settings and in situations of chronic hardship. By promoting the sharing of practical advice and resources on both proven and promising interventions, MHPSS intends to improve the effectiveness and sustainability of services provided to vulnerable people experiencing the immediate, short-term, and long-term social and mental health consequences of natural disasters, armed conflict, chronic poverty, and devastating epidemics such as HIV/AIDS and Ebola. Groups and forums discuss real-time emergencies, such as the Nepal Earthquake in 2015; this allows those on the ground and in-country to give and share up-to-date information, while also getting support from those with expertise and previous relevant experience elsewhere. See: http://www.mhpss.net

Mental Health Europe

This European umbrella NGO has a mission to promote mental health, prevent mental health problems, and protect and advance the interests of all people with mental health problems and their carers. It does this by lobbying the European Union, the WHO, and the Council of Europe, and sharing information through conferences and publications. See: https://mhe-sme.org

Mental Health Innovation Network

Established in 2013 through funding from Grand Challenges Canada, and supported by teams at the Centre for Global Mental Health and

MHNGOs represented on MHIN by region

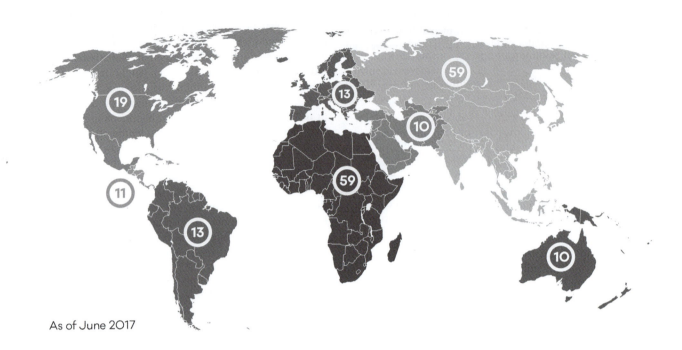

As of June 2017

Fig. 51.1 Mental Health Innovation Network-derived map of mental health non-governmental organizations and activity.

WHO, the Mental Health Innovation Network (MHIN) is a network for the global mental health community to communicate and share knowledge, experiences, and resources to improve the quality and coverage of care. Users sign up to become MHIN members and contribute actively to the site. Its aim is to enable learning, build partnerships, disseminate knowledge, and leverage resources.

As of June 2018, MHIN has over 4500 individual members and nearly 280 live organization profiles. MHIN has developed a unique database of innovations, which catalogues comprehensive summaries of mental health programmes and projects currently showcasing over 150 examples from around the world. The map in Fig. 51.1 shows the spread of mental health NGOs in 2017 registered on the network. On the website, you can further break down the work being undertaken in each region by specific population groups supported (e.g. children and adolescents, minority populations) and the type of work they are undertaking (e.g. advocacy, task sharing). See: http://www.mhinnovation.net

CitiesRISE (formerly mhNOW)
Initially branded mhNOW, CitiesRISE is a multi-stakeholder initiative to catalyse, connect, and support cities committed to driving change in the field of mental health. CitiesRISE has built its approach around four core programmes: Local Collective Action; Young people and Youth Leadership; Innovation and Acceleration; Learning Collaborative.[18]

UK Perspective: public mental health and prevention
Despite the UK's strong international presence in many health areas, there are currently only a few UK-based international NGOs that focus on mental health or include mental health as part of their wider remit. These include Voluntary Service Overseas, BasicNeeds, and International Medical Corps. There are several initiatives underway to increase the number of UK international NGOs working on mental health. One such initiative is the recently established mental health subgroup of the Bond Disability and Development group. Bond is the UK membership body for NGOs working in international development, which promotes, supports, represents, and (on occasion) leads the work and interests of UK international development organizations that are united by the common goal to rededicate global poverty. The subgroup was established to influence UK stakeholders to do more on mental health and share learning and good practice between those already working on mental health and those who are interested in doing more.[19]

Domestically, the UK has a strong mental health charity sector although, as in the rest of the world, the focus is generally on service provision and advocacy. Several strong coalitions and alliances have been established to move forward the mental health agenda in the UK, detailed in Table 51.1.

---

[18] CitiesRISE: http://cities-rise.org/

[19] Bond Disability and Development Group: https://www.bond.org.uk/groups

Table 51.1 List of current mental health coalitions and alliances within the UK

Coalition/alliance	Description	Area covered
Alliance for Mental Health Research Funders (http://www.amhrf.org.uk/)	15 charities and foundations working to improve and increase mental health research in the UK	UK
Association for Mental Health Providers (https://amhp.org.uk)	The leading voice representing voluntary sector mental health service providers across England	England
Children and Young People's Mental Health Coalition (http://www.cypmhc.org.uk/)	A coalition of charities launched in 2010 that come together and speak as one on behalf of children and young people's mental health	England
Health and Social Care Alliance Scotland (https://www.alliance-scotland.org.uk)	An alliance of over 1700 organizations, NGOs, and individuals working together to ensure the voice of people who are disabled, living with long-term conditions, or delivering unpaid care are heard	Scotland
Heads Together (https://www.headstogether.org.uk/)	Heads Together brings together a team of charities working on mental health issues driven by an interest of The Duke and Duchess of Cambridge and Prince Harry	UK
Human Rights Alliance (https://www.bihr.org.uk/alliance)	A network of over 150 organizations from across the UK committed to protecting human rights and the Human Rights Act	UK
Maternal Mental Health Alliance (http://maternalmentalhealthalliance.org/)	A coalition of national professional and patient organizations committed to improving the mental health and well-being of women and their children during pregnancy and the first postnatal year	UK
MEAM (Making Every Adult Matter) (http://meam.org.uk/)	A coalition of Clinks, Homeless Link, and Mind, formed to improve policy and services for people facing multiple needs	England
Mental Health Alliance (http://www.mentalhealthalliance.org.uk)	A coalition of 75 organizations working together to advocate for fair implementation of the Mental Health Act in England and Wales	England and Wales
Mental Health and Smoking Partnership (http://smokefreeaction.org.uk/smokefree-nhs/smoking-and-mental-health/)	A coalition of mental health and public health organizations initiated to drive forward the recommendations in the Smoking and Mental Health Action report 'The Stolen Years' [31]	UK
Mental Health Challenge (http://www.mentalhealthchallenge.org.uk/)	A coalition set up to support and encourage local authorities to take a proactive approach in implementing a mental health strategy and improving mental health in their communities by becoming mental health champions	England
Mental Health Policy Group [32]	Six national mental health charities working together to improve mental health by influencing policy	England
National Survivor User Network (NSUN) (http://www.nsun.org.uk/)	A user-led network of individuals, groups, and allies that allows members to network, access information, share examples, and contribute to policy and practice debates and issues	England
National Voices (http://www.nationalvoices.org.uk/)	A coalition of health and social care charities calling for health and care systems to be person centred	England
The Scottish Mental Health Partnership [33]	The Scottish Mental Health Partnership provides a collective, strategic voice calling for radical change to mental health in Scotland	Scotland
The Wales Alliance for Mental Health (http://www.mentalhealthwales.net/mhw/voluntary_sector.php)	The collective voice of the 12 national voluntary organizations in Wales working in the field of mental health	Wales
Together For You (http://www.togetherforyou.org.uk/)	10 NGOs engaged in public mental health programme collaboration and policy advocacy	Northern Ireland
Voices Of eXperience (VOX) (http://voxscotland.org.uk/about-vox-scotland/)	A member-led organization representing members' views to Scotland's politicians and health professionals to make sure Scotland's laws and mental health services reflect service user needs and interests	Scotland
We Need to Talk Coalition	A coalition of mental health charities, professional organizations, Royal Colleges, and service providers who campaign for better access to therapies for people with mental health problems.	England, Wales

Note. NGO: non-governmental organization.

Contribution of non-governmental organizations

NGOs make significant contributions to mental health beyond the activities already described: service provision, capacity building, advocacy, expertise, research, stigma, and discrimination campaigns. Their character, as defined earlier, means that they make important interventions in disrupting and challenging common discourses about mental health to reframe the conventional viewpoints and re-focus discussions on finding solutions. These are practices that engage and transform relationships and structures of power, most obviously between legal systems, clinicians, people with lived experiences, and their families and carers.

Working from a social justice ethos, NGOs:

◆ draw on the expertise of beneficiaries, their families/carers, workers and volunteers;

◆ employ new and novel evidence collected from seldom-heard and often disempowered individuals and communities, including refugees, migrants, trafficked people, and destitute groups;

◆ dynamically evolve innovative practice, research, and advocacy;

◆ interpret and transmit their knowledge and lessons to decision-makers;

◆ inform public discourse through awareness raising and campaigning activities.

The ethos and character of NGOs creates opportunities to influence public mental health in socially and culturally specific ways that engage and respond to the context, and are therefore more effective. Rather than simply replicating Global North models of mental health provision and public mental health, NGOs promote localized solutions that are often founded on human rights and solidarity. These include peer support (person to person and community to community) and self-management. In places where public services are limited or absent, NGOs are critical, but even where services exist NGOs can model innovation that connects co-created interventions to the people they are intended to benefit.

Such approaches are uniquely grounded in social movements, including lived experience/psychiatric survivor/service-user movements and movements of at-risk populations. One key element of the approach of NGOs is their focus on distinct populations, who are often at the margins of society and not easily accessed by conventional health services. These include people with physical or intellectual disabilities; indigenous peoples; women; lesbian, gay, and bisexual people; transgender people; refugees and asylum seekers; black, Asian, and minority ethnic communities; homeless and trafficked people; Travellers; religious minorities; victims of violence; people who have experienced trauma or abuse; families and carers of people with mental health problems; and people with mental health problems themselves. Transnational social movements are particularly important for groups experiencing marginalization, discrimination, and violence within their own countries; and these groups benefit from NGOs' ability to lever protection and change through human rights advocacy and legal challenge.

Human rights

There has been a welcome shift towards a rights-based approach to health in the last decade, which has given NGOs a strong position, owing to their longstanding and established role advocating for the use of human rights as guiding principles in the development of policy, programmes, and practice. Taking a human rights-based approach involves empowering the marginalized and vulnerable in society to know and claim their rights; ensuring developments do no undermine or constrain human rights; actively ending practices that are discriminatory; and increasing accountability [19].

There has been welcome UN focus on mental health through the selection of depression as the theme for World Mental Health Day 2017. The statement by the Special Rapporteur, Mr Dainius Pūras, on the right of everyone to the enjoyment of the highest attainable standard of physical and mental health, noted the recognition of mental health as a human development imperative in the Sustainable Development 2030 Agenda and highlighted that a human rights' lens is increasingly being used to scrutinize legal, policy, and service-level responses to mental health. He stated that:

> There can be no health without mental health and everyone is entitled to an environment that promotes health, well-being, and dignity [20].

This echoes his appeal on World Mental Health Day 2016 that 'dignity must prevail' [21]. In his report to the Human Rights Council (June 2017), the Special Rapporteur called on States to 'take immediate measures to establish inclusive and meaningful participatory frameworks in the design and decision-making around public policy, to include (…) users of services, civil society and those living in poverty and in the most vulnerable situations' [20].

Currently, a primary role for many mental health NGOs involves combating serious human rights violations from the extremes of chaining and caging to the more institutional issues around choice and freedom [22]. Once a person is diagnosed as having a mental health problem, that person often loses the autonomy to make decisions about his/her care and treatment, unlike with physical health problems. User-led NGOs are often leaders in emphasizing basic human rights, such as the right to be safe, the right to a home and family life, the right to health care, and the right to work. The Central Gauteng Mental Health Society in South Africa[20] and the Voices Of eXperience (VoX) in Scotland[21] are two examples of service user-led organizations that help empower people with lived experience by ensuring they are aware of their rights under national and international legislation.

Key challenges for non-governmental organizations

Mental health is an extremely heterogeneous health issue, which also translates to mental health NGOs, whose diverse beliefs, priorities, understandings, and approaches can make it difficult to develop a coordinated approach to public mental health.

There are many challenges that can hinder NGOs in their missions to support good mental health, related to funding, competing priorities, and the complexity of mental health.

Limited reach

Because many NGOs are based in urban settings, there can often be a lack of presence in rural and hard-to-reach areas. Many NGOs

---

[20] Central Gauteng Mental Health Society: http://www.mhinnovation.net/organisations/central-gauteng-mental-health-society

[21] Voices of eXperience (VoX) Scotland: http://voxscotland.org.uk/

have started to tackle this by expanding services to cover rural areas, partnering and capacity-building with local organizations already in place and using advances in technology. For the last 10 years, Rural and Remote Mental Health has been delivering mental health programmes and services to people living and working in rural and remote Australia to fill the gap in available support.[22]

Lack of prioritization

Globally, mental health is still not seen as a priority health condition by governments and health systems, despite its huge global burden, with physical health still dominating, although this is beginning to change slightly in high-income countries, illustrated by references to parity of esteem for mental health in almost all political party manifestos in the 2015 and 2017 UK general elections. The lack of visibility of people with mental health problems, because of being inpatients or being afraid to speak out because of stigma, means it is often absent from public discourse, except in extreme cases of self-harm and suicide, and therefore the burden on individuals, families, and communities goes unseen.

Lack of mental health services and professionals

Mental health NGOs are often left to fill the gap in mental health services, but often do not have adequate resources to employ specialist mental health staff, especially in countries already experiencing shortages of trained mental health human resources, such as India. A move toward community mental health-using task sharing, peers, and community champions is often the only viable option, as training psychiatrists and skilling-up nurses is a slow process [23], and, for the most part, charities have been left with this task owing to a lack of prioritization by governments and their access to those in low-income communities who are marginalized from mainstream services.

Funding

As with all NGOs, those working in mental health are reliant on often-unstable funding streams that hinder their ability to support fully or plan long-term. There are also the complications of competing issues, with funding streams and charitable giving often diverting unexpectedly to emerging issues and crises, which leave ongoing and stable mental health support a lower-priority area.

Traditionally, most NGOs have been dependent on the general public for their financial support and the limited group of funders that will support mental health programmes. The process of receiving funding from these sources is highly competitive. Currently, the main UK funders of international mental health work are the Department for International Development (DFID) and the Wellcome Trust, although their funding tends to be geared towards medically orientated research and evaluation. The All-Party Parliamentary Group report on 'Mental Health for Sustainable Development' called on DFID to support countries to implement the WHO Action Plan by conducting a review of its current strategies to consider its role in achieving the plan's objectives; to incorporate mental health impact metrics into its

existing programmes; and to commit to 'programme funding to scale up mental health projects that prove successful as part of DFID-funded research' [14].

The Canadian government took the unprecedented decision in 2012 to begin funding mental health programmes globally through Grand Challenges Canada. They have invested $39 million in 71 innovations across 28 countries.[23] The National Institute for Mental Health in the USA has also taken steps to increase the funding available to mental health charities worldwide, although it is often restricted to funding research.[24] The Gates Foundation, a prominent funder in global health, has been slow to get involved in funding mental health projects, and although the foundation has awarded nearly $600,000 for domestic mental health projects in the USA, and a similar amount to projects providing emotional and physiological support to children in Haiti after the 2010 earthquake, these are very small pots compared with the money the foundation is spending in other areas [24].

The origins of funding can have serious implications for the legitimacy of a mental health NGO, and there is an ongoing debate about accepting funding from donors such as the pharmaceutical industry, who can be seen by many as having a vested interest, even when there are no obvious conditions attached. This can be further complicated by NGOs sometimes not being aware of the source of the funding. Greater transparency from funding bodies is required to ensure mental health NGOs are making a conscious decision about where they take funding from. The Research Councils of the UK issued a joint statement on cross-disciplinary mental health research in August 2017, and in their first funding call to establish mental health research consortia required substantial involvement of NGOs [25].

Two of the major funders of the work done by mental health NGOs in the UK are Comic Relief[25] and the Big Lottery Fund.[26] MQ is a more recently established mental health charity in the UK that funds mental health research to be undertaken by scientists, universities and NGOs.[27]

However, with traditional funding streams from government and public bodies, charitable giving, and funders on the decline, many NGOs are now turning to research funding, and expanding their research capacity to access this. Others are introducing a social enterprise element to their programmes, such as subscriptions, as has been introduced by Big White Wall (UK)[28] or selling products, such as Mental Health First Aid, who deliver training on a large scale.[29]

Public trust

Historically, NGOs enjoyed a high degree of public trust and were seen as having an unbiased legitimacy to represent the concerns of stakeholders. However, recent controversies and scandals across the globe, including the misuse of funding and misuse of power, have damaged the sector's reputation in the public's eye. More regulation is being introduced to eliminate these issues, but it is to be seen if the damage can be undone.

---

[22] Rural and Remote Mental Health: http://www.rrmh.com.au/

[23] Grand Challenges Canada: http://www.grandchallenges.ca/who-we-are/
[24] NIH National Institute of Mental Health: https://www.nimh.nih.gov/index.shtml
[25] Comic Relief: http://www.comicrelief.com
[26] Big Lottery Fund: https://www.biglotteryfund.org.uk/
[27] MQ Mental Health: https://www.mqmentalhealth.org/
[28] Big White Wall: https://www.bigwhitewall.com/
[29] Mental Health First Aid England: http://mhfaengland.org/

Next steps to achieving non-governmental organization potential

Mental health is currently in the limelight, both across the UK and internationally, and NGOs have a key role to play in making the most of the opportunity to ensure the advancement of the public's mental health by playing their part as advocates, service providers, and innovators. There are some very concrete steps that NGOs working directly or peripherally on mental health can take to ensure parity for mental health within public strategies and investment.

Expand perspective to tackle the root causes of mental health problems

In the last two decades, the understanding of mental health has expanded from the traditional, biomedical model that dominated historically, to a broader perspective that considers the social, environmental, and economic determinants of mental health. NGOs must also update their thinking to ensure that factors such as experiences of violence, educational exclusion, homelessness, and unemployment as all considered within the remit of mental health, given the dynamic interaction between these and mental health.

For NGOs to have a lasting impact on the levels of good and poor mental health in the societies within which they operate, their work needs to help people to avoid or exit cycles of poverty and discrimination that compound mental health issues. This is likely to require capacity building, co-production practice and skill building, building on different cultural strengths in peer support, self-management, and community solidarity. An example of this is 'Zeebags', an income-generation component of the Friendship Bench Project in Zimbabwe. A group of women with mental health problems meet for peer support and during these sessions they make bags out of recycled plastic, which are sold in Harare and internationally. The proceeds go to the women to help them buy food and pay for other living expenses.[30]

NGOs whose work is focused on physical health, equality, human rights, social rights, empowerment, or economic security are all likely to be contributing to improving mental health, but the impact in this domain is not generally monitored or measured. It is important for NGOs to be aware that prevention, promotion, and treatment of mental health can also be a significant help for them to achieve their wider goals. Studies have shown the impact of mental health interventions in low-income countries in preventing social drift and supporting the economic well-being of the families concerned [26]. It is important that NGOs understand the interconnections of these issues and advocate for strategies that will address mental health and the economic, legal, and environmental circumstances that influence the key mental health inequalities within the societies they operate in. It is equally important that mental health professionals assist NGOs to implement community-based interventions and to institute public mental health programmes that are practical and pragmatic, particularly for communities where public services are scarce or non-existent.

The WHO Mental Health Action Plan [12] and the UN Resolution on Mental Health and Human Rights [27] are both potentially powerful advocacy tools to ensure governments follow through on their commitments to improving public mental health. One key element is for NGOs to ensure that service users and their family carers are involved as advocacy partners, in a meaningful way, in the development of mental health promotion, prevention, treatment, and recovery service development and improvement.

The WHO has developed a key resource for NGOs called the Mental Health Gap Action Programme (mhGAP), which is a set of non-specialized guidelines developed to reduce the mental health treatment gap in many countries and is currently being used in over 90 countries. Examples of NGOs using mhGAP include CBM and BasicNeeds [28].

Collaborate

It is important for NGOs to come together at local, national and international levels to share learnings, to present common concerns and to support each other. This will allow MHNGOs to increase awareness about mental health among others from outside the field and to allow opportunities for the exploration of avenues to integrate mental health into existing programmes and projects.

Public–private partnerships and task forces are common in other public health fields, such as HIV and cancer, but are not so common in mental health. For mental health NGOs to increase their impact it will be important to cross boundaries and begin to work in a coordinated way with the rest of civil society; with the business sector; with research institutions; and with academics. Pooling resources and expertise will expand the knowledge base and the impact of mental health initiatives. In 2015–16, the Global Agenda Council on Mental Health was convened by the World Economic Forum to do just that. The individuals involved all have experience in treating, investigating, and combating poor mental health, and used this to develop a seven-step guide for building mentally healthy workplaces [29].

ThriveNYC is a key example of collaboration at a local level. In 2015 the city of New York Mayor Bill de Blasio and First Lady of New York City Chirlane McCray initiated a mental health roadmap for New York; a comprehensive plan involving numerous stakeholders across the city, working toward six principles:[31]

1. Change the culture.

2. Act early.

3. Close treatment gaps.

4. Partner with communities.

5. Use data better.

6. Strengthen government's ability to lead.

This led to the Cities Thrive Coalition, a network of more than 185 cities across the USA coming together to develop innovate ways to address mental health challenges, and the model has since been adapted for London with ThriveLDN launched in summer 2017.[32]

---

[30] Friendship Bench Zimbabwe: https://www.friendshipbenchzimbabwe.org

[31] ThriveNYC: https://thrivenyc.cityofnewyork.us/
[32] ThriveLDN: http://thriveldn.co.uk/

Increase visibility of mental health

Mental health is often secondary to physical health in public policy and investment. NGOs have a big part to play in advocating for the visible prioritization of mental health within governments' agendas and among the public. Stigma, and the complexity of the causation and solutions to mental health problems, can both contribute to limited political attention. Using public health advocacy campaigns, information sharing, and the voices and experiences of people with lived experience of mental health problems can all help to raise awareness of the issue. The Time to Change campaign in England and Wales, and the See Me campaign in Scotland, are two key NGO-led anti-stigma campaigns aiming to do this by packaging compelling and valid information to change public attitudes, increase accurate media reporting, and demystify mental health.[33,34]

Continue to make the case for investing in mental health

Given the limited money in mental health, NGOs should ensure they monitor and evaluate their programmes to understand what is effective in impact and costs. This means making the case in funding applications for adequate evaluation budgets and using measures that will be meaningful for key audiences. In this way pilots developed by NGOs and shown to be high quality and successful can be more readily adopted by public sector services and government for replicability and scale up. CHeW is a relatively new evaluation community of practice and peer support for evaluation and research managers in the third sector, which is working to improve the monitoring and evaluation being done by NGOs.[35] A variety of tools and resources, such as return on investment analyses, are available, which can be used to show how investment in good public mental health practice pays off [30].

Mental health NGOs have a vital role in meeting the mental health needs of individuals, families, and communities. But to continue being effective there is a need for NGOs to be innovative and develop deeper relationships and stronger partnerships, outside of health and social care, with those working in the wider sectors, to ensure sectors are aligned with the social, economic, and environmental determinants of mental health, and to ensure sustainability, increase reach, and achieve change.

Acknowledgements

To ensure this chapter was as representative as possible, the authors reached out to a number of stakeholders to gather their views on the role of NGOs on mental health. We would like to thank the following for sharing thoughts, suggestions, and resources with us: Lord Nigel Crisp; Grace Ryan, Mental Health Innovation Network; Ellen Morgan, Grand Challenges Canada; Mark Jordans, War Child; Vikram Patel, Sangath; Tatiana Los, Basic Needs; Hannah Loryman, Bond.

[33] Time to Change: http://www.time-to-change.org.uk/
[34] See me Scotland: https://www.seemescotland.org/
[35] Charity Evaluation Working Group (ChEW): https://www.linkedin.com/groups/8266095/profile

References

1. OECD. How DAC members work with civil society organisations. Available at: https://www.oecd.org/dac/peer-reviews/Final_How_DAC_members_work_with_CSOs%20ENGLISH.pdf (accessed 28 March 2018).
2. Funk M. Mental Health and Development: Targeting People with Mental Health Problems as a Vulnerable Group. Geneva: WHO/Mental Health and Poverty Project, 2010. Available at: http://www.who.int/mental_health/policy/mhtargeting/en/ (accessed 28 March 2018).
3. #FundaMentalSDG. Mental Health Indicators for the UN Sustainable Development Goals (SDGs). Available at: http://www.fundamentalsdg.org/ (accessed 28 March 2018).
4. Expert Citizens. INSIGHT Evaluation ©2015. Available at: http://www.expertcitizens.org.uk/insight-standards/ (accessed 28 March 2018).
5. NHS England. The Five Year Forward View for Mental Health. Available at: https://www.england.nhs.uk/wp-content/uploads/2016/02/Mental-Health-Taskforce-FYFV-final.pdf (accessed 28 March 2018).
6. Mental Health Foundation. Research strategy and approach. Available at: https://www.mentalhealth.org.uk/our-work/research/strategy-and-approach (accessed 28 March 2018).
7. Patel V, Thara R (eds). *Meeting Mental Health Needs in Developing Countries: NGO Innovations in India.* New Delhi: Sage, 2003.
8. The British Institute of Human Rights. Mental Health Advocacy and Human Rights. Available at: https://www.bihr.org.uk/mental-health-advocacy-and-human-rights-your-guide (accessed 28 March 2018).
9. Harker K, Cheeseman H. The Stolen Years: The Mental Health and Smoking Action Report. Available at: http://ash.org.uk/information-and-resources/reports-submissions/reports/the-stolen-years/ (accessed 28 March 2018).
10. Stuart H. United Nations convention on the rights of persons with disabilities: a roadmap for change. *Curr Opin Psychiatry* 2012; 25: 365–369.
11. United Nations. Convention on the Rights of Persons with Disabilities (CRPD). Available at: https://www.un.org/development/desa/disabilities/convention-on-the-rights-of-persons-with-disabilities.html (accessed 28 March 2018).
12. World Health Organization. Mental health action plan 2013–2020. Available at: http://www.who.int/mental_health/publications/action_plan/en/ (accessed 28 March 2018).
13. United Nations. Millennium Development Goals and Beyond 2015. Available at: http://www.un.org/millenniumgoals/ (accessed 28 March 2018).
14. De Silva M, Roland J. *Mental Health for Sustainable Development.* London: All Party Parliamentary Group on Global Health, 2014.
15. United Nations Statistics Division. Resolution adopted by the General Assembly on 6 July 2017. 7/313. Work of the Statistical Commission pertaining to the 2030 Agenda for Sustainable Development. Available at: http://ggim.un.org/meetings/2017-4th_Mtg_IAEG-SDG-NY/documents/A_RES_71_313.pdf (accessed 28 March 2018).
16. World Bank. Mental Health. Available at: http://www.worldbank.org/en/topic/mental-health (accessed 28 March 2018).
17. DeSilva M, Roland J. *Mental Health for Sustainable Development.* London: Joint All-Party Parliamentary Group on Global Health and Mental Health, 2014. Available at: http://www.appg-globalhealth.org.uk/download/i/mark_dl/u/4009611296/4616433442/APPG_Mental-Health_Report.pdf (accessed 28 March 2018).
18. Lancet Global Mental Health Group. Scaling up services for mental disorders—a call for action. *Lancet* 2007; 370: 1241–1252. Available at: https://www.thelancet.com/journals/lancet/article/PIIS0140-6736(07)61242-2/abstract (accessed 28 March 2018).
19. Mental Welfare Commission for Scotland. *Human Rights in Mental Health Care in Scotland: A Report on Progress Towards Meeting Commitment 5 of the Mental Health Strategy for Scotland: 2012–2015.* Edinburgh: Mental Welfare Commission for Scotland, 2015.
20. United Nations Human Rights Office of the High Commissioner. Special Rapporteur on the right of everyone to the enjoyment of the

highest attainable standard of physical and mental health. Available at: http://www.ohchr.org/EN/NewsEvents/Pages/DisplayNews.aspx?NewsID=21480&LangID=E (accessed 28 March 2018).

21. United Nations Human Rights Office of the High Commissioner. "Dignity must prevail" – An appeal to do away with non-consensual psychiatric treatment World Mental Health Day – Saturday 10 October 2016. Available at: http://www.ohchr.org/EN/NewsEvents/Pages/DisplayNews.aspx?NewsID=16583&LangID=E (accessed 28 March 2018).

22. Persaud A, Bhui K, et al. Careif Global Position Statement: Mental Health, Human Rights and Human Dignity "Magna Carta for people living with mental illness". Available at: http://www.careif.org/assets/pdfs/CAREIF-PS-Mental-Health-Human-Rights-and-Human-Dignity.pdf (accessed 28 March 2018).

23. Kakuma R, Minas H, van Ginneken N, et al. Human resources for mental health care: current situation and strategies for action. *Lancet* 2011; 378: 1654–1663. Available at: https://www.ncbi.nlm.nih.gov/pubmed/22008420 (accessed 5 April 2018).

24. Mackenzie J, Kesner C. Mental health funding and the SDGs: what now and who pays? Available at: https://www.odi.org/publications/10423-mental-health-funding-and-sdgs-what-now-and-who-pays (accessed 28 March 2018).

25. Research Councils UK. UK Research Councils join forces on mental health. Available at: http://www.cso.scot.nhs.uk/uk-research-councils-join-forces-on-mental-health/ (accessed 5 April 2018).

26. Lund C, De Silva M, Plagerson S, et al. Poverty and mental disorders: breaking the cycle in low-income and middle-income countries. *Lancet* 2011; 378: 1502–1514. Available at: https://www.ncbi.nlm.nih.gov/pubmed/22008425 (accessed 28 March 2018).

27. United Nations General Assembly Human Rights Council (32nd session) Mental Health and human rights. Available at: http://ap.ohchr.org/documents/dpage_e.aspx?si=A/HRC/32/L.26 (accessed 28 March 2018).

28. World Health Organization. mhGAP Intervention Guide - Version 2.0. Available at: http://www.who.int/mental_health/mhgap/mhGAP_intervention_guide_02/en/ (accessed 28 March 2018).

29. MQ. Seven actions towards a mentally healthy organization. Available at: https://www.mqmentalhealth.org/articles/global-agenda-council-mental-health-seven-actions (accessed 28 March 2018).

30. Chisholm D, Sweeny K, Sheehan P, et al. Scaling up treatment of depression and anxiety: a global return on investment analysis. *Lancet Psychiatry* 2016; 3: 415–424. Available at: https://www.thelancet.com/journals/lanpsy/article/PIIS2215-0366%2816%2930024-4/abstract (accessed 28 March 2018).

31. Harker K, Cheeseman H. *The Stolen Years: The Mental Health and Smoking Action Report*. London: Action on Smoking and Health, 2016. Available at: http://www.ash.org.uk/stolenyears (accessed 28 March 2018).

32. Mental Health Policy Group. A manifesto for better mental health. Available at: https://www.centreformentalhealth.org.uk/a-manifesto-for-better-mental-health (accessed 28 March 2018).

33. Mental Health Foundation. Why Mental Health Matters to Scotland's Future. Available at: https://www.mentalhealth.org.uk/publications/why-mental-health-matters-scotlands-future (accessed 28 March 2018).

34. Culter P, Hayward R, Tanasan G. Supporting User Led Advocacy in Mental Health. Available at: https://www.opensocietyfoundations.org/sites/default/files/cutler.pdf (accessed 28 March 2018).

CHAPTER 52

Public health and terrorism

Kamaldeep Bhui

Introduction

In 2015, there were over 11,000 terrorist attacks around the world; over 28,000 people were killed. Most attacks took place in Iraq and most casualties were in Iraq [1]. This data source found bombs and explosions were the most common type of incident; most attacks were on private citizens and property. Terrorism has a long history, although the types of attacks have changed over time; for example, incidents have included assassinations, shootings, and hostage-taking to produce political change [2]. McCauley and Moskalenko [2] suggest 12 processes that they report in many varieties of terrorism over the ages. They summarize these as:

◆ personal experiences of victimization and political grievances;

◆ a slippery slope of developing more extreme ideas and actions and rationalizing each stage before moving onto the next;

◆ the love, trust, and support of like-minded individuals;

◆ competitiveness for the same resources and condensation of ideas and desires;

◆ fissuring within groups leading to polarizations being sustained and extended;

◆ ju-jitsu (attack and counterattack) positioning involving action and counteractions to destabilize and undermine the other;

◆ hatred and prejudice;

◆ martyrdom as a legitimized act.

Linden and Klandermans [3] put forward several psychological processes in radicalization and suggested these could be continuous, moving from political protest and right-wing activism to terrorism, or they could include sudden conversion and commitment, and, in accord with the findings of McCauley and Moskalenko [2], compliance follows group pressures and charisma. These processes act in a complex way with cultural identity, experiences of grievance and perceived discrimination, and lack of power [4]. Terrorist acts include bombings, some hostage-taking, and political defiance, with threats to attack democratic society and related cultures [5]. Often those considered terrorists do not see themselves as criminals or terrorists, but frame their identity as freedom fighters, or they perceive they are tackling an injustice. However, the use of violence and the killing of innocent citizens is intolerable to state security and stability; any actions that produce mass killings through organized groups that adopt violence as political protest are labelled as terrorism. These labels can be contested, depending on the perspective taken, of the state or of the political campaign; these labels are often reinforced when a known or accepted terrorist organization claims responsibility for homicide in the name of their sacred, political, or social cause. An essential component is that there is an attempt to overthrow or undermine a state and its laws and governance, and cultural practices and economic and political systems of government. Extremist groups often foster a specific ideology, and this can claim religious, political, territorial, or some social cause for which they must fight. However, extremism includes right- and left-wing groups, social protesters, and Islamist-based terror organizations that seem to have captured the attention of the world.

The first use of the term 'terrorism' was at the time of the French revolution in 1789, to challenge the system of terror enforced by the French government. What has changed over the generations is the speed of telecommunications, the sophistication of the plots, and the globalization of motives and actors in such acts, either through formal terrorism organizations or through their influence to recruit individual or isolated groups with no formal connection to the terrorist organization [6, 7]. The use of social media, digital communications, and the rapid circulation of video materials designed to persuade people to join a terrorist cause are visible and well-established influences seen to impact on young people and adults involved in terrorist causes [7].

Terrorism defined and state responses

The current definition of terrorism from the British government is: *an action that endangers or causes serious violence to a person/people; causes serious damage to property; or seriously interferes with or disrupts an electronic system. The use or threat must be designed to influence the government or to intimidate the public and is made for the purpose of advancing political, religious or ideological cause* [8].[1]

What is especially challenging for governments is when citizens born and raised in a country then turn on that country, claiming closer association with other countries or causes, and kill innocent civilians or attack the military or official personnel of that country. The term radicalization was proposed to explain this process, of apparently ordinary people undergoing a social and psychological process and turning against their home country, perhaps with a migrant or Islamic history, or perhaps even people with British or American heritage and born and raised by White British (in the UK) or American (USA) parents.

---

[1] Reproduced from Section 1 of the Terrorism Act, Copyright (2000), reproduced under the Open Government Licence v3.0.

That is, migrants and Muslims are not the only ones suspected of becoming radicalized, although empirical evidence is largely in the form of case reports.

The main response of governments has been to signal harsh penalties, the commitment of resources to pursue terrorists, and efforts to ensure prosecution through the criminal justice system. The aim is to keep those at risk or suspected of terror network associations under surveillance, and ensuring those charged are convicted and 'made safe' before the leave prisons or restricted environments. Less attention has been paid to what leads to apparently intelligent and rational people to act in this way. Firstly, we do not have enough information to be sure what processes radicalization includes, and there is nothing to suggest the forms of persuasion are any different to what takes place at times of war and in marketing and recruitment campaigns for soldiers, except the integrity of information and the adherence to orthodox religious texts is questioned; that is, there is little accountability in the form of public and societal redress for failures of justice and governance. Radicalization may not be a linear and natural series of steps rather than random or sporadic. Case studies of individual terrorists invariably throw up a range of very idiosyncratic lives, with unusual pressures and dangerous decisions and choices. Whether learning about these unusual lives and their trajectories can be applied to whole populations is a question that might be addressed using existing theories of public health prevention efforts for severe and rare outcomes [9–11]. Even though we are uncertain about the process and lack evidence, the desire to signal strength and certainty in fighting a powerful but amorphous enemy has led to calls for public servants in health and social care, and teachers, to now have responsibilities for identifying at-risk individuals and acting on suspicions of radicalization, even though the science of risk prediction for rare outcomes is strongly critical of any potential predictive potential [12–14].

Public health definitions and values

The Faculty of Public Health defines public health as 'The science and art of promoting and protecting health and well-being, preventing ill-health and prolonging life through the organised efforts of society' [15]. The approach is population based; it emphasizes collective responsibility for health, its protection and disease prevention; it recognizes the key role of the state, linked to a concern for the underlying socio-economic and wider determinants of health, as well as disease; it emphasizes partnerships with all those who contribute to the health of the population (see Chapter 19). This approach has been applied to violence prevention in general [16], and to behaviours such as suicide, violence, drug taking, crime, and now also to radicalization and terrorism [17].

These approaches have been applied to violence prevention in general, to teenage pregnancy, to gun and violent crime, as well as to smoking and other societal ills that, if unaddressed, consume significant healthcare resources [16, 18–20]. The purpose of a population-level intervention is to shift the risk factor profile of any early indicator towards the left so reducing the likelihood of adverse outcomes. However, to reduce the incidence of radicalization and violent protest, we need to better understand the social and psychological conditions that lie on the pathway.

Public health applied to radicalization

Several countries have adopted public health approaches to tackle radicalization and terrorism, using lessons for countering violence [17, 21–23]. The National Academy of Sciences in the USA held a workshop inviting experts evidence on radicalization and terrorism [24]. This showed that extremist actions were not restricted to Islamist-based terrorist organizations (15%), but were dominated by far-right (43%), far-left (21%), and single-issue extremists (21%). Previous criminal activity was common among far-right groups, with Islamist groups showing least previous criminal activity, but this was not uncommon, so shattering the notion of radicalization affecting ordinary citizens. Islamist and far-right groups were 2–3 times more likely to be violent than other groups. The presence of a mental illness increased the chances of violence, although we know people with mental illness are more likely to be victims of violence rather than perpetrators. Nonetheless, it may be that people with severe mental illness act, but without belonging to an organized gang or terrorist group, or perhaps following contact with prisons or just adopting views from the Internet or social groups encountered.

An advantage of making radicalization and terrorism a public health issue, as well as a criminal justice one, is that the whole community is engaged in finding solutions, including all public services and all organizations, local and national government, schools, health, social care, police, teachers, and so on. The risk is, of course, that we still do not know enough about prevention or intervention to make this engagement effective or informed, and it may stigmatize, or terrify, or just alienate the very people we try and engage [4].

Community actions

Public engagement, discourse, and research are essential to what works and for whom. It is likely that approaches may have much in common with preventing gun crime or gang membership, or other adverse outcomes for troubled young people, and for alienated older people. The challenges are captured by a European Union report, which not only lists different types of de-radicalization programmes, but also ways to prevent radicalisation [25]. The place of civic, community, and political engagement and action are highlighted. Specifically, ensuring young people and adults feel invested in society and communities, and are empowered to change their lives through political and social action, and that pessimism and contact with radical groups offering simplistic but dangerous propositions to secure meaning and sacred fulfillment are avoided [26, 27]. This also means developing better social cohesion and cultural integration policies and practices [28], not least as migration and cultural segregation of communities appear to foster more violence in society and greater perceived discrimination and failure to make use of social and political action for change [29, 30]. However, social capital may act in a paradoxical way by providing those at risk of radicalization better confidence, resources, and networks to organize their actions [31].

Beginnings rather than conclusions

The response of local and national security agencies, and local community agencies including those considered at risk is essential. This means mapping existing violence prevention strategies and community cohesion policies, and locating actions on terrorism within these. It is difficult to test interventions for rare outcomes, but we can measure extremist attitudes, crime and violence in general, and then specific threats to see if all shift in response to moves to counter violence extremism. In reality, these programmes are being set up on a trial-and-error basis, prototypes of what might work for whom, but definitive evidence is lacking. It is unlikely a single intervention will work for all terrorist groups or actors, and interventions will need adaptation to address the many motivations that are expressed when terrorists are convicted, or threats are made, or incidents claimed. The importance of religious beliefs is not consistent, and social and political contexts may be more important for some. For example, see the dilemmas faced in Canada for de-radicalization clinics around how much religious or cultural emphasis is needed or helpful. However, in the Middle East, religious-based programmes seem essential. The social and cultural and political fabric of each country and its citizens' needs careful deliberation in proposing solutions that risk more harm than good if they do not make sense to the public or are seen as a draconian and harsh form of persecution of some communities. Alternatively, seeking advice from those who have left terror networks is seen as a progressive way forward, but trust is difficult to establish. Public health approaches offer much, yet much needs to be developed to ensure that the approach is truly inclusive, community focused, universal, and can be scaled without creating unexpected consequences or additional risks. The approach must also be in harmony with other sectors, especially state security and criminal justice agencies.

References

1. Statistica.com. Terrorism - Statistics and Facts. Available at: https://www.statista.com/topics/2267/terrorism/ (2017, accessed 20 March 2018).
2. McCauley C, Moskalenko M. *How Radicalization Happens to Them and Us*. Oxford: Oxford University Press, 2011.
3. Linden A, Klandermans B. Stigmatization and repression of extreme-right activism in the Netherlands. *Mobilization* 2006; 11: 213–228.
4. Parliamentary Office of Science and Technology. Addressing Islamic Extremism. Available at: http://researchbriefings.parliament.uk/ResearchBriefing/Summary/POST-PN-0526 (2016, accessed 20 March 2018).
5. McCauley C, Moskalenko S. Understanding political radicalization: the two-pyramids model. *Am Psychol* 2017; 72: 205–216.
6. Bhui K, Ibrahim Y. Marketing the 'radical': symbolic communication and persuasive technologies in jihadist websites. *Transcult Psychiatry* 2013; 50: 216–234.
7. Baines PR, O'Shaughnessy NJ, Moloney K, et al. The dark side of political marketing: Islamist propaganda, Reversal Theory and British Muslims. *Eur J Market* 2010; 44: 478–495.
8. Canterbury Christ Church University. Government Definitions of extremism, radicalisation and terrorism. Available at: https://www.canterbury.ac.uk/university-solicitors-office/docs/government-definitions-of-extremism-radicalisation-and-terrorism.pdf (2016, accessed 20 March 2018).
9. Mastors E, Siers R. Omar al-Hammami: a case study in radicalization. *Behav Sci Law* 2014; 32: 377–388.
10. McGilloway A, Ghosh P, Bhui K. A systematic review of pathways to and processes associated with radicalization and extremism amongst Muslims in Western societies. *Int Rev Psychiatry* 2015; 27: 39–50.
11. European Commission's Expert Group on Violent Radicalisation. Radicalisation Processes Leading to Acts of Terrorism. Available at: http://www.rikcoolsaet.be/files/art_ip_wz/Expert%20Group%20Report%20Violent%20Radicalisation%20FINAL.pdf (2008, accessed 20 March 2018).
12. Bhui K. Flash, the emperor and policies without evidence: counter-terrorism measures destined for failure and societally divisive. *Br J Psych Bull* 2016; 40: 82–84.
13. Szmukler G. Risk assessment for suicide and violence is of extremely limited value in general psychiatric practice. *Aust N Z J Psychiatry* 2012; 46: 173–174.
14. Szmukler G, Everitt B, Leese M. Risk assessment and receiver operating characteristic curves. *Psychol Med* 2012; 42: 895–898.
15. The UK's Faculty of Public Health. What is public health. Available at: http://www.fph.org.uk/what_is_public_health (accessed 20 March 2018).
16. Mikton CR, Butchart A, Dahlberg LL, et al. Global status report on violence prevention 2014. *Am J Prev Med* 2016; 50: 652–659.
17. Bhui KS, Hicks MH, Lashley M, et al. A public health approach to understanding and preventing violent radicalization. *BMC Med* 2012; 10: 16.
18. Mikhail JN, Nemeth LS. Trauma center based youth violence prevention programs: an integrative review. *Trauma Violence Abuse* 2016; 17: 500–519.
19. Massetti GM, Holland KM, Gorman-Smith D. Implementation measurement for evidence-based violence prevention programs in communities. *J Community Health* 2016; 41: 881–894.
20. Henry DB, Farrell AD, Multisite Violence Prevention P. The study designed by a committee: design of the Multisite Violence Prevention Project. *Am J Prev Med* 2004; 26(1 Suppl.): 12–19.
21. Kennedy MS. Gun Violence as a Public Health Problem. *Am J Nurs* 2016; 116: 7.
22. Sood AB, Berkowitz SJ. Prevention of youth violence: a public health approach. *Child Adolesc Psychiatr Clin N Am* 2016; 25:243–256.
23. Eisenman DP, Wold C, Setodji C, et al. Will public health's response to terrorism be fair? Racial/ethnic variations in perceived fairness during a bioterrorist event. *Biosecur Bioterror* 2004; 2: 146–156.
24. The National Academies of Sciences, Engineering and Medicine. Countering violent extremism through public health practice: Proceedings of a workshop. Available at: https://www.ncbi.nlm.nih.gov/books/NBK424492/pdf/Bookshelf_NBK424492.pdf (accessed 20 March 2018).
25. EU RAN. Proposed policy recommendations for the high level conference from the . Available at: https://ec.europa.eu/home-affairs/sites/homeaffairs/files/what-we-do/networks/radicalisation_awareness_network/ran-high-level-conference/docs/proposed_policy_recommendations_ran_derad_en.pdf (accessed 20 March 2018).
26. Atran S. Genesis of suicide terrorism. *Science* 2003; 299: 1534–1539.
27. Alderdice JT. Sacred values: psychological and anthropological perspectives on fairness, fundamentalism, and terrorism. *Ann N Y Acad Sci* 2009; 1167: 158–173.
28. Bhugra D, Ventriglio A, Bhui K. Acculturation, violent radicalisation, and religious fundamentalism. *Lancet Psychiatry* 2017; 4: 179–181.
29. Galea S, Karpati A, Kennedy B. Social capital and violence in the United States, 1974–1993. *Soc Sci Med* 2002; 55: 1373–1383.
30. Fitzpatrick KM, Piko BF, Wright DR, et al. Depressive symptomatology, exposure to violence, and the role of social capital among African American adolescents. *Am J Orthopsychiatry* 2005; 75: 262–274.
31. Bhui K, Warfa N, Jones E. Is violent radicalisation associated with poverty, migration, poor self-reported health and common mental disorders? *PLOS ONE* 2014; 9: e90718.

CHAPTER 53

Resilience and well-being

Sarah Stewart-Brown

Introduction

Well-being has a long pedigree in that its meaning and origins have been reflected on and written about by philosophers and spiritual leaders in both the East and West for many millennia, but the word itself—even the way it is written (wellbeing, well-being, well being, and wellness)—is used today in different ways in different countries, by different disciplines, and even by different groups within those disciplines.

Resilience derives from the Latin word *resilio*—to spring back. It is a concept that that is recognized as important in many different contexts from material science, through ecosystems to individuals, organizations, and societies. It may be defined differently in these different settings.

As is fitting to new ideas, the nature of well-being and resilience is being explored, debated, and in some cases disputed in both public health and psychiatry. Yet among the patients and the public, which these disciplines aim to serve, both words are part of common parlance, obviously related and obviously relevant to public mental health [1]. Indeed, some of the concern to include concepts of well-being and resilience in psychiatric services is coming from users of those services [1]. Examining these concepts and the ways in which they relate to one another is an important endeavour in a textbook of public mental health.

Well-being history and definition

Well-being was first placed at the centre of the modern health stage when, in 1946, the World Health Organization (WHO) defined health as 'physical, mental and social wellbeing, not merely the absence of disease' [2]. More recently the WHO has defined mental health as 'a state of wellbeing in which every individual realises his or her own potential can cope with the normal stresses of life can work productively and fruitfully and is able to make a contribution to his or her community' [3]. Defining health as a positive concept enabled the emergence of the discipline of health promotion from health education and disease prevention, and influenced public health practice on the ground in schools and communities. Defining health as well-being, however, created confusion because the word 'health' is so ubiquitously linked to health services and disease. As a result, most people—scholars, professionals, and the public—now use well-being to describe the positive end of the spectrum of health, with illness at the other end.

Well-being is a holistic concept that implicitly recognizes the interplay between the physical, mental, social, and—in some circles—spiritual self. It is sometimes broken down into different components (e.g. mental well-being, physical well-being), and at the same time often used to refer to its mental health components alone. So the subject is plagued with inconsistencies. Historically, discourses on well-being have been influenced by the subtleties of different languages, which, in turn, reflect societal interests and understandings. Translation of ancient texts into modern languages and cultures is a complex discipline that depends on the translator's understanding of the concepts. Simple words like happiness and pleasure have been used by some to translate texts relating to concepts that others translate as the more complex concept of well-being [4]. Psychologists have used the term positive mental health in the place of mental well-being [5]. The two are usually regarded as synonymous.

In terms of the present discourse in the academic literature, it is the mental health components of well-being that have proved most controversial, perhaps because the topic of mental well-being exists in an interdisciplinary context (see Chapter 15). The social or relational components are often considered as part of the mental component. Spiritual components have yet to be comprehensively addressed across contemporary academic disciplines, although aspects of well-being often regarded as part of the spiritual domain—for example a feeling of purpose in life, and the capacity to grow, learn, and develop—are considered part of mental well-being by most authorities so there is some overlap. This chapter focuses on mental well-being and the various approaches to and understanding of the topic.

Social science views

Broadly speaking, the social scientists and economists have adopted simple definitions of well-being, using measures of happiness and life satisfaction in their studies [6, 7]. They make the distinction between these outcomes, which they refer to as subjective well-being and objective well-being, which focuses on the social circumstances and structures they regard as necessary for well-being. Their research interests lie in demonstrating how the latter impact on well-being and how these circumstances and structures can be changed. For this, very simple measures seem to suffice. The *Concise Oxford English Dictionary* definition of well-being—'the state of being comfortable, healthy, or happy'—echoes this approach. Using the language of the ancient Greek philosophers, this view corresponds to hedonic well-being [8]. It is a feeling, a state of mind, that comes and goes, often determined by circumstances beyond the control of the individual.

Psychology and philosophy views

The underlying belief system of social scientists—that society, rather than individuals themselves, holds the trump cards when it comes to determining well-being—contrasts with that of the psychologists, philosophers, and spiritual leaders [5, 9, 10] whose interests have related to helping people develop the insights, personal characteristics, and behaviours that enable positive functioning and well-being. Different schools of thought have offered different labels and slightly different perspectives to describe this aspect of well-being. These include 'psychological well-being' [11, 12], which addresses self-acceptance, environmental mastery or agency, autonomy, purpose in life, personal growth, positive relations with others, and engagement with existential challenges of life. Several of these characteristics are also central to 'self-determination' theory [13], which holds that autonomy, competence, and relatedness enable intrinsic motivation and engagement, which bring a sense of well-being. Positive psychologists have introduced the concept of 'flourishing' to the well-being debate [14]. Although definitions of the key contributors are not identical, all conceived of this as a composite of positive psychological and social functioning. Broadly speaking, psychological well-being and flourishing correspond to the concept of eudaimonic well-being described by Aristotle [10], which he suggested is achieved through the cultivation of the character traits and behaviours that maximize happiness for self and other. The traits he described map closely onto those of psychological well-being, flourishing, and self-determination. Although in the past psychological traits have been regarded as genetic, these character traits are now recognized to be developmental and can be honed even in adulthood through a variety of personal development practices. Embedded in the concept of eudaimonic well-being is the recognition that personal well-being is related to the well-being of others and that the pursuit of the former needs to encompass concern for the latter.

The literature on well-being in childhood is written primarily from the perspective of educational psychologists and tends to refer to emotional and social well-being rather than mental well-being. Emotional intelligence [15], and the closely related concept of emotional literacy, key skills for positive relationships with others, are recognized as important for well-being in childhood, but, interestingly, not much is written with regard to adult well-being. Childhood emotional and social well-being have not been as heavily disputed or debated as mental well-being in adulthood. Examining research on this topic suggests that they are defined in ways that relate to adult mental well-being but in a rather more restricted way [16]. Instruments used to measure emotional and social well-being in childhood include measures of self-esteem and positive relationships. Perhaps the most common measurement instruments are measures of emotional and behavioural problems, which allow well-being to be defined as the absence of problems, an approach that belies the definition of well-being as more than the absence of disease. Increasingly, researchers and practitioners interested in mental health in schools are calling for and using measures of mental well-being in place of these older measures [17].

Well-being scholars are coming to believe that mental well-being comprises both positive functioning (eudaimonic well-being) and positive feelings (hedonic well-being) [4, 8]. This approach has the merits of complementing current understanding of mental illness where diagnosis is based on the observation and reporting of a combination of negative feelings (affect) and impaired functioning. Feelings are influenced on a moment-to-moment basis by things that are not under the control of the individual, but they are also influenced by the individual's response to those happenings, and this is dependent on their psychological functioning. Psychological functioning is perceived as a process of development. In this model, many of these skills are developed in adolescence and are available to be drawn on throughout life. They can also be developed in adulthood through therapeutic intervention and personal development, for example using a variety of approaches like anger management; emotional literacy; cognitive approaches challenging negative beliefs and attitudes; and mindfulness.

While seemingly derived from different approaches, the feeling and functioning aspects of mental well-being are inextricably linked and it can be surprisingly difficult, faced with the items in mental well-being inventories to decide whether an item measures feeling or functioning [17]. For example, self-acceptance is as an aspect of psychological functioning often measured by items like 'I feel confident in myself'. At the same time, this is a feeling that can fluctuate depending on external circumstances. Similarly, optimism is both a way of looking at the world or character trait and a feeling that comes and goes, depending on external circumstances. The personal development required in enhancing psychological functioning is difficult to achieve when someone has negative feelings about their capabilities, but when it is achieved the accomplishment brings pleasure and the new skills increases emotional resilience to negative life events.

Resilience history and definition

In the ecological literature resilience is defined as the 'capacity to absorb perturbations and disturbances before fundamental changes occur in the state of the system' [18]. This view is prevalent in writings about humans, but it is not the only perspective. Typical definitions include: 'the amount of stress an individual can withstand without a fundamental change in capacity to pursue aims that give life meaning' [18]. The concept in humans has been looked at in various ways: as a process, an outcome, a dynamic steady state in the face of adversity, and defiance of risk [19]. Originally viewed as an innate characteristic of remarkable individuals, resilience is now seen as a dynamic and developmental process; a result of the interplay between stress and the ability to cope. Models of resilience now emphasize the dynamic interaction between risk and protective factors on the level of individual, family, and environment, and that resilience is a process that empowers the individual to shape their environment and be shaped by it [20]. The idea of overcoming stress or adversity is common in the resilience literature [21], as is successful adaptation in the face of adversity [22]. In these definitions resilience is 'predicated on exposure to significant threat or adversity, and on the attainment of good outcomes *despite* this exposure' [19, emphasis added].

Other definitions encompass the idea that challenging or threating circumstances are necessary to human growth, moving the definition towards a belief that the attainment of good outcomes is achieved *because* of adversity. For example, Richardson et al. [23] defined resilience as 'the process of coping with disruptive stressful or challenging life events in a way that provides the individual with *additional* protective and coping skills' (emphasis added). In this model, resilience is developed by meeting adversity successfully and becomes an essential skill for personal growth. Instead of being seen as a process of bouncing back, as in the Latin origins of the word, resilience is seen as bouncing forward.

Resilience has been studied in both adults [24] and children [25], and the research settings and aspects of interest vary in both.

Adults

Three distinct fields of study arising in different disciplines—social science, psychology, psychiatry and gerontology—are all contributing to the development of understanding of resilience in adult populations.

Sense of coherence

One major contributor, Aaron Antonovsky, was stimulated into thinking about resilience in his study of holocaust survivors [26]. He was intrigued to find that almost a third of women who survived Nazi concentration camps had positive mental health, not that much less than the general population in which half were categorized as having positive mental health. In investigating what it was that enabled people to survive such circumstances in a psychologically healthy way he identified a characteristic he called 'sense of coherence' as a key protective factor. This he defined as 'a global orientation that expresses the extent to which someone has a pervasive, enduring though dynamic feeling of confidence such that:

- the stimuli deriving from one's internal and external environments in the course of living are structured, predictable and explicable;

- the resources are available to one to meet the demands posed by these stimuli; and

- these demands are challenges, worthy of investment and engagement'.[1]

He wrote about sense of coherence thus: 'Beyond the specific stress factors that one might encounter in life, and beyond your perception and response to those events, what determines whether stress will cause you harm is whether or not the stress violates your sense of coherence.' This finding led him to develop the 'salutogenic' or health-generating model, which he refined down to a capacity to comprehend, manage, and find meaning. Meaningfulness was considered the most important attribute.

Antonovsky's concept of 'salutogenesis' provided valuable impetus for the developing discipline of health promotion. And the concept of sense of coherence is currently proving valuable in studies of resilience relating to both mental and physical health outcomes. Recently, for example, a strong sense of coherence has been shown to protect against relapse in delusional psychiatric patients [27]. Community-based studies looking at the characteristics of people with a strong sense of coherence show that this concept is also related to that of mental well-being [28]. In the latter study psychological well-being and some of its components, including self-esteem, perceived control (mastery), and coping were all correlated with sense of coherence. Sense of coherence has also been shown to protect against the premature

[1] Reproduced from Antonovsky, A, Unravelling The Mystery of Health - How People Manage Stress and Stay Well, Copyright (1987), with permission from John Wiley and Sons

mortality attributable to work-related stressors [29], illustrating the holistic effects.

Post-traumatic stress disorder

The identification of post-traumatic stress disorder (PTSD) as an illness triggered by a terrifying event, either experiencing it or witnessing it, has given rise to a further body of work on resilience. This work is supported by the interest of the armed forces, where triggering events are common, but only a proportion of survivors are affected. Interest focuses on identifying precursors that protect those at risk from exposure and on the pathophysiology of the condition. Other populations of interest include refugees. These populations have usually witnessed or experienced terrifying events, but prevalence rates of PTSD vary widely, from 4% to 86%, in different populations [30]. Paramedics are another high-risk population that has been studied. But terrifying events can affect people living in comparative safely doing very safe jobs.

Studies of resilience to PTSD usually focus on high-risk groups or groups seeking treatment. The results of these studies are influenced in the first case by survivor bias; only those whose health was not so compromised that they died can be studied. The second type of study tends to underestimate population levels of resilience, because resilient individuals do not present to services for treatment with the same frequency as those who are not resilient [31]. These studies, more often based on cross-sectional than longitudinal designs, which are inherently weak in terms of unravelling possible causative factors, are also influenced by the interests of researchers who include only the variables they are curious about.

In the context of weak study designs, recent reviews and meta-analyses have concluded that preceding circumstances are less influential in terms of resilience than those surrounding the event or recovery period [32]. The preceding factors that play a part are pre-morbid trauma experiences, including childhood abuse and the factors with which it is associated—low educational achievement and general childhood adversity, female gender, and relationship status at the time of deployment, with the married faring better. Relationship difficulties more generally, including with romantic partners, family cohesion, social support, and social functioning were identified as important in one review of combat-related PTSD predictors [33]. Studies of people who have been held captive found, as might be expected, the most predictive variables to be the subjective experience of captivity and prior experience of war; but negative life events during childhood were also predictive. [34]. These later studies largely mirror the findings of earlier reviews [35], which singled out child abuse, and personal or family history of mental illness as 'uniformly' predictive; more general childhood adversity, education, and previous trauma as 'consistently' predictive; and suggested other factors such as gender, age at trauma, and ethnicity to be predictive in some populations but not in others.

A small number of other studies of relevance to a review of the ways in which resilience and well-being are related have shown sense of coherence to protect against PTSD in paramedics [36]; self-compassion, mediated by emotional regulation, to be protective in women seeking treatment for PTSD [37]; and general spiritual beliefs to be predictive in a community sample [38]. The role of positive emotional outlook as a protective factor has been highlighted more recently [39]. The psychologically healthy survivors of an environmental stressor were characterized in a further study by a challenge-oriented and humorous attitude towards stress [40].

A number of studies, many in animals, have found specific changes in the brains of trauma victims that throw light on the ways PTSD limits resilience and well-being [41]. On the basis of these studies effects have been postulated in the response of the locus coeruleus to stress. The locus coeruleus reacts to stress by triggering the release of norepinephrine in the amygdala, which is involved in the neural circuitry of fear and emotion regulation, and in the nucleus acumbens, which is involved in the neural circuitry of reward, as well as the prefrontal cortex and hippocampus. Altered reward processing has been reported in addictive behaviours, major depression, and history of childhood maltreatment, as well as PTSD. The amygdala triggers the fight-and-flight reaction to stress predisposing to violence as a response. Chronically hyperresponsive locus coeruleus–norepinephrine pathways are thus one of the pathways thought to predispose the organism to heightened anxiety and cardiovascular problems.

Successful ageing

A third body of literature relevant to adult resilience is presented in the research on optimal ageing. A study from the 1980s [42] presented healthy ageing as a process of resilience covering both recovery from adverse events (bouncing back) and maintenance of development in the face of cumulative risks (bouncing forward). This study proposed a model of resilient ageing as selection, optimization, and compensation. According to Bowling [43], the psychological attributes of healthy ageing include many of those familiar from definitions of both mental well-being and resilience: positive outlook, self-worth, sense of control over life, autonomy, and effective coping and adaptive strategies in the face of changing circumstances. Sustained enjoyment of life seems to increase longevity in this population.

Children

Resilience has been of interest in to child psychologists and psychiatrics since the middle of the last century. John Bowlby's 1951 WHO monograph [44] has been heralded as introducing an era of interest in resilience. His descriptions of the family origins of psychopathology gave rise to the inevitable question: 'How do some children survive the circumstances that lead to problems in others?' Much interest has been devoted to investigating the extent to which resilience was an innate, possibly genetic trait, or a dynamic process. Although genetic factors are once again of interest in this literature, this is in the context of epigenetics, the interaction between genes and the environment, rather than as a predetermined characteristic with which individuals are born. A recent review [45] stresses that resilience is a dynamic developmental process predicated around exposure to adversity and positive adjustment outcomes in the context of an interactive, ecological, transactional model where stressors of different origins interact with one another. Thus, both risk and protective factors can operate cumulatively and in different contexts within individuals, families, and the environment [20]. Socio-economic and cultural factors contribute to the environment, as well as neighbourhood factors, and may be studied as risk factors in their own right. At the same time, animal models suggest that manageable stressors in early development are valuable, leading to positive physiological and behavioural adaptations [46]. Resilience in childhood is studied as relevant to

a much wider range of aspects of health and well-being as adult resilience, including educational and social outcomes, criminality, violence, physical health, and a broad range of psychopathologies.

Schools

Early quantitative research on resilience focused on factors that enabled children from adverse environments to succeed academically in school. Rutter's study [47, 48] of children of parents with mental illness living on the Isle of Wight, UK, made an important contribution, highlighting the role of school environments, meaningful involvement in school, social success with peers, holding positions of responsibly, and academic achievement as the factors that protected children. He also drew attention to the importance of success in non-academic areas, for example sport or music. His findings echoed those of Garmezy [49] studying children of parents with schizophrenia, who highlighted the importance of good peer relationships, academic achievement, commitment to education, and purposive life goals, as well as an early successful work history. Latterly, the overarching importance of a caring, supportive environment in school has been emphasized [50]. Werner's influential study on the Island of Kauai, Hawaii [51, 52], showed that a single caring and supportive teacher could enable a child from a difficult background to succeed.

Families

The importance of a caring, supportive environment in the family, the factor that had been highlighted by Bowlby [44], has been more difficult to study, but has been proven to be a more important predictor [22]. Long-term follow-up of the children in the Isle of Wight study has also thrown the spotlight back on the home and community relational environment, showing that perceptions of parental caring, the quality of peer relationships in adolescence, and successful romantic attachments in adulthood, as well as personality factors and social functioning, were key to resilience to psychopathology in later life [53]. Werner and Smith [52] concluded in their study on the children of Kauai that although resilience and protective factors were multifaceted and cumulative, a range of family-based factors—maternal caregiving particularly in infancy, family support, family rules during adolescence, family cohesion, and adult role models who provide additional support—were key. Caring, supportive relationships in infancy and childhood enable the development of trust in others and underpin the capacity for healthy relationships in adulthood [54]. The earliest relationships are the most influential, but the presence of any trusting relationship in adulthood is protective.

Post-traumatic stress disorder in children

The childhood trauma literature [55], based both on careful psychotherapeutic observation of humans and animals in experimental situations, serves to complement understanding of the childhood origins of resilience based on quantitative observational studies described earlier. Rather than studying the circumstances in which the chances of trauma are increased, for example poverty, parental mental illness, this literature homes in on the nature of the trauma—sexual, physical, or emotional abuse; loss or abandonment; chronic and severe neglect; and exposure to family or community violence, terrorism, or war. This literature has found that these traumatic experiences have the potential to derail the neurological basis for psychological development, with profound implications for the future functioning of essential self-regulatory processes. The effects are manifest in problems with self-regulation of emotion and bodily processes, information processing, impulse control, and goal-directed behaviour, as well as in some severe psychopathology and personality disorders. Observations of the effect of trauma during sensitive developmental periods has led researchers and therapists to define a condition called 'complex PTSD' [56, 57]. The brains of children with complex PTSD have been described as focusing on survival instead of on learning [58]. They manifest affect dysregulation [58], threat-biased perceptions [59], and dissociation [60]. Biological dysregulation with regard to a range of psychoneuroimmunological processes is now well established [58, 61], together with studies showing how these processes track though to incidence of physical illness both in childhood and adulthood [62, 63]. The individuals' perception of trauma has an effect on the sequelae and so differs at different stages of cognitive development. The infant is thus relatively unprotected and particularly vulnerable to developing a world view dominated by feeling of helplessness, pessimism, guilt, and lack of trust. This conditioned response results in feelings of helpless in the face of future traumas, Because of their vulnerability infants are more likely to trigger and condition the reptilian freeze, dissociative response to trauma [64, 65]. The older child, especially in the presence of a caring, supportive adult, is more capable of making cognitive sense of what is happening to them and may be less vulnerable to persistent effects of trauma than infants and young children.

Physiology and neurology of resilience and well-being

With the advent of neuroimaging and non-invasive approaches to studying the functioning of different parts of the brain, and both animal and human models for studying the physiology and pathophysiology, aspects of the science of well-being and resilience are becoming clearer [41, 66]. But the findings are complex, ranging from epigenetic effects [67] and discovery of genetic polymorphisms [68] to the effects of mindfulness on specific neural pathways and brain regions [69], and a great deal remains to be understood. In terms of this chapter, it is helpful to be aware of the research on neuroendocrine pathways, polyvagal theory, and neuroplasticity.

Neuro-endocrine pathways

The body of research related to the key pathway involved in response to threat has been well reviewed [67, 70]. The hypothalamic–pituitary–adrenal (HPA) axis and adrenocorticotropic hormone (ACTH) and cortisol (and associated glucocorticoids and mineralocorticoids) have been well studied in humans and animals at different life stages, and these studies contribute to understanding of the ways in which resilience and well-being develop. The effects of stress differ at various life stages. The infant HPA system is quite labile, and sensitive parental care buffers the stress response and enables the programming of self-regulation. It is associated with smaller increases in or less prolonged activation of the HPA axis to everyday perturbations. Stressors vary in intensity along a wide spectrum and can be acute or chronic. The more severe effects of separation and deprivation in infancy, based partly on animal studies, extend beyond the HPA axis to include reducing the size and connectivity of the hippocampus (the seat

of memory), increasing the size of parts of the amygdala (which orchestrates response to threat), and reducing the size and connectivity of the prefrontal cortex involved in emotional regulation and positive affect. The hippocampus plays a role in inhibiting the hypothalamus from releasing ACTH and this damage can therefore lead to dysregulation of the HPA axis. In severe deprivation or abuse in very early childhood, low basal levels of glucocorticoids are observed, suggesting that this stress response is down-regulated perhaps superseded by the fold-and-freeze response. Exposure to stress in adolescence results in greater HPA axis activation than in adulthood, and adolescents with early adverse experiences show more pronounced activation. There are indications that this may have long-lasting effects on the prefrontal cortex and anterior cingulate involved in the processing of positive emotions and the regulation of the response to threat. Exposure to stress in adolescence impacts negatively on learning and susceptibility to drugs of abuse in adulthood. In adulthood, acute stressors have different responses. Small increases in glucocorticoids are associated with enhanced hippocampal-mediated learning and memory. Larger prolonged elevations are associated with impaired hippocampal function. In normal adults, in contrast to children, these effects are reversible, but reductions in the size of the hippocampus are regularly reported in adult PTSD. Two different mechanisms have been proposed to explain this reduced hippocampal volume seen in adults with PTSD, which are not mutually exclusive. The first suggests that it is the result of prolonged exposure to glucocorticoids in adulthood; the second, that reduced hippocampal size has childhood origins and as such is a pre-existing risk factor for PTSD induced by early exposure to stress.

Polyvagal theory

Understanding of the effects of stress, threat, and trauma in humans has advanced with Porges description of the two distinct autonomic responses to stress [64]. The first, the sympathetic fight-and-flight response mediated by the HPA axis, is well known and well studied. The second, the dorso-vagal, unmyelinated parasympathetic pathway, which is responsible for the freeze-and-fold response, is less well known. This second pathway is important in understanding trauma because it comes into play when mammals are overwhelmed or immobilized in a state of HPA arousal. When this system is triggered, bradycardia and hypoventilation ensue and the bowels are evacuated, as they are, for example, in fetal distress during labour. Early childhood trauma tends to illicit this response, which may manifest as dissociation. The phylontologically newer, more familiar, myelineated, ventro-vagal parasympathetic pathway, which promotes rest, digestion, and repair, is not well developed at birth. It is highly likely that it is the conditioning of this system through responsive, attuned caregiving that enables the infant to develop the capacity to self-sooth and, subsequently, to regulate their emotional responses to threat, including the HPA axis response. If this is the case the essential toxicity of the failure of caregiving in early life becomes clear, together with its negative impact throughout life. Poor functioning of this pathway would render the developing child and adult vulnerable to the negative impact of stressors that children with a capacity to self-soothe are protected from. And conditioning of the freeze response with its incumbent emotions of overwhelm and inadequacy would place severe restrictions on the capacity to bounce forward in response to trauma.

Neuroplasticity throughout life

The brain is a self-organizing set of interconnections between neurons, determined, in large part, by experience. Although neural pathways tend to become potentiated or suppressed in ways that progressively fix and dictate an individual's personality, behaviour, and approach to life, the brain remains plastic and can be influenced to the end of life [71, 72]. In early life, when the rate of growth is greatest [73], the infant's undeveloped cognitive functioning and lack of capacity to direct awareness mean it has little or no control over its experience and thus the creation of new pathways. At older ages, and particularly in adolescence when there is another phase of rapid brain development, it is possible to influence which parts of the brain grow and develop most by consciously choosing where to place our attention [69]. Thus, plasticity depends, in part, on the capacity to focus attention, which is the skill of mindfulness—defined as paying attention on purpose in the present moment. Increasing appreciation of the positive in life, as in the recommendations of positive psychologists, and paying attention to positive emotions, will enhance feelings of well-being. Neurophysiological studies show the left prefrontal cortex functioning (key in the manifestation of positive emotions) is enhanced in individuals who often experience well-being [66]. They also show enhanced pathways between the prefrontal cortex and the amygdala, the area of the brain involved in reaction to threat, in these individuals. These are the pathways responsible for healthy self-regulation of emotional states triggered by threat, which are deficient in children and adults exposed to trauma.

Together these bodies of literature are consistent with other literature suggesting that resilience and well-being are dependent on what happens in very early life. In the context of attuned, sensitive care, the infant develops the capacity for self-regulation, which protects against everyday stressors and enables the positive responses to challenge the characteristic of resilience. In the absence, to variable degrees, of such care and/or the presence of more extreme stressors, this capacity does not develop well, children are susceptible to being overwhelmed by their stress responses, and pathological neurophysiological responses are programmed with long-term consequences on development and health. Adolescence represents another period of vulnerability in which neurophysiological pathways can be programmed or not to support resilience and well-being, dependent, in part, of the relational support available to the adolescent and their early life experiences. But the brain remains plastic throughout life and studies provide evidence that meditative and cognitive practices effect neural patterns and pathways in a way that is compatible with increases in resilience and well-being, and are entirely consistent with descriptions of both mental well-being and resilience as including the capacity for personal growth and development.

Relationship to physical well-being

This chapter would not be complete without reference to studies showing the interplay between mental and physical health and the profound role that psychological resilience plays in protection from physical disease. The very high risk of premature mortality in people suffering severe and enduring mental illness can be partly attributed to unhealthy lifestyles, which tend to be adopted by such groups to mitigate stress, but this does not explain all the variation in mortality risk. The gap is very likely to be explained by the way mental illness disturbs the functioning of the autonomic nervous system and resilience to environmental and social stress. Friedman and McEwen coined the term allostatic load to describe the elevations in physiological indicators concomitant with failure to down-regulate following a stress response and restore homeostasis [74].

There is ample literature showing that positive emotions and psychological well-being in adulthood enhance longevity and reduce the risk of disease [75, 76]. And there is a growing body of research showing that adverse experience of childhood, known as ACEs, which, when encountered in the absence of supportive caring relationships, have the potential to disrupt resilience and the development of well-being and predispose to chronic illness in middle life [62, 63]. Relatively minor problems with the parent–child relationship in normal populations increase risk [77].

Building resilience and well-being

Resilience and well-being are thus clearly interrelated. Resilience is derived from the capacity to draw on the support of others, face challenges with a positive mindset, and the growth and development that ensues. Some have argued that its development is actually dependent on the experience of challenge and adversity. Development in infancy and childhood is dependent on meeting stressors in the context of high levels of relational support. It would seem that children who missed out early on can develop resilience in later childhood or adult life if they encounter challenges at a time when they also have the backing of nurturing supportive relationships. However, early experience of relationships, because it dictates the capacity to trust others, will play a part in determining the extent to which it is possible to draw on the support of others in later life. Early support for resilience means that setbacks and challenges can be met with the following question: 'Why has this happened to me now and what is it trying to teach me?' When these are not sufficient, the help and support of others can be sought to rebuild a state of well-being. Coming into adulthood without the resource of resilience places individuals at risk of being overwhelmed in adulthood by stressful events and unable to grow and learn through the experience.

Well-being describes both a state and a capacity. Day to day, in the absence of challenges, a positive optimistic frame of mind will be associated with mental well-being. But resilient response to challenges is a hallmark of well-being and one which, in the long run, enables continuing enhancement of well-being by promoting personal growth and development.

Both mental well-being and resilience are profoundly important to public mental health. So what can be done to promote these and are they different things or the same?

Parenting support

Approaches that enhance sensitive, responsive parenting—the sort of parenting that can help children meet challenges constructively—must be the starting point, as if it is possible to achieve this, later problems in the form of stress response conditioning, dysfunctional coping, and lack of capacity to trust others can be prevented. There are now a range of programmes that can influence care giving [78]. The effect sizes of programmes in the very-high-risk groups to which they are usually offered are relatively small, and the work is challenging, highly skilled, and time consuming. Because a high proportion of children are affected to some degree, a small investment in the general population—upskilling of midwives and health visitors, support for third-sector public provision—might achieve more in the longer term. While investment of resources in parenting support is likely to yield a very large return on investment in terms of future health and social problems avoided, some of the gains are far into the future, making it difficult to fund programmes in times of adversity.

Schools

Schools have long been recognized to provide opportunities to enhance resilience. A range of programmes are now evidence based and available [79]. Effective programmes have at least two components: (i) a universal component, including staff well-being, behaviour policies, and bullying prevention; and (ii) a targeted component offering more intensive support to the least resilient and most challenging children. Some programmes also reach out to parents and the community aiming to increase relational support at home.

Adult and adolescent programmes

On the whole, approaches to enhance well-being in adolescence and adulthood are likely to yield dividends in a shorter time period than parenting programmes, but the dividends are likely to be smaller. Programmes to support adults severely damaged in childhood will be labour intensive and costly. Obvious places for provision are prisons, hostels for the homeless, and mental illness service. But, as for children, much can be achieved by enhancing resilience and well-being in the middle ground. Here, a change in mindset alone is helpful and achievable by public education. Tackling the negative and dismissive media responses to well-being enhancement policies and programmes would be a valuable start. Dissemination the UKs 'Five Ways to Wellbeing' programme [80] alongside the USA's top-10 tips for developing resilience (develop signature strengths; positive attitude; reframing; sense of purpose; social support; find mentor or friend who can support and practice, etc.) [81] is possible. Supporting the widespread provision of community and workplace activities and programmes to teach, for example mindfulness or mindful movement like yoga and tai chi or participation in the arts [82], would be of low cost and effective. Enabling asset-based community development [83] and programmes to enhance social support and reduce isolation and loneliness in old age [84], and development of the medical education and continuing professional development of doctors to embrace the concepts of well-being and resilience would enable a sea change in public understanding. In the longer term, upskilling the psychology workforce to better support adolescents and adults with complex PTSD through the new approaches such as eye movement desensitization reprocessing [83] and trauma release and somatic experiencing [84] could prove valuable.

References

1. Crepaz-Keay D. *Mental Health Today.... And Tomorrow: Exploring Current and Future Trends in Mental Health.* Hove: Pavilion Publishing and Media, 2015.
2. World Health Organization (WHO). *Preamble to the Constitution of the World Health Organization.* Geneva: WHO, 1948.
3. World Health Organization (WHO). *The World Health Report—Mental Health: New Understanding New Hope.* Geneva: WHO, 2001.
4. Stewart-Brown S. Population level: wellbeing in the general population. In: Slade M, Oades L, Jarden A (eds). *Wellbeing, Recovery and Mental Health.* Cambridge: Cambridge University Press, 2015, pp. 215–230.
5. Jahoda M. *Current Concepts of Positive Mental Health.* New York; Basic Books, 1958.
6. Kahneman D, Diener E, Schwarz N (eds). *Well-being: Foundations of Hedonic Psychology.* New York: Russell Sage Foundation, 1999.
7. Clark A E, Flèche S, Layard R, Powdthavee N, Ward G. *The Origins of Happiness: The Science of Well-Being Over the Life Course.* Princeton, NJ: Princeton University Press, 2018.
8. Ryan RM, Deci EL. On happiness and human potentials: a review of research on hedonic and eudaimonic well-being. *Annu Rev Psychol* 2001; 52: 41–166.
9. Albee GW. Preventing psychopathology and promoting human potential. *Am Psychol* 1982; 37: 1043–1050.
10. Schoch R. *The Secrets of Happiness: Three Thousand Years of Searching for the Good Life.* New York: Simon and Schuster, 2008.
11. Ryff CD. Happiness is everything, or is it. *J Person Soc Psychol* 1989; 57: 1069–1081.
12. Ryff C, Keyes C. The structure of psychological well-being revisited. *J Person Soc Psychol* 1995; 69: 719–727.
13. Ryan RM and Deci EL. *Self-Determination Theory: Basic Psychological Needs in Motivation, Development, and Wellness.* New York: Guilford Press, 2017.
14. Hone LC, Jarden A, Schofield GM, Duncan S. Measuring flourishing: the impact of operational definitions on the prevalence of high levels of wellbeing. *Int J Wellbeing* 2014; 4: 62–90.
15. Salovey P, Mayer JD. Emotional intelligence. *Imagin Cogn Person* 1989; 9: 185–211.
16. Stewart-Brown S, Edmunds L. Assessing emotional and social competence in early years and primary school settings. *Perspect Educ* 2003; 21: 17–41.
17. Rose T, Joe S, Warren Brown G, et al. Measuring mental wellbeing among adolescents: a systematic review of instruments. *J Child Fam Stud* 2017; 26: 1–14.
18. Zautra AJ, Hall JS, Murray KJ. Resilience: a new definition of health for people and communities. In: Reich JW, Zautra AJ, Stuart J (eds). *Hall Handbook of Adult Resilience.* New York: Guilford Press, 2010, pp. 3–34.
19. Luthar SS, Cicchetti D, Becker B. The construct of resilience: a critical evaluation and guidelines for future work. *Child Dev* 2000; 71: 543–562.
20. Gamezy N. Resiliency and vulnerability to adverse developmental outcomes associated with poverty. *Am Behav Sci* 1991; 34: 416–430.
21. Rutter MJ Implications of resilience concepts for scientific understanding. Ann N Y Acad Sci 2006; 1094: 1–12.
22. Masten AS, Best KJ, Garmezy N. Resilience and development: contributions from the study of children who overcome adversity. *Dev Psychopathol* 1990; 2: 425–444.
23. Richardson GE, Neiger BL, Jensen S, Kumpfer KL The resiliency model. *Health Educ* 1990; 21: 33–39.
24. Reich JW, Zautra AJ, Hall JS. *Handbook of Adult Resilience.* New York: Guilford Press, 2010.
25. Goldstein S, Brooks RB. *Handbook of Resilience in Children.* New York: Springer, 2012.
26. Antonovsky A. *Unravelling The Mystery of Health—How People Manage Stress and Stay Well.* San Francisco, CA: Jossey-Bass Publishers, 1987.
27. Bergstein M, Weizman A, Solomon Z. Sense of coherence among delusional patients: prediction of remission and risk of relapse. *Compr Psychiatry* 2008; 49: 288–296.
28. Pallanta JF, Laeb L. Sense of coherence, well-being, coping and personality factors: Further evaluation of the sense of coherence scale. *Person Indiv Differ* 2002; 33: 39–48.
29. Nilsen C, Andel R, Fritzell J. Work-related stress in midlife and all-cause mortality: can sense of coherence modify this association? *Eur J Public Health* 2016; 26: 1055–1061.

30. Hollifield M, Warner TD, Lian N, et al. Measuring trauma and health status in refugees: a critical review. *JAMA* 2002; 288: 611–621.

31. Bonanno GA. Loss, trauma, and human resilience: have we underestimated the human capacity to thrive after extremely aversive events? *Am Psychol* 2004; 59: 20–28.

32. Lebens ML, Lauth GW. Risk and resilience factors of post-traumatic stress disorder: a review of current research. *Clin Exp Psychol* 2016; 2: 120.

33. Xue C, Ge Y, Tang B, et al. A meta-analysis of risk factors for combat-related PTSD among military personnel and veterans *PLOS ONE* 2015; 10: e0120270.

34. Solomona Z, Horesh D, Ein-Dorc T, Ohryd A. Predictors of PTSD trajectories following captivity: a 35-year longitudinal study. *Psychiatry Res* 2012; 199: 188–194.

35. Brewin CR, Andrews B, Valentine JD: Met-analysis of risk factors for posttraumatic stress disorder in trauma-exposed adults. *J Consul Clin Psych* 2000; 68: 756.

36. Streb M, Häller P, Michael T. PTSD in paramedics: resilience and sense of coherence. *J Behav Cogn Psychother* 2014; 42: 452–463.

37. Scoglio AAJ, Rudat DA, Garvert D, Jarmolowsik M, Jackson C, Hermans JL. Self compassion and responses to trauma: the role of emotion regulation. *J Interpers Violence* 2015 (Epub ahead of print).

38. Connor KM, Davidson JRT, Lee LC. Spirituality, resilience and anger in survivors of violent trauma: a community survey. *J Trauma Stress* 2003; 16: 487–494.

39. Ong AD, Bergeman CS, Chow S-M. Positive emotion as a basic building block of resilience in adulthood. In: Reich JW, Zautra AJ, Hall JS (eds). *Handbook of Adult Resilience*. New York: Guilford Press, 2010, pp. 81–93.

40. Tran US, Glück TM, Lueger-Schuster B. Influence of personal and environmental factors on mental health in a sample of Austrian survivors of World War II with regard to PTSD: Is it resilience? *BMC Psychiatry* 2013; 13: 47.

41. Baltes PB, Baltes MM. Psychological perspectives on successful aging: the model of selective optimization with compensation. In: Baltes PB, Baltes MM (eds). *Successful Aging: Perspectives from the Behavioral Sciences*. Cambridge: Cambridge University Press, 1990, pp. 1–34.

42. Federa Nestler EJ, Westphal M, Charney DS. Psychobiological mechanisms of resilience to stress. In: Zautra AJ, Hall JS, Murray KJ (eds). *Handbook of Adult Resilience*. New York: Springer, 2010, pp. 35–54.

43. Bowling A. *Ageing Well: Quality of Life in Old Age*. Maidenhead: Open University Press, 2005.

44. Bowlby J. Maternal care and mental health. *Bull World Health Organ* 1951; 3: 355–534.

45. Luthar SS, Cicchetti D. Resilience in development: a synthesis of research across five decades. In: Cohen DJ (eds). *Developmental Psychopathology: Risk, Disorder, and Adaptation*, Vol. 3, 2nd ed. Hoboken, NJ: John Wiley & Sons, 2006, pp. 739–795.

46. Lyons DM, Parker KJ. Stress inoculation-induced indications of resilience in monkeys. *J Trauma Stress* 2007; 20: 423–433.

47. Rutter M. Protective factors in the children's responses to stress and disadvantage. In: Kent MW, Rolf JE (eds). *Primary Prevention in Psychopathology: Social Competence in Children*. Hanover, NH: University Press of New England, 1979, pp. 49–74.

48. Rutter M. Isle of Wight revisited: twenty-five years of child psychiatric epidemiology. *J Am Acad Child Adolesc Psychiatry* 1989; 28: 633–653.

49. Garmezy N. Vulnerability research and the issue of primary prevention. *Am J Orthopsychiatry* 1971; 411: 101–116.

50. Henderson N, Milstein M. *Resiliency in Schools*. Thousand Oaks, CA: Corwin Press, 1996.

51. Werner EE, Smith RS. *Vulnerable but not Invincible: A Longitudinal Study of Resilient Children and Youth*. New York: RR Donnelley and Sons, 1982.

52. Werner EE, Smith RS. *Journeys from Childhood to Midlife: Risk Resilience and Recovery*. London: Cornell University Press, 2001.

53. Collishaw S, Pickles Am Messer J, Rutter M, Shearer C, Maughan B. Resilience to psychopathology following childhood maltreatment: evidence from a community sample. *Child Abuse Negl* 2007; 31: 211–229.

54. Erickson E. *Childhood and Society*. New York: W.W. Norton, 1993.

55. Cicero SD, Nooner K, Silva R Vulnerability and resilience in childhood trauma and PTSD. In: Ardino V (ed.). *Post Traumatic Syndromes in Childhood and Adolescence: A Handbook of Research and Practice*. Hoboken, NJ: John Wiley and Sons, 2011, pp. 43–60.

56. Ford JD. Future directions in conscpetualising complex post-traumatic stress disorder syndromes in childhood and adolescence: towards a developmental trauma disorder diagnosis. In: Ardino V (ed.). *Post Traumatic Syndromes in Childhood and Adolescence: A Handbook of Research and Practice*. Hoboken, NJ: John Wiley and Sons, 2011, pp. 433–448.

57. Cook A, Spinazzola J, Ford JD, et al Complex trauma in children and adolescents. *Psychiatr Annu* 2005; 161: 390–398.

58. Ford JD. Treatment implications of altered neurobiology, affect regulation and information processing following child maltreatment. *Psychiatry Annu* 2005; 35: 410–419.

59. Pollack S, Toley-Schell S. Selective attention to facial emotions in physically abused children. *J Abnorm Psychol* 2003; 112: 323–338.

60. Van de Kolk BA. Developmental trauma disorder. *Psychiatr Annu* 2005; 35: 439–448.

61. De Bellis M. Developmental traumatology. *Psychoneuroimmunology* 2001; 27: 155–170.

62. Felletti V, Anda R, Nordenberg D, et al. Relationship of childhood abuse and household dysfunction to many of the leading causes of death in adults. *Am J Prev Med* 1998; 14: 245–258.

63. Bellis MA, Hughes K, Leckenby N, Hardcastle KA, Perkins C, Lowey H. Measuring mortality and the burden of adult disease associated with adverse childhood experiences in England: a national survey. *J Public Health* 2015; 37: 445–454.

64. Porges SW. *Polyvagal Theory: Neurophysiological Foundations of Emotional Attachment Communication Self Regulation*. New York: W.W. Norton, 2011.

65. Lanius RA, Vermetten E, Loewenstein RJ, et al. Emotion modulation in PTSD: clinical and neurobiological evidence for a dissociative subtype. *Am J Psychiatry* 2010; 167: 640–647.

66. Davidson RJ. Well-being and affective style: neural substrates and biobehavioural correlates. In: Huppert FA, Bayliss N, Kervines B (eds). *The Sciences of Well-being*. Oxford: Oxford University Press, 2005.

67. Lupien SJ McEwen BS Gunnar MR, Heim C. Effects of stress throughout the lifespan on the brain behaviour and cognition. *Nature* 2009; 110: 434–445.

68. Rutter M, Moffitt TE, Caspi A. Gene–environment interplay and psychopathology: multiple varieties but real effects. *J Child Psychol Psychiatry* 2006; 47: 226–261.

69. Siegel DJ. *The Mindful Brain: Reflection and Attunement in the Cultivation of Well-being*. New York: W.W. Norton, 2007.

70. Lai M-C, Hauang L-T. Effects of early life stress on neuroendocrine and neurobehaviour: mechanisms and implications. *Pediatr Neonatol* 2011; 52: 122–128.

71. Doidge N. *The Brain that Changes Itself: Stories of Personal Triumph from the Frontiers of Brain Science*. New York: Penguin Books, 2007.

72. Begley S. *Train Your Mind, Change your Brain: How a New Science Reveals Our Extraordinary Potential to Transform Ourselves*. New York: Ballantine Books, 2007.

73. National Research Council. From Neurons to Neighborhoods: The Science of Early Childhood Development. In: Shonkoff JP, Phillips DA (eds) *Committee on Integrating the Science of Early Childhood Development, Board on Children, Youth, and Families*. Washington, DC: National Research Council, 2000.

74. Friedman MJ, McEwen BS. PTSD, allostatic load and medical illness. In: Schnurr PP, Green BL (eds). *Trauma and Healing: Physical Consequences of Exposure to Extreme Stress*. Washington, DC: American Psychological Association, 2004, pp. 157–189.

75. Chida Y, Steptoe A. Positive psychological well-being and mortality: a quantitative review of prospective observational studies *Psychosom Med* 2008; 70: 741–756.

76. Pressman SD, Cohen S. Does positive affect influence health? *Psychol Bull* 2005; 131: 925–971.

77. Stewart-Brown SL Fletcher L, Wadsworth MEJ. Parent child relationships and health problems in adulthood in three national birth cohort studies. *Eur J Publ Health* 2005; 15: 640–646.

78. Stewart-Brown S, Schrader-McMillan A. Parenting for mental health: what does the evidence say we need to do? Report of Workpackage 2 of the DataPrev project. *Health Promot Int* 2011; 26: i10–i28.

79. Weare K, Mind M. Mental health promotion and problem prevention in schools: what does the evidence say? *Health Promot Int* 2011; 26: i29–i69.

80. Mind. Five ways to wellbeing. Available at: http://www.mind.org.uk/workplace/mental-health-at-work/taking-care-of-yourself/five-ways-to-wellbeing/ (accessed 20 March 2018).

81. American Psychological Association. 10 Tips to Build Resilience. Available at: https://psychcentral.com/lib/10-tips-to-build-resilience/ (accessed 20 March 2018).

82. Faculty of Public Health. Better Mental Health For All: A public health approach to mental health improvement. Available at: http://www.fph.org.uk/uploads/Better%20Mental%20Health%20For%20All%20FINAL%20low%20res.pdf (accessed 20 March 2018).

83. National Institute for Health and Care Excellence. Post-traumatic stress disorder: management. Available at: https://www.nice.org.uk/guidance/cg26 (accessed 20 March 2018).

84. Levine P. *In an Unspoken Voice: How the Body Releases Trauma and Restores Goodness*. Berkely, CA: North Atlantic Books, 2010.

CHAPTER 54

Resilience and the role of spirituality

Christopher C. H. Cook and Nathan H. White

Introduction

What is resilience? How, if in any way, is spirituality related to it? The answers to these questions will be relevant to mental and public health professionals, as well as commissioners of services. They are also vital to clinicians and chaplains in their daily work. These vocations involve an acknowledgement of the brokenness of many individuals' human experience paired with a hope that such brokenness might be mended. The intersection of 'resilience' and 'spirituality', then, may not be as unexpected as at first it may seem. As will become evident, the two concepts are closely related. Yet both in clinical practice and in public health promotion, the resources found in spirituality often are not adequately recognized as a means of understanding and inculcating resilience.

Mental health clinicians, at both individual and public policy levels, necessarily take into account the personal history, cultural influences, and self-understanding of their patients [1]. For many, spirituality is a significant aspect of their own history, culture, and self-understanding. It can thus exert a considerable influence on self-identity and systems of meaning at both an individual and communal level. This suggests that spirituality can play a significant role in resilient adaptation to adversity.

Resilience

Definitions and conceptions of resilience abound within psychology and medicine. This may be because, although it is intuitively understood, resilience is difficult to define concisely [2]. (Also see Chapter 53.) Resilience may be understood through a systems theory approach, as in Ann Masten's [3] conception of resilience as the 'capacity of a dynamic system to adapt successfully to disturbances that threaten system function, viability, or development' (p. 6). For the purposes of this chapter, resilience is defined as the 'process of harnessing biological, psychosocial, structural, and cultural resources to sustain wellbeing' [4, p. 333].

Despite varying definitions of resilience, several integral components of the concept must be acknowledged: (i) confrontation of significant adversity or risk; (ii) use of internal and external resources to adapt despite adversity; and (iii) a positive outcome [5]. These criteria introduce several distinct characteristics for the concept of resilience. Firstly, the adversity an individual faces must exceed normal everyday stressors. Managing normal difficulties would largely fall within the realm of 'coping'. Secondly, an individual may use various 'resources', 'assets', or 'strengths' to sustain well-being, despite adversity. These resources may be either internal or external to the individual, and may encompass a wide variety of types of assets. Finally, resilient adaptation should result in a good outcome, generally understood in terms of human well-being or health.

Because of the complexity of the construct, a multiple-levels-of-analysis approach is necessary for understanding resilience [6]. In this schema, spirituality may aid both in gaining a clearer idea of the concept of resilience and in promoting resilient adaptation. With regard to the latter, spirituality should be understood as a psychosocial and cultural resource that may foster well-being.

Spirituality

Spirituality is notoriously difficult to delimit and define. There is little consensus regarding the boundaries of this concept both within a clinical context, and, more broadly, at a colloquial level. This difficulty is especially pronounced in a healthcare environment. To clarify the boundaries of good practice in clinical settings, the Royal College of Psychiatrists provided a Position Statement, *Recommendations for Psychiatrists on Spirituality and Religion*, which defines spirituality as [7]:

> … a distinctive, potentially creative, and universal dimension of human experience arising both within the inner subjective awareness of individuals and within communities, social groups and traditions. It may be experienced as a relationship with that which is intimately 'inner', immanent and personal, within the self and others, and/or as relationship with that which is wholly 'other', transcendent and beyond the self. It is experienced as being of fundamental or ultimate importance and is thus concerned with matters of meaning and purpose in life, truth, and values [8].

While this expansive definition is not easily applied in research settings, it illustrates the broad nature of the concept. Several fundamental aspects of spirituality are apparent here [1]. Spirituality is concerned with private, individual experiences, as well as with relationships to community and the world more broadly. Spirituality includes both elements that are transcendent (above and beyond the individual), and aspects that are immanent (experientially immediate to the individual). The heterogeneity of the concept is unified by a fundamental concern with questions of meaning, purpose, and ultimate value.

Some would question whether the construct of spirituality is significant beyond the conglomeration of sub-constructs associated with it. Kenneth Pargament [9] maintains that the 'sacred core' of spirituality makes it a unique construct distinct from mental health or associated concepts. Harold Koenig [10] and Chris Cook [11] consider transcendence to be the distinctive aspect of spirituality. This may differentiate accounts of 'implicit spirituality' and related modes of human meaning and purpose from accounts of spirituality that highlight the uniqueness of the construct.

Religion

Religion, despite having clearer visible manifestations than spirituality, is also difficult to define [12]. John Bowker [12] proposes that religions serve as systems that promote human survival and protect human flourishing. Spirituality may serve similar purposes in promoting mental health, but its role must be distinguished from that of religion [13]. Spirituality is not synonymous with religion, yet neither is it unrelated [13]. Religion is commonly understood to be concerned with the liturgical practices of particular faith groups. Alternatively, in modern Western society spirituality is thought to encompass the private expression of subjective devotional experience that is inherent to all human beings [13]. In a Western context, individuals may consider themselves spiritual and religious, spiritual but not religious, or neither spiritual nor religious. While there is also discussion about religion devoid of spirituality, it seems to be less common that people self-identify as religious but not spiritual [13].

Generally, individuals who understand themselves as spiritual and religious perceive their spirituality to be derivative from religion rather than the other way around. Religion, for them, may provide the content of their faith, whereas spirituality is more closely related to individual practice. This group holds most closely to a traditional understanding of the relationship between these two concepts [13]. The individuals who identify as 'spiritual but not religious' are a growing demographic in many Western nations for whom transcendence, community, and the goodness of human nature are important, but the belief in a personal and world-intervening God is not [14]. These individuals may see religion as negative and authoritarian while embracing spirituality as an unencumbered expression of the human spirit and locating spiritual authority within each person. Conversely, an individual who self-identifies as 'religious but not spiritual' may put great stock in particular religious expressions of faith but may be more uneasy with a particular perception of 'spirituality'. Finally, those who see themselves as 'neither spiritual nor religious' may not perceive a need for anything beyond the secular in their search for meaning.

Assessing spirituality and religion

Numerous instruments for assessing and measuring spirituality and religion (S/R) have been developed [15]. These include, for instance, the Multidimensional Measure of Religiousness/Spirituality (MMRS) [16], the Functional Assessment of Chronic Illness—Spiritual Well-Being (FACIT-Sp) [17], the Royal Free Interview for Religious and Spiritual Beliefs [18], and the Spiritual Well-Being Scale [19]. Such measures enable clinicians to assess patients' spirituality and researchers to gauge the effect of S/R upon multiple aspects of human experience, including differentiation between various components of S/R.

Because conceptions of S/R differ in various cultures and contexts [20], a contextually based approach will recognize that a Western understanding of these concepts may not be appropriate in other contexts. Questions of ultimate purpose and meaning should be addressed through the substance of particular belief systems. Many other expressions of spirituality are possible and may provide meaning for individuals and faith communities.

Spirituality and resilience

Resilience is a complex concept that creates difficulties for both measuring and understanding the aetiology of the construct [21]. Yet the concept of spirituality may give a particular awareness of difficulties inherent in standard accounts of resilience and provide possible solutions. For instance, what could, at first glance, seem to be a patient treatment situation with straightforward solutions, may, in fact, contain more complex issues. While the clinician may suggest, for example, freedom from anxiety as a beneficial patient treatment goal, a more complex question underlies this assumption: 'Is being anxious universally harmful in every circumstance?' Furthermore, 'Can an anxious individual ever be considered resilient in any meaningful sense?' The answers to these questions necessitate a deeper understanding of human well-being and mental health, a perspective that spirituality can provide. Would there be any situation in which anxiety could be a beneficial and resilient response? A 'resilient' individual may have bouts of anxiety but cope successfully through them. By being spurred to continued growth of character, this individual is more resilient than one who is 'cured' of anxiety and consequently no longer sees a need for further growth. Thus, resilience cannot be equated either with lack of psychopathology or lack of vulnerability [22]. Here a distinction must be made between a 'healthy' individual and a 'resilient' individual. The two are not always synonymous. Could it be that a currently 'unhealthy' yet 'resilient' person will have greater long-term well-being than a currently 'healthy' yet 'un-resilient' person? The answer to this question may determine the trajectory and scope of care by the clinician and the policies implemented by the public health official.

Beyond questioning assumptions that a spiritual viewpoint may enable, spirituality can provide distinctive insights into the processes of positive adaptation found in resilience. For example, a spiritual point of view may suggest otherwise unnoticed, potentially beneficial, aspects of adverse situations. While in no way affirming adversity as good in itself, a perspective that takes into account the transcendent may find meaning even in dire circumstances. This 'spiritual' viewpoint provides insight beyond a purely immanent and secular understanding of human experience, thus enabling one to place the reality of evil and suffering within a larger framework of meaning. Such higher-level questions of meaning are useful for interrogating the relationship between resilience and spirituality, but further evidence is needed to establish the contours of this relationship.

Mental health

For some, discussing spirituality and resilience in the context of public mental health is problematic. Jeff Levin [23] notes 'That religion might have something to say about mental health, for good or bad, has been a sensitive and contentious issue within psychiatry, dating to Freud, as familiarity with the history of psychiatry attests' (p. 103). Additionally, practical theologian Don Browning suggests that psychiatry in the USA risks alienating the general population because of an antagonism toward S/R [24]. But this trend is changing. Modifications, such as those made to the *Diagnostic and Statistical Manual of Mental Disorders, Fifth Edition* (DSM-5) [25], signal a new openness to recognizing the role that S/R may play in human health and well-being. Nonetheless, some scholars are adamant in maintaining the divide between professional mental health care and spirituality [26, 27], in part highlighting shortcomings in the research methodology of studies linking spirituality and health. Certainly, some studies are lacking in good design and methodology. Yet others, such as those by Koenig and colleagues, are methodologically more robust. If spirituality has a role in promoting health and well-being, as many reputable studies indicate, it would be unwise to dismiss it indiscriminately.

The role of spirituality in promoting mental health is perhaps seen nowhere more clearly than in fostering resilient adaptation to adversity. Research indicates that S/R is among the most significant resources that many individuals use to cope through adverse circumstances. For example, a representative national survey in the USA indicated that 90% of surveyed Americans coped using religion following the 9/11 attacks [28]. Research conducted in various geographical, cultural, and religious demographics suggests that the use of spiritual coping resources is widespread, although particular spiritual and religious coping methods may vary [20, 29, 30]. Furthermore, a World Health Organization (WHO) study indicated that S/R was significantly positively correlated with quality of life for individuals across 18 countries [31]. A separate WHO report [32] indicates the importance of spirituality as a category of resources available to the individual that is 'essential to psychological wellbeing' (p. piii). Because of the significance of spirituality for resilience, Andrew Hatala proposes a model that views resilience as the 'dynamic interaction' of physical, psychological, interpersonal, and spiritual capabilities [33]. There is a growing body of research to support the supposition that spirituality plays an important role in resilience [10, 34, 35].

Evidence for the health-promoting effects of spirituality

Studies, on the whole, indicate an inverse relationship between spirituality and psychopathology—a finding consistent with research on the positive health benefits of spirituality more generally.[1] In the most complete review of the literature to date, Koenig lists more than 2100 quantitative studies related to religion, spirituality, and health from 2000 to 2010. He estimates this to represent approximately 75% of the total available quantitative research [10]. Furthermore, he suggests that the number of qualitative studies concerning the role of S/R in health is too numerous to include in the already massive volume. Studies show that S/R patients are less likely to develop depression or depressive symptoms and that

religion both protects individuals from depression and acts as an aid in recovery [36, 39, 40].[2] There is ample research to suggest positive correlations between spirituality and length of life, speedy recovery after major surgery, and lack of substance abuse, just to name a few other indicators of health [10]. Not all evidence points to supremely positive outcomes and associations, however. For example, one meta-analysis of research on the correlation of religion and depression found merely a mild association between the two, with positive religiosity making only a small difference in the depressive symptoms [40]. Additionally, some research suggests that spirituality untethered from religious affiliations is associated with negative health outcomes [42].

Research indicates that the positive effects of S/R can be most clearly seen in situations of significant adversity [43, 44]. As an example, studies demonstrate the significance of spirituality for helping patients with cancer [45, 46]. Studies also suggest that S/R provides resources for individuals to deal with severe and/or chronic pain [47–49]. Significantly, spiritual resources are particularly important for those whose ailments are beyond the scope of modern medicine to help [50].

Recent research is more clearly able to delineate the relationship between spirituality and resilience due to technological advances, as well as accumulation of data from many studies. The advance in understanding this relationship is especially prominent in the fields of neurobiology and genetics.

Neurobiology, genetics, and resilience

Technological advances, such as functional magnetic resonance imaging (fMRI), used while a patient is conscious, enable greater understanding of the neurobiology of resilience [51, 52]. For instance, fMRI studies indicate that the experience of pain is significantly influenced by beliefs, expectations, and the interpretation of experience [53]. Spiritual practices such as mindfulness [54] and religious belief [49] may elicit similar effects.

These studies suggest a particularly complex relationship between relatively stable characteristics of the person, such as genetics; changeable physical and mental constructs, such as brain circuitry and belief systems; and environmental factors. This dynamic relationship enables the promotion of resilience through altering environmental and/or biological influences [51].

Here the confluence of several dynamic factors are evident in their effect upon resilience. Research indicates that resilience is partially genetically influenced and mildly heritable, roughly equivalent to the heritability of depression [21]. Similarly, stressful life events may modify genetic expression through biological stress reactions [55]. Thus, genetic and environmental factors dynamically interact to impact resilient adaptation [56].

Neuroplasticity, the ability of the adult brain to adapt so as to mitigate the negative effects of trauma [51], also has significant potential for resilience [6, 52]. Just as negative environmental stimuli may detrimentally alter the brain, so too can positive environmental influences bring about positive physiological changes

[1] Koenig [36] notes that most studies examining the correlation between S/R and health found a 'significant positive association' (p. 35), a conclusion reached by other reviews of the literature [37]. While association does not necessarily imply causation [13], longitudinal research suggests that there may be a causative relationship between S/R and resilience [38].

[2] Much research indicates that S/R protects against and aids in recovery from depression, but there are indications that this relationship is complex with no clear one-to-one correlation [41].

in neural circuitry [57]. This suggests that physical changes to the brain may be precipitated by the environment [21, 58].

Environment

Environmental factors, including familial support, physical exercise, cognitive therapy, and contemplative practices [58], are significant in shaping resilience outcomes [6, 56]. Researchers suggest a threefold division among factors that influence resilience in children: individual characteristics, the familial environment, and the wider social environment [59]. More broadly, environmental considerations are significant for resilience and spirituality as spirituality may affect resilience as an environmental factor working at all of these levels. Thus, several components of spirituality, both 'internal' and 'external' to the individual, must be distinguished and assessed for their role in promoting resilient adaptation. But, first, further distinction must be made between S/R coping and resilience.

Spiritual coping

The concept of 'coping' is closely related to resilience in that both concern adaptation to adversity. They differ, however, in that coping does not necessitate significant adversity and does not imply a positive outcome. Thus, coping may be either positive or negative, depending on both the means of coping and the result achieved.

In relation to spirituality, scholars propose the concept of 'spiritual coping' to describe the use of spiritual resources in the coping process.[3] As with coping more generally, both positive and negative results are associated with corresponding modes of positive and negative spiritual coping [60]. Significant benefits are associated with positive spiritual coping for patients experiencing chronic pain [47, 48] and those diagnosed with cancer [46]. Spiritual resources are one among many means of coping with adversity, and, as with other means of coping, all research does not point to supremely good outcomes for the use of spiritual coping. Personal values associated with spirituality can be both positively and negatively correlated with post-traumatic stress disorder in soldiers following deployment [65]. Furthermore, some studies indicate that individuals who consider spiritual values important, such as the search for meaning and understanding adversity in life, have a higher incidence of psychiatric disorders, especially in the absence of a religious framework [42, 61].[4]

Some of the variation in outcomes may be owing to the fact that spirituality can be used and abused in a negative manner. For example, spirituality may be used to foster hatred towards others or

oneself, to increase irrational and unnecessary guilt, or to condone uncharitable or harmful actions [66].

Self-efficacy

Research shows the importance of self-efficacy, choice, and control in positive health outcomes and, alternatively, the role of uncertainty and feelings of loss of control in negative health outcomes [67, 68]. S/R can provide an important means of control, both by direct and indirect means, and thereby increase feelings of self-efficacy. Pargament links his understanding of religious coping methods with the construct of control. He notes four types of methods of religious coping: self-directing, collaborative, deferring, and pleading [69]. Researchers found that '[c]ollaborative religious coping methods were especially linked to positive religious outcomes and greater coping efficacy' [69, p. 676]. Some propose 'spiritual struggle' as an aspect of negative spiritual coping [70]. Additional clarity is needed to understand the relationship between 'struggle' and resilience.

Components of spirituality

Spirituality is a multidimensional construct, encompassing a variety of diverse and complementary facets. Owing to its complex nature, the same event in an individual's life may have both positive and negative spiritual implications; it may be good for someone in one way and not in another. An individual may beneficially use aspects of spirituality while at the same time use other parts negatively. The relationship between spirituality and resilience must therefore be understood in terms of individual constructs that together compose the concept of spirituality. These components, and their effect on resilience, now need to be addressed more fully.

These represent only a limited number of constructs associated with spirituality that may influence resilient adaptation. One could also include forgiveness, altruism, and self-regulation among the many other concepts within this list.

Purpose

Many individuals find purpose through spiritual experiences and views of the world informed by spirituality. Such feelings of purpose may be rooted in finding fulfilment through something outside of oneself, being 'caught up' in a cause greater than oneself, or another means significant to the individual.

Research demonstrates that a sense of purpose plays a substantial role in positive health outcomes [71–73]. Purpose may also be significant for resilient adaptation. While not all discussions of 'purpose' contend with meanings of ultimate (or spiritual) purpose, scholars often see purpose and spirituality as related. One scholar introduced the concept of ultimacy as a means of differentiating ultimate purpose from more ordinary conceptions of purpose [71], yet ultimate and mundane purpose are not always easy to differentiate. The sense of purpose involved in giving direction and hope in everyday life is of the same kind, although different in scale, than 'ultimate' purpose. Additionally, 'ultimate' purpose may very well play itself out in the details of everyday life. Spirituality is concerned with the purposive nature of human existence—a pursuit that has significant implications for resilience.

Meaning

Also associated with the construct of spirituality, research indicates that meaning and meaning-making are important in positive

---

[3] Similarly, some scholars suggest 'religious coping' as an appropriate description for the use of religious resources in dealing with adversity [36].
[4] Regarding religion, Pargament [62] suggests a 'stress mobilization theory' as a way to account for the seeming negative outcome associated with some religious coping. He proposes that negative outcomes in such studies are due to their cross-sectional nature. They are a snapshot of times when individuals facing adversity turn to religion as a means of coping. This creates an apparent positive correlation between religion and distress. If these individuals were studied in a longitudinal manner, he suggests, religiosity would be found to correlate with reduced distress. Several studies seem to confirm this theory [63, 64]. Similar reasoning could be applied to the relationship between spirituality and coping.

mental health outcomes [74–76]. Ann Masten [77] suggests that 'meaning-making systems of belief, and organizations and cultural practices that nurture these systems, such as schools and religions' are protective factors that increase positive resilience outcomes (p. 579). Theological and philosophical understandings of suffering and evil, 'theodicies', have long been a part of the work of theologians and philosophers. Although the relationship between S/R beliefs and response to difficulty is somewhat ambiguous, those who experience trauma seek to find meaning for their traumatic experiences [75, 78], and, for many, S/R beliefs provide the framework in which these experiences can be understood [74]. However, in certain circumstances traumatic experiences can weaken religious faith [78].

Research suggests that cognitive processing ('rumination') is linked to meaning-making and post-traumatic growth [79]. Reappraisal allows an individual to reframe his or her circumstances and emotional reactions in a way that enables positive coping [80]. In the context of spirituality, this could often mean 'reframing' the apparent paradox of a good God and suffering [81]. S/R coping also can take place at a community level, in particular through the meaning-making process of creating a community narrative [82].

The creation of a narrative, which can be part of the meaning-making process, is intricately tied to the belief systems that underlie the perception and interpretation of reality. Froma Walsh argues that belief systems are the 'heart and soul of resilience' [83]. She writes, 'We cope with crisis and adversity by making meaning of our experience: linking it to our social world, to our cultural and spiritual beliefs, to our multigenerational past, and to our hopes and dreams for the future' (p. 49). An individual's beliefs about the world have a significant impact on his or her assessment of the world and, ultimately, upon health and ability to be resilient.

Transcendence

For many, connection with the transcendent is not only fundamental to spirituality, but also may provide a common reference point for chaplains and mental health clinicians [11]. Transcendence can be understood in various ways, such as 'God,' 'nature,' or the 'numinous Other', but remains essential to expression of spirituality 'as being both distinctive and characteristic of spirituality' [11, p. 143]. What is common to these understandings is that the transcendent provides a perspective beyond that of the individual—one that supersedes the supremacy of the *ego*.

Connection with the transcendent supports resilient adaptation through a number of different avenues. Belief in that which is transcendent can provide stability despite change or perception of change [72, 74]. Thus, external sources of input associated with the transcendent, such as sacred writings, may offer guidance in the midst of adversity. Additionally, for many, the transcendent includes recognition of an agent who can act on behalf of the individual, especially during adverse circumstances. This is particularly true, though not exclusively so, of those who believe in God or gods.

In the midst of adversity many turn to an external source to find hope, purpose, and meaning [28–30]. These are often provided by a viewpoint beyond the individual—a source of transcendent vision. The connection between the individual and that which is outside of the self, however, often necessitates more than a cursory encounter.

Relationship

As an aspect of spirituality, social support is a predictor for resilience [84, 85]. Some scholars suggest that this correlation is owing, in part, to the social support received within a faith community [50, 86, 87].[5] Similarly, Walsh suggests that family belief systems including the ability to make meaning out of adversity, have a positive outlook, and use transcendence and spirituality to deal with difficulty are key to family resilience [83]. This highlights the prominent role that relationships and interpersonal connectedness play in spirituality and its promotion of health.

In like manner, studies show the powerful relationship between attachment and well-being [88, 89]. In terms of relationship to the Divine, research suggests that an individual's beliefs about God have significant implications for both attachment and health [90, 91]. Thus, relationship, both with the Transcendent and with others in community, figures significantly in the connection between resilience and spirituality.

Case study

While much research highlights the significance of spirituality for resilience, such abstracted data is not able to describe fully the role that spirituality plays in resilience. For a more complete picture that is also relevant and useful in clinical settings, additional personal insight is needed. Here a case study is provided to fill that need.

Mary

Mary (not her real name) was not a practising member of any religion when one of the authors (NW) met her. Despite being raised in a culture with strong religious influences, when religious topics came up in conversation she would politely change the subject. Her disposition changed, however, when she went through a divorce. In the midst of this crisis she reached out to a pastor, received support, and became a part of a Christian faith community. Mary found strength in her faith and enthusiastically joined Bible studies and worship services in this new community, which became like family to her. She made scripture reading and prayer a part of her daily routine and commented that she did not know how she could get through a day without the help of Jesus. Mary continued growing in this newfound life of faith when, less than 2 years after beginning her faith journey, she was diagnosed with an advanced stage of an aggressive form of cancer. She received the news with a calm and resolve that had not been present during her divorce, nor before. Through the crisis of divorce her faith had comforted and strengthened her, and she received support through her faith community. Reliance upon her faith had developed resilience in her during the years following the trauma of divorce. Throughout chemotherapy treatment Mary displayed a love and a peace that others noticed. Certainly, there were moments of tears, but for her these were tempered by an overwhelming sense of God's love, even in the experience of this disease. Facing the prospect of her own death, she was more concerned for the welfare of her teenage son and ailing mother than for herself. After nearly a year of battling

---

[5] Some suggest, however, that the association of church attendance with health cannot simply be reduced to a function of social support [87].

cancer Mary died, at peace with herself, her God, and the world—a change she would have attributed to her faith.

Clinical applications

The role of spirituality in promoting resilience indicates the need for understanding how these insights can be used in public mental health and clinical settings. The application of these insights must go beyond a simple step-by-step or 'how to' mentality of prescribed treatment protocols. Instead, this relationship suggests a framework within which a number of specific applications may take place. While a growing body of research assesses the relationship between spirituality and resilience, less work has developed a framework within which these concepts may be understood and insights applied. Because of this, Levin [23] proposes that more is needed than simply collection of data on this relationship: a framework for making sense of the empirical data is vital.

One aspect of this framework could include viewing resilience through the lens of environment (sometimes called a 'social-ecological model of resilience' [2, p. 441]). This would enable practitioners to see spiritual resources as one environmental resource among many that may help promote resilient adaptation to adversity. Both external and internal spiritual resources, such as relationship, purpose, meaning, and transcendence, are available to the individual and community to foster resilient adaptation.

Professional mental health organizations are recognizing the possibilities in spirituality for the promotion of mental health. For example, the World Psychiatric Association recently issued a Position Statement on Spirituality and Religion in Psychiatry [92] that sets forth guidelines for the beneficial use of S/R in clinical settings. This position statement suggests the importance of clinicians taking a spiritual assessment of patients and seeing the patient's spirituality as a resource for supporting coping rather than dismissing it or ignoring it altogether [7].

Beyond simply appreciating spirituality as a potentially significant factor in patients' lives and mental health, clinicians should be cognisant of the ways spirituality may affect patient coping ability both in clinical [93] and public health [94] settings. Psychiatrists and clinicians would do well to persevere with individuals in their struggles, realizing that for many adversity could have a potentially transformative, or even spiritual, component. Adversities should not be accepted blindly or wholesale, but this viewpoint suggests that there may be beneficial treatment goals beyond a surface-level 'non-pathology'. In this regard, narrative is a useful tool both for assessing patient history and for partnering with individuals towards treatment goals owing to the close relationship among narrative, belief, and hope [95].

Public mental health policymakers should be aware of the potential health benefits associated with spirituality and support integration of spirituality into a comprehensive approach to health promotion when possible. This could involve promoting spiritual care through chaplaincy and spiritual care services, encouraging clinician engagement with wider community and faith-based organizations, and implementing policies and codes of conduct that address issues that arise in the context of practice. For instance, policymakers should understand that clinical staff may face opposition to the use of spirituality in a clinical setting and are vulnerable in many regards, including in legal matters [96]. Furthermore, additional attention should be paid to the role of faith communities in

public health crises such as natural disasters, disease pandemics, and economic crises [94, 97, 98]. In many instances, a local faith community is among the first to respond to such crises, is already intimately integrated into the community in crisis, and is a continuing presence once aid organizations depart.

Cautions

Several cautions for understanding the role of spirituality in resilient adaptation must be mentioned. Some scholars suggest that a purely utilitarian use of S/R distorts its true nature [99]. From this perspective, the distortion of spirituality as solely a utilitarian means to the goal of health cannot be rectified by any outcome. Such use misrepresents the essence of spirituality and disfigures it until it is nearly unrecognizable. Spirituality must be taken on its own terms and accepted as such without subjecting it to a foreign purpose or end. Put simply, the goal of spirituality is not the promotion of health. Good health may well be a by-product of spirituality, certainly, but not the ultimate goal.

Additionally, it should be recognized that resilience may not always be a goal to be pursued. Some social scientists argue that a focus upon resilience can paradoxically lead to an emphasis on narratives of disempowerment and insecurity as the status quo of human existence, thereby creating a nihilistic and meaningless existence [100]. Given these observations, the concept of resilience should be embraced with a degree of caution, recognizing assumptions inherent in the concept and the way they may shape broader understandings of the world. Resilience is not a panacea to all human ills, but it can be useful for understanding positive human adaptation to adversity. The person informed by a spiritual vantage point may be better able to distinguish between beneficial and unhelpful forms of resilience.

Conclusions

The positive benefits of spirituality in supporting resilient adaptation to adversity suggested by research warrant the inclusion of spiritual practices as a valuable part of broader efforts in the promotion of public mental health. Such efforts should proceed attentive to the pitfalls inherent in this undertaking, yet sensitive to the powerful influence exerted by spirituality on many individuals and communities. Perhaps the most compelling evidence for the role of spirituality in resilience is the lives of people such as Mary, illustrative of countless individuals throughout nearly every culture, socio-economic class, time, and place that are enabled to face adversity resiliently through the aid of spiritual resources.

References

1. Cook CCH. Religion and spirituality in clinical practice. *BJPsych Adv* 2015; 21: 42–50.
2. Panter-Brick C. Health, risk, and resilience: interdisciplinary concepts and applications. *Annu Rev Anthropol* 2014; 43: 431–448.
3. Masten AS. Global perspectives on resilience in children and youth. *Child Dev* 2014; 85: 6–20.
4. Panter-Brick C, Leckman JF. Editorial Commentary: Resilience in child development—interconnected pathways to wellbeing. *J Child Psychol Psychiatry* 2013; 54: 333–336.
5. Windle G. What is resilience? A review and concept analysis. *Rev Clin Gerontol* 2011; 21: 152–169.

6. Cicchetti D, Blender JA. A multiple-levels-of-analysis perspective on resilience: implications for the developing brain, neural plasticity, and preventive interventions. *Ann N Y Acad Sci* 2006; 1094: 248–258.

7. Cook CCH. Recommendations for psychiatrists on spirituality and religion (Position Statement PS03/2013). Available at: http://www.rcpsych.ac.uk/pdf/ps03_2013.pdf (2013, accessed 10 March 2016)

8. Cook CCH. Addiction and spirituality. *Addiction* 2004; 99: 539–551.

9. Pargament KI. The psychology of religion and spirituality? Yes and no. *Int J Psychol Relig* 1999; 9: 3–16.

10. Koenig HG, King DE, Carson VB. *Handbook of Religion and Health*, 2nd ed. Oxford: Oxford University Press, 2012.

11. Cook CCH. Transcendence, immanence and mental health. In: Cook CCH (ed.). *Spirituality, Theology and Mental Health: Multidisciplinary Perspectives*. London: SCM Press, 2013, pp. 141–159.

12. Bowker JW. Religion. In: Bowker JW (ed.). *The Oxford Dictionary of World Religions*. Oxford: Oxford University Press, 1997, pp. xv–xxiv.

13. Casey P. 'I'm spiritual but not religious': implications for research and practice. In: Cook CCH (ed.). *Spirituality, Theology and Mental Health: Multidisciplinary Perspectives*. London: SCM Press, 2013, pp. 20–39.

14. Mercadante LA. *Belief Without Borders: Inside the Minds of the Spiritual but not Religious*. New York: Oxford University Press, 2014.

15. Monod S, Brennan M, Rochat E, Martin E, Rochat S, Büla CJ. Instruments measuring spirituality in clinical research: a systematic review. *J Gen Intern Med* 2011; 26: 1345–1357.

16. Fetzer Institute, National Institute on Aging Working Group. Multidimensional Measurement of Religiousness, Spirituality for Use in Health Research. Available at: http://fetzer.org/resources/multidimensional-measurement-religiousnessspirituality-use-health-research (2003, accessed 4 June 2018).

17. Brady MJ, Peterman AH, Fitchett G, Mo M, Cella D. A case for including spirituality in quality of life measurement in oncology. *Psychooncology* 1999; 8: 417–428.

18. King M, Speck P, Thomas A. The Royal Free interview for religious and spiritual beliefs: development and standardization. *Psychol Med* 1995; 25: 1125–1134.

19. Ellison CW. Spiritual well-being: conceptualization and measurement. *J Psychol Theol* 1983; 11: 330–340.

20. Ganga NS, Kutty VR. Influence of religion, religiosity and spirituality on positive mental health of young people. *Ment Health Relig Cult* 2013; 16: 435–443.

21. Amstadter AB, Myers JM, Kendler KS. Psychiatric resilience: longitudinal twin study. *Br J Psychiatry* 2014; 205: 275–280.

22. Yehuda R, Flory JD. Differentiating biological correlates of risk, PTSD, and resilience following trauma exposure. *J Trauma Stress* 2007; 20: 435–447.

23. Levin J. Religion and mental health: theory and research. *Int J Appl Psychoanal Stud* 2010; 7: 102–115.

24. Browning DS. *Reviving Christian Humanism: The New Conversation on Spirituality, Theology, and Psychology*. Minneapolis, MN: Fortress Press, 2010.

25. American Psychiatric Association. Diagnostic and Statistical Manual of Mental Disorders. Fifth Edition. Available at: http://psychiatryonline.org/doi/book/10.1176/appi.books.9780890425596 (2013, accessed 14 March 2016).

26. Poole R, Higgo R, Strong G, et al. Religion, psychiatry and professional boundaries. *Psychiatr Bull* 2008; 32: 356–357.

27. Sloan RP, Bagiella E, Powell T. Religion, spirituality, and medicine. *Lancet* 1999; 353: 664–667.

28. Schuster MA, Stein BD, Jaycox LH, et al. A national survey of stress reactions after the September 11, 2001, terrorist attacks. *N Engl J Med* 2001; 345: 1507–1512.

29. Büssing A, Ostermann T, Koenig HG. Relevance of religion and spirituality in German patients with chronic diseases. *Int J Psychiatry Med* 2007; 37: 39–57.

30. Büssing A, Abu-Hassan WM, Matthiessen PF, Ostermann T. Spirituality, religiosity, and dealing with illness in Arabic and German patients. *Saudi Med J* 2007; 28: 933–942.

31. WHOQOL SRPB Group. A cross-cultural study of spirituality, religion, and personal beliefs as components of quality of life. *Soc Sci Med*. 2006; 62: 1486–1497.

32. Friedli L. Mental health, resilience and inequalities. Available at: http://www.euro.who.int/__data/assets/pdf_file/0012/100821/E92227.pdf (2009, accessed 18 November 2014).

33. Hatala AR. Resilience and healing amidst depressive experiences: an emerging four-factor model from emic/etic perspectives. *J Spiritual Ment Health* 2011; 13: 27–51.

34. Connor KM, Davidson JR, Lee L-C. Spirituality, resilience, and anger in survivors of violent trauma: a community survey. *J Trauma Stress* 2003; 16: 487–494.

35. Peres JFP, Moreira-Almeida A, Nasello AG, Koenig HG. Spirituality and resilience in trauma victims. *J Relig Health* 2007; 46: 343–350.

36. Koenig HG. *Spirituality in Patient Care: Why, How, When, and What*, 3rd ed. West Conshohocken, PA: Templeton Foundation Press, 2013.

37. Wong YJ, Rew L, Slaikeu KD. A systematic review of recent research on adolescent religiosity/spirituality and mental health. *Issues Ment Health Nurs* 2006; 27: 161–183.

38. Kasen S, Wickramaratne P, Gameroff MJ, Weissman MM. Religiosity and resilience in persons at high risk for major depression. *Psychol Med* 2012; 42: 509–519.

39. Miller L, Wickramaratne P, Gameroff MJ, Sage M, Tenke CE, Weissman MM. Religiosity and major depression in adults at high risk: a ten-year prospective study. *Am J Psychiatry* 2012; 169: 89–94.

40. Smith TB, McCullough ME, Poll J. Religiousness and depression: evidence for a main effect and the moderating influence of stressful life events. *Psychol Bull* 2003; 129: 614–636.

41. Maselko J, Gilman SE, Buka S. Religious service attendance and spiritual well-being are differentially associated with risk of major depression. *Psychol Med* 2009; 39: 1009–1017.

42. King M, Marston L, McManus S, Brugha T, Meltzer H, Bebbington P. Religion, spirituality and mental health: results from a national study of English households. *Br J Psychiatry* 2013; 202: 68–73.

43. Kim J. The protective effects of religiosity on maladjustment among maltreated and nonmaltreated children. *Child Abuse Negl* 2008; 32: 711–720.

44. Koenig HG, Larson DB, Larson SS. Religion and coping with serious medical illness. *Ann Pharmacother* 2001; 35: 352–359.

45. Balboni TA, Vanderwerker LC, Block SD, et al. Religiousness and spiritual support among advanced cancer patients and associations with end-of-life treatment preferences and quality of life. *J Clin Oncol* 2007; 25: 555–560.

46. Holt CL, Schulz E, Caplan L, Blake V, Southward VL, Buckner AV. Assessing the role of spirituality in coping among African Americans diagnosed with cancer. *J Relig Health* 2012; 51: 507–521.

47. Büssing A, Michalsen A, Balzat H-J, et al. Are spirituality and religiosity resources for patients with chronic pain conditions? *Pain Med* 2009; 10: 327–339.

48. Wachholtz AB, Pearce MJ, Koenig H. Exploring the relationship between spirituality, coping, and pain. *J Behav Med* 2007; 30: 311–318.

49. Wiech K, Farias M, Kahane G, Shackel N, Tiede W, Tracey I. An fMRI study measuring analgesia enhanced by religion as a belief system. *Pain* 2008; 139: 467–476.

50. Koenig HG. An 83-year-old woman with chronic illness and strong religious beliefs. *JAMA* 2002; 288: 487–493.

51. Karatoreos IN, McEwen BS. Annual research review: the neurobiology and physiology of resilience and adaptation across the life course. *J Child Psychol Psychiatry* 2013; 54: 337–347.

52. Southwick SM, Charney DS. The science of resilience: implications for the prevention and treatment of depression. *Science* 2012; 338: 79–82.

53. Tracey I. Getting the pain you expect: mechanisms of placebo, nocebo and reappraisal effects in humans. *Nat Med* 2010; 16: 1277–1283.

54. Gard T, Holzel BK, Sack AT, et al. Pain attenuation through mindfulness is associated with decreased cognitive control and increased sensory processing in the brain. *Cereb Cortex* 2012; 22: 2692–2702.

55. Yehuda R, Daskalakis NP, Desarnaud F, et al. Epigenetic biomarkers as predictors and correlates of symptom improvement following psychotherapy in combat veterans with PTSD. *Front Psychiatry* 2013; 4: 118.

56. Rende R. Behavioral resilience in the post-genomic era: emerging models linking genes with environment. *Front Hum Neurosci* 2012; 6: 50.

57. Cicchetti D, Valentino K. Toward the application of a multiple-levels-of-analysis perspective to research in development and psychopathology. In: Masten AS (ed.) *Multilevel Dynamics in Developmental Psychopathology: Pathways to the Future*. Mahwah, NJ: Lawrence Erlbaum Associates, 2007, pp. 243–284.

58. Davidson RJ, McEwen BS. Social influences on neuroplasticity: stress and interventions to promote well-being. *Nat Neurosci* 2012; 15: 689–695.

59. Luthar, SS, Cicchetti, D, Becker, B. The construct of resilience: a critical evaluation and guidelines for future work. *Child Dev* 2000; 71: 543–562.

60. Gall TL. Spirituality and coping with life stress among adult survivors of childhood sexual abuse. *Child Abuse Negl* 2006; 30: 829–844.

61. Baetz M, Bowen R, Jones G, Koru-Sengul T. How spiritual values and worship attendance relate to psychiatric disorders in the Canadian population. *Can J Psychiatry* 2006; 51: 654–661.

62. Pargament KI. *The Psychology of Religion and Coping: Theory, Research, Practice*. New York: Guilford Press, 1997.

63. Hebert RS, Dang Q, Schulz R. Religious beliefs and practices are associated with better mental health in family caregivers of patients with dementia: findings from the REACH study. *Am J Geriatr Psychiatry* 2007; 15: 292–300.

64. Pargament KI, Ishler K, Dubow EF, et al. Methods of religious coping with the Gulf War: cross-sectional and longitudinal analyses. *J Sci Study Relig* 1994; 33: 347–361.

65. Zimmermann P, Firnkes S, Kowalski JT, et al. Personal values in soldiers after military deployment: associations with mental health and resilience. *Eur J Psychotraumatology* 2014; 5.

66. Crowley N, Jenkinson G. Pathological spirituality. In: Cook CCH, Powell A, Sims A (eds). *Spirituality and Psychiatry*. London: RCPsych Publications, 2010, pp. 254–272.

67. Kay AC, Whitson JA, Gaucher D, Galinsky AD. Compensatory control achieving order through the mind, our institutions, and the heavens. *Curr Dir Psychol Sci* 2009; 18: 264–268.

68. Jackson BR, Bergeman CS. How does religiosity enhance well-being? The role of perceived control. *Psychol Relig Spiritual* 2011; 3: 149–161.

69. Pargament KI, Magyar-Russell GM, Murray-Swank NA. The sacred and the search for significance: religion as a unique process. *J Soc Issues* 2005; 61: 665–687.

70. McConnell KM, Pargament KI, Ellison CG, Flannelly KJ. Examining the links between spiritual struggles and symptoms of psychopathology in a national sample. *J Clin Psychol* 2006; 62: 1469–1484.

71. Emmons RA. *The Psychology of Ultimate Concerns: Motivation and Spirituality in Personality*. New York: Guilford Press, 1999.

72. Schaefer SM, Morozink Boylan J, van Reekum CM, et al. Purpose in life predicts better emotional recovery from negative stimuli. *PLOS ONE* 2013; 8: e80329.

73. Schnitker SA, Emmons RA. Spiritual striving and seeking the sacred: religion as meaningful goal-directed behavior. *Int J Psychol Relig* 2013; 23: 315–324.

74. Murphy SA, Johnson LC, Lohan J. Finding meaning in a child's violent death: a five-year prospective analysis of parents' personal narratives and empirical data. *Death Stud* 2003; 27: 381–404.

75. Park CL, Folkman S. Meaning in the context of stress and coping. *Rev Gen Psychol* 1997; 1: 115–144.

76. Wexler LM, DiFluvio G, Burke TK. Resilience and marginalized youth: making a case for personal and collective meaning-making

as part of resilience research in public health. *Soc Sci Med* 2009; 69: 565–570.

77. Masten AS. Risk and resilience in development. In: Zelazo PD (ed.). *The Oxford Handbook of Developmental Psychology*. Oxford: Oxford University Press, 2013, pp. 579–607.

78. Fontana A, Rosenheck R. Trauma, change in strength of religious faith, and mental health service use among veterans treated for PTSD. *J Nerv Ment Dis* 2004; 192: 579–584.

79. Calhoun LG, Cann A, Tedeschi RG, McMillan J. A correlational test of the relationship between posttraumatic growth, religion, and cognitive processing. *J Trauma Stress* 2000; 13: 521–527.

80. Gross JJ. Antecedent-and response-focused emotion regulation: divergent consequences for experience, expression, and physiology. *J Pers Soc Psychol* 1998; 74: 224–237.

81. McCann RA, Webb M. Enduring and struggling with God in relation to traumatic symptoms: the mediating and moderating roles of cognitive flexibility. *Psychol Relig Spiritual* 2012; 4: 143–153.

82. Tuval-Mashiach R, Dekel R. Religious meaning-making at the community level: the forced relocation from the Gaza Strip. *Psychol Relig Spiritual* 2014; 6: 64–71.

83. Walsh F. *Strengthening Family Resilience*, 2nd ed. New York: Guilford Press, 2006.

84. Nuttman-Swartz O. Macro, meso, and micro-perspectives of resilience during and after exposure to war. In: Ungar M (ed.) *The Social Ecology of Resilience*. New York: Springer, 2012, pp. 415–424.

85. Southwick SM, Sippel L, Krystal J, Charney D, Mayes L, Pietrzak R. Why are some individuals more resilient than others: the role of social support. *World Psychiatry* 2016; 15: 77–79.

86. Harris JI, Erbes CR, Winskowski AM, Engdahl BE, Nguyen XV. Social support as a mediator in the relationship between religious comforts and strains and trauma symptoms. *Psychol Relig Spiritual* 2014; 6: 223–229.

87. Pargament KI. The sacred character of community life. *Am J Community Psychol* 2008; 41: 22–34.

88. Belavich TG, Pargament KI. The role of attachment in predicting spiritual coping with a loved one in surgery. *J Adult Dev* 2002; 9: 13–29.

89. Kirkpatrick LA. Attachment theory and the evolutionary psychology of religion. *Int J Psychol Relig* 2012; 22: 231–241.

90. Bradshaw M, Ellison CG, Flannelly KJ. Prayer, God imagery, and symptoms of psychopathology. *J Sci Study Relig* 2008; 47: 644–659.

91. Kirkpatrick LA. God as a substitute attachment figure: a longitudinal study of adult attachment style and religious change in college students. *Pers Soc Psychol Bull* 1998; 24: 961–973.

92. Moreira-Almeida A, Sharma A, van Rensburg BJ, Verhagen PJ, Cook CCH. WPA position statement on spirituality and religion in psychiatry. *World Psychiatry* 2016; 15: 87–88.

93. Cook CCH, Breckon J, Jay C, Renwick L, Walker P. Pathway to accommodate patients' spiritual needs. *Nurs Manag (Harrow)* 2012; 19: 33–37.

94. McCabe OL, Semon NL, Lating JM, et al. An academic-government-faith partnership to build disaster mental health preparedness and community resilience. *Public Health Rep* 2014; 129(Suppl. 4): 96–106.

95. Cook CCH, Powell A, Sims A. *Spirituality and Narrative in Psychiatric Practice: Stories of Mind and Soul*. London: RCPsych Publications, 2016.

96. Eagger S, Richmond P, Gilbert P. Spiritual care in the NHS. In: Cook CCH, Powell A, Sims A (eds). *Spirituality and Psychiatry*. London: RCPsych Publications, 2010, pp. 190–211.

97. Aten JD, O'Grady KA, Milstein G, Boan D, Schruba A. Spiritually oriented disaster psychology. *Spiritual Clin Pract* 2014; 1: 20–28.

98. Brenner GH, Bush DH, Moses J (eds). *Creating Spiritual and Psychological Resilience: Integrating Care in Disaster Relief Work*. New York: Routledge, 2009.

99. Shuman JJ, Meador KG, Hauerwas SM. *Heal Thyself: Spirituality, Medicine, and the Distortion of Christianity*. Oxford: Oxford University Press, 2002.

100. Evans B, Reid J. Dangerously exposed: the life and death of the resilient subject. *Resilience* 2013; 1: 83–98.

CHAPTER 55

Innovations in the area of social media

Annisa Lee and Stephan Stiller

Introduction

Innovations in the area where mental health meets social media include computerized self-help strategies, online psychotherapy and support groups, websites with medical information, forums, blogs, web applications, mobile apps, games, and online social media networking platforms such as Facebook, Instagram, Google+, Snapchat, Twitter, Flickr, YouTube, Pinterest, and Reddit. Online social networking is the process of developing and engaging with a virtual network of people with whom one has articulated a personal or professional connection within the online environment of a social networking site (SNS) [1]. In 2017, 2.46 billion people used SNSs worldwide [2]. These innovations have transformed the way people communicate with each other, as screen time has substituted for real-life, face-to-face interactions and as a virtual presentation replaces authentic expressions of oneself. Because social media are so widely used all over the world, any concern, issue, or defect has the potential to be amplified into a global public mental health issue. Broadly speaking, over the last decade, empirical evidence shows that these new communicative habits, acting like a two-edged sword, have profound diametric harms and benefits effects on the general public. More specifically, research into addictive technological behaviours has revealed a prevalence of addiction to SNSs and co-morbidity between behavioural addictions and various types of psychiatric disorders. Many studies suggest a complex relationship between online social networking and mental illness involving specific factors that can mediate or moderate this relationship. However, these new technologies can provide efficient interventions for psychiatric diseases. This chapter will investigate the essential factors in the context of the two dynamic effects with respect to major mental health-related topics.

Methodology

A list of common mental health conditions and concepts was generated. Entries include expressions such as 'ADD/ADHD', 'anxiety', 'bereavement/grief', 'depression', 'drug abuse', 'loneliness', 'mindfulness', 'OCD', 'social anxiety/phobia', and 'stress'. All medical subject headings (MeSH) in the PubMed database covering these mental health conditions and concepts were identified. Thus, the search terms identified were conjoined (i.e. AND'ed together) with

'Social Media' [MeSH] in order to narrow properly the scope of the investigation to the intersection of the concept of 'mental health' and the concept of 'social media'. The search was restricted to the preceding 5 years (as of the beginning of 2017). To the resulting list of PubMed articles for each topic, articles from the major journals about social media and health were added: *Health Communication* (2010–present), *Journal of Computer-Mediated Communication* (all issues), *Journal of Health Communication* (2010–present), *Journal of Interactive Advertising* (all issues), *New Media & Society* (all issues), and *Translational Behavioral Medicine* (all issues). The time ranges considered were determined by first going through the past 7 years and then going further, if it seemed that such a search might be fruitful. The resulting list of articles for each topic was perused and narrowed to those which can properly be said to describe a recent innovation in the intersection of the areas of mental health and social media.

Negative effects of social media on mental health

Associations and co-morbidity

In a large cross-sectional online survey with 23,533 adults (mean age 35.8 years), correlations between symptoms of addictive uses of social media and video games and symptoms of attention deficit hyperactivity disorder (ADHD), obsessive–compulsive disorder (OCD), anxiety, and depression were all positive and significant; there were also weak associations between the two addictive technological behaviours [3]. In a meta-analysis of 30 empirical studies, five found a positive correlation between engagement in SNSs and symptoms of depression [4]. In Singapore, in a study with 1110 college students, the co-morbidity rates of SNS addiction and affective disorders were 21.0% for depression, 27.7% for anxiety, and 26.1% for mania. Students' SNS addiction (29.5%) was also found to co-occur with food addiction and shopping addiction [5]. Obsessive and compulsive behaviours have been observed in pathological Internet users. OCD is an anxiety disorder characterized by obsessive thoughts and compulsive behaviours to reduce the anxiety caused by those thoughts [6]. A study assessed the relationship between problematic media use and compulsion, looking at compulsive buying, compulsive Internet use, and compulsive mobile phone use, and found that

that these behaviours are not carried out to feel pleasure, but to relieve anxiety [7].

Demographics

There are generational differences in the degree of familiarity and problematic use of social media. ADHD and social anxiety disorder were associated with high problematic Internet uses in young participants aged 25 years or younger, whereas generalized anxiety disorder and OCD were associated with highly problematic Internet use among participants aged 55 years and older [8]. In a large online survey, symptoms of addictive use of social media and of video games and symptoms of mental disorder for ADHD and OCD were all related, with age being inversely related to the addictive use of these technologies. In the study, the authors argue that the two types of computer addictions are distinct. Interesting correlations exist (i) between social networking and being female, single, and younger; and (ii) between video-gaming and being male, single, and younger [3]. As glucocorticoids are stress hormones that moderate the brain's development during adolescence, Julia Morin-Major's team discovered that the systemic output of cortisol was positively associated with the number of Facebooks friends and negatively associated with Facebook peer interactions among adolescent boys and girls [9]. College students with an SNS addiction reported higher co-morbidity rates with other behavioural addictions and with affective disorders [5]. In addition, adolescents who use social media more—both overall and at night—and adolescents who are more emotionally invested in social media experience poorer sleep, lower self-esteem, and higher levels of anxiety and depression. After controlling for anxiety, depression, and self-esteem, night-time-specific social media use predicted poorer sleep quality [10]. Another study found that users with self-identified sleep issues were more active during typical sleeping hours, which may suggest that they were having sleep problems. They were significantly less active on Twitter, in general, and had fewer friends and followers. They also exhibited significantly lower sentiment in their tweets, suggesting an association between the lack of sleep and psychosocial issues [11].

Sex was also found to influence the relationship between online social networking and depression [12–14]. Females reported higher co-morbidity rates of SNS addiction and affective disorders than males [5]. Emerging evidence suggests that social media use may increase the risk of poor well-being, including depression, anxiety, and concerns about body image among pregnant women [15]. In adolescent girls, emotional engagement in SNSs has been linked to lower self-esteem and a depressed mood, and for boys it was anxiety that triggered higher SNS involvement for the fear of missing out [16]. Exposure to SNSs that emphasize appearance, such as Instagram, has been linked to an increased body-image disturbance [17].

Personality was found to influence the relationship between online social networking and depression. Giota and Kleftaras [18] found that female participants with higher neuroticism had significantly higher levels of problematic SNS use and exhibited more depressive symptoms than those who scored lower on measures of neuroticism. They found a negative correlation between problematic SNS use and agreeableness, and no correlations between problematic SNS use and conscientiousness, openness to experience, or extraversion. In a study with 945 participants (790 Facebook users and 155 Facebook non-users), Facebook users were found to score significantly higher on narcissism, self-esteem, and extraversion than non-users. They also had more social support, life satisfaction, and perceived happiness, whereas Facebook non-users have higher values of depression symptoms [19]. In a study about investigating personality factors as predictors for Facebook usage, the factor and path analyses of the traits and usages of 654 Italian Facebook users show that openness was a predictor of Facebook adoption, conscientiousness was with sparing use, extraversion was with long sessions and abundant friendships, and neuroticism was with high frequency of sessions [20].

The manner of using social networking sites

Usage variables include frequency, quality, and the type of SNS use. In terms of frequency, positive correlations were found between depression and Facebook addiction, Facebook intrusion, and compulsive and prolonged SNS use [21–23]. Frequent posting on Facebook was associated with depression via rumination [24]. In a study that examined the use of the most popular professional social network, LinkedIn, and emotional distress, there was evidence to show that, compared with those who did not use LinkedIn, young adult participants (aged 19–32 years) using LinkedIn at least once per week had significantly greater odds of increased depression [25].

Alvarez-Jimenez et al. [26] argue that the Internet is suited to patients with psychosis because it offers anonymity and eases difficulties in social interaction. Kalbitzer et al. [27] believes that 'Twitter may have a high potential to induce psychosis in predisposed users'. This might have to do with Twitter's limitation of 280 characters, resulting in messages that are cryptic to outsiders and hence highly susceptible to misinterpretation. In a case study presented in the article, Twitter's addictive potential is a contributing factor.

As for different online social networking behaviours, depression was found to be significantly correlated with Facebook profiling management [28], frequent negative status updates, and negative comparison with others, leading to increased rumination [29]. Passive use of SNSs by browsing others' social events without posting one's own updates and frequent Facebook surveillance trigger resentment, jealousy, and loneliness [30, 31]. There are also associations between the display of symptoms of depression on Facebook and self-reported symptoms of depression among university students. Over 200 public Facebook profiles of undergraduates from two US universities were analysed in accordance with their owners' completed patient health questionnaires of clinical screen for depression. The results showed that self-disclosed references to depression symptoms in Facebook were associated with self-reported depression in real life [32]. Another study of 238 US college students discovered the same association exists between psychological distress and display of depressive symptoms in Facebook but not to self-reported negativity in status updates. In fact, most status updates were generally positive, regardless of the psychological distress status. Students with distress are more concerned with their self-presentation to their friends than those without distress [33]. The ambivalence to show both depression by being authentic and happiness to avoid others' unfavourable judgement becomes a tensed current flowing underneath 'smiling depression' in social media.

Lack of social support

A study found out that having a larger number of Facebook friends predicted more clinical symptoms of bipolar mania, narcissism, and histrionic personality disorder but fewer symptoms of dysthymia and schizoid personality disorder [28]. Positive correlations were found between depression and negative social networking interactions in Facebook [4]. More frequent Instagram use has significant associations with social comparisons and depressive symptoms for people who follow more strangers [34]. Being single was positively related to both addictive social networking and video gaming [3].

Online support groups gather anonymous people of similar health conditions who disclose their own struggles and share useful health information to gain support and understanding of their problems. Xu and Zhang [35] used linguistic analysis and social network analysis to find out that there was an intensive use of 'self-focus words' and 'negative affect words' in a major online group about depression. The members are self-preoccupied and share negative thought content, showing landmark characteristics of depression. Using a new Facebook Measure of Social Support Scale to measure the effectiveness of social support online, McCloskey et al. discovered that negative support in a Facebook social support group was correlated with depressive symptoms and poorer quality of life [36]. The authors suggested that online support might not translate to significant therapeutic benefits with a measurable reduction in depressive symptoms and an improvement of one's quality of life [36]. Regarding key-opinion leaders, a content analysis of Sina Weibo (the most popular social media platform in China) shows that public opinion leaders' stereotypical presentations of depressed people promotes stigmatization and reduces support for depressed individuals among their followers. Sharing information related to treatment reduces stigmatization and decreases support among followers. People's association between crime and depression increases stigmatization, whereas discussing depression in a health context helps increase support [37].

Cyberbullying

'The most common definitions of cyberbullying include the three basic components of traditional bullying, namely: repetition, power imbalance and deliberate intent to harm' [38]. Cyberbullying may be, in part, a shifting of existing aggressive tendencies to the online world [39]. Examples of modalities for cyberbullying are telephone calls, text messages, chats and chatrooms, online posts, emails, instant messages, and communication and interactions in online gaming, and so on [40]. Modes of cyberbullying include anonymous calls; messages (e.g. textual, visual, audio, or video content) that disturb as a result of to their pointless, annoying, insulting, threatening, obscene, libellous, or vilifying nature (e.g. gossip, rumours, or voting in a defamatory online poll); the spread of malware; exclusion from online communities; and relational aggression such as teasing, 'outing' of private information, impersonation, or undesired name tagging [40–43]. Cyberbullying differs from traditional bullying in that perpetrators can act anonymously, that the potential audience is very large, and that content can spread virally and is potentially permanent [44, 45], thereby making it harder for the cybervictim to find a bully-free retreat.

Jeffrey Lin, at the video game company Riot Games, which produces the world's leading online multiplayer battle game *League of Legends* (with 100 million players in 2016 [46], describes that harassment and toxic behaviour among players is rampant in online games and takes the form of malicious in-game chatting and behaviour-based manipulation during the game. Brendan Maher

[47] reports that '[r]acist, sexist and homophobic language is rampant; aggressors often threaten violence or urge a player to commit suicide; and from time to time, the vitriol spills beyond the confines of the game' and causes more psychological damage.

In a case study about participants' exposure to hate speech online, Oksanen et al. [39] report that their resulting mental health problems are likely effected by concurrent causal factors, such as pre-existing 'low levels of [family] attachment'. Hamm et al. [43] report in their review that 'the most common reason for cyberbullying is relationship issues'. They further list 'lack of confidence', 'desire to feel better about [oneself]', 'desire for control', 'finding it entertaining', and 'retaliation' as motivations for cyberbullying. Heirman et al. [44] use social network analysis to analyse cyberbullying. Their results show that 'in classes featured by high closeness centralization in the offline and online friendship network, more cyberbullying happens' and that 'in classes featuring a high global clustering coefficient in the online network, less cyberbullying occurs'.

Suicide

Among cases of suicide that are investigated, in more than 95% there is a diagnosable mental disorder. Mood disorders, especially depression (accounting for 35.8% of suicide cases), are highly associated with suicide [48]. An estimated 2–15% of persons who have been diagnosed with major depression die by suicide, whereas 3–20% of persons who have been diagnosed with bipolar disorder die by suicide. Suicide is the leading cause of death in those diagnosed with schizophrenia. The co-morbidity of substance abuse, anxiety disorders, schizophrenia, and bipolar disorder puts persons with depression at an even higher risk for suicide [49].

Suicide is the third leading cause of death among adolescents in the USA. Thom et al. [50] were not sure whether the net influence of online technologies on suicidality is positive or negative: while '[the Internet] can normalize self-harm and provide access to suicide content and [...] can create a forum for bullying and harassment [it can also] provide a support network, helping those who are socially isolated to form connections' [51]. Analyses of a nationally representative sample of adolescents showed that a 10% increase in suicide attempts by family members were associated with a 2.13% and 1.23% increase in adolescent suicidal ideation and attempts. The study also showed a 10% increase in peer suicidal ideation and attempts would lead to a 0.7% and 0.3% increase in such behaviours among peers. However, such associations became insignificant after environmental confounders were considered [52]. Giordano [53] explained the concept of suicide contagion as the transformation of the distant idea of suicide into a more familiar method to adopt when coping with stress, sorrow, or alienation after one's exposure to the suicide attempts of significant others. As such, when a friend attempts suicide, suicide becomes a more legitimized solution for distress coping that the adolescents may try to deploy. A study found evidence of emotional contagion and suicide contagion: emotional participants who know about their friends' suicide attempts, are significantly associated with their emotional distress, suicide ideation, and attempts [54]. In another study, Bailin et al. [55] report that use of new media is associated with higher mortality and correlation between the time spent on SNSs and various indicators of poor mental health, including suicidality, for adolescents. The interpersonal–psychological theory of suicidal behaviour [56] proposes that an individual will contemplate suicide if he or she has both the desire to die and the ability to carry out a suicide. The desire to die includes two psychological states: a low sense of belonging and perceived burdensomeness. Moberg and Anestis found out in an exploratory study involving 305 undergraduates that higher levels of negative interactions on SNSs significantly predict thwarted belongingness, which can impact on suicidal desire [57].

Mental health benefits of social media

Social networking platforms

Many studies have presented opposite results in terms of positive impact of social networking on health benefits [34]. Benefits of Facebook use have been found to arise from increased social contact, social capital, and self-esteem. Quality of feedback plays a role, with positive feedback enhancing self-esteem and well-being, and negative feedback producing the opposite result in users [31]. Negative correlations were found between depression and location tagging, and frequent posting of positive Facebook status updates leading to reduced rumination and less depression [4]. Grieve and Watkinson [58] showed that authentic self-presentation, a stronger coherence between one's true self and one's Facebook self, was associated with better social connectedness and less stress.

Treatment-resistant major depressive disorder (MDD) is a complex condition with low remission rates. Interventions based on cognitive–behavioural therapy (CBT) and psychodynamic psychotherapy have been administered to patients with MDD via the Internet, and results have been promising. Results show that Facebook groups had a decrease in 17-item Hamilton Depression Scale (HAM-D-17) and Beck Depression Inventory-II (BDI-II) scores, as well as higher remission and response rates than the control group. Therefore, in treatment-resistant MDD, Facebook can be used as an effective enhancement therapy, together with pharmacological therapy, especially if the psychiatrist is the patient's online 'friend' on Facebook [59].

Support groups

In face-to-face interaction, strong social support reduces stress and improves psychological well-being, and some studies have shown that the same holds true for online communication. Benefits of Facebook use have been found to arise from increased social contact and social capital (one's ability to stay connected with members of a previously inhabited community) [60]. A survey of 401 undergraduate Facebook users showed that the number of Facebook friends is the strongest predictor of stronger perceived social support, reduced stress, and better well-being [61]. Negative correlations were also found between depression and Facebook social support satisfaction, positive social comparison, and perceived social connectedness on Facebook [4]. A study of 2400 postings in two online forums for patients with bipolar disorder and their relatives found that 'group cohesion', 'emotional support', and 'exchange of information' were the major self-help mechanisms. The users discussed useful topics such as 'social network', 'symptoms of the illness', 'medication', 'illness-related aspects', 'social aspects', and 'financial and legal issues' in order to support each other [62]. Emotional support for hospice caregivers in case their patient dies is of varied quality in the USA, because it is obligatory but unfunded. In order to address this issue, Wittenberg-Lyles et al. [63] have experimented with a Facebook support group for hospice caregivers. There, people could discuss 'triggers' of emotional memories of the bereaved and share stories and coping strategies. Participation in the Facebook group was at least 3 months and in most cases longer than 6 months in duration. The intervention successfully lowered caregiver anxiety and depression. The authors state that 'there remains a strong need to establish guidelines for hospice bereavement care and to minimize the resources used to provide bereavement services'.

Psychotherapy websites

The Internet can provide resources around the clock every day; it can target specific, hard-to-reach groups with a specific intervention at a relatively low cost. Strong evidence exists for the effectiveness of a variety of online psychotherapy sites, with potential application both as an alternative to traditional healthcare delivery and as an addendum to face-to-face treatment [34]. Internet interventions using CBT and psychodynamic psychotherapy were applied to patients with major depressions and the results were promising. Yet, 'Internet and mobile technologies [have] been rarely applied to the treatment of psychotic disorders'. Most applications of online/mobile technologies merely transfer offline methods (doctor–patient conversations, conversations between patients, informative leaflets, questionnaires, etc.) to the online world. Exceptions that stood out were feedback 'supplemented with videoclips with actors modelling communication strategies' and 'personalized cognitive behavioural interventions in real time through text messaging' [64].

Mobile apps

There is a proliferation of mental health-related apps on the market, with 'an estimated 100,000 mHealth apps on iTunes and Google Play' [65]. They have been employed casually by smartphone users, as well as in clinical settings. Mobile apps have entered many different areas of health, ranging from exercise [66] to breast cancer [67] to depression [68] to the treatment of chronic diseases [69] to elderly care [70]. For example, the online website PsychiatryAdvisor.com [71] offers a list of 'Top 10 Mental Health Apps', broadly covering the ailments of depression, stress, anxiety, and post-traumatic stress disorder, and employing approaches such as connecting people with therapists, discussion boards, meditation, and CBT. These apps provide tailor-made support for numerous mental health conditions:

1. Code Blue—provides teenagers struggling from depression or bullying with a support group when they need it.

2. Breathe2Relax—developed for stress management and walks users through breathing exercises.

3. Lantern—combines techniques from CBT with advice from real experts.

4. PTSD Coach—provides a self-assessment tool that allows users to track symptoms over time and manage symptoms.

5. Optimism—focuses on self-tracking as a tool with a customized plan for coping with mental illnesses, including depression, bipolar disorder, anxiety, and post-traumatic stress disorder.

6. Talkspace—makes therapy more available by connecting users with one of over 200 licensed therapists via messaging.

7. Big White Wall—a community application where people suffering from mental illnesses come together and talk about their problems with support from trained therapists.

8. SAM—helps people manage anxiety by recording their anxiety levels and identifying triggers.

9. IntelliCare—This is a suite of apps developed by researchers at Northwestern University to target symptoms of depression and anxiety. The apps were developed as part of a national research study funded by the National Institutes of Health. The suite includes the IntelliCare Hub app and 12 mini apps. The Hub helps users manage their preferences and recommends apps based on their concerns.

10. Equanimity—a meditation timer that features simple graphics to minimize distractions during meditation and emits chime sounds at certain intervals.

Self-help apps offer many advantages. Many of them are 'meet[ing] an important need', owing to the prevalence of mental health issues and the ubiquity of mobile phones. They are very accessible, and hence using them may, owing to stigma around mental health issues, be a better first step than seeing a doctor [72]. They can be used whenever convenient or necessary [73]; for example, sufferers of post-traumatic stress disorder may need help at a moment's notice. They can monitor one's smartphone usage patterns as an early-warning system [72]. There is also an app that supplies time-appropriate reminders (or 'ecological momentary interventions') to not engage in risky sexual behaviour. Patients might even personify an app [68]. For example, one study [74] goes beyond the administration of questionnaires and make algorithm-based recommendations in the app (based on the responses to the questionnaires administered via the app). Users often prefer to have the interactions with the app be customized, that is, tailored to the emotional preferences of the user [68] and sometimes share data with their therapists as well [73].

In a Korean study, researchers developed the EmotionDiary app to evaluate users' depressive symptoms and provide information and tips about ways of coping with depression while measuring their responses. They found that Facebook activities had predictive power in distinguishing depressed and non-depressed individuals. Participants' responses (measured as the number of app tips viewed and via points), had a positive correlation with a scale measuring depression, whereas the number of friends and location tags had a negative correlation with it [75]. Oh and DeVylder [76] make an excellent suggestion for applying online/mobile technologies to treating psychosis, namely to use 'mobile technologies [to] monitor psychotic experiences'. The resulting data could be used for further analysis and for a warning system when interventions are urgently needed.

However, evidence-based clinical guidelines are often not observed in app design [65]. While 'smartphone apps claim to help conditions from addiction to schizophrenia', "most apps haven't been tested at all". Not only do we not know about their efficacy, but 'some may even be harmful'. An example would be an app meant to estimate one's blood alcohol concentration based on one's consumption of alcoholic drinks. This app seemed to increase the frequency of drinking and has the potential to promote drinking games. Ironically, this app was sponsored by the Swedish government, showing that even scientific endeavours with the best intentions may need care and testing [72]. Some apps pose a privacy risk due to Internet security issues. Mental health apps are regulated by the US Food and Drugs Administration only if they seem to be high

risk. Commercial apps tend to lack scientific backing, whereas more scientific ones take a long time to be produced [65, 72]. Apps may need to be adapted to the cultural environment of the users [72, 77], but many apps are merely an electronic interface for printed materials and serve a purely informative purpose (e.g. one app is essentially an interface for the DSM-5), presenting text (sometimes in a structured way) and audio clips [78]. Some apps are merely electronic tools for conducting surveys without much interactive capability or capacities for data analysis [79]. In order to maximize the potential of apps, evidence-based clinical guidelines should be developed accordingly.

Games

In a literature review of 15 game studies, Eichenberg and Schott [80] found that most 'serious' games use CBT modules as major interventions. Games include psychoeducation, cognitive restructuring, relaxation techniques for anxiety and anger management, and depression reduction. They discovered that such serious games are effective both as a standalone intervention and as part of psychotherapy, and appeal to patients, independent of age and sex. Some turned out to be as good as (offline) treatment. They are helpful tools for increasing one's motivation and for strengthening a therapeutic relationship. Alvarez-Jimenez et al. [64] mention the idea of evaluating psychosis treatment outcomes via social network analysis. They propose 'social gamification': the use of quizzes and team games to get participants with psychosis to get to know each other and to interact in a more engaging way.

Reducing cyberbullying

There are many anti-cyberbullying programmes and strategies [41, 81]. Lin's League of Legends team experimented with messages that would be displayed to players, advising them to be civil to each other. Messages differed in their wording (positive or negative framing), colour, and time of being displayed in the game. Overall, there were 216 conditions to test against a control, in which no tips were given. Lin discovered that warnings about harassment reduced different types of negativity if presented in red. In order to give players more power, Riot Games 'introduced the Tribunal, which gives players a chance to serve as judge and jury to their peers. In it, volunteers review chat logs from a player who has been reported for bad behaviour, and then vote on whether the offender deserves punishment'. They discovered that 'homophobic and racial slurs … triggered the most rebukes'. Lin's team experimented with different types of 'reform cards' that gave feedback about the rationale for their ban. Those that contained more details and Tribunal judgements were the most effective, with a 'reform rate' of 70%. In order to be more effective, Lin used machine learning to give automatic feedback to players 'within 5–10 minutes of an offence', with a reform rate of 92%. 'Since that system was switched on, Lin says, verbal toxicity among so-called ranked games, which are the most competitive—and most vitriolic—dropped by 40%. Globally, he says, the occurrence of hate speech, sexism, racism, death threats and other types of extreme abuse is down to 2% of all games.'

A very similar study was conducted by Anderson et al. [82] about weight-based cyberbullying. When dissenting comments were presented, 'participants' comments were significantly more positive or supporting for the victim'. 'This effect was more pronounced for men than for women.' Meter and Bauman [83] warn against children sharing passwords with friends. Hilt [84] writes that:

> [p]arents need to specifically tell their children that they will not revoke their phone or online privileges if they are cyber bullied, as this is a common fear preventing disclosures to parents. Parents should actively monitor their children's online media use through practices such as checking out their child's home page or viewing password-protected areas, particularly with young children (p. 481).

He also provides concrete advice such as to 'delete [the bully's messages] without reading them'. Doan et al. [85] caution patients to not read comments and to 'not engage in social media discussions' in the context of online stories about them. Klein et al. [40] advise: 'Physicians should also recognize that a patient's hesitancy to use or converse about electronic media may be evidence of undisclosed cyberbullying … They should educate parents about the phenomenon and empower them to supervise their children, to discuss cyberbullying, and to set limits on their children's media use.' Aboujaoude et al. [45] write about 'anonymous social networks' as a technical innovation that did not exist before 2014 and that serve as a novel platform for cyberbullying. They 'are made possible by mobile and geolocalization technologies [and] allow anonymous attacks from within a very narrow radius'. They have 'already been linked to several suicides and led to the "geofencing" of many schools to prevent access to certain apps from school grounds'.

Suicide prevention

Social media presents a contemporary opportunity for friends and family to recognize changes in their loved ones' moods and emotions, which lets them intervene before the irreversible happens.

Tracking and identification

Social media help to track and identify symptoms and signs of suicides. Ahuja et al. [86] describe a case where social media was used to (i) create an exact timeline of the attempt (important for treatment); (ii) convince the patient of the severity (thereby gaining his consent to inpatient treatment); and (iii) demonstrate the negative effects of his attempt on others. How important social media are nowadays is clear from the fact that 'studies show that 50% of suicide attempters disclose their plan to family or friends before the attempt'. Fu et al. [87] present a case study using network analysis to track the reactions to a suicide-related post on Sina Weibo (a Chinese microblogging platform). The authors found that, surprisingly,

> loose acquaintances, known as 'weak ties' … might be more helpful than a closed group within an interpersonal network in terms of responding to emergencies such as suicide attempts. …Therefore, if suicide prevention professionals or organizations can build up an online social media platform, it would be helpful to build up a network of gatekeepers or spectators who are able to contribute to early identification of people at risk from the population at large (p. 6).

Woo et al. [88] use natural language processing to track how often the general public used words expressing negative emotions on Twitter after the well-known tragedy of many Koreans dying when a ferry capsized in 2014, in an attempt to track the national public mood. Examples of the words tracked are 'anger', 'pain', and 'despair' (in Korean). The authors suggest that natural language processing methods can be used to 'monitor … the public mood',

thereby providing 'novel opportunities for policy makers to monitor the mental health of the general population'. In another study, Won et al. [89] used two blog-derived measures together with national statistical data to predict national suicide rates in South Korea with high correlations (above 0.7). The two variables in question are the number of blogs mentioning the Korean words for 'suicide' and 'to be exhausted' during the preceding 3 days.

A qualitative research study suggested using Twitter to surveil public mental health; the participants shared a positive view of using public domain Twitter data as a resource for public mental health monitoring [90]. O'Dea et al. [91] attempted to use machine learning to classify tweets with potentially suicide-related content into the three categories of being ignorable, problematic, or alarming. The data were preselected to contain certain suicide-related phrases, such as 'go to sleep forever' and 'better off without me'. Cash et al. [92] analysed public statements on MySpace for suicidal content. Their analysis discussed 'themes' such as reasons and methods of suicide that were referenced.

Intervention

Some studies suggested methods of suicide interventions, for example Haim et al. [93] looked at whether one's Google search history would influence subsequent results for suicide-related search queries. Their result was negative, but they discovered that a 'helpline box' for suicide prevention was among the results shown only in some cases, suggesting that its presence was determined algorithmically. The authors suggest that 'the helpline box should be presented in more search results for an increase in beneficial preventive effects'. Facebook has been experimenting with an intervention in response to suicidal posts. Basically, once a post has been reported or automatically flagged as suicide-related, Facebook will provide the user with a phone number for distress counselling and with links to support videos.

A simple, but highly effective, assessment and intervention was developed by Haas et al. [94]. They advertised an anonymous online, questionnaire-based assessment for depression and suicidality to college students via email. All students were given a personalized evaluation by a counsellor; the higher-risk ones were encouraged to engage in anonymous follow-up counselling. The programme seemed to noticeably reduce the number of suicides on campus. Rice et al. [95] organized and analysed three specific Internet-based interventions for suicidal young people with the goal of improving 'feelings of connectedness', which would (according to the interpersonal theory of suicide) reduce suicidality.

Young et al. [96] discuss news guidelines about reporting about suicides. They show that such guidelines are often not followed by the US media, even though research has shown that they are 'associated with a decrease in the number of suicides'. Guidelines include advice to avoid sensationalizing language, to avoid attributing the suicide to a single cause, and to avoid disclosure of certain details about the case. In addition to protecting the privacy of the family and the deceased, such guidelines are intended to raise awareness, point readers to resources, and avoid suicide contagion.

Conclusion

Water can float a boat as it can capsize it. In general, social media usage generates unprecedented benefits and conveniences for the users but using social media excessively in everyday life will create profoundly unhealthy mental conditions for the abusers. Many social media tools are effective intervention implements to tackle only part of the problem, which is now becoming a worldwide public health epidemic. The most effective way, however, is for the users to have a disciplined usage of the technology and to enjoy more real life face-to-face time.

References

1. Boyd DM, Ellison NB. Social network sites: definition, history, and scholarship. *J Comput Mediat Commun* 2007; 13: 210–30.
2. Statistica. Number of social network users worldwide. Available at: https://www.statista.com/statistics/278414/number-of-worldwide-social-network-users/ (assessed 10 May 2018).
3. Andreassen CS, Billieux J, Griffiths MD, et al. The relationship between addictive use of social media and video games and symptoms of psychiatric disorders: a large-scale cross-sectional study. *Psychol Addict Behav* 2016; 30: 252–262.
4. Baker DA, Algorta GP. The relationship between online social networking and depression: a systematic review of quantitative studies. *Cyberpsychol Behav Soc Netw* 2016; 19: 638–648.
5. Tang CS-K, Koh YYW. Online social networking addiction among college students in Singapore: comorbidity with behavioral addiction and affective disorder. *Asian J Psychiatry* 2017; 25: 175–178.
6. American Psychiatric Association (APA). *Diagnostic and Statistical Manual of Mental Disorders*, 4th Edition, Text Revision. Washington, DC: APA, 2000.
7. Billieux J, Gay P, Rochat L, Van der Linden M. The role of urgency and its underlying psychological mechanisms in problematic behaviours. *Behav Res Ther* 2010; 48: 1085–1096.
8. Ioannidis K, Treder M, Chamberlain S, et al. Problematic internet use as an age-related multifaceted problem: evidence from a two-site survey. *Addict Behav* 2018; 81: 157–166.
9. Morin-Major JK, Marin M-F, Durand N, Wan N, Juster R-P, Lupien SJ. Facebook behaviors associated with diurnal cortisol in adolescents: Is befriending stressful? *Psychoneuroendocrinology* 2016; 63: 238–246.
10. Woods HC, Scott H. #Sleepyteens: social media use in adolescence is associated with poor sleep quality, anxiety, depression and low self-esteem. *J Adolesc* 2016; 51: 41–49.
11. McIver DJ, Hawkins JB, Chunara R, et al. Characterizing sleep issues using Twitter. *J Med Internet Res* 2015; 17: e140.
12. Davila J, Hershenberg R, Feinstein BA, Gorman K, Bhatia V, Starr LR. Frequency and quality of social networking among young adults: Associations with depressive symptoms, rumination, and corumination. *Psychol Pop Media Cult* 2012; 1: 72–86.
13. Feinstein BA, Bhatia V, Hershenberg R, Davila J. Another venue for problematic interpersonal behavior: the effects of depressive and anxious symptoms on social networking experiences. *J Soc Clin Psychol* 2012; 31: 356–382.
14. Simoncic TE, Kuhlman KR, Vargas I, Houchins S, Lopez-Duran NL. Facebook use and depressive symptomatology: investigating the role of neuroticism and extraversion in youth. *Comput Hum Behav* 2014; 40: 1–5.
15. Hicks S, Brown A. Higher Facebook use predicts greater body image dissatisfaction during pregnancy: the role of self-comparison. *Midwifery* 2016; 40: 132–140.
16. Oberst U, Wegmann E, Stodt B, et al. Negative consequences from heavy social networking in adolescents: the mediating role of fear of missing out. *J Adolesc* 2017; 55: 51–60.
17. Meier EP, Gray J. Facebook photo activity associated with body image disturbance in adolescent girls. *Cyberpsychology Behav Soc Netw* 2014; 17: 199–206.
18. Giota KG, Kleftaras G. The role of personality and depression in problematic use of social networking sites in Greece. *Cyberpsychology J Psychosoc Res Cyberspace* 2013; 7(3), article 6.
19. Brailovskaia J, Margraf J. Comparing Facebook users and Facebook non-users: relationship between personality traits and mental health variables – an exploratory study. *PLOS ONE* 2016; 11: 1–17.
20. Caci B, Cardaci M, Tabacchi M, et al. Personality variables as predictors of Facebook usage. *Psychol Rep* 2014; 114: 528–539.
21. Koc M, Gulyagci S. Facebook addiction among Turkish college students: the role of psychological health, demographic, and usage characteristics. *Cyberpsychology Behav Soc Netw* 2013; 16: 279–284.
22. Hanprathet N, Manwong M, Khumsri J, Yingyeun R, Phanasathit M. Facebook addiction and its relationship with mental health among Thai high school students. *J Med Assoc Thail Chotmaihet Thangphaet* 2015; 98(Suppl. 3): S81–S90.
23. Błachnio A, Przepiórka A, Pantic I. Internet use, Facebook intrusion, and depression: results of a cross-sectional study. *Eur Psychiatry* 2015; 30: 681–684.
24. Locatelli SM, Kluwe K, Bryant FB. Facebook use and the tendency to ruminate among college students: testing mediational hypotheses. *J Educ Comput Res* 2012; 46: 377–394.
25. Jones JR, Colditz JB, Shensa A, et al. Associations between Internet-based professional social networking and emotional distress. *Cyberpsychol Behav Soc Netw* 2016; 19: 601–608.
26. Alvarez-Jimenez M, Alcazar-Corcoles MA, González-Blanch C, Bendall S, McGorry PD, Gleeson JF. Online, social media and mobile technologies for psychosis treatment: a systematic review on novel user-led interventions. *Schizophr Res* 2014; 156: 96–106.
27. Kalbitzer J, Mell T, Bermpohl F, Rapp MA, Heinz A. Twitter psychosis: a rare variation or a distinct syndrome? *J Nerv Ment Dis* 2014; 202: 623.
28. Rosen LD, Whaling K, Rab S, Carrier LM, Cheever NA. Is Facebook creating 'iDisorders'? The link between clinical symptoms of psychiatric disorders and technology use, attitudes and anxiety. *Comput Hum Behav* 2013; 29: 1243–1254.
29. Feinstein BA, Hershenberg R, Bhatia V, Latack JA, Meuwly N, Davila J. Negative social comparison on Facebook and depressive symptoms: Rumination as a mechanism. *Psychol Pop Media Cult* 2013; 2: 161–170.
30. Tandoc EC, Ferrucci P, Duffy M. Facebook use, envy, and depression among college students: Is facebooking depressing? *Comput Hum Behav* 2015; 43: 139–146.
31. Lup K, Trub L, Rosenthal L. Instagram #Instasad?: Exploring associations among Instagram use, depressive symptoms, negative social comparison, and strangers followed. *Cyberpsychol Behav Soc Netw* 2015; 18: 247–252.
32. Moreno MA, Christakis DA, Egan KG, et al. A pilot evaluation of associations between displayed depression references on Facebook and self-reported depression using a clinical scale. *J Behav Health Serv Res* 2012; 39: 295–304.
33. Bazarova N, Choi Y, Whitlock J, et al. Psychological distress and emotional expression on Facebook. *Cyberpsychology Behav Soc Netw* 2017; 20: 157–163.
34. Parikh SV, Huniewicz P. E-health: an overview of the uses of the Internet, social media, apps, and websites for mood disorders. *Curr Opin Psychiatry* 2015; 28: 13–17.
35. Xu R, Zhang Q. Understanding online health groups for depression: social network and linguistic perspectives. *J Med Internet Res* 2016; 18: e63.
36. McCloskey W, Iwanicki S, Lauterbach D, Giammittorio DM, Maxwell K. Are Facebook 'friends' helpful? Development of a Facebook-based measure of social support and examination of relationships among depression, quality of life, and social support. *Cyberpsychol Behav Soc Netw* 2015; 18: 499–505.
37. Wang W, Liu Y. Discussing mental illness in Chinese social media: the impact of influential sources on stigmatization and support among their followers. *Health Commun* 2016; 31: 355–363.
38. Dredge R, Gleeson J, de la Piedad Garcia X. Cyberbullying in social networking sites: an adolescent victim's perspective. *Comput Hum Behav* 2014; 36: 13–20.

39. Oksanen A, Hawdon J, Holkeri E, Näsi M, Räsänen P. Exposure to online hate among young social media users. *Soc Stud Child Youth* 2014; 18: 253–273.

40. Klein DA, Myhre KK, Ahrendt DM. Bullying among adolescents: a challenge in primary care. *Am Fam Physician* 2013; 88: 87–92.

41. Tanrıkulu T, Kınay H, Arıcak OT. Sensibility development program against cyberbullying. *New Media Soc* 2015; 17: 708–719.

42. Vandebosch H, Van Cleemput K. Cyberbullying among youngsters: profiles of bullies and victims. *New Media Soc* 2009; 11: 1349–1371.

43. Hamm MP, Newton AS, Chisholm A, et al. Prevalence and effect of cyberbullying on children and young people: a scoping review of social media studies. *JAMA Pediatr* 2015; 169: 770–777.

44. Heirman W, Angelopoulos S, Wegge D, Vandebosch H, Eggermont S, Walrave M. Cyberbullying-entrenched or cyberbully-free classrooms? A class network and class composition approach. *J Comput Mediat Commun* 2015; 20: 260–277.

45. Aboujaoude E, Savage MW, Starcevic V, Salame WO. Cyberbullying: review of an old problem gone viral. *J Adolesc Health* 2015; 57: 10–18.

46. Statistica. Number of League of Legends monthly active users from 2011 to 2016 (in millions). Available at: https://www.statista.com/statistics/317099/number-lol-registered-users-worldwide/ (assessed 10 May 2018).

47. Maher B. Can a video game company tame toxic behaviour? *Nature* 2016; 531: 568–571.

48. Bertolote JM. Suicide and mental disorders: do we know enough? *Br J Psychiatry* 2003; 183: 382–383.

49. University of Washington, School of Social Work. Facts about mental illness and suicide. Available at: http://depts.washington.edu/mhreport/facts_suicide.php (accessed 21 March 2018).

50. Thom K, Edwards G, Nakarada-Kordic I, McKenna B, O'Brien A, Nairn R. Suicide online: portrayal of website-related suicide by the New Zealand media. *New Media Soc* 2011; 13: 1355–1372.

51. Church EJ. Examining suicide: imaging's contributions. *Radiol Technol* 2015; 86: 275–295.

52. Ali M, Dwyer D, Rizzo J. The social contagion effect of suicidal behaviour in adolescents: does it really exist? *J Ment Health Policy Econ* 2011; 14: 3–12.

53. Giordano P. Relationships in adolescence. *Annual Rev of Sociology* 2003; 29: 252–281.

54. Mueller A, Abrutyn S. Suicidal disclosures among friends: using social network data to understand suicide contagion. *J Health Soc Behav* 2015; 56: 131–148.

55. Bailin A, Milanaik R, Adesman A. Health implications of new age technologies for adolescents: a review of the research. *Curr Opin Pediatr* 2014; 26: 605–619.

56. Joiner TE. *Why People Die by Suicide*. Cambridge, MA: Harvard University Press, 2007.

57. Moberg FB, Anestis MD. A preliminary examination of the relationship between social networking interactions, internet use, and thwarted belongingness. *Crisis* 2015; 36: 187–193.

58. Grieve R, Watkinson J. The psychological benefits of being authentic on Facebook. *Cyberpsychol Behav Soc Netw* 2016; 19: 420–425.

59. Mota P. Facebook enhances antidepressant pharmacotherapy effects. *Sci World J* 2014.

60. Ellison N, Steinfield C, Lampe C. 2007. The benefits of Facebook 'friends': social capital and college students' use of online social network sites. *J Comput Mediat Commun* 2007; 12: 1143–1168.

61. Nabi R, Prestin A, So J. Facebook friends with (health) benefits? Exploring social network site use and perceptions of social support, stress, and well-being. *Cyberpsychol Behav Soc Netw* 2013; 16: 721–727.

62. Bauer R, Bauer M, Spiessl H, Kagerbauer T. Cyber-support: An analysis of online self-help forums (online self-help forums in bipolar disorder). *Nord J Psychiatry* 2013; 67: 185–190.

63. Wittenberg-Lyles E, Washington K, Oliver DP, et al. 'It is the 'starting over' part that is so hard': using an online group to support hospice bereavement. *Palliat Support Care* 2015; 13: 351–357.

64. Alvarez-Jimenez M, Alcazar-Corcoles MA, Gonzalez-Blanch C, Bendall S, McGorry PD, Gleeson JF. Online social media: new data, new horizons in psychosis treatment. *Schizophr Res* 2015; 166: 345–346.

65. Lobelo F, Kelli H, Tejedor S. The Wild Wild West: A framework to integrate mhealth software applications and wearables to support physical activity assessment, counseling and interventions for cardiovascular disease risk reduction. *Prog Cardiovasc Dis* 2016; 58: 584–594.

66. Martin S, Feldman D, Blumenthal R, et al. mActive: a randomized clinical trial of an automated mHealth intervention for physical activity promotion. *J Am Heart Assoc* 2015; 4: 11.

67. Keohane D, Lehane E, Rutherford E, et al. Can an educational application increase risk perception accuracy amongst patients attending a high-risk breast cancer clinic? *J Breast* 2017; 32: 192–198.

68. Shrier L, Spalding A. "Just take a moment and breathe and think": Young women with depression talk about the development of an ecological momentary intervention to reduce their sexual risk. *J Pediatr Adolesc Gynecol* 2017; 30: 116–122.

69. Kennelly M, Ainscough K, Lindsay K, et al. Pregnancy, exercise and nutrition research study with smart phone app support (Pears): study protocol of a randomized controlled trial. *Contemp Clin Trials* 2016; 46: 92–99.

70. Chen Y, Schulz P. The effect of information communication technology interventions on reducing social isolation in the elderly: a systematic review. *J Med Internet Res* 2016; 18: 1.

71. PsychiatryAdvisor. Top 10 Mental Health Apps. Available at: http://www.psychiatryadvisor.com/top-10-mental-health-apps/slideshow/2608/ (accessed 5 July 2017).

72. Anthes E. Mental health: There's an app for that. *Nature* 2016; 532: 20–23.

73. Kazdin A, Fitzsimmons-Craft E, Wilfley D. 2017. Addressing critical gaps in the treatment of eating disorders. *Int J Eat Disord* 2017; 50: 170–189.

74. Maulik PK, Tewari A, Devarapalli S, Kallakuri S, Patel A. The Systematic Medical Appraisal, Referral and Treatment (SMART) mental health project: development and testing of electronic decision support system and formative research to understand perceptions about mental health in rural India. *PLOS ONE* 2016; 11: e0164404.

75. Park S, Lee SW, Kwak J, Cha M, Jeong B. Activities on Facebook reveal the depressive state of users. *J Med Internet Res* 2013; 15: e217.

76. Oh H, DeVylder J. Possibilities and challenges of online, social media, and mobile technologies for psychosis treatment. *Schizophr Res* 2015; 166: 347–348.

77. Povey J, Mills P, Dingwall K, et al. Acceptability of mental health apps for aboriginal and Torres Strait Islander Australians: a qualitative study. *J Med Internet Res* 2016; 18: e65.

78. Morganstein J. Mobile applications for mental health providers. *Psychiatry* 2016; 79: 358–363.

79. Hashemi B, Ali S, Awaad R, et al. Facilitating mental health screening of war-torn populations using mobile applications. *Soc Psychiatry Psychiatr Epidemiol* 2017; 52: 27–33.

80. Eichenberg C, Schott M. Serious games for psychotherapy: a systematic review. *Games Health J* 2017; 6: 127–135.

81. Garaigordobil M, Martínez-Valderrey V. Effects of Cyberprogram 2.0 on 'face-to-face' bullying, cyberbullying, and empathy. *Psicothema* 2015; 27: 45–51.

82. Anderson J, Bresnahan M, Musatics C. Combating weight-based cyberbullying on Facebook with the dissenter effect. *Cyberpsychol Behav Soc Netw* 2014; 17: 281–286.

83. Meter DJ, Bauman S. When sharing is a bad idea: the effects of online social network engagement and sharing passwords with friends on cyberbullying involvement. *Cyberpsychol Behav Soc Netw* 2015; 18: 437–442.

84. Hilt RJ. Cyber bullying: what's a parent to do? *Pediatr Ann* 2013; 42: 481.

85. Doan AP, Yung K, Bishop F, Klam WP. Cyberbullying of mental health patients: ethical and professional considerations for publication of case reports in the digital age. *Addict Behav* 2015; 42: A1–A2.

86. Ahuja AK, Biesaga K, Sudak DM, Draper J, Womble A. Suicide on Facebook. *J Psychiatr Pract* 2014; 20: 141–146.

87. Fu K, Cheng Q, Wong PWC, Yip PSF. Responses to a self-presented suicide attempt in social media: a social network analysis. *Crisis* 2013; 34: 406–412.

88. Woo H, Cho Y, Shim E, Lee K, Song G. Public trauma after the Sewol ferry disaster: the role of social media in understanding the public mood. *Int J Environ Res Public Health* 2015; 12: 10974–10983.

89. Won H-H, Myung W, Song G-Y, et al. Predicting national suicide numbers with social media data. *PLOS ONE* 2013; 8: e61809.

90. Mikal J, Hurst S, Conway M. Ethical issues in using Twitter for population-level depression monitoring: a qualitative study. *BMC Med Ethics* 2016; 17: 22.

91. O'Dea B, Wan S, Batterham PJ, Calear AL, Paris C, Christensen H. Detecting suicidality on Twitter. *Internet Interv* 2015; 2: 183–188.

92. Cash SJ, Thelwall M, Peck SN, Ferrell JZ, Bridge JA. Adolescent suicide statements on MySpace. *Cyberpsychol Behav Soc Netw* 2013; 16: 166–174.

93. Haim M, Arendt F, Scherr S. Abyss or shelter? On the relevance of web search engines' search results when people Google for suicide. *Health Commun* 2017; 32: 253–258.

94. Haas A, Koestner B, Rosenberg J, et al. An interactive web-based method of outreach to college students at risk for suicide. *J Am Coll Health* 2008; 57: 15–22.

95. Rice S, Robinson J, Bendall S, et al. Online and social media suicide prevention interventions for young people: a focus on implementation and moderation. *J Can Acad Child Adolesc Psychiatry* 2016; 25: 80–86.

96. Young R, Subramanian R, Miles S, et al. Social representation of cyberbullying and adolescent suicide: a mixed-method analysis of news stories. *Health Comm* 2017; 32: 1082–1092.

CHAPTER 56

Telemental health
A public mental health perspective

Maryann Waugh, Matthew Mishkind, and Jay H. Shore

Introduction

Telemental health is a rapidly growing mode of mental health delivery service that offers viable solutions to care access problems associated with growing mental health need, provider shortages, and patient obstacles, especially as related to geography, mobility, and stigma [1]. Telemental health has the capacity to make a significant and positive impact on public mental health by its ability to not only increase access to care, but also more effectively tailor mental health services to individual or community-wide healthcare needs. Using the virtual care modality can promote a public health-oriented, stepped-care approach by providing healthcare beneficiaries with a range of increasingly specialized and intensive services. It allows patients to more readily access web-based services for mild-to-moderate concerns using a range of technologies. This mild-to-moderate level of service may be sufficient for the majority of patients seeking care, and in addition to helping to alleviate existing symptoms, reduces the potential for escalating symptoms and related, unnecessary office visits. For patients with more severe needs, telemental health provides for a direct person-to-person connection with a mental health provider and helps to mitigate a variety of care access and care disparity challenges.

This chapter describes ways that telemental health is currently being used to impact mental health promotion, prevention, and treatment, summarizes the evidence base for these applications, and highlights some practical considerations for providers and systems implementing this newer virtual care delivery system.

What is telemental health?

Telemental is a subset of a larger umbrella term known as telehealth, or telemedicine, which uses communication networks to provide health care or medical services. More specifically, telemental health is a term for health care that leverages audio and video telecommunications technologies such as video-teleconferencing, computers, mobile devices, the Internet, telephones, and broadband connectivity to provide mental health services across time and physical distance [2]. Telemental health is not a discreet clinical service but rather a mode of service used to provide a range of clinical, educational, and other healthcare options when patients and providers are geographically distant. Other terms include sub-specialties such as telepsychology and telepsychiatry, and other broader terms like telebehavioural health, or virtual care.

There are both synchronous and asynchronous applications of telemental health. Synchronous interactions include a patient and provider interacting in real time using two-way audio and video communications. Connecting with a provider to conduct a live therapy session using video-teleconferencing equipment is a form of synchronous mental health. Asynchronous applications, also known as 'store and forward', consist of healthcare information that is collected and later sent and reviewed electronically by a specialist provider. For example, a psychiatrist who views video footage of a patient and emails consultative notes to the patient's primary care physician hours or days after the video was recorded is a form of asynchronous telemental health [3]. Other applications may include a hybrid of both synchronous and asynchronous applications. Some web-based services or mobile phone applications allow patients to conduct asynchronous self-assessments and then connect with a provider if they have elevated symptoms or additional questions.

Clinical telemental health services are wide ranging and are provided in a variety of settings to include inpatient and outpatient clinics, correctional facilities, schools, nursing homes, and patient homes. The setting location may be considered unlimited assuming that connectivity, safety, and privacy requirements are met. Non-clinical applications include administrative work, distance learning, and research.

The ability of telemental health to impact public mental health challenges

Increased care access to reduce the burden of untreated mental illness

High rates of mental illness, low rates of seeking and receiving treatment, and the high costs associated with untreated mental illness across the USA demonstrate an ongoing need for improved access to mental health services. The Centers for Disease Control estimates that about half of all Americans will suffer some form of mental illness across their lives [4], and the Substance Abuse and Mental Health Services Administration (SAMHSA) found that every year 10 million US adults suffer from a serious, functionally debilitating, mental illness [5]. Despite the prevalence of mental health concerns and the public's need for services, the National Institute of Mental Health (NIMH) estimated that, in 2010 alone, of the 7.9 million US adults with serious mental illness, 40% with schizophrenia and 51% with bipolar were left untreated [6].

Untreated mental illness should be viewed as a significant public health concern that manifests in significant direct and indirect costs to society. NIMH notes that in addition to direct treatment costs (estimated at US$57.5 billion in 2006 [7]) the largest contributors to the economic burden of mental illness are indirect costs associated with loss of income due to unemployment, publicly funded supports, and untreated chronic disability that begins early in life [6]. Other outcomes of untreated mental illness are homelessness, incarceration, and a variety of common physical co-morbidities with additional and compounding treatment costs [7]. By providing care from a distance and thus reaching beyond traditional clinic locations, telemental health offers a way to reduce some of these societal costs by providing improved access to care for different populations.

Efforts to quantify this economic burden highlight the pressing need for improved behavioural healthcare access. The National Comorbidity Study, conducted three times since 1985, estimates the annual and lifetime individual and societal cost of mental illness upon earnings. Using DSM criteria and a diagnostic interview structure, the survey collects data about serious mental illness, physical illness, and role-based earnings, for a large, representative US adult sample. These survey data have consistently found 'massive losses of productive human capital' associated with mental disorders, with the most recent, 2008 estimate, at US$193.2 billion after controlling for factors such as age, race, and gender—those factors historically and most significantly associated with earnings. This measured impact does not include social security or other public expenditures that likely further exacerbate the true societal dollar cost [8]. While correlational, these data raise substantial concerns given the rates of mental illness and low rates of treatment. Kessler et al. [8] note that despite these trends, US healthcare expenditures for mental health remain low (6.2% in 2008) compared with equally debilitating physical disorders.

Access to and completion of efficacious mental health treatment effectively lowers both health and societal cost burdens, including reduced work impairment, medical disability, workers' compensation claims and employee absenteeism, and increased employee productivity [9]. Telemental health has documented efficacy to increase care access to such evidence-based treatments. While the field still needs more return-on-investment analyses that include long-term outcomes related to not just symptom reduction, but also increased earnings/savings to individuals, systems, and society, there are increasing numbers of studies documenting the association between telemental health and cost savings. Improving health equity and reducing health disparities is a core tenet of public health [10]. As such, sub-populations with particularly disparate rates of mental illness, or particularly low rates of care access, are of particular concern.

Telemental health is also playing an important role in helping systems shift to models of care that have greater impact on populations. An example is its increasing use in integrated care—providing mental health treatments within primary care clinics using a virtual team-based approach. Integrated care, typically enabled through technology, shifts the model of treatment from individual care for only those with severe need, to a more population based approached, that provides preventative to intervention-level behavioural health care and consultation across the full patient census in a primary care clinic. This improves the overall health of a clinic population and helps avoid medical costs incurred by untreated mental health diagnosis in a primary care setting. Later we discuss in more detail specific telepsychiatry integrated care models as illustrations of the impact of this virtual medium in shifting models of care to population approaches [11].

Improving continuity of care

In addition to increasing care access overall, and reducing costs related to untreated mental illness, telemental health has the potential to improve care continuity by changing healthcare providers or changing systems to improve the outcomes for patients transitioning from one location or system to another. Suicide is the second-leading cause of death for people aged 10–34 years, and the fourth leading cause of death for those aged 35–54 years [12]. Patients likely to attempt suicide are at particularly high risk following transitions from the emergency department (ED), making the successful connection to an outpatient provider a significant public health concern. Across all age groups, the strongest predictor of suicide is a past suicide attempt, or expressed suicide ideation, resulting in hospitalization or visit to the ED. And, in this high-suicide-risk group, risk for suicide attempts and death is highest immediately following discharge from an emergency department or an inpatient psychiatric unit. An estimated 1 in 10 suicide victims were in the ED within 2 months of dying, and almost 4 in 10 suicide victims were in the ED in the year before their death (15% for self-harm behaviours). With estimates of mental health-related ED visits surpassing 5.3 million each year; this is a substantial public health concern [13] and a case example for where telemental health offers viable solutions.

The most effective way to reduce post-discharge suicide risk is to get patients actively engaged in evidence-based outpatient care immediately following ED release. Given current rates of outpatient follow-up for this high-risk group (data show that 70% of persons who attempt suicide will never even attend their first scheduled outpatient visit), effective patient-engagement strategies are crucial to saving lives. A report commissioned by the Suicide Prevention Resource Center, in collaboration with SAMHSA, recommends the following engagement strategies: (i) increase skilled clinical screening in the ED for suicide risk and urgent mental health needs; (ii) include a therapeutic and pharmacological component to outpatient treatment that begins a maximum of 48–72 hours following discharge; (iii) implement frequent, low-intensity check-ins with an empathetic, caring, and consistent provider; and (iv) use a continuity-of-care framework that includes shared intake data and a shared care plan and ongoing data integration across physical and mental health care [13].

While these are challenging recommendations to implement, there is research to support the use of virtual technology to mitigate some of these challenges. The South Carolina Department of Mental Health implemented 24-hour, 7-day-a-week psychiatric coverage for 18 hospital EDs using six full-time and one part-time psychiatrists who were physically located in dispersed locations across the state [14]. As part of the programme workflow, psychiatrists provided case/intake review, provided direct emergent patient evaluation and treatment, participated in treatment plan formulation, and were responsible for facilitating discharge to community outpatient treatment for patients. The psychiatrist and the ED team scheduled initial appointments for patients discharging to community mental health or other behavioural health centres to facilitate immediate patient engagement in outpatient services. In a final sample of over

7000 psychiatric ED patients who participated in the telepsychiatry intervention and a matched sample of psychiatric ED patients who were treated at non-participating South Carolina hospitals, findings favoured telepsychiatry. The telepsychiatry patients were significantly and substantially more likely to attend both 30- and 90-day outpatient follow-up visits, and were less likely to be admitted to the hospital during the ED visit, and, when admitted, had a significantly shorter stay [14]. While this intervention did not include all recommendations noted earlier, it did use skilled clinical screening in the ED, and a continuity-of-care framework that included shared data and focus on immediate outpatient engagement, and these were associated with patient outcomes that were significantly better than treatment as usual.

A report on telemental health in rural Minnesota noted improved continuity of care benefits related to the implementation of telemental health into primary care settings [15]. Primary care settings serve as the first point of contact for many individuals seeking mental health care and serves as the sole form of health care used by more than one-third of patients with a mental health diagnosis. Patients who seek care beyond the primary care setting must navigate a fragmented system of general and specialist providers who do not share records or communication about patients and care plans [9]. In Minnesota, this fragmented care, which has gaps, duplications, and involves long waiting times and high no-show rates for behavioural health care, was avoided for patients whose primary care providers were able to access psychiatric consultation via telehealth. Because of the telepsychiatry, patients were able to experience continuous physical and mental health care with their single provider, and the patients and systems were able to optimize the benefits of early intervention and higher patient engagement [15].

Accommodating provider and patient mobility

Telemental health applications can also be used flexibly to support provider needs and are well suited to mitigate care access challenges for rural patients. They are also a flexible solution for systems, particularly those in rural areas, who may otherwise struggle to provide continuous coverage for population treatment during provider absences. Rural providers are often isolated from collegial support, and face particular challenges finding coverage for training, vacations, and/or health reasons—including unexpected illness, maternity, and short- and long-term situations [16]. Researchers in Maryland completed a short-term study of telepsychiatry as a medium to address these challenges and provide coverage to a rural general hospital psychiatric unit. The virtual coverage had high ratings of patient and provider satisfaction and allowed the hospital to avoid costs previously spent on not just travel, but also lodging for short-term psychiatric providers. Furthermore, a hearing for one patient on an involuntary hold included psychiatrist testimony via video, based on record review and interactive video assessment of the patient—with no objection from judge or defence attorney [16]. While not intended specifically for public health, this study demonstrated how telemental health can impact public health care by allowing providers schedule flexibility without loss of access for patients.

Increased health equity

Reduced social inequalities

The offender population is a group with higher rates of mental illness than the general population. Of about seven million incarcerated Americans, half are diagnosed with a mental illness [17]. A review article by Deslich et al. [1] noted that with few exceptions, telemental health was associated with increased care access and decreased care costs for inmate populations across a variety of studies. Untreated mental illness in this population is associated with a variety of negative outcomes, including increased rates of violent behaviour and fighting-related injuries, which come at high costs to both the individuals involved and the correctional facilities and systems, and the overall public. Appropriate behavioural health treatment is associated with reduced risks for violent behavioural in mentally ill populations [18], and in-person or virtual applications can improve facility safety and save costs associated with correctional staff time spent on security and administrative tasks related to violent incidences. Telemental health can help with additional travel time and cost savings as virtual treatment eliminates the need to transport offenders to off-site treatment locations. In addition to actual travel costs and staff time, offender off-site transport represents unmeasured public safety costs en route, and during offender treatment at sites unlikely to have adequate security [1], so avoided travel is of particular value to correctional systems and the communities in which they are located.

Another population significantly less likely to receive any, or minimally adequate, mental health care, are rural residents [19]. A randomized controlled trial of a telemedicine-based collaborative depression care intervention found that depressed, rural patients enrolled with the Veterans Health Administration (VHA) had higher quality-adjusted life-year ratios when treated by a depression team (including a psychiatrist, pharmacist, nurse, and depression care manager). These life-year ratios were associated with lower 12-month healthcare expenditures across both depression-related, and co-morbid health issues [19]. In an evaluation of telemental health in rural Minnesota, researchers found that more than 85% of patients seen via telemedicine were able to remain in their local communities for outpatient treatment, as opposed to travelling to distant, usually urban, outpatient settings, escalating to needing inpatient treatment, or accessing no treatment at all. This led to lower costs of care for the individuals and the local healthcare systems, and contributed to the financial viability of the rural community more than in years prior to telemental health availability [15].

A number of studies have demonstrated the capacity of telemental health to reduce disparities for minority and underserved population by improving both access and quality of care. A series of clinics targeting rural native veterans have wedded cultural models of care and outreach with telepsychiatry services to reach this population with significant needs. Rural native veterans serve at the highest rate per capita of any minority group, are the most rural, and suffer higher rates of services-related mental health disorders. In addition to obvious geographical access issues this population also faces cultural, resource, and provider availability challenges in accessing optimal care. These native veteran clinics have been shown to reduce travel costs, have reliable and effective treatments, and provide culturally relevant psychiatric care for this population [20].

Some within the US Military Health System (MHS) face unique challenges in accessing available mental health care because of the nature of their occupations, deployments to and permanent duty at stations in isolated geographies, and discontinuity of services. In 2009, a pilot study was conducted to evaluate the use of a telehealth-modified shipping container to provide telemental health services to MHS beneficiaries on American Samoa [2]. American Samoa is the most remote territory of the USA, and at the time of this pilot study its population of approximately 68,000 served the US military in great numbers, and had reported gaps in access to medical care, with high costs of delivering care. The shipping container was placed on American Samoa through a joint project with the local Veterans Affairs Pacific Islands Healthcare System Community Based Outpatient Clinic, which had network communications in place that ran directly to the MHS/VHA Tripler Army Medical Center on Honolulu, Hawaii. Results from the pilot study suggested that the shipping container was a safe and appropriate place to receive care. From a public health perspective, the use of the shipping containers and, more broadly, telemental health, meant that beneficiaries did not have to the make the choice between flying 2500 miles to Hawaii or going without MHS-delivered care. Although return-on-investment was not calculated for this pilot, a substantial cost saving was likely given that at the time of the evaluation a single trip to Hawaii to receive care was estimated to cost, at minimum, US$2600. Finally, all 28 participants in the pilot reported that they were better able to access a provider using telemental health, and the vast majority agreed that this service saved them time traveling to another clinic [2].

Beyond the issues of care access, there can be care inequities based on language barriers. Some research shows that asynchronous telemental health applications may help mitigate such barriers. Yellowlees et al. [21] conducted a study with English- and Spanish-speaking patients in primary care settings, using an asynchronous telepsychiatry platform for language translation. Spanish-speaking patients were interviewed in Spanish, and using an electronic medical record-like technical platform with added video data capabilities, the clinical interview video, and patient history were recorded for later psychiatrist review. A Spanish-speaking psychiatrist reviewed the records and wrote diagnostic assessments and treatment plans for the referring primary care doctor. Medical interpreters translated the Spanish patient records to English for review, diagnosis, and treatment plans from English-speaking psychiatrists. Researchers measured inter-rater reliability between the English and Spanish-speaking psychiatrists and concluded that the asynchronous platform was feasible and effective for increasing access to care for non-English-speaking patients and, similarly, non-Spanish-speaking providers. They further concluded that the clinical process had a unique advantage over real-time care because translation after the fact widened the pool of providers who could provide the psychiatric assessment and consult with the primary care physician. This disruptive technology identified a process of care that was more cost-effective than either in-person or synchronous psychiatric consultation [21].

Reduced perceptions of stigma

Unfortunately, stigma surrounding behavioural care access through traditional clinical settings still persists. This is particularly relevant in rural communities where patients may have dual, non-clinical relationships with providers and support staff at community and other mental health centres, and have no anonymity from community members, to include employers, who may see and recognize patients or their cars at such known sites [22]. Telemental health applications can reduce perceptions of stigma by allowing patients to access the same quality mental health care with some increase in anonymity. As noted previously, many individuals initially seek mental health care from their primary care providers, and a

significant subset of patients will continue only to access mental health care through this venue [9]. Mental health specialists are often not available in rural communities, which exacerbates the overall concerns with access and stigma. One solution is to use telemental health virtually to integrate mental health providers into primary care settings thus allowing patients to access quality mental health care in a familiar and less stigmatizing environment, and access providers from outside of their home communities, thereby minimizing the duality of relationships.

Telemental health consultation models allow patients to remain in the care of their primary care doctor and receive care at their familiar primary care sites. Even patients who have televisits directly with a psychiatrist for diagnostic and medication assessments typically do so from their primary care office. The consultative model is developing an increasing evidence base for efficacy and improved care quality. A review article by Hilty et al. [23] note that this consultative model is associated with improved diagnoses and psychotropic prescription choices, clinical improvements in a large number of patients, and increases in primary care provider mental health knowledge and skills, particularly in rural setting. The consultative primary care model is also associated with cost savings and increased patient anonymity.

Children and adolescents are able to access integrated primary and paediatric care settings, and, increasingly, also have options for less stigmatizing care access within their school settings. School-based health clinics are a natural fit for telemental health strategies, allowing psychiatric providers to consult with on-site physicians responsible for ongoing medication management, whereas other behavioural health professionals provide virtual care plan consultative and even direct group and individual care. Many school-based models incorporate virtual mental health professionals within a multidisciplinary school treatment team. This team may include parents, teachers, nurses, occupational therapists, and school-based mental health professionals such as school psychologists [24].

While more research is still needed, school-based telemental health models appear effective and acceptable. Telemental health in the school setting helps to reduce scheduling demands for families, allows parents to participate in virtual sessions from work or home, gets medical and educational professionals on board with one shared care plan, and leverages parents' and young people's existing comfort and trust with school personnel to help them feel more comfortable about a new mental health professional. These may all help reduce perceived stigma. While the school-based model can also help reduce stigma by allowing families to avoid visits to known mental health centres and to potentially see virtual providers from distal communities, there are some potential disadvantages, too. Some families may perceive reduced privacy because a multidisciplinary school team becomes involved their child's mental health care. Also, telemental health provider may worry about limited parent engagement in the care plan, and the challenge of practising not just virtually, but also within the unfamiliar culture of a school—particularly when those providers are from distal communities [24].

Telemental health across the public mental health continuum

Mental health promotion and prevention

Van Voorhees et al. [24] note the significant potential for prevention-focused efforts to make a positive impact on global public health. This potential is maximized by efforts that are scalable and easily disseminated using telemental health technologies and services. Web- and other technology-based delivery modalities boast benefits such as limited need for professional time and clinical space, patient autonomy/reduced stigma in access, and the ability of patients to self-pace learning and participation. Other benefits include the ability of professionals to offer inexpensive programmes to prevent the onset of illness to individuals who fall below the diagnostic threshold and may not be eligible for treatment coverage. Using telemental health technology, providers can design flexible programmes for full patient populations, population subsets such as those screened for disorder risk factors, or for patients with early disorder symptoms. Van Voorhees et al. [24] use the term 'behavioral vaccine' for such models, and describe growing evidence of prevention efficacy across the life span, from young people to older adults. Web-based programmes show comparable effects to similar in-person delivery, and progress maintenance has been measured up to a year after program conclusion. These results have been achieved in primary care, school, and home settings—with the majority of home-based programmes having initial visits in school or primary care settings. A noted advantage of web-based interventions is fidelity of treatment implementation, although adult supervision is highly recommended for young patients navigating these applications [25].

Mental health treatment

Telemental health treatment has application across the mental health continuum—from emergent and inpatient settings, community mental health centres, primary care settings, and even outpatient services delivered to patient homes. Virtual mental health services delivered to children and adults across a variety of outpatient settings have demonstrated clinical outcomes related to depression, global assessment of function, reduced utilization of emergent services, treatment adherence, and patient satisfaction that mirror those of in-person intervention [23]. While some studies have reported increased costs related to telehealth infrastructure development and service utilization for previously untreated populations, the majority of studies link telemental health with cost savings. Cost savings are related to patient and provider travel, greater optimization of provider time (i.e. using store and forward and on-demand availability during patient no-show time), as well as overall reduced healthcare costs for participating patients [23]. A 2013 rural survey found that of 52 organizational survey respondents, academic medical centres were most frequently implementing telemental health programmes (28%). Nine per cent were community mental health centres, 9% were acute care hospitals, 8% were private vendors, 6% federally qualified health centres, and 6% rural health centres. Psychiatrists were the most frequent mental health specialty provider, followed by clinical psychologists, clinical social workers, and psychiatric nurse practitioners [26].

Increasing outpatient applications

There is a dearth of licensed mental health clinicians, and community mental health centres are no exception, with a particular need for child services and psychiatrists. The literature shows that patients can be reliably assessed, diagnosed, and treated via therapeutic and medical intervention in outpatient applications using a variety of videoconferencing and electronic communications

[27]. Telemental health solutions are particularly critical in rural areas, where, historically, residents have been not only less likely to access care, but also less likely to receive evidence-based behavioural health care when accessed. This is generally attributed to professional shortages, lack of collegial support for existing professionals, and lack of connection to universities and other sources of ongoing research and efficacy information [28]. Rates of suicide, substance abuse, and untreated mental illness are particularly high in rural areas [29]. Not surprisingly, the state of Alaska reports rates of suicide and substance abuse that exceed national averages. In response, Alaska's Medicaid system has embraced telemental health, allowing for full reimbursement for psychiatric and substance abuse assessment, psychotherapy, and medical management services delivered virtually. Further, to maximize effective use of professional expertise and optimize timely care to a historically underserved population, Alaska Medicaid allows a broad definition of telemental health that includes store and forward and other e-solutions in addition to real-time audio-video care delivery. The agency also allows full flexibility on originating site, including no restrictions that limit the patients' location during service delivery [30]. These changing policies reflect a growing awareness of the need to leverage technology to address long standing, and still persistent, public health gaps and disparities.

Inpatient applications

Telemental health has been used across a variety of inpatient settings from medical hospitals to long-term care facilities. The addition of virtual mental health evaluation services has been linked to improved outcomes in hospital emergency departments. Outcomes previously noted include improved patient engagement and continuity of care following discharge [14], as well as shorter wait times for patient intake to evaluation, intake to treatment, and shorter in-patient stays for virtually evaluated patients (whether inpatient or outpatient status prior to inpatient admission) [31]. A 2015 meta-analysis found 23 studies of telepsychiatry used in acute care applications and additionally found clinical outcomes comparable to in-person psychiatry and strong indices of cost efficacy [32]. DeVido et al. [33] summarize a variety of successful inpatient applications, including the use of videoconference, to complete—quickly and accurately—psychiatric intake interviews for psychiatric inpatient patients, to evaluate ED patients presenting with health complaints with equal diagnostic accuracy and disposition/treatment recommendations to in-person evaluation, to improve care access for nursing home patients, and to improve inpatient unit care planning at a reduced cost for a rural, inpatient psychiatry unit.

Primary care/integrated care applications

Telemental health is also growing in application across primary care settings. High rates of behavioural and physical health comorbidities and the large proportion of the population who seek behavioural health support in the primary care setting is driving care integration efforts [34]. In the primary care setting, telemental health can take a variety of forms. Fortney et al. [11] describe these applications in terms of increasing behavioural health resource intensity. Less intense models include curbside consultation, when primary care physicians provide full care with case consultation from a virtual psychiatrist, and consultation–liaison models in which a psychiatrist conducts an e-consultation with patients and provide diagnosis and treatment recommendations to primary care. More resource-intense models include behavioural health consultation, leveraging team-based care that includes mental health providers embedded virtually into the primary care team, and a more intense application of this team model—telepsychiatry collaborative care—in which the care team also includes mental health professionals who conduct virtual outreach to patients who are treatment resistant/non-adherent [11]. Care managers often support team-based care and work to coordinate across primary and specialist providers. Clinical trials and meta-analyses show positive results for a variety of these virtual applications, with rural trials even expanding to virtual care management [11]. Online asynchronous applications of telemental health are also increasing as primary care interventions are augmented by patient-driven, web-based resources for depression and other chronic care management [34].

Applications in non-clinical settings

While many publicly funded healthcare systems, and some private healthcare payers still limit delivery of virtual mental health services to patients located in their homes, or other community-based settings [35], there are increasing broad applications of telemental health to these non-clinical settings. As noted earlier, Alaska represents an example where Medicaid patients may receive services from any location. As patients across the globe become 'e-patients', defined as patients who are 'equipped, enabled, empowered, and engaged in their health and healthcare decisions' [36], they demand easier access to healthcare data and expect care access via laptops, tablets, and phones. Consequently, telemental health is expanding into homes and other non-clinical settings to provide a wider variety of care services. In an analysis of the role of technology in changing the patient–provider relationship, Yellowlees and Nafiz [36] list online/televideo-based patient support groups, multimedia educational materials for both patients and providers, personal electronic health records and tools for self-directed chronic disease management, store and forward options for assessments and other data, as well as telepsychiatry for direct patient care and provider to provider consultation, as some of the more recent strategies used to treat an increasingly tech and health savvy patient population.

Store and forward technology is being leveraged to improve care efficiency and competency—for example having a non-specialist provider collect clinical information via documents, audio, and/or video clinical information and electronically transmitting this information to a distal psychiatrist. Not only does this maximize the professional capacity of the psychiatrist who focuses time on specialized assessment (not clinical information collection or travel), but it also expands opportunities for culturally competent care across an increasingly diverse public. A clinical interview can be conducted in a patient's native language by another native speaker, translated to the psychiatrist's language, and transmitted to wherever that psychiatrist is located [36].

Literature regarding the safety and efficacy of direct telemental health care delivered to patients at home and in other non-clinical settings is still limited. A 2010 review found only nine published studies of this application. Based on this small sample, reviewers concluded that safety was manageable, that safety plans were a particularly important care delivery component in clinically unsupervised settings, and that standard delivery protocols were likely forthcoming as patient demand for telemental health increases [37]. Despite reimbursement challenges from many healthcare payers,

home-based telepsychiatry is starting to expand, particularly for Millenials and younger generations, who are described as 'digital natives'. Members of these sub-populations increasingly demand convenient, technology-based care solutions [38]. Gloff et al. [39] provide recommendations from a group of child and adolescent psychiatrists who completed a home-based care pilot. They note that providers must be very aware of home-based safety concerns that cannot be mitigated by on-site staff like in clinical telemental health applications. Providers must also consider privacy and technology concerns based on less robust home-based broadband, and increased risk of young people getting distracted and wandering away from a home tele-session to siblings, toys, and other factors that do not compete for youth attention in clinic settings. Recommendations include the development of collaborative back-up plans with patients prior to in-home sessions. These may include planning to continue visits via the phone if the Internet connection becomes unstable, and having parents support youth attention, as well as having safety plans in the event of expressed and immediate suicide ideation or other emergencies [39].

The VHA is in the midst of a 3-year clinical trial to further assess home-based telemental health for service members and veterans with depression. They are currently conducting a randomized controlled trial to compare the safety, feasibility, and clinical efficacy of behavioural activation for depression delivered via web-based video technology to patients either in-office or at home [40]. Hopefully, these, and future, studies will help inform evidence-based practice and public health policy for non-clinical applications.

Conclusions

The world continues to get smaller with the gaps in human space continuing to shrink and the ability to connect anytime from anywhere continuing to increase. Unfortunately, the prevalence of mental illness and chronic health conditions such as diabetes and obesity are also increasing, with many individuals unable to access the care they need. This is especially true for individuals with mobility issues and stigma concerns, and communities that are geographically and culturally isolated. Telemental health utilizes a vast array of technologies and offers great promise to provide access to high-quality healthcare for those who were previously unable to receive the care they need. Practitioners and systems wishing to address this public health concern efficiently have a variety of technology-supported options well suited to prevention and intervention across diverse populations. Some practical considerations involve carefully assessing the needs and existing resources that exist within the population or community of concern, and identifying opportunities where telemental health technology can support care quality, access, and continuity most efficiently. Care models such as primary care-based integration may help reduce perceptions of stigma and provide a wider pool of patients with mental health expertise. Collaborative and consultative models also represent more cost-efficient ways to use and pay for more limited, but impactful, psychiatric provider time. Store and forward models can make use of local and familiar on-site personnel to collect evaluative information for additional time and personnel efficiencies. Home-based care is an area that is growing—and while it offers great convenience, flexibility, and patient anonymity, it must be considered in light of concerns related to patient safety, home technology adequacy, and billing and reimbursement.

Overall, an ever-growing variety of technology-based mental health treatment applications and models are expanding the opportunities to address the ongoing public health burden of untreated mental illness. The literature base associated with telemental health shows promising results across a myriad of populations and telemental health applications, and it is anticipated that future research will help practitioners and systems align need with more efficient uses of resources within individualized local context.

References

1. Deslich SA, Stec B, Tomblin S, Coustasse A. Telepsychiatry in the 21st century: transforming healthcare with technology. *Perspect Health Inf Manag* 2013; 10: 1–17.

2. National Center for Telehealth & Technology. *Introduction to Telemental Health*. Available at: http://t2health.dcoe.mil/sites/default/files/cth/introduction/intro_telemental_health_may2011.pdf (accessed 21 March 2018).

3. Butler TN, Yellowlees P. Cost analysis of store-and-forward telepsychiatry as a consultation model for primary care. *J Telemed E Health* 2012; 8: 74–77.

4. Centers for Disease Control and Prevention. CDC Report identifies need for increased monitoring of adult mental illness. Available at: http://www.cdc.gov/media/releases/2011/a0901_adult_mental_Illness.html (accessed 9 May 2016).

5. SAMHSA. Behavioral Health Trends in the United States: Results from the 2014 National Survey on Drug Use and Health. Available at: http://www.samhsa.gov/data/sites/default/files/NSDUH-FRR1-2014/NSDUH-FRR1-2014.pdf (accessed 6 June 2016).

6. Insel TR. Assessing the economic costs of serious mental illness. *Am J Psychiatry* 2008; 165: 703–711.

7. Soni A. The Five Most Costly Conditions, 1996 and 2006: Estimates for the U.S. Civilian Noninstitutionalized Population. Available at: http://www.meps.ahrq.gov/mepsweb/data_files/publications/st248/stat248.pdf (accessed 9 May 2016).

8. Kessler RC, Heeringa S, Lakoma MD, et al. Individual and societal effects of mental disorders on earnings in the United States: results from the national comorbidity survey replication. *Am J Psychiatr* 2008; 165: 703–711.

9. American Hospital Association. Bringing behavioral health into the care continuum: opportunities to improve quality, costs and outcomes. Available at: http://www.aha.org/research/reports/tw/12jan-tw-behavhealth.pdf (accessed 6 June 2016).

10. American Public Health Association. Health equity. Available at: https://www.apha.org/topics-and-issues/health-equity (accessed 24 May 2016).

11. Fortney JC, Pyne JM, Turner EE, et al. Telepsychiatry integration of mental health services into rural primary care settings. *Int Rev Psychiatry* 2015; 27: 525–539.

12. National Vital Statistics System, National Center for Health Statistics, CDC. 10 Leading Causes of Death by Age Group, United States – 2014. Available at: http://www.cdc.gov/injury/wisqars/pdf/leading_causes_of_death_by_age_group_2014-a.pdf (accessed 19 May 2016).

13. Knesper DJ, American Association of Suicidology, & Suicide Prevention Resource Center. Continuity of Care for Suicide Prevention and Research. Available at: http://www.sprc.org/sites/sprc.org/files/library/continuityofcare.pdf (accessed 6 June 2016).

14. Narasimhan M, Druss BG, Hockenberry JM, et al. Quality, utilization, and economic impact of a statewide emergency department telepsychiatry program. *Psychiatr Serv* 2015; 66: 1167–1172.

15. Office of Rural Health and Primary Care, Minnesota Department of Health. Rural Health Advisory Committee's Report on Telemental Health in Rural Minnesota. Available at: http://www.health.state.mn.us/divs/orhpc/pubs/rhac/tmh.pdf (accessed 19 May 2016).

16. Grady B, Singleton M. Telepsychiatry 'coverage' to a rural inpatient psychiatric unit. *J Telemed E Health* 2011;17: 603–608.

17. Kaeble D, Glaze L, Tsoutis A, Minton T. Correctional Populations in the United States, 2014. Available at: https://www.bjs.gov/content/pub/pdf/cpus14.pdf. (accessed 9 May 2016).

18. Rueve ME, Welton RS. Violence and mental illness. *Psychiatry* 2008; 5: 34–38.

19. Pyne JM, Fortney JC, Tripathi SP, Maciejewski ML, Edlund MJ, Williams DK. Cost effectiveness analysis of a rural telemedicine collaborative care intervention for depression. *Arch Gen Psychiatry* 2010; 67: 812–821.

20. Shore J, Kaufmann LJ. Brooks E, et al. Review of American Indian veteran telemental health. *Telemed E Health* 2012; 18: 87–94.

21. Yellowlees PM, Odor A, Parish MB. Cross-lingual asynchronous telepsychiatry: disruptive innovation? *Psychiatr Serv* 2012; 63: 945.

22. Weiss Roberts L, Battaglia J, Epstein RS. Frontier ethics: mental health care needs and ethical dilemmas in rural communities. *Psychiatr Serv* 1999; 50: 497–503.

23. Hilty DM, Ferrer DC, Parish MB, Johnston B, Callahan EJ, Yellowlees PM. The effectiveness of telemental health: a 2013 review. *Telemed J E Health* 2013; 19: 444–454.

24. Van Voorhees BW, Mahoney N, Mazo R, et al. Internet-based eepression prevention over the life course: A call for behavioral vaccines. *Psychiatr Clin North Am* 2011; 34: 167–183.

25. Myers K, Comer JS. The case for telemental health for improving the asccessibility and quality of children's mental health services. *J Child Adol Psychopharmacol* 2016; 26: 186–191.

26. Lambert D, Gale DJ, Hansen AY, Croll Z, Hartley D. Telemental health in today's rural health system. Available at: http://muskie.usm.maine.edu/Publications/MRHRC/Telemental-Health-Rural.pdf (accessed 13 June 2016).

27. Grady B, Myers KM, Nelson E, et al. Evidence based practice for telemental health. *J Telemed E Health* 2011; 17: 131–148.

28. Myers KM, Valentine JM, Melzer SM. Feasibility, acceptability, and sustainability of telepsychiatry for children and adolescents. *Psychiatr Serv* 2007; 58: 4.

29. Clay RA. Reducing rural suicide. *Monitor Psychol* 2014: 45: 36.

30. American Telemedicine Association. State Medicaid Best Practice: Telemental and Behavioral Health. Available at: http://old.ndcrc.org/sites/default/files/telemental_and_behavioral_health.pdf (accessed 21 March 2018).

31. Southard EP, Neufeld JD, Laws S. Telemental health evaluations enhance access and efficiency in a critical access hospital emergency department. *J Telemed E Health* 2014; 20: 664–668.

32. Salmoiraghi A, Hussain S. A systematic review of the use of telepsychiatry in acute settings. *J Psychiatr Pract* 2015; 21: 389–393.

33. DeVido J, Glezer A, Branagan L, Lau A, Bourgeois JA. Telepsychiatry for inpatient consultations at a separate campus of an academic medical center. *J Telemed E Health* 2016; 22: 572–576.

34. Myers KM, Lieberman D. Telemental health: responding to mandates for reform in primary healthcare. *J Telemed E Health* 2013; 19: 438–443.

35. Waugh M, Voyles D, Thomas M. Telepsychiatry: benefits and costs in a changing health-care environment. *Int Rev Psychiatr* 2015; 27: 558–568.

36. Yellowlees P, Nafiz N. The psychiatrist–patient relationship of the future: anytime, anywhere? *Harv Rev Psychiatry* 2010; 18: 96–102.

37. Luxton DD, Sirotin AP, Mishkind MC. Safety of telemental healthcare delivered to clinically unsupervised settings: a systematic review. *J Telemed E Health*. 2010; 16: 705–711.

38. Chan S, Parish M, Yellowlees P. Telepsychiatry today. *Curr Psychiat Rep* 2015; 17: 89.

39. Gloff NE, LeNoue DR, Novins DK, Myers K. Telemental health for children and adolescents, *Int Rev Psychiatry* 2015; 27: 513–524.

40. Luxton DD, Pruitt LD, O'Brien K, et al. Design and methodology of a randomized clinical trial of home-based telemental health treatment for U.S. military personnel and veterans with depression. *Contemp Clin Trials* 2014; 38: 134–144.

CHAPTER 57

Policy and public mental health in low- and middle-income countries

Laura Shields, Soumitra Pathare, Pallavi Karnatak, and Keshav Desiraju

Introduction

There was clear agreement in the three sites [Mexico, Nicaragua, and Chile] regarding the importance of fostering access to mental health and addiction services, with an emphasis on primary health care and the full continuum from health promotion to rehabilitation and recovery...Some of the challenges of collaborative mental health care on which there was agreement across the three sites were lack of financial resources and training of health professionals and limited access to psychotropic and evaluation. These limitations were said to affect access and quality of care [1].[1]

That is where the biggest gap is. The gap between the wonderful legislation, Bill of Rights and ... the resourcing, the providing, the infrastructure for people to access services. That is either seriously lacking, or is, in fact, absent [2].

As these quotes show, low- and middle-income countries (LAMICs) face struggles with the development and implementation of mental health policy. In general, mental health policy is a complex concept with many influential factors, stakeholders, and unique circumstances; the World Health Organization (WHO) states that:

A mental health policy can be broadly described as an official statement by government or health authority that provides the overall direction for mental health by defining a vision, values, principles and objectives, and by establishing a broad model of action to achieve that vision [3].

A mental health policy, therefore, is a document (or set of documents) that guides mental health care in a given country or region; these documents signal a government's intent to address the mental health needs of its population [4]. The goal of a policy dedicated to mental health is to describe a country or region's vision for mental health. Subsequently, a policy outlines priorities related to mental health care for a specific time horizon and the ways in

which the policy should be carried out by local policymakers, organizations, and healthcare workers. This work is based on policy objectives across sectors and stakeholders, which, in turn, state how and what will be done to address the needs of people with mental health problems [5].

In this chapter, we set out to explore and describe the role of mental health policy in LAMICs,[2] using examples from the literature and from experience in research and practice in LAMICs. We will then explore ways in which stakeholders in LAMICs can improve the development and implementation of mental health policy to improve care systems, care delivery, and the lives of those with a mental health problem.

Policy context in low- and middle-income countries

Within the international health policy community, there has been growing interest in the support, development, and implementation of mental health policy in LAMICs. Historically, efforts were made to encourage mental health policy development in LAMICs. For instance, in 1988 and 1990, Member States in the African WHO region adopted two resolutions (AFR/RC39/R1 and AFR/RC40/R9) to improve mental health; the expectation was that each Member State was to formulate a mental health policy, programme, and action plan [6]. Unfortunately, a 2-year evaluation revealed that little progress had been made [6, 7]. Since then, several countries in the African region have drafted a mental health policy, and published some research on the policy development and implementation process [4, 8–10]. In Latin America, the majority of countries have national and local initiatives to improve

[1] Reproduced from *Health Expect*, 19(1), Sapag JC, Rush B, Ferris LE, Collaborative mental health services in primary care systems in Latin America: contextualized evaluation needs and opportunities, pp. 152–69, Copyright (2016), with permission from John Wiley and Sons.

[2] The World Bank defines LAMICs using the following criteria: for the 2017 fiscal year, low-income economies are defined as those with a gross national income (GNI) per capita, calculated using the World Bank Atlas method, of $1025 or less in 2015; lower middle-income economies are those with a GNI per capita of between $1026 and $4035; upper middle-income economies are those with a GNI per capita between $4036 and $12,475; high-income economies are those with a GNI per capita of $12,476 or more. A full list of LAMICs can be found here: https://data.worldbank.org/income-level/low-and-middle-income.

delivery of mental health services, particularly in light of the Caracas Declaration, which set the foundation for mental health reforms throughout Latin America from the 1990s onwards. Of particular focus in the Caracas Declaration was the commitment to transition mental health care away from hospital-based settings to community-based settings [11]. In 2008, eight Commonwealth of Independent States countries came together to sign the Merano Declaration on Mental Health, which identified shared challenges and areas of action for joint work—one domain of which included defining effective mechanisms for implementing policy and legislation [12].

More recently, an important step forward in mental health policy at a global scale was taken in May 2013 when the World Health Assembly adopted the Comprehensive Mental Health Action Plan (2013–2020), which secured the commitment of United Nations (UN) Member States to take actions to reach the identified targets set out in the plan (Box 57.1) [13–15].

Many non-governmental organizations, researchers, implementation specialists, and policy advocates have been working to support the development, implementation, customization, and evaluation of mental health policy documents in LAMICs. These efforts have resulted in the majority of LAMICs initiating the development of mental health policy [3, 16]. However, these policies may need updating, revision, or support in order to be effectively implemented. The 2014 WHO Mental Health Atlas shows that of 68% of (global) Member States have a standalone policy or plan for mental health [3, 16]. The Atlas further reports that many policies are not fully aligned with human rights treaties and conventions, and the implementation of the policies remains weak [3, 16]. For example, while a mental health policy may exist in a certain country or region, the policy may not be compliant with conventions and treaties that the country has ratified, such as the UN Conventions on the Rights of Persons with Disabilities (UNCRPD). In other places, a mental health policy may be well written and based on consensus from stakeholders in the country but may have been written in such a way that it is not measurable or implementable, resulting in a knowledge–action gap in policy implementation [4, 5]. Some countries have outdated mental health policies in

need of reformulation, particularly to enshrine human rights and community-based approaches to providing mental health care, whereas other countries revisit and update their policies regularly.

An obstacle to improving care in LAMICs is a lack of practical mental health policies, which are needed to direct comprehensive, coordinated mental health care efforts and facilitate implementation of services [17]. At the policy level, there has been consensus that mental health is a neglected public health issue [18]. Despite substantial efforts to create consensus about the importance of mental health at policy level, this consensus has not transcended the abstract policy level into practical realities in many LAMICs. This is evidenced by the most recently published version of the WHO's Mental Health Atlas (2014), which found that 68% of countries have a mental health policy and/or plan. Of those that had a mental health policy or plan, the policy/plan is often not drafted in line with human rights instruments, and is followed by weak implementation where a critical stakeholder such as the family is not involved in the implementation process [3].

Policy development process

Theoretical frameworks and guides exist to explain the policy development process, such as the step-by-step guide outlined in the WHO Mental Health Service Guidance Package (Box 57.2) [19].

While a review of such frameworks is not the focus of this chapter, it is important to note that these theoretical frameworks depict policy development as a linear process. In practice, policy development is often not linear and there are often challenges that arise that can delay, reduce commitment for, or impact the quality of a mental health policy.

Policy processes can often take many years before a policy document is finalized [20]. It is not uncommon for post-implementation revisions to occur after a policy has been developed. This usually reflects the practical implementation process for policies. Therefore, it is important to reserve a time frame in the policy development process solely dedicated to testing and revisions.

Box 57.1 Objectives laid out by the Comprehensive Mental Health Action Plan (2013–2020)

The four objectives of the Comprehensive Mental Health Action Plan were [13–15]:

- to strengthen effective leadership and governance for mental health;
- to provide comprehensive, integrated, and responsive mental health and social care services in community-based settings;
- to implement strategies for promotion and prevention in mental health;
- strengthen information systems, evidence, and research for mental health.

Source: Data from Mental Health Action Plan 2013–2020, World Health Organization. Available at: http://www.who.int/mental_health/action_plan_2013/en/

Box 57.2 Process for mental health policy development (World Health Organization's Mental Health Service Guidance Package)

The WHO's Mental Health and Policy Service Guidance package outlines the following process for mental health policy development [19]:

- assess population needs;
- gather evidence for effective policy;
- consultation and negotiation;
- exchange with other countries;
- set out the vision, values, principles, and objectives;
- determine areas for action;
- identify major roles and responsibilities of different sectors;
- conduct pilot projects.

Source: Data from Mental Health Policy and Service Guidance Package, World Health Organization. Available at http://www.who.int/mental_health/policy/essentialpackage1/en/

The rationale to commit to development of a mental health policy differs depending on the country's context. Policies can be demand-driven when there is a need to address identified weaknesses in routine performance or assessment reports of mental health care, or the policy could be initiated by decision-makers, as a result of being informed about evidence that suggests an urgent change, or the decision-makers are politically motivated.

For a mental health policy process to be initiated, it is important that mental health is high on the political agenda, and can garner strong political will to ensure good mental health for the population [4, 21]. In many LAMICs, competing priorities and/or misunderstanding of mental health puts mental health as a low priority on the agenda [4, 22]. Compounding this problem is often the lack of local, contextualized data to inform policy priorities in mental health, inaccurate data, or data difficult to generalize to the broader country context [4, 23]. Internationally, there is a substantial evidence base to draw upon for policy; however, it is often too difficult to extrapolate this information in the local context and inform decision-makers on how to address problems that exist in that particular country context [4, 23].

It is important to note that a standalone mental health policy is not always necessary if it has been well covered and sufficiently addressed in a general health policy, for instance in the case of Austria and Finland [24]. Unfortunately, this is not the case in numerous LAMICs, where mental health is covered as a separate topic from physical health. Furthermore, it is easier to advocate for a separate mental health policy with ministries [19], as there may be a focal point for mental health who is able to initiate the policy process, but may not have sufficient traction in the ministry to influence for a substantial part of a general health policy to be dedicated towards mental health.

In some countries, prioritization of mental health by international donors led LAMICs to put mental health on their policy agenda [4]. International donors can also influence governments to develop a policy in a shorter time span, for example to fulfil requirements for receiving external funding from a donor in the context of a project. This is in contrast to countries where there exists an internal impetus to develop or update a mental health policy, such as India. An internal impetus to develop a mental health policy may come from a public governmental response to a recent case in the media or a report concerning human rights violations of person with mental health problems, a response to recent data showing the treatment gap or gaps in service provision, or increasing population needs for care. Some countries, such as Zambia, faced an internal push in the form of local lobbying to develop a mental health policy, which led to a mental health policy being developed within 2 years [4]. In Central and Eastern Europe, some governments were influenced by international organizations to formulate a mental health policy, one that particularly prioritized the development of community-based alternatives to mental health care provided in large-scale psychiatric institutions [12]. Some of these policies were developed to fulfil criteria for an international project and thus did not have sufficient substance and context as to how to develop, implement, or evaluate the set-up of these community-based mental health services. Consequently, policy implementation suffered greatly as governments could not develop or finance the scale-up of these pilot initiatives without external support [12], and many mental health services continued to operate as before the policy.

Once there is a commitment to develop a mental health policy, it is important to ensure that each of the following parts of the policy development process are addressed sufficiently, in order to have a widely consulted, well-formulated policy that is measurable and meets the needs of the population. The following section outlines the steps of policy development, using examples from both the literature and from our experiences in policy development in various LAMICs.

Collect information and data to inform a situational analysis of the state or country

Well-formulated policies should have an in-depth understanding of the mental health needs of the target population. This includes not only the prevalence and incidence of mental health problems (informed by epidemiological studies), but also the current functioning of the mental health system, knowledge about what services are offered in both public and private sector for people with mental health problems, and information on who provides these services. This information is collected by conducting a needs assessment and/or situational analysis; data collection for a needs assessment exercise can be done by collecting scientific research that has been carried out in the country, such as epidemiological studies, economic evaluations, or health services research, or can be done through secondary analysis of data from existing information systems, as well as with interviews with a broad range of stakeholder groups [19]. The focal point for the mental health policy process should commission the work of the situational analysis to a team of researchers, from a knowledge institute or university, or even a research department of the Ministry of Health. Scientific evidence is important in policy formulation; however, findings need to be actively brought to the attention of decision-makers [20]. Many decision-makers have limited time to review emerging evidence or to conduct an in-depth review of an evidence base [20]. For instance, in Uganda, decision-makers found that the policy development process was much easier when policy development was preceded by a situational analysis and other evidence showcasing the need for a policy [25]. Other research has shown that while mental health policies may exist, these policies do not provide advice or guidance for populations with specific care needs, such as children, refugees, or pregnant women. A situational analysis of maternal mental health care in Ethiopia, India, Nepal, South Africa, and Uganda revealed that the mental health policies in Ethiopia and Uganda, both low-income countries, did not include specific information about maternal mental health [26]. It becomes imperative for a comprehensive situational analysis to not only addresses key topics and populations in mental health, but also to facilitate the subsequent steps in the policy development process.

After the needs assessment and situational analysis has been completed, strategies to address those needs should be identified. To identify potentially useful strategies, local knowledge and good practices should be utilized, along with reviewing international good practices and literature [20]. Local knowledge and good practices can include any evaluations that have been carried out of previous mental health policies or plans (e.g. using the WHO Mental Health Policy Checklist) [27], any recommendations or evaluations of health system assessments of community-based programmes led by non-profit organizations (NGOs). Such information can be very useful in pointing strategies or highlighting key components for strategies that work in that particular country's context.

This step also involves learning from good practices in other countries with respect to well-formulated, feasible, mental health policies. Ideal sources of information would come from evaluations conducted of previous policy, plans or programmes in other countries with a similar cultural or socio-economic profile [19]. This helps not only in avoiding reinventing the wheel, but can also build a bilateral relationship between two countries to collaborate in the future on sharing knowledge and good practices in policy development and implementation, or in other domains related to mental health. Additionally, the learnings can help avoid falling in the traps of situations where ready-made policy solutions do not necessarily tackle the fragmented policy problems specific to various LAMICs. In Uganda, the policy drafting committee consulted mental health policies from other countries that had mental health policies in place (Santa Lucia, Gambia, Nigeria, and Australia) and could serve as useful examples for their own policy structure and content [25].

Consultative process for input on draft mental health policy

A policy process is more consultative and participatory where a broad range of stakeholders are engaged *before* the policy process begins. Those in charge of the mental health policy process should brief stakeholders about the aim/scope, target audience, and timeframe of the policy development process, as well as inform the stakeholders on when they can expect to be consulted.

Having a comprehensive consultative process for input on a draft mental health policy is essential in ensuring that the policy is feasible, is pragmatic and reflects the needs of the targeted population. The consultative process should be coordinated by a high-level focal point at the Ministry of Health (or by the commissioning body of the mental health policy development process). In many countries, including LAMICs, there is a technical working group or a drafting committee set up to draft the policy content and is responsible for responding to the input of the stakeholder consultation, and incorporating changes into the draft policy. For example, in Uganda, the Ministry of Health developed a new mental health policy and set up a five-member drafting committee consisting of both civil society experts and mental health professionals [25]. In India, the mental health policy working group consisted of national experts working in mental health promotion, service delivery, and advocacy, including service user representatives, mental health professionals, social workers, and civil servants.

In many LAMICs, people with mental health problems face substantial discrimination [28–30]. This is compounded by the fact that mental health in a number of LAMICs is given limited priority and results in people with mental health problems seldom included in the very policy-making process that affects them the most [2]. Service users and their carers are best placed to represent their perspective and inputs in the policy process, being the ultimate beneficiaries of the policy actions [31, 32]. If a policy is solely a top-down process (e.g. originated by decision-makers at ministerial level) it usually is not inclusive and thus it might be difficult to implement the policy actions in practice [20].

In South Africa, policy development for mental health has incorporated actions that would encourage people with mental

> **Box 57.3** Involvement of people with mental health issues in mental health policy-making
>
> **(I):** Who should create awareness about mental health as a priority?
> **(R):** *One, the first, is those that are being affected ... because they know their needs ... The second is the community organisations or the NGOs, because they are in the community and they are an entry-point ... much of government policies have been influenced by what is coming from the community.* Female national policy maker, Department of Housing [2].
>
> *Source:* Reproduced from *BMC International Health and Human Rights*, 13(17), Kleintjes S, Lund C, Swartz L, Barriers to the participation of people with psychosocial disability in mental health policy development in South Africa: a qualitative study of perspectives of policy makers, professionals, religious leaders and academics, Copyright (2013), BioMed Central Ltd, reproduced under the Creative Commons License 2.0.

health problems to get involved and play a role in policy development (see Box 57.3).

In addition to service users as a crucial stakeholder in reviewing the draft policy document, stakeholders outside the health sector (e.g. religious organizations, social policy and gender experts, etc.) also play an important role in shaping housing, employment, and social care opportunities for people with mental health problems. In some LAMICs, governments are not able to, or have not chosen to, consult stakeholders outside the health sector [4].

Examples of stakeholders:

- service user associations and/or networks;
- carer association and/or networks;
- providers of mental health care (from both the health sector, social care sector, and, if relevant, faith-based or alternative medicine sector, e.g. traditional healers or traditional health workers);
- professional associations (e.g. National-level Primary Care Association, Association of Psychiatrists, Association of Psychologists), and, if relevant, national counterpart for World Psychiatric Association or similar, regional networks;
- government agencies;
- academia;
- NGOs;
- for-profit organizations involved in mental health;
- religious organizations;
- local community influencers (local business owners);
- special interest groups;
- unions;
- healthcare payers (e.g. a national insurance company or separate health insurance companies, depending on the health system).

Policy content

The content of a policy is usually drafted by a technical working group appointed by the coordinator of the mental health policy process. The situational analysis carried out, as well as any local or international research or project data relevant to mental health, can be used as sources of data to draft the content of the policy [20]. In principle, the structure and content of a mental health policy does not differ from other health policies.

Setting a vision

Policies start with a clear vision statement that state what the future of mental health will look like in the state or country; and sets the stage for targets in the short- and long-term horizons that the country or state/province plans to achieve through an action plan. Setting a vision is an important but challenging process, as it means reaching consensus on a shared vision for mental health care, which requires obtaining consensus from a diverse set of actors with different interests and power dynamics. A vision statement is often the first part of a policy document, and having a clear, feasible, and concise vision that imbibes the policy's values, principles, and objectives is important [33] in providing an overall direction for the policy. When formulating a vision, it should be ambitious in its expectations for improving mental health, and state what success would look like in mental health for a country or region. At the same time, a lofty vision that could never be achieved or contributed to within the timeframe of the policy is also not helpful; therefore, the vision should be realistic for the particular resources and state of play of that particular region or country (Box 57.4). The latter vision statement is poorly formulated as it does not have an inspiration or a positive vision for the future, and is too broad. Another pitfall to avoid when formulating vision statements is to use too much jargon that may sound impressive but that is difficult to inspire the reader or give a concrete sense of what is meant with the vision statement. An example of such a lofty vision statement is: *[a country] that adopts a participatory, inclusive, community-based approach to mental health care, treatment, and support where people with severe and enduring mental ill health can realize an optimal quality of life, satisfaction with care, and be empowered to exercise their rights.*

Defining underlying principles that reflect the ethos of the policy

After setting the vision for a mental health policy, principles that underpin policy provisions should be determined and made explicit early on in the policy document. Such values and principles are specific to each country context, and need to be defined through a consensus-building procedure among key stakeholders. These values and principles cannot be defined in one meeting; rather, it is an open, consultative process where different stakeholders should reflect on what is meaningful for them in mental health care. Principles often mentioned in policy documents include adopting evidence-based approaches to care and upholding and respecting the rights of person with mental health problems and their carers [23].

Developing policy goals and objectives

Once the underlying principles have consensus by the policy working group, policy goals need to be established. Policy goals are context-driven; the country or state must describe the range of desired outcomes that ought to be achieved in a certain time frame in the country. In contrast, policy objectives, which follow policy goals, should be measurable statements that assess/measure policy goals.

The key strategy in developing a policy objective is the meticulous use of clear and effective language; any ambiguous phrasing in a policy goal or objective poses a risk in adhering to or delivering upon the policy objectives and, consequently, making a weak policy in the region or country. For instance, if we take the example in Box 57.5, we see a concrete policy goal and objective. If the objective did not have a desired proportion to reduce suicides by, or a timeframe for when such a desired outcome is expected, it would be difficult to translate this objective into a series of actions that stakeholders (health and social care professionals, users and carers, decision-makers) could carry out.

It also makes it difficult to allocate resources (human and financial) if the objective is left vague. This renders the objective less likely to be achieved, which results in stagnated progress of the mental health system in the country. An objective could be even further strengthened if it has a 'by' statement at the end of the objective, such as in the following example:

> Reduce the number of suicides in the state by 20% by 2020 through implementing a multi-pronged suicide prevention strategy that reduces access to means, promotes an anti-stigma campaign, and raises awareness in schools and workplaces.

After the policy objectives have been agreed upon, they need to be translated in priority areas for action. These broad areas for action vary by each country's context; however, we list some areas that have been included in the majority of policies developed [20]:

- financing;
- legislation and human rights;
- mental health services development (organization);

Box 57.4 What a mental health vision statement should look like

Example of a well-formulated mental health vision statement:

> An Ireland where people experiencing mental health difficulties can recover their well-being and live a full life in their community [63].

Example of a poorly formulated mental health vision statement:

> Ensure that people with mental health problems get care.

Source: Data from A United Voice for Reform of Mental Health Supports. Strategic Plan Summary 2015–17, Copyright (2015), Mental Health Reform Ireland.

Box 57.5 Example showcasing a clear policy goal and objective

Example:
Policy goal:

- Reduce the number of suicides in the state through suicide prevention efforts.

Policy objective:

- Reduce the number of suicides in the state by 20% by 2020.

♦ capacity building and human resources;

♦ information systems;

♦ intersectoral collaboration;

♦ research;

♦ promotion, prevention treatment, and recovery.

Once these areas for action are defined, the content for each need to be developed. Some LAMICs such as South Africa have cited that the WHO recommendations for policy content was very useful for developing their own mental health policy [34]. The recent Comprehensive Mental Health Action Plan adopted by the 66th World Health Assembly [13] has also been useful for countries like South Africa to base its strategic directions and areas for action on [15].

Content depends on what the local priorities and contextual factors are. For instance, in India, there had never been a national mental health policy in place before the introduction of the 2012 National Mental Health Policy. The old Mental Health Act (1987) was a regressive law that enabled institutions and legal bodies that 'took care' of many choices for people with mental illness, removing autonomy, responsibility, and self-direction [35, 36]. The national mental health policy group (consisting of civil servants, clinicians, researchers, service user representatives, and civil society organizations) spent a substantial amount of time meeting in person to discuss the time frame in which the policy should be written. In light of the fact that India has ratified the UN Convention on the Rights of Persons with Disabilities, a rights-based approach was agreed upon to frame the new mental health policy. The policy has since been celebrated as being progressive for embedding the rights of people with mental health problems throughout the policy document, as well as addressing the complex interplay between social disadvantage and mental health problems [37]. India is among one of the countries that has made progress in ensuring the inclusion of people with mental health problems in society, and upholding their rights. However, a number of countries do not yet see organization of care and treatment for people with mental health problems as a human rights issue. This results in limited political momentum to make the linkages between mental health and human rights and reflects the connection in a policy document in a meaningful and actionable way [5]. Incorporating human rights means that policies and their subsequent plans and programmes contribute to the fulfilment of human rights, and, improve outcomes [38].

Another issue frequently surfacing in mental health policies in LAMICs is having strategies to address the shortage of mental health professionals [39–42]. A recent review found that in LAMICs, mental health care could be improved by adopting a stepped-care approach, having sufficient mental health specialists for the needs of the population, having an infrastructure that supports mental health care in the community, increasing mental health literacy, including those with chronic mental health problems in the community, and using a collaborative, community-based mental health care model [43]. For example, in India, there will likely never be enough mental health professionals to cater to a population of 1.2 billion [44]. To tackle this scarcity of human resources for mental health, countries have included policy actions related to integrating mental health into primary care [20, 41, 45–48], task-shifting [39, 49–53] and strengthening the capacity of existing community members to provide basic mental health supports [54]. This body of research

looking at strategies for reducing the gap in mental health care provision have been carried out in LAMICs (e.g. Zimbabwe, South Africa, India, Pakistan, Chile), and thus provide a more relevant, localized evidence base to draw upon for policy.

Mental health policy implementation

(R): What we have said is people must get out of psychiatric institutions and be back in the community … with whom? I'm saying this Act is such a good Act but … the resources to make the implementation viable and see it happen, they are not there [2].

In LAMICs, sometimes the hardest part of the policy process in mental health care is the implementation of the policy. There are several reasons for the difficult in implementation. In many LAMICs there is a triple burden of disease (non-communicable, communicable, accidents, and injuries), which means that all health conditions are competing for healthcare financing. This can be a competitive process, and can result in other priorities being funded ahead of mental health priorities [4, 17]. Policymakers often do not perceive mental health as amenable to being defined, easily costed, readily understood, and easily implemented solutions [55]. Another reason for poor policy implementation can stem as a result of vague policy provisions and actions, policy lacking concrete steps, or unclear budget allocation [9]. The vague and unstructured design results in difficulty in translating policies into strategic, operational plans [4].

Countries with a devolved health system structure (e.g. India) can also have a situation where there is confusion between priorities of regional state governments versus national government, the latter of which administer the policy. There are often disagreements about whether to follow state policies and guidelines versus differing priorities and policy provisions in the national policy [56]. In India, health is a state subject [57]; even though the national Ministry of Health and Family Welfare has released a national mental health policy, two states have their own mental health policies (Gujarat, Kerala). Given the vast population in each State of India and health being a state subject, it is a positive step for the states to develop state-specific mental health policy, yet the state and the national policies ought to work on being coherent and converge targeting a common goal..

Finally, many LAMIC governments may have the budget allocated for policy implementation but do not have the sufficient human resources required for the implementation of policy provisions [40, 56]. The lack of human resources could be at the governance level (e.g. difficulty in appointing a coordinating body to take leadership and oversee implementation of the policy) [4]. It could also be difficult in human resources capacity at the local level. In India, the national mental health policy recommended that the flagship national programme for community mental health, the District Mental Health Programme, be scaled up from 182 districts in India to all 648 [37, 58]. Implementing this in practice translates to an enormous increase in capacity building efforts (as the programme entails training primary care workers to provide community mental health services) [37].

Strategies to enhance policy implementation in low- and middle-income countries

For the uptake of programmes or provisions specified in policies in practice, there are a number of factors that are important; these include effective leadership, strong strategic alliances, and an (expedited) institutionalization process that ensures sustainability of programmes over time in the country [20].

Strategies to enhance implementation can already be utilized before a mental health policy is drafted. Involving all stakeholders in the process of policy development helps to create a policy that has broad consensus and therefore has a greater chance of being implemented. Other advantages of an inclusive process of policy development is that implementation problems will be identified long before the policy is announced, it facilitates intersectoral alliances among different stakeholders working in mental health, and is likely to result in a policy that is of relevance to the ultimate beneficiaries—service users and carers.

Furthermore, efforts need to be made by policy implementers that show how the public health system can be strengthened, given that a mental health policy governs primarily the public health system rather than the private healthcare system and/ or NGOs. This requires consideration of the budgetary alloca-tion for mental health within the public health system, current gaps in human resources, an analysis of existing services and programmes, and an understanding of service user needs and caseloads of existing care providers. This analysis should be synthesized into a workable action plan presented to decision-makers, as any new programmes that fit within policy priorities require a business case or viable proposal for their sustainability into the public health system [20]. Here, working together with health economists to carry out health economic evaluations of existing mental health interventions or programmes is extremely useful in preparing a business case or proposal for scale-up of an intervention [59–61]. Cost-effectiveness studies carried out in Chile and India have been useful to provide a proposal to gov-ernment about the importance of integrating mental health into primary care, or on task-shifting, in reducing the treatment gap [20, 62]. However, limited international investment in mental health systems reform, including mental health infrastructure (e.g. information systems) makes it difficult to build a compelling business case for continued implementation of mental health programmes to ministers of health and ministers of finance [55]. Private providers and NGOs play an important and valuable role in promotion, prevention, and treatment of mental health problems in many LAMICs and are certainly implicated in policy provisions stated, and a part of the key stakeholder groups in a country that work together to realize the vision stipulated in the policy document.

Support for mental health policies has also been difficult for many stakeholders in LAMICs. A review of the mental health policies of Latin American countries, many of which are categorized as LAMICs, found that 'the mental health budget allocation in most Latin American countries continues to be far below the level that would reflect the population's health needs according to the current epidemiological evidence'[11].

When the policy specifies programmes or actions related to capacity building in mental health, in an effort to tackle the scar-city of mental health professionals, human resource planning efforts are needed for implementation of these policy actions to be successful. Numerous strategies have been employed in countries like India, Mozambique, Malawi, and Tanzania that span from scholarships to contracts for placement in rural areas with higher financial incentives to contracts mandating in-country service after

education (which has been subsidized/financed, accommodation, and food provision for staff) [55].

Changes in a mental health system are challenging; consequently, dedicating efforts to change management processes is essential, coordinated by the body that is in charge of the implementation of the policy, such as the Ministry of Health. For instance, those implicated in policy implementation may perceive that some of the policy priorities threatens or compromises their positions. In countries where the deinstitutionalization process is underway, a policy that aims at downsizing psychiatric hospitals or closing beds in psychiatric hospitals may lead directors or staff of those hospitals to perceive the implementation of that policy as a negative change and may resist or block its implementation. To mitigate this, emphasizing new and positive roles within this process of change are important for hospital staff, as is capacity building in how to work as a hospital in the deinstitutionalization process and how to work in community-based settings.

Another crucial aspect of the policy implementation process is dissemination of the information that will influence the target audi-ence of the policy. The dissemination procedure differs according to (i) the kind of policy solution that is being adopted; (ii) to whom this solution targets; and (iii) where the information needs to be disseminated. Various policy instruments could be used for dis-semination. For example, if the policy has a legal focus and involves technical nuances with a smaller set of stakeholders, advocating for a legal change in the mental health policy requires specific en-gagement; therefore, usage of authority-based instruments where the information will be distributed in the form of guidelines and awareness-raising events will be useful. When the policy solu-tion is focused on structural changes, such as establishing more community-based mental health care centres in a country, a treasure-based policy instrument is needed to help secure funds required for such infrastructural changes. Lastly, if the policy is long term and seeks a change in mindset, the stakeholder engage-ment becomes very wide yet focused, such policy solution demands mostly an information-based policy instrument that concentrates on disseminating the information. This could take the form of policy dialogues, where decision-makers and other key stakeholders come together to debate and reach consensus on one specific policy ask. It could also be the case that a policy solution needs a combination of the three policy instruments to be fully viable.

Conclusions

Evidently, mental health policy processes are complex, and a myriad of factors affect its development and implementation. LAMICs face competing priorities vying for the same attention and resources, and mental health has historically been low on the pol-itical agenda. Mental health policies are an important process and document when countries recognize that mental health problems are important in their population and commit to taking action in addressing these problems.

In our view, there are three elements fundamental to a good mental health policy development process. The first is to create an inclusive policy process, which involves all stakeholders that play a role in or are affected by mental health. Stakeholders need to be included in shaping the content and direction of the policy, particu-larly beneficiaries of the policy. Secondly, a mental health policy, to have an impact across sectors, should be harmonized with other health and social policies. Thirdly, the policy should state a specific time frame for when its implementation should be realized.

Implementation of the policy is essential to making any sustainable changes and improvements in a regional or national mental health system. Dedicated human and financial resources, political will and commitment at the highest level, evaluation and monitoring mechanisms for policy implementation, policy dialogue, and communication between stakeholders are all important enablers for policy implementation. Evaluation of mental health policies is as important as drafting a mental health policy and therefore time and effort should be devoted to evaluation mechanisms so that it forms the basis for revision and refinement of the policy.

Finally, dissemination of the policy is important. Often, key stakeholders may be unaware of the existence of the policy or the policy goals. Policy messages should be tailored for different audiences in a format in which is accessible and appropriate. When a policy development process is inclusive, involving a diverse set of stakeholders in mental health, it is less likely that stakeholders will be uninformed about the policy or its intentions.

Acknowledgements

The authors would like to acknowledge Dr Bethany Hipple Walters for her helpful edits of this chapter.

References

1. Sapag JC, Rush B, Ferris LE. Collaborative mental health services in primary care systems in Latin America: contextualized evaluation needs and opportunities. *Health Expect* 2016; 19: 152–169.
2. Kleintjes S, Lund C, Swartz L. Barriers to the participation of people with psychosocial disability in mental health policy development in South Africa: a qualitative study of perspectives of policy makers, professionals, religious leaders and academics. *BMC Int Health Hum Rights* 2013; 13: 17.
3. World Health Organization. Mental Health Atlas 2014. Available at: http://www.who.int/mental_health/evidence/atlas/mental_health_atlas_2014/en/ (accessed 22 March 2018).
4. Omar MA, Green AT, Bird PK, et al. Mental health policy process: a comparative study of Ghana, South Africa, Uganda and Zambia. *Int J Ment Health Syst* 2010; 4: 24.
5. Knapp M, Mcdaid D, Mossialos E, Thornicroft G. Mental health policy and practice across Europe. Available at: http://www.euro.who.int/__data/assets/pdf_file/0007/96451/E89814.pdf (accessed 22 March 2018).
6. Gureje O, Alem A. Mental health policy development in Africa. *Bull World Health Organ* 2000; 78: 475–482.
7. Uznanski A, Roos J. The situation of mental health services of the World Health Organisation, African region, in the early 1990s. *South African Med J* 1997; 87: 1743–1749.
8. Awenva AD, Read UM, Ofori-Attah AL, et al. From mental health policy development in Ghana to implementation: What are the barriers? *Afr J Psychiatry* 2010; 13: 184–191.
9. Faydi E, Funk M, Kleintjes S, et al. An assessment of mental health policy in Ghana, South Africa, Uganda and Zambia. *Health Res Policy Syst* 2011; 9: 17.
10. Draper CE, Lund C, Kleintjes S, Funk M, Omar M, Flisher AJ. Mental health policy in South Africa: development process and content. *Health Policy Plan* 2009; 24: 342–356.
11. Minoletti A, Galea S, Susser E. Community mental health services in Latin America for people with severe mental disorders. *Public Health Rev* 2012; 34(2).
12. Petrea I. Mental health in former Soviet countries: from past legacies to modern practices. *Public Health Rev* 2013; 34: 1–21.
13. World Health Assembly. Comprehensive mental health action plan 2013–2020. Available at: http://www.who.int/mental_health/action_plan_2013/en/ (accessed 22 March 2018).
14. Saxena S, Funk M, Chisholm D, Whiteford H, et al. World Health Assembly adopts Comprehensive Mental Health Action Plan 2013–2020. *Lancet* 2013; 381: 1970–1971.
15. Stein DJ. A new mental health policy for South Africa. *South African Med J* 2014; 104: 115–116.
16. World Health Organization. WHO Mental Health Atlas 2014: Executive Summary. Available at: http://www.who.int/mental_health/evidence/atlas/executive_summary_en.pdf?ua=1 (accessed 22 March 2018).
17. Monteiro NM, Ndiaye Y, Blanas D, Ba I. Policy perspectives and attitudes towards mental health treatment in rural Senegal. *Int J Ment Health Syst* 2014; 8: 9.
18. Menil V De. Missed Opportunities in Global Health : Identifying New Strategies to Improve Mental Health in LMICs. Available at: www.cgdev.org/publication/missed-opportunities-global-health-identifying-new-strategies-improve-mental-health (accessed 22 March 2018).
19. World Health Organization. Mental Health Policy, Plans and Programmes. Available at: http://www.who.int/mental_health/policy/services/2_policy plans prog_WEB_07.pdf (22 March 2018).
20. Araya R, Alvarado R, Sepúlveda R, Rojas G. Lessons from scaling up a depression treatment program in primary care in Chile. *Rev Panam Salud Publica* 2012; 32: 234–240.
21. Jenkins R. Supporting governments to adopt mental health policies. *World Psychiatry* 2003; 2: 14–19.
22. Khenti A, Fréel S, Trainor R, et al. Developing a holistic policy and intervention framework for global mental health. *Health Policy Plan* 2016; 31: 37–45.
23. Patel V, Eaton J. Princípios para orientar as políticas de saúde mental em países de baixa e média rendas. *Rev Bras Psiquiatr* 2010; 32: 345–346.
24. European Commission. Mental Health Systems in the European Union Member States, Status of Mental Health in Populations and Benefits to be Expected from Investments into Mental Health. Available at: https://ec.europa.eu/health//sites/health/files/mental_health/docs/europopp_full_en.pdf (accessed 22 March 2018).
25. Ssebunnya J, Kigozi F, Ndyanabangi S. Developing a national mental health policy: a case study from Uganda. *PLOS Med* 2012; 9: e1001319.
26. Baron EC, Hanlon C, Mall S, et al. Maternal mental health in primary care in five low- and middle-income countries: a situational analysis. *BMC Health Serv Res* 2016; 16: 53.
27. World Health Organization. Checklist for Evaluating a Mental Health Policy. Available at: http://www.who.int/mental_health/policy/WHOPolicyChecklist_forwebsite.pdf (accessed 22 March 2018).
28. Egbe CO, Brooke-Sumner C, Kathree T, Selohilwe O, Thornicroft G, Petersen I. Psychiatric stigma and discrimination in South Africa: perspectives from key stakeholders. *BMC Psychiatry* 2014; 14: 191.
29. Ngui EM, Khasakhala L, Ndetei D, Weiss L. *Int Rev Psychiatry* 2011; 22: 235–244.
30. Mascayano F, Armijo JE, Yang LH. Addressing stigma relating to mental illness in low- and middle-income countries. *Front Psychiatry* 2015; 6.
31. Sweeney DA, Wallcraft DJ, 2010 J. WHO-EC Partnership Project on User Empowerment in Mental Health Quality Assurance / Monitoring of Mental Health Services by Service Users and Carers. Available at: http://www.scie.org.uk/publications/guides/guide45/files/WHO_paper_final_draft.pdf?res=true (accessed 22 March 2018).
32. Semrau M, Evans-Lacko S, Alem A, et al. Strengthening mental health systems in low- and middle-income countries: the Emerald programme. *BMC Med* 2015; 13: 79.
33. Lund C. What are the principles that should guide mental health policies in low and middle-income countries? *Rev Bras Psiquiatr* 2010; 32: 348.

34. Draper CE, Lund C, Kleintjes S, et al. Mental health policy in South Africa: development process and content. *Health Policy Plan* 2009; 24: 342–356.

35. Pathare S, Shields L. Supported decision-making for persons with mental illness: a review. *Public Health Rev* 2012; 34: 1–40.

36. Srebnik D, Livingston J, Gordon L, King D. Housing choice and community success for individuals with serious and persistent mental illness. *Community Ment Health J* 1995; 31: 139–152.

37. Sharma DC. India's new policy aims to close gaps in mental health care. *Lancet* 2014; 384: 1564.

38. Gruskin S, Bogecho D, Ferguson L. 'Rights-based approaches' to health policies and programs: articulations, ambiguities, and assessment. *J Public Health Policy* 2010; 31: 129–145.

39. Chibanda D, Bowers T, Verhey R, et al. The Friendship Bench programme: a cluster randomised controlled trial of a brief psychological intervention for common mental disorders delivered by lay health workers in Zimbabwe. *Int J Ment Health Syst* 2015; 9: 21.

40. Rao M, Rao KD, Kumar AKS, Chatterjee M, Sundararaman T. Human resources for health in India. *Lancet* 2011; 377: 587–598.

41. Petersen I, Lund C, Bhana A, Flisher AJ. A task shifting approach to primary mental health care for adults in South Africa: human resource requirements and costs for rural settings. *Health Policy Plan* 2012; 27: 42–51.

42. Saxena S, Thornicroft G, Knapp M, Whiteford H. Resources for mental health: scarcity, inequity, and inefficiency. *Lancet* 2007; 370: 878–889.

43. Petersen I, Lund C, Stein DJ. Optimizing mental health services in low-income and middle-income countries. *Curr Opin Psychiatry* 2011; 24: 318–323.

44. van Ginneken N, Jain S, Patel V, Berridge V. The development of mental health services within primary care in India: learning from oral history. *Int J Ment Health Syst* 2014; 8: 30.

45. Hailemariam M, Fekadu A, Selamu M, et al. Developing a mental health care plan in a low resource setting: the theory of change approach. *BMC Health Serv Res* 2015; 15.

46. Ngo VK, Rubinstein A, Ganju V, et al. Grand challenges: integrating mental health care into the non-communicable disease agenda. *PLOS Med* 2013; 10: e1001443.

47. Araya R, Flynn T, Rojas G, Fritsch R, Simon G. Cost-effectiveness of a primary care treatment program for depression in low-income women in Santiago, Chile. *Am J Psychiatry* 2006; 163: 1379–1387.

48. Petersen I, Ssebunnya J, Bhana A, Baillie K. Lessons from case studies of integrating mental health into primary health care in South Africa and Uganda. *Int J Ment Health Syst* 2011; 5: 8.

49. dos Santos P., Wainberg M., Caldas de Almeida J., Saraceno B, de Jesus Mari J. Overview of the mental health system in Mozambique: addressing the treatment gap with a task-shifting strategy in primary care. *Int J Ment Health Syst* 2016; 10(1).

50. Joshi R, Alim M, Kengne AP, et al. Task shifting for non-communicable disease management in low and middle income countries—a systematic review. *PLOS ONE* 2014; 9: e103754.

51. Patel V, Goel DS, Desai R, Singh D. Scaling up services for mental and neurological disorders in low-resource settings. *Int Health* 2009; 1: 37–44.

52. Mendenhall E, De Silva MJ, Hanlon C, et al. Acceptability and feasibility of using non-specialist health workers to deliver mental health care: Stakeholder perceptions from the PRIME district sites in Ethiopia, India, Nepal, South Africa, and Uganda. *Soc Sci Med* 2014; 118C: 33–42.

53. Patel V, Weiss H, Chowdhary N, et al. Effectiveness of an intervention led by lay health counsellors for depressive and anxiety disorders in primary care in Goa, India (MANAS): a cluster randomised controlled trial. *Lancet* 2010; 376: 2086–2095.

54. Shields-Zeeman L, Pathare S, Hipple Walters B, Kapadia-Kundu N, Joag K. Promoting wellbeing and improving access to mental health care through community champions in rural India: The Atmiyata intervention approach. *Int J Ment Health Syst* 2016; 11: 6.

55. Jenkins R, Baingana F, Ahmad R, McDaid D, Atun R. International and national policy challenges in mental health. *Ment Health Fam Med* 2011; 8: 101–114.

56. University of Cape Town. Policy brief 3 Challenges of implementing mental health policy and legislation in South Africa. Available at: http://www.who.int/mental_health/policy/development/MHPB3.pdf (accessed 22 March 2018).

57. Khandelwal SK, Jhingan HP, Ramesh S, Gupta RK, Srivastava VK. India mental health country profile. *Int Rev Psychiatry* 2004; 16: 126–241.

58. van Ginneken N, Jain S, Patel V, Berridge V. The development of mental health services within primary care in India: learning from oral history. *Int J Ment Health Syst* 2014; 8: 30.

59. Knapp M, Evers S, Salvador-carulla L. Cost-effectiveness and mental health. Available at: http://eprints.lse.ac.uk/4276/1/MHEEN_policy_briefs_2_cost-effectiveness(LSERO).pdf (accessed 22 March 2018).

60. Siskind D, Araya R, Kim J. Cost-effectiveness of improved primary care treatment of depression in women in Chile. *Br J Psychiatry* 2010; 197: 291–296.

61. Chisholm D, Sweeny K, Sheehan P, et al. Scaling-up treatment of depression and anxiety: a global return on investment analysis. *Lancet Psychiatry* 2016; 366: 1–10.

62. Buttorff C, Hock RS, Weiss HA, et al. Economic evaluation of a task-shifting intervention for common mental disorders in India. Available at: http://www.who.int/bulletin/volumes/90/11/12-104133/en/ (accessed 22 March 2018).

63. Mental Health Reform Ireland. A united voice for reform of mental health supports. Available at: https://www.mentalhealthreform.ie/wp-content/uploads/2015/07/MHR_Strategic-Plan-summary-2015-16-PDF-for-website.pdf (accessed 22 March 2018).

CHAPTER 58

Managing research and evaluation for public mental health

Sarah Stewart-Brown

Introduction

Public mental health is of interest to a wide variety of disciplines each with their own preferences and belief systems around what constitutes research evidence. These include the research approaches developed:

- in public health—including the quantitative science of epidemiology;
- at the interface between public health and clinical medicine—including the randomized controlled trial (RCT) and systematic review;
- in psychiatry—including detailed observation of clinical signs, symptoms, patterns of behaviour, and responses to intervention together with careful classification;
- in social science
  - o both the regression modelling and evaluation of 'natural experiments' done by the quantitative branch, including the economists
  - o and the observational and qualitative methodologies of the other branch of the discipline;
- in psychology—often in laboratory experiments that aim to replicate experiences in the wider world;
- in the laboratory studies of neuroscientists and psychologists, sometimes on animals, examining neural and neuroendocrine pathways and their development and plasticity.

Once developed and proven to be useful, the methods can spread beyond the discipline in which they were developed and become accepted in other disciplines. RCTs and epidemiological studies are now very familiar and well regarded in all medical disciplines and increasingly in other areas of service provision. However, some silos remain and these can be important in an interdisciplinary field like public mental health because new ideas and approaches to health improvement and disease prevention are more readily accepted if they can be verified by familiar research methodologies. In making the case for public mental health most of the listed disciplines need to be convinced that the endeavour is worthwhile and each discipline

may need to verify the new ideas using its preferred methods. This means that the spread of ideas is likely to be very slow. Of all the branches of research listed, that of the neuroscientists is the most complex for those working in other disciplines to grasp, requiring as it does detailed contemporary knowledge of neuroanatomy and neurophysiology, each with their own complex nomenclatures, together with an understanding of electromagnetic and biochemical techniques that can be used to investigate brain structure and functioning. Yet, arguably, this field has been the one that has been able to most strongly challenge the mindsets that limit public mental health. One of these mindsets, which, although now very outdated, still holds sway in some quarters, believes that brain growth and development occurs in childhood and that brains do not change in adulthood. Another believes that brain growth and development is primarily genetically determined. Research that is confronting these mindsets and enabling awareness of the full potential of public mental health to improve human health and social functioning includes demonstration of:

- the phenomenon of life-course neural plasticity [1, 2];
- that this can be brought, to some extent, under the control of the individual [3];
- the profound influence of the environment, particularly the relational environment in childhood, on the architecture and functioning of the adult brain [4–8].

This chapter looks at some of the research methods commonly used in public mental health and identifies the strengths and limitations of these methods for advancing knowledge in this field. A review of the neuroscientific and psychology research is beyond the scope of the current chapter, but some of the former is reviewed and discussed in Chapter 53.

Epidemiology

Origins

Public health research has its origins in statistics relating to death. Firstly, simple counts of numbers of deaths showing the course of an epidemic, then, secondly, counts of deaths from different causes and then mortality rates (see Chapter 1) played a very important part in enabling policy and legislation to combat communicable diseases in the eighteenth and nineteenth centuries. From these origins developed the quantitative science of epidemiology on which a high proportion of medical knowledge is now based. Epidemiology is steeped in the mindset that was developing during the nineteenth century that individual diseases were caused by specific agents that could be identified and then treated, and it is at its most efficient when investigating specific diseases and agents, for example scurvy caused by lack of vitamin C, cholera caused by the *Vibrio cholerae* bacterium, mesothelioma caused by asbestos exposure, and diabetes caused by lack of insulin. The job of the epidemiologist was to find the agent. The job of the public health doctor, sometimes the same person, was to take this evidence to policymakers and persuade them that it was worth investing in prevention. Together, these disciplines and their research have made a huge impact on morbidity rates and on longevity.

Lifestyles

The identification of smoking as a cause of lung cancer in the mid-twentieth century heralded a change in the focus of epidemiology. Firstly, because the problem was something individuals did to themselves and state interference was not necessarily welcomed; secondly, because it rapidly became clear that smoking increased the risk of a wide range of diseases; and, thirdly, because it turned out that smoking was only one of a number of lifestyle factors (alcohol, drugs, diet, physical inactivity) that increased the risk of the diseases related to smoking. These factors were often associated with one another and for some diseases like heart disease they all contributed a bit and sometimes potentiated the impact of one another. While the mindset of a single agent causing a single disease was clearly not applicable in these circumstances, the latter was such an attractive way of viewing diseases and medicine that it has lingered on long after its principle purpose has been served. The principles of establishing causality from epidemiological studies (see Chapter 1) still in use today are based on this mindset.

Social factors

During this period epidemiologists also became interested in social factors as a cause of disease and started to demonstrate social inequalities—poor health related to poor social status. Like lifestyle factors, low social status increased the risk of dying from a wide range of diseases. Low social status was often associated with adverse lifestyle factors and with other adverse social factors—unemployment, low levels of education, poor housing. Regression analyses became the methodology of choice at this stage aiming to partial out the impact of the different social or lifestyle risk factors, adjust for those which were not considered causal (confounding factors) (see Chapter 1), and identify key agents or factors for the prevention of that disease. These analyses focused on causes of death or disease, both binary outcomes, estimated by logistic regression and reported as relative risks.

Mental health

Regression analysis has been applied to psychiatric disorder and mental illness more generally, and valuable information about prevalence, incidence, and co-morbidity (see Chapter 1) is now routinely collected in Westernized societies. However, because mental illness is not a common cause of death—people with mental illness

have reduced longevity, but it is nearly always physical illness that causes the death—psychiatric epidemiology is based on surveys or cohort studies. Because much mental illness goes undiagnosed and because it carries a stigma, people may be unable or reluctant to self-disclose. Therefore, the collection of data for psychiatric epidemiology often requires expensive clinical examination surveys. The search for causes of mental illness has provided evidence that lifestyle choices like smoking increase the risk of common mental disorders, excessive alcohol consumption can cause psychotic illness, and vitamin deficiency can play a role in some psychiatric disorders. However, the search for specific agents for specific psychiatric disorders has not been as fruitful as it has been in physical diseases. Many well-recognized risk factors like attachment insecurity in infancy [9, 10] and parental mental illness [11] increase risk for many different mental illness. Indeed, the experience of a single psychiatric illness is relativey rare, co-morbidity being the norm [12]. Even the demonstration of clear patterns of prevalence related to social status is not readily interpretable because the relationship is often bidirectional: lack of social status adds to stress and so increases the incidence of disease, but the onset of mental illness interrupts learning, education, and productivity, and so is often association with a reduction in social status. So while epidemiology has yielded valuable insights into mental illness and psychiatric disorder, its limitations are evident.

Well-being

Epidemiology has its origins in the study of disease—the negative aspects of the health spectrum. Although epidemiological methods can be applied to investigating the positive—well-being, resilience, longevity—it is only recently that they have been. Regression studies, grounded in the linear, hierarchal thinking of twentieth-century epidemiology, aiming to separate out the impact of different agents or factors and identify that which is most important are even more ill fitted to investigating the complex causal pathways (see Chapter 1) of mental well-being than they are of mental illness. In both cases it is clear that many different factors or agents interact to create the conditions in which illness arises in people who are susceptible, or well-being develops in those who are resilient, and the same agents or factors create conditions in which either mental or physical illness or both may arise (see Chapter 1 for discussion of holism). It is also clear from Chapter 53 that the same event can predispose to illness, or support the development of resilience, depending on the relational environment. If we add to this mix the fact that the factors that are important in the development of well-being are rarely amenable to simple measurement or interventions, it is very difficult to establish the final criterion for demonstrating causality (see Chapter 1)—that changing the putative cause changes the outcome of interest. However, because mental well-being is a new concept in public health it is important to try to apply the tried-and-trusted epidemiological methods to identifying both causes and consequences of mental well-being as best as can be. Studies showing the extent to which mental well-being enhances longevity [13], coercive parenting is an important causal factor in conduct disorder [14], child abuse increases the risk for a range of mental disorders [10], minor issues with the parent–child relationship increase the risk of adult mental illness [15], and supportive family and social relationships [16, 17] are predictive of resilience in the face of trauma are all examples of the successful application of epidemiology to the study of mental illness and mental well-being.

Randomized controlled trials and systematic reviews

The RCT was proposed in the latter half of the twentieth century by a famous professor of public health [18] as the best way of rationalizing health care so that provision could be based on objective evidence of what works. The theory is compelling—comparison of the effects of a new treatment in two groups of people chosen at random gives a precise quantified measure of the value of the treatment. It has proved so compelling that a doctrine of 'evidence-based medicine' has grown up around the RCT. Escalation of research using this method demonstrated quite quickly that these trials can give conflicting results and to overcome this problem a research industry has grown up undertaking systematic reviews and meta-analyses of the results of trials. Both government-funded [19] and non-government-funded organizations [20] have been formed to undertake reviews and disseminate evidence, and the methodology of the RCT and systematic review has spread to be regarded as the gold standard in other publically funded services.

Randomized controlled trials in mental health

Psychiatry has embraced the doctrine of evidence-based medicine and aspires to ensure that all interventions are backed by RCT evidence. Other mental health practitioners—notably psychotherapists—have been reluctant to engage with this methodology, maintaining that RCTs present problems for evaluation of talking therapies [21]. Practitioners and academics in public health [22] have flagged up multiple issues that arise in trying to apply this methodology to public health interventions, and, famously, the World Health Organization declared in 1996 that for evaluating health promotion, 'RCTs were inappropriate, misleading and unnecessarily expensive' [23]. As the evidence-based medicine doctrine has dominated the discourse about evaluation, dissenters in disciplines like psychotherapy are often accused of lacking the courage to test whether what they do has value and their very valid concerns are swept aside. In the meantime, it has become extremely difficult to find funding for interventions that lack an RCT evidence base.

Criticisms of randomized controlled trials

The criticisms that have been raised against RCTs in these disciplines include the following.

- *The difficulty in providing interventions 'blind' so that neither the receiver nor the 'prescriber' know what is being delivered.* Blinding is the way expectation biases and placebo effects can be eliminated, and the approach is appropriate and helpful in evaluating pharmaceutical interventions but has proven unworkable for obvious reasons in areas of medical practice like surgery or in the talking therapies, and areas of public health that involve practitioners engaging patients or the public. Separating the process of data collection from provision of the intervention helps to overcome some of this bias and would now be regarded as necessary Cluster- or area-based RCTs in which geographical areas or services are randomized rather than individual participants can also address some of these problems, but cluster RCTS are,

necessarily, very large and the encounter issues relating to the second and third bullet points below.

- *The methodological issues that arise in evaluating the very small effects that can provide important health gain when implemented at a population level [22].* Enormous trials may be required and that means consistent implementation of the intervention across a range of services or areas and many service providers. This may not be achievable in practice or in the time span for which funding has been provided.

- *The myriad of issues that arise in trying to implement complex interventions to order in the context of an RCT [24].* People and organizations differ and do not respond in exactly the same way to new ideas or approaches meaning that the new intervention may have to implemented differently in different places and standardization of the intervention is sacrificed

- *Undertaking RCTs where implementation requires a policy development that is achieved as part of the democratic process.* This is particularly challenging as the process cannot be controlled.

- *The impact of recruiting and consenting participants to RCTs, which influences who is recruited and thus the external validity of the trial [25, 26].* Behaviour change or personal development happens when the individual is 'ready to change'. At this point the individual is ready to take some personal responsibility for the change and engages with the process. The development of autonomy and agency are often key components of mental well-being interventions and depend on the exercise of choice. The process of recruitment to a trial involves giving up autonomy and agency as the participant allows their treatment to be randomly allocated. Once someone is ready to change they are likely to be reluctant to be randomized to no-intervention, especially if help is available outside the trial, which it often is. This process means that individuals recruited to the trial are less likely to be people who are in the optimum state of mind to succeed in making the necessary changes. Indeed, effective clinicians intuitively assess readiness to change and do not waste scarce supportive services on people who are not. Given this phenomenon, it is not surprising that RCTs often demonstrate lower levels of effectiveness than non-controlled studies.

- *The potential for providing higher-quality interventions and intervention support in the context of research than can be provided in practice.* The provision of mental health interventions often involves the training, development, and ongoing supervision of staff. Funding for these in the trials setting is often much greater than when programmes are rolled out into routine practice.

Ways round many of these issues have been found and can be put in place [27], but the net effect can be such a complex, cumbersome, over-controlled setting that the intervention takes second place and is not properly implemented.

Therapeutic relationships

It is notable that the disciplines in which objections to RCTs have been raised most often are those where successful outcome is dependent on the quality of the relationship established between the practitioner, and patient or member of the public. The development of a therapeutic relationship is an art and skill, and cannot be provided because a protocol specifies this. The necessary quality is similar to that which can enable challenging events or situations to result in personal growth and resilience (see Chapter 53). What needs to be offered by the practitioner to enable the active engagement of the participant in the process of their development varies from one patient or client to another. Success is likely to involve a change in neural pathways and therefore intention, awareness, and practice. The pharmaceutical approaches, where RCTs are at their best and have been most readily embraced, are those in which treatments can be applied passively and relationship quality is not of primary importance. The evidence-based doctrine is tending to bias healthcare provision towards that which can be evaluated in RCTs.

Randomized controlled trials for well-being interventions

Public mental health interventions that address well-being encounter many of the difficulties identified earlier. Mental well-being interventions are almost always complex; often involved policy development, cannot be offered blinded, and may need to be offered on very large scale. In addition, success often depends on development of practitioners and enhancing their ability to establish therapeutic or healthy relationships. Personal engagement and the development of autonomy and agency are usually key components.

In both therapeutic and public health settings improvements in well-being can take many forms. The outcome often depends on what is the most appropriate developmental step for any individual at that particular stage in their lives and may thus vary from one individual to another. It may be manifested in improvements in mental or physical health. The RCT methodology demands that a primary outcome be defined at the trial design stage and sample size calculations are based around this measure. But given the difficulties mentioned above, it is rarely possible to find a single measure that captures all positive outcomes effectively. This means that positive change can go undetected and the effects of the intervention are under estimated. The issue of appropriate outcomes is further addressed later in the chapter (see 'Outcome measurement').

Linear regression modelling

Quantitative social scientists often research large national datasets collected for the purpose of generating routine statistics and enabling multiple comparisons across different parts of the world [28, 29]. These studies make a great contribution to knowledge and have an important and often quite immediate influence on policy. Multiple independent variables are entered into a regression equation and those which are most significantly associated with the factor of interest (dependent variable or outcome), after adjusting for all others, are considered causal. Outcomes are continuous in linear regression rather than binary, as in logistic regression studies. The impact of drawing inappropriate conclusions from these studies is not so immediate and personal as it is for health and disease-related research and it may be for this reason that social scientists have not developed or adopted strict criteria for establishing causality in the same way as has happened for epidemiology (see Chapter 1). Causal assumptions have been made on much weaker grounds, for example from cross-sectional rather than longitudinal studies. As economists become more interested in health and well-being [30], their approach is beginning to change and they are identifying and using cohort and panel study data more often [31].

Secondary data analysis and categorization of variables

Secondary data analyses—in which data collection has not been designed with the specific research question in mind—make use of variables in which data were gathered with other purposes or analyses in mind. Categories of, for example, educational achievement, income levels, or social class, can vary, but the impact of the way data items have been measured is rarely considered. The correlation with the outcome under study of a variable measuring social class in six categories may be different from one measuring it in two, and the extent of statistical adjustment will differ in the two cases. Studies of alcohol consumption and mental health can be effected by classification problems. Light drinking (< 7 units a week) is often associated with positive physical, emotional, and mental health [32], whereas high levels of consumption are associated with mental illnesses [33]. Study findings will therefore depend on where the cut points for alcohol consumption are placed.

The regression models used by quantitative social scientists can be very complex, with a myriad of variables considered. Because the data are available for analysis, they can be used without consideration of the literature relating to all the variables and thus the implications of different cut points and approaches to classification. However, the conclusions of these studies are often presented as precise quantitative estimates that bely the uncertainty involved in the model.

Well-being studies

As might be expected for social scientists' studies, both outcomes and the possible causal variables often focus on income, employability, productivity, social status, and the effects of government and government-funded services. Gross domestic product (GDP) at country level or income at the individual level is a common focus, following the belief that these are the primary drivers of citizens' quality of life. Recently, economists have started to study quality of life more directly and are undertaking studies looking at happiness and life satisfaction [34]. As both of the latter are components of mental well-being this research is making an important contribution to public mental health and influencing policy decisions about allocation of resources. Happiness and life satisfaction are described in the economists' literature as measures of 'subjective' well-being and contrasted with the 'objective' measures of income and GDP. Well-being is thus conceptualized in terms of current feeling states. These studies do not embrace or address the developmental or functioning components of the well-being definitions of other disciplines (see Chapters 15 and 53). These distinctions are important in interpreting conflicting findings from studies in different disciplines, but when studies from the different disciplines, each using their preferred research approaches, present findings that are consistent with each other the evidence base is strengthened. This is particularly valuable when the research is challenging commonly held beliefs. Regression models using life satisfaction as an outcome [34] and logistic regression models using the Warwick-Edinburgh Mental Well-being Scale (WEMWBS; see Fig. 58.1) [35] both find educational achievement to be a poor predictor of mental well-being in adulthood. This finding is both important and counterintuitive because of the strong association between educational underachievement and mental illness.

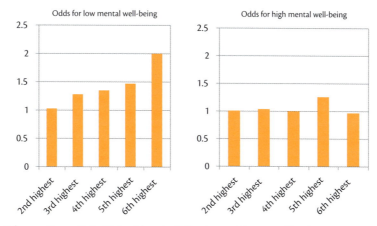

Fig. 58.1 Education as a predictor of mental well-being (Warwick-Edinburgh Mental Well-being Scale).
Source: Data from *Br J Psych*, 206(6), Stewart-Brown S, Chandimali PC, Taggart F, et al., Socio-economic Gradients and Mental Health: Implications for Public Health, pp.461-465, Copyright (2015), The Royal College of Psychiatrists.

Path analyses, structural equation modelling, and latent variable models

Regression analyses may attribute shared correlation between two independent variables as belonging to the variable entered first in the equation or partial out correlations that are shared between different variables and add this to the correlation that is not shared. Whichever approach is used, the variables are then ranked according to their overall correlation in a hierarchy, which is taken to indicate which are the most important contributors to causality. It is possible to examine and estimate statistical interactions between variables in which the correlation between one variable and the outcome changes according to the level of the other variable. But while there are statistical approaches to assessing whether a variable is mediating the effect of another, both mediator and moderator effects are not displayed in an intuitive visual way. In public mental health both mediators and moderators are important. A mediator is a variable through which some or all of the effect of the independent variable is exerted on the dependent variable or outcome. A moderator is a variable that influences the effect of one variable on another. Taking the example of resilience (see Chapter 53)—a challenging negative life event or situation can have a positive or negative effect on child development depending on the extent of relational support available to the child. Both mediators and moderators are very common in mental health research.

Path analysis [36] is a form of multiple regression modelling that provides a more sophisticated picture of possible causal relationships. In statistical terms it describes the directed dependencies among a set of variables. Path analysis is also a particular approach to structural equation modelling. Other terms used to refer to path analysis include causal modelling, analysis of covariance structures, and latent variable models. In the example shown in Fig. 58.2 [37], parenting is one of the mediator variables through which economic stresses impact on child outcomes. The implication of this analysis is that economic stresses only impact child outcomes if parenting is adversely effected. They suggest that it would be worthwhile (especially if the economic stressors cannot

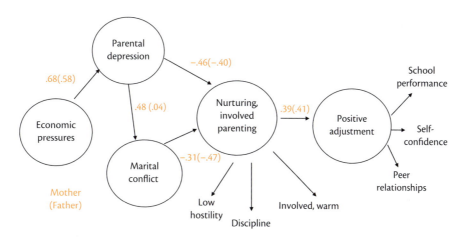

Fig. 58.2 Parenting as a mediator of the effect of family economic stress on adjustment (boys).
Reproduced from Child Dev., 63(3), Conger RD, Conger KJ, Elder GH Jr, et al., A family process model of economic hardship and adjustment of early adolescent boys, pp. 526-41, Copyright (1992) with permission from John Wiley and Sons.

be influenced) to offer parenting support at this time to protect children's development.

There are many other approaches to analysing data in which complex causal pathways operate, including structural equation modelling, latent growth curve models, and time series analyses, to examine whether the change in level of one variable is correlated with the change in level of another. These are often more appropriate to public mental health research because they recognize that multiple factors at individual, family, community and society level interact with each other in a dynamic way over the course of a lifetime to influence individual and collected mental health.

Outcome measurement

The selection of the outcome or dependent variable in a study defines the purpose and focus of the study. In an investigation of the causes of bipolar disorder, for example, the outcome is a measurement of the presence or absence of bipolar disorder. In a study assessing whether mindfulness prevents recurrence in depression, a measure of depression is the outcome.

Objective versus subjective

The medical research literature has addressed at some length the pros and cons of 'objective' versus subjective outcomes. Objective measures are made without the involvement of the person who is being measured—exam results and clinical assessments of mental health, for example. A subjective measure is one reported by the person with the condition or outcome of issue. Although often still regarded as inferior to objective measures by the research community, patient-reported outcome measures (PROMS) are now required in applications for research funding by many UK research funding bodies. Both objective, as in clinical examination, and subjective, as in PROMS, measures depend on observation and awareness, which will vary between observers. In psychiatry, patients may be more accurate observers of how they feel and clinicians more accurate observers of how their patients are functioning. Clear criteria for the development of PROMS have now been agreed [38], starting with qualitative studies (see section 'Qualitative approaches') to ensure that the measure covers the concerns of participants or patients, moving to reviews of the contents and parameters of existing measures, and then both quantitative (are the measurement properties robust) and qualitative (does the measure feel appropriate and acceptable, and understood by participants) evaluation.

Quantitative evaluation

The quantitative evaluation of outcome measures whether patient-, clinician-, or third party reported is a science in its own right (psychometrics) developed first by psychologists. Public mental health measures vary greatly in their length, breadth, and sophistication from single-item life satisfaction or happiness measures favoured by the economists to the multidimensional instruments of psychologists [39, 40]. Each has its place, but not all will work in all circumstances. Single-item measures are often not sensitive to change, that is, there are not enough categories to detect subtle improvement or deterioration. A recent review of music, singing, and well-being [41], for example, found that intervention studies using life satisfaction as an outcome measure were less likely to show effectiveness than those using more sophisticated measures. Multidimensional scales allow researchers to investigate differences in the prevalence of different components of well-being in different countries [40]; which risk or protective factors impact on which components; and what treatments or interventions influence which. In between these two extremes sit the multi-item single-dimensional measures.

A good outcome measure collects data that are good enough for the purpose of the study with the minimum of cost and effort. Good enough includes:

- The face validity—the instrument make sense to the participants as a measure of mental health.

- The content validity—when the scale is administered as self-report all the items get answered and all the levels of response options are used.

- The criterion validity—the measure correlates with measures of related outcomes and varies in different populations in the predicted way. The scale may be assessed against a gold standard, e.g. a clinical diagnosis, where one exists.

- The factor structure is consistent with the hypothesized structure, i.e. single or multidimensional.

- The scaleability of the measure is demonstrated.

- The responsiveness of the measure has been assessed—is there a change in scores among people who report that they have improved or got worse (anchor method), for example.

But good enough may be viewed differently by different disciplines. Commissioners of mental health promotion interventions used to ask practitioners to evaluate their programmes using suicide rates because, for them, this was a concrete, robust measure. However, the incidence of suicide is so low that a community-based intervention could not have the statistical power to show reliably differences on this outcome. Social scientists find life satisfaction and single-item happiness measures good enough for purpose, even though these measures have not been demonstrated to fulfil the criteria given in the aforementioned list. The General Health Questionnaire (GHQ) [42] is a self-report measure developed to identify common mental disorder in the general population. It is now very widely used because it works very well at an epidemiological level in examining associations and predictors. It can do this even though it classifies a significant proportion of people differently with regard to the presence or absence of psychiatric disorder from psychiatrists.

Well-being measurement

Until recently, mental health research has focused on disease, and outcome measures have been created to capture different psychiatric disorders, both clinician and patient report. Mental health promotion practitioners had few options when it came to evaluating their projects. The GHQ-12 was the instrument most widely recommended, but many found this instrument—in which the items were about problems—far from ideal for programmes or projects that aimed to improve health. The advent of measures whose contents were positive [43–45] like the Warwick-Edinburgh Mental Well-being Scale (WEWMBS) has made an important contribution to research and evaluation in this area, and new measures continue to be developed [46].

Warwick-Edinburgh Mental Well-being Scale (WEMWBS)

The psychometric properties of the WEMWBS have been compared with those of the GHQ-12 [47], and it has been shown that the items in these instruments assess mainly the same construct. This does not come as a great surprise because the items in the two instruments are similar except in that they are couched in the positive or the negative. The performance of WEMWBS in a therapy population [48] has also proved very similar to other commonly used measures like the Patient Health Questionnaire (PHQ-9) and Generalized Anxiety Disorder (GAD-7), although the latter two measures were more sensitive at the clinical end of the population and WEWMBS at the well-being end. But the overlap between measures does raise the question of why it is important to have measures focusing on the positive when there are well tried-and-tested measures focusing on the negative. These theoretical considerations contrast with statistics on usage. Registrations for use of WEMWBS have risen at a rapid pace to over one new registration a day in 2016, and the number of published studies using WEMWBS as an outcome measure is also increasing rapidly [49]. Translations of WEMWBS into Scandinavian, European, and languages of the East demonstrate that the appetite for measuring mental well-being is not restricted to the UK. WEMWBS has also become popular among users and carers of mental health services [50], and while it was not developed for this purpose, recent validation studies have shown WEMWBS works well in this context [51].

It would appear that positive measures like WEMWBS are meeting a need that goes beyond the purely statistical. It is likely that positively focused measures support positively focused interventions and it would seem that by being better suited to these interventions and enabling their evaluation, WEMWBS is enabling change to happen in service provision.

Response shift

Widely accepted definitions of well-being (see Chapter 15) include personal development and personal development often involves changes in self-awareness. Interventions in mental illness may also include development of self-awareness. Self-report instruments depend on self-awareness for their accuracy, particularly of emotional or feeling states. However, if during the course of a therapeutic or community-based intervention self-awareness changes scores at the end of the project will not be based on the same ground as those at the beginning. A fall in score in someone who has become aware of their depression or anxiety could be a good outcome. This phenomenon is called response shift. It is an issue for which there is as yet no easy solution.

Health economic measures

The EQ-5D [52] is an important outcome for health service commissioners because it can be used to create a common metric across very different interventions or different conditions or problems. So, for example, it can be used to assess whether an intervention to improve mental health is more cost-effective than an intervention to replace a damaged hip joint. Unfortunately, this particular measure—which is the only one available at present—is poor at capturing quality of life due to mental illness and mental well-being [47]

Qualitative approaches

Qualitative research remains less highly regarded that quantitative research in health-service evaluation. It aims to understand how things look from the perspective of study participants and often demonstrates that these are different from the perspective of professionals or practitioners. It is fundamentally reflexive, requiring both participants and researchers to reflect on their current perspectives and the way in which these might differ from those of others. In a relatively new field like mental health promotion it is also fundamentally important. Mental well-being has not received much attention until recently and reflection is a very important part of finding out what it is.

Qualitative methods have been used to investigate perceptions of mental well-being and how these differ in different cultural groups [53]. These have highlighted differences in meaning of happiness and differences in perceptions of the causes of well-being. The Chinese, for example, prioritze harmonious interpersonal and family relationships over autonomy as the basis for well-being. Pakistani communities share this attitude and recognize the fundamental contribution of a quiet mind. Family relationships and quiet minds would also feature in Western perspectives of mental well-being, but autonomy and agency would be more prominent.

Qualitative research can investigate how change comes about, what helps this process and what hinders, and develop a theory of change. It can show that the process of change and what helps/hinders can be very different in different individuals. It is in qualitative research that the importance of the therapeutic relationship was established. Qualitative research can help to develop understanding of new approaches to identifying the way in which these have their effect. As an example complementary and alternative medicine is something of an enigma in health care because it is clearly valued by a significant proportion of the public for its contribution to well-being, but the evidence base, although sometimes suggestive, is far from robust [54, 55]. Qualitative research is able to show that complementary and alternative medicine approaches contribute to mental health by enabling self-awareness and greater engagement in health development, as well as the more typical outcomes such as reduction in anxiety or pain [56]. These are valuable outcomes in terms of health gain but not covered in existing PROMS at present and so the full impact of these therapies is underestimated.

While qualitative research contributed little to twentieth-century medical practice with its belief in single external causes for single diseases, it has a great deal to contribute to understanding well-being and to the development of methods to enhance health and well-being.

Conclusions

Research and evaluation matter in that they aid understanding at many levels. But research is not neutral. It is heavily influenced by the mindsets of the researchers and what they regard as good evidence. In an interdisciplinary field like public mental health these mindsets need to become explicit and be discussed openly in order for understanding of their implications to be appreciated.

Public mental health is a new area of practice and many of its attributes—the need for a focus on the positive, complexity, and holism—demand new approaches to research. As, to paraphrase the words of Albert Einstein, 'problems cannot be solved with the same level of consciousness as that in which the problem was created', there is a strong need for disciplines to work together to develop research methods that can contribute to solving problems in this new way of looking at the world. At the same time a new area of practice like public mental health needs research and evaluation to develop and test the effectiveness of new approaches and interventions. For the next decade it is likely that we will need to use the old tried-and-tested methods as best we can to do this.

References

1. Doidge N. *The Brain that Changes Itself. Stories of Personal Triumph from the Frontiers of Brain Science.* New York: Penguin Books, 2007.
2. Begley S. *Train Your Mind Change Your Brain: How a New Science Reveals Our Extraordinary Potential to Transform Ourselves.* New York: Ballantine Books, 2007
3. Siegel DJ. *The Mindful Brain: Reflection and Attunement in the Cultivation of Well-being.* New York: W.W. Norton, 2007.
4. National Research Council, Institute of Medicine. *From Neurons to Neighborhoods: The Science of Early Childhood Development.* Washington, DC: National Academy Press.]
5. Erickson E. *Childhood and Society.* New York: W.W. Norton.
6. Luthar SS, Cicchetti D. Resilience in development: a synthesis of research across five decades. In: Cohen DJ (ed.). *Developmental Psychopathology: Risk, Disorder, and Adaptation*, Vol. 3, 2nd ed. Hoboken, NJ: John Wiley & Sons, 2006, pp. 739–795.
7. Porges SW. *Polyvagal Theory: Neurophysiological Foundations of Emotional Attachment Communication Self Regulation.* New York: W.W. Norton, 2011.
8. Rutter M, Moffitt TE, Caspi A. Gene–environment interplay and psychopathology: multiple varieties but real effects. *J Child Psychol Psychiatry* 2006; 47: 226–261.
9. Sroufe LA. Attachment and development: a prospective, longitudinal study from birth to adulthood. *Attach Hum Dev* 2005; 7: 349–367.
10. Weich S, Patterson J, Shaw R, Stewart-Brown S. Family relationships in childhood and common psychiatric disorders in later life: systematic review of prospective studies. *Br J Psychiatry* 2009; 194: 392–398.
11. Beardslee WR, Versage EM, Gladstone TR. Children of affectively ill parents: a review of the past 10 years. *J Am Acad Child Adolesc Psychiatry* 1998; 37: 1134–1141.
12. McManus S, Meltzer H, Brugha T, Bebbington P, Jenkins R. Adult Psychiatric Morbidity in England – 2007, Results of a household survey. Available at: http://content.digital.nhs.uk/catalogue/PUB02931/adul-psyc-morb-res-hou-sur-eng-2007-rep.pdf (accessed 22 March 2018).
13. Chida Y, Steptoe A. Positive psychological well-being and mortality: a quantitative review of prospective observational studies *Psychosom Med* 2008; 70: 741–756.
14. Patterson GR. *Coercive Family Process.* Eugene, OR: Castalia, 1982.
15. Morgan Z, Fryers T, Brugha T, Stewart-Brown S. The effects of parent-child relationships on later life mental health status in two national birth cohorts. *Soc Psychiatry Psychiatr Epidemiol* 2012; 47: 1707–1715.
16. Collishaw S, Pickles Am Messer J, Rutter M, Shearer C, Maughan B. Resilience to psychopathology following childhood maltreatment: Evidence from a community sample. *Child Abuse Neglect* 2007; 31: 211–229.
17. Brewin CR, Andrews B, Valentine JD. Meta-analysis of risk factors for posttraumatic stress disorder in trauma-exposed adults. *J Consult Clin Psychol* 2000; 68: 748–766.
18. Cochrane AL Effectiveness and efficiency: random reflections on health services. Report on randomised controlled trials (RCTs). Available at: https://www.nuffieldtrust.org.uk/research/effectiveness-and-efficiency-random-reflections-on-health-services (accessed 22 March 2018).
19. National Institute for Health and Clinical Excellence. Available at: https://www.nice.org.uk/ (accessed 22 March 2018).
20. Early Intervention Foundation. Available at: http://www.eif.org.uk/ (accessed 22 March 2018).
21. Carey TA, Stiles WB. Some problems with randomized controlled trials and some viable alternatives. *Clin Psychol Psychother* 2016; 23: 87–95.
22. Fischer AJ, Threlfall A, Meah S, Cookson R, Rutter H, Kelly MP. The appraisal of public health interventions: an overview. *J Public Health (Oxf)* 2013; 35: 488–494.
23. WHO Regional Office for Europe. Health promotion evaluation: recommendations to policy makers: report of the WHO European Working Group on Health Promotion Evaluation. Available at: http://apps.who.int/iris/bitstream/handle/10665/108116/E60706.pdf;jsessionid=D688144C5480D1ECAB6C03F6C3370049?sequence=1 (accessed 22 March 2018).
24. Pawson R. Evidence based policy: In search of a method. *Evaluation* 2002; 8: 157–181.
25. Stewart-Brown S, Anthony R, Wilson L, et al. Should randomized controlled trials be the 'gold standard for research on preventive interventions for children. *J Child Serv* 2011; 6: 228–235.
26. Britton A, Mckee M, Black N, McPerson K, Sanderson C, Bain C. Choosing between randomised and non randomised studies. *Health Technol Assess* 1998; 2: 1–124.
27. Black N. Why we need observational studies to evaluate the effectiveness of healthcare. *BMJ* 1996; 312: 1215–1218.
28. Kelly M, Moore T. The judgement process in evidence-based medicine and health technology assessment. *Soc Theory Health* 2012; 10: 1.
29. Helliwell JF, Fortin N, Wang S. How does subjective wellbeing vary around the world by gender and age? In: Helliwell J, Layard R, Sachs J (eds). *World Happiness Report 2015.* Washington, DC: United Nations Sustainable Development Solutions Network, 2015, pp. 42–74.
30. Blanchflower DG, Oswald AJ, Stewart-Brown S. Is psychological well-being linked to the consumption of fruit and vegetables? *Soc Indic Res* 2013; 114: 785.
31. Mujcic R, Oswald AJ. Evolution of well-being and happiness after increases in consumption of fruit and vegetables. *Am J Public Health* 2016; 106: pp. 1504–1510.
32. Baum-Baicker C. The psychological benefits of moderate alcohol consumption: a review of the literature. *Drug Alcohol Depend* 1985; 15: 305–322.
33. Mental Health Foundation. Cheers Understanding the relationship between alcohol and mental health. Available at: http://www.drugsandalcohol.ie/15771/1/cheers_report%5B1%5D.pdf (accessed 22 March 2018).
34. Clark A, Fleche S, Layard R, Powdthavee N, Ward S. *The Origins of Happiness—How New Science can Transform Our Priorities.* Princeton, NJ: Princeton University Press, 2017.
35. Stewart-Brown S, Chandimali Samaraweera P, Taggart F, Stranges S. Socio-economic gradients and mental health: implications for public health. *Br J Psychiatry* 2015; 206: 461–465.
36. Dodge Y. *The Oxford Dictionary of Statistical Terms.* Oxford: Oxford University Press, 2003.
37. Conger RD, Conger KJ, Elder GH Jr, Lorenz FO, Simons RL, Whitbeck LB. A family process model of economic hardship and adjustment of early adolescent boys. *Child Dev* 1992; 63: 526–541.
38. U.S. Department of Health and Human Services, Food and Drug Administration. Guidance for Industry: Patient-Reported Outcome Measures: Use in Medical Product Development to Support Labeling Claims. Available at: https://www.fda.gov/downloads/drugs/guidances/ucm193282.pdf (accessed 22 March 2018).
39. Ryff CD, Keyes CLM. The structure of psychological well-being revisited. *J Person Soc Psychol* 1995; 69: 719–727.
40. Huppert FA, So TTC. Flourishing across Europe: application of a new conceptual framework for defining well-being. *Soc Indic Res* 2013; 110: 837–861.
41. What Works for Wellbeing Centre. Music, singing and wellbeing in healthy adults. Available at: https://www.whatworkswellbeing.org/product/music-and-healthy-adults/ (accessed 22 March 2018).

42. Goldberg DP, Williams P. *A User's Guide to the General Health Questionnaire*. Windsor: NFER-Nelson, 1988.

43. Bech P. Measuring the dimensions of psychological general well-being by the WHO-5. *QoL Newsletter* 2004; 32: 15–16.

44. Keyes CLM. The subjective well-being of America's youth: toward a comprehensive assessment. *Adolesc Fam Health* 2005; 4: 3–11.

45. Tennant R, Hiller L, Fishwick R, et al. The Warwick-Edinburgh Mental Well-being Scale (WEMWBS): development and UK validation. *Health Qual Life Outcomes* 2007; 5: 63.

46. Rose T, Joe S, Brown GW, et al. Measuring mental wellbeing among adolescents: a systematic review of instruments. *J Child Fam Stud* 2017; 26: 1–14.

47. Bohke JR, Croudace TJ. Calibrating well-being, quality of life and common mental disorder items: psychometric epidemiology in public mental health research. *Br J Psychiatry* 2016; 209: 162–168

48. Shah N, Cadir M, Andrews WP, Stewart-Brown SL. Short Warwick-Edinburgh Mental Well-being Scale (SWEMWBS): performance in a clinical sample in relation to PHQ-9 and GAD-7. *Health Qual Life Outcomes* 2018 (in press).

49. Shah N, Steiner D, Petrou S, Johnson R, Stewart-Brown S. Exploring the impact of the Warwick-Edinburgh Mental Well-being scales on public health research and practice. *J Health Serv Res Policy* 2018 (in press).

50. Crawford MJ, Robotham D, Thana L, et al. Selecting outcome measures in mental health: the views of service users. *J Ment Health* 2011; 20: 336–346.

51. Trousselard M, Steiler D, Dutheil F, et al. Validation of the Warwick-Edinburgh Mental Well-being Scale (WEMWBS) in French Psychiatric and General Populations. *Psychiatry Res* 2016; 245: 282–290.

52. Brooks R, Robin R, de Charro F (eds). *The Measurement and Valuation of Health Status Using EQ5-D: A European Perspective*. Norwell, MA: Kluwer Academic Publishers, 2003.

53. Newbigging K, Bola M, Shah A. Scoping exercise with black and minority ethnic groups on perceptions of mental wellbeing. Available at: http://www.healthscotland.com/documents/2803.aspx (accessed 22 March 2018).

54. MacPherson H, Richmond S, Bland M, Brealey S, Gabe R, Hopton A, et al. Acupuncture and counselling for depression in primary care: a randomised controlled trial. *PLOS Med* 2013; 10: e1001518.

55. Maheswaran H Weich S Powell J Stewart-Brown S. Evaluating the responsiveness of the Warwick Edinburgh Mental Well-Being Scale (WEMWBS): group and individual level analysis. *Health Qual Life Outcomes* 2012; 10: 156.

56. Brough N, Lindenmeyer A, Thistlethwaite J, Lewith G, Stewart-Brown S. Developing awareness. Exploring clients' experiences of craniosacral therapy: what happens and why? A qualitative study. *Eur J Integr Health Care* 2015; 7: 172–183.

CHAPTER 59

Working with traditional healers to reduce the mental health treatment gap in low- and middle-income countries

David M. Ndetei, Christine W. Musyimi, Erick S. Nandoya, Lydia Matoke, and Victoria N. Mutiso

Introduction

Traditional health practice means:

> the utilization of traditional medicine or practice on other persons with the objective of diagnosis, treatment or prevention of a physical or mental illness of that person but excludes acts of a person acting pursuant to the Medical Practitioners and Dentists Act, the Pharmacy and Poisons Act, the Nurses Act or any other written law [1].

Although this definition comes from the Kenyan legal system, similar definitions abound elsewhere. Traditional healers mainly use traditional means to improve the mental well-being of their patients. Although little has been done to evaluate the efficacy of their treatment, their availability, accessibility, their consideration of sociocultural perspectives during treatment, and relationship with the patient and family [2, 3] provides a pool of resources that could be utilized to reduce the huge mental health treatment gap. As a matter of fact, their patients know them very well as they reside in their communities and they have been known to treat health problems that are likely to be linked to their culture.

They are also affordable as compared with allopathic physicians. Payment for their services is sometimes made after patients have recuperated, in installments, or in kind, and therefore patients are not afraid of visiting the healers, regardless of their financial status. However, one cannot visit the hospital without money, a key factor that is likely to cause severe mental disorders if untreated at an early stage. Out of the total patients that visit traditional healers, 95% of them are often satisfied with the services and only visit primary healthcare settings as a temporary measure, mostly for pain relief or as a last resort [3, 4].

Classification of traditional healers

There are different categories of healers, each with a specific role but they mostly focus on the physical, spiritual, cultural, psychological, emotional, and social elements of illness [5]. The most common categories are outlined in the following, as discussed in various studies [6–8]:

1. Diviners who mainly act as the medium with the ancestral spirits and interpret their messages while trying to understand the causes of a problem. It is assumed that 90% of these healers are female and do not choose to become diviners but instead are mostly 'called' by the ancestors. However, this 'calling' is open to either gender. Their mystical powers and leadership make them very respectable healers in the society.

2. Herbalists use herbal medicine, such as plants (mostly the leaf, root, bark or the whole plant), or medicines from animal sources, such as cow's milk, to improve the effectiveness of the remedy. They prepare most remedies through boiling, but they also pound, burn, macerate, steam, fry, crush, squeeze, or administer the plant as raw. It is believed that the ancestors confirm the effectiveness of their medication. Ninety per cent of herbalists are male.

3. Faith healers or prophets heal through prayer, using holy water or ash, or by laying hands on the patient. Their interpretation of illness is made through the patient's world view or perception. Faith healers integrate Christian, Islam, and African traditional beliefs in their healing.

4. Traditional birth attendants are elderly and respected women in the society, especially in the rural areas. Having at least two babies and being apprenticed for a period ranging between 15 and 20 years is a condition for being a traditional birth attendant. They mostly do not charge their patients, but they accept gifts. Although they interact with individuals who have mental illness or neurological disorders such as epilepsy [9], they may not have the skills to provide the necessary treatment and therefore refer patients to either another healer or to healthcare settings for further treatment.

Most healers acquire their knowledge from fellow healers or from family members such as parents or grandparents. They treat physical problems and mental illnesses such as depression, psychosis, and epilepsy [7, 10].

Non-pharmacological and unwarranted mental health practices used by traditional healers

One of the challenges of working with traditional healers has been due to biomedical personnel's genuine concern that traditional healer practice may harm patients, which may not always be the case [11]. Previous studies have also confirmed that traditional healers feel that they are not respected and are stereotyped as 'dirty' by allopathic physicians [4, 12]. On the contrary, traditional healers come across and interact with people suffering from mental disorders [12]. They use counselling, divination (involving the acquisition of supernatural revelation through consultation with the spirits), herbal preparations, and the driving away of evil spirits or exorcism as modes of treatment for their patients [3, 8].

Many traditional healers immensely believe the cause of mental illness is attributed to witchcraft [3, 12] and allopathic physicians cannot treat the supernatural causes. In the process, they use harmful methods to treat their patients [13]. Their intention is to do no harm; however, the consequence is perceived as harming the patient. Our experience with traditional healers has revealed the following strategies that could be harmful to their patients if not dealt with at the initial stages of collaboration.

1. **Quackery:** These are ignorant medical practices and sometimes traditional healers may practise pseudo-medicine or incorrect treatment, resulting in death instead of recovery. This is sometimes performed through incorrect medication, dosage, frequency, and storage—a phenomenon not entirely absent in some practitioners of allopathic medicine. For instance, some traditional healers require epileptic patients to inhale some types of herbal medicine that are considered therapeutic, although their effectiveness has not been evaluated.

2. **Driving evil spirits from the patient (exorcism of evil spirits):** This is the most common form of treatment, especially for psychosis owing to its bizarre symptoms, and includes;

   a. Throwing sand or flour to remove a spell. This could be directed to any part of the body, including the eyes.

   b. Whipping a patient with a stick with the aim of sending away demons.

3. **Biting their patients:** This is interpreted as removing obnoxious substances that are assumed to have been inserted in the body of the patients through witchcraft.

4. **Making body incisions on the patient:** The incisions are made with sharp objects, such as a knife or a razor blade, in order to administer herbs, cleanse those bewitched, and prevent further bewitchment or curse. This method is also used to drive away evil spirits from their patients.

Most of the these practices are also used to treat mental illness in other African countries such as Uganda [14]. Rather than throwing the baby out with the bath water, we could engage with the traditional healers in a mutually respectable dialogue on these harmful practices, given that their primary motive is not to harm but to do good.

Beliefs about mental illness

Factors such as spirit possession, witchcraft, breaking of religious taboos, divine retribution, and the capture of the soul by a spirit have been considered as very vital in management of patients with mental health conditions in the African setting, making it difficult to define mental illness without taking into account social and religious factors [15]. In addition, mental illness has for a long time been attributed to supernatural phenomena, such as witchcraft and possession by evil spirits [16–19]. Some traditional healers believe that mental illnesses are inherited or due to the ancestors' displeasure with one's failures, mistakes, or being cursed [3].

In terms of identification, traditional healers are not able to correctly recognize mental disorders because they lack formal training [20]. This lack of knowledge and understanding contributes to their inability to use a correct psychiatric label in diagnosing the signs and symptoms of mental health conditions [21]. Majority of traditional healers therefore use physical, spiritual, and cultural factors with minimal consideration on biological and psychosomatic deductions to identify mental health problems [22].

Their mode of treatment is often based on the cultural beliefs related to causes [19]. Diseases resulting from natural causes such as malaria or fever manifestation could easily lead to a hospital referral as compared to those attributed to supernatural causes, which would require consulting with the ancestral spirits. Considering the perceptions about the cause of mental illness among this category of providers, a large clientele still prefer to use their services. A study conducted in rural Haiti showed that suicidal individuals were nearly eight times more likely to prefer community-based providers, including traditional healers, than health care workers, whereas those that were found to have severe depression were associated with increased odds of ever having been to a traditional healer [23]. Although some of the treatment modalities used by the healers include the use of herbs and products from animal parts to treat psychotic conditions, and the use of non-medication therapies such as prayers/divination, counselling, and religious rituals [3]., some of them develop their skills while caring for the mentally ill [12]. This paradox leaves a gap that needs to be addressed. Therefore, utilizing the available and preferred resources at the community level could meet the needs of populations in resource-limited settings.

Knowledge and practices of traditional healers towards mental illness

The majority of traditional healers have no formal education or training on how to identify and treat patients with mental illnesses. Even though traditional healers have a strong belief in the supernatural powers as a causative factor for mental illness, they are able to recognize most symptoms of mental illness except undue sadness [24]. A recent study conducted in rural Kenya also showed that they can identify depression, schizophrenia, bipolar disorder, and drug addiction as mental conditions. However, stress and grief were misdiagnosed as mental problems by more than three-quarters of the healers. The treatment modalities used by traditional healers for mental illness such as psychosis include counselling, herbs, appeasing the spirits, and divination [3, 8, 24–26]. A qualitative study conducted in South Africa found that community members prefer traditional healers because when they visit health facilities they do not see improvement and the doctors do not explicitly explain the cause of their ailments like the healers, who are readily available with shorter waiting lines. As a matter of fact, 70% believed that traditional healers are more holistic in their approach to health [27]. Therefore, the use of information, education, and communication intervention techniques could lead to more positive and less hazardous forms of practice [24] as a result of increased mental health literacy.

Traditional healers constitute an untapped resource with enormous potential to be effective agents of change owing to their ability to command authority in their communities, acting as psychologists, marriage and family counsellors, physicians, legal, and political advisors [28]. The cultural acceptability and accessibility, the healers' holistic approach to care, and less stigma could be used as a task-shifting model to integrate mental health services while adapting their cultural acceptability to deliver evidence-based treatments [29]. Gureje et al. [29] have also suggested the need to train traditional healers not only on identification and treatment of mental illnesses, but also with regard to education on collaboration, ways of engagement and referral, and the need for mutual respect and trust. In addition, investigations on the efficacy of traditional healing practices for mental illness should be conducted and the mental health literacy increased to reduce incorporation of potentially toxic modern ingredients in treating psychosis and other ailments [30]. Poor knowledge, negative attitudes, and stigma affect the help-seeking behaviour of individuals, whereas education has positive implications on their mental health situation [31, 32].

Attitudes of traditional healers towards mental illness

About 50% of patients seeking formal mental health care in Africa choose healers as their first care provider [33]. Traditional healers have a basic idea of the definition of mental illness and describe them as behaving abnormally [4, 12]. Seeking help within community settings has been shown to be related to beliefs about the causes of mental illness, the nature of service delivery, accessibility, cost, and stigma [34]. As mental illness is often considered to be due to supernatural causes, traditional healers shoulder a large burden of these patients [25]. A study conducted by James and Peltzer [35] of psychiatric patients in Jamaica showed that a number of patients felt that their problems did not concur with the Western practitioners and this caused them distress; however, those that sought a traditional healers' care were happy about their interaction and the treatment they received from the healers. The healers also believe that mental illness is caused by witchcraft [12] and thus makes the mode of treatment dependent on ancestral consultation.

Traditional healers often feel unappreciated by allopathic physicians who consider their mode of treatment inappropriate [4, 12, 36]. Establishing respectful collaborative relationships between traditional healers and allopathic physicians, and better understanding of sociocultural factors that may influence accessibility, engagement, and collaboration with traditional healers and conventional practitioners, are required to promote an equitable collaboration in the interests of improved patient care [34, 36].

Addressing traditional healer attitudes could also be a way of reducing the mental health treatment gap. The theory of planned behaviour could be used to predict traditional healer referral practices of patients with mental illnesses in order to design interventions that provide relevant information and skills to traditional healers so as to appropriately refer patients with mental illnesses [37]. The World Health Organization (WHO) has requested governments to promote the inclusion and integration of traditional healers in national healthcare delivery systems and donor-specific health programmes [38], as healers and patients have been shown to agree with psychiatrists in the diagnosis and identification of 'serious' symptoms of mental illness [39].

Roles of traditional healers in mental health

Traditional healers are often preferred and their services sought more than Western medicine in many parts of Africa. A study conducted in Ghana showed a greater delay in presenting to health centres if the patients had previously visited a traditional or faith healer [40]. This demonstrates the importance of engaging the healers in improving mental health care. Although there is considerable debate on whether they should be legally allowed to practice or not, their role in mental health care is pivotal in reducing the huge treatment gap, largely related to insufficient human resources.

Promotion of advocacy by building individual and community capacity for change

Collaboration and training of traditional healers have provided an opportunity for them to take a role in advocating for enforcement or development of public and/or institutional policies that address individual or community mental health needs. Studies have demonstrated that supporting traditional healers through training and dialogue can be one of the channels to engage community members to build knowledge and skills for self-directed change and community development [12, 41]. Many traditional healers in Africa are registered under various associations and the traditional health practitioners' bill governs and regulates their practice. Therefore, the umbrella associations could be used to integrate mental health programmes and enhance sustainability. The involvement of traditional healers in mental health has also promoted mobilization of community-owned resources and actions for scaling up mental health services [42]. This suggests that the community-led needs assessment and owned services tend to build a strong capacity for community sustained services.

There is ample evidence to show the widespread of healers in rural low- and middle-income countries (LAMICs). They are available and fairly affordable, making them the first choice of alternative healthcare system to be accessed by persons with mental health conditions, before conventional care. They tend to have a first-hand understanding of social, cultural, economical, and structural barriers affecting access to services for their beneficiaries. It is apparent that their participation can potentially contribute to more culturally competent services, personal empowerment of beneficiaries of mental health services, and greater community control of mental health. Their participation in community mental health services therefore raises hope for engendering community-led public health actions to bring to perspective some of the social determinants of mental ill health.

Promotion of access by facilitating effective linkages between the community and conventional healthcare system

Many LAMICs have poor health infrastructure and are economically unstable, thus limiting the access of the majority of patients in rural settings to quality mental health services. Traditional healers have therefore helped to bridge this gap by bringing health services closer to their consumers. Some studies in Africa have shown that informal health practitioners help patients by assessing their eligibility for health services provided within their community [43]. They have provided either direct or indirect assistance to patients, such as psychosocial support [44], thus serving as a link between the community and local health facility.

There is a growing emphasis on 'task shifting', where traditional healers play a central role in delivering expanded services in resource-poor contexts with few trained personnel. Studies in developing countries have indicated their usefulness in mental health as their sustainable contact with patients could enhance strong links between the community and conventional health systems, and ensure continuity of care if well trained [36, 45] as they also conduct home visits to ensure persons identified as being at risk access quality services [3].

A study by Campbell and Burgess [46] revealed that most patients who visit local health facilities in rural settings are likely to be referred or seen by either a traditional, faith healer, or local community health worker [46]. During the initial assessment, traditional healers provide psychosocial support and identify critical patient health needs of high priority to biomedical practitioners. It is evident that traditional healers have, in one way or another, enhanced patient's timely access to health systems through referrals and coordination of care [19].

Attitude, behaviour, and intention to refer have been shown to be predictors of traditional healer referral practices [37]. As such, traditional healers' role in increasing access to mental health care through referral is imperative as many individuals with severe mental illness, such as psychosis and epilepsy have been shown to visit traditional healers, whose ability to handle such cases has been questioned [9, 47]. Therefore, collaboration between traditional healers and biomedical mental health practitioners can be achieved and can benefit patients whose access to mental health care is limited.

With adequate human resources; better access to medication through referral from healers; and improved training, support, compensation, and supervision in the LAMIC community, the task-sharing approach in mental health care is perceived to be acceptable and feasible, and could be a channel to plan interventions while focusing on the sociocultural context of the communities [48].

Provision of health education and information

Traditional healers have acted as agents who are readily available to teach basic concepts of health promotion and disease prevention [20]. Given their patronage, evidence shows that they are knowledgeable and skilled, and that their practices are based on theories, beliefs, and experiences indigenous to different cultures [46]. This then allows them to better understand the sociocultural aspects of the local population. Therefore, a continuous dialogue with traditional healers can improve the healthcare system by developing culturally sensitive educational material that would be instrumental in promoting health education for non-communicable diseases such as mental health.

Provision of direct care to patients

The literature on some countries in sub-Saharan Africa has shown that alternative health practitioners have helped provide routine screening of some selected conditions such as depression and HIV [36]. A recent study conducted in Kenya showed estimates of depression (nearly 23%) similar to those found in healthcare settings are detected by traditional healers [49]. Another study has revealed that some alternative or traditional practitioners have provided direct medical translation and interpretation to patients during receipt of care services provided within their area or institutions. The study also indicated that they helped provide informal counseling and social support to individuals and groups [46].

Traditional healers also live with the patients in the community and therefore tend to be best situated to provide practical, emotional, and material support to patients, to help them cope with the condition and address social stigma. Traditional healers have been suggested to offer an important human resource for mental health care in LAMICs [50].

Contribution of traditional healers in mental health care

Many countries in Africa do not have a national policy on traditional healers. However, some countries have or are in the process of developing laws that include regulation of the practice of traditional healers such as registration of such persons. This will ensure their practice does minimal harm to patients and will create an opportunity for evidence-based training, as their diagnoses of mental disorders are based primarily on consulting the ancestral spirits [3].

Training traditional healers has been shown to improve significantly their knowledge on mental illness [49, 51]. These are therefore some channels that could be used to provide knowledge and elaborate on the causes and identification of mental illness before training the healers on the interventions. Traditional healers have been shown to be responsive to training and collaboration [12, 52]. Therefore, working with traditional healers is one of the solutions to reducing barriers to accessing mental health services as most studies in Africa have revealed a preference for traditional healers for the treatment of mental disorders [53, 54]. Moreover, the patients of traditional healers report improvements [55], which tend to be high, although not significant, when compared with patients attending primary healthcare clinics [56].

There is ample evidence to suggest that traditional healers can provide an effective psychosocial intervention [57, 58], an approach that could be adapted from the WHO Mental Health Gap Action Programme, developed for use in non-specialized healthcare settings, and non-specialist healthcare providers could use it with necessary adaptation to increase coverage [59]. Therefore, this could be an appropriate channel for tackling the huge treatment gap inherent as a result of inadequately skilled human resources.

Another challenge likely to be experienced while working with traditional healers is legitimacy as some of them are not registered. However, collaborative initiatives have stated that one of the most useful ways of identifying genuine and committed healers is

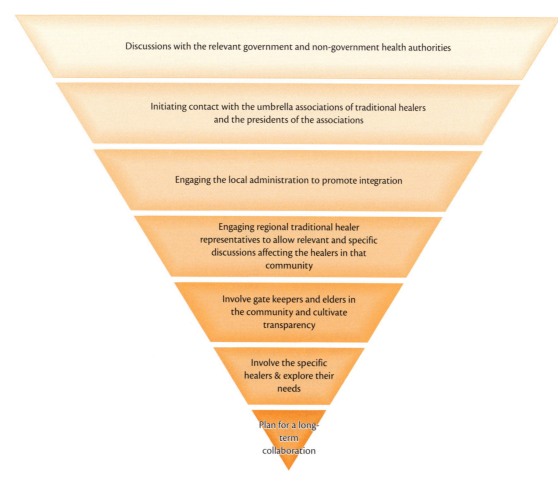

Fig. 59.1 Steps to build trust and respect before starting up initiatives in community settings.
Source: Data from Africa Mental Health Foundation, 2016.

recognizing through the community their competence in tackling diseases, being trustworthy, and spending time together and having discussions [60]. This strategy has been employed, in part, in some African settings [12, 61].

It is also imperative to involve traditional healers at the initial steps of planning, in order to build trust and respect. Through our experience in conducting such studies in a low- and middle-income setting, we recommend a systematic process that involves either a top-down or bottom-up approach, depending on the context. Either way, the starting point would involve participatory theory of change development to map out progress. This process can be summarized in the pyramid shown in Fig. 59.1.

Successful collaboration is based on mutual understanding through dialogue, emphasizing the importance of complementarities of both traditional and allopathic physicians by referral from one health system to another in order to improve the lives of patients and the community [12, 61, 62]. A step-by-step process is also imperative in initiating and enhancing collaboration, and reducing the mistrust inherent between the two systems [12].

Making traditional healers complementary providers in mental health care is a solution to reducing the burden of mental illnesses in the family as healers are prevalent in the communities and see a large number of patients. The need to develop models of collaboration to promote a workable relationship between conventional and traditional health practitioners in treating mental illness has been suggested in several studies [3, 33, 35, 52].

Future plans

While there is a Traditional Health Practitioners' Bill to provide for traditional healer and other practitioner training, registration, and licensing, so as to regulate their practice in some countries [1, 63, 64], most of traditional healers operate outside formal health structures. It is therefore crucial to put in place mechanisms to ensure that traditional health practice complies with universally accepted healthcare norms and values as stated in the bill. The available human resources in the communities that have served a large number of individuals in the past represent a resourceful pool of people who could provide complementary services, hence strengthening the mainstream healthcare system in resource-limited settings.

Traditional healers have been known to refer only severe cases of conditions and measures to prohibit their practice may destabilize their system or lead to malpractice for fear of losing their patients or their jobs. As such, they should be encouraged to engage in open discussions with relevant authorities such as those in governmental and non-governmental institutions, as well as community groups and follow-up to monitor their competency after training. Their roles also need to be clearly defined to avoid overlap with the conventional workers.

Additionally, traditional healing systems have demonstrated efficacy in areas such as mental health, disease prevention, treatment of non-communicable diseases, and improvement of the quality of life of persons living with chronic diseases, as well as for the ageing population [64]. However, there is need for further research to evaluate scientifically traditional healer treatments and evidence-based treatment to cater holistically for the needs of their patients. The identified treatments should be piloted and their efficacy established through proven evaluation methods before scaling them to other regions. One of the areas to enhance this process is to build an atmosphere of trust and respect between the formal and the informal sectors while monitoring any successes and shortcomings that would have an impact on the initiative.

Conclusions

In summary, collaborative initiatives between traditional and conventional health practitioners should be contextually developed in order to increase access to mental health services and reduce the mental health treatment gap through promoting the mental wellbeing and prevent the recurrence of mental health problems among patients, in settings with limited resources. Existing initiatives should also be evaluated to reduce duplicate negative impact and enhance successful collaborations while emphasizing trust-building and respect between the two sectors.

References

1. Republic of Kenya. Traditional Health Practitioners' Bill. *Kenya Gaz Suppl* 2014; 59: 2457–2482.
2. Buchwald D, Panwala S, Hooton TM. Use of traditional health practices by Southeast Asian refugees in a primary care clinic. *West J Med* 1992; 156: 507–511.
3. Mbwayo A, Ndetei D, Mutiso V, Khasakhala L. Traditional healers and provision of mental health services in cosmopolitan informal settlements in Nairobi, Kenya. *Afr J Psychiatry* 2013; 16: 134–140.
4. Sorsdahl K, Stein DJ, Flisher AJ. Traditional healer attitudes and beliefs regarding referral of the mentally ill to Western doctors in South Africa. *Transcult Psychiatry* 2010; 47: 591–609.
5. Zuma T, Wight D, Rochat T, Moshabela M. The role of traditional health practitioners in Rural KwaZulu-Natal, South Africa: generic or mode specific. *BMC Complement Altern Med* 2016; 16(304).
6. Kale R. Traditional healers in South Africa: a parallel health care system. *BMJ* 1995; 310: 1182–1185.
7. Semenya SS, Potgieter MJ. Bapedi traditional healers in the Limpopo Province, South Africa: their socio-cultural profile and traditional healing practice. *J Ethnobiol Ethnomed* 2014; 10(4).
8. Truter I. African traditional healers: cultural and religious beliefs intertwined in a holistic way. *SA Pharm J* 2007; 74: 56–60.
9. Bucher K, Liechty G, Gisore M, et al. Self-reported practices among traditional birth attendants surveyed in western Kenya a descriptive study. *BMC Pregnancy Childbirth* 2016; 16: 1–7.
10. Abbo C, Ekblad S, Waako P, Okello E, Musisi S, Abbo C. The prevalence and severity of mental illnesses handled by traditional healers in two districts in Uganda. *Afr Health Sci* 2009; 9(Suppl. 1): S16–S22.
11. Makundi EA, Malebo HM, Mhame P, Kitua AY, Warsame M. Role of traditional healers in the management of severe malaria among children below five years of age: the case of Kilosa and Handeni Districts, Tanzania. *Malar J* 2006; 5(58).
12. Musyimi CW, Mutiso VN, Nandoya ES, Ndetei DM. Forming a joint dialogue among faith healers, traditional healers and formal health workers in mental health in a Kenyan setting: towards common grounds. *J Ethnobiol Ethnomed* 2016; 12(4).
13. Keikelame MJ, Swartz L. 'A thing full of stories': traditional healers' explanations of epilepsy and perspectives on collaboration with biomedical health care in Cape Town. *Transcult Psychiatry* 2015; 52: 659–680.
14. Ovuga E, Boardman J, Oluka E. Traditional healers and mental illness in Uganda. *Psychiatr Bull* 1999; 23: 276–279.
15. Dein S. Mental health in a multiethnic society. *BMJ* 1997; 315: 473–476.
16. Snow LF, Michigan LE. Traditional health beliefs and practices among lower class black Americans. *West J Med* 1983; 139: 820–828.
17. King M, Smith A, Gracey M. Indigenous health part 2: the underlying causes of the health gap. *Lancet Public Health* 2009; 374: 76–85.
18. Raguram R, Venkateswaran A, Ramakrishna J, Weiss MG. Traditional community resources for mental health : a report of temple healing from India. *BMJ* 2002; 325: 38–40.
19. Thirthalli J, Zhou L, Kumar K, et al. Traditional, complementary, and alternative medicine approaches to mental health care and psychological wellbeing in India and China. *Lancet Psychiatry* 2016; 3: 660–672.
20. Jorm AF. Mental health literacy: public knowledge and beliefs about mental disorders. *Br J Psychiatry* 2000; 177: 396–401.
21. Shankar BR, Saravanan B, Jacob KS. Explanatory models of common mental disorders among traditional healers and their patients in rural south India. *Int J Soc Psychiatry* 2006; 52: 221–233.
22. Aidoo M, Harpham T. The explanatory models of mental health amongst low-income women and health care practitioners in Lusaka, Zambia. *Health Policy Plan* 2001; 16: 206–213.
23. Wagenaar BH, Kohrt BA, Hagaman AK, McLean KE, Kaiser BN. Determinants of care seeking for mental health problems in rural Haiti: culture, cost, or competency. *Psychiatr Serv* 2013; 65: 366–372.
24. Adelekan ML, Makanjuola AB, Ndom RJE. Traditional mental health practitioners in Kwara State, Nigeria. *East Afr Med J* 2001; 78: 190–196.
25. Abbo C. Profiles and outcome of traditional healing practices for severe mental illnesses in two districts of Eastern Uganda. *Glob Health Action* 2011; 4.
26. Puckree T, Mkhize M, Mgobhozi Z, Lin J. African traditional healers: what health care professionals need to know. *Int J Rehabil Res* 2002; 25: 247–251.
27. Mathibela MK, Egan BA, Du Plessis HJ, Potgieter MJ. Socio-cultural profile of Bapedi traditional healers as indigenous knowledge custodians and conservation partners in the Blouberg area, Limpopo Province, South Africa. *J Ethnobiol Ethnomed* 2015; 11: 49.
28. Rudolph MJ, Ogunbodede EO, Mistry M. Management of the oral manifestations of HIV/AIDS by traditional healers and care givers. *Curationis* 2007; 30: 56–61.
29. Gureje O, Nortje G, Makanjuola V, Oladeji BD, Seedat S, Jenkins R. The role of global traditional and complementary systems of medicine in the treatment of mental health disorders. *Lancet Psychiatry* 2015; 2: 168–177.
30. Sorsdahl KR, Flisher AJ, Wilson Z, Stein DJ. Explanatory models of mental disorders and treatment practices among traditional healers in Mpumulanga, South Africa. *African J Psychiatry (South Africa)* 2010; 13: 284–290.
31. Sorsdahl K, Stein DJ, Grimsrud A, et al. Traditional healers in the treatment of common mental disorders in South Africa. *J Nerv Ment Dis* 2009; 197: 434–441.
32. Peltzer K, Mngqundaniso N, Petros G. HIV/AIDS/STI/TB knowledge, beliefs and practices of traditional healers in KwaZulu-Natal, South Africa. *AIDS Care* 2006; 18: 608–613.
33. Burns JK, Tomita A. Traditional and religious healers in the pathway to care for people with mental disorders in Africa: a systematic review and meta-analysis. *Soc Psychiatry Psychiatr Epidemiol* 2015; 50: 867–877.

34. Nsereko JR, Kizza D, Kigozi F, et al. Stakeholder's perceptions of help-seeking behaviour among people with mental health problems in Uganda. *Int J Ment Health Syst* 2011; 5: 5.

35. James C, Peltzer K. Traditional and alternative therapy for mental illness in Jamaica: patients' conceptions and practitioners' attitudes. *Afr J Tradit Complement Altern Med* 2012; 9: 94–101.

36. Campbell-Hall V, Petersen I, Bhana A, Mjadu S, Hosegood V, Flisher JA. Collaboration between traditional practitioners and primary health care staff in South Africa: developing a workable partnership for community mental health services. *Transcult Psychiatry* 2010; 47: 610–628.

37. Sorsdahl K, Stein D, Flisher A. Predicting referral practices of traditional healers of their patients with a mental illness: an application of the Theory of Planned Behaviour. *Afr J Psychiatry* 2013; 16: 35–40.

38. Wreford J. 'Sincedisa—We Can Help!' A literature review of current practice involving traditional African healers in biomedical HIV/AIDS interventions in South Africa. *Soc Dyn* 2005; 31: 90–117.

39. Kapur RL. The role of traditional healers in mental health care in rural India. *Soc Sci Med Part B Med Anthropol* 1979; 13: 27–31.

40. Appiah-Poku J, Laugharne R, Mensah E, Osei Y, Burns T. Previous help sought by patients presenting to mental health services in Kumasi, Ghana. *Soc Psychiatry Psychiatr Epidemiol* 2004; 39: 208–211.

41. Al-Krenawi A, Graham JR. Culturally sensitive social work practice with arab clients in mental health settings. *Health Soc Work* 2000; 25: 9–22.

42. Petersen I, Baillie K, Bhana A. Understanding the benefits and challenges of community engagement in the development of community mental health services for common mental disorders: lessons from a case study in a rural South African subdistrict site. *Transcult Psychiatry* 2012; 49: 418–437.

43. Hodes RM. Cross-cultural medicine and diverse health beliefs. Ethiopians abroad. *West J Med* 1997; 166: 29–36.

44. Jenkins R, Kiima D, Okonji M, Njenga F, Kingora J, Lock S. Integration of mental health into primary care and community health working in Kenya: context, rationale, coverage and sustainability. *Ment Health Fam Med* 2010; 7: 37–47.

45. Keikelame JM, Swarts L. 'A thing full of stories'. Traditional healers' explanations of epilepsy and perspectives on collaboration with biomedical health care in Cape Town. *Transcult Psychiatry* 2015; 52: 659–680.

46. Campbell C, Burgess R. The role of communities in advancing the goals of the Movement for Global Mental Health. *Transcult Psychiatry* 2012; 49: 379–395.

47. Ensink K, Robertson B. Patient and family experience of Psychiatric Services and African Indegeniou Healers. *Transcult Psychiatry* 1999; 36: 23–43.

48. Mendenhall E, De Silva MJ, Hanlon C, et al. Acceptability and feasibility of using non-specialist health workers to deliver mental health care: stakeholder perceptions from the PRIME district sites in Ethiopia, India, Nepal, South Africa, and Uganda. *Soc Sci Med* 2014; 118: 33–42.

49. Musyimi CW, Mutiso VN, Musau AM, Matoke LK, Ndetei DM. Prevalence and determinants of depression among patients under the care of traditional health practitioners in a Kenyan setting: policy implications. *Transcult Psychiatry* 2017; 54: 285–303.

50. Saraceno B, van Ommeren M, Batniji R, et al. Barriers to improvement of mental health services in low-income and middle-income countries. *Lancet* 2007; 370: 1164–1174.

51. Bruni A. Assessing the efficacy of the Mental Health Gap Action Programme (mhGAP) training for non-specialized health workers in Ethiopia. Available at: https://run.unl.pt/bitstream/10362/13220/1/Bruni%20Andrea%20TM%202014.pdf (accessed 22 March 2018).

52. Ndetei D, Khasakhala L, Kingori J, Oginga A, Raja S. The complementary role of traditional and faith healers and potential liaisons with western-style mental health services in Kenya. Available at: http://erepository.uonbi.ac.ke/handle/11295/26392 (accessed 22 March 2018).

53. Ayonrinde O, Gureje O, Lawal R. Psychiatric research in Nigeria: bridging tradition and modernisation. *Br J Psychiatry* 2004; 184: 536–538.

54. Tumbwene M, Outwater AH. Perceived barriers on utilization of mental health services among adults in Dodoma Municipality—Tanzania. *J Public Ment Health* 2015; 14: 79–93.

55. Kleinman A, Gale JL. Patients treated by physicians and folk healers: A comparative outcome study in Taiwan. *Cult Med Psychiatry* 1982; 6: 405–423.

56. Patel V, Todd C, Winston M, et al. Outcome of common mental disorders in Harare, Zimbabwe. *Br J Psychiatry* 1998; 172: 53–57.

57. Nortje G, Oladeji B, Gureje O, Seedat S. Effectiveness of traditional healers in treating mental disorders: a systematic review. *Lancet Psychiatry* 2016; 3: 154–170.

58. Musyimi CW, Mutiso V, Ndetei DM, Henderson DC, Bunders J. Mental Health outcomes of psychosocial intervention among traditional health practitioner depressed patients in Kenya. *Cult Med Psychiatry* 2017; 41: 453–465.

59. World Health Organization. Mental Health Gap Action Programme: mhGAP Intervention Guide for Mental, Neurological and Substance Use Disorders in Non-specialized Health Settings. Available at: http://www.who.int/mental_health/publications/mhGAP_intervention_guide/en/ (accessed 22 March 2018).

60. Joint United Nations Programme on HIV/AIDS (UNAIDS). Collaborating with Traditional Healers for HIV Prevention and Care in sub-Saharan Africa: suggestions for Programme Managers and Field Workers. Available at: http://data.unaids.org/publications/IRC-pub07/jc967-tradhealers_en.pdf (accessed 22 March 2018).

61. King R. *Collaboration with Traditional Healers on Prevention and Care in Sub Saharan Africa: A Practical Guideline for Programs.* Geneva: UNAIDS, 2005.

62. Musyimi CW, Mutiso VN, Ndetei DM, et al. Mental health treatment in Kenya : task-sharing challenges and opportunities among informal health providers. *Int J Ment Health Syst* 2017; 11: 45

63. Republic of South Africa. Research agenda 2014–2017. Available at: http://www.dhet.gov.za/Gazette/DHET Research Agenda 19 Aug 2014 Final edited [1].pdf (accessed 22 March 2018).

64. World Health Organization. Legal Status of Traditional Medicine and Complementary/Alternative Medicine: A Worldwide Review. Available at: http://apps.who.int/medicinedocs/en/d/Jh2943e/ (accessed 22 March 2018).

SECTION V

Conclusions

CHAPTER 60

Conclusion

Dinesh Bhugra, Kamaldeep Bhui, Samuel Y. S. Wong, and Stephen E. Gilman

Mental ill health places a considerable burden on society, as well as on individuals who develop mental illness, their families, and their carers. The case for prevention is significant not only for economic reasons, but also for the functioning of society as a whole. There is evidence to indicate that the burden of mental illness cannot be reduced simply by treating mentally ill individuals [1]. It has been argued that the only sustainable method of reducing the burden of disease is prevention [2].

It is well recognized that positive mental health can result in better educational attainment, greater productivity, reduced mortality, and reduce risky behaviour [3]. All these factors will contribute to a successful, safe, and happy society. Both mental health promotion at all levels and mental illness prevention strategies are needed. As the evidence presented in this volume has illustrated, interventions from parenting skills and support during pregnancy itself can provide clear evidence that these work. Promotion of mental health and well-being in schools is essential. What these interventions also highlight is that mental health promotion and prevention have to work across areas of education, employment, families, and the judicial system. The relationship between mental health promotion and prevention of mental ill health is important and deserves further exploration as to how and to which levels these are to be linked. We recognize that as clinicians are trained in managing mental illness and mental ill health they may feel that they do not possess the expertise to deliver public mental health, but it must be noted that they are well placed in advocating for their patients, their families, and carers.

Risk factors for mental ill health are genetic, behavioural, and environmental. As we understand more about epigenetics and genetic contributions to mental illness, it should be possible to reduce if not completely eliminate these risks. Behavioural risks, such as smoking, bad diet, lack of exercise, and substance and alcohol use, are easily preventable. These vulnerability factors in childhood are of three types: those relating to the child, those relating to the family, and those related to the household itself. These have been addressed in this volume. To reiterate, factors such as maternal stress, substance abuse during pregnancy, child (physical, sexual, and emotional) abuse, lone parents, low income, poor housing, overcrowding, debt, violence, unemployment, and so on, all play a role. Vulnerable groups such as looked-after children (those in care); the elderly; women; lesbian, gay, bisexual, and transgender (LGBT) people; and prisoners are all at a higher risk of developing mental ill health. Broader social and cultural factors such as poverty, overcrowding, lack of green spaces, and poor access to public transport have to be considered and dealt with at national policy levels. Cultural variations should be remembered in exploring the variations of mental ill health and the potential for successful interventions.

Mental health and physical health should be promoted together and not in isolation from each other. Mental health promotion can be focused on whole populations and societies and vulnerable families, as well as individuals. At each level different strategies are needed. Individuals must be encouraged and trained if necessary to develop personal ability to deal with the social environment and that of the individual's internal world. The entire population as a whole should be seen as the base of a pyramid. When distressed, most individuals will seek help first from their personal, social, and folk sector, and seek professional help only if that does not work. Depending upon health care systems and resources a small proportion will seek help in primary care and of these only a few may be referred on to secondary care. Those being referred to tertiary care will further be filtered out at the secondary care level. Thus, different interventions and health promotion strategies have to focus on different levels in order to be successful. Kalra et al. [4] recommend that mental health promotion is to be targeted at different vulnerable groups.

What should clinicians and policymakers do? First and foremost, public mental health is about highlighting and identifying social inequalities and their impact on the individual's physical and mental health. Education about types of stress and managing stress must start at an early age in schools. It must be directed at parents and children as well as at teachers. Preschool and school-based health education can help prevent conduct and emotional disorders, as can prevention of violence and abuse. Promoting physical and mental health through parenting skill interventions, home visits in the postpartum period, and peer support may help reduce the likelihood of developing mental ill health.

Early interventions for mental ill health such as conduct disorders, psychosis, and addictions can be helpful in reducing long-term illness and problems. For specific at-risk groups, it is important to build information portals that can be used appropriately. With telemental health and e-mental health these become useful tools for educating younger people, in particular. Teaching reduction in risk-taking behaviours (e.g. ceasing smoking, substance, and alcohol abuse) can reduce the likelihood of developing complex co-morbidities.

Promoting strength and resilience through various activities such as school-based programmes, workplace-based promotion, promoting well-being individually, as well as environmentally improving housing, increasing access to better and affordable transport, and green spaces can all contribute to improved mental health. Suicide prevention programmes have been shown to be extremely successful in many settings, taking into account the local and cultural factors. Early identification, diagnosis, and therapeutic interventions in managing physical illness can also be helpful in reducing the onset of mental ill health.

As this volume has illustrated, there is considerable evidence that confirms the value of mental health promotion, but there is an urgent need to translate this not only into education and interventions, but also into policies. Education and empowerment are critical in engaging populations and in helping to improve public mental health.

References

1. Andrews G, Issakidis C, Sanderson K, Corry J, Lapsley H. Utilising survey data to inform public policy: comparison of the cost-effectiveness of treatment of ten mental disorders. *Br J Psychiatry* 2004; 184: 526–533.
2. Saxena S, Jané-Llopis E, Hosman C. Prevention of mental and behavioural disorders: implications for policy and practice. *World Psychiatry* 2006; 5: 5–14.
3. Campion J, Bhui K, Bhugra D; European Psychiatric Association. European Psychiatric Association (EPA) guidance on prevention of mental disorders. *Eur Psychiatry* 2012; 27: 68–80.
4. Kalra G, Christodoulou G, Jenkins R, et al. Mental health promotion: guidance and strategies. *Eur Psychiatry* 2012; 27: 81–86.

Index

Notes: Tables, figures and boxes are indicated by an italic *t*, *f* or *b* following the page number. Abbreviations used in the index can be found on page xi-xii *vs.* indicates a comparison